Caplan's
Stroke: A Clinical Approach

Caplan's Stroke: A Clinical Approach

Fourth Edition

Louis R. Caplan, MD

Professor of Neurology, Harvard Medical School
Senior Neurologist and Member Stroke Service
Beth Israel Deaconess Medical Center
Boston, Massachusetts

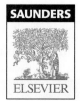

SAUNDERS

ELSEVIER

SAUNDERS
ELSEVIER

1600 John F. Kennedy Blvd.
Ste 1800
Philadelphia, PA 19103-2899

CAPLAN'S STROKE: A CLINICAL APPROACH, FOURTH EDITION   ISBN: 978-1-4160-4721-6

Notice

Neither the Publisher nor the Author assumes any responsibility for any loss or injury and/or damage to persons or property arising out of or related to any use of the material contained in this book. It is the responsibility of the treating practitioner, relying on independent expertise and knowledge of the patient, to determine the best treatment and method of application for the patient.

The Publisher

Library of Congress Cataloging-in-Publication Data

Caplan, Louis R.
  Caplan's stroke : a clinical approach / Louis R. Caplan. — 4th ed.
      p. ; cm.
  Includes bibliographical references and index.
  ISBN 978-1-4160-4721-6 (alk. paper)
  1. Cerebrovascular disease. I. Title. II. Title: Stroke.
  [DNLM: 1. Stroke—diagnosis. 2. Stroke—therapy. 3. Cerebrovascular
Disorders—diagnosis. 4. Cerebrovascular Disorders—therapy. WL 355
C244c 2009]
  RC388.5.C33 2009
  616.8'1—dc22

                                        2009007599

Acquisitions Editor: Adrianne Brigido
Developmental Editor: John Ingram
Project Manager: Mary Stermel
Design Direction: Karen O'Keefe Owens

Printed in the United States of America

Working together to grow libraries in developing countries

www.elsevier.com | www.bookaid.org | www.sabre.org

ELSEVIER   BOOK AID International   Sabre Foundation

Last digit is the print number: 9 8 7 6 5 4 3 2 1

This is the fourth edition of *Caplan's Stroke: A Clinical Approach*. It is the last edition that I will write as a single-author monograph. The topic of clinical stroke has become far too vast for one person to provide up-to-date, concise but thorough coverage in a single book format. The stroke literature has expanded exponentially since the first edition appeared in 1984. During the last decade alone, there are more journals, many more reports, more monographs, more meetings, many more physicians caring for stroke patients, more clinical trials, more new diagnostic technology, and more new treatments and therapeutic strategies. This major growth in interest and activity has been triggered and stimulated by the advent of diagnostic technology that can show the brain and its vasculature rapidly, safely, and accurately and by potential treatment of conditions that physicians felt powerless to effectively manage in the past.

I take this opportunity to herein review past editions and place them in perspective. In the early 1980s, representatives from Butterworth book publishing approached Dr. Robert Stein, my former stroke fellow and then junior staff colleague in the Neurology Department at the Michael Reese Hospital in Chicago, to write a clinical book about stroke. At that time the first edition of the large stroke multiauthored compendium edited by Henry Barnett, Jay P. Mohr, Frank Yatsu, and Ben Stein was nearing publication by Churchill-Livingstone Publishers. I had contributed a long, detailed chapter on posterior circulation brain ischemia for that multiauthored volume. The Churchill-Livingstone stroke compendium was intended to serve as a reference text. Butterworth had in mind a smaller book that would serve more as a primer for medical students, trainees, and nonstroke experts as an introductory *how-to* monograph about the burgeoning field of stroke.

At that time I was the Neurologist-in-Chief at the Michael Reese Hospital, having moved from Boston to that very large urban hospital and the University of Chicago in 1978. Dr. Mohr and I, as well as others, had recently published data from a large collection of patients studied in Boston—the Harvard Stroke Registry. Dr. Stein approached me to help him with the writing and creation of the book, and I, at first, declined. I was very occupied with taking care of patients

and with stroke clinical research, teaching, and administration. I wasn't convinced about the need for the book.

Later having thought about the offer and concept more thoroughly, I decided to join Robby Stein in creating the then first edition of *Stroke: A Clinical Approach*. The book was planned to differ considerably from the Churchill-Livingstone stroke compendium. It would (1) be clinical and include only the most relevant basic science aspects needed by clinicians to care for stroke patients; (2) be organized as a didactic course meant to be read in full from the beginning to the end rather than serving solely as a reference source; (3) be aimed at novitiates as a primer about stroke; (4) use a case method expounding principles and clinical findings, diagnosis, and management in reference to individual patient scenarios; (5) be well illustrated using only drawings (radiographs were much more expensive to publish then); (6) be easy to read and understand; and (7) contain personal guidance to the care of stroke patients rather than a repository of information. We asked Dr. Juan Sanchez-Ramos, an MD, PhD who had recently completed his Neurology residency at the University of Chicago in addition to being an accomplished artist, to render the cartoons and illustrations of the brain and vascular images. We were very fortunate that he agreed to work with us in the creation of the book.

It took Robby Stein, Juan Sanchez-Ramos, and me much more time than expected to get the book into print. The first edition of *Stroke: A Clinical Approach* by Caplan and Stein was finally published by Butterworth in 1986. It contained 15 chapters, 343 pages, 24 tables, and 61 illustrations. By the time the book was published, I had already moved back to Boston in 1984 to become the Neurologist-in-Chief at the New England Medical Center and Chair of the Neurology Department at Tufts University. Stein had moved to Penobscott Bay, Maine, where he still lives and practices Neurology.

At the time the first edition was being written in the early 1980s, computed tomography had become generally available, but accurate vascular imaging required catheter-based dye angiography. Magnetic resonance imaging was in its infancy. Personal computers were becoming popular, but e-mail was not yet used. I did the writing of the first edition on yellow lined paper and the typing was laboriously performed by my all-suffering secretaries who had to change multiple renditions by typewriter—Pam Helder at Michael Reese and Pauline Dawley at the New England Medical Center. The absence of computer files made it very laborious to update previously written chapters, so by the time of publication, many of the earliest written chapters were out of date.

The book proved (to my surprise) to be much more popular than expected, and so Susan Pioli, who was then working for the publisher (now Butterworth-Heinemann), pressed for a second edition circa 1990. By that time Stein was very busy with clinical practice and had left academia, and we both agreed that I would write the second edition of *Stroke: A Clinical Approach* alone. Dr. Sanchez-Ramos agreed to again do the illustrations. The aim of the second edition was broader than the first. The popularity of the first edition with stroke neurologists stimulated me to try to make the second edition both a primer for trainees and junior staff and a relatively up-to-date source of information for experienced clinicians.

The second edition was published in 1993. It contained 19 chapters—4 more than the first edition—a new introductory chapter conveying a historical background and perspective, and chapters on stroke in children and young adults, spinal cord strokes, and surgery. Most other stroke texts included a great deal of information about trials and tried to maintain a balanced view on many controversial topics. Instead, I purposely strove to share my own views about treatment of various conditions and other issues. This volume (a maroon cover) was 562 pages long and included 36 tables and 93 figures. Some figures of CT scans and primitive MRIs and MRAs were included. The second edition proved to be much more popular than the first edition.

The third edition (a blue cover)—now entitled *Caplan's Stroke: A Clinical Approach* at the suggestion of the publisher, Butterworth-Heinemann—was published in the year 2000—7 years after the second edition and 14 years after the first edition. The major changes from the second edition were more figures and descriptions of cerebral venous anatomy; a new chapter on cerebral dural sinus and venous thrombosis (in retrospect I was embarrassed that previous editions had so little information about this subject); and much expanded coverage of brain and vascular imaging, treatment, nonatherosclerotic conditions, brain embolism, and aneurysms and vascular malformations. Although the page numbers (556) were about the same as the second edition, this volume was printed with two columns on each page and so contained almost double the amount of text. As in the second edition, I strove to include material useful for novitiates, neurologists, and other clinicians and general neurologists, as well as stroke specialists. The third edition had 59 tables (23 more than the second edition) and 176 figures (nearly double that in the previous edition). The text was also more heavily referenced. The third edition was translated into Italian and Chinese and was even more widely read than prior editions.

This fourth edition will appear nearly a decade after the third edition. It proved much more difficult to produce and keep up to date due to the great proliferation of activity and literature in the expanding stroke field. I had to frequently update previously written chapters. This time the publisher was Elsevier, a very large international organization that had purchased Butterworth-Heinemann, as well as other smaller publishing companies. I began to plan the volume with Susan Pioli but the bulk of the later interface with Elsevier was with the very able hands of Adrianne Brigido and John Ingram—Susan Pioli having moved on to work with other organizations. In order to produce a volume that contained very consistent figures, all art was drawn by Elsevier artists. This was the only edition not illustrated by Dr. Juan Sanchez-Ramos. I strove to also include state-of-the-art images in this edition. My recent stroke fellows Drs. Manu Mehdiratta, Adnan Safdar, and David Eric Searls, as well as my neurosurgical colleague Dr. Ajith Thomas, were very helpful in helping me to choose appropriate figures and to convert them from hospital imaging files.

In this edition, I have greatly expanded Chapters 4 (Imaging and Laboratory Diagnosis) and 5 (Treatment). I have eliminated the chapter on surgery (Chapter 16 in the third edition titled Strokes, Cerebrovascular Disease, and Surgery) and integrated discussions of surgical treatment into Chapter 5 and into discussions of treatment of specific conditions in Chapters 6 through 13. I have extensively revised the chapters on stroke prevention (Chapter 17) and on rehabilitation (Chapter 19), now concentrating the latter chapter on recovery. I have expanded and updated the references for all of the chapters. In addition to there being more words on each page, this volume now contains 666 pages, 85 tables, and 282 figures. I believe that the coverage of cerebrovascular disease and stroke is broader and more thorough than in previous editions, but, as before, I have strived to continue to provide personal opinions and my own modus operandi related to diagnosis and management.

I thank Adrianne Brigido and John Ingram of Elsevier and Megan Greiner of Graphic World Inc. for shepherding this volume into print. The book would not have been possible without the help and advice of my present colleagues at Beth Israel Deaconess Medical Center, Harvard University, and past co-workers at the Michael Reese Hospital, University of Chicago, and the Tufts-New England Medical Center, Tufts University. Most of all I am indebted to the stroke patients and their families that I have cared for during the past 40 years. They have taught me much about stroke and cerebrovascular diseases but also about life and dealing with illness, adversity, and handicaps. I hope that in some small measure their experiences and this volume will help physicians to better care for the stroke patients of the future.

Louis R. Caplan, MD

Boston, Massachusetts

January 2009

Contents

General Principles I

It was then that it happened. To my shock and incredulity, I could not speak. That is, I could utter nothing intelligible. All that would come from my lips was the sound ab which I repeated again and again.... Then as I watched it, the telephone handpiece slid slowly from my grasp, and I, in turn, slid slowly from my chair and landed on the floor behind the desk.... At 5:15 in that January dusk I had been a person; now at 6:45 I was a case. But I found it easy to accept my altered condition. I felt like a case.

—ERIC HODGINS[1]

Cheshire puss ... Would you tell me please which way I ought to go from here?
That depends a great deal on where you want to get to, said the cat.
I don't much care where, said Alice.
Then it doesn't matter which way you go, said the cat.
So long as I get somewhere, Alice added.
Oh, you're sure to do that, said the cat, if you only walk long enough.

—LEWIS CARROLL[2]

The past is always with us, never to be escaped; it alone is enduring; but amidst the changes and chances which succeed one another so rapidly in life, we are apt to live too much for the present and too much in the future.

—WILLIAM OSLER[3]

NUMBERS

In the United States, nearly three fourths of a million individuals have a stroke and 150,000 (90,000 women and 60,000 men) die from stroke each year.[4] At any one time, there are approximately 2 million stroke survivors living in the United States. In China, approximately 1.5 million people die each year because of stroke.[5] Someone in the United States has a stroke every 45 seconds, and every 3.1 minutes someone dies of stroke. Stroke affects three times as many women as breast cancer and yet receives much less public attention. For a long time, stroke has been the third leading cause of death in most countries in the world, surpassed as a killer only by heart disease and cancer. Strokes are an even more important cause of prolonged disability. Survivors of strokes are often unable to return to work or to assume their former effectiveness as spouses, parents, friends, and citizens. The economic, social, and psychological costs of stroke are enormous. In the United States, each ischemic stroke costs on average $140,000, and costs related to stroke nationwide were expected to reach $65.5 billion in 2008.[5a]

IMPORTANT MEDICAL AND HISTORICAL FIGURES WHO HAD STROKES

The history of the world has undoubtedly been altered by stroke. Many important leaders in science, medicine, and politics have had their productivity cut prematurely short by stroke. Marcello Malpighi, discoverer of capillaries and the microscopic anatomy of the lungs, kidneys, and spleen, died of an apoplectic right hemiplegia.[6] Louis Pasteur, at age 46, had a stroke that caused a left hemiparesis, although he continued to make important advances until additional strokes impaired his function at age 65.[6]

Three important figures in 20th-century neurology—Russell DeJong,[7] the first editor of the journal *Neurology*; Raymond Escourolle, the French neuropathologist; and Houston Merritt, longtime Columbia professor and writer of *Merritt's Neurology*—were severely disabled by multiple strokes in their later years. Two important political leaders during the early 20th century, Vladimir Lenin and Woodrow Wilson, had intellectual impairment owing to stroke while they were at the helms of their countries at critical times in history. Lenin, at age 52 years, had the sudden onset of dysarthria and right hemiparesis. An observer noted that "often as he spoke, the words were slurred, and he paused several times like a man who has lost the thread of his argument."[8] Wilson, the architect of the League of Nations, had a series of small strokes that left him pseudobulbar and with a left hemiparesis at a time when he was ardently working for world peace and cooperation. The heads of state who met at Yalta and elsewhere to divide up the spheres of influence after World War II—Franklin Roosevelt, Winston

Churchill, and Josef Stalin (Fig. 1-1)—all had severe cerebrovascular disease at the time.[8] Roosevelt subsequently died of a fatal stroke after years of severe hypertension.[9] History might have been different if the brains of these leaders had not been addled by strokes. Public awareness of stroke increased dramatically when President Dwight Eisenhower developed acute dysarthria, when Richard Nixon died after a large embolic cerebral hemisphere infarction, and when Israeli Prime Minister Ariel Sharon was left unconscious after a series of cerebrovascular events.

PERSONAL TRAGEDY OF STROKE

The mortality, morbidity, and economic toll of stroke are impressive. Knowledge that government leaders may have brains damaged and even riddled with brain infarcts and hemorrhages is undoubtedly sobering. Yet even more important, in my own opinion, is the effect of stroke on the individual. What could be worse than the sudden inability to speak, move a limb, stand, walk, see, read, or feel or becoming unable to understand spoken language, write, think clearly, or remember? Loss of function is often instantaneous and totally unanticipated; impairments may be transient or permanent, slight or devastating. The first common term for stroke, *apoplexy,* literally meant in Greek "struck suddenly with violence."[10] The word *stroke* refers to being suddenly stricken. Stroke patients tell graphically about the personal tragedy of their illness. Eric Hodgins, the popular author of *Mr. Blandings Builds His Dream House,* wrote an autobiographic account of his stroke that he titled *Episode,* from which I quoted at the beginning of this chapter.[1] He changed from a functioning human in one moment to a helpless, dumb invalid, "a case" in the next instant. Imagine an articulate author dependent for his

livelihood on his use of language becoming totally unable to speak. Surely, the brain is wholly responsible for intelligence, capability, character, wit, humor, personality, and most of the characteristics that make us recognizable as individuals and as humans. Losing brain function can be dehumanizing and often makes individuals dependent on others. For these reasons, most individuals fear stroke more than any other disease, with the possible exception of cancer. Everyone would like to exit this life with their capabilities and mind intact, despite the inevitable aging of their bodies.

When I conjure in my own mind the personal tragedy of stroke, I picture one of my own patients, Dr. Herman Blumgart, an extremely gifted physician, teacher, and investigator. He was, for many years, physician-in-chief at the Beth Israel Hospital in Boston.[11] His early investigations in coronary artery disease were landmark advances in the understanding of vascular disease of the heart.[12,13] He gave the annual introductory lecture to incoming Harvard Medical School students about the joys and responsibilities of being a physician. I recall his vivid, articulate lectures and bedside demonstrations. He was, in many ways, the model physician. He was also a vocal advocate on behalf of patients. His lecture "Caring for the Patient," presented in 1963 and reported in the *New England Journal of Medicine,* remains a model exposition on doctoring, as valid today as when it was originally delivered.[14] Tragically, this master of communication became in an instant, severely aphasic. His Wernicke-type aphasia was so severe that he could barely communicate verbally his basic needs and could hardly understand the queries and spoken and written statements of others. He could no longer read, eliminating one of his lifelong joys. As a junior staff neurologist, I was one of his physicians. The angst and frustration of his plight showed clearly on his face each time I saw him. This personal disaster was palpable and dramatic.

BRIEF HISTORY OF STROKE

In any human endeavor, the future is heavily influenced by the past. As the Wonderland dialogue between Alice and the Cheshire Cat (quoted at the beginning of this chapter)[2] teaches, if you want to get somewhere, you must know where you are going. If clinicians are to know where they are headed, they must know where they are and where they and their predecessors have been. History adds an important dimension to knowledge. The past helps focus and broaden the perspective of the present and the future.

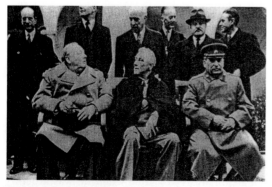

Figure 1-1. A photograph taken at the Yalta conference after World War II showing (from left to right in the front row) Winston Churchill, Franklin Delano Roosevelt, and Joseph Stalin. (From Toole JF: Cerebrovascular Disorders, 4th ed. New York: Raven Press, 1990.)

Osler, and most other important medical innovators, was aware of his debt to history and of his inevitable entanglement with the past, as well as the present and future.[3] I begin with a review of the history of stroke. Space necessitates inclusion of only a brief review of a few important people and milestones to convey a sense of the historical context of the present state of knowledge about stroke. Of course, the following view of history is eclectic and personal and should be recognized as such.

Early Observers: Hippocrates to Morgagni

Hippocrates (circa 400 BC) was probably the first to write about the medical aspects of stroke.[6,10] He and his followers were mostly interested in prognosis, predicting for the patient and family the outcome of an illness.[15-17] Hippocrates was a keen observer and urged careful observation and recording of phenomenology. Hippocrates wrote in his aphorisms on apoplexy, "persons are most subject to apoplexy between the ages of forty and sixty"[16] and attacks of numbness might reflect "impending apoplexy."[10] He astutely noted that "when persons in good health are suddenly seized with pains in the head and straightaway are laid down speechless and breathe with stertor, they die in seven days when fever comes on."[6,17] This description of subarachnoid hemorrhage shows the Hippocratic emphasis on observation and prognosis. Hippocrates also observed that there were many blood vessels connected to the brain, most of which were "thin," but two (the carotid arteries) were stout. The Greeks recognized that interruption of these blood vessels to the brain could cause loss of consciousness, and so they named the arteries carotid, from the Greek word *Karos*, meaning "deep sleep."

A few hundred years after Hippocrates, Galen (131 to 201 AD) described the anatomy of the brain and its blood vessels from dissections of animals. Although his early writings emphasized observation and experimentation, much of his later works combined mostly theorizing and speculation, in which he attributed disease to a disequilibrium between putative body humors and secretions such as water, blood, phlegm, bile, and so forth.[15] Galen and his voluminous writings dominated the 1300 years after his death. During the ensuing Dark and Middle Ages, persons who called themselves physicians gained their knowledge solely from studying the Galenic texts, considered at the time to be the epitome of all medical wisdom. Dissection, experimentation, and personal observations were discouraged and not considered scholarly.

Andreas Vesalius (1514-1564) challenged the Galenic tradition by dissecting humans and relying on his own personal observations instead of Galen's writings. Vesalius could not find the *rete mirabile* of blood vessels that Galen had described (presumably in a lower animal).[15] Vesalius's dissections were published in a volume entitled *De Humani Corpis Fabrica* (usually referred to as the *Fabrica*), which contained the detailed drawings that his young artist and collaborator Jan Kalkar reproduced as woodcuts and copper plates.[6,18] The seventh book of the *Fabrica* contains 15 diagrams of the brain. These were the most detailed neuroanatomic studies up to that time.[6] By all accounts, Vesalius had a great flair for lecturing and teaching, and his works and passion stimulated much interest in anatomy and in the brain.[15]

During the last half of the 17th century, two important physicians, Johann Jakob Wepfer (1620-1695) and Thomas Willis (1621-1675), made further anatomic and clinical observations. Wepfer wrote a popular treatise on apoplexy that was originally published in 1658 and had five subsequent editions.[6,19] Wepfer performed meticulous examinations of the brains of patients dying of apoplexy. He described the appearance of the carotid siphon and the course of the middle cerebral artery in the sylvian fissure. Obstruction of the carotid and vertebral arteries was recognized as a cause of apoplexy (the blockage preventing sufficient blood from reaching the brain).[19,20] Wepfer was the first to show clearly that bleeding into the brain was an important cause of apoplexy. Thomas Willis (Fig. 1-2), a physician and neuroanatomist best known for his *Cerebri Anatome*, which contained a description of a circle of anastomotic vessels at the base of the brain, was also a well-known clinician and an astute observer. Willis was born soon after the deaths of William Shakespeare and Queen Elizabeth when Great Britain was still basking in the artistic bloom of Elizabethan England. Willis recognized transient ischemic attacks and the phenomenology of embolism, as well as the existence of occlusion of the carotid artery.[20-25] Willis described clearly the collateral circulation in the head and neck: "[T]he cephalic arteries, whether they be carotid or vertebrals, communicate one with the other reciprocally in various ways.... This we have demonstrated by injecting dark substances in only one branch and observing that the whole brain becomes colored."[22] Willis was able to recruit a remarkable group of coworkers to Oxford, England including the illustrator and architect Christopher Wren, and the physicists

1

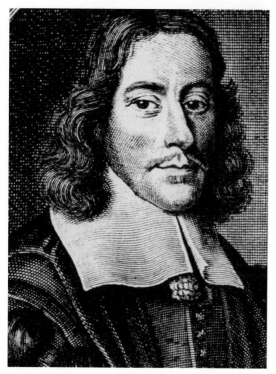

Figure 1-2. Sir Thomas Willis (1621-1675).

Robert Hooke and Robert Boyle.[24,25] These investigators were an important stimulus for science in post-Elizabethan England.[24]

During the 18th century, one of the true giants in medical history, Giovanni Battista Morgagni (1682-1771), was able to focus attention on pathology and the cause of disease. Up to that time, anatomy and prognostic formulas had prevailed. Morgagni, a distinguished professor of anatomy at the University of Padua, had a vision that the secret to understanding disease was to carefully perform necropsies on humans with illnesses and then to correlate the pathologic findings with their symptoms during life.[15] Although the clinicopathologic method is now taken for granted, this was a new approach for physicians in the 18th century. Morgagni labored his entire career to meticulously collect material for his epic work, *De Sedibus et Causis Morborum per Anatomen Indagatis*, which was published when he was 79 years old.[15,26] *De Sedibus* is a five-volume work organized in the form of 70 letters to a young man describing the cases collected. The first volume was titled *Disease of the Head*. Morgagni's clinical descriptions of patients were detailed but contained no formal physical or neurologic examinations because these were not performed during his lifetime.

One of Morgagni's descriptions illustrates the style and content of the book. "A certain man, who was a native of Genoa, blind of one eye, and

liv'd by begging, being drunk, and quarreling with other drunken beggars, receiv'd two blows by their sticks; one on his hand which was slight, and another violent one at the left temple so that blood came out of the left ear. Yet soon after, the quarrel being made up, he sat down at the fire with them ... and again fill'd himself with a great quantity of wine, by way of pledge of friendship being renewed; and not long after, on the same night, he died."[15] Necropsy showed a large epidural hematoma. Morgagni also described cases of intracerebral hemorrhage and recognized that paralysis was on the side of the body opposite to the brain lesion. Morgagni's work shifted the emphasis from anatomy alone to inquiry about diseases and their pathology, causes, and clinical manifestations during life.

Nineteenth and Early Twentieth Centuries: Atlas Makers, Virchow and Foix

During the early years of the 19th century, an influential treatise on apoplexy was written by a prominent Irish physician John Cheyne (1777-1836). Cheyne's book, which appeared in 1812, was titled *Cases of Apoplexy and Lethargy with Observations upon the Comatose Diseases*.[27] In *Cases*, he sought to separate the phenomenology of lethargy and coma from apoplexy. Cheyne's description of the neurologic abnormalities was more detailed than those of his predecessors, and the "morbid appearances" of the patients' brains were emphasized after the example of Morgagni. One illustrative patient was a woman of 32 years who was near the end of her pregnancy. After a headache she became less responsive. Cheyne found that "she preserved the power of voluntary motion of the left side, but the right was completely paralytic. She seemed perfectly conscious, attempted to speak, but could not articulate; she signified by pointing with her left hand that she desired to drink."[27] After describing her case history, Cheyne discussed the available treatments (bloodletting, emetics, purges, and external applications) and then described 23 other cases. The pathologic findings included clear descriptions of brain softenings and intracerebral and subarachnoid hemorrhages.[27] After Cheyne, developments were made concurrently in the clinical, anatomic, and pathologic aspects of stroke.

John Abercrombie contributed a more detailed clinical classification of apoplexy in his general text published in 1828.[28] Abercrombie used the presence of headache, stupor, paralysis, and outcome to separate apoplectics into three clinical groups. In the first group, which he termed primary apoplexy, the onset was sudden, unilateral paralysis; rigidity and stupor were present, and the outcome was poor. These patients probably had large intracerebral hemorrhages or large brain infarcts. In the second group, patients had the sudden onset of headache, vomiting, and either faintness or falling but no paralysis. Undoubtedly, these patients had subarachnoid hemorrhages. In the third group, there was unilateral paralysis, often with abnormal speech, but neither stupor nor headache was present. This group must have had small infarcts or parenchymatous hemorrhages. Abercrombie also speculated on etiologic mechanisms, mentioning spasm of vessels, interruption of the circulation, and rupture of diseased vessels causing hemorrhage.[10,28]

During the middle of the 19th century, dissemination of knowledge about the pathology of stroke came with the publication of four atlases, each containing plates showing brain and vascular lesions. Hooper's atlas, published in 1828, clearly illustrated pontine and putaminal hemorrhages and a subdural hematoma.[29] Cruveilhier (1835-1842),[30] Carswell (1838),[31] and Bright (1831)[32] also published atlases containing lithographs of systemic and neuropathologic lesions. Bright, better known for his work on nephritis, collected more than 200 neuropathologic cases and specimens[10] and included illustrations of 25 nervous system specimens, including cerebrovascular cases, in his volume on nervous system disorders.[32]

During the latter half of the 19th century, the most important experimental and pathologic information about vascular disease was published by Rudolf Virchow (1821 to 1902) (Fig. 1-3), a pathologist working in Berlin.[15] He described the phenomenology of in situ antemortem thrombosis with subsequent embolism. In a remarkable series of observations and experiments, Virchow analyzed the relationship between thrombi and infarction, locally and at a distance. Among 76 necropsies performed in 1847, Virchow found thrombi in extremity veins in 18 patients and within the pulmonary arteries in 11 and reasoned that the bloodstream emanating from these veins must have been the conduit for transportation of the thrombi to distant sites such as the arteries of the lung.[33,34] Virchow then used animal experiments to study the fate of foreign materials placed in veins. He later sought and found obstruction of brain, splenic, renal, and limb arteries at necropsy in patients who had cardiac valve disease and left atrial thrombi. Virchow showed systematically that in situ thrombosis and embolism were the cause of infarction and that the process was unrelated to inflammation, the predominant

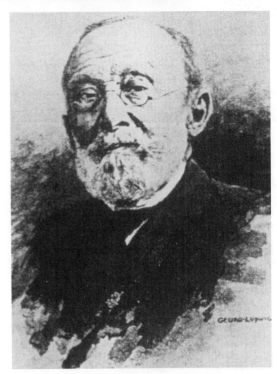

Figure 1-3. Rudolf Ludwig Karl Virchow (1821-1902).

theory at that time. Virchow described his classic triad of vascular thrombosis: (1) stasis of blood in a vessel, (2) injury to the wall of the blood vessel, and (3) an abnormality in the balance between blood procoagulant and anticoagulant factors. Before Virchow's studies and reports, blood factors and thrombosis were given little attention.

During the latter part of the 19th and the early years of the 20th centuries, the anatomic details of the arteries supplying the brain were studied carefully. Detailed observations of the distribution of the arteries and veins in the cranium were made by Düret, a French neurosurgeon, first working in Charcot's laboratory[35,36]; by Stopford in Britain[37]; and later by Foix, who dissected pathologic specimens at the Salpetriere in France.[38-41] Foix (Fig. 1-4) made many key anatomic and clinical observations. Also during this same period, clinicians gathered more information on the clinical findings in patients with strokes that involved various brain regions. The bulk of these data involved clinical descriptions, with little interest concerning pathogenesis, laboratory confirmation, or treatment. The general medical and neurologic texts of Osler,[42] Gowers,[43] and Wilson[44] contained detailed descriptions of the clinical findings and prognosis of many stroke syndromes. Sir William Osler (Fig. 1-5), a famous internist, writer, and teacher, noted in detail the neurologic findings in patients with bacterial endocarditis and described brain embolism in patients with rheumatic carditis. Osler first described the findings in patients with hemorrhagic telangiectasia (Osler, Weber, Rendu disease). The clinicopathologic method culminated in descriptions by Foix and his colleagues of the syndromes of infarctions in the regions of the middle cerebral artery,[40,41] posterior cerebral artery,[41,45] anterior cerebral artery,[41,46] and vertebrobasilar arteries.[39,41]

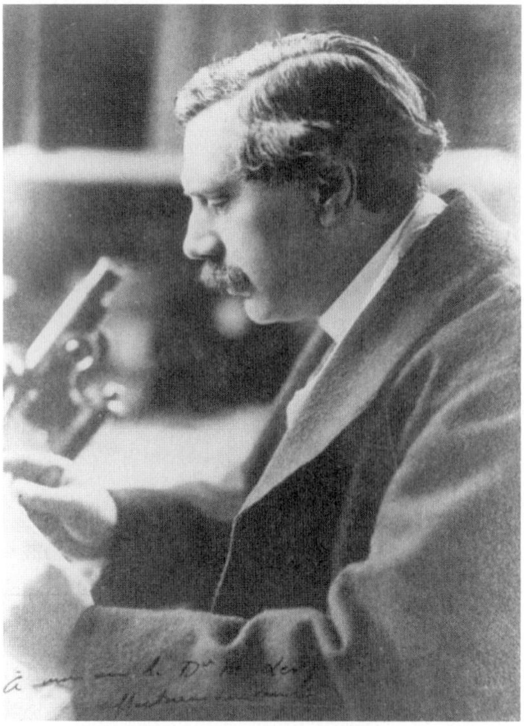

Mid-Twentieth Century and Miller Fisher

After Foix, a Canadian and American neurologist, C. Miller Fisher (Figures 1-6 to 1-8), did much to awaken clinical interest in stroke. Fisher enlisted in the Canadian army during World War II and was captured and spent years in a prisoner-of-war

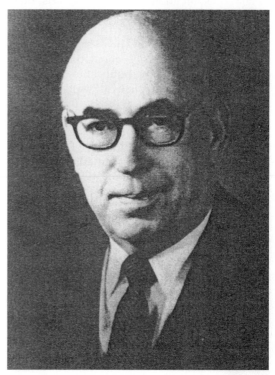

Figure 1-6. Charles Miller Fisher.

Figure 1-4. Charles Foix (1882-1927).

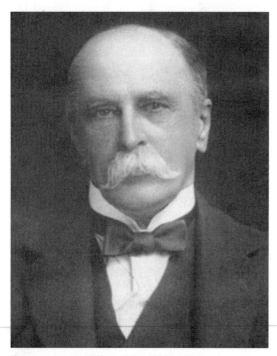

Figure 1-5. Sir William Osler (1849-1919).

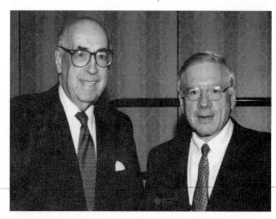

Figure 1-7. Miller Fisher with Louis Caplan.

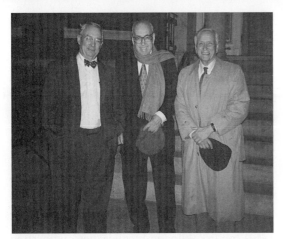

Figure 1-8. Jay P. Mohr, Miller Fisher, and Robert Ackerman.

camp. After the war, he was determined to make important contributions to medicine. His interest in stroke was tweaked by encounters with patients. One particular patient described in detail his episodes of transient monocular blindness that had heralded a hemisphere stroke. Fisher reviewed the literature and found scant reference to transient episodes before stroke. Fisher took meticulous thorough histories from patients hospitalized with stroke at a veterans hospital in Canada and found that transient prodromal episodes were quite common. In patients with transient monocular blindness preceding stroke, Fisher reasoned that the causative occlusive process was likely in the internal carotid artery in the neck or head. A patient with transient monocular blindness then died suddenly. After death, Fisher dissected the neck and found, as predicted, that the internal carotid artery was occluded.[47] He then collected and reported series of patients with internal carotid artery occlusions and described in detail the clinical histories and neurologic findings.[48,49] Fisher emphasized the frequent occurrence of warnings before stroke that he later dubbed transient ischemic attacks. "Prodromal fleeting attacks of paralysis, numbness, tingling, speechlessness, unilateral blindness, or dizziness" often preceded and warned of impending strokes in patients with carotid artery disease.[9]

Fisher, like Foix, was both a pathologist and a clinician. During his early career in Canada, and later in Boston, he thoroughly examined at necropsy the neck and cranial arteries and their microscopic-sized branches. He obtained specimens of arteries from their origins from the aorta to their major intracranial branches. During the period between 1950 and 1990, Fisher made many major pathologic and clinical observations on the pathologic and clinical features of carotid artery disease,[48-52] the pathologic and clinical

aspects of intracerebral hemorrhage,[53-56] the pathologic and clinical syndromes related to lacunar brain infarction,[57-59] and the clinical and pathologic features of various posterior circulation neurologic signs and brain and vascular lesions.[60-66] Before Fisher's major stroke publications, Raymond Adams, his mentor, had written a classic clinicopathologic descriptive report with Charles Kubik on basilar artery occlusion.[67] Fisher developed the first stroke fellowship in the United States and mentored many now senior stroke neurologists. I was fortunate to serve as his stroke fellow during 1969-1970. Figure 1-7 shows a recent picture of Fisher and I. J.P. Mohr, who worked with me in developing and maintaining the Harvard Stroke Registry in the early 1970s, and a leader in the field of stroke trials, was another of Fisher's stroke fellows. Robert Ackerman, a pioneer in the early field of PET scanning and stroke, and in the noninvasive evaluation of stroke risk, was a trainee and later colleague of Fisher, and the organizer of the Boston Stroke Society for 3 decades. Mohr, Fisher, and Ackerman are shown in Figure 1-8. Ackerman also trained stroke fellows including several future leaders in the field (Geoffrey Donnan and Steven Davis, Australia; Jean-Claude Baron, France and UK; and James Grotta and Viken Babikian, United States).

Fisher's reports contained meticulous descriptions of the signs and symptoms found in patients with infarcts and hemorrhages in various vascular and brain distributions. Elegant and thorough as these descriptions were, their limitations included (1) reliance on only the fatal cases because precise diagnosis was not possible during life; (2) predominance of anecdotal cases, with few data on the incidence and frequency of findings in large series of patients with the specific described conditions; (3) insufficient availability of technology to allow accurate diagnosis or clarification of the pathogenesis or pathophysiology of the vascular lesions and their effects on the brain; and (4) little information about the effectiveness of various treatments.

1975 to Present

During the last quarter of the 20th century, there was an explosive growth of interest in and knowledge about stroke. Advances in technology allowed better visualization of the anatomy and functional aspects of the brain and of vascular lesions during life. Databases and registries of large numbers of well-studied stroke patients helped identify and quantify the most common clinical and laboratory findings in patients with various stroke syndromes. Epidemiologic studies identified more accurately the risk factors for stroke-prevention strategies. New surgical and medical treatments were now possible. Therapeutic trials began to evaluate systematically the efficacy and safety of some of these treatments. Physicians began to explore the use of devices that could be introduced through the arterial system to treat various arterial lesions including atherosclerotic stenoses, aneurysms, and vascular malformations. Thrombolysis became a reality, and strokes were considered a medical emergency requiring urgent attention. Stroke units were formed in many hospitals and greatly improved the care of stroke patients.

Technological Advances

The technological revolution probably began with the work of the Portuguese neurosurgeon Egaz Moniz (1874-1955). Moniz surgically exposed and temporarily ligated the internal carotid artery in the neck and then rapidly injected by hand a 30% solution of sodium iodide, taking skull films later at regular time intervals.[68] He first used the technique for studying patients suspected of having brain tumors, but he later studied stroke patients. By the time of his monograph on angiography in 1931,[69] Moniz had studied 180 patients; switched to another opaque-contrast agent, Thorotrast, because of convulsions that occurred after the injection of sodium iodide; and demonstrated the occurrence of occlusion of the internal carotid artery during life.[68,69] Modern angiography began with the work of Seldinger in Sweden, who devised a technique by which a small catheter could be inserted into an artery over a flexible guide-wire after withdrawing the needle.[70,71] Catheter angiography of selected vessels in the carotid and vertebral circulations was then possible without surgical incisions. Newer dyes and filming techniques have since made angiography safer and more definitive.

Hounsfield of the British Electrical Musical Instruments (EMI) research laboratories originated the concept of computed tomography (CT) during the mid-1960s. The instrument was first used at the Atkinson-Morley Hospital in London.[6] CT scanners were first used in North America in 1973. Films from first-generation scanners were quite primitive, but by the late 1970s, third-generation scanners had made CT a useful, almost indispensable, diagnostic technique. By the mid-1980s, CT was readily available throughout North America and most of Europe. CT allowed clear distinction between brain ischemia and hemorrhage and allowed definition of the size and location of most brain

infarcts and hemorrhages. The advent of magnetic resonance imaging (MRI) into clinical medicine in the mid-1980s was a further major advance. MRI proved superior to CT in showing old hemosiderin-containing hemorrhages and in imaging vascular malformations, lesions abutting on bony surfaces, and posterior fossa structures. MRI also made it easier to visualize lesions in different planes by providing sagittal, coronal, and horizontal sections. Improved filming techniques have made it possible to image the brain vasculature through the techniques of magnetic resonance angiography[72] and CT angiography.[73]

Ultrasound was introduced to medicine in 1961 by Franklin and colleagues, who used Doppler shifts of ultrasound to study blood flow in canine blood vessels.[6,74] B-mode ultrasound was soon used to noninvasively provide images of the extracranial carotid arteries. By the early 1980s, B-mode, continuous-wave, and pulsed-Doppler technology could reliably detect severe extracranial vascular occlusive disease in the carotid and vertebral arteries in the neck. Sequential ultrasound studies allowed physicians to study the natural history of the development and progression of these occlusive lesions and to correlate the occurrence and severity of disease with stroke risk factors, symptoms, and treatment. In 1982, Aaslid and colleagues introduced a high-energy, bidirectional, pulsed-Doppler system that used low frequencies to study intracranial arteries, termed "transcranial Doppler ultrasound" (TCD).[75] TCD made possible noninvasive detection of severe occlusive disease in the major intracranial arteries during life, as well as sequential study of these lesions.[76]

Introduction of echocardiography and ambulatory cardiac rhythm monitoring in the 1970s and 1980s greatly improved cardiac diagnoses and detection of cardiogenic sources of embolism. By the early 1990s, clinicians could safely define the nature, extent, and localization of most important brain, cardiac, and vascular lesions in stroke patients. Accurate diagnosis using modern technology facilitated clinical-imaging correlations in patients with nonfatal strokes, and this paved the way for monitoring the effects of various treatments. By the end of the 20th century, advanced brain imaging with CT, MRI, and newer magnetic resonance (MR) modalities, including fluid-attenuating inversion recovery (FLAIR) images, diffusion, perfusion, and functional MRI, and MR spectroscopy, were able to show clinicians the localization, severity, and potential reversibility of brain ischemia. Vascular lesions could be quickly and safely defined using CT angiography, MR angiography, and extracranial and transcranial ultrasound. Cardiac and aortic sources of stroke were studied using trans-esophageal echocardiography. More sophisticated hematologic testing led to new insights into the role of altered coagulability in causing or contributing to thromboembolism. Clinicians were finally able to recognize and quantify quickly and accurately the key data elements needed to logically treat patients with brain ischemia and hemorrhage.

DATA BANKS AND STROKE REGISTRIES

During the middle years of the 20th century, clinicians had advanced knowledge of clinical phenomenology by personally studying and describing small groups of patients. In 1935, Aring and Meritt studied a group of patients coming to necropsy at the Boston City Hospital to clarify the differential diagnosis between brain hemorrhages and infarcts.[77] Fisher and his colleagues and students studied and described the clinical findings in small numbers of patients with various cerebrovascular syndromes. During the 1970s and 1980s, the technological advances described made it possible to define the clinical and laboratory features of nonfatal, even minor, strokes and prestroke vascular lesions. With better knowledge of clinical and morphologic features, clinicians naturally sought more quantitative data. How often did intracerebral hemorrhages or lacunar infarcts occur? How often did each of the clinical symptoms and signs occur in each subtype of stroke? Clinicians recognized that valid, statistically meaningful data could not be collected unless large numbers of patients with a wide spectrum of representative cases were studied and analyzed. The advent of computers in medicine in the 1970s greatly facilitated the storage and analysis of large quantities of complex data. Collection of data on large numbers of stroke patients began with the series of Dalsgaard-Nielsen in Scandinavia[78] and with series of patients seen by clinicians at the Mayo Clinic in Rochester, Minnesota.[79,80]

The Harvard Cooperative Stroke Registry in the early 1970s was the first computer-based registry of prospectively studied stroke patients.[81] Other stroke registries and databases were developed around the world and provided more quantitative information about clinical and laboratory phenomena and diagnoses.[82-89] Community-based studies in South Alabama[90]; Framingham, Massachusetts,[91] Oxfordshire in Great Britain,[92] the Lehigh Valley in Pennsylvania,[93] and various regions in North Carolina, Oregon, and New York[94] generated important epidemiologic data. Computer-based registries and data banks have undoubtedly assisted collection and analysis of a wide variety of clinical, radiologic, pathologic, and epidemiologic information.[95,96] Recognition of various risk factors that predispose to stroke has been especially important. The present text relies heavily on data from these studies, especially those in which I was personally involved.[81,83,85]

Stroke Units, Stroke Specialists, and Stroke Nurses

During the 19th and first two thirds of the 20th century, nearly all acute stroke patients were cared for in the general wards and rooms of hospitals. There were very few stroke specialists and no stroke nurse specialists. Some rehabilitation units, almost entirely outside of acute hospitals, did specialize in stroke rehabilitation. During the 1960s and 1970s, neurology departments began to be split off from departments of internal medicine within academic medical centers in the United States and Europe. When this occurred, hospitals with neurology departments began to place stroke patients and other patients with neurologic diseases on neurology wards and private rooms while other stroke patients continued to be treated on medical services scattered throughout the hospitals. During the 1970s and 1980s, hospitals placed very sick patients, requiring frequent monitoring and care, into specialized intensive care units (ICUs). Cardiac, surgical, and medical ICUs were first formed. Neurosurgeons and neurologists in large medical centers were successful in creating neuroscience ICUs staffed with nurses specially trained to care for very ill and acute neurologic disorders including stroke. A new neurologic specialty—neurology intensivists—began to grow.

A number of factors during the 1980s and 1990s conspired to promote the development and proliferation of specialized stroke units. CT, MRI, ultrasound, and vascular imaging capabilities made it clear that strokes were complex and composed of very diverse etiologies and pathophysiologies. Moreover, specific diagnosis could be made rather quickly and safely but required special training, expertise, and experience. Funding for trials made it possible in academic medical centers to hire nursing coordinators. The development of managed care strategies in hospitals in the United States forced more rapid and efficient care and throughput of stroke patients. Newer therapies, surgeries, percutaneous interventions, and especially thrombolysis made it advantageous to segregate stroke patients in ICUs and specialized stroke units.

These specialized units were composed of nurses with experience and training in stroke, internists, and stroke neurologists. These stroke units were able to deliver specialized nursing care; attention to management of blood pressure, fluid volumes, and other physiologic and biochemical factors; protocols and practices to facilitate rapid and thorough evaluation and treatment, monitor treatment, carry out randomized therapeutic trials, and prevent complications; and educate about stroke and its prevention to patients and their families and caregivers.[97-100] They also promoted an up-beat optimistic view of stroke recovery in contrast to the previous situation on medical wards where stroke patients were often considered undesirable patients with hopeless outcomes.

Once these units began to proliferate, especially in Europe, it became clear that they were an important major advance. Dedicated stroke units have been convincingly shown to decrease mortality, limit stroke morbidity, and allow more patients to retain their independence and to return home after stroke.[101-103] Between the carrying out of the two large European thrombolytic trials (ECASS I and ECASS II),[104,105] neurologists in the hospitals engaging in these trials developed dedicated stroke units. These units attended to the general medical care of the stroke patients and prevention of complications. As a result, the morbidity in both the thrombolytic treatment group and the placebo groups improved dramatically in the ECASS II trial, and the good results in the placebo-treated group exceeded that of any prior thrombolytic trial. The milieu and the care in dedicated stroke units lead to better outcomes. Mortality is reduced. More patients return home, and less are transferred to chronic hospitals and nursing homes. Short-term and long-term functional outcomes are also improved. There is no longer any doubt that stroke units work. One of the most important therapeutic advances during the last decades of the 20th century in the treatment of patients with acute stroke was the development of stroke services, stroke nurses, stroke specialists, and stroke units.

Advances in Medical and Surgical Therapy and Randomized Trials

During the first half of the 20th century, researchers discovered the anticoagulant effects of warfarin and heparin compounds. McLean, a medical student at Johns Hopkins, first isolated an anticoagulant compound from body tissues.[6,106] Howell and Holt extended McLean's research and named the new compound heparin.[6,107] Link and colleagues found that a natural coumarin compound found in hay was transformed during spoilage into a substance that led to bleeding in cattle.[6,108] Link crystallized dicumarol in 1939, and soon thereafter many laboratories synthesized related warfarin-type compounds that could be used therapeutically.[6] During the 1950s, clinicians began to give these anticoagulants to patients with various clinical syndromes mostly based on the tempo of brain ischemia-transient ischemic attacks, progressing stroke, completed stroke, and so on.

One of the first randomized therapeutic trials concerned the effectiveness of anticoagulant therapy in patients with various ischemic syndromes.[109] This trial, which was reported in 1962, contained only 443 patients, 219 of whom were anticoagulated.[109] The methodology and analysis used in this trial would be considered rather primitive by today's standards. Treatment was open label, not blinded, the number of patients in each ischemic group of ischemia was very few, and the end points varied depending on the nature of the group; for example, in patients entered in the group thrombosis-in-evolution (128 patients), the investigators analyzed progression of infarction and mortality. This study preceded CT scanning so that estimates of progression of infarction were only clinical. During the last decades of the 20th century, many trials studied the utility of anticoagulation in a variety of causes of brain ischemia, especially prevention of stroke in patients with atrial fibrillation.[110-113]

Sparked by clinical observations, clinicians in the mid-20th century turned to drugs that affect platelet functions as an alternative to heparin and coumadin. Probably the first clinical observations on the potential anticoagulant functions of aspirin were made by Craven, who noted that dental patients bled more if they had used aspirin.[6] He urged friends and patients to take one or two aspirin tablets a day and later published the effectiveness of this strategy in preventing coronary and cerebral thrombosis among 8000 men in articles during the mid-1950s in the *Mississippi Valley Medical Journal*,[114,115] Case reports from the United States and Britain on the effectiveness of aspirin in preventing attacks of transient monocular blindness brought the subject to more general attention.[116,117] The American[118] and Canadian[119] aspirin trials soon followed during the 1970s. These studies were the first of many trials of various antiplatelet agents almost invariably studied in large numbers of patients lumped together as having transient ischemic attacks or minor strokes.

Miller Fisher, in his seminal reports on carotid artery disease in the early 1950s, predicted that, in the future, surgery would be feasible on the internal carotid artery to prevent stroke.[48,49] During the 1950s, surgeons reported their experience with surgery on the internal carotid[120-123] and other extracranial arteries.[6,124-126] In order to study the effectiveness of surgery on the extracranial arteries, a host of neurologists and adventurous surgeons led by Bill Fields organized and carried out a large surgical trial in the 1960s.[127,128] The trial was entitled the Joint Study of Extracranial Arterial Occlusions and was supported by the National Heart Institute. This was the first surgical versus medical treatment trial carried out in the United States in which 6535 patients were randomly assigned to surgical versus nonsurgical treatment. Mortality in this trial was equal in the medical and surgical groups and death was most often cardiac. William S. Fields (Fig. 1-9) was a pioneer in the study of cerebrovascular diseases, hosted and published many conferences in Houston about various stroke conditions, and was the principal investigator and organizer of pioneering stroke trials.[6,129,130]

During the 1960s and early 1970s, Donaghy and colleagues devised a microsurgical technique to anastamose small arteries together.[131,132] One of their trainees, Gazi Yasargil, was mostly responsible for bringing this technique into clinical practice when he created surgical extracranial to intracranial shunts to treat patients with occlusive vascular disease who had brain ischemia.[133,134] By 1977, bypass procedures usually anastamosing the superficial temporal artery to branches of the middle cerebral artery were being performed widely in the United States and Europe. Henry Barnett (Fig. 1-10) organized and performed a trial of these extracranial to intracranial (EC-IC) bypass procedures and showed that the procedure as performed at the time was less successful than medical treatment.[135] Trial results, published in 1985, drastically reduced the number of procedures performed.

Alarmed that the number of carotid endarterectomy cases was growing out of hand, Henry Barnett organized a trial of surgical versus medical treatment for patients with symptomatic carotid artery disease. This North American Symptomatic Carotid Endarterectomy Trial (NASCET)[136,137] and the concurrent European Carotid Surgery Trial (ECST)[138,139] showed the effectiveness of carotid endarterectomy in selected patients with selected lesions performed by surgeons who had low surgical mortality and morbidity results. Trials of carotid surgery in patients who had no related symptoms soon followed in both the United States[140] and Europe.[141,142]

During the last decades of the 20th century, there was an almost religious zeal for randomized clinical trials. Some enthusiasts saw the future dominated by doctors searching computer

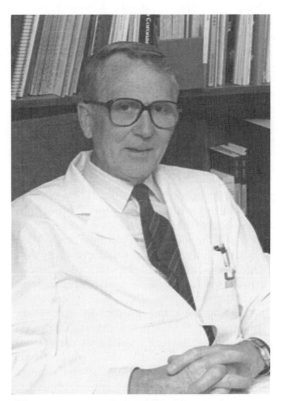

Figure 1-10. Sir Henry J.M. Barnett. (From Barnett HJM (ed): Neurologic Clinics, vol 1, no 1, Cerebrovascular Disease. Philadelphia: WB Saunders, 1983.)

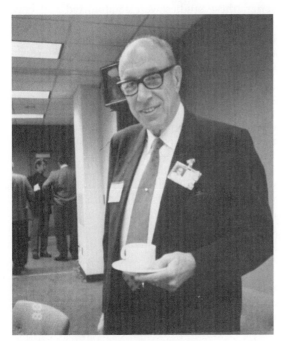

Figure 1-9. William S. Fields (1913-2004).

databases of trials to select treatment for their individual patients,[143-145] while some clinicians, including myself, were very skeptical about this vision of the future.[146]

THROMBOLYSIS

Beginning in the late 1950s, a few clinicians reported very small series of thrombolytic treatment of stroke patients.[147-150] These early investigators used bovine or human thrombolysins or streptokinase. During the early 1960s, John Sterling Meyer and his colleagues in Detroit randomized 73 patients with progressing strokes to receive streptokinase intravenously and/or concomitant anticoagulants within 3 days of stroke onset.[151,152] Clots were lysed in some patients, but 10 patients treated with streptokinase died, and some patients developed brain hemorrhages. After these studies, streptokinase and other thrombolytics were considered to be too dangerous to use, and the use of streptokinase for systemic and cardiac thromboembolism was considered contraindicated in the presence of brain lesions or past strokes.

The successful use of thrombolytic agents for the treatment of coronary artery thrombosis reawakened an interest in stroke thrombolysis during the 1980s. A group of neurologists in Aachen, Germany, led by Klaus Poeck, Hermann Zeumer, Werner Hacke, Andreas Ferbert, Berndt Ringelstein, and Helmut Bruckmann, began to treat patients with both anterior and posterior circulation thromboembolism using intra-arterial thrombolytic agents.[153,154] The early results were published in neuroradiology journals. Then Hacke and colleagues published a landmark paper in the journal *Stroke* in 1988 that convincingly showed the benefit of intra-arterial thrombolysis in patients with acute basilar artery thromboembolism when the artery was successfully recanalized.[155] Following this a consortium of investigators that included Hacke and the Aachen group, Michael Pessin and I at the New England Medical Center in Boston, Tony Furlan at the Cleveland Clinic, Gregory del Zoppo at the Scripps Clinic in La Jolla, California, and Etsuko Mori in Japan began studies, one of which was sponsored by the Burrows-Welcome group, on intravenous thrombolysis.[156,157] These investigators and others during the late 1980s and early 1990s preformed many usually small observational studies concerning the utility and risk of intravenous and intra-arterial thrombolysis. In these studies, an angiogram was performed after a CT scan had excluded hemorrhage and the catheter was not removed from the patient;

the thrombolytic drugs—streptokinase, urokinase, or rt-PA—were then given either intravenously or intra-arterially to patients whose arteriogram had shown an intracranial arterial occlusion. A follow-up angiogram was then performed after thrombolysis to determine if the occluded artery had recanalyzed. In most studies, thrombolytic drugs were given within 6 to 8 hours or longer after symptom onset. The results of these preliminary observational, nonrandomized studies were reviewed by Drs Pessin, del Zoppo, and Furlan at the 19th Princeton Vascular Disease Conference.[158]

In 1990, a group of investigators convened the first meeting on stroke thrombolysis in Heidelberg, Germany.[159] The proceeding of this meeting was published and succeeding international stroke thrombolytic meetings have occurred, at first every 2 years and more recently annually. The results of these early angiographically controlled series showed that recanalization correlated with outcome; patients who recanalized often improved; recanalization was better after IA treatment than IV treatment; manipulation of the clot during IA treatment abetted recanalization, and brain hemorrhage was an important complication, more commonly noted after intravenous treatment, which involved a larger dose of thrombolytic agent.

Stimulated by these early encouraging results, studies were planned and launched in the United States (supported by the National Institute of Neurological Disease and Stroke [NINDS] and aided by Genentech)[160] and in Europe.[104,105] In contrast to the previous smaller observational series, these studies were randomized and controlled, had larger patient numbers, had no suggested or mandated vascular studies, and shorter time intervals from symptom onset were used—90, 180, and 360 minutes. Publication of the positive results of the NINDS study in the prestigious *New England Journal of Medicine*[160] gave momentum to a movement in the United States to quickly introduce intravenous thrombolysis into the treatment of patients with acute ischemic strokes. During the summer of 1996, about half a year after the publication of the NINDS rt-PA study, the U.S. Food and Drug Administration (FDA) approved the use of rt-PA for the treatment of stroke patients when the drug was given within the first 3 hours. Subsequent published treatment protocols adopted by committees of the American Heart Association[161] and the American Academy of Neurology[162] recommended intravenous administration of rt-PA according to the methods and inclusion–exclusion criteria of the NINDS trial. The drug authorization authorities in Canada and Europe released rt-PA for clinical use much later than the FDA.

During the 1990s, clinicians and investigators launched randomized controlled trials of intra-arterial thrombolysis using prourokinase. These trials were carried out in the United States and Canada.[163],[164] The larger Proact II study included 180 patients with angiographically shown middle cerebral artery occlusions treated intra-arterially within 6 hours.[164] The study showed unequivocally that the treatment was effective, but inexplicably, the FDA failed to approve intra-arterial thrombolysis. Clinicians, however, were impressed by the results and continued to treat selected patients intra-arterially.

During the last few years of the 20th century, clinicians and investigators began to use intra-venous and intra-arterial thrombolysis and to accrue results. Unfortunately, less than 5% of acute stroke patients were treated. Clinicians began to explore ways to establish more stroke centers, ways to get patients to these stroke centers more quickly, and protocols for more rapid evaluation and treatment. They also explored ways to extend the window of treatment by using modern brain and vascular imaging (MRI/MRA, CT/CTA, and neck and transcranial ultrasound) to identify the presence and extent of infarction and the presence and nature of occluded supply arteries.

Mechanical Devices

The two most popular treatment-related buzz words used during the last quarter of the 20th century were *evidence based* and *minimally invasive surgery*. During the 1970s, physicians began to explore nonsurgical means of obliterating cerebral aneurysms and vascular malformations. Much credit should go to Fedor Serbinenko, a Russian neurosurgeon who pioneered the use of detachable latex balloons introduced through the arterial system.[165] Serbinenko used the balloons to obliterate arteries feeding aneurysms and to occlude aneurysms sparing the feeding artery. He also used the balloons to occlude arteries supplying arteriovenous malformations (AVMs). Later, interventionalists began to use silicone detachable balloons.[166] Balloons however had limited utility in treating aneurysms since many of the balloons were unable to conform to the shape of the lumens of aneurysms, and they exerted force on the walls of the aneurysm. A major advance was the development of fibered platinum coils that could be delivered through the neck of the aneurismal sacs to obliterate aneurysms. Guglielmi, an Italian radiologist, deserves credit for developing electrolytically detachable coils, which are still used frequently

today to obliterate aneurysms.[167] Observational studies and trials later showed that interventional treatment of aneurysms was at least as effective as surgery and was associated with less mortality and morbidity. Neurosurgeons began to train in interventional treatment as the 20th century ended.

During the last half of the 20th century, physicians also explored a variety of techniques to treat brain vascular malformations.[168] Luessenhop used silastic beads introduced from extracranial intra-arterial catheters to try and obliterate arteries that fed AVMs and reported the first case in 1960.[169] Subsequently, neurosurgeons and interventional radiologists began to use a wide variety of materials introduced through intra-arterial catheters to obliterate AVMs—microcatheters, glues and tissue adhesives, beads and other particles, microcoils, sutures, and balloons.[168] During the last decade of the 20th century, interventional treatment, radiation, and surgery were often used sequentially and selectively, depending on the features of the malformations.

During the 1960s and early 1970s, researchers explored the use of catheter systems that dilated arteries in animals. Andreas Gruentzig deserves great credit for introducing angioplasty into clinical practice in man. In 1978, Gruentzig reported the results from the first 5 coronary balloon angioplasties,[170] and a year later, he reported the results from the first 50 patients so treated.[171] Stimulated by the successful use of angioplasty in the coronary arteries, researchers and clinicians began to explore angioplasty in the arteries that supplied the brain. Endovascular treatment of carotid artery disease with balloon angioplasty began in 1980.[172] Kerber and colleagues reported the first use of angioplasty for treatment of carotid artery stenosis.[173] A second small series was later published in 1983 by Bockenheimer and Mathias.[174] In 1987, Theron published the first sizable series of extracranial stenosis patients treated with angioplasty (48 patients); the technical success rate was 94%, and the major stroke morbidity was 4.1%.[175] Carotid artery angioplasty became quite popular, and by 1995, it was possible to publish a review that included a worldwide experience among 523 patients.[172],[176] The development of stenting in conjunction with balloon angioplasty for carotid artery stenosis was based on studies that showed improved outcomes during coronary percutaneous interventions when stents were used.

By the end of the 20th century, stenting for extracranial carotid artery stenosis threatened to supplant surgical endarterectomy, and trials began to compare the two treatment strategies. Interventionalists also began to use angioplasty

1

and stents to treat intracranial arterial stenotic lesions[177] and to angioplasty vasoconstricted arteries in patients with subarachnoid hemorrhages. Devices began to be made and employed that could help retrieve clots. In patients with acute stroke related to thromboemboli, interventionalists could use chemical (thrombolytics) or mechanical means to retrieve thrombi within arteries, and angioplasty and stenting could be performed during the same procedure to maintain arterial patency. Many different specialists, including neurologists, neuroradiologists, neurosurgeons, vascular surgeons, and cardiologists, were trained to perform interventional treatments. The equipment available to the interventionalist looked more like a hardware store than a usual medical equipment tray. At the end of the century, physicians also explored the use of filters placed in the aorta to catch aortic and other debris generated during cardiac surgery and to use balloons placed in the aorta to augment cerebral blood flow in patients with brain ischemia due to occlusive cerebrovascular disease and vasoconstriction after subarachnoid hemorrhage.

STROKE AS A MODEL EXAMPLE OF BRAIN AND VASCULAR DISEASE

Stroke is the prototype of a focal, well-circumscribed brain lesion. C. Miller Fisher is fond of saying that neurology is learned "stroke by stroke." Knowledge of the symptoms and signs in patients with focal brain infarcts and hemorrhages has been instrumental in developing an understanding of the functioning of various brain structures and regions. Awareness of the clinical findings in patients with frontal-lobe hemorrhages has undoubtedly helped clinicians to recognize tumors, focal infections, atrophies, and other disease processes located in the frontal lobes. The ability to localize infarcts and hemorrhages precisely with CT and MRI has greatly facilitated study of anatomic-physiologic correlations. Study of stroke patients and stroke animal models has improved understanding of brain electrophysiology, chemistry, pharmacology, and overall physiology.

Stroke also provides a model for the study of vascular diseases. Atherosclerosis, embolism, and thrombosis are all usually systemic disorders that affect many critical organs in addition to the brain. Information about the morphology, development, and etiology of lesions in the cerebrovascular bed has undoubtedly influenced knowledge of vascular conditions that affect the coronary, renal, and limb arteries. Of course, the corollary

is also true; stroke clinicians clearly can and should gain from clinicians and researchers who study vascular diseases affecting these other body regions. Similarly, study of patients with cardioembolic strokes has advanced knowledge about the heart and its diseases.[178] Stroke patients often have abnormalities of blood coagulation. Elucidation of clotting and bleeding dysfunction underlying stroke has advanced general knowledge about the formed and serologic elements of the blood and the vascular endothelium and about their functions in coagulation.

STROKE CARE

It is not possible to overemphasize that the care of strokes is not the same as the care of individual stroke patients. Most strokes result from systemic illnesses such as hypertension, atherosclerosis, cardiac diseases, and coagulopathies. These conditions profoundly affect other body organs and general health, as well as the brain and central nervous system. Specialists sometimes only see and treat one portion of the body and ignore the general problem, similar to the proverbial blind men feeling isolated parts of the elephant. As physicians, we must be sure that the general systemic disorders, such as hypertension and atherosclerosis, receive deserved detailed and long-term attention. As entry portals into the healthcare system, clinicians seeing stroke patients can and should become key figures in preventing disease and in correcting unhealthy practices.

Strokes create other health problems. These include not only the acute complications that are discussed in Chapter 18, but also problems such as increased wear and tear on the joint structures of the hip, knee, and ankle because of altered gait; aspiration and recurrent bronchopulmonary infections; and poor bladder emptying, with an increased frequency of urinary-tract infections. Strokes also have profound social, psychological, and economic effects on stroke patients and their families and friends. Physicians caring for stroke patients must consider all of the multiple facets of the condition and must liberally use other medical and ancillary health personnel. The family often needs as much attention, education, and compassion as the patient. In another book, I have devoted considerable attention to the general approach toward and care of patients, especially those with neurologic illnesses.[179]

The other organs exist to keep the brain functioning normally. Any change in the brain's function and activity profoundly affects living. No medical task exists that is more complex, more multifaceted, more important, and potentially more rewarding than caring for a stroke patient.

References

1. Hodgins E: Episode: Report on the Accident Inside My Skull. New York: Atheneum, 1964.
2. Carroll L: Alice's Adventures in Wonderland. New York: Dutton, 1929.
3. Osler W: Aequanimitas with Other Addresses to Medical Students, Nurses and Practitioners of Medicine. Philadelphia: Blakiston, 1932.
4. Broderick J, Brott T, Kothari R, et al: The Greater Cincinnati/Northern Kentucky Stroke Study. Preliminary first-ever and total incidence rates of strokes among blacks. Stroke 1998;29:415-421.
5. Chen ZM, Xu Z, Coillins R, et al: Blood pressure, blood cholesterol and stroke mortality in a population with low mean cholesterol level. Cerebrovasc Dis 1998;8(suppl 4):1.
5a. Rosamond W, Flegal K, Furie A, et al: Heart disease and stroke statistics—2008 update: A report from the American Heart Association Statistics Committee and Stroke Statistics Committee. Circulation 2008;117:e25-e146.
6. Fields WS, Lemak NA: A History of Stroke: Its Recognition and Treatment. New York: Oxford University Press, 1989.
7. Gilman S, Russell N: DeJong, 1907-1990. Ann Neurol 1991;29:108-109.
8. Friedlander WJ: About three old men: An inquiry into how cerebral atherosclerosis has altered world politics. Stroke 1972;3:467-473.
9. Bruenn HG: Clinical notes on the illness and death of president Franklin D. Roosevelt. Ann Intern Med 1970;72:579-591.
10. McHenry Jr LC: Garrison's History of Neurology. Springfield, Ill: Charles C. Thomas, 1969.
11. Linenthal AJ: First a Dream: The History of Boston's Jewish Hospitals, 1896 to 1928. Boston: Beth Israel Hospital, 1990:276-294.
12. Blumgart HL, Schlesinger MJ, Davis D: Studies on the relation of the clinical manifestations of angina pectoris, coronary thrombosis, and myocardial infarction to the pathological findings. Am Heart J 1940;19:1-9.
13. Blumgart HL, Schlesinger MJ, Zoll PM: Angina pectoris, coronary failure, and acute myocardial infarction. JAMA 1941;116:91-97.
14. Blumgart HL: Caring for the patient. N Engl J Med 1964;270:449-456.
15. Nuland S: Doctors: The Biography of Medicine. New York: Knopf, 1988.
16. Adams F: The Genuine Works of Hippocrates: Translated from the Greek. Baltimore: Williams & Wilkins, 1939.
17. Clark E: Apoplexy in the Hippocratic writings. Bull Hist Med 1963;37:301-314.
18. Vesalius A: De Humani Corporis Fabrica. Basileae, Italy: J Oporini, 1543.
19. Wepfler JJ: Observationes Anatomicae, ex Cadaveribus Eorum, quos Sustulit Apoplexia, cum Exercitatione de Ejus Loco Affecto. Schaffhausen, Germany: Joh Caspari Suteri, 1658.
20. Gurdjian ES, Gurdjian ES: History of occlusive cerebrovascular disease: I. From Wepfer to Moniz. Arch Neurol 1979;36:340-343.
21. Willis T: The London Practice of Physick. London: Printed for Thomas Basset at the George in Fleet Street and William Crooke at the Green-Dragon without Temple-Bar 1685.
22. Willis T: Cerebri anatome: Cui accessit nervorum descriptio et usus. J Flesher, London, 1664.
23. Willis T: Instructions and prescripts for curing the apoplexy. In Portage S (ed): The London Practice of Physic. London: 1679.
24. Carl Zimmer: Soul Made Flesh: The Discovery of the Brain and How It Changed the World. New York: William Heinemann (Random House), 2004.
25. Caplan LR: Posterior circulation ischemia: Then, now, and tomorrow. The Thomas Willis lecture—2000. Stroke 2000;31:2011-2023.
26. Morgagni GB: The Seats and Causes of Disease Investigated by Anatomy. Translated by B Alexander. London: Millar and Cadell, 1769. Birmingham: Classics of Medicine Library, 1983.
27. Cheyne J: Cases of Apoplexy and Lethargy with Observations upon the Comatose Diseases. London: J Moyes Printer, 1812.
28. Abercrombie J: Pathological and Practical Researches on Diseases of the Brain and Spinal Cord. Edinburgh: Waugh and Innes, 1828.
29. Hooper R: The Morbid Anatomy of the Human Brain Illustrated by Coloured Engravings of the Most Frequent and Important Organic Diseases to Which That Viscus Is Subject. London: Rees, Orme, Brown, and Green, 1831.
30. Cruveilhier J: Anatomie Pathologique du Corps Humain: Descriptions Avec Figures Lithographiées et Caloriées des Diverses Alterations Morbides Dont le Corps Humain Est Susceptible. Paris: JB Bailliere, 1835-1842.
31. Carswell R: Pathological Anatomy: Illustrations of the Elementary Forms of Disease. London: Longman, 1838.
32. Bright R: Reports of Medical Cases, Selected with a View of Illustrating the Symptoms and Cures of Diseases by a Reference to Morbid Anatomy. London: Longman, Rees, Orme, Brown, and Green, 1831.
33. Fisher CM: The history of cerebral embolism and hemorrhagic infarction. In Furlan A (ed): The Heart and Stroke. Berlin: Springer-Verlag, 1987, pp 3-16.
34. Virchow R: Ueber die akut entzundung der arterien. Virchows Arch Pathol Anat 1847;1:272-378.
35. Duret H: Sur la distribution des arteres nouricieres du bulbe rachidien. Arch Physiol Norm Pathol 1873;2:97-113.
36. Duret H: Recherches anatomiques sur la circulation de l'encephale. Arch Physiol Norm Pathol 1874;3:60-91, 316-353.
37. Stopford JS: The anatomy of the pons and medulla oblongata. J Anat Physiol 1928;50:225-280.
38. Foix C, Hillemand P: Irrigation de la protuberance. C R Soc Biol (Paris) 1925;92:35-36.
39. Foix C, Hillemand P: les Arteres de l'axe encephalique jusqu'au diencephale inclusivement. Rev Neurol (Paris) 1925;41:705-739.

40. Foix C, Levy M. Les Ramollissements sylviens. Rev Neurol (Paris) 1927;43:1-51.

41. Caplan LR: Charles Foix—The first modern stroke neurologist. Stroke 1990;21:348-356.

42. Osler W: The Principles and Practice of Medicine, 5th ed. New York: D Appleton, 1903.

43. Gowers WR: A Manual of Disease of the Nervous System. London: J and A Churchill, 1893.

44. Wilson SAK, Bruce AN: Neurology, 2nd ed. London: Butterworth-Heinemann, 1955.

45. Foix C, Masson A: Le Syndrome de l'artere cerebrale posterieure. Presse Med 1923;31:361-365.

46. Foix C, Hillemand P: Les Syndromes de l'artere cerebrale anterieure. Encephale 1925;20:209-232.

47. Estol CJ: Dr C. Miller Fisher and the history of carotid artery disease. Stroke 1996;27:559-566.

48. Fisher CM: Occlusion of the internal carotid artery. Arch Neurol Psychiatry 1951;65:346-377.

49. Fisher M: Occlusion of the carotid arteries. Arch Neurol Psychiatry 1954;72:187-204.

50. Fisher CM, Ojemann RG: A clinico-pathologic study of carotid endarterectomy plaques. Rev Neurol 1986;142:573-589.

51. Fisher CM: Observations of the fundus oculi in transient monocular blindness. Neurology 1959;9:333-347.

52. Fisher CM: Facial pulses in internal carotid artery occlusion. Neurology 1970;20:476-478.

53. Fisher CM: The pathology and pathogenesis of intracerebral hemorrhage. In Fields WS (ed): Pathogenesis and Treatment of Cerebrovascular Disease. Springfield, Ill: Charles C Thomas, 1961, pp 295-317.

54. Fisher CM: Clinical syndromes in cerebral hemorrhage. In Fields WS (ed): Pathogenesis and Treatment of Cerebrovascular Disease. Springfield, Ill: Charles C Thomas, 1961, pp 318-342.

55. Fisher CM: Pathological observations in hypertensive cerebral hemorrhage. J Neuropathol Exp Neurol 1971;30:536-550.

56. Fisher CM, Picard EH, Polak A, et al: Acute hypertensive cerebellar hemorrhage: Diagnosis and surgical treatment. J Nerv Ment Dis 1965;140:38-57.

57. Fisher CM: Lacunes: Small deep cerebral infarcts. Neurology 1965;15:774-784.

58. Fisher CM: The arterial lesions underlying lacunes. Acta Neuropath (Berlin) 1969;12:1-15.

59. Fisher CM: Pure motor hemiparesis of vascular origin. Arch Neurol 1965;13:30-44.

60. Fisher CM, Karnes W, Kubik CS: Lateral medullary infarction. The pattern of vascular occlusion. J Neuropath Exp Neurol 1961;20:323-379.

61. Fisher CM: A new vascular syndrome - "the subclavian steal". N Engl J Med 1961;265:912.

62. Fisher CM, Caplan LR: Basilar artery branch occlusion: A cause of pontine infarction. Neurology 1971;21:900-905.

63. Fisher CM: The posterior cerebral artery syndrome. Can J Neurol Sci 1986;13:232-239.

64. Fisher CM: Ocular bobbing. Arch Neurol 1964;11:543-546.

65. Fisher CM: Some neuro-opthalmological observations. J Neurol Neurosurg Psychiatry 1967;30:383-392.

66. Fisher CM: The 'herald hemiparesis' of basilar artery occlusion. Arch Neurol 1988;45:1301-1303.

67. Kubik CS, Adams RD: Occlusion of the basilar artery: A clinical and pathological study. Brain 1946;69:73-121.

68. Moniz E: l'Encephalographie artèrielle, son importance dans la localizationdes tumeurs cérébrales. Rev Neurol (Paris) 1927;2:72-90.

69. Moniz E: L'Angiographie Cérébrale. Paris: Masson, 1931.

70. Gurdjian ES, Gurdjian ES: History of occlusive cerebrovascular disease. II. After Moniz with special reference to surgical treatment. Arch Neurol 1979;36:427-432.

71. Seldinger SI: Catheter replacement of the needle in percutaneous arteriography. Acta Radiol 1953;39:368-376.

72. Edelman RC, Mattle HP, O'Reilly GV, et al: Magnetic resonance imaging of flow dynamics in the circle of Willis. Stroke 1990;21:56-65.

73. Knauth M, von Kummer R, Jansen O, et al: Potential of CT angiography in acute ischemic stroke. Am J Neuroradiol 1997;18:1001-1010.

74. Franklin DL, Schlegel WA, Rushner RF: Blood flow measured by Doppler frequency shift of back-scattered ultrasound. Science 1961;134:564-565.

75. Aaslid R, Markwalder TM, Nornes H: Non-invasive transcranial Doppler ultrasound recording of flow velocity in basal cerebral arteries. J Neurosurg 1982;57:769-774.

76. Caplan LR, Brass LM, DeWitt LD, et al: Transcranial Doppler ultrasound: Present status. Neurology 1990;40:696-700.

77. Aring CD, Meritt HH: Differential diagnosis between cerebral hemorrhage and cerebral thrombosis. Arch Intern Med 1935;56:435-456.

78. Dalsgaard-Nielsen T: Survey of 1000 cases of apoplexia cerebri. Acta Psychiatr Neurol Scand 1955;30:169-185.

79. Whisnant JP, Fitzgibbons JP, Kurland LT, et al: Natural history of stroke in Rochester, Minnesota, 1945 through 1954. Stroke 1971;2:11-22.

80. Matsumoto N, Whisnant JP, Kurland LT, et al: Natural history of stroke in Rochester, Minnesota, 1955 through 1969. An extension of a previous study 1945 through 1954. Stroke 1973;4:20-29.

81. Mohr JP, Caplan LR, Melski JW, et al: The Harvard Cooperative Stroke Registry: A prospective registry. Neurology 1978;28:754-762.

82. Kunitz S, Gross CR, Heyman A, et al: The Pilot Stroke Data Bank: Definition, design, and data. Stroke 1984;15:740-746.

83. Caplan LR, Hier DB, D'Cruz I: Cerebral embolism in the Michael Reese Stroke Registry. Stroke 1983;14:530-536.

84. Chambers BR, Donnan GA, Bladin PF: Patterns of stroke: An analysis of the first 700 consecutive admissions to the Austin Hospital Stroke Unit. Aust N Z J Med 1983;13:57-64.

85. Foulkes MA, Wolf PA, Price TR, et al: The Stroke Data Bank: Design, methods, and baseline characteristics. Stroke 1988;19:547-554.

86. Bogousslavsky J, Mille GV, Regli F: The Lausanne Stroke Registry: An analysis of 1,000 consecutive patients with first stroke. Stroke 1988;19:1083-1092.

87. Moulin T, Tatu L, Crepin-Leblond T, et al: The Besancon Stroke Registry: An acute stroke registry of 2,500 consecutive patients. Eur Neurol 1997;38(1):10-20.

88. Heuschmann PU, Kolominsky-Rabas PL, Misselwitz B, et al: Predictors of in-hospital mortality and attributable risks of death after ischemic stroke: The German Stroke Registers Study Group. Arch Intern Med 2004;164: 1761-1768.

89. Vemmos KN, Takis CE, Georgilis K, et al: The Athens stroke registry: Results of a five-year hospital-based study. Cerebrovasc Dis 2000;10: 133-141.

90. Gross CR, Kase CS, Mohr JP, et al: Stroke in south Alabama: Incidence and diagnostic features—a population based study. Stroke 1984;15:249-255.

91. Wolf PA, Kannel WB, Dauber TR: Prospective investigations: The Framingham study and the epidemiology of stroke. Adv Neurol 1978;19:107-120.

92. Oxfordshire Community Stroke Project: Incidence of stroke in Oxfordshire: First year's experience of a community stroke registry. BMJ 1983;287:713-717.

93. Alter M, Sobel E, McCoy RC, et al: Stroke in the Lehigh Valley: Incidence based on a community-wide hospital registry. Neuroepidemiology 1985;4:1-15.

94. Yatsu FM, Becker C, McLeroy K, et al: Community hospital-based stroke programs: North Carolina, Oregon, and New York. I. Goals, objectives, and data collection procedures. Stroke 1986;17:276-284.

95. Mohr JP: Stroke data banks [editorial]. Stroke 1986;17:171-172.

96. Caplan LR: Stroke data banks, then and now. In R Courbier (ed): Basis for a Classification of Cerebrovascular Disease. Amsterdam: Excerpta Medica, 1985, pp152-162.

97. Caplan LR: Caplan's short rendition of stroke during the 20th century: Part 2. A short history. Int Stroke J 2006;1:28-234.

98. Indredavik B, Bakke F, Solberg R, et al: Benefit of a stroke unit: A randomized controlled trial. Stroke 1991;22:1026-1031.

99. Indredavik B, Slordahl SA, Bakke F, et al: Stroke unit treatment. Long-term effects. Stroke 1997;28:1861-1866.

100. Diez-Tejedor E, Fuentes B: Acute care in stroke: Do stroke units make the difference? Cerebrovasc Dis 2001;11(suppl 1):31-39.

101. Birbeck GL, Zingmond DS, Cui X, Vickrey BG: Multispecialty stroke services in California hospitals are associated with reduced mortality. Neurology 2006;66:1527-1532.

102. Stroke Unit Trialists' Collaboration: Collaborative systematic review of the randomized trials of organised in-patient (stroke unit) care after stroke. BMJ 1997;314:1151-1159.

103. Stroke Unit Trialists' Collaboration: How do stroke units improve patient outcomes? A collaborative systematic review of the randomized trials. Stroke 1997;28:2139-2144.

104. Hacke W, Kaste M, Fieschi C, et al: Intravenous thrombolysis with recombinant tissue plasminogen activator for acute hemispheric stroke. The European Cooperative Acute Stroke Study (ECASS). JAMA 1995;274:1017-1025.

105. Hacke W, Kaste M, Fieschi C, et al for the Second European-Australasian Acute Stroke Study Investigators. Randomised double-blind placebo-controlled trial of thrombolytic therapy with intravenous alteplase in acute ischaemic stroke (ECASS-II). Lancet 1998;352:1245-1251.

106. McLean J: The thromboplastic action of cephalin. Am J Physiol 1916;41:250-257.

107. Howell WH, Holt E: Two new factors in blood coagulation—Heparin and pro-antithrombin. Am J Physiol 1918;47:328-341.

108. Link KP: The discovery of dicumarol and its sequels. Circulation 1959;19:97-107.

109. Baker RN, Broward JA, Fang HC, et al: Anticoagulant therapy in cerebral infarction. Report on cooperative study. Neurology 1962;12:823-835.

110. The Boston Area Anticoagulation Trial for Atrial Fibrillation Investigators: The effect of low-dose warfarin on the risk of stroke in patients with nonrheumatic atrial fibrillation. N Engl J Med 1990;323:1505-1511.

111. Petersen P, Godtfredsen J, Boysen G, et al: Placebo-controlled, randomized trial of warfarin and aspirin for prevention of thromboembolic complications in chronic atrial fibrillation: The Copenhagen AFASAK Study. Lancet 1989;1:175-179.

112. The Stroke Prevention in Atrial Fibrillation Investigators: The stroke prevention in atrial fibrillation study: Final results. Circulation 1991;84: 527-539.

113. EAFT (European Atrial Fibrillation Trial) Study Group: Secondary prevention in non-rheumatic atrial fibrillation after transient ischaemic attack or minor stroke. Lancet 1993;342:1255-1262.

114. Craven LL: Experiences with aspirin (acetylsalicylic acid) in the nonspecific prophylaxis of coronary thrombosis. Mississippi Valley Med J 1953;75:38-44.

115. Craven LL: Prevention of coronary and cerebral thrombosis. Mississippi Valley Med J 1956;78: 213-215.

116. Mundall J, Quintero P, von Kaulla K, et al: Transient monocular blindness and increased platelet aggregability treated with aspirin—A case report. Neurology 1971;21:402.

117. Harrison MJG, Marshall J, Meadows JC, et al: Effect of aspirin in amaurosis fugax. Lancet 1971;2:743-744.

118. Fields WS, LeMak NA, Frankowski RF, Hardy RJ: Controlled trial of aspirin in cerebral ischemia. Stroke 1977;8:301-316.

119. The Canadian Cooperative Study Group: A randomized trial of aspirin and sulfinpyrazone in threatened stroke. N Engl J Med 1978;299:53-59.

120. Lin PM, Javid H, Doyle EJ: Partial internal carotid artery occlusion treated by primary resection and vein graft. J Neurosurg 1956;13:650-655.

121. Eastcott HHG, Pickering GW, Rob CG: Reconstruction of internal carotid artery in a patient with intermittent attacks of hemiplegia. Lancet 1954;2:994-996.

122. DeBakey ME: Successful carotid endarterectomy for cerebrovascular insufficiency. Nineteen years follow-up. JAMA 1975;233:1083-1085.

123. Carrea R, Molins M, Murphy G: Surgical treatment of spontaneous thrombosis of the internal carotid artery in the neck. Carotid-carotideal anastomosis. Acta Neurol Latinoam 1955;1:71-78.

124. Cooley DA, Al-Naaman YD, Carton CA: Surgical treatment of arteriosclerotic occlusions of common carotid artery. J Neurosurg 1956;2:1265-1267.

125. Cate WR Jr, Scott HW: Cerebral ischemia of central origin. Relief by subclavian-vertebral artery thromboendarterectomy. Surgery 1959;45:19-31.

126. Thompson JE: The evolution of surgery for the treatment and prevention of stroke: The Willis lecture. Stroke 1996;27:1427-1434.

127. Fields WS, North RR, Hass WK, et al: Joint study of extracranial arterial occlusion as a cause of stroke: Organization of study and survey of patient population. JAMA 1968;203:955-960.

128. Hass WK, Fields WS, North R, et al: Joint study of extracranial arterial occlusion. II. Arteriography, techniques, sites, and complications. JAMA 1968;203:961-968.

129. Fields WS (ed): Pathogenesis and Treatment of Cerebrovascular Disease. Springfield, Ill: Charles C Thomas, 1961.

130. Fields WS, Sahs AL (eds): Intracranial aneurysms and subarachnoid hemorrhage. Springfield, Ill: Charles C Thomas, 1965.

131. Maroon JC, Donaghy RMP: Experimental cerebral revascularization with autogenous grafts. J Neurosurg 1973;38:172-179.

132. Hunter KM, Donaghy RMP: Arterial micrografts. An experimental study. Can J Surg 1973;16:23-27.

133. Yasargil MG, Krayenbuhl HA, Jacobson JH: Microneurosurgical arterial reconstruction. Surgery 1970;67:221-233.

134. Yasargil MG (ed): Microsurgery applied to neurosurgery. Stuttgart: George Thieme Verlag, 1969.

135. EC/IC Bypass Study Group: Failure of extracranial-intracranial arterial bypass to reduce the risk of ischemic stroke: Results of an international randomized trial. N Engl J Med 1985;313:191-200.

136. North American Symptomatic Carotid Endarterectomy Trial (NASCET) Collaborators: Beneficial effects of carotid endarterectomy in symptomatic patients with high-grade carotid stenosis. N Engl J Med 1991;325:445-453.

137. Barnett HJM, Taylor DW, Eliasziw M, et al for the North American Symptomatic Carotid Endarterectomy Trial Collaborators. Benefit of carotid endarterectomy in patients with symptomatic moderate or severe stenosis. N Engl J Med 1998;339:1415-1425.

138. European Carotid Surgery Trialists' Collaborative Group: MRC European Carotid Surgery trial: Interim results of symptomatic patients with severe (70–99%) or with mild (0–29%) carotid stenosis. Lancet 1991;1:1235-1243.

139. European Carotid Surgery Trialists' Collaborative Group: Randomized trial of endarterectomy for recently symptomatic carotid stenosis: final results of the MRC European Carotid Surgery Trial (ECST). Lancet 1998;351:1379-1387.

140. Asymptomatic Carotid Atherosclerosis Study Group: Carotid endarterectomy for patients with asymptomatic carotid artery stenosis. JAMA 1995;273:1421-1428.

141. Halliday AW, Thomas DJ, Mansfield AO: The Asymptomatic Carotid Surgery Trial (ACST). Int Angiol 1995;14:18-20.

142. Halliday A, Mansfield A, Marro J: Prevention of disabling and fatal strokes by successful carotid endarterectomy in patients without recent neurological symptoms: Randomised controlled trial. Lancet 2004;363:1491-1502.

143. Meinert CL: Clinical Trials: Design, Conduct, and Analysis. New York: Oxford University Press, 1986.

144. Sackett DL: Evidence-based medicine: What it is and what it isn't. BMJ 1996;312:71-72.

145. Sackett DL, Rosenberg W: On the need for evidence-based medicine. Evid Based Med 1995;1:5-6.

146. Caplan LR: Editorial. Evidence-based medicine: Concerns of a clinical neurologist. J Neurol Neurosurg Psychiatry 2001;71:569-576.

147. Sloan MA: Thrombolysis and stroke: Past and future. Arch Neurol 1987;44:748-768.

148. Sussman BJ, Fitch TSP: Thrombolysis with fibrinolysin in cerebral arterial occlusion. JAMA 1958;167:1705-1709.

149. Herndon RM, Meyer JS, Johnson JF, et al: Treatment of cardiovascular thrombosis with fibrinolysin. Am J Cardiol 1960;30:540-545.

150. Clark RL, Clifton EE: The treatment of cerebrovascular thrombosis and embolism with fibrinolytic agents. Am J Cardiol 1960;30:546-551.

151. Meyer JS, Gilroy J, Barnhart ME, et al: Anticoagulants plus streptokinase therapy in progressive stroke. JAMA 1963;189:373.

152. Meyer JS, Gilroy J, Barnhart ME, et al: Therapeutic thrombolysis in cerebral thromboembolism. Randomized evaluation of intravenous streptokinase. In Millikan CH, Siekert R, Whisnant JP (eds): Cerebral Vascular Diseases. New York: Grune and Stratton, 1964, pp 200-213.

153. Zeumer H, Hacke W, Ringelstein EB: Intra-arterial thrombolysis in vertebrobasilar thromboembolic disease. Am J Neuroradiol 1983;4:401-404.

154. Zeumer H, Hundgen R, Ferbert A, et al: Local intra-arterial fibrinolyic therapy in inaccessible internal carotid occlusion. Neuroradiology 1984;76:315-317.

155. Hacke W, Zeumer H, Ferbert A, et al: Intra-arterial thrombolytic therapy improves outcome in patients with acute vertebrobasilar occlusive disease. Stroke 1988;19:1216-1222.

156. del Zoppo GJ, Poeck K, Pessin MS, et al: Recombinant tissue plasminogen activator in acute thrombotic and embolic stroke. Ann Neurol 1992;32:78-86.

157. Wolpert SM, Bruckmann H, Greenlee R, et al: Neuroradiologic evaluation of patients with acute stroke treated with recombinant tissue plasminogen activator. The rt-PA Acute Stroke Study Group. AJNR Am J Neuroradiol 1993;14:3-13.

158. Pessin MS, del Zoppo GJ, Furlan AJ: Thrombolytic treatment in acute stroke: Review and update of selected topics. In Cerebrovascular Diseases, 19th Princeton Conference, 1994. Boston: Butterworth-Heinemann, 1995, pp 409-418.

159. Hacke W, del Zoppo GJ, Hirschberg M (eds): Thrombolytic Therapy in Acute Ischemic Stroke. Berlin: Springer-Verlag, 1991.

160. The National Institute of Neurological Disorders, Stroke rt-PA Study Group: Tissue plasminogen activator for acute ischemic stroke. N Engl J Med 1995;333:1581-1587.

161. Adams HP, Brott TG, Furlan AJ, et al: Use of thrombolytic drugs. A supplement to the guidelines for the management of patients with acute ischemic stroke. A statement for health care professionals from a special writing group of the Stroke Council American Heart Association. Stroke 1996;27:1711-1718.

162. Quality Standards Subcommittee of the American Academy of Neurology: Practice advisory: Thrombolytic therapy for acute ischemic stroke—Summary statement. Neurology 1996;47:835-839.

163. del Zoppo GJ, Higashida RT, Furlan AJ, et al: PROACT: A phase II randomized trial of recombinant pro-urokinase by direct arterial delivery in acute middle cerebral artery stroke. PROACT Investigators. Prolyse in Acute Cerebral Thromboembolism. Stroke 1998;29:4-11.

164. Furlan AJ, Higashida RT, Wechsler L, et al: Intra-arterial Prourokinase for acute ischemic stroke. The PROACT II Study: A randomized controlled trial. JAMA 1999;282:2003-2011.

165. Serbinenko FA: Balloon catheterization and occlusion of major cerebral vessels. J Neurosurg 1974;41:125-145.

166. Introcaso JH, Uske A: Endovascular treatment of intracranial aneurysms. In Batjer HH, Caplan LR, Friberg L, et al (eds): Cerebrovascular Disease. Philadelphia: Lippincott-Raven, 1996, pp 915-927.

167. Guglielmi G, Viñuela F, Sepetka I, et al: Electrothrombosis of saccular aneurysms. Neurosurgery via endovascular approach. I. Electrochemical basis, technique, and experimental results. J Neurosurg 1991;75:1-7.

168. Latchaw RE, Madison MT, Larsen DW, Silva P: Intracranial arteriovenous malformations: Endovascular strategies and methods. In Batjer HH, Caplan LR, Friberg L, et al (eds): Cerebrovascular Disease. Philadelphia: Lippincott-Raven, 1996, pp 707-725.

169. Luessenhop AJ, Spence WT: Artificial embolization of cerebral arteries. Report of use in a case of arteriovenous malformation. JAMA 1960;172:1153-1155.

170. Gruentzig A: Transluminal dilatation of coronary artery stenosis. Lancet 1978 1;263.

171. Gruentzig AR, Senning A, Siegenthaler WE: Nonoperative dilatation of coronary artery stenosis: Percutaneous transluminal coronary angioplasty. N Engl J Med 1979;301:61-68.

172. Meyers PM, Schumacher HC, Higashida RT, et al: Use of stents to treat extracranial cerebrovascular disease. Ann Rev Med 2006;57:437-454.

173. Kerber CW, Cromwell LD, Loehden OL: Catheter dilatation of proximal carotid stenosis during distal bifurcation endarterectomy. AJNR Am J Neuroradiol 1980;1:348-349.

174. Bockenheimer SA, Mathias K: Percutaneous transluminal angioplasty in arteriosclerotic internal carotid artery stenosis. AJNR Am J Neuroradiol 1983;4:791-792.

175. Theron J, Raymond J, Casasco A, Courtheoux F: Percutaneous angioplasty of atherosclerotic and postsurgical stenosis of carotid arteries. AJNR Am J Neuroradiol 1987;8:495-500.

176. Kachel R: Results of balloon angioplasty in the carotid arteries. J Endovasc Surg 1996;3:22-30.

177. Meyers PM, Schumacher HC, Higashida RT, Caplan LR: Intracranial revascularization. Ann Rev Med 2007;58:107-122.

178. Caplan LR, Manning W (eds): Brain Embolism. New York: Informa Healthcare, 2006.

179. Caplan LR, Hollander J: The Effective Clinical Neurologist, 2nd ed. Boston: Butterworth-Heinemann, 2001.

2

Basic Pathology, Anatomy, and Pathophysiology of Stroke

Stroke is anything but a homogeneous entity. Disorders as different as rupture of a large blood vessel that causes flooding of the brain with blood and occlusion of a tiny artery with softening in a small but strategic brain site both qualify as strokes. These two pathologic caricatures of stroke subtypes are as divergent as grapes and watermelons, two very different substances that fit in the general category of fruit. Stroke refers to any damage to the brain or the spinal cord caused by an abnormality of the blood supply. The term *stroke* is typically used when the symptoms begin abruptly, whereas *cerebrovascular disease* is a more general term that carries no connotation as to the tempo of brain injury. Of course, many patients with severely diseased blood vessels have no injury to brain tissue. A blood or cardiovascular abnormality precedes and subsequently leads to the brain injury. Recognition of the cardiac or cerebrovascular lesion or hematologic disorder before the brain becomes damaged offers clinicians a window of opportunity during which brain damage can be prevented. At times, even when brain injury has occurred, the patient is unaware of any symptoms and neurologists may not be able to detect any abnormality on neurologic examination. Sophisticated neuroimaging techniques have taught clinicians that such "silent strokes" are common.

Diagnosis and treatment of stroke patients require a basic understanding of the anatomy, physiology, and pathology of the major structures involved—the brain and spinal cord, the heart and blood vessels that supply blood to these structures, and the blood itself. To be effective, clinicians caring for stroke patients must be intimately familiar with (1) the appearance of the normal brain and its various lobes and regions; (2) the appearance of brain tissue damaged by various vascular disorders; (3) the usual locations and course of arteries supplying the brain and spinal cord and veins that drain blood from these regions; and (4) the frequency, location, and appearance of diseases of the cerebrovascular system. Note that this discussion includes a number of words related to vision. Many of the diagnostic tests used, especially imaging of the brain and blood vessels, produce pictures. Clinicians must be able to visualize what the structures and diseases look like. For this reason, this chapter relies heavily on illustrations.

This chapter offers succinct and basic coverage of the topics just mentioned. I begin the chapter by introducing the various mechanisms of brain damage in stroke. These stroke mechanisms are the major players, the key actors in the drama of stroke. Their characterization, recognition, and treatment form the core of this book. Normal vascular anatomy and distribution are then described and illustrated. Next, the usual distribution and frequency of these various mechanisms in the blood vessels and in the brain are discussed and diagrammed. The chapter closes with a discussion of stroke pathophysiology, the dynamics of the functional response of the vascular system and brain to the primary injuries.

PATHOLOGY: MECHANISMS OF CEREBROVASCULAR DAMAGE TO BRAIN TISSUE

The first questions that the clinician should ask about a stroke patient are "What caused the brain dysfunction?" and "What pathologic process is active in this patient?" There are two major categories of brain damage in stroke patients: (1) ischemia, which is a lack of blood flow depriving brain tissue of needed fuel and oxygen; and (2) hemorrhage, which is the release of blood into the brain and into extravascular spaces within the cranium. Bleeding damages the brain by cutting off connecting pathways and by causing localized or generalized pressure injury to brain tissue; biochemical substances released during and after hemorrhage also may adversely affect nearby vascular and brain tissues.[1,2]

Ischemia

Ischemia can be further subdivided into three different mechanisms: thrombosis, embolism, and decreased systemic perfusion. An analogy to a simple plumbing situation illustrates the differences among the mechanisms. Suppose that a homeowner calls a plumber and tells her that when the faucet in the second-floor bathroom at the right is turned on, water does not flow (Fig. 2-1). The

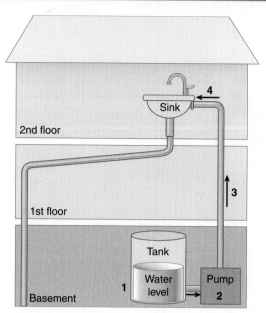

Figure 2-1. Cartoon of home plumbing illustrating possible problem areas: (1) insufficient water in the tank, (2) low pump pressure, (3) low water pressure in the pipes, and (4) rust buildup or blockage in a pipe leading directly to the sink.

plumber finds that the pipe feeding the sink is rusty and has become blocked. The plumber repairs the local pipe, and water flow is restored. The local occlusive process in the pipe, in vascular terms, would qualify as thrombosis, meaning a process that occurs in situ within a blood vessel. Suppose instead that the pipe had been blocked by material that originated in the water tank and simply became lodged in the pipe to the sink, occluding the pipe. This obstruction by material originating from afar is referred to as embolism. Fixing the local pipe would not prevent additional material from getting into the system and blocking other pipes. Suppose instead that the plumber finds that the water pressure is intermittently low and the flow to all the sinks and showers is deficient because of a leak in the water tank or low water pressure in the house's entire plumbing system. This situation is akin to systemic hypoperfusion; there is no local problem with the pipe to a single sink but instead a general circulatory problem. Clearly, these three situations dictate different management by the plumber, and that is the main reason for separating them into three mechanisms. I return to this analogy when treatment is discussed in Chapter 5.

Thrombosis

By convention, *thrombosis* refers to an obstruction of blood flow due to a localized occlusive process within one or more blood vessels. The lumen of the vessel is narrowed or occluded by an alteration in the vessel wall or by superimposed clot formation. Figure 2-2A shows a normal artery, Figure 2-2B shows plaque encroaching on the arterial lumen, and Figure 2-2C shows occlusion of the artery by superimposed white and red thrombi. The most common type of vascular pathology is atherosclerosis, in which fibrous and muscular tissues overgrow in the subintima, and fatty materials form plaques that can encroach on the lumen. Next, platelets adhere to plaque crevices and form clumps that serve as nidi for the deposition of fibrin, thrombin, and clot.[3,4] Figure 2-3 is a cartoon that shows the development of plaque in a carotid artery in the neck with subsequent occlusion of the artery by thrombi and embolization of the thrombus intracranially, causing a large brain infarct in the distribution of that carotid artery. Figure 2-4 is a photograph of a necropsy specimen that shows a large thrombus in an internal carotid artery; the lumen of the artery was nearly occluded by atherosclerotic plaque. Atherosclerosis affects chiefly the larger extracranial and intracranial arteries.[5,6] Occasionally, a clot forms within the lumen because of a primary hematologic problem, such as polycythemia, thrombocytosis, or a systemic hypercoagulable state. The smaller, penetrating intracranial arteries and arterioles are more often damaged by hypertension than by atherosclerotic processes.[7,8] In such cases, increased arterial tension leads to hypertrophy of the media and deposition of fibrinoid material into the vessel wall, a process that gradually encroaches on the already small lumen. Atheromatous plaques, often referred to as *microatheromas*, can obstruct the orifices of penetrating arteries.

Less common vascular pathologies leading to obstruction include (1) fibromuscular dysplasia,[9] an overgrowth of medial and intimal elements that compromises vessel contractility and luminal size; (2) arteritis, especially of the Takayasu[10] or giant-cell type[11]; (3) dissection of the vessel wall,[12] often with a luminal or extraluminal clot temporarily obstructing the vessel; and (4) hemorrhage into a plaque,[13] leading to acute or chronic luminal compromise. At times, the focal vascular abnormality is a functional change in the contractility of blood vessels. Intense focal vasoconstriction can lead to decreased blood flow and thrombosis. Dilatation of blood vessels also alters local blood flow and clots often form in dilated segments.[14]

Embolism

In embolism, material formed elsewhere within the vascular system lodges in an artery and blocks blood flow. Blockage can be transient or

2

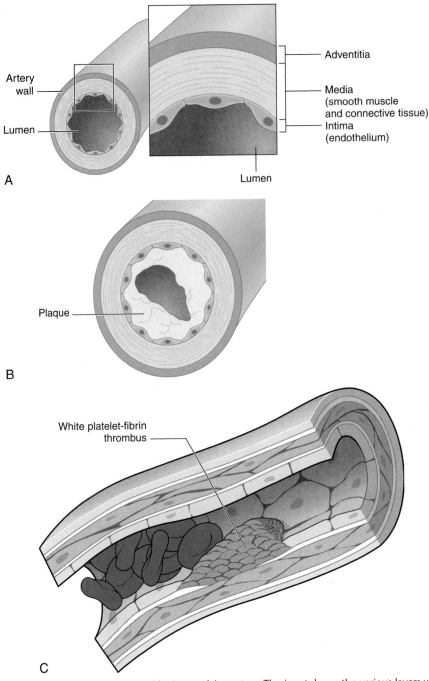

Figure 2-2. (**A**) The cartoon shows a normal brain-supplying artery. The *insert* shows the various layers within a normal artery. (**B**) Atherosclerotic plaque within an artery narrowing the lumen. (**C**) White and red thrombi occluding a longitudinal segment of an artery.

may persist for hours or days before moving distally. In contrast to thrombosis, embolic luminal blockage is not caused by a localized process originating within the blocked artery. The material arises proximally, most commonly from the heart; from major arteries such as the aorta, carotid, and vertebral arteries; and from systemic veins (Fig. 2-5). Cardiac sources of

embolism include the heart valves and clots or tumors within the atrial or ventricular cavities.[15] Artery-to-artery emboli are composed of clots, platelet clumps, or fragments of plaques that break off from the proximal vessels.[16] Clots originating in systemic veins travel to the brain through cardiac defects such as an atrial septal defect or a patent foramen ovale, a process

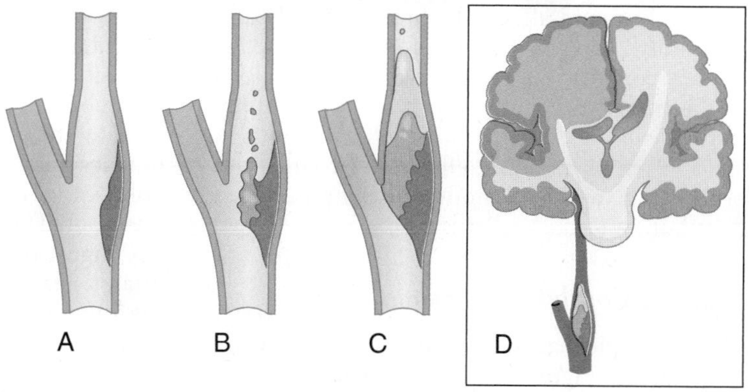

Figure 2-3. Internal carotid artery atherosclerotic lesions: (**A**) plaque; (**B**) plaque with platelet-fibrin emboli; (**C**) plaque with occlusive thrombus; (**D**) recent ischemic cerebral infarct due to embolization of the internal carotid artery thrombus.

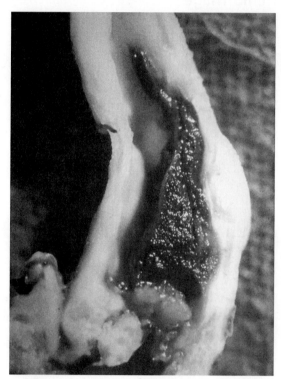

Figure 2-4. Carotid artery removed at necropsy. The internal carotid artery origin is nearly occluded by an atherosclerotic plaque. A long thrombus protrudes from the plaque and extends far rostrally within the arterial lumen. A part of this thrombus had embolized intracranially to cause a fatal brain infarct.

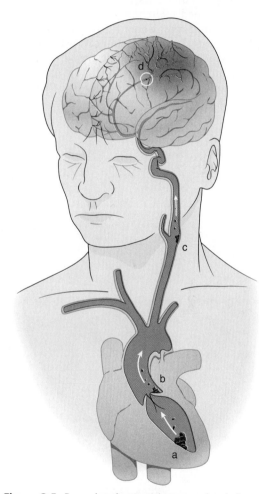

Figure 2-5. Examples of potential sources of embolism: (**a**) cardiac mural thrombus; (**b**) vegetations on heart valve; (**c**) emboli from carotid plaque. (**d**) shows infarcted cortex in area supplied by terminal middle cerebral artery due to embolism.

termed *paradoxical embolism*.[17] Also, occasionally air, fat, plaque material, particulate matter from injected drugs, bacteria, foreign bodies, and tumor cells enter the vascular system and embolize to brain arteries.[18]

Decreased Systemic Perfusion

In decreased systemic perfusion, diminished flow to brain tissue is caused by low systemic perfusion pressure. The most common causes are cardiac pump failure (most often due to myocardial infarction or arrhythmia) and systemic hypotension (due to blood loss or hypovolemia). In such cases, the lack of perfusion is more generalized than in localized thrombosis or embolism and affects the brain diffusely and bilaterally. Poor perfusion is most critical in border zone or so-called watershed regions at the periphery of the major vascular supply territories (Fig. 2-6, compare B with both A and C).[19-21] Asymmetric effects can result from preexisting vascular lesions causing an uneven distribution of underperfusion.

Damage Caused by Ischemia

The three mechanisms of brain ischemia are illustrated in Figure 2-7. All may lead to temporary or permanent tissue injury. Permanent injury is termed *infarction*. Capillaries or other vessels within the ischemic tissue may also be injured, so that reperfusion can lead to leakage of blood into the ischemic tissue, resulting in a hemorrhagic infarction.[22] The extent of brain damage depends on the location and

duration of the poor perfusion and the ability of collateral vessels to perfuse the tissues at risk. The systemic blood pressure, blood volume, and blood viscosity also affect blood flow to the ischemic areas. Brain and vascular injuries may lead to brain edema during the hours and days after stroke. In the chronic phase, glial scars form, and macrophages gradually ingest the necrotic tissue debris within the infarct, leading to shrinkage of the volume of the infarcted tissue or to formation of a frank cavity.

Hemorrhage

Hemorrhage can be further subdivided into four subtypes: subarachnoid, intracerebral, subdural, and epidural (Fig. 2-8). These subtypes have different causes, pose different clinical problems, and have different management.

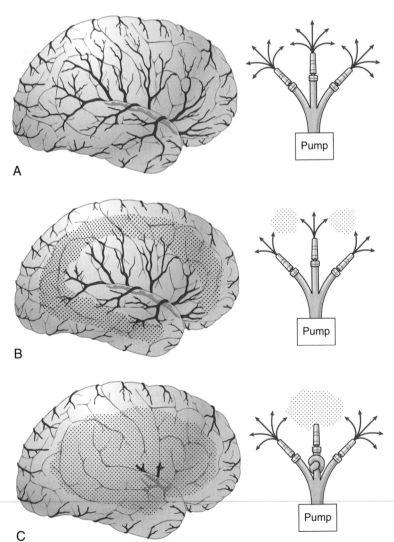

A

B

C

Figure 2-6. In heart (pump) failure and watershed infarction: (**A**) normal pump and arterial circulation; (**B**) low pump pressure and border-zone ischemia. Water goes to the center of hoses (arteries), and stippled areas show poor flow. In contrast, with (**C**) "blocked hose" and middle cerebral-artery infarction, water flow is deficient in the center of supply (stippled area).

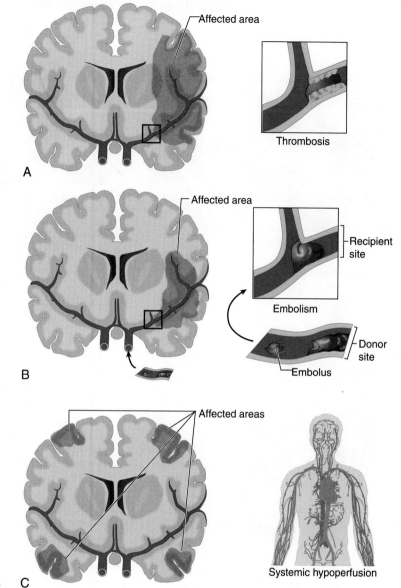

Figure 2-7. Illustrations of the three major causes of brain ischemia. **(A)** Thrombosis. The *insert* shows a thrombus in an atherosclerotic artery leading to a brain infarct, **(B)** Embolism. A thrombus that originated in a donor source embolized to the recipient site (shown in the insert) causing an embolic brain infarct, and **(C)** systemic hypoperfusion. Infarcts are in border-zone regions.

Subarachnoid Hemorrhage

In subarachnoid hemorrhage, blood leaks out of the vascular bed onto the brain's surface and is disseminated quickly via the spinal fluid pathways into the spaces around the brain (see Fig. 2-8, top right).[23,24] Bleeding most often originates from aneurysms or arteriovenous malformations, but bleeding diatheses or trauma can also cause subarachnoid bleeding. A ruptured aneurysm releases blood rapidly at systemic blood pressure, suddenly increasing intracranial pressure, whereas bleeding from other causes is usually slower and at lower pressures. The blood within the subarachnoid space often contains substances that promote vasoconstriction of the basal arteries that are bathed in cerebrospinal fluid.

Intracerebral Hemorrhage

The terms *intracerebral* and *parenchymal hemorrhage* describe bleeding directly into the brain substance. The cause is most often hypertension, with leakage of blood from small intracerebral arterioles damaged by the elevated blood pressure.[25-29] Bleeding diatheses, especially from the iatrogenic prescription of anticoagulants or from trauma, drugs, vascular malformations, and vasculopathies (such as cerebral amyloid angiopathy), can also cause bleeding into the brain. Parenchymatous hemorrhages occur in a localized region of the brain (see Fig. 2-8, top left). The degree of damage depends on the location, rapidity, volume, and pressure of the bleeding.

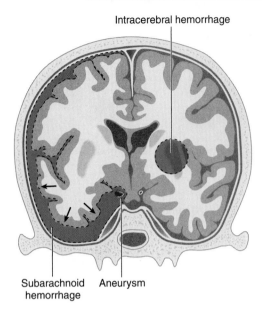

Intracerebral hemorrhage

Subarachnoid   Aneurysm
hemorrhage

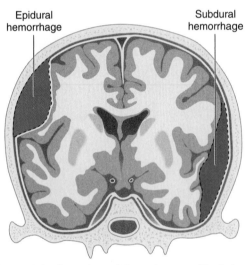

Epidural   Subdural
hemorrhage   hemorrhage

Figure 2-8. Illustrations of the main types of brain hemorrhages: intracerebral, subarachnoid, subdural, and epidural.

Intracerebral hemorrhages are at first soft and dissect along white matter fiber tracts. When bleeding dissects into the ventricles or onto the surface of the brain, blood is introduced into the cerebrospinal fluid. The blood in the hematoma clots and solidifies, causing swelling of adjacent brain tissues. Later, blood is absorbed, and after macrophages clear the debris, a cavity or slit forms that may disconnect brain pathways (Fig. 2-9). The intracranial cavity is a closed system. The bony skull and dura matter act as a fortress protecting the brain from outside injury. In adverse situations, such as swelling or hemorrhage arising inside the fortress, these structures can function as a prison, restricting and strangulating their

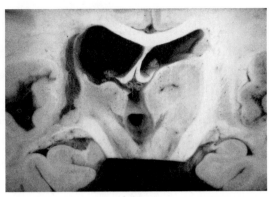

Figure 2-9. Brain specimen showing a slit-like cavity adjacent to the lateral ventricle. A large putaminal hematoma had been present at this site. There is also a butterfly-shaped infarct adjacent to the third ventricle that resulted from herniation caused by the mass effect of the putaminal hemorrhage. The patient survived for some time after the hemorrhage.

enclosed contents and forcing herniation of tissue from one compartment to another.[30-32]

Subdural and Epidural Hemorrhages

These hemorrhages are almost always caused by head trauma. Subdural hemorrhages arise from injured veins that are located between the dura mater and the arachnoid membranes. The bleeding is most often slow and accumulates during days, weeks, and even a few months. When a large vein is lacerated, bleeding can develop more rapidly over hours to days. Epidural hemorrhages are caused by tearing of meningeal arteries, most often the middle meningeal artery. Blood accumulates rapidly over minutes to hours between the skull and the dura mater. Both subdural and epidural hemorrhages cause symptoms and signs by compressing brain tissue and increasing intracranial pressure (see Fig. 2-8, bottom).

STROKE MECHANISM GUIDES TREATMENT

The problems in these five major subtypes of stroke—thrombosis, embolism, decreased systemic perfusion, subarachnoid hemorrhage, and intracerebral hemorrhage—are quite distinct and require different treatment strategies. Some therapies suitable for ischemia would be disastrous if the problem were hemorrhage (e.g., using anticoagulants or opening a blood vessel to diminish supposed ischemia would augment hemorrhage). Even within the various subcategories of ischemia, treatment depends on the subtype. For example, in a patient with embolism arising from the heart, operating on a recipient artery for supposed local thrombosis would certainly be ineffective in preventing subsequent embolism. The origin of an embolus also affects treatment: Embolism arising from the heart requires different therapeutic strategies than embolism arising from localized vessel plaques. In regard to systemic hypoperfusion, pump failure or hypovolemia owing to intestinal bleeding needs urgent attention, which would be needlessly delayed by inappropriate angiography or a futile search for a localized extracranial vascular lesion. In subarachnoid hemorrhage, the major aim of treatment is to prevent the next aneurysmal leak, whereas in intracerebral hemorrhage, rebleeding is rare and treatment is aimed at controlling and limiting the bleeding and pressure effects of the hemorrhage. When subdural and epidural hemorrhages are sizable, surgical drainage is the main treatment.

To treat the stroke patient optimally, the physician must identify the correct mechanism of stroke. Because it is not always possible to be absolutely certain of the single true mechanism, the clinician often must consider the possibility of more than one mechanism, such as thrombosis and embolism, and must evaluate for each. At times, more than one mechanism is operant. For example, in subarachnoid hemorrhage, the blood may cause spasm of blood vessels and thus induce local ischemia, and a thrombus obstructing a carotid artery can also fragment and lead to distal artery-to-artery embolism.

ANATOMY: COMMON ANATOMIC SITES OF VASCULAR AND BRAIN LESIONS

Clinical neurology differs from most medical specialties in its emphasis on, and even obsession with, anatomy. To localize and repair damage to water pipes, the effective plumber must be aware of exactly where the pipes are, what they supply, and where they are most likely to be damaged by various hazards. Abnormal neurologic signs and symptoms depend more on the localization of the brain injury than on its mechanism. Although all portions of the lung or liver look and function identically, different regions within the brain appear and act differently. The nervous system is a world of uncountable individual nerve cells and networks, each with quite different and unique characteristics and chemical messengers. Each of the various mechanisms of stroke just reviewed has its own preferences for anatomic brain locations. Identification of the location of the stroke depends on analysis of the abnormal neurologic symptoms and signs and on interpretation of

brain imaging. A major important question in every stroke patient is—where is the brain and vascular problem located?

This section reviews the important anatomic facts about the extracranial and intracranial arteries,[33] their normal regions of supply, and the most common locations for various vascular pathologies. Differences in the anatomy of extracranial and intracranial arteries are outlined. Next, the anatomic predilections of the major stroke mechanisms within the brain are discussed. Aspects of the anatomy and localization of various lesions are reviewed more extensively in the second part of this book, where specific stroke syndromes are addressed.

Normal Vascular Anatomy
Arterial Circulation

The common carotid arteries (CCAs) bifurcate in the neck, usually opposite the upper border of the thyroid cartilage, into the internal carotid arteries (ICAs), which are located posteriorly as a direct extension of the CCA, and into the external carotid arteries (ECAs), which course more anteriorly and laterally. The ICAs travel behind the pharynx; they give off no branches in the neck. Figure 2-10A shows the carotid arteries in the neck. Figure 2-10B shows the branches of the external carotid artery, which supplies the face and major cranial structures except for the brain. The ICAs then enter the skull through the carotid canal within the petrous bone and form an S-shaped curve. The ICA within this curve is usually referred to as the *carotid siphon*. There are three divisions of the ICA within the siphon—an intrapetrous portion, an intracavernous portion within the cavernous sinus, and a supraclinoidal portion[34] (see Fig. 2-10C). The siphon portion of the ICAs (usually the clinoidal segment but occasionally the intracavernous segment) gives rise to ophthalmic artery branches that exit anteriorly. The ICAs then penetrate the dura mater and give rise to anterior choroidal and posterior communicating arteries, which arise and course posteriorly from their proximal supraclinoid portions. The termination of the intracranial ICAs (the so-called T-portion because of its shape) is the bifurcation into the anterior cerebral arteries (ACAs), which course medially, and the middle cerebral arteries (MCAs), which course laterally. Figure 2-11 shows the major intracranial branches of the ICA.

The ECAs have two major vascular channels that ordinarily supply the face that can act as collateral circulation if the ICAs occlude: the facial arteries, which course along the cheek toward the nasal bridge, where they are termed the *angular*

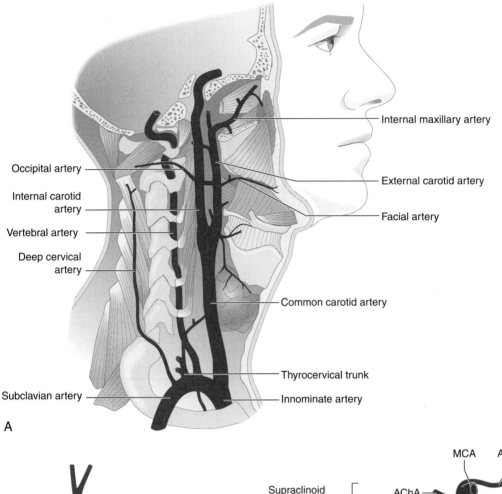

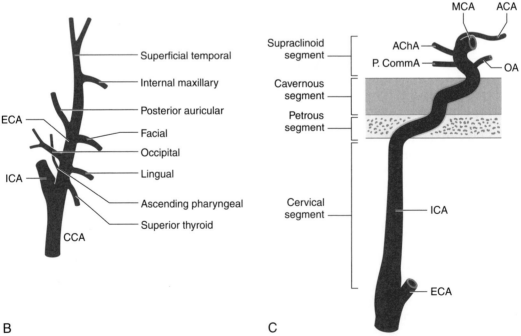

Figure 2-10. Drawings of the major right-sided neck arteries. (**A**) The innominate artery gives rise to subclavian and common carotid artery branches. The right vertebral artery is shown originating from the right subclavian artery. The common carotid artery bifurcation into internal and external carotid arteries is also shown. The external carotid artery and its branches (**B**), and (**C**) the segments of the internal carotid artery are shown in relation to their relationships with the adjacent skull structures.

A-P view

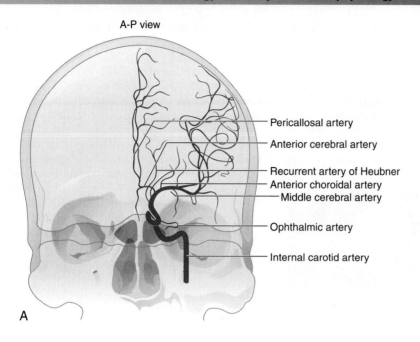

- Pericallosal artery
- Anterior cerebral artery
- Recurrent artery of Heubner
- Anterior choroidal artery
- Middle cerebral artery
- Ophthalmic artery
- Internal carotid artery

A

Lateral view

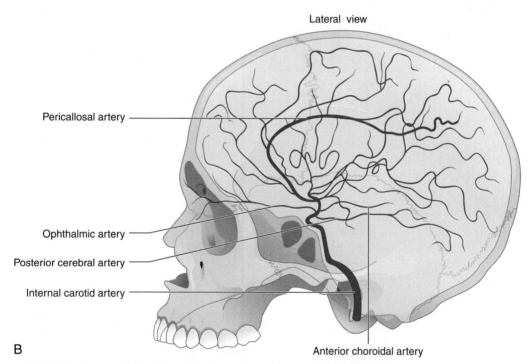

Pericallosal artery

Ophthalmic artery

Posterior cerebral artery

Internal carotid artery

B

Anterior choroidal artery

Figure 2-11. The intracranial branches of the internal carotid artery. (**A**) Anteroposterior view and (**B**) lateral view.

arteries, and the preauricular arteries, which terminate as the superficial temporal arteries. The internal maxillary artery and ascending pharyngeal branches of the ECAs also can contribute to collateral circulation when an ICA occludes. The internal maxillary arteries give off the middle meningeal artery branches, which penetrate into the skull through the foramen spinosum. Another important arterial supply of the

face involves the frontal and supratrochlear branches that originate from the ophthalmic arteries (ICA system), which supply the medial forehead above the brow. When an ICA occludes, these ECA branches can be an important source of collateral blood supply.

The ACAs course medially until they reach the longitudinal fissures and then run posteriorly over the corpus callosum. They supply the

2

anterior medial portions of the cerebral hemispheres and give off deep branches to the caudate nuclei and the basal frontal lobes. Figure 2-12 shows the small artery branches of the ACAs. The first portion of the ACA is sometimes hypoplastic on one side, in which case the ACA from the other side supplies both medial frontal lobes. The anterior communicating artery connects the right and left ACAs and provides a means of collateral circulation from the anterior circulation of the opposite side when one ACA is hypoplastic or occludes.

The main stem of the MCAs course laterally, giving off lenticulostriate artery branches to the basal ganglia and internal capsule (Fig. 2-13). Although most often the lenticulostriate penetrating branches arise from the mainstem MCA, when the mainstem is short, the lenticulostriate branches may arise from the superior division branch. As they near the sylvian fissures, the MCAs trifurcate into small anterior temporal branches and large superior and inferior divisions. The superior division supplies the lateral portions of the cerebral hemispheres above the sylvian fissures, and the inferior division supplies the temporal and inferior parietal lobes below the sylvian fissures. Figure 2-14 is a view of the lateral surface of the left cerebral hemisphere showing the MCA branches and the supply of the superior and inferior divisions of the left MCA. Figure 2-15 is a drawing of the paramedian sagittal surface of the cerebral hemispheres showing the distribution of the ACA and posterior cerebral artery (PCA) branches.

The anterior choroidal arteries (AChAs) are relatively small arteries that originate from the internal carotid arteries after the origins of the ophthalmic and posterior communicating arteries. The ophthalmic artery projects anteriorly into the back of the orbit, whereas the anterior choroidal and posterior communicating arteries project posteriorly from the ICA. The AChAs course posteriorly and laterally running

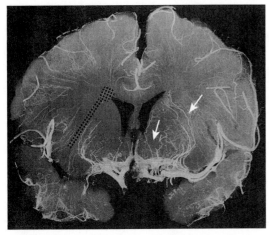

Figure 2-12. Coronal postmortem angiogram showing the branches of the anterior cerebral arteries *(white arrows)*. The *black dot* region (L of drawing) indicates the internal border-zone region. (From Pullicino P: Lenticulostriate arteries. In Bogousslavsky J, Caplan LR (eds): Stroke Syndromes, 2nd ed. Cambridge: Cambridge University Press, 2001, pp 428-437.)

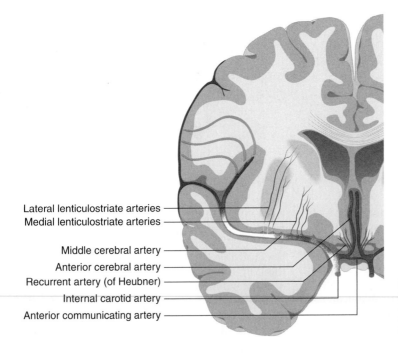

Lateral lenticulostriate arteries
Medial lenticulostriate arteries

Middle cerebral artery
Anterior cerebral artery
Recurrent artery (of Heubner)
Internal carotid artery
Anterior communicating artery

Figure 2-13. Drawing of a coronal section of the cerebral hemispheres showing one mainstem middle cerebral artery and its lenticulostriate artery branches.

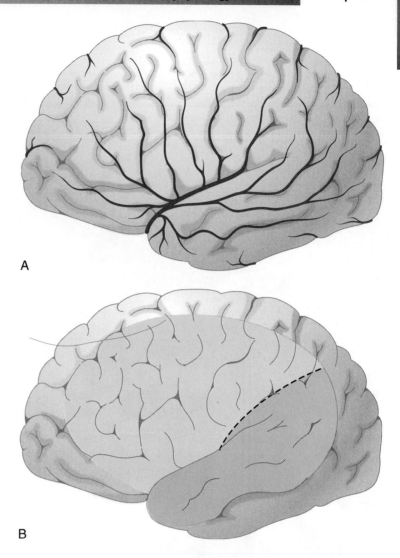

Figure 2-14. (**A**) Drawing of the lateral surface of the left cerebral hemisphere showing the usual branches of the MCA. (**B**) The superior division MCA supply is mainly suprasylvian *(pink)* and the inferior division mainly infrasylvian supply is shown in *darker pink*.

along the optic tract. They straddle territory between components of the anterior (internal carotid) and posterior circulations (vertebrobasilar system).[35] The AChAs give off penetrating artery branches to the globus pallidus and posterior limb of the internal capsule. They then give branches laterally to the medial temporal lobe, and medial branches supply a portion of the midbrain and the thalamus. The AChAs end in the lateral geniculate body where they anastamose with lateral posterior choroidal artery branches of the posterior cerebral arteries and in the choroid plexus of the lateral ventricles near the temporal horns. Figure 2-16 is a drawing of the course of the AChA. Figure 2-17 shows a drawing of a coronal section of the cerebral hemispheres showing the distribution of the supply of these cerebral arteries and the AChA. More detailed maps of the distribution of the blood supply in the cerebral hemispheres have been published.[36]

Traditionally, by convention, the carotid artery territories just described are referred to as the *anterior circulation* (front of the brain), whereas the vertebral and basilar arteries and their branches are termed the *posterior circulation* (because they supply the back of the brain). Each ICA supplies roughly two fifths of the brain by volume, whereas the posterior circulation accounts for approximately one fifth of the total. Despite its much smaller size, the posterior circulation contains the brainstem, a midline strategically critical structure without which consciousness, movement, and sensations cannot be preserved. The posterior circulation is constructed quite differently from the anterior circulation and consists of vessels from each side (the vertebral and anterior spinal artery branches), which unite to form midline arteries that supply the brainstem and spinal cord. Within the posterior circulation, there is a much higher incidence of asymmetric,

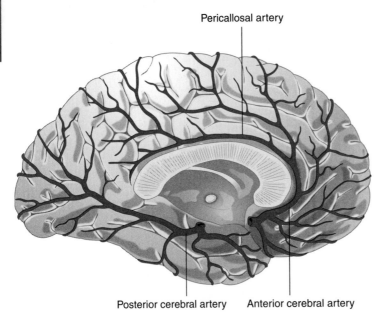

Pericallosal artery

Posterior cerebral artery   Anterior cerebral artery

Figure 2-15. Drawing of sagittal-section paramedian view of cerebral hemispheres showing branches of the anterior (ACA) and posterior (PCA) cerebral arteries.

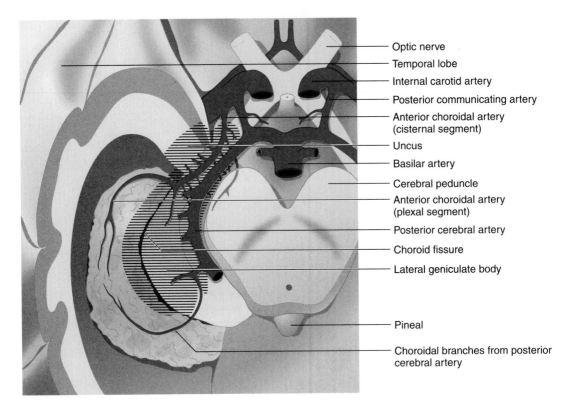

Optic nerve

Temporal lobe

Internal carotid artery

Posterior communicating artery

Anterior choroidal artery (cisternal segment)

Uncus

Basilar artery

Cerebral peduncle

Anterior choroidal artery (plexal segment)

Posterior cerebral artery

Choroid fissure

Lateral geniculate body

Pineal

Choroidal branches from posterior cerebral artery

Figure 2-16. Drawing of vascular supply of the anterior choroidal artery.

hypoplastic arteries; of variability of supply; and of retention of fetal circulatory patterns.[37,38] The proximal portions of the posterior circulation on the two sides differ. On the right, the subclavian artery arises from the innominate artery, a common channel supplying the anterior and posterior circulations. On the left side,

the subclavian artery usually arises directly from the aortic arch after the origin of the left CCA.

The first branch of each subclavian artery is the vertebral artery (VA) (Fig. 2-18; see also Fig. 2-10). The VAs course upward and backward until they enter the transverse foramens of the sixth or fifth cervical vertebra and run

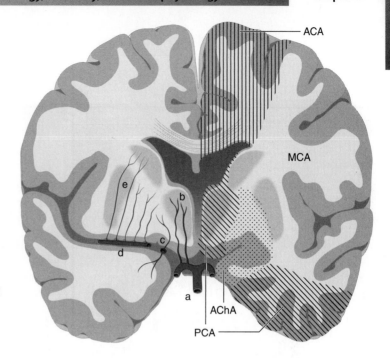

Figure 2-17. Drawing of a coronal view of the cerebral hemispheres showing the vascular supply territories: The *right* side depicts territories supplied by the anterior cerebral artery (ACA), middle cerebral artery (MCA), posterior cerebral artery (PCA), and anterior choroidal artery (AChA). The *left* side depicts individual vessels: (**a**) basilar artery; (**b**) thalamo-perforators, which originate in the PCA; (**c**) AChA; (**d**) MCA; (**e**) lenticulostriate arteries.

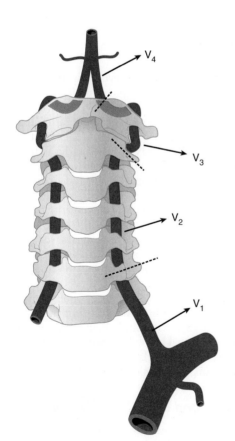

Figure 2-18. Drawing showing portions of the vertebral artery and their relation to the bony vertebral column.

within the intravertebral foramina, exiting to course behind the atlas before piercing the dura mater to enter the foramen magnum. Their intracranial portions end at the medullopontine junction, where the two VAs join to form the basilar artery. Figure 2-18 shows the divisions of the VAs: the first portion before entry into the bony vertebral column (V1), the portion within the vertebral columns (V2), the portion of the artery after exit from the vertebral column that arches behind the atlas and before entry into the cranium (V3), and the intracranial portion (V4). In the neck, the VAs have many small muscular and spinal branches.

The intracranial portions of the VAs give off posterior and anterior spinal artery branches, penetrating arteries to the medulla and the large posterior inferior cerebellar arteries (PICAs). The basilar artery runs in the midline along the clivus, giving off bilateral anterior inferior cerebellar artery (AICA) and superior cerebellar artery (SCA) branches before dividing at the pontomesencephalic junction into terminal PCA branches (Fig. 2-19). Figure 2-20 is a drawing that shows the major arterial branches of the intracranial vertebral and basilar arteries as they appear on angiograms.

The vascular supply of the brainstem has been worked out by Foix,[39-41] Stopford,[42] Gillilan,[43] and Duvernoy[44] and is illustrated in Figure 2-21. Large paramedian arteries and smaller, short circumferential arteries penetrate through the basal portions of the brainstem into

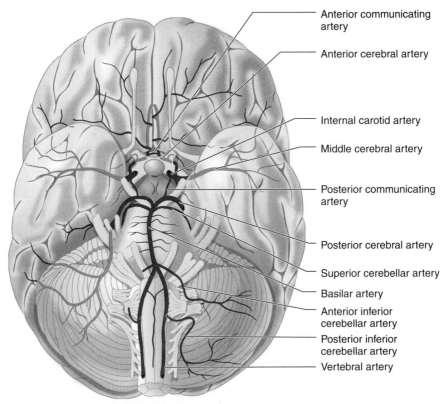

Anterior communicating artery

Anterior cerebral artery

Internal carotid artery

Middle cerebral artery

Posterior communicating artery

Posterior cerebral artery

Superior cerebellar artery

Basilar artery

Anterior inferior cerebellar artery

Posterior inferior cerebellar artery

Vertebral artery

Figure 2-19. Drawing of a basal view of the brain showing the intracranial branches of the vertebral and basilar arteries and the basal branches of the circle of Willis and the carotid arteries.

the tegmentum. Long circumferential arteries course around the brainstem giving off branches to the lateral tegmentum. The PCAs give off penetrating arteries to the midbrain and thalamus, course around the cerebral peduncles, and then supply the occipital lobes and inferior surface of the temporal lobes (Fig. 2-22). The circle of Willis allows for connections between the anterior circulations of each side, through the anterior communicating artery, and between the posterior and anterior circulations of each side through the posterior communicating artery (Fig. 2-23).

The blood supply of the spinal cord will be covered in Chapter 15, which deals with spinal cord strokes.

Composition of Cervico-Cranial Artery Walls

The walls of the extracranial arteries consist of three well developed coats; intima, media, and elastica[45,46] (see Fig. 2-2A). The intima is composed of a single row of endothelial cells that forms a continuous barrier between the arterial wall and the circulating blood. The endothelium sits on a basal membrane that is separated from the internal elastic lamina and the media by a space that contains a noncellular matrix containing collagen, elastin, and glycoproteins. The internal elastic lamina is a thick fenestrated layer of elastin that separates the intima from the media. The media is the thickest component of the arterial wall and is composed of smooth muscle, elastic fibers, and an extracellular matrix. The external elastic lamina separates the media and adventitia. The outermost layer of the arterial wall, the adventitia, is composed of loose connective tissue and adipose cells. Nerves and vessels (so-called *vasa vasorum*) penetrate the adventitia and may extend into the media.

Intracranial arteries are morphologically different from extracranial arteries. Intracranial arteries have no external elastic membrane and have a thinner intimal layer. The media and adventitia are relatively poor in elastic fibers when compared to extracranial arteries of comparable size.[45,46]

Venous and Dural Sinus Anatomy

The veins within the cranium contain approximately 70% of the cerebral blood volume. The intracranial veins are usually divided into the

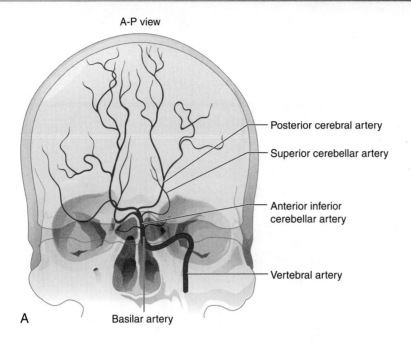

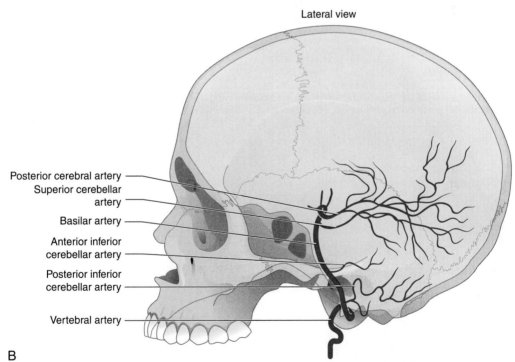

Figure 2-20. Large intracranial posterior circulation arteries as they appear on arteriograms. (**A**) Anteroposterior view and (**B**) lateral projection.

venous dural sinuses and the superficial and deep venous drainage systems.[33,44,47]

The dural venous sinuses are trabeculated, endothelial-lined channels whose fibrous walls are formed by the inner and outer layers of the dura mater. The sinuses are situated at the junctions and edges of the falx cerebri and the tentorium cerebelli. The intracranial veins drain into the dural sinuses, which in turn empty into the neck veins to drain into the superior vena cava. A system of venous lakes within the skull also drains into the dural sinuses.

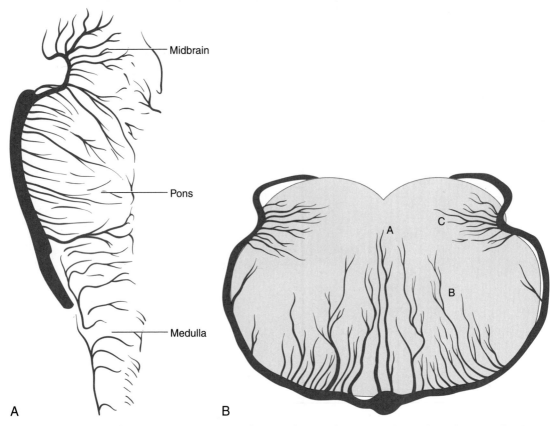

Figure 2-21. Drawing of the penetrating arteries to the pons showing the pattern of arterial supply. (**A**) Midline large median arteries, (**B**) paramedian penetrators, (**C**) penetrating arteries into the lateral tegmentum of the pons.

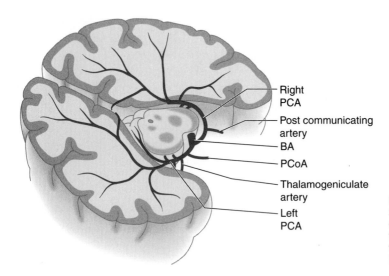

Right PCA

Post communicating artery

BA

PCoA

Thalamogeniculate artery

Left PCA

Figure 2-22. Artist's drawing shows the course and branching of the PCAs as they course around the midbrain, and branches to the temporal and parieto-occipital lobes.

The paired cavernous sinuses are located on the lateral surface of the body of the sphenoid bone and are connected to each other by the anterior and posterior intercavernous sinuses (Fig. 2-24). The cavernous sinuses reach the superior orbital fissure anteriorly and posteriorly extend to the petrous apices. The ophthalmic and facial veins drain into the cavernous sinuses. The internal carotid arteries lie on the medial walls of the cavernous sinuses.

The superior sagittal sinus courses in an arc from anteriorly to far posteriorly in the superior margin of the falx cerebri and ends

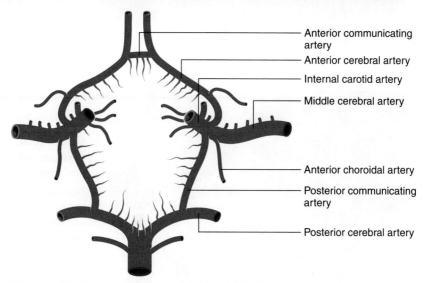

Figure 2-23. Drawing of the arterial "circle of Willis."

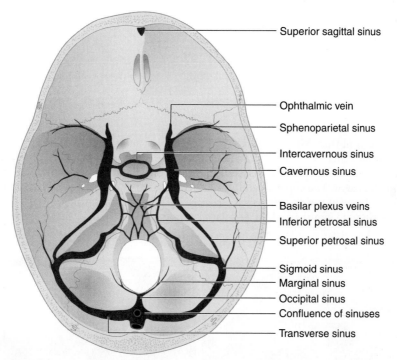

Figure 2-24. Drawing of the base of the skull with the brain removed showing the various dural sinuses.

at the internal occipital protuberance by draining into the confluens of the sinuses (torcula herophili) (Fig. 2-25). The superior sagittal sinuses drain most of the blood from the cerebral hemispheres. The posterior portion of the superior sagittal sinus is better developed than the anterior portion. The inferior sagittal sinus is smaller and shorter than the superior sagittal sinus and runs in the inferior margin of the falx until it joins with the great cerebral vein of Galen to form the straight sinus.

The paired transverse sinuses originate at the torcula and course anterolaterally along the skull between the attachments of the tentorium cerebelli. At the petrous portion of the temporal bones, the transverse sinuses empty into the sigmoid sinuses, which course medially and inferiorly to reach the jugular foramina where they become the jugular

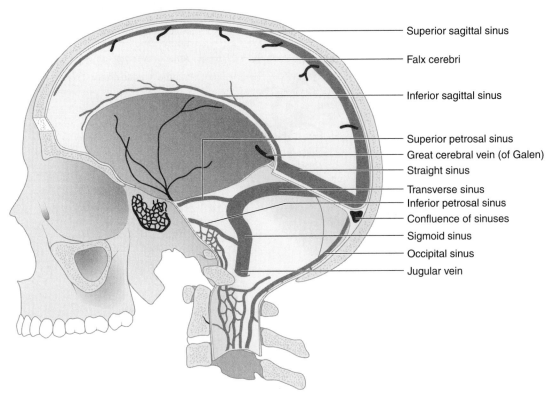

Superior sagittal sinus

Falx cerebri

Inferior sagittal sinus

Superior petrosal sinus
Great cerebral vein (of Galen)
Straight sinus
Transverse sinus
Inferior petrosal sinus
Confluence of sinuses
Sigmoid sinus
Occipital sinus
Jugular vein

Figure 2-25. Drawing of a midsagittal view of the skull showing the major large veins and dural sinuses.

veins. Figure 2-26 is a normal MR venogram that shows the major dural sinus structures. One of the transverse sinuses (most often the left) is sometimes hypoplastic or absent. The superior and inferior petrosal sinuses begin at the cavernous sinuses and drain into the sigmoid sinuses and the jugular

veins. The majority of the venous blood flow within the cranium flows posteriorly and drains into the sigmoid sinuses into the jugular veins and from there into the superior vena cava.

The superior group of cerebral veins drains most of the medial surface, the superior parts

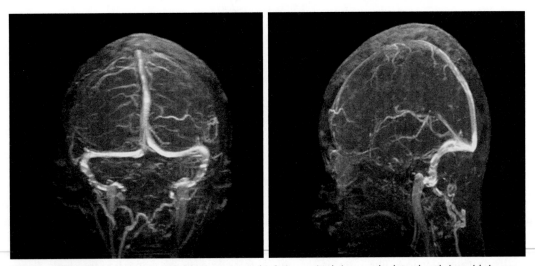

Figure 2-26. MR venogram showing the superior and inferior sagittal sinuses, the lateral and sigmoid sinuses, and the jugular veins.

of the lateral surfaces, and the anterior portions of the ventral surfaces of the cerebral hemispheres. The veins empty into the frontal and parietal regions of the superior sagittal sinus. The middle cerebral veins consist of a superficial and a deep vein. The superficial middle cerebral veins drain the sylvian fissures and the opercula and empty into the cavernous sinuses. The deep middle cerebral veins form on the insular surfaces and drain into the basal veins of Rosenthal. The basal veins arise on the ventral surface of the brain lateral to the optic chiasm and course posteriorly to the cerebral peduncles where the interpeduncular vein connects the two basal veins. The basal veins then course around the cerebral peduncles with the posterior cerebral arteries and empty into the great cerebral vein of Galen. The inferior cerebral veins drain from the inferior and lateral surfaces of the temporal and occipital lobes into the transverse sinuses.

Some large veins are often readily identified on cerebral angiography. The superficial middle cerebral veins course in the sylvian fissure. The veins of Trolard anastamose with the posterior ends of the middle cerebral veins and course superiorly to empty into the superior sagittal sinus. The veins of Labbe anastamose with the middle cerebral veins and empty into the transverse sinuses. Figure 2-27 shows the major veins on the lateral surface of the cerebral hemispheres. The veins of Trolard and Labbe are quite variable in size and location.

The deep venous system veins drain into structures at or near the midsagittal plane. The paired internal cerebral veins originate behind the foramina of Monro and course posteriorly side by side near the midline. The thalamostriate veins course with the stria terminalis between the caudate nucleus and the thalamus on each side to drain into the internal cerebral veins. The two internal cerebral veins and the basal veins of Rosenthal join below or behind the splenium of the corpus callosum to form the great cerebral vein of Galen. Figure 2-28 shows the deep venous drainage system.

The veins that drain the brainstem and cerebellum are divided into three groups. The superior group drains the superior portions of the cerebellum and the rostral and dorsal brainstem. They empty into the vein of Galen, the basal veins of Rosenthal, or the petrosal veins, which drain into the petrosal sinuses. One of the superior veins, the precentral vein, is an important anatomic landmark because it separates the pons, which lies below the vein, from the midbrain, which lies above the vein. The petrosal group of veins drains the ventral surface of the brainstem, the superior and inferior surfaces of the cerebellar hemispheres, and the lateral recesses of the fourth ventricle. They drain into the superior petrosal sinuses or their tributaries. The tentorial group of veins is posteriorly located and drains the inferior vermis and the medial portions of the cerebellar hemispheres. They drain into the straight sinus or lateral sinuses near the torcula.[33,44] Figure 2-29 shows the major posterior fossa venous structures.

Distribution of Vascular Pathology

Thrombosis

Atherosclerotic narrowing most often occurs at the origins of the ICAs in the neck. The remaining nuchal ICAs are seldom affected, but

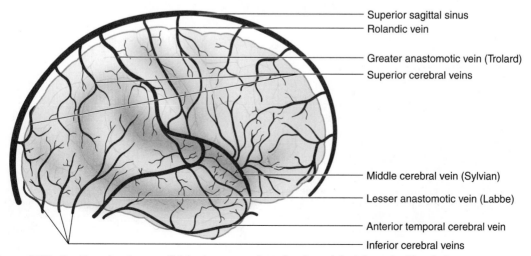

Figure 2-27. Drawing of major superficial veins seen on lateral surface of the left cerebral hemisphere.

- Superior sagittal sinus
- Rolandic vein
- Greater anastomotic vein (Trolard)
- Superior cerebral veins
- Middle cerebral vein (Sylvian)
- Lesser anastomotic vein (Labbe)
- Anterior temporal cerebral vein
- Inferior cerebral veins

2

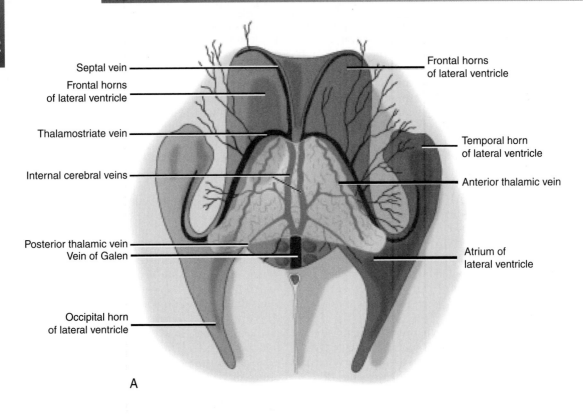

Septal vein

Frontal horns
of lateral ventricle

Thalamostriate vein

Internal cerebral veins

Posterior thalamic vein
Vein of Galen

Occipital horn
of lateral ventricle

Frontal horns
of lateral ventricle

Temporal horn
of lateral ventricle

Anterior thalamic vein

Atrium of
lateral ventricle

A

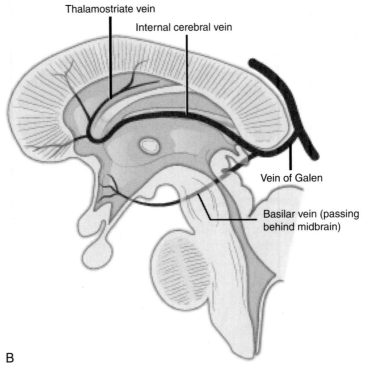

Thalamostriate vein

Internal cerebral vein

Vein of Galen

Basilar vein (passing
behind midbrain)

B

Figure 2-28. Drawing of the deep venous drainage system: (**A**) Axial section showing the veins and their relations to the lateral ventricles; (**B**) sagittal section.

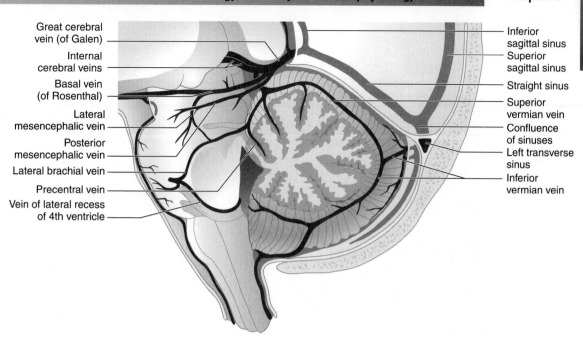

Figure 2-29. Drawing in a sagittal plane showing the brainstem and cerebellum and the major posterior fossa veins.

Labels (clockwise):
- Great cerebral vein (of Galen)
- Internal cerebral veins
- Basal vein (of Rosenthal)
- Lateral mesencephalic vein
- Posterior mesencephalic vein
- Lateral brachial vein
- Precentral vein
- Vein of lateral recess of 4th ventricle
- Inferior sagittal sinus
- Superior sagittal sinus
- Straight sinus
- Superior vermian vein
- Confluence of sinuses
- Left transverse sinus
- Inferior vermian vein

the carotid siphon is a frequent site for atheromas. The supraclinoid carotid arteries and the mainstem MCAs and ACAs are affected less often than the ICAs in the neck and the siphon in the general population,[6,48,49] although in black, Chinese, and Japanese patients, MCA disease is more common than disease of the ICAs.[50-54]

Sites of predilection for atherosclerotic narrowing in the posterior circulation include the proximal origins of the VAs and the subclavian arteries, the proximal and distal ends of the intracranial vertebral arteries, the basilar artery, and the origins of the PCAs.[6,38] Figure 2-30 shows the most frequent locations of atherosclerosis. Atherosclerotic narrowing rarely affects the distal superficial branches of the cerebral (ACA, MCA, PCA) or cerebellar (PICA, AICA, SCA) arteries.

Lipohyalinosis and medial hypertrophy secondary to hypertension affect mainly (1) penetrating lenticulostriate branches of the MCAs (see Fig. 2-13); (2) anterior perforating artery branches of the ACA, often referred to as the recurrent artery of Heubner (Fig. 2-31; see also Fig. 2-12); (3) penetrating arteries originating from the AChAs (see Figs. 2-16 and 2-31); (4) thalamoperforating and thalamogeniculate penetrators from the PCAs (see Fig. 2-31); and (5) paramedian perforating vessels to the pons,

midbrain, and thalamus from the basilar artery.[7,55] At times, atheromatous plaques within parent arteries or microatheromas within the orifices of branches cause blockage of penetrating arteries[56] (Fig. 2-32). The distribution of atheromatous branch disease is the same as that of lipohyalinosis except that atheromatous branch disease may also obstruct larger branches (e.g., the anterior choroidal artery branches of the ICAs and the thalamogeniculate pedicles from the PCAs).

Dissection—traumatic or spontaneous tearing of a vessel wall with intramural bleeding—usually involves the pharyngeal portion of the carotid arteries and the vertebral arteries between their origin and penetration into the intravertebral foramina and in their third portion as they wind around the rostral cervical vertebrae before penetrating the dura mater to enter the cranium.[12,38,57,58] In these regions, the neck arteries are mobile and not anchored to other arteries or bony structures. Tearing of neck arteries is most often due to sudden stretching of the arteries or direct trauma. Less common are dissections of the intracranial ICAs, MCAs, VAs, and basilar arteries.[38,59,60] Temporal arteritis characteristically affects the ICAs and VAs just before they pierce the dura to enter the cranial cavity, as well as the branches of the ophthalmic arteries before they pierce the globe.[11,61]

2

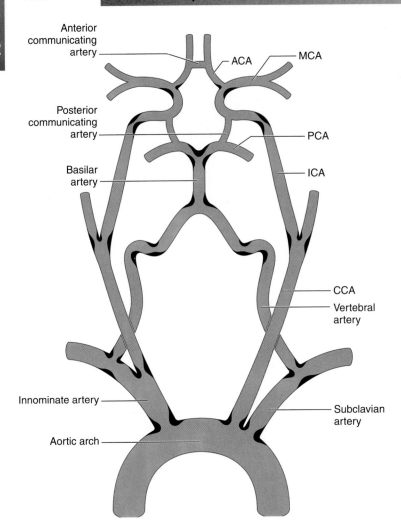

Anterior
communicating
artery

ACA

MCA

Posterior
communicating
artery

PCA

Basilar
artery

ICA

CCA

Vertebral
artery

Innominate artery

Subclavian
artery

Aortic arch

Figure 2-30. Cartoon showing sites of predilection for atherosclerotic narrowing; *black areas* represent plaques.

Embolism

Emboli can block any artery depending on the size and nature of the embolic material.[62] Large emboli, often clots formed within the heart, can block even large extracranial arteries, such as the innominate, subclavian, carotid, and vertebral arteries in the neck. More often, smaller thrombi formed in the heart or the proximal arteries embolize to block intracranial arteries, such as the ICAs, ACAs, VAs, basilar arteries, PCAs, and especially the MCAs and their superior and inferior trunks.[62] Within the anterior circulation, there is a strong predilection for emboli to go to the MCAs and their branches. Small balloons released into the ICAs in experimental animals consistently follow flow patterns to travel to MCA branches.[63] Within the posterior circulation, emboli preferentially block the intracranial VA, the distal basilar artery, and the PCAs.[38] Smaller fragments, such as tiny or fragmented thrombi, platelet-fibrin clumps, cholesterol crystals or other fragments

from atheromatous plaques, and calcified fragments from heart valves and arterial surfaces, tend to embolize to superficial small branches of the cerebral and cerebellar arteries and the ophthalmic and retinal arteries.

Intracerebral Hemorrhage

Intracerebral hemorrhage is most often caused by hypertension and has the same vascular distribution as lipohyalinosis (Fig. 2-33).[28,29] In 1872, Charcot and Bouchard originally described microaneurysms, which they believed had ruptured, causing intracerebral hemorrhage.[26,27] Sudden increases in blood pressure and blood flow can also cause these same penetrating arteries to break, even in the absence of chronic hypertensive changes.[28,29] Vascular malformations can occur anywhere within the brain. Cerebral amyloid angiopathy involves small arteries and arterioles within the subarachnoid space and within the cerebral cortex.[64,65]

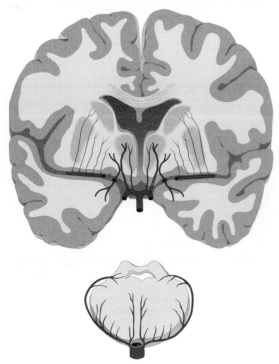

Figure 2-31. Cartoon showing penetrating arteries that supply the basal ganglia and thalamus

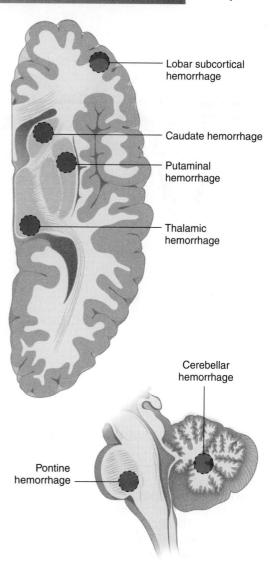

Lobar subcortical hemorrhage

Caudate hemorrhage

Putaminal hemorrhage

Thalamic hemorrhage

Cerebellar hemorrhage

Pontine hemorrhage

Figure 2-33. Drawings of horizontal cerebral section and sagittal brainstem section, showing most common sites of intracerebral hemorrhage.

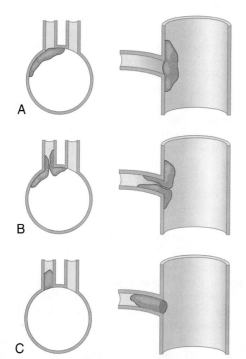

A

B

C

Figure 2-32. Drawing showing the arterial pathology in atheromatous branch disease: (**A**) plaque in parent artery obstructing a branch, (**B**) junctional plaque extending into the branch, (**C**) microatheroma formed at the orifice of a branch.

Subarachnoid Hemorrhage

Aneurysms most often affect junctional regions of the larger arteries of the circle of Willis. The ICA-posterior communicating artery junction, anterior communicating artery-ACA junction, and the MCA trifurcations are the most common sites. The supraclinoid ICAs, pericallosal arteries, vertebral-PICA junctions, and apex of the basilar artery are also frequent sites (Fig. 2-34).[23,46,66,67] Arteriovenous malformations that cause the syndrome of subarachnoid hemorrhage are either located in the brain, abutting on pial or ventricular surfaces, or situated within the ventricular system or the subarachnoid space. Some large

2

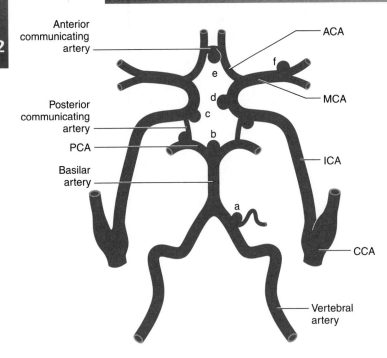

Anterior communicating artery — ACA

f

e

Posterior communicating artery — MCA

d

c

b

PCA

Basilar artery — ICA

a

CCA

Vertebral artery

Figure 2-34. Cartoon illustrating the most common sites of intracranial aneurysms; **(a)** PICA, **(b)** basilar artery, **(c)** posterior communicating artery, **(d)** ICA, **(e)** anterior communicating artery, and **(f)** bifurcation of the MCA.

malformations are located entirely within the subarachnoid cerebrospinal fluid compartment.

Distribution of Brain Pathology

Ischemia

The distribution of brain lesions caused by thrombosis is not easily distinguished from that owing to embolism, because in many patients thrombosis of an artery can lead to distal artery-to-artery embolism. Usually, the region of ischemia tends to lie in the center of the supply of the occluded artery. The extent and size of the infarct depends on the location of the occlusion, rate of occlusion, adequacy of collateral circulation, and resistance of brain structures to ischemia. In patients with angiographically documented occlusion of the ICA in the neck, Ringelstein and colleagues separated those patients with an intra-arterial embolus to the MCA and its branches ("occlusio supra occlusionem") from those who had cortical and subcortical infarcts that were considered related to diminished blood flow secondary to the ICA occlusion.[68] Figure 2-35 shows common patterns of infarction in patients with ICA occlusions. In a separate study, Ringelstein and colleagues studied the distribution of lesions in the brain in patients with cardiogenic cerebral embolism. Figure 2-36, derived from their report, illustrates their findings; A through F are patterns associated with intra-arterial embolism, while H through M are attributable to hypoperfusion often with microembolism and failure to wash out the microemboli.[69]

In patients who have systemic hypoperfusion, in contrast, the regions most vulnerable to ischemia are located in the border zones between major vessel supply zones (see Fig. 2-6). The situation has been likened to a watering system for a field.[20,70] If a hose is blocked and the pressure of water in the pump remains constant, the portion of the field least well supplied is at the center of the blocked hose (see Fig. 2-6B). More water flows through the open hoses to supply the edges of territory supplied by the blocked hose. However, if pump pressure is reduced, water trickles out each hose, and only the center of supply of each hose receives water (see Fig. 2-6C). Low pressure reduces flow to the border-zone regions or watersheds between hoses. Some border zones are cortical or cortical-subcortical while others are deep; the latter are usually referred to as internal border-zones. Another way to consider the distribution of damage in patients with low flow is the concept of distal fields.[20] The regions that receive the least blood are those farthest from the center of the longest vessels. These distal fields are situated at the edges of the major vessel distributions and most often are located in the posterior portions of the cerebral

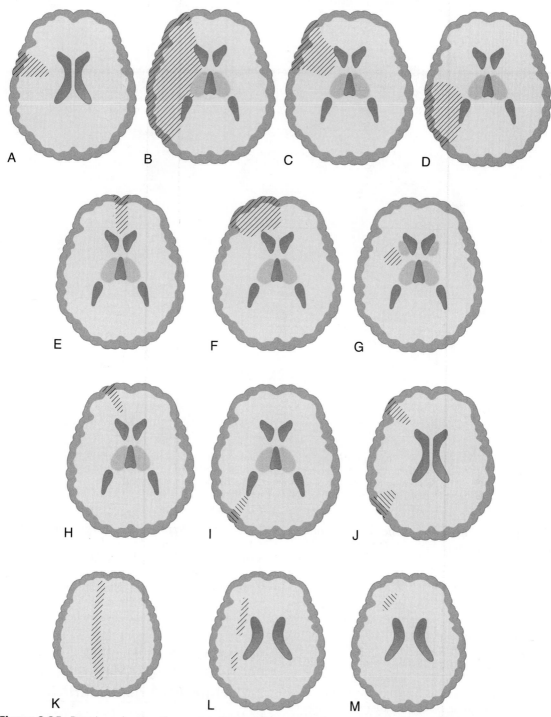

Figure 2-35. Drawings showing the most common CT locations of infarcts in the anterior circulation in patients with ICA occlusions; infarcts are shown by *hatched gray*: (**A**) wedge-shaped MCA infarct; (**B**) entire MCA territory; (**C**) superior division MCA; (**D**) inferior division MCA; (**E**) ACA; (**F**) ACA and MCA; (**G**) striatocapsular infarct; (**H**) wedge-shaped, anterior watershed infarct; (**I**) wedge-shaped, posterior watershed infarct; (**J**) anterior and posterior watershed infarcts; (**K**) linear internal watershed infarct; (**L**) oval-shaped, deep watershed infarct; (**M**) small white-matter watershed infarct. (Adapted from Ringelstein E, Zeumer H, Angelou D: The pathogenesis of strokes from internal carotid artery occlusion. Stroke 1983;14:867-875.)

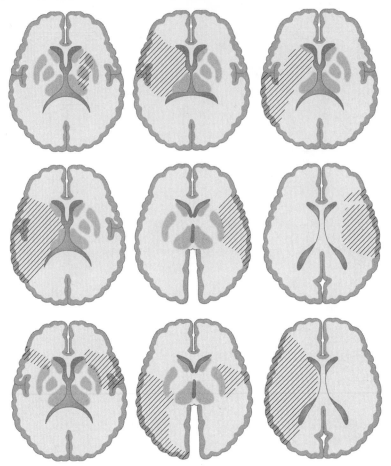

Figure 2-36. Drawings showing the most common infarct patterns in patients with embolic strokes. (Adapted from Ringelstein EB, Koschorke S, Holling A, et al: Computed tomographic pattern of proven embolic brain infarctions. Ann Neurol 1989;26:759-765.)

hemispheres. The common border-zone infarct regions are shown in Fig. 2-35H to M.

Intracerebral Hemorrhage

The most common brain locations for hypertensive intracerebral hemorrhages are as follows: lateral ganglionic and capsular (40%), thalamus (12%), lobar white matter (15% to 20%), caudate nucleus (8%), pons (8%), and cerebellum (8%)[29,71] (see Fig. 2-33). Hemorrhages owing to vascular malformations have no special predilection sites but are most often either subcortical or near the brain surface. Hemorrhages caused by amyloid angiopathy also are usually lobar, often occipital, and seldom affect the basal ganglia or posterior fossa structures.[65,72]

Hemorrhages related to illicit drug use, especially cocaine and amphetamines, have the same general distribution as hypertensive hemorrhages, probably because the mechanism of bleeding is an acute increase in blood pressure. Patients who develop intracranial hemorrhages after using cocaine have a much higher frequency of aneurysms and vascular malformations than hemorrhages that develop after amphetamine use.[73] Hemorrhages in patients who are being treated with anticoagulants preferentially involve the cerebral white matter and the cerebellum.[74,75]

PHYSIOLOGY AND PATHOPHYSIOLOGY OF BRAIN ISCHEMIA AND HEMORRHAGE

Ischemia

Normal Metabolism and Blood Flow

The brain is a metabolically active organ. Despite its relatively small size, the brain uses about one quarter of the body's energy supply. Brain cells depend mainly on oxygen and sugar to survive. Unlike other body organs, the brain uses glucose as its sole substrate for energy metabolism. Glucose is oxidized to carbon dioxide (CO_2) and water (H_2O). Glucose metabolism leads to conversion of adenosine diphosphate (ADP) into adenosine triphosphate (ATP). A constant supply of ATP is needed to maintain neuronal integrity and to keep the major extracellular cations Ca^{++} (calcium ions) and Na^+ (sodium ions) outside the cells and the intracellular cation K^+ (potassium ions) within the cells. Production of ATP is much more efficient in the presence of oxygen. Although in the absence of oxygen anaerobic glycolysis leads to formation of ATP and lactate, the energy yield is relatively small, and lactic acid accumulates within and outside of cells.[76] The brain requires and uses approximately 500 mL of oxygen and 75 to 100 mg of glucose each minute, a total of 125 g of glucose each day.[77]

These requirements for oxygen and glucose translate into a need for lots of oxygenated blood containing adequate sugar. Even though the brain is a relatively small organ, accounting for only 2% of adult body weight, the brain uses approximately 20% of the cardiac output when the body is resting.[76] Cerebral blood flow (CBF) is normally approximately 50 mL for each 100 g of brain tissue per minute, and cerebral oxygen consumption, usually measured as the cerebral metabolic rate for oxygen ($CMRO_2$), is normally approximately 3.5 mL/100 g per minute.[78] By increasing oxygen extraction from the bloodstream, compensation can be made to maintain $CMRO_2$ until CBF is reduced to a level of 20 to 25 mL/100 g per minute.[76] Positron emission tomography (PET) can measure CBF, $CMRO_2$, and oxygen extraction fraction (OEF) and the cerebral metabolic rate for glucose (CMRgl) in various brain regions of interest.[78,79] PET scanning is discussed in more detail in Chapter 4.

Brain energy use and blood flow depend on the degree of neuronal activity. In 1890, Roy and Sherrington first demonstrated the ability of the brain to increase local blood flow in response to regional changes in neuronal activity.[80,81] PET and functional magnetic resonance imaging (MRI) show that using the right hand increases metabolism and CBF in the left motor cortex. Clearly, it is critical for survival of brain tissue that there be systems to maintain CBF despite changes in systemic blood pressure. The capacity of the cerebral circulation to maintain relatively constant levels of CBF despite changing blood pressure has traditionally been termed *autoregulation*. CBF remains relatively constant when mean arterial blood pressures are between 50 and 150 mm Hg.[76] When blood pressure is chronically raised, both the upper and lower levels of autoregulation are raised, indicating a higher tolerance to hypertension but also increased sensitivity to hypotension.[82]

Mean blood flow velocities as measured by transcranial Doppler (TCD) within the intracranial arteries range from 35 to 75 cm per second but vary considerably with age, blood pressure, hematocrit, and blood vessel location.[83] When CBF increases or an artery narrows, the velocity in that segment of artery increases. At first glance, increased velocity in response to a reduction in luminal diameter seems paradoxical. One must try, however, to visualize a simple everyday example of velocity of liquid flow—an ordinary garden hose. When using a hose to wash off a pavement or a patio, to generate a high pressure jet of water, the nozzle is turned to reduce the luminal diameter. The narrower the nozzle lumen, the more pressure in the stream until the lumen is nearly effaced, at which time water dribbles out, and velocity becomes greatly reduced. This analogy will be useful to recall in Chapter 4, when I discuss transcranial Doppler measurements of blood flow velocities in segments of the major intracranial arteries.

Local Brain Effects of Ischemia

When blood flow to a brain region is reduced, survival of the at-risk tissue depends on the intensity and duration of the ischemia and the availability of collateral blood flow. Animal experiments provide estimates of thresholds of brain ischemia (Fig. 2-37).[76] At blood flow levels of approximately 20 mL/100 g per minute, electroencephalographic (EEG) activity is affected. $CMRO_2$ also begins to fall when CBF is diminished below 20 mL/100 g per minute. At levels below 10 mL/100 g per minute, cell

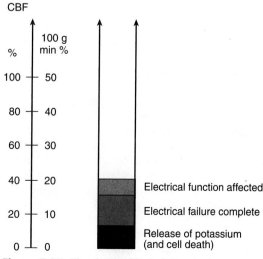

Figure 2-37. Thresholds of brain ischemia.

membranes and functions are severely affected. Neurons cannot survive for long at blood flows below 5 mL/100 g per minute.

When neurons become ischemic, a number of biochemical changes potentiate and enhance cell death: K^+ moves across the cell membrane into the extracellular space, and Ca^{++} moves into the cell, where it greatly compromises the ability of intracellular membranes to control subsequent ion fluxes and causes mitochondrial failure[78]; normally, there is a 10-fold gradient difference between extracellular and intracellular (cytosolic) Ca^{++}. Decreased oxygen availability leads to production of oxygen molecules with unpaired electrons, termed *oxygen-free radicals*. These free radicals cause peroxidation of fatty acids in cell organelles and plasma membranes, causing severe cell dysfunction.[84,85] With decreased oxygen availability, anaerobic glycolysis leads to an accumulation of lactic acid and a decrease in pH. The resulting acidosis also greatly impairs cell metabolic functions.

The activity of neurotransmitters, often referred to as *excitatory neurotransmitters* (glutamate, aspartate, and kainic acid), is significantly increased in regions of brain ischemia.[85-88] Hypoxia, hypoglycemia, and ischemia all contribute to cause energy depletion and an increase in glutamate release but a decrease in glutamate uptake. This increased availability of glutamate causes vulnerable neurons to receive toxic exposure to glutamate, thereby increasing the likelihood of cell death. Glutamate entry opens membranes and increases Na^+ and Ca^{++} influx into cells. Large influxes of Na^+ are followed by entry of chloride ions and water, causing cell swelling and edema. Glutamate is an agonist at both N-methyl-D-aspartate (NMDA) and non-NMDA (kainate and quisqualate) receptor types, but only NMDA receptors are linked to membrane channels with high calcium permeability.[87] Knowledge of these changes in the neuronal and extracellular spaces is important to recall when treatment of acute stroke patients is discussed in Chapter 5.

These aforementioned local metabolic changes cause a self-perpetuating cycle of changes that lead to increasing neuronal damage and cell death. Changes in ionic concentrations of Na^+, K^+, and Ca^{++}; release of oxygen-free radicals; acidosis; and release of excitatory neurotransmitters further damage cells, leading to more local biochemical changes, which in turn cause more neuronal damage.[87,88] At some point, the process of ischemia becomes irreversible, despite reperfusion of tissues with adequate oxygen and glucose-rich blood. At times, although the severity of ischemia is insufficient to cause neuronal necrosis, ischemia may nevertheless set in

motion a process of programmed cell death referred to as *apoptosis*.[89]

The degree of ischemia caused by blockage of an artery varies in different zones supplied by that artery. In the center of the zone, blood flow is lowest and ischemic damage is most severe. This region of the most severe damage is often referred to as the *core* of the infarct. On the periphery of blood supply, collateral blood flow allows continued delivery of blood, although at a rate lower than normal. Referring to Figure 2-37, metabolism at the center of blood supply may be reduced sufficiently to cause cell necrosis (0 to 10 mL/100 g/minute), whereas at the periphery, supplies of 10 to 20 mL/100 g per minute might stun the brain, causing electrical failure but not permanent cell damage. The zone of dysfunctional, but not dead, brain surrounding the center of infarction has traditionally been referred to as the *ischemic penumbra* (Fig. 2-38). Garcia and Anderson eloquently describe this region as follows: "Penumbral neurons are thought to be paralyzed in a shadowy state between life and death, merely awaiting the restoration of either adequate blood flow or other as yet unknown conditions before resuming full life."[85] Some neurons are thought to be more vulnerable to hypoxia and decreased fuel supply than other neurons, termed *selective vulnerability*.[86]

Arterial Occlusion and Reaction to the Occlusive Process

Brain ischemia should not be viewed as a static anatomic-pathologic process. It is a dynamic, often unstable, condition. Brain tissue, in imminent danger of irreversible death, nevertheless often recovers remarkably well, leaving no trace of its previous precarious situation. To treat patients optimally, physicians must understand the various factors that affect outcome. The discussion of pathophysiology has so far centered on the function and metabolism of local regions of brain tissue. To understand the variety of factors affecting outcome, I now turn to a more macroscopic view of both the process of arterial occlusion and the way in which occlusive changes are handled by the body.

Vascular occlusion most often begins with formation of atherosclerotic plaques within extracranial and large intracranial arteries. These plaques contain a mixture of lipid, smooth muscle, fibrous and collagen tissues, macrophages, and inflammatory cells. Plaques may enlarge quickly when hemorrhages occur within the plaques. When a critical plaque size and significant encroachment on the lumen develop, the atherosclerotic process often accelerates. Reduced

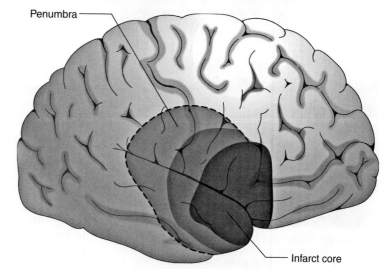

Penumbra

Infarct core

Figure 2-38. Cartoon showing core and penumbra of a brain infarct. The darkest region represents the core—tissue already infected. The surrounding grey zones represent areas with decreased blood flow but capable of recovery if the blood supply improves. In the most peripheral grey zone, the blood supply decrement is least severe.

luminal area and the bulk of the protruding plaque alter the physical and mechanical properties of blood flow and create regions of local turbulence and stasis. Platelets often adhere to irregular plaque surfaces. Secretion of chemical mediators within platelets and within the underlying vascular endothelium causes aggregation and further adherence of platelets to the endothelium. ADP, epinephrine, and collagen can all increase platelet aggregation.[90] Activated platelets release ADP and arachidonic acid. In the presence of the enzyme cyclooxygenase, arachidonic acid is metabolized to prostaglandin endoperoxides, which can be converted by thromboxane synthetase to thromboxane A_2, a potent vasoconstrictor and inducer of further platelet aggregation and secretion.[3] At the same time, the vascular endothelium may secrete prostacyclin, a potent vasodilator and inhibitor of platelet aggregation.[91] Both vascular patency and the formation of platelet fibrin clots are influenced by the balance between thromboxane A_2, prostacyclin, and other factors. Platelets begin to stick together and adhere to the endothelial lining of the plaque. A "white clot" composed of platelets and fibrin develops (Fig. 2-39; see also Fig. 2-2C).

Plaques often interrupt the endothelial lining of arteries and ulcerate. Figure 2-40 shows ulcerated irregular plaques within specimens of carotid arteries removed at surgery. Breaches in the endothelium allow cracks and fissures to form, allowing contact of the constituents of the plaque with the blood within the lumen. Tissue factor, an important stimulator of the body's coagulation system, is released. The coagulation cascade is activated by this contact and a "red thrombus" composed of erythrocytes and fibrin forms within the lumen (Fig. 2-41; see also

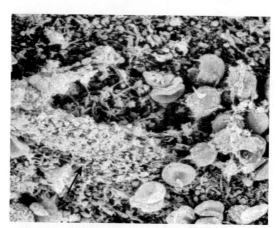

Figure 2-39. Phase microscope image of a white fibrin-platelet thrombus formed in a high-flow system. (Courtesy of S.H. Hanson and Ch. Kessler, Emory University, Division of Hematology.)

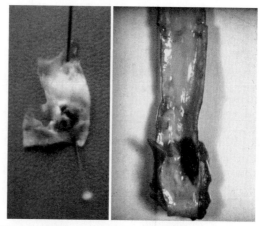

Figure 2-40. Ulcerated internal carotid artery plaques in specimens of arteries removed at surgery.

2

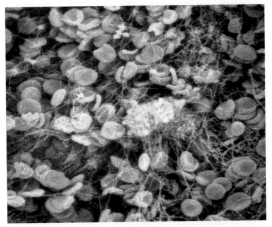

Figure 2-41. Phase microscope image of a red thrombus, composed of fibrin and erythrocytes, formed in a thrombogenic system, in a vessel with a low flow rate. (Courtesy of S.H. Hanson and Ch. Kessler, Emory University, Division of Hematology.)

Fig. 2-2C). Platelet secretion can also activate the serine proteases that form the body's coagulation system and also promote the formation of red clots. When white or red thrombi first form, they are poorly organized and only loosely adherent. They often propagate and embolize. Figure 2-4 shows an occluded carotid artery found at necropsy. The specimen contains a large mobile red thrombus, a part of which had embolized to the brain. Within a period of 1 to 2 weeks, thrombi organize and become more adherent and fragments are less likely to break off and embolize. A variety of different materials—cholesterol crystals, calcified plaque fragments, white clots, and red thrombi—can form the substance of intra-arterial emboli.

Atherosclerotic plaques and vascular stenosis cause brain ischemia in a variety of ways. Progressive intimal thickening leads to stenosis or occlusion of the artery, resulting in reduced distal blood flow. Stasis of blood flow enhances the formation of thrombi that often embolize. Physical factors are clearly important in the formation, lysis, clearance, and washout of thromboemboli. Blood flow at arterial bifurcations is complex even in normal nonstenotic arteries. Eddies, turbulence, flow separation, and vortices are common and vary with location along the arteries.[92] As an artery narrows, blood flow velocity increases within the center of the artery and flow separation becomes more prominent.[92] Flow is reduced in some parts of the artery, especially on the outer perimeter of the residual lumen. When subtotal or complete occlusion of an artery develops, the bloodstream flow diminishes because of reduced volume of flow, and blood flow velocity also is

decreased.[92-94] Antegrade perfusion becomes less effective. This reduced perfusion and pressure decreases washout and throughput of emboli, especially in remote border-zone portions of the brain circulation.[95-97] Hypoperfusion and embolism interact and complement each other to promote and enhance brain infarction.[93,94]

Thrombus Formation

Thrombi form in situ when the body's coagulation system has been activated and the blood is hypercoagulable. In some patients with hypercoagulability, red thrombi form simultaneously or sequentially in multiple, systemic extracranial and intracranial arteries and veins. In other patients with arterial lesions (e.g., arterial atherosclerotic plaques or dissections), the process of occlusive thrombosis is accelerated at sites of vascular disease. Hypercoagulability can be a lifelong hereditary problem. Systemic diseases, such as cancer, regional enteritis, and thrombocytosis, can cause increased clotting. The process of atherothrombosis (e.g., in the coronary or cerebrovascular systems) can also activate serologic coagulation factors that promote further thrombosis.[98-102]

Much of the treatment of patients with thromboembolic stroke concerns attempts to affect or reverse the coagulation process or to facilitate clot lysis or removal. Clinicians treating patients with ischemia should be familiar with the general features of blood coagulation to effectively choose and monitor antithrombotic and thrombolytic therapies.

The final step in the coagulation cascade is the conversion of the soluble protein fibrinogen into insoluble polymers termed *fibrin*. These strands of fibrin form a network of fibers that entangle formed blood elements (i.e., platelets and erythrocytes) into a clot. Fibrin is quite adhesive and has the capability of contracting. The fibrinogen-to-fibrin reaction occurs when factor II, prothrombin, is converted to thrombin. The amounts of circulating fibrinogen and prothrombin are important in these reactions.

Prothrombin can be activated in two different ways: In the so-called extrinsic system of coagulation, a tissue or endothelial injury releases thromboplastic substances, known as tissue factors, which in turn cause both platelet activation and activation of some of the blood serine protease coagulation factors, especially factors V and VII. Tissue factor forms a complex with factor VIIa; the tissue factor-VIIa complex converts factor X to Xa. Factor Xa activates a prothrombinase complex composed of activated factor V, Ca^{++}, and phospholipids, which in turn with factor Xa catalyzes the reaction of prothrombin to thrombin. Activation of platelets causes them to agglutinate, to adhere to the injured vessel wall, and to release various intracellular substances, which in turn activate the coagulation system.[98-100]

The complementary intrinsic coagulation system refers to blood-coagulation factors that circulate in inactive forms (factors V, VIII [antihemophilic globulin], IX, X, XI, XII) and are intrinsic to the blood. Activation of factor XII from an inert precursor form to an activated form triggers a series of reactions, described as the *coagulation cascade* in which the various blood-clotting factors are sequentially converted to their active enzymatic forms. Ultimately, these reactions lead to activation of factor X, which catalyzes the prothrombin → thrombin reaction.[100-102] Figure 2-42 is a simplified diagram of the coagulation reactions. Thrombin, in turn, in addition to converting fibrinogen to fibrin, has an important influence on blood platelets, causing them to swell, aggregate, and release substances that affect vascular tone and blood coagulability.

Also important are various natural inhibitors of coagulation: antithrombin III, protein C, and protein S. Deficiencies in any of these serum proteins can cause increased coagulability. Genetically transmitted disorders can also lead to hypercoagulability. One common inherited disorder leads to functional resistance to the anticoagulant effects of activated protein C.[103]

This genetic defect is termed the *Leiden factor V mutation* and is caused by a point mutation in factor V.[104] Another genetic disorder that predisposes to thrombosis is caused by a mutation in the prothrombin gene.[105] These mutations in the prothrombin and factor V genes are common in patients who develop cerebral venous thrombosis and phlebothromboses, especially if they also take oral contraceptives.[106]

Key components in the coagulation system are factor Xa, prothrombin, and thrombin. Factor Xa is especially important since it is the focal point at the intersection of both the intrinsic and extrinsic portions of the coagulation cascade. Heparins cause a conformational change in antithrombin III, which increases its ability to inactivate factor Xa. Warfarins inhibit the action of vitamin K necessary for the biosynthesis of prothrombin and factor X. Researchers and clinicians are now exploring the potential for using other agents that inactivate factor Xa or directly inhibit thrombin generation and function.

Naturally occurring factors also exist that act to lyse clots once they are formed. Tissue plasminogen activator and other substances activate plasminogen to form plasmin, a potent fibrinolytic enzyme. Plasminogen is also activated by various coagulation factors, such as factor XII, so that the process of coagulation itself activates the thrombolytic system. Various plasmin inhibitors ("antiplasmins") are also present.[102,107]

Pathologists and hematologists recognize and describe three types of thrombi[101]:

1. Red thrombi are composed mostly of red blood cells and fibrin, and they form in areas of slowed blood flow. Their formation does not require an abnormal vessel wall or tissue thromboplastin (see Fig. 2-41).
2. White thrombi, in contrast, are composed of platelets and fibrin and do not contain red blood cells (see Fig. 2-39). White clots form almost exclusively in areas in which the arterial wall or endothelial surface is abnormal, characteristically in fast-moving bloodstreams.
3. Disseminated fibrin deposition in small vessels.

These types of thrombi are distinct and are affected by different therapeutic agents. In many cases, the thrombus begins as a white platelet fibrin clot and then a red thrombus is laid down as a cap over the initial platelet mass.[101]

When a major artery occludes, a crisis ensues. Pressure drops distal to the occlusion, and the brain region supplied by that vessel is acutely deprived of blood. Diminished blood flow in turn activates protective mechanisms that help restore

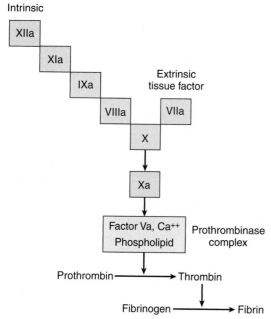

Figure 2-42. Diagrammatic scheme of extrinsic and intrinsic coagulation systems.

needed blood flow to the ischemic region. Low pressure helps to draw blood from higher pressure regions. Collateral circulation increases. Ischemic cell damage causes release of lactic acid and other metabolites. The resulting local tissue acidosis leads to vasodilation, augmenting regional CBF.[108] If brain tissue is deprived of blood and needed nourishment for too long, it dies. At times, there are varying grades of ischemia, ranging from irreversible cell death in the most deprived zone to a reversible situation of diminished electrical activity but normal or only slightly elevated extracellular potassium concentration in the threatened ischemic penumbral zone.[71,85,86,108,109] The severity of the ischemic crisis depends on the rate of vascular occlusion. A vessel that gradually occludes may already have stimulated abundant collateral circulation so that final occlusion produces less stress on the system.

Factors Affecting Tissue Survival

The survival of the brain regions at risk depends on a number of factors: (1) the adequacy of collateral circulation, (2) the state of the systemic circulation, (3) serologic factors, (4) changes within the obstructing vascular lesion, and (5) resistance within the microcirculatory bed.

ADEQUACY OF COLLATERAL CIRCULATION

Congenital deficiencies in the circle of Willis and prior occlusion of potential collateral vessels decrease the available collateral supply. Hypertension or diabetes diminishes blood flow in smaller arteries and arterioles and thus reduces the potential of the vascular system to supply blood flow to the needy region.

STATE OF THE SYSTEMIC CIRCULATION

Cardiac pump failure, hypovolemia, and increased blood viscosity all reduce CBF. The two most important determinants of blood viscosity are the hematocrit and the fibrinogen levels.[110-112] In patients with hematocrits in the range of 47% to 53%, lowering of the hematocrit by phlebotomy to below 40% can increase cerebral blood flow by as much as 50%.[112] Blood pressure is also very important. Elevation of blood pressure except at malignant ranges increases CBF. Surgeons take advantage of this fact by injecting catecholamines to raise blood pressure and flow during the clamping phase of carotid endarterectomy. Low blood pressure significantly reduces cerebral blood flow. In some patients, the balance is so tenuous that simply sitting in bed or standing lowers collateral pressure enough to induce symptoms.[113,114] Low blood and fluid volume also limit available blood flow in collateral channels.

Many older individuals limit their fluid intake, especially in the evening, to avoid getting up at night to urinate. After the stroke, there may not have been any fluid intake because of swallowing difficulty or lack of feeding during the trip to the hospital and hospital encounters.

SEROLOGIC FACTORS

The blood functions as a carrier of needed oxygen and other nutrients. Hypoxia is clearly detrimental because each milliliter of blood delivers a less-than-normal oxygen supply.[115] Low blood sugar similarly increases the risk of cell death. Higher-than-normal blood sugar also can be detrimental to the ischemic brain.[116,117] Elevated serum calcium levels[118,119] and high blood-alcohol content[120] are also potential important detrimental variables.

CHANGES WITHIN THE OBSTRUCTING VASCULAR LESION

Embolic occlusive thrombi do not adhere to the vessel wall of the recipient artery and frequently move on. The moving embolus can block a more distal intracranial artery, causing added or new ischemia, or it may fragment and pass through the vascular bed. Clot formation activates an endogenous thrombolytic system that includes tissue plasminogen activator (tPA).[102,107] Inhibitors of tPA are also present. Sudden obstruction of a vascular lumen can cause reactive vasoconstriction (spasm), which in turn causes further luminal compromise. Thrombolysis, passage of clots, and reversal of vasoconstriction all promote reperfusion of the ischemic zone. If reperfusion occurs quickly enough, the stunned, reversibly ischemic brain may recover quickly. The occlusive clot may propagate further proximally or distally along the vessel, blocking potential collateral channels. The distal end of the thrombus can also break loose and embolize to an intracranial receptive site. Hypercoagulable states promote such extension of thrombi.

RESISTANCE WITHIN THE MICROCIRCULATORY BED

The vast majority of CBF does not occur in the large macroscopic arteries at the base of the brain or along the surface. Most flow occurs through microscopic-sized vessels: the arterioles, capillaries, and venules.[102] Resistance to flow in these small vessels is affected by prior diseases, such as hypertension and diabetes, which often cause thickening of arterial and arteriolar walls. Experimental animals and patients that have been hypertensive before a vascular occlusion fare worse than individuals previously normotensive, presumably because of these microcirculatory changes. Both hyperviscosity and diffuse thromboses within the capillaries and microvessel bed greatly reduce flow through the microcirculation. Ischemic insults may produce biochemical changes that lead to platelet activation, clumping of erythrocytes, and plugging of the microcirculation. Ames referred to these changes as causing a "no reflow" state in the microvascular bed, even when large arteries are reperfused.[121] In general, studies of CBF are sensitive to changes in resistance in the microcirculatory bed. Remember that flow is inversely proportional to resistance in the vascular bed, the majority of which is microcirculatory.

BRAIN EDEMA AND INCREASED INTRACRANIAL PRESSURE

Edema and pressure changes within the brain and cranial cavity also influence survival of brain tissue and patient recovery after vascular occlusions. There are two types of brain edema: (1) water accumulation inside cells, termed *cytotoxic edema;* and (2) fluid within the extracellular space, often termed *vasogenic edema.*[122] Extracellular edema is also often referred to as *wet edema* because in such cases, the cut surface of the brain oozes edema fluid, whereas intracellular (cytotoxic) edema is termed *dry edema.*[122] Cytotoxic edema is caused by energy failure, with movement of ions and water across the cell membranes into cells. Extracellular edema is influenced by hydrostatic pressure factors, especially increased blood pressure and blood flow, and by osmotic factors. When proteins and other macromolecules enter the brain extracellular space because of breakdown of the blood-brain barrier, they exert an osmotic gradient pulling water into the extracellular space. This vasogenic edema accumulates more in the cerebral and cerebellar white matter because of the difference in compliance between gray and white matter.

Brain swelling caused by cytotoxic edema means a large volume of dead or dying brain cells, which implies a bad outcome. On the other hand, edema within the extracellular space does not necessarily imply neuronal injury, and fluid in the extracellular compartment can potentially be mobilized and removed. In any case, severe edema may cause gross swelling of the brain; shifts in position of brain tissue, with potential pressure damage; and herniation of brain contents from one compartment to another.

Intracranial pressure may also be increased, leading to increased morbidity and decreased CBF. When intracranial pressure is increased, the pressure in the venous sinuses and draining veins must also increase if blood is to be drained normally from the cranium. There must be a gradient between venous pressure and intracranial pressure for drainage to occur. Also, for tissue perfusion to occur, arterial pressure must exceed venous pressure. Blood flow is compromised in the presence of arterial and venous occlusions. When the intracranial venous system contains occlusions, venous pressure is increased. The limited drainage often causes fluid to back up into the brain, causing vasogenic edema. Increased intracranial pressure places an additional stress on the system, forcing even higher the flow values required for tissue survival. Brain edema and increased intracranial pressure also cause headache, decreased consciousness, and vomiting.[123] Pressure shifts and herniation cause pressure-related damage to adjacent tissues and signs of dysfunction of the compressed structures.[32,123,124] Because pressure shifts and herniations are more common after intracerebral hemorrhage, due to the additional presence in the brain of an extra mass of tissue (hematoma), I discuss herniations further in the discussion of intracerebral hemorrhage.

Events during the First Three Weeks after Vascular Occlusion

Experience shows that the tenuous balance created by occlusion of a major artery is temporary and usually resolves in 2 to 3 weeks at most. During this period, any systemic changes, such as decrease in fluid volume or positional or pharmacologically mediated drops in blood pressure, can cause worsening of symptoms. By 3 weeks, either the brain tissue has died, causing a brain infarct, or collateral sources of blood flow develop that adequately supply the region at risk. By 2 to 3 weeks, collateral circulation stabilizes, and the patient is less vulnerable to positional or circulatory changes. In addition to causing ischemia through low perfusion, the occlusive thrombus, which at first loosely adheres to the vessel wall, can propagate distally or can fragment and embolize to a distal artery. By 2 to 3 weeks, the clot has become more adherent and has much less tendency to embolize. Most studies of patients with anterior[125,126] and posterior circulation ischemia[38,127-131] show a low frequency of progression of acute ischemic deficits after 2 weeks.

During the hours, days, and early weeks after a vascular occlusion, the question of death or survival of at-risk brain tissue can be viewed as a clash between factors acting to worsen ischemia and natural body responses that prevent or limit ischemia. Table 2-1 summarizes these "good guys" versus "bad guys" responses, which are useful to keep in mind when treatment is discussed. Clinicians hope to build on the body's natural defenses and counteract the factors that promote ischemia.

2

Table 2-1.	**Balancing of Factors after Vascular Occlusion**

Factors Promoting Ischemia	Responses Limiting Ischemia
Decreased blood flow due to occlusion	Opening of collateral vascular channels
Embolization of clot	Passing and fragmentation of emboli
Activation of coagulation factors and inhibitors of thrombolysis	Activation of thrombolytic factors
Propagation of clot	Lysis of clot
Decreased blood flow due to hypotension, hypovolemia, low cardiac output	Improvement in general medical condition, especially after correction of abnormalities

This process of shifting vulnerability translates clinically into fluctuating variable symptoms and signs during the early period after a vascular occlusion. Acute blockage of an artery often translates into the sudden onset of symptoms. After vascular occlusion, a weighing of the balance of positive and adverse factors toward the adverse side causes transient deficits or causes fluctuating, stepwise, or gradual worsening of neurologic symptoms and signs. Sudden worsening is often related to distal embolization.

Intracerebral Hemorrhage

Hemorrhage into the brain parenchyma is often preceded by hypertensive damage to small cerebral penetrating arteries and arterioles. Small aneurysmal dilatations, first hypothesized by Charcot and Bouchard in the 1870s, pepper the penetrating vascular territories of hypertensive patients[26,27] and in some patients represent weak points that rupture under increased arterial tension. In the majority of patients, abrupt elevation in blood pressure causes rupture of small penetrating arteries that had no prior vascular damage.[28,29] Leakage from these small vessels produces a sudden but local pressure effect on surrounding capillaries and arterioles, causing them in turn to break.[132] An avalanche-type effect ensues, in which vessels at the circumference break, adding volume to the gradually enlarging hemorrhage (Fig. 2-43). The accumulation of blood along the circumference of the hematoma is like a snowball rolling downhill, gathering volume along its outer surfaces as it descends. High blood pressure and this avalanche effect enlarge the hemorrhage, while mounting local tissue pressure acts as a tamponade to the bleeding.

Trauma, bleeding disorders, and degenerative changes in congenitally abnormal blood vessels within vascular malformations also may initiate intracerebral bleeding, which then progresses in a manner similar to hypertensive intracerebral hemorrhage. The gradual increase in size of the hematoma translates clinically into gradual worsening

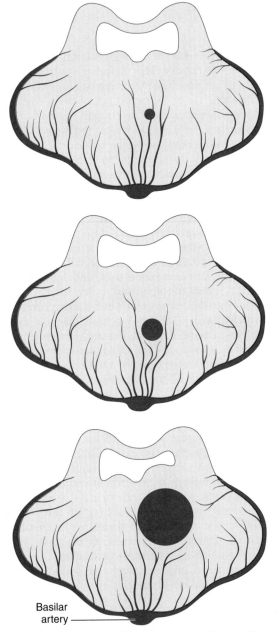

Basilar
artery

Figure 2-43. Drawing illustrating avalanche-type effect in pontine hemorrhage, showing gradual development of hemorrhage due to rupture of small vessels on the periphery of the hemorrhage.

of symptoms and signs until the hematoma attains its final size. Hematomas can stop enlarging and may drain themselves by emptying into the ventricular system or the cerebrospinal fluid (CSF) at the pial surface.

If the hemorrhage becomes sizable, the increase in intracranial volume must increase intracranial pressure. When intracranial pressure rises, the venous pressure in the draining dural sinuses increases pari passu. To perfuse the brain, the arterial pressure must rise to produce an effective arteriovenous difference. Thus, the patient with intracerebral hemorrhage may have a markedly elevated blood pressure merely because of the hemorrhage, not necessarily reflecting the true level of premorbid blood pressure. Although lowering this pressure does help to stop bleeding, caution must be exercised because the elevated pressure also serves to perfuse the areas of the brain not damaged by the hemorrhage.

Patients with intracerebral hemorrhage often worsen during the first 24 to 48 hours after their initial symptoms. This worsening can be explained by continued bleeding but most often is related to the development of edema around the lesion,[132,133] to the effects of the lesion on blood flow and metabolism, and, in large hemorrhages, to shifts in brain contents and herniations. Effects caused by masses in patients with hematomas are more common than in patients with ischemia because an extra volume of substance has been added (blood in the hematoma) in addition to the surrounding edema. Most often, pressure effects in hemispheral hematomas result in a shift of the midline without herniation of brain contents. The brain is compartmentalized by bony fortresses (anterior, middle, and posterior fossas) and by dural structures (falx cerebri and tentorium cerebelli), which, under normal circumstances, contain their usual contents. When mass effects are severe, brain tissue bulges or spills out of its usual abode into a different compartment—a process called *herniation*.[30-32,124]

Brain shifts and herniations and their effects are shown in Figure 2-44. The most common are (1) herniation of the temporal lobe through the tentorial notch, to compress the midbrain (see Fig. 2-44A); (2) symmetric, downward pressure by the swollen cerebral hemispheres on the rostral brainstem, causing elongation (see Fig. 2-44B); (3) herniation of the anterior medial frontal lobe, usually of the cingulate gyrus, under the falx cerebri (see Fig. 2-44C); (4) herniation of the cerebellum upward through the tentorial notch, to compress the brainstem (see Fig. 2-44D); and (5) downward herniation of the cerebellar tonsils through the foramen magnum, compressing the medulla and upper cervical spinal cord (see Fig. 2-44E).

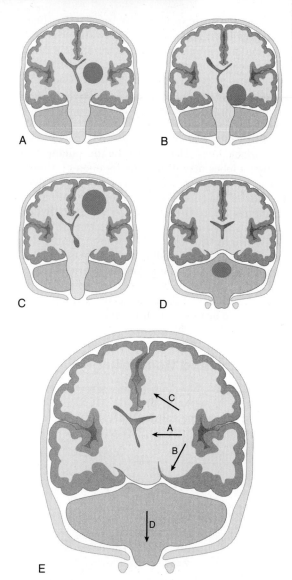

Figure 2-44. Drawings illustrating shifts and herniations. Displacement of brain tissues due to mass-producing strokes is illustrated by patients with hematomas. (**A**) Basal ganglionic hematoma causes compression of the ipsilateral ventricle and shift of the midline to the opposite side. (**B**) Deep hematoma causes uncal herniation. The medial temporal lobe exerts pressure on the upper brainstem. (**C**) Frontal hematoma causes herniations of the cingulum under the falx cerebri. (**D**) Cerebellum hematoma causes increased posterior fossa pressure with herniation of the cerebellum (**E**) through the foramen magnum. These patterns are also illustrated in **E**.

Shifts in brain contents can also lead to compression or stretch of arteries and infarction in areas of supply and secondary hemorrhages. The most common loci of secondary vascular changes leading to infarction involve the PCAs where they pass between the tentorium and the medial temporal lobe and the ACAs adjacent to the falx (Fig. 2-45). Distortion of the upper brainstem at

2

the tentorial opening often leads to secondary hemorrhages in the brainstem. These usually involve the midline and paramedian vessels and are called *Düret hemorrhages,* after the French clinician and researcher who first described them.[134] A necropsy specimen of a Düret hemorrhage is shown in Figure 2-46 and a drawing of another Düret hemorrhage is shown in figure 2-47B.

The ventricular system may also be compressed at variable sites. Hematomas in the putamen or cerebral lobes may distort the foramen of Monro, causing dilatation of the contralateral lateral ventricle. Thalamic hematomas often obstruct and compress the third ventricle, leading to hydrocephalus of both lateral ventricles. Cerebellar hemorrhages can compress the forth ventricle or cerebral aqueduct, leading to obstructive hydrocephalus of the third and lateral ventricles. Shifts in brain contents, herniations, and secondary infarctions, as well as Düret hemorrhages and hydrocephalus, all cause clinical worsening of signs and symptoms.

Subarachnoid Hemorrhage

Subarachnoid bleeding nearly always abruptly increases intracranial pressure (ICP). Systemic blood pressure and volume must be maintained or

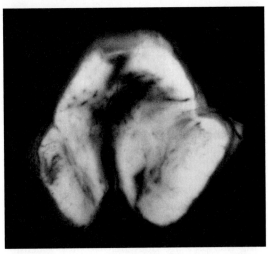

Figure 2-46. A necropsy specimen of a Düret midbrain hemorrhage. A left subdural hematoma was present on the lateral surface of the cerebral hemisphere.

augmented to preserve brain perfusion in the face of the increased ICP. After the initial bleeding, three major risks affect subsequent events: rebleeding, vasoconstriction, and hydrocephalus. Once the outer wall of abnormal blood vessels, most often aneurysms and vascular malformations, has been breached, the vessels are vulnerable

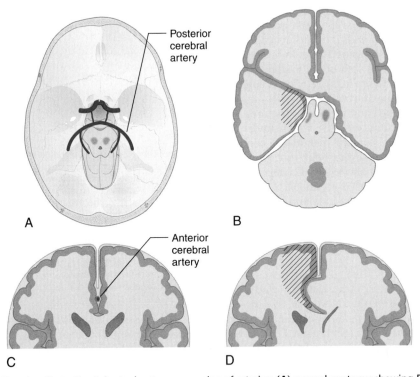

A

B

C

D

Figure 2-45. Drawing illustrating infarcts due to compression of arteries: (**A**) normal anatomy showing PCA crossing up and over the edge of the tentorium; (**B**) infarction of medial temporal lobe due to compression of PCA between herniated uncus and tentorium; (**C**) anatomy showing ACA in relation to falx; (**D**) infarction of medial frontal lobe, due to compression of ACA against the falx cerebri.

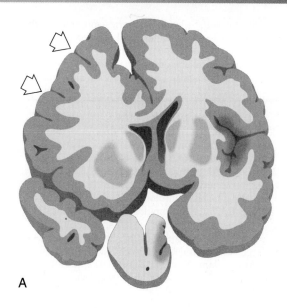

A

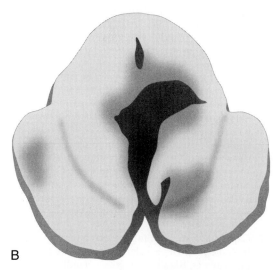

B

Figure 2-47. Drawings of autopsy findings in patients who died of lesions that increased intracranial pressure. **A,** A subdural hematoma was present in the region shown by the *open arrows*. The underlying brain is flattened and compressed in contrast to the opposite cerebral hemisphere. The extrinsic pressure on the brain has caused compression of the ipsilateral lateral ventricle and a shift in midline structures. The increased pressure forced the midbrain against the contralateral tentorium, causing injury to the contralateral cerebral peduncle—"Kernohan's notch." **B,** A Düret hemorrhage in the midbrain that developed in a patient with a large intracerebral hemorrhage.

to rebleeding. Clearly, a second or third bleed poses substantial threats for survival because each bleed increases ICP and the amount of blood in the CSF. Arteries bathed in bloody CSF often become constricted.[135,136] Vasoconstriction can be local or more diffuse and frequently leads to

ischemia, brain edema, and infarction.[136-138] Blood within the CSF can clog the absorptive membranes, leading to communicating hydrocephalus and dilation of all of the ventricular system. At times, the initial bleed or subsequent bleeds are into the brain, as well as on its surface. In these patients, the discussion of intracerebral hemorrhage also applies because they have both intracerebral and subarachnoid hemorrhages.

Having presented the basic building blocks for understanding the mechanisms of stroke, I proceed directly to clinical diagnosis at the bedside and then laboratory diagnosis in the following chapters.

References

1. Wagner KR, Xi G, Hua Y, et al: Early metabolic alterations in edematous perihematomal brain regions following experimental intracerebral hemorrhage. J Neurosurg 1998;88:1058-1065.
2. Bullock R, Brock-Utne J, van Dellen J, Blake G: Intracerebral hemorrhage in a primate model: effect on regional cerebral blood flow. Surg Neurol 1988;29:101-107.
3. Weiss H: Platelet physiology and abnormalities of platelet function. N Engl J Med 1975;293:531-540, 580-588.
4. Ashby B, Daniel JL, Smith JB: Mechanisms of platelet activation and inhibition. Hematol Oncol Clin North Am 1990;4:1-26.
5. Baker A, Iannone A: Cerebrovascular disease. I. The large arteries of the circle of Willis. Neurology 1959;9:321-332.
6. Fisher CM, Gore I, Okabe N, et al: Atherosclerosis of the carotid and vertebral arteries-extracranial and intracranial. J Neuropathol Exp Neurol 1965;24:455-476.
7. Fisher CM: Lacunes: Small deep cerebral infarcts. Neurology 1965;15:774-784.
8. Fisher CM: The arterial lesions underlying lacunes. Acta Neuropathol 1969;12:1-15.
9. Luscher TF, Lie JT, Stanson AW, et al: Arterial fibromuscular dysplasia. Mayo Clin Proc 1987; 62:931-952.
10. Shinohara Y: Takayasu disease. In Bogousslavsky J, Caplan LR (eds): Uncommon Causes of Stroke. Cambridge: Cambridge University Press, 2001, pp 37-42.
11. Davis SM: Temporal arteritis. In Bogousslavsky J, Caplan LR (eds): Uncommon Causes of Stroke. Cambridge: Cambridge University Press, 2001, pp 10-17.
12. Mokri B: Cervicocephalic arterial dissections. In Bogousslavsky J, Caplan LR (eds): Uncommon Causes of Stroke. Cambridge: Cambridge University Press, 2001, pp 211-229.
13. Imparato A, Riles T, Mintzer R, et al: The importance of hemorrhage in the relationship between gross morphologic characteristics and cerebral symptoms in 376 carotid artery plaques. Ann Surg 1983;197:195-203.

14. DeGeorgia M, Belden J, Pao L, et al: Thrombus in vertebrobasilar dolichoectatic artery treated with intravenous urokinase. Cerebrovasc Dis 1999;9:28-33.

15. Caplan LR, Manning W: Cardiac sources of embolism: The usual suspects. In Caplan LR, Manning WJ (eds): Brain Embolism. New York: Informa Healthcare, 2006, pp 129-159.

16. Caplan LR: Arterial sources of embolism. In Caplan LR, Manning WJ (eds): Brain Embolism. New York: Informa Healthcare, 2006, pp 203-222.

17. Gautier JC, Durr A, Koussa S, et al: Paradoxical cerebral embolism with a patent foramen ovale. A report of 29 patients. Cerebrovasc Dis 1991;1:193-202.

18. Caplan LR: Embolic particles. In Caplan LR, Manning WJ (eds): Brain Embolism. New York: Informa Healthcare, 2006, pp 259-275.

19. Caplan LR: Cardiac arrest and other hypoxic-ischemic insults. In Caplan LR, Hurst JW, Chimowitz M (eds): Clinical Neurocardiology. New York: Marcel Dekker, 1999, pp 1-34.

20. Mohr J: Neurological complications of cardiac valvular disease and cardiac surgery including systemic hypotension. In Vinken P, Bruyn G (eds): Handbook of Clinical Neurology, vol 38. Amsterdam: North Holland, 1979, pp 143-171.

21. Romanul F, Abramowicz A: Changes in brain and pial vessels in arterial boundary zones. Arch Neurol 1964;11:40-65.

22. Fisher CM, Adams RD: Observations on brain embolism with special reference to hemorrhagic infarction. In Furlan A (ed): The Heart and Stroke. London: Springer-Verlag, 1987, pp 17-36.

23. Weir B: Aneurysms affecting the nervous system. Baltimore: Williams & Wilkins, 1987.

24. Chicoine MR, Dacey RG: Clinical aspects of subarachnoid hemorrhage. In Welch KMA, Caplan LR, Reis DJ, et al (eds): Primer on Cardiovascular Diseases. San Diego: Academic Press, 1997, pp 425-432.

25. Kaufman HH (ed): Intracerebral Hematomas.. New York: Raven Press, 1992.

26. Cole F, Yates P: Intracerebral microaneurysms and small cerebrovascular lesions. Brain 1967; 90:759-768.

27. Rosenblum W: Miliary aneurysms and "fibrinoid" degeneration of cerebral blood vessels. Hum Pathol 1977;8:133-139.

28. Caplan LR: Intracerebral hemorrhage revisited. Neurology 1988;38:624-627.

29. Caplan LR: Hypertensive intracerebral hemorrhage. In Kase C, Caplan LR (eds): Intracerebral Hemorrhage. Boston: Butterworth-Heinemann, 1993, pp 99-116.

30. Finney L, Walker A: Transtentorial Herniation. Springfield, Ill: Thomas, 1962.

31. Fisher CM: Observations concerning brain herniation. Ann Neurol 1983;14:110.

32. Ropper AH: Lateral displacement of brain and level of consciousness in patients with acute hemispheral mass. N Engl J Med 1986;314: 953-958.

33. Stephens R, Stilwell D: Arteries and Veins of the Human Brain. Springfield, Ill: Thomas, 1969.

34. de Oliveira E, Tedeschi H, Rhoton Jr AL, Peace DA: Microsurgical anatomy of the internal carotid artery: Intrapetrous, intracavernous, and clinoidal segments. In Carter LP, Spetzler RF, Hamilton MG (eds): Neurovascular Surgery. New York: McGraw-Hill, 1995, pp 3-10.

35. Helgason C, Caplan LR, Goodwin J, Hedges T: Anterior choroidal artery-territory infarction. Arch Neurol 1986;43:681-686.

36. Tatu L, Moulin T, Bogousslavsky J, Duvernoy H: Arterial territories of the human brain: Cerebral hemispheres. Neurology 1998;50:1699-1708.

37. Lie T: Congenital malformations of the carotid and vertebral arterial systems, including the persistent anastomoses. In Vinken P, Bruyn G (eds): Handbook of Clinical Neurology, vol 12. Amsterdam: North Holland, 1972, pp 289-339.

38. Caplan LR: Posterior Circulation Disease: Clinical Findings, Diagnosis, and Management. Boston: Blackwell, 1996.

39. Foix C, Hillemand P: Contributions a l'etude des ramollissements protuberentiels. Rev Med 1926; 43:287-305.

40. Foix C, Hillemand P: Les Arteres de l'axe encephalique jusqu'a diencephale inclusivement. Rev Neurol 1925;32:705-739.

41. Caplan LR: Charles Foix—The first modern stroke neurologist. Stroke 1990;21:348-356.

42. Stopford J: The arteries of the pons and medulla oblongata. J Anat Physiol 1915,1916;50:131-164, 255-280.

43. Gillilan L: Anatomy and embryology of the arterial system of the brainstem and cerebellum. In Vinken P, Bruyn G (eds): Handbook of Clinical Neurology, vol 11. Amsterdam: North Holland, 1972, 24-44.

44. Duvernoy HM: Human brainstem vessels. Berlin: Springer-Verlag, 1978.

45. Capron L: Extra-and intracranial atherosclerosis. In Toole JF (ed): Vascular Diseases. Part 1, vol 53, PJ, Bruyn G, Klawans HL (eds): Handbook of Clinical Neurology. Amsterdam: Elsevier Science, 1988, pp 91-106.

46. Stehbens WE: Pathology of the Cerebral Blood Vessels. St Louis: Mosby, 1972.

47. Taveras JM, Wood EH: Diagnostic neuroradiology. Baltimore: Williams & Wilkins, 1964.

48. Moosy J: Morphology, sites, and epidemiology of cerebral atherosclerosis in research publications. Assoc Res Nerv Ment Dis 1966;51:1-22.

49. Caplan LR: Cerebrovascular disease: Large artery occlusive disease. In Appel S (ed): Current Neurology, vol 8. Chicago: Yearbook Medical, 1988, pp 179-226.

50. Gorelick PB, Caplan LR, Hier DB, et al: Racial differences in the distribution of anterior circulation occlusive cerebrovascular disease. Neurology 1984;34:54-59.

51. Caplan LR, Gorelick PB, Hier DB: Race, sex, and occlusive cerebrovascular disease: A review. Stroke 1986;17:648-655.

52. Caplan LR: Cerebral ischemia and infarction in blacks. Clinical, autopsy, and angiographic studies. In Gillum RF, Gorelick PB, Cooper ES (eds): Stroke in Blacks. Basel: Karger, 1999, pp 7-18.

53. Kieffer S, Takeya Y, Resch J, et al: Racial differences in cerebrovascular disease: Angiographic evaluation of Japanese and American populations. AJR Am J Roentgenol 1967;101:94-99.

54. Feldmann E, Daneault N, Kwan E, et al: Chinese-white differences in the distribution of occlusive cerebrovascular disease. Neurology 1990;40:1541-1545.

55. Mohr JP: Lacunes. Stroke 1982;13:3-11.

56. Caplan LR: Intracranial branch atheromatous disease. Neurology 1989;39:1246-1250.

57. Caplan LR, Zarins C, Hemmatti M: Spontaneous dissection of the extracranial vertebral artery. Stroke 1985;16:1030-1038.

58. O'Connell BF, Towfighi J, Brennan RW, et al: Dissecting aneurysms of head and neck. Neurology 1985;35:993-997.

59. Caplan LR, Baquis GD, Pessin MS, et al: Dissection of the intracranial vertebral artery. Neurology 1988;38:868-877.

60. Chaves C, Estol C, Esnaola M, et al: Spontaneous intracranial internal carotid artery dissection. Arch Neurol 2002;59:977-981.

61. Wilkinson I, Russell R: Arteries of the head and neck in giant cell arteritis. Arch Neurol 1972;27:378-391.

62. Caplan LR: Recipient artery: Anatomy and pathology. In Caplan LR, Manning WJ (eds): Brain Embolism. New York: Informa Healthcare, 2006, pp 31-59.

63. Gacs G, Merei FT, Bodosi M: Balloon catheter as a model of cerebral emboli in humans. Stroke 1982;13:39-42.

64. Vinters HV, Gilbert JJ: Cerebral amyloid angiopathy: Incidence and complications in the aging brain. II. The distribution of amyloid vascular changes. Stroke 1983;14:924-928.

65. Kase CS: Cerebral amyloid angiopathy. In Kase C, Caplan LR (eds): Intracerebral Hemorrhage. Boston: Butterworth-Heinemann, 1993, pp 179-200.

66. Bull J: Contribution of radiology to the study of intracranial aneurysms. BMJ 1922;2:1701-1708.

67. Alpers B: Aneurysms of the circle of Willis. In WS Fields (ed): Intracranial Aneurysms and Subarachnoid Hemorrhage. Springfield, Ill: Thomas, 1965, 5-24.

68. Ringelstein E, Zeumer H, Angelou D: The pathogenesis of strokes from internal carotid artery occlusion. Stroke 1983;14:867-875.

69. Ringelstein EB, Koschorke S, Holling A, et al: Computed tomographic pattern of proven embolic brain infarctions. Ann Neurol 1989;26:759-765.

70. Zulch K, Behrends R: The pathogenesis and topography of anoxia, hypoxia, and ischemia of the brain in man. In Meyer J, Gastant H (eds): Cerebral Anoxia and the EEG. Springfield, Ill: Thomas, 1961, 144-163.

71. Caplan LR: Clinical features at different sites. In Kase C, Caplan LR (eds): Intracerebral Hemorrhage. Boston: Butterworth-Heinemann, 1993, pp 305-308.

72. Smith EE, Eichler F: Cerebral amyloid angiopathy and lobar intracerebral hemorrhage. Arch Neurol 2006;63:148-151.

73. Caplan LR: Drugs. In Kase C, Caplan LR (eds): Intracerebral Hemorrhage. Boston: Butterworth-Heinemann, 1993, pp 201-220.

74. Kase CS: Bleeding disorders. In Kase C, Caplan LR (eds): Intracerebral Hemorrhage. Boston: Butterworth-Heinemann, 1993, pp 117-152.

75. Kase C, Robinson K, Stein R, et al: Anticoagulant-related intracerebral hemorrhage. Neurology 1985;35:943-948.

76. Jafar JJ, Crowell RM: Focal ischemic thresholds. In Wood JH (ed): Cerebral Blood Flow. New York: McGraw-Hill, 1987, pp 449-457.

77. Toole JF: Cerebrovascular Disorders, 4th ed. New York: Raven Press, 1990.

78. Frackowiak R, Lenzi G, Jones T, et al: Quantitative measurements of regional cerebral blood flow and oxygen metabolism in man using 150 and positron emission tomography: Therapy, procedure, and normal values. J Comput Assist Tomogr 1980;4:722-736.

79. Baron J-C: Positron emission tomography. In Babikian VL, Wechsler LR, Higashida RT (eds): Imaging Cerebrovascular Disease. Philadelphia: Butterworth-Heinemann, 2003, pp 115-130.

80. Roy CS, Sherrington CS: On the regulation of the blood-supply of the brain. J Physiol (London) 1890;11:85-108.

81. Friedland RP, Iadecola C: Roy and Sherrington (1890): A centennial reexamination of "On the regulation of the blood-supply of the brain." Neurology 1991;41:10-14.

82. Symon L: Pathological regulation in cerebral ischemia. In Wood JH (ed): Cerebral Blood Flow. New York: McGraw-Hill, 1987, pp 413-424.

83. Tong DC, Albers GW: Normal values. In Babikian VL, Wechsler LR (eds): Transcranial Doppler Ultrasonography, 2nd ed. Boston: Butterworth-Heinemann, 1999, pp 33-46.

84. Kontos HA: Oxygen radicals in cerebral ischemia: The 2001 Willis Lecture. Stroke 2001;32:2712-2716.

85. Garcia JH, Anderson ML: Pathophysiology of cerebral ischemia. Crit Rev Neurobiol 1989;4:303-324.

86. Collins RC, Dobkin BH, Choi DW: Selective vulnerability of the brain: New insights into the pathophysiology of stroke. Ann Intern Med 1989;110:992-1000.

87. Choi DW: Excitotoxicity and stroke. In Caplan LR (ed): Brain Ischemia: Basic Concepts and Clinical Relevance. London: Springer, 1995, pp 29-36.

88. Garcia JH: Mechanisms of cell death in ischemia. In Caplan LR (ed): Brain Ischemia: Basic Concepts and Clinical Relevance. London: Springer, 1995, pp 7-18.

2

89. Mattson MP, Barger SW: Programmed cell life: Neuroprotective signal transduction and ischemic brain injury. In Caplan LR (ed): Cerebrovascular Diseases, Nineteenth Princeton Stroke Conference, Moskowitz MA. Boston: Butterworth-Heinemann, 1995, pp 271-290.

90. Nurden AT, Duperat V-G, Nurden P: Platelet function and pharmacology of antiplatelet drugs. Cerebrovasc Dis 1997(suppl 6):2-9.

91. Moncada S, Higgs E, Vane J: Human arterial and venous tissues generate prostacyclin (prostaglandin 4) a potent inhibitor of platelet aggregation. Lancet 1977;1:18-20.

92. Schmid-Schonbein H, Perktold K: Physical factors in the pathogenesis of atheroma formation. In Caplan LR (ed): Brain Ischemia: Basic Concepts and Clinical Relevance. London: Springer, 1995, pp 185-213.

93. Caplan LR, Hennerici M: Impaired clearance of emboli (washout) is an important link between hypoperfusion, embolism, and ischemic stroke. Arch Neurol 1998;55:1475-1482.

94. Caplan LR, Wong KS, Gao S, Hennerici MG: Is hypoperfusion an important cause of strokes? If so, how? Cerebrovasc Dis 2006;21:145-153.

95. Masuda J, Yutani C, Ogata J, et al: Atheromatous embolism in the brain: A clinicopathologic analysis of 15 autopsy cases. Neurology 1994; 44:1231-1237.

96. McKibbin DW, Bulkley BH, Green WR, et al: Fatal cerebral atheromatous embolization after cardiac bypass. J Thorac Cardiovasc Surg 1976; 71:741-745.

97. Pollanen MS, Deck JHN: The mechanism of embolic watershed infarction: Experimental studies. Can J Neurol Sci 1990;17:395-398.

98. Fisher M, Francis R: Altered coagulation in cerebral ischemia. Arch Neurol 1990;47: 1075-1079.

99. Tohgi H, Kawashima M, Tamura K, et al: Coagulation-fibrinolysis abnormalities in acute and chronic phases of cerebral thrombosis and embolism. Stroke 1990;21:1663-1667.

100. Feinberg WM: Coagulation. In Caplan LR (ed): Brain Ischemia: Basic Concepts and Clinical Relevance. London: Springer, 1995, 85-96.

101. Deykin D: Thrombogenesis. N Engl J Med 1967;276:622-628.

102. del Zoppo GJ: Vascular hemostatsis and brain embolism. In Caplan LR, Manning WJ (eds): Brain Embolism. New York: Informa Healthcare, 2006, pp 243-258.

103. Svensson PJ, Dahlback B: Resistance to activated protein C as a basis to venous thrombosis. N Engl J Med 1994;330:517-522.

104. Bertina RM, Koelman BPC, Rosendall FR, et al: Mutation in the blood coagulation factor V associated with resistance to activated protein C. Nature 1994;369:64-67.

105. Poort SR, Rosendaal FR, Reitsma PH, Bertina RM: A common genetic variation in the 3' untranslated region of the prothrombin gene is associated with elevated plasma prothrombin levels and an

increase in venous thrombosis. Blood 1996;88: 3698-3703.

106. Martinelli I, Sacchi E, Landi G, et al: High risk of cerebral vein thrombosis in carriers of a prothrombin-gene mutation and in users of oral contraceptives. N Engl J Med 1998;338: 1793-1797.

107. Sloan M: Thrombolysis and stroke. Arch Neurol 1987;44:748-768.

108. Raichle M: The pathophysiology of brain ischemia. Ann Neurol 1983;13:2-10.

109. Astrup J, Siesjo B, Simon L: Thresholds in cerebral ischemia: The ischemic penumbra. Stroke 1981;12:723-725.

110. Thomas D, du Boulay G, Marshall J, et al: Effect of hematocrit on cerebral blood flow in man. Lancet 1977;2:941-943.

111. Thomas D, Marshall J, Russell RW, et al: Cerebral blood flow in polycythemia. Lancet 1977;2: 161-163.

112. Tohgi H, Yasmanouchi H, Murakami M, et al: Importance of the hematocrit as a risk factor in cerebral infarction. Stroke 1978;9:369-374.

113. Caplan LR, Sergay S: Positional cerebral ischemia. J Neurol Neurosurg Psychiatry 1976;39:385-391.

114. Toole J: Effects of change of head, limb, and body position on cephalic circulation. N Engl J Med 1968;279:307-311.

115. Kim HY, Singhal AB, Lo EH: Normobaric hyperoxia extends the reperfusion window in focal cerebral ischemia. Ann Neurol 2005;57: 571-575.

116. Ginsberg M, Welsh F, Budd W: Deleterious effect of glucose pretreatment on recovery from diffuse cerebral ischemia in the cat. Stroke 1980;11:347-354.

117. Plum F: What causes infarction in ischemic brain? Neurology 1983;33:222-233.

118. Siesjo BK, Kristian T, Katsura K: The role of calcium in delayed postischemic brain damage. In Caplan LR (ed): Cerebrovascular Diseases, the Nineteenth Princeton Stroke Conference, Moskowitz MA. Boston: Butterworth-Heinemann, 1995, pp 353-370.

119. Gorelick PB, Caplan LR: Calcium, hypercalcemia and stroke. Curr Concepts Cerebrovasc Dis (Stroke) 1985;20:13-17.

120. Hillbom M, Kaste M: Ethanol intoxication: A risk factor for ischemic brain infarction in adolescents and young adults. Stroke 1981;12:422-425.

121. Ames III A, Wright RL, Kouada M, et al: Cerebral ischemia. II. The no-reflow phenomenon. Am J Pathol 1968;52:437-453.

122. O'Brien MD: Ischemic cerebral edema. In Caplan LR (ed): Brain Ischemia: Basic Concepts and Clinical Relevance. London: Springer, 1995, pp 43-50.

123. Ropper AH: Brain edema after stroke, clinical syndrome and intracranial pressure. Arch Neurol 1984;41:26-29.

124. Ropper AH: A preliminary MRI study of the geometry of brain displacement and level of

consciousness with acute intracranial masses. Neurology 1989;39:622-627.

125. Barnett H: Delayed cerebral ischemic episodes distal to occlusion of major cerebral arteries. Neurology 1978;28:769-774.

126. Fisher CM: Occlusion of the internal carotid artery. Arch Neurol Psychiatry 1951;65:346-377.

127. Caplan LR: Occlusion of the vertebral or basilar artery. Stroke 1979;10:277-282.

128. Glass TA, Hennessey PM, Pazdera L, et al: Outcome at 30 days in the New England Medical Center Posterior Circulation Registry. Arch Neurol 2002;59(3):369-376.

129. Caplan LR, Wityk RJ, Glass TA, et al: New England Medical Center Posterior Circulation Registry. Ann Neurol 2004;56:389-398.

130. Savitz SI, Caplan LR: Current concepts: Vertebrobasilar disease. N Engl J Med 2005; 352:2618-2626.

131. Jones H, Millikan C, Sandok B: Temporal profile of acute vertebrobasilar system infarction. Stroke 1980;11:173-177.

132. Fisher CM: Pathological observations in hypertensive cerebral hemorrhage. J Neuropathol Exp Neurol 1971;30:536-550.

133. Herbstein D, Schaumberg H: Hypertensive intracerebral hematoma: An investigation of the initial hemorrhage and rebleeding using Cr 51 labeled erythrocytes. Arch Neurol 1974;30: 412-414.

134. Duret H: Traumatismes Cranio-Cerebaux. Paris: Librarie Felix Alcan, 1919.

135. Fisher CM, Kistler JP, Davis JM: Relation of cerebral vasospasm to subarachnoid hemorrhage visualized by computerized tomographic scanning. Neurosurgery 1980;6:1-9.

136. MacDonald RL: Cerebral Vasospasm. In Welch KMA, Reis DJ, Caplan LR, et al (eds): Primer on Cerebrovascular Diseases. San Diego: Academic Press, 1997, pp 490-497.

137. Hijdra A, van Gijn J, Nagelkerke NJD, et al: Prediction of delayed cerebral ischemia, rebleeding, and outcome after aneurysmal subarachnoid hemorrhage. Stroke 1988;19:1250-1256.

138. Aygun N, Perl II J: Subarachnoid hemorrhage. In Babikian VL, Wchsler LR, Higashida RT (eds): Imaging Cerebrovascular Disease. Philadelphia: Butterworth-Heinemann, 2003, pp 241-269.

3   Diagnosis and the Clinical Encounter

A 36-year-old man, JH, becomes confused at work. His wife was called, and she came to the workplace and brought him to the hospital. On arrival about 4 hours after symptom onset, it is obvious that his left limbs are weak. He is very sleepy and at times barely arousable. The nurse in the emergency ward at the hospital calls you, his physician, and relates that your patient is having a stroke.

INFORMATION USED FOR STROKE DIAGNOSIS

The preceding brief patient vignette describes a seriously ill man, presumably an acute stroke patient. The clinician's first task is to decide what is happening to the patient. This chapter follows the process of diagnosis by a stepwise consideration of the facts in his case. Before proceeding with the specific case example, however, I will review the general process of stroke diagnosis. Clinical diagnosis is often difficult, but the process becomes easier and more logical if approached systematically. I routinely follow several steps and rules and urge each individual clinician to become familiar with the diagnostic methods that he or she uses. Routines and thoroughness prevent errors made by snap guesses or impulsive diagnoses. I have elaborated elsewhere in much more detail on the subject of clinical neurologic diagnoses[1,2] and only summarize briefly the main points here.

First, the clinician must decide on the key questions to ask. Answers are difficult unless the questions are clearly framed. The most general questions should be asked first, followed by the more specific ones. In neurology, two diagnostic questions always require answers: (1) *What* is the disease mechanism, that is, the pathology and pathophysiology? and (2) *Where* is the lesion(s), that is, the anatomy of the disorder? Regarding the stroke patient, the "what" question concerns which of the five stroke mechanisms (hemorrhage-subarachnoid or intracerebral; ischemia-thrombotic, embolic, or decreased global perfusion) is present. Of course, before distinguishing among stroke mechanisms, clinicians should first ask whether the findings could be caused by a nonvascular process, such as a brain tumor, metabolic disorder, infection, intoxication, or traumatic injury that mimics stroke. The "where" question concerns the anatomic location of the disorder, both in the brain and in the vascular system.

Different data are used to answer these two quite different questions. In determining stroke mechanism—the "what" question—the following clinical bedside data are most helpful:

1. Ecology—the past and present personal and family illnesses
2. Presence and nature of past strokes or transient ischemic attacks (TIAs)
3. Activity at the onset of the stroke
4. Temporal course and progression of the findings (Was the stroke onset sudden with the deficit maximal at onset? Did the deficit improve, worsen, or remain the same after onset? If it worsened, did this occur in a stepwise, remitting, or gradually progressive fashion? Were there fluctuations between normal and abnormal?)
5. Accompanying symptoms such as headache, vomiting, and decreased level of consciousness

Information about these items can all be gleaned from a thorough and thoughtful history from the patient, a review of physician and medical records, and data collected from observers, family members, and friends. These data are primarily historical and require little sophisticated knowledge of neurology. The general physical examination, which uncovers disorders not known from the history, adds to the data used for diagnosing the stroke mechanism. Elevated blood pressure, cardiac enlargement or murmurs, and vascular bruits are examples of physical findings that influence identification of the stroke mechanism.

Diagnosis of stroke location—the "where" question—is made using very different information:

1. Analysis of the neurologic symptoms and their distribution
2. Findings on neurologic examination

The history and knowledge of general systemic diseases tells the clinician *what* is wrong; the neurologic examination provides more information on *where* the disease process is located.

Mechanism and anatomic diagnoses are not absolute. More realistic are estimates of probabilities. In one patient, intracerebral hemorrhage may be by far the most likely diagnosis, but embolism and thrombosis are also possible and should not be eliminated from consideration. In another patient, there might be an apparent toss-up between thrombosis and embolism.

The process of diagnosis involves two basic techniques: (1) hypothesis generation and testing and (2) pattern matching.

The Inductive Method: Sequential Hypothesis Generation and Testing

Hypothesis generation should begin as soon as the first information about the patient becomes available. This may come from a call to the doctor (e.g., by an emergency room nurse as in the vignette at the beginning of the chapter) or when the patient is first seen. As the patient or another individual relates the history, the clinician should be thinking of possible diagnoses. It is best to first let the patient (or other historian) give an overview of the events while the doctor listens without interrupting. The information conveyed should generate hypotheses and queries. Ask the patient and available others questions whose answers should help confirm or refute the hypotheses. For example, an elderly patient with known coronary and peripheral limb atherosclerosis has a left hemiparesis noted on awakening. In such a case, considering the patient's risk factors and time of onset, I would first think of thrombosis because that would be a common stroke mechanism. I would then ask whether there had been prior transient episodes of left limb symptoms. Their presence would strongly favor thrombosis.

Anatomic hypotheses are also generated. A left hemiparesis raises the possibility of a right cerebral or brainstem lesion, so I ask about accompanying visual, sensory, or brainstem symptoms that would help generate a more specific anatomic localization. The process of anatomic diagnosis is much like locating a missing person. First, the clinician must determine whether the person is in the United States before narrowing the locale to Massachusetts, and then the Boston vicinity, and a specific street in the Brookline neighborhood. Similarly, regarding the diagnosis of mechanism, the physician must decide on ischemia versus hemorrhage before hypothesizing about subtypes of ischemia. The physician must identify thrombosis versus embolism versus global hypoperfusion

before distinguishing subtypes of thrombosis, such as lacunar or large artery, anterior or posterior circulation. Thus, the clinician proceeds systematically from the more general to the more specific. Clearly, the amount of available data may limit reasonable hypotheses to the most general inferences. For some patients, little historical data are available.

Pattern Matching

The other technique used by most clinicians is pattern matching. For example, I recognize the person I call "Jim" by comparing the individual in front of me with a mental image of Jim that I conjure up in my mind's eye. I do not ordinarily list individual features (e.g., height, glasses, hair style). Similarly, clinicians try to identify a constellation of findings that match their mental images of patterns of stroke mechanisms and pathology and anatomy. For example, the diagnosis of Parkinsonism may become readily obvious to you even as you walk with a new patient into your office because of the resemblance of the patient's facial expression, posture, gait, and tremor to other Parkinsonian patients whom you have seen in the past.

Although the diagnostic analysis should be pursued sequentially, diagnosis of the "what" and "where" questions should proceed concurrently. While obtaining the patient's history, have the patient describe information that will allow prediction of the probability of various stroke mechanisms and locations. At the end of the history, be prepared to list these and to assign rough probability estimates. Next, think about and plan the examination. In this patient, what additional findings are important and help to confirm or refute the preliminary diagnoses? What data will allow more specificity? In the patient with left hemiparesis, the presence of a left visual field deficit or left visual neglect would localize the lesion to the right cerebral hemisphere. Nystagmus or a gaze palsy to the right or an internuclear ophthalmoplegia would favor a brainstem site. A right carotid bruit or a cholesterol crystal found on examining the retina of the right eye would favor a right carotid artery site. After the general and neurologic examinations, reexamine the original hypotheses and their probabilities. New or unexpected findings from the examinations might stimulate new hypotheses or might confirm or refute prior hypotheses. A blood pressure of 260/140 mm Hg would clearly increase the likelihood of hemorrhage. The absence of a pulse or presence of papilledema on examination would change prior estimated probabilities.

3

Next, proceed to ask what laboratory tests might help refine the hypotheses generated at the end of the history and the examinations. Also, initial laboratory test results help determine the need for other tests. Laboratory tests should also be planned, reviewed, and ordered sequentially (this topic is elaborated in Chapter 4). Overall, the process of diagnosis should be logical, systematic, and sequential.

PROCEDURE FOR DIAGNOSIS OF STROKE MECHANISM AND BRAIN LOCALIZATION

Mimicking a Computer

Computers have taught clinicians to be more aware of the process and mechanics of diagnosis. In an individual patient, how would a computer estimate the most likely stroke mechanism diagnosis? Physicians can emulate the logic and methodology of the computer process for a more systematic diagnostic strategy. One technique of computer diagnosis is the use of Bayes theorem.[3,4] Information needed for this methodology include knowledge of (1) the incidence of each illness (in this case, stroke mechanism) in the population studied and (2) the incidence of a given finding in each illness (stroke mechanism). Armed with this information and the findings in the individual patient, the computer calculates the probability of a given stroke mechanism. The use of probabilities mimics the way that clinicians usually approach a diagnostic problem. Seldom is a single diagnosis absolutely certain (100%). More often, a given diagnosis (e.g., brain embolism) is considered most likely (perhaps 70% probable); but thrombotic occlusion also should be considered (perhaps 20%), and intracerebral hemorrhage, although unlikely (10%), still enters into the differential diagnosis.

Knowing the frequencies of the various stroke mechanisms provides what is often called *a priori odds*. An analysis of data from large stroke studies and registries[5-23] (Table 3-1) shows that approximately 80% of all strokes are ischemic and 20% are hemorrhagic. Therefore, if no other specific information was available about a stroke patient, the diagnosis of ischemic stroke would be correct four out of five times, but subarachnoid hemorrhage would be correct for only about 1 in 10 patients. The remainder of the computer prediction uses individual factors (e.g., headache preceding stroke, presence of TIAs, activity at onset, prior evidence of atherosclerosis) to predict the likely stroke mechanism. For example, Table 3-2 presents the relative frequency of headache during the days or weeks preceding stroke. Relatively few patients had

headaches preceding stroke, but the finding was slightly more common in patients with thrombotic stroke and intracerebral hemorrhage and less common in patients with either subarachnoid hemorrhage or brain embolism. In this example, the difference in frequency is small. In contrast, headache at or near the onset of stroke (Table 3-3) invariably occurred in patients with subarachnoid hemorrhage but was clearly less often present in patients with other mechanisms of stroke.

These data can also be presented in graphic form, as seen in Figure 3-1, which derives from a study of patients seen at the stroke service at the Michael Reese Hospital and the University of Illinois.[24] The figure shows the frequency—by stroke subtype—of headache preceding stroke (often called *sentinel headache*) at onset. Computer software and the alert physician sum the individual data items, factor in the a priori odds, and arrive at a total probability for a given stroke mechanism in each stroke patient. During the discussion of individual topics in the remainder of this chapter, I include important data results selected from stroke registry experience.

Ecology

Included within ecology are prior medical diseases and demographic data that might predispose the patient to have one or more of the various stroke mechanisms. When called to see a patient with stroke, the physician usually has some background information available from the family, another physician, or the clinician's own experience with the patient. For example, a call from the hospital emergency room might describe a "65-year-old man with angina pectoris, two prior heart attacks, diabetes, and hypertension who arrived here today with...." This information leads the physician to consider the probability of particular stroke mechanisms in the patient who is about to be seen. In this example, the presence of diabetes and coronary artery disease strongly favors a diagnosis of associated atherosclerosis of the extracranial cervical arteries and a thrombotic (or artery-to-artery embolus) mechanism of stroke. The presence of prior heart disease raises the possibility of arrhythmia, mural thrombosis, ventricular aneurysm, and valvular heart disease—all potential sources of brain embolism. The presence of hypertension increases the probability of intracerebral hemorrhage (ICH), especially if the hypertension is severe, a determination that can be made quickly when the patient is seen. An alert physician would also be sure to inquire whether the patient was being treated with anticoagulants

Table 3-1. Frequency and Types of Stroke in Various Studies

Study	Year	n	T	LA	Lac	ICU	Emb	ICH	SAH	Isc Total	Hem Total
Aring-Merritt[5]	1935	407	81	—	—	—	3	—	—	84	15
Whisnant et al[8]	1971	548	75	—	—	—	3	10	5	78	15
Matsumoto et al[9]	1973	993	71	—	—	—	8	10	6	79	16
Harvard Stroke Registry[7]	1978	694	53	34	19	—	31	10	6	84	16
Michael Reese Stroke Registry[10]	1983	472	31	18	13	30	17	14	8	78	22
Austin Hospital[11]	1983	700	68	45	23	18	8	6	Excl	94	6
South Alabama[17]	1984	160	19	6	13	40	26	8	6	85	14
Lausanne Stroke Registry[13]	1988	1000	56	43	13	8	20	11	Excl	89	11
Stroke Data Bank[12]	1988	1805	25	6	19	32	14	13	13	71	26
Lehigh Valley Stroke Registry[21]	1989	2639	60	—	9	—	20	9	Excl	91	9
Oxfordshire Community Stroke Project[19]	1990	675	—	—	—	—	—	10	5	81	15
Taiwan Stroke Registry[22]	1997	676	46	17	29	20	29	Excl	Excl	100	Excl
Community Hospital Stroke Program[23]	1990	4129	32	—	—	—	11	5	2	60	10

Emb, embolism; Excl, excluded from study; Hem, hemorrhage; ICH, intracerebral hemorrhage; Isc, ischemia; LA, large artery; Lac, lacune; SAH, subarachnoid hemorrhage; T, thrombosis (sum of large artery and lacune)

Table 3-2. Headache Preceding Stroke

	Thrombosis	Embolism	ICH	SAH
yes	27 (8.2%)	8 (4%)	6 (8%)	1 (3%)
no	291 (89%)	177 (87%)	61 (77%)	27 (87%)
other	9 (2%)	18 (9%)	12 (15%)	3 (10%
totals	327	203	79	31

ICH, intracerebral hemorrhage; SAH, subarachnoid hemorrhage.

From Mohr JP, Caplan LR, Melski JW, et al: The Harvard Cooperative Stroke Registry: A prospective registry. Neurology 1978;28:754-762.

for his cardiac disease, a factor that would greatly increase the chance of ICH.

The clinician uses the presence of individual risk factors to alter the likelihood that an individual patient has a particular stroke mechanism. Perhaps another example will help clarify this statement. On average, 60% of strokes are considered thrombotic (including intra-arterial embolism) 20% are cardioembolic, 12% are ICH, and 8% are due to subarachnoid hemorrhage (SAH). The presence of severe hypertension (e.g., 220/130 mm Hg) would certainly make

Table 3-3. Headache at Onset of Stroke (%)

Registry	T	Lac	Emb	SAH	ICH	ICU
HSR	12	3	9	78	33	—
MRSR	29	16	17	98	80	13

Emb, embolism; HSR, Harvard Stroke Registry; ICH, intracerebral hemorrhage; ICU, infarct cause unknown; Lac, lacune; MRSR, Michael Reese Stroke Registry; SAH, subarachnoid hemorrhage; T, thrombosis.

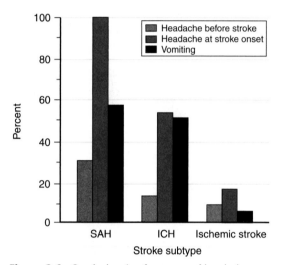

Figure 3-1. Graph showing frequency of headache patterns and vomiting in patients with ischemic strokes and hemorrhages in the Michael Reese and University of Illinois stroke registries. (From Gorelick PB, Hier DB, Caplan LR, et al: Headache in acute cerebrovascular disease. Neurology 1986;36:1445-1450.)

hemorrhage, especially ICH, much more likely. This factor would significantly shift the odds toward ICH and slightly to SAH. If another factor, such as age, is then added (e.g., if the severely hypertensive patient were a 23-year-old woman), this would make the major alternative diagnosis, thrombotic stroke, much less likely and would further increase the likelihood of a hemorrhagic mechanism. This shift of probabilities can be described as "loading on" or "detracting from" a specific diagnosis. For example, severe hypertension loads heavily on ICH (+ + + +), and youthfulness detracts from thrombosis. Data from prior experience, such as those found in registries, can help determine quantitatively the relative shift of odds.

Table 3-4 lists the frequencies of diabetes, hypertension, and coronary artery disease in the various subtypes of stroke in the Harvard Stroke Registry (HSR)[7] and the frequencies of other similar variables in the Michael Reese Stroke Registry (MRSR).[10] Note that hypertension was more common in all groups in the MRSR and atherosclerosis more prominent in the HSR. The populations in these two registries were quite different: The HSR included a predominantly white, middle- and upper-class population with a high incidence of atherosclerosis, whereas the MRSR had more young, black, hypertensive individuals with a lower prevalence of atherosclerosis. Black, Chinese, and Japanese populations have a higher incidence of ICH and intracranial occlusive disease than white populations.[25-34] Table 3-5 lists

Table 3-4. Incidence of Various Risk Factors in Each Type of Stroke (%)

	T	Lac	Emb	ICH	SAH
HSR					
Atherosclerosis*	56	37	34	11	5
Diabetes	26	28	13	15	2
Past hypertension	55	75	40	72	19
MRSR					
Angina pectoris	13	8	20	5	0
Past MI	23	16	40	12	0
Recent MI	7	12	12	3	0
Past hypertension	75	55	55	68	44

*Includes peripheral vascular disease, coronary artery disease, and neck bruits.

Emb, embolism; HSR, Harvard Stroke Registry; ICH, intracerebral hemorrhage; Lac, lacune; MRSR, Michael Reese Stroke Registry; SAH, subarachnoid hemorrhage; T, thrombosis.

Table 3-5.   Weighting of Ecologic Factors

	T	Lac	Emb	ICH	SAH
Hypertension	++	+++		++	+
Severe hypertension		+		++++	++
Coronary disease	+++		++		
Claudication	+++		+		
Atrial fibrillation			++++		
Sick sinus syndrome			++		
Valvular heart disease			+++		
Diabetes	+++	+	+		
Bleeding diathesis				++++	+
Smoking	+++		+		+
Cancer	++		++		
Old age	+++	+	+	+	
Black or Asian ethnic origin	+	+		++	

Emb, embolism; ICH, intracerebral hemorrhage; Lac, lacune; SAH, subarachnoid hemorrhage; T, thrombosis.

estimated loading weights that could be assigned to various risk factors. At times, the effect of a condition is indirect; for example, the presence of diabetes increases the chance of myocardial infarction, which in turn increases the likelihood of a cardiac-origin embolism.

I now return to the patient JH discussed at the beginning of this chapter. I continue to discuss his case and its analysis during the remainder of the discussion of clinical diagnosis.

After the call from the emergency room, before leaving for the hospital, the doctor asked her secretary to pull JH's office chart. He had last been seen 1 year ago, at age 35 years, because of bronchitis. Notes indicate that he smoked three packs of cigarettes a day, had always had normal blood pressures, and had no history of cardiac or neurologic symptoms. He had described, however, a high incidence of heart attacks in his family. He had been overweight, and his blood cholesterol level last year was 295. He was advised to pursue a weight-reduction program, to reduce his intake of fats and cholesterol-containing foods, to stop smoking, and to return for a recheck. He had not returned.

When leaving for the hospital, think about the information known, based on the emergency room nurse's call and on JH's records. The illness was said to have begun rather suddenly, and the brain lesion must be focal because he has an obvious left limb paralysis. Abrupt-onset focal brain lesions are most often strokes, but his youth serves as a reminder to be certain to consider focal brain lesions other than stroke. Brain tumors, abscesses, trauma, and encephalitis can cause focal findings, and without other information, it is not yet clear how abruptly the symptoms began and progressed. If the process is a stroke, as would be statistically most likely, review the background information regarding risks for the different stroke mechanisms. His past smoking, family history of cardiac disease, and high blood-cholesterol level suggest to you the possibility of premature atherosclerosis, with large-artery occlusive disease as the mechanism of the stroke. An unusual type of cardiac disease with brain embolism is another mechanism that is suggested by the family history of cardiac disease. ICH could also cause left-sided paralysis and sleepiness, but the absence of past hypertension makes this less likely, unless he had recently developed hypertension. Make a mental note to quickly check his blood pressure and seek signs of organ damage due to hypertension on examination. The first hypothesis regarding preliminary stroke mechanism is large artery atherosclerosis with embolism; cardiac-origin embolism and ICH are also to be seriously considered. Systemic hypoperfusion and SAH seldom cause severe hemiplegia at outset.

Thus far, little detail about neurologic symptoms are available that could help localize the lesion. The patient is said to have a left-sided paralysis, and so the right cerebral hemisphere and right pons are the most likely sites of pathology. The report of confusion at work favors a cerebral hemispheric lesion. Plan to ask questions that will promote more precise localization.

Having used the ecologic data to shift the usual stroke mechanism probabilities, carry these probabilities into an investigation of the next data items, such as prior cerebrovascular symptoms, course of illness, accompanying symptoms, and so on—each of which then further modifies the probabilities.

When you arrive at the emergency room, the nurse says that the patient's pulse and blood pressure are normal. The patient is awake but cannot give any account of his illness. He seems unaware that his left limbs are paralyzed. The coworker who was with him when he became ill says that he suddenly seemed dazed and quickly became hemiplegic, falling to the ground. His wife says that he did not follow previous dietary advice and was still smoking heavily. She said he had not been ill, but a week before he told her that for 10 minutes one morning, his left arm and face had temporarily felt numb, symptoms he attributed to a draft from an air conditioner in the office.

Prior Cerebrovascular Symptoms, Especially Transient Ischemic Attacks

Although not especially common, prior cerebrovascular events so heavily load probabilities that they should be given considerable importance. TIAs in the same vascular territory are frequent precursors of thrombotic stroke, so their presence, especially when multiple, is virtually diagnostic of that stroke mechanism. If a patient presenting to the hospital with aphasia and right limb weakness had had an attack of transient right-handed weakness 3 weeks earlier and an attack of right-face and right-hand numbness and weakness 1 week earlier, the clinician could be relatively certain that the stroke was a result of thrombotic occlusive disease within the left anterior circulation. If, in addition, that same individual had also had a black shade descending over the left eye, causing temporary blindness, the location could be further refined, and it would seem certain that the occlusive lesion involved the internal carotid artery before its ophthalmic artery branch.

The presence, nature, and duration of TIAs are important. Information about the presence of TIAs must be vigorously and repeatedly sought. Many patients are quite naive about the functions of the body, especially the nervous system. Some stroke patients attribute their weakness, lack of feeling, and visual deficits to the local limbs or to the eyes; they often do not understand that the central nervous system (CNS) control of these functions has been damaged. They often wonder why the head is being studied and imaged rather than the arm or leg, where surely the trouble resides. Patients usually do not volunteer information that they think is unrelated to their present trouble. A woman with visual difficulty will not tell her eye doctor about a vaginal discharge, considering the latter problem in the province of her gynecologist. Similarly, a patient with hand weakness might not tell the physician about prior leg weakness, not realizing that the conditions are related. The same individual will surely not tell the doctor about temporary visual dysfunction, considering the eye problem to belong to the ophthalmologist. Patients often attribute their temporary symptoms to banal causes in the environment (e.g., an air conditioner draft, as in the case of JH). Symptoms of TIA must be elicited specifically: "Have you ever had temporary weakness of your right hand, your right leg, your face? Have you had difficulty speaking, seeing, and so forth?"

On entry to the hospital, or during the early physician encounters, patients are often not at their optimum performance levels. They may be sick, frightened, tired, or worried and therefore suboptimal observers and witnesses. Many patients have told me on the third or even sixth day of stroke about prior TIAs, having denied their presence when queried on admission.

Physicians should acquire as much detail as possible about the TIAs. Some features of TIAs are helpful in diagnosing a subtype of brain ischemia, as will be discussed below. When there were multiple attacks, when was the first and when was the last? Are they getting more frequent or is the interval between attacks becoming longer? Are the episodes stereotyped and nearly identical in all attacks? How long do the TIAs last? What is the shortest, longest, and average duration? Are attacks becoming longer or shorter? Are TIAs provoked by standing or activity? Are they positional? Neck positioning can occasionally temporarily occlude stenotic vertebral arteries.

Some patients cannot provide information about a TIA because of aphasia, altered level of consciousness, amnesia, and so on. Some patients with right hemisphere dysfunction do not realize when things go wrong. Other observers, such as family, hospital visitors, and friends, should be queried because the patient may have told them about prior symptoms, or these individuals may have observed altered function in the patient. Caution must be exercised in exploring symptoms at the patient's work site, because knowledge about a patient's neurologic problem might adversely affect job status. Clearly, permission should be sought before approaching employers or coworkers for health information. In this case, the coworker and wife were present and could provide useful data when the patient could not.

Many studies in various populations have shown that TIAs carry a very substantial risk of imminent brain infarction and should be handled emergently.[35-41] Johnston and colleagues analyzed outcomes among 1707 patients with TIAs who presented to emergency departments in 16 hospitals in the San Francisco Bay area in California.[35] During the 90 days after emergency room presentation, 180 patients (10.5%) returned with a stroke, occurring in half the patients within the first 2 days.[35] Kleindorfer et al. performed a population-based study of TIAs occurring in the Cincinnati-northern Kentucky region during 1 year.[37] During the year, 1023 TIA events occurred among 927 patients. Within 6 months of the index TIA, 144 patients had an ischemic stroke and 77 died. The median time for stroke to develop was 12 days.[37] Rothwell and Warlow used a different approach.[39] They retrospectively reviewed data from 2146 stroke admissions in the UK. A preceding TIA was present in 23%; 17% of TIAs occurred on the day of the stroke, 9% on the preceding day, and 43% during the preceding week.[39]

The designation TIA should mean what it says. *Transient* implies temporary, although not stating how temporary; it at least is not permanent; *ischemic* identifies the cause, lack of blood flow; and *attack* implies a suddenness and limited time duration of a discrete event, although again not stating the duration of the attack or the rapidity of onset. The two key words are *ischemic,* conveying an etiology, and *transient,* meaning not permanent and not causing irreversible cell death or infarction. According to the old definition created by the Committee on Cerebrovascular Disease in 1975, "[T]ransient ischemic attack is defined as a cerebral dysfunction of ischemic nature lasting no longer than 24 hours with a tendency to recur."[42] This definition is outdated and should no longer be used. The 24-hour duration was arbitrarily chosen without data. Studies have shown that, in fact, most TIAs last only a few minutes, and the great majority last less than an hour. Those lasting longer than 1 hour are often associated with brain infarction on modern brain imaging.[43] The new definition that I strongly favor is "a TIA is a brief episode of neurological dysfunction caused by focal brain or retinal ischemia, with clinical symptoms typically lasting less than an hour, and without evidence of acute infarction."[43]

Although the term *TIA* designates ischemia, it does not differentiate between an embolic and a thrombotic mechanism or between a small artery and a large artery site. Brain embolism can produce a transient disorder that would qualify as a TIA. Some evidence supports the notion that embolism is more likely to produce less frequent but longer attacks, whereas low flow states produce briefer but more frequent attacks. Shotgun-like repeated episodes of ischemia in the same vascular territory virtually always indicate a critical degree of vessel narrowing. Single but longer attacks are more often associated with an ulcerated plaque or another embolic source.

In patients with penetrating artery disease (lacunar infarction), TIAs occur but are less common. In the HSR, TIAs occurred in 23% of patients with lacunar disease, compared with 50% of patients with large artery arteriosclerosis.[7] When present, TIAs in patients with lacunar disease are more likely to be stereotyped (e.g., weakness of face, arm, and leg in each attack) and are usually limited to a period of days. In contrast, patients with occlusion of larger arteries, such as the internal carotid artery (ICA) in the neck, may have TIAs during a period of weeks or months. It takes longer for a large vessel (8 to 15 mm in diameter) to occlude than for a small artery (several hundred microns in diameter) to do so. In large artery disease, TIAs may be less stereotyped, with weakness of a hand in one attack and aphasia and facial numbness in another. The larger the vascular territory, the more opportunity there is for variety. In Table 3-6, note that in carotid artery occlusion, the initial TIA most often occurred months before the stroke, whereas the last TIA often preceded the stroke by less than a week. As an artery occludes, TIAs may become more frequent. Thus, a TIA occurring yesterday is much more ominous than a single TIA that occurred 3 months ago, and the recent TIA would demand more urgent evaluation and treatment.

Occasionally, a patient gives a history of transient deficits in different vascular territories. Such a patient was DB, who awakened one night with numbness of his left arm and leg, symptoms that were gone by morning, when he told his wife. Two nights later, while on his way to the

| | **First TIA** | **Last TIA** |
Time	*n*=59	*n*=56*
<1 day	2	16
1 day-1 week	9	25
1 week-1 month	14	7
>1 month	34	8

Table 3-6. TIAs in Patients with Severe Carotid Artery Occlusive Disease

*In three patients, the timing of the last TIA was unknown.

TIA, transient ischemic attack.

From Mohr JP, Caplan LR, Melski JW, et al: The Harvard Cooperative Stroke Registry: A prospective registry. Neurology 1978;28:754-762.

bathroom, he noted weakness and numbness of his right limbs. In the morning, his physician could still document slight weakness of the right hand but noted no other abnormalities on examination. Had this patient confused his left and right sides and mislocalized the initial night symptoms? A week later, the same patient suddenly developed a cold, painful right leg, and investigations confirmed bacterial endocarditis as the source of his multiple embolizations.

In the patient JH, the single TIA provided an important clue in predicting the most probable stroke mechanism. The symptoms involved the left arm and face, making it unlikely that the cause was a local disturbance in these parts of the body. This must have been a transient brain event and one localized to the same side of the brain, probably the same vascular territory as the stroke. A thrombotic event seems the most likely mechanism. TIAs do not usually precede ICH. If the mechanism was cardiac-origin embolism, emboli would have hit the same general target twice in a row, an unusual occurrence. It would help if he were alert enough to tell whether there had been more transient attacks because many attacks in the same territory make cardiac-origin embolism quite unlikely.

A history of past strokes also helps the alert clinician pinpoint a stroke mechanism. A patient with three prior strokes during the past year involving the vertebrobasilar, left carotid, and right carotid artery systems has a high probability of brain embolism. A normotensive patient with several prior ICHs in different loci has a high probability of having a bleeding diathesis or cerebral amyloid angiopathy as the cause of a propensity for ICH. JH had no history of a prior stroke.

Activity at Onset

Traditional teaching states that most thrombotic strokes occur when the circulation is least active and most sluggish (e.g., during the night or during a nap, with the deficit usually noticed on arising). Embolism and hemorrhage, in contrast, would be more likely to occur when the circulation is more active or when blood pressure rises. New data show that most ischemic[44] and hemorrhagic strokes[45] actually occur during the morning hours, especially between 10 AM and noon after the patient has awakened and begun daily activities. Table 3-7 contains data from the MRSR[10] on the frequencies of the various stroke mechanisms in relationship to activity at onset. A significant number of hemorrhages do occur at night, and thrombotic deficits can occur during activity. It is, however, unusual for a thrombotic stroke or a lacune to develop during vigorous physical activity or during sex. A particularly common time for embolism to occur is on arising at night to urinate, the so-called matudinal (morning) embolus. Coughing or a vigorous sneeze can also shake loose an embolic particle, resulting in brain embolism. The onset in JH was during relatively sedentary activities at work.

Early Course of Development of the Deficit

Table 3-8 contains data from the HSR,[7] MRSR,[10] and Lausanne[13] Stroke Registries concerning the temporal course of the neurologic deficit. Often, the early course gives important information about the stroke mechanism. I encourage clinicians to construct "course of illness" graphs that show the temporal pattern of the findings.[1,46] A few examples may serve to illustrate.

> WC, a previously hypertensive man, suddenly became aphasic and hemiplegic while eating lunch with his family. When initially examined in the emergency room, he was mute and had a severe right hemiplegia. Two hours later, he was much improved and could lift his right leg and say a few words. Four hours after the symptoms began, he had returned to normal except for minor weakness of the right hand and arm.

Figure 3-2 illustrates the course of illness in patient WC. The improvement shortly after onset of the deficit argues strongly against an ICH. The deficit, which was maximal at onset and was unassociated with headache, is most compatible

Table 3-7.	Activity at Onset in Subtypes of Stroke (%)					
Activity at Onset	T	Emb	Lac	ICU	ICH	SAH
On arising	40	17	50	31	13	15
Stress	1	5	1	5	10	15
ADL	54	68	47	50	64	64
Unknown	5	10	2	14	13	6

ADL, activities of daily living; Emb, embolism; ICH, intracerebral hemorrhage; ICU, infarct cause unknown; Lac, lacune; SAH, subarachnoid hemorrhage; T, thrombosis.

From Caplan LR, Hier DB, D'Cruz I: Cerebral embolism in the Michael Reese Stroke Registry. Stroke 1983;14:530-536.

Table 3-8.   Early Course of Deficit in Various Registries (%)

	T			Lac			Emb			ICH			SAH	
	HSR	MR SR	LSR	HSR	MR SR	LSR	HSR	MR SR	LSR	HSR	MR SR	LSR	HSR	MR SR
Maximal at onset	40	45	66	38	40	54	79	89	82	34	38	44	80	64
Stepwise/ stutter	34	30		32	28		11	10		3	9		3	14
Gradual, smooth	13	14	27	20	24	40	5	1	13	63	51	52	14	18
Fluctuating	13	11	7	10	8	5	5	0	5	0	2	4	3	4

Emb, embolism; HSR, Harvard Stroke Registry; ICH, intracerebral hemorrhage; Lac, lacune; LSR, Lausanne Stroke Registry; MRSR, Michael Reese Stroke Registry; SAH, subarachnoid hemorrhage; T, thrombosis.

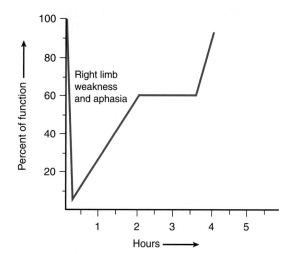

Figure 3-2. Course of illness for patient WC.

with an embolic mechanism. The next patient illustrates a different scenario.

RP was admitted to the hospital, and the intern called to say that RP had developed a gradually progressive hemiplegia throughout the day. On closer questioning, RP related the following account: At 9:30 AM, while eating breakfast, her left hand became clumsy, and she dropped a piece of bread. When she climbed the stairs to go to her room, she noticed a slight limp in her left foot. Worried about her problem, she rested for an hour and was comforted when, on rising, she could walk down the stairs without any difficulty and clear the table without a trace of left-hand awkwardness. Thirty minutes later while sitting on the couch, her left limbs became weak and she could not lift her left arm or leg. Twenty minutes or so after this worsening, her left limb function improved and remained the same until her arrival in the hospital about 3 hours after the first onset of symptoms. When she was seen at the hospital 3 hours after onset, the left limbs were slightly weak.

This course of illness in RP (Fig. 3-3) was typical of a stuttering onset, with improvement in the deficit, followed by worsening and a second improvement. Again, this course would be difficult to understand if the initial deficit had been caused by ICH; the tempo was most compatible with a thrombotic process.

I call the process of eliciting the historical details from RP "walking through" the course of illness with the patient. Most patients have difficulty quantifying their deficits and estimating the course of their illness. When patients are asked to describe their activities, an alert observer can often better gauge the course of development of the deficit. Inspection of these course-of-illness graphs (see Figs. 3-2 and 3-3) helps to predict stroke mechanism. Such a graph (Fig. 3-4) would also aid diagnosis in the following case.

BK was admitted to the hospital with a note that said that she had the sudden onset of left hemiplegia while shopping. A review of the events

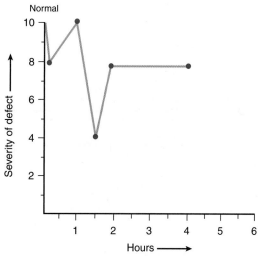

Figure 3-3. Course of illness for patient RP.

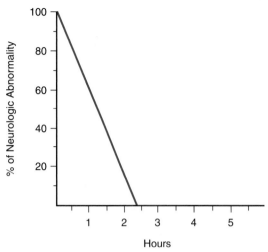

Figure 3-4. Course of illness for patient BK.

mechanisms with the highest probability thus far—atherosclerosis with thrombosis and later embolism and cardiac-origin embolism—each has a tendency to begin abruptly and to have maximal deficit at or near onset. Recall from the discussion in Chapter 2 that when atherosclerotic large artery lesions critically reduce the size of the residual lumen, an occlusive thrombus often develops. Because the thrombus is initially not adherent, portions may break loose and embolize. Sudden, maximal-at-onset deficits in patients with large artery occlusions are presumed to be caused by artery-to-artery embolism from the donor site of thrombosis to a recipient intracranial artery. Thus, the onset and course to date of JH do not help choose between the two mechanisms being considered most strongly, but the preceding TIA in the same vascular territory favors artery-to-artery embolism over cardiac origin embolism.

Accompanying Symptoms

Headache is an invariable symptom of SAH. Sudden release of blood into the subarachnoid space increases intracranial pressure and usually leads to severe headache, vomiting, and a decrease in the level of consciousness. In ICH, the focal deficit usually develops progressively, and only later, when there has been enlargement of the hematoma, do headache, vomiting, and decreased consciousness develop. Loss of consciousness is common in SAH and is rare in ischemic stroke unless the ischemia involves the brainstem bilaterally. Seizures are rare in the early period after stroke onset; their presence argues for embolic stroke or ICH. Table 3-9 lists the frequency of accompanying features by stroke mechanism.

Combining two pieces of information often adds greatly to the accuracy of the probabilities. An example of this is seen in Table 3-10, which analyzes the presence of vomiting for each stroke mechanism in relation to the location of the stroke in the anterior or posterior circulation. Vomiting is

with her sister who accompanied her and a call to the shopkeeper revealed a different story. While the patient was trying on a hat in a store, the shopkeeper had noted a droop of the face and had called for an ambulance, against the patient's wishes. The shopkeeper recalled the patient walking to the next room and gesturing with both hands. When the ambulance arrived 10 minutes later, the patient could walk to the ambulance but had a limp and less swing of the left arm. On arrival at the hospital 30 minutes after onset, she had a severe left hemiplegia, eyes and head were deviated to the right, and she vomited and reported a headache. During the next 2 hours she continued to worsen and became comatose.

The gradual development of a progressive focal deficit, accompanied by gradually developing symptoms of increased intracranial pressure (ICP) suggested ICH, a diagnosis confirmed by computed tomography (CT). In this case, a more detailed account of the early course of illness helped suggest the correct diagnosis.

In patient JH, the onset was abrupt and presumably maximal at onset because he fell with a hemiplegia. Between the two stroke

Table 3-9.	**Frequency of Accompanying Symptoms At or Near Onset by Stroke Subtype (%)**													
	Thrombosis			Lacune			Embolus			ICH			SAH	
	HSR	LSR	SDB	HSR	LSR	SDB	HSR	LSR	SDB	HSR	LSR	SDB	HSR	SDB
Decreased consciousness	15	13	14	20	12	29	3	3	2	39	50	57	68	48
Vomiting	11	—	8	6	—	5	3	—	1	46	—	29	48	45
Seizures	0.3	1	3	4	0	3	0	0	1	7	7	9	7	7
Headache	12	17	11	9	18	10	3	7	5	33	40	41	78	87

HSR, Harvard Stroke Registry; ICH, intracerebral hemorrhage; LSR, Lausanne Stroke Registry; SAH, subarachnoid hemorrhage; SDB, stroke data bank.

Table 3-10.	**Vomiting and Location and Type of Stroke**
Intracerebral hemorrhage	
Anterior circulation	19/29 (48.5%)
Posterior circulation	8/12 (67%)
Thrombosis	
Anterior circulation	3/141 (2%)
Posterior circulation	24/83 (29%)
Embolism	
Anterior circulation	4/198 (2%)
Posterior circulation	6/21 (29%)

From Mohr JP, Caplan LR, Melski JW, et al: The Harvard Cooperative Stroke Registry: A prospective registry. Neurology 1978;28:754-762.

common in posterior circulation strokes, presumably because of involvement of the so-called vomiting center in the floor of the fourth ventricle. Vomiting is rare in ischemic strokes in the anterior circulation, however, whether thrombotic or embolic. In the anterior circulation, ICH was accompanied by vomiting, presumably because of the associated increase in ICP. Thus, vomiting and anterior circulation location usually equals ICH. A patient with a right hemiparesis and aphasia who vomits early during the stroke has a high likelihood of harboring an ICH.

Patient JH denied headache but did have lethargy, qualifying as some decrease in level of consciousness. Decrease in level of consciousness is very rare in lacunar infarction, one subtype of thrombotic stroke. He had not vomited. These features do not, in his case, help differentiate between thrombosis with embolism and cardiogenic embolism.

LOCALIZATION AND DETECTION OF THE VASCULAR LESION

Having pursued the history as thoroughly as possible, the clinician should be ready to perform a general and neurologic examination. While proceeding, the principal aims should be kept in mind. They are (1) to detect vascular and cardiac abnormalities that aid in determining stroke mechanism and localization of vascular lesions and (2) to localize the process within the central nervous system. Once the clinician knows where the lesion is in the brain, knowledge about the anatomy of the vascular supply, the risk factors in the patient, and the results of the vascular examination help the clinician predict the most likely vascular location and process in the patient.

Findings from Heart Examination

The diagnosis of cardiogenic embolism is important because its evaluation and treatment differ from intrinsic disease of the extracranial and intracranial arteries. A careful detailed history of possible cardiac symptoms, angina, myocardial infarction, palpitations or arrhythmia, congestive heart failure, and rheumatic heart disease is as important as the neurologic history. The heart should be examined thoroughly, taking time to estimate size, character, and quality of heart sounds and gallops; listening for murmurs is not enough.

Findings from Vascular System Examination

Examination of the available systemic and extracranial arteries may give clues to the presence of atherosclerosis or diminished flow not detectable by history. Note the pulse for at least a minute, seeking any irregularities. Feel the radial pulses simultaneously, looking for a significant difference in the strength of the pulses or a delay on one side. In all reported examples of subclavian steal, the diminished blood flow to the arm related to subclavian artery occlusive disease produced a definite pulse alteration.[47,48] The radial pulse is smaller and delayed on the ischemic side. If the pulses are equal and synchronous, it is not necessary to check the blood pressures in each arm. Feel the femoral and foot pulses and listen to the femoral region for an arterial bruit. Remember that some patients with a hyperdynamic circulation (e.g., fever, anemia, or hyperthyroidism) have bruits over many peripheral vessels. When a femoral bruit is present, listen over the antecubital and supraclavicular fossas to determine whether bruits are a generalized phenomenon and do not necessarily indicate focal disease.

Next, gently palpate the carotid artery in the neck. Recall that you are feeling the common carotid artery (CCA) until you reach the bifurcation high in the neck. The ICA then proceeds posteriorly and usually cannot be felt; the external carotid artery (ECA) projects slightly forward and laterally and can be traced. The left carotid artery is positioned more posteriorly and deeper, so that the carotid pulses rarely feel equal. Feeling a carotid pulse in the neck tells the examiner that the CCA is patent; it gives no information about the ICA. Even if the proximal ICA is occluded, a pulse can often be seen and felt along the ICA because of propagation of the pulse wave from the CCA. All too often, a bounding carotid pulse is falsely considered evidence against an ICA occlusion. Listening to the carotid artery beginning low in the neck and progressing cranially is important.

The stethoscope used to listen over arteries should have a relatively small diameter bell. Most new stethoscopes (Litman types) have too-large flat bells and diaphragms and are not very suitable for listening to arteries or examining blood vessels in children. The bell of an old-fashioned stethoscope is usually superior to the diaphragm or flat bell of the newer stethoscopes for bruit detection and analysis.

Recall that many nonstenosing processes can cause carotid bruits. The most common of these are transmitted cardiac murmurs, especially aortic stenosis, tortuous vessels, dilated aortas, and hyperdynamic circulatory states. Transmitted heart and aortic murmurs and hyperdynamic states produce bruits usually heard over the entire artery, often loudest at the base of the neck. These bruits are usually low-pitched, relatively short, and are invariably heard best over the supraclavicular fossa, perhaps because of the presence of lung tissue just beneath this region, which better transmits the sound. The auscultatory features of a focal vascular constriction can be compared with that of mitral stenosis because each impedes flow and creates a pressure differential beyond the area of blockage. The bruit caused by local constriction of a carotid or vertebral artery is usually:

1. Focal. The bruit is often loudest at the bifurcation high in the neck and inaudible at the base. Osler said that the murmur of mitral stenosis is often limited to the region of a dime; the same explanation is valid for the focality of a localized region of carotid artery stenosis.
2. Long. It takes longer for blood to course across a constricted vessel; the diastolic murmur of tight mitral stenosis is also long.
3. High-pitched. The blood flow velocity is often increased in regions of arterial stenosis. The increased velocity is associated with a high-pitched sound.

At times, stenosis at the origin of the ECA produces a bruit that can be confused with an ICA-origin lesion. When the lesion is in the ECA, the bruit can sometimes be traced forward toward the area of the facial artery. In addition, blockage of the major ECA branches by finger pressure reduces or obliterates an ECA bruit but does not alter a bruit of ICA origin.[49]

After examining the carotid arteries, listen over the supraclavicular fossa and then follow the course of each vertebral artery (VA), first within the posterior cervical triangle and then up the sternocleidomastoid muscle to the mastoid region. Sometimes, a unilateral vertebral artery bruit is a reflection of augmented flow to compensate for a contralateral VA occlusion; the bruit is then on the "wrong side" for the symptoms.

Clues to the patency of the carotid system arteries can also be obtained by careful palpation of the ECA branches on the face. The most readily palpable arteries in normal individuals are the facial artery along the edge of the lower jaw; the preauricular artery just anterior to the ear; and the superficial temporal artery in the temple region. It is important to feel both sides simultaneously to detect a delay or asymmetry of the pulses. When the ECA or CCA on one side is occluded or severely stenosed, the facial, preauricular, and superficial temporal pulses are diminished on that side, and the regions of supply may feel cool to the touch. When the ICA is occluded before its ophthalmic artery branch, the ECA may supply critical collateral vessels, usually about the orbit.

The augmented flow can often be felt as brisk increased pulsation at the cheek, brow, or inner angle of the eye. Fisher designated these pulses ABC (angular, brow, cheek) for easy recall (Fig. 3-5).[50] At times, the superficial temporal artery provides collateral supply to the supraorbital and supratrochlear branches of the ophthalmic artery feeding the low-pressure, ophthalmic-carotid system.[51] In the normal situation, blood flows from the ICA to the ophthalmic artery to the supraorbital (frontal artery) and supratrochlear branches cephalad up the brow. In the normal situation, obliteration of these arteries at the brow blocks the distal pulse above it. When there is low pressure in the ophthalmic system, flow goes down these vessels from superficial temporal artery collaterals into the orbit. In that circumstance, obliteration of the brow pulse does not block the forehead pulses, but a finger on the forehead pulses stops the pulsation in the brow, a reversal of the usual normal pattern of flow (Fig. 3-6). This finding is called the *frontal artery sign*.[51]

Remember that there is alternative rich collateral circulation at the circle of Willis, especially through the anterior communicating and posterior communicating arteries, which bring collaterals from the opposite cerebral hemisphere and posterior circulation, respectively. Thus, the absence of augmented facial collateral vessels does not mean that the ICA system is not obstructed. On the other hand, the presence of collateral flow through the orbit is diagnostic of a low-pressure, ophthalmic-carotid artery system and so is important clinically. The technique for detecting this is easy to master at the bedside.

Also feel for the occipital artery behind the mastoid process. This branch of the ECA often provides collateral circulation to the distal

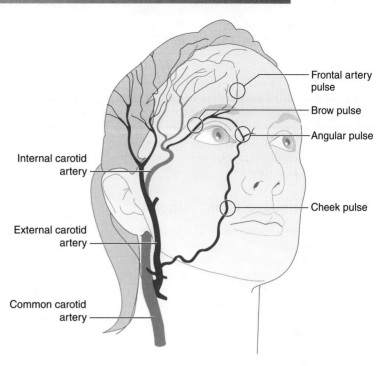

Figure 3-5. *Lateral* view showing internal (ICA) and external (ECA) carotid arteries. ECA branches supply collateral circulation after ICA occlusion. Circles show the areas to palpate the angular, brow, cheek, and frontal artery pulses.

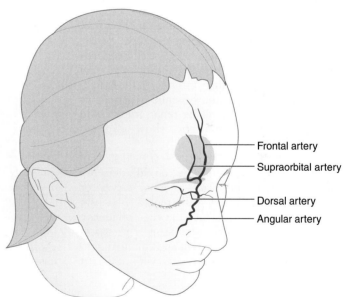

Figure 3-6. Drawing shows the major arterial branches about the eye. The shaded region is supplied by the frontal and supraorbital branches of the ophthalmic artery.

extracranial VA in the neck when the VA is occluded at its origin. A bounding occipital artery pulse on one side provides some evidence of VA occlusive disease.

In temporal arteritis, the superficial temporal and occipital arteries are often tender, nodular, and pulseless. Compression of these arteries in patients who have temporal arteritis often reveals firm arterial walls in contrast to the normal situation. Unless a clinician gains experience by routinely palpating these arteries, they will not be able to recognize pathological changes when they occur.

Be sure to feel the femoral and pedal pulses and to inspect the fingers and toes. Claudication and peripheral vascular occlusive disease highly correlate with atherostenosis of the carotid and VAs in the neck.[7] Cyanosis, coldness, or frank gangrene of digits usually means either embolism from the heart or the aortoiliac region blocking the distal digital arteries or in situ thrombosis of digital arteries owing to a coagulopathy or severe occlusive peripheral vascular disease. Endocarditis is often associated with tender small nodules in the pulp of the fingers and toes.

JH had a normal-sized heart and rhythm. There were no cardiac murmurs. Blood pressure was 130/70 mm Hg. All pulses were palpable, and there were no vascular bruits. The facial pulses were normal and symmetric.

The results of the cardiac and vascular examinations provided no new clues in JH. The absence of a carotid artery bruit and the presence of normal facial pulses do not exclude severe carotid artery disease in the neck but offers no positive evidence for its occurrence.

Findings from Eye Examination

The eyes provide a window into the body's vascular system and can yield clues concerning stroke mechanism. Subhyaloid hemorrhages (Fig. 3-7), large round hemorrhages with a fluid level, represent sudden bleeding below the retina and almost always reflect a sudden change in intracranial pressure. They are often seen in patients with SAH and also occur in acutely developing large ICHs.

The severity of hypertensive retinopathy and arteriosclerotic changes is important to note. In long-standing stenosis of the ICA, the reduced pressure in the ophthalmic artery tributaries may minimize hypertensive changes ipsilateral to the stenosis. The same phenomenon is well known as the Goldblatt phenomenon in experimental renal artery stenosis. The kidney arteries on the side of the ligature are spared the systemic hypertensive effects, whereas the opposite renal arteries and arterioles and systemic arteries show advanced hypertension.

Examination of the retina can also yield signs of embolism, most often from the carotid artery but sometimes from the heart and its valves or the aorta. Some patients with retinal embolism have had attacks of transient monocular blindness, but some give no history of transient or persistent visual loss. The most important and common ophthalmoscopic finding in patients with transient monocular blindness is the presence of embolic particles within retinal arteries. The most common particles seen are cholesterol crystals (Hollenhorst plaques), which are white but may appear bright, often glinting, and yellow-orange in color (Fig. 3-8A and B). These crystals are usually small (10 μm to 250 μm in diameter). They most often lodge at bifurcations of retinal arteries and do not ordinarily block flow. They can move or disappear rapidly, but they may injure the vascular wall leading to sheathing of the artery. Compressing the orbit may cause crystals to move, flip over, or "flash," making them more visible with the ophthalmoscope. Platelet-fibrin emboli ("white clots") are longer gray-white columns that gradually progress through small retinal arteries with distal fragments breaking off as the column moves[52-54] (Fig. 3-9).

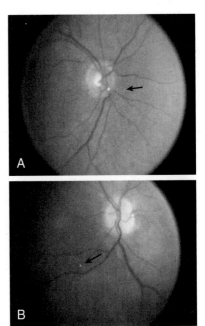

Figure 3-8. Retinal photographs (**A** and **B**) showing cholesterol crystal emboli (*black arrows* point to the emboli).

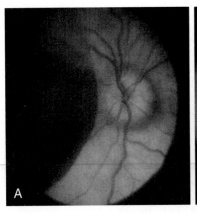 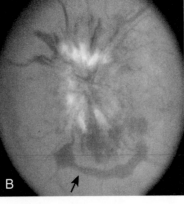

Figure 3-7. Retinal photographs showing subhyaloid hemorrhages. The *left* photograph shows a very large sphere-shaped hemorrhage with a fluid level. The retinal veins are dilated. In the *right* photograph, the subhyaloid hemorrhage (bottom, *black arrow*) is scaphoid in shape. Papilledema and multiple retinal flame-shaped hemorrhages are also present *(black arrow)* in the retina of the left eye. (Courtesy of Kathleen Digre, MD.)

Other embolic materials occasionally seen on ophthalmoscopy are calcium fragments that appear chalky white and usually remain in one location obstructing blood flow, and talc, cornstarch, and other foreign-body emboli in patients who inject intravenously mashed-up pills intended for oral use after dissolving the tablets in water.

In some patients, ophthalmoscopy will show retinal artery occlusions (Fig. 3-10) or branch retinal artery occlusions. Retinal infarcts and focal cotton-wool spots called *cytoid bodies* that represent retinal microinfarcts are often seen. Patients with carotid artery occlusions sometimes develop a condition that has been called venous stasis retinopathy.[55,56] The diagnosis of venous stasis retinopathy is made on the basis of small-blot and dot hemorrhages (especially at the midperiphery of the retina), darkening and dilatation of retinal veins,

disc edema, and retinal edema (Fig. 3-11). These findings provide evidence of low pressure in the ophthalmic-ICA system. In chronic ocular ischemia, the optic disc may be revascularized and the retina show cotton-wool spot infarcts (Fig. 3-12). The iris is also supplied by tributaries of the ophthalmic artery and can reveal ischemic damage in patients with ICA disease.[56] In occasional patients, the pupil on the side of chronic severe ICA disease can be dilated in relation to iris ischemia.[57]

Occlusion of the central retinal vein often produces very dramatic abnormalities on ophthalmoscopy. There are often florid hemorrhages in

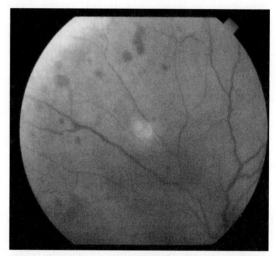

Figure 3-11. Retinal photograph showing peripheral blot hemorrhages and dilated central veins in a patient with venous stasis retinopathy due to a carotid artery occlusion. The optic disc is obscured. (Courtesy of Kathleen Digre, MD.)

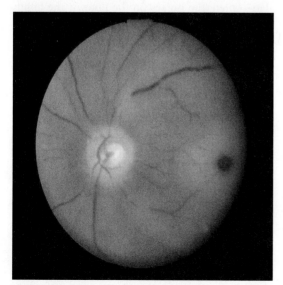

Figure 3-9. Retinal photograph showing a long white, platelet-fibrin plug *(black arrow)* impacted in two arterial branches.

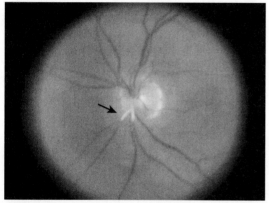

Figure 3-10. Retinal photograph in a patient with a central retinal artery occlusion. Few arteries are seen and the veins are dilated. The retina is pale.

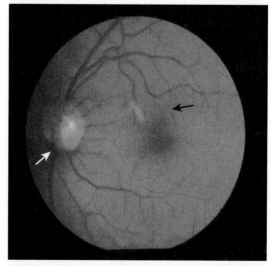

Figure 3-12. Retinal photograph showing neovascularization of the optic disc *(white arrow)* and retina, and a cotton-wool spot retinal infarct *(black arrow)*. (Courtesy of Kathleen Digre, MD.)

the peripapillary region and the retinal veins become dilated and tortuous. Central retinal vein occlusion is often a clue to the presence of a coagulopathy.[58,59]

STROKE LOCALIZATION

Findings from Neurologic Examination

Clinical localization of the brain lesion is primarily from the patient's description of neurologic symptoms and the findings on neurologic examination.[1,60] It would be impossible and probably unprofitable to review here the full details of the neurologic examination. Many non-neurologists feel uncomfortable when confronted with a stroke patient because they feel ill-equipped to detect neurologic signs and to explain them in anatomic detail. Actually, the neurologic findings do not have much impact on the diagnosis of stroke mechanism, although the findings do help with the anatomic location of the lesion. Useful anatomic data for practical diagnosis can, in fact, be summarized rather briefly. Rather than systematically reviewing the examination, I comment here only on important, practical, and useful features. More detailed discussions of the neurologic examination are published elsewhere.[1,60]

I have been impressed that the most important and most frequently missed signs of brain dysfunction involve abnormalities of (1) higher cortical function, (2) level of alertness, (3) the visual and oculomotor systems, and (4) gait. These are parts of the examination most often overlooked by non-neurologists, which provide key clues to anatomic localization.

Bedside Tests of High-Level Cortical Function

Cognitive function testing should always include examination of language function, especially if the patient has symptoms or signs referable to the right limbs or the right visual field. A good screening test is the writing of a brief paragraph describing the stroke or TIA. Alternatively, ask the patient to write a few lines about the town where they live. Asking the patient to read a paragraph from a newspaper or a magazine is also helpful. Ask the patient to name objects in the environment and to repeat spoken language. Remember that there is a large difference between dysarthria (an abnormality of speech articulation and pronunciation) and aphasia (altered content, expression, and understanding of language). If patients are mute and do not write, it is often difficult to be sure whether they are aphasic unless they follow commands or select objects or words from choices in a clearly erroneous manner.

When symptoms or signs of dysfunction are present in the left limbs or visual field, it is especially important to test visual spatial functions and to look for neglect of the left side of space.[1,60-62] Ask the patient to draw a clock or a house and to copy a single two-dimensional figure. Patients with right hemispheral cortical lesions will often omit the left side of their figures and their drawings contain abnormal angles and proportions. Ask the patient to read a brief paragraph or headline or to look at a picture with the examiner. Left neglect is manifested by omitting words, phrases, or people on the left side of the page. Also note how the patient responds to environmental stimuli to the right and left sides.

Memory can also be affected by a focal CNS lesion, usually involving the posterior cerebral artery (PCA) territories. The clinician can test memory by asking patients to recall the material contained in the paragraph they read, a picture they were shown, or details of the paragraph that they wrote earlier. Alternatively, patients may be asked to recall three or more items or a story that they were given to recall later.

Level of Alertness

Decreased level of consciousness is an important sign of increased ICP or lesions of the brainstem reticular activating system or bilateral cerebral hemispheres.[2,63-66] Nonetheless, often there is no comment in the record regarding whether the patient was bright and alert or drowsy or delirious. Does the patient require frequent prodding to stay alert? Often, the nurses on the floor or the family who are with the patient for much of the day can best answer this question. They should always be interrogated about the patient's alertness and the appropriateness of mental performance or deviations from behavior before the stroke.

Visual and Oculomotor Function

Much of the mammalian brain is concerned with visual interpretation and exploration, looking and seeing. Large lesions of the posterior hemispheres may produce only visual dysfunction and may leave speech, movement, and other sensations unscathed. Not to test the visual fields in a stroke patient is a cardinal sin, similar to failing to palpate the abdomen in a patient with unexplained shock. Test the visual fields by presenting a visual stimulus, usually a finger or pin in the peripheral portion of each visual field in each eye, and determine on confrontation when the patient sees it. Also ask the patient to look at something—a picture, a paragraph, or the scene outside the window. Is there consistent omission of objects on one side? Is the individual scanning the materials presented and visual environment normally?

Probably the most common eye movement abnormality in patients with stroke is a conjugate-gaze paralysis. The eyes may be deviated to one side, usually the side of the hemispheral lesion, and both eyes fail to look toward the opposite side. This abnormality usually means a frontal or deep hemispheral lesion in the hemisphere opposite to the gaze palsy[60,66,67] or a lesion in the pontine tegmentum on the same side as the gaze palsy. Nystagmus, a rhythmic oscillation of the eyes on horizontal or vertical gaze, is usually diagnostic of a vertebrobasilar location of the stroke, as are dysconjugate palsies or paralysis of movement of one eye or one eye muscle.

Gait

Some patients with cerebellar lesions have a normal examination when recumbent or seated but cannot walk. These patients are too often discharged from the emergency room only to return later, desperately ill from cerebellar hemorrhage or infarction. Observation of gait also gives a great deal of information about motor function and its symmetry. Is there dragging of one foot, delay in hip flexion on one side, or less arm swing on one side? Are tremors or odd posturing of a limb seen as the patient walks?

Aspects of Motor Function

Having covered the usual omissions, I now turn to an evaluation of the motor system. Be sure to test each limb proximally and distally. In central lesions, the most important weakness is usually in the shoulder abductors, arm extensors, finger extensors and abductors, thigh flexors, leg flexors, and foot and toe dorsiflexors and everters. Check for drift of the outstretched hands. Try to estimate the relative motor strength in face, arms, hands, and legs. In hemiparetic patients, are any of these regions disproportionately affected or preserved? Test coordination of each limb by the finger-nose, toe-object maneuvers. Deep tendon reflexes are of little importance in central lesions during the acute stroke, but it is informative to elicit the Babinski responses.

Somatosensory Functions

In patients with cerebral lesions, higher sensory functions—such as position sense, object recognition, and extinction—are more often affected than elementary pin or touch perception. A useful single screening test is (1) have the patient close the eyes; (2) touch a specific spot on the patient's fingers, hand, or foot; and then (3) direct the patient to touch precisely the same spot with the opposite hand. This test requires no equipment and is an excellent measure of point-position localization, a good reflection of higher sensory tactile function. Of course, at the same time, you are also testing fine touch because if patients cannot feel the touch, they fail the test. Also, with the patient's eyes still closed, touch both arms, both hands, and then both legs simultaneously, to see whether the patient fails to recognize the touch consistently on one side of the body. Again, try to assess the relative sensory involvement in face, arms, hands, and legs for disproportionately severe involvement or sparing.

When you have tabulated in your mind the neurologic abnormalities, step back from the bedside and *think*. Where is the lesion likely to be? If there is more than one possible or probable location, you may consider further bedside testing that could distinguish among these possibilities. Do not leave the bedside before you feel confident in your clinical localization.

Common Localization Patterns

Neurologic signs most often fall into recognizable patterns that predict the likely anatomic localization of the brain lesion. The neurologic symptoms and signs can usually be placed in one of seven general categories. The process is simply one of pattern recognition—that is, matching the patient's clinical deficit with that of patients with known lesions in one of the following regions. In addition, are there expected findings that are absent or unexpected added findings beyond those described among these patterns?

1. Left hemisphere lesion (in the anterior hemisphere in the territory of the ICA and its middle cerebral artery [MCA] and anterior cerebral artery [ACA] tributaries)—Aphasia, right limb weakness, right limb sensory loss, right visual field defect, reduced right conjugate gaze, difficulty reading, writing, and calculating

2. Right hemisphere lesion (in ICA-ACA-MCA distribution)—Neglect of the left visual space, difficulty drawing and copying, left visual field defect, left limb motor weakness, left limb sensory loss, reduced left conjugate gaze, extinction of the left stimulus of two simultaneously given visual or tactile stimuli

3. Left PCA lesion—Right visual field defect, difficulty reading with retained writing ability, difficulty naming colors and objects presented visually, normal repetition of spoken language, numbness and sensory loss in the right limbs

4. Right PCA lesion—Left visual field defect, often with neglect, left limb numbness, and sensory loss

5. Vertebrobasilar territory infarction[68]—Spinning dizziness; diplopia; weakness or numbness of all four limbs or bilateral regions; crossed motor or sensory findings (e.g., numbness or weakness of one side of the face and the opposite side of the body); ataxia; vomiting; headache in the occiput, mastoid, or neck; bilateral blindness or dim vision; on examination, nystagmus or dysconjugate gaze, gait or limb ataxia out of proportion to weakness, recently acquired bilateral weakness or numbness (i.e., one side not due to an old stroke or other defect), crossed signs, bilateral visual-field defects, amnesia

6. Pure motor stroke (internal capsule or basis pontis) or ataxic hemiparesis—Weakness of face, arm, and leg on one side of the body, without abnormalities of higher cortical function, sensory or visual dysfunction, or reduced alertness. Included in this category are patients with mixed weakness and incoordination or ataxia on the same side of the body

7. Pure sensory stroke (thalamus)—Numbness or decreased sensibility of face, arm, and leg on one side of the body, without weakness, incoordination, visual, or higher cortical function abnormalities

In some patients, the findings are quite limited and do not represent the full clinical syndrome. For example, the abnormality may be limited to aphasia, yet this is sufficient to place the patient in the category of left hemisphere anterior circulation disease because no other pattern includes aphasia. Similarly, nystagmus and ataxia are diagnostic of a brainstem or cerebellar process in the category of vertebrobasilar disease. In other patients, the findings are not sufficient to allow definite localization but suggest a number of possibilities. Acute decrease in activity level and motivation are found in patients with caudate nucleus,[69-71] thalamic,[72-74] and frontal lobe infarction.[75,76] Weakness limited to a single limb could fit into a number of these categories depending on other neurologic signs (numbers 1 to 6 in the preceding list).

The neurologic findings also may help predict the stroke mechanism. An example would be a hypertensive patient with pure motor stroke on the right. This lesion is invariably due to a small lacunar infarct in the internal capsule or pons or a small hemorrhage in these areas. A patient with sudden onset of Wernicke-type fluent aphasia without accompanying weakness or motor signs has a left temporal embolus or a small posterior putaminal hemorrhage undercutting the left temporal lobe. We now return to the patient JH who had a different presentation.

JH was very sleepy. He could not cooperate for tests of drawing or copying. He was not aware of his left limb paralysis. He did not notice visual stimuli to his left. His eyes were deviated to the right but moved fully to the left with passive head rotation. There was severe paralysis of the left face, arm, and leg, with virtually no movement to pinch or other stimulation. He did not feel touch on his left limbs and could not reliably tell whether his fingers and toes were moved up or down. Pin and pinch were felt as a general discomfort, which he could not localize. Deep tendon reflexes were reduced on the left, and the left plantar response was extensor.

The neurologic findings in JH clearly localize the process to the right cerebral hemisphere (category 2 above). The severe motor, somatosensory, and vision loss and lack of awareness of the deficit point to a large lesion involving the frontal and paracentral regions. The decreased level of alertness and the involvement of multiple systems (motor, somatosensory, visual) suggest a large area of brain abnormality or a deep lesion involving subcortical structures and the internal capsule. Conjugate eye deviation is especially common in deep lesions.

I now review my hypotheses about stroke mechanisms and localization in JH. The site of brain dysfunction is surely the frontal and central portions of the right cerebral hemisphere. The vascular pathway supplying this region involves blood coming from the heart to the aorta to the right innominate, internal carotid, and middle cerebral arteries. Vascular examination has offered no evidence for disease at any of these locations. The ecology suggests the possibility of large artery occlusive disease, which would be statistically most commonly located at the origin of the ICA in the neck. Atherostenosis of the ICA within the siphon and within the proximal MCA are less likely but possible sites of disease.

Probable stroke mechanisms can be listed, in order of likelihood, as (1) premature atherosclerotic occlusive disease with thrombosis and distal intra-arterial embolization of clot, (2) cardiogenic embolism, and (3) ICH. The clinical findings on neurologic examination exclude the possibility of lacunar infarction. The focality of findings and absence of headache exclude SAH. ICH is possible, given the reduction in alertness and the likelihood of a large, deep hemispheral lesion, but the absence of risk factors (e.g., hypertension, bleeding abnormality, anticoagulation, and drug use) and the presence of a preceding TIA argue strongly against ICH. The absence of any history of cardiac disease and the normal cardiac findings place cardiogenic embolism below thrombosis as a probable stroke mechanism. I am now ready to test and refine these hypotheses by laboratory and imaging investigations, which are discussed in the next chapter.

USING INFORMATION FROM A STROKE REGISTRY OR DATA BANK

Early in the discussion of clinical diagnosis, I introduced the computer so that the clinician could emulate computer logic. I now return to the computer. Suppose that data were available from detailed analyses of patients with stroke. The registry could be the clinician's own data, collected from patients seen at a single institution, or it could be data gleaned by others or pooled from many registries. I have cited information from such databases and registries throughout this chapter.[5-23] Ideally, these registries should include information from each of

the categories discussed so far (i.e., demography, risk factors, past TIAs and strokes, onset and course of the deficit, accompanying symptoms, cardiac and vascular abnormalities on examination, and localization from the clinical and imaging tests). The clinician could then search the registry data for patients with characteristics matching his or her cases. The final diagnosis in these matching cases would help the clinician to estimate more accurately the probability of particular stroke mechanisms and causative vascular lesions in his or her own patients.

I now illustrate the use of such a registry. First is a patient who is agitated and has Wernicke's aphasia as the only abnormality on neurologic examination. Tables 3-11, 3-12, and 3-13 document a search on a patient with Wernicke's aphasia, using data from the HSR.[7] From among all testable patients with information about aphasia (469 patients), 54 had Wernicke's aphasia. The distribution of diagnoses in patients with and without Wernicke's aphasia is tabulated in Table 3-11. The Wernicke's aphasia group differs from patients without Wernicke's aphasia because they include more patients with emboli and ICH and fewer examples of thrombosis. However, there are significant numbers of patients showing all stroke mechanisms, so that this information only suggests probabilities. Next, I think of a way to make the groups more

Table 3-11.	**Diagnosis in Patients with and without Wernicke's Aphasia**				
	Thrombosis	Embolism	Intracerebral Hemorrhage	Subarachnoid Hemorrhage	Total
With Wernicke's aphasia	8 (15%)	35 (65%)	8 (15%)	3 (6%)	54
Without Wernicke's aphasia	222 (53%)	124 (30%)	39 (9%)	30 (7%)	415

From Mohr JP, Caplan LR, Melski JW, et al: The Harvard Cooperative Stroke Registry: A prospective registry. Neurology 1978;28:754-762.

Table 3-12.	**Diagnosis: No Motor Weakness with and without Wernicke's Aphasia**				
	Thrombosis	Embolism	Intracerebral Hemorrhage	Subarachnoid Hemorrhage	Total
With Wernicke's aphasia	0 (0%)	12 (75%)	3 (19%)	1 (6%)	16
Without Wernicke's aphasia	56 (58%)	24 (25%)	2 (2%)	14 (15%)	96

From Mohr JP, Caplan LR, Melski JW, et al: The Harvard Cooperative Stroke Registry: A prospective registry. Neurology 1978;28:754-762.

Table 3-13.   Diagnosis: No Motor Weakness and No Hypertension with and without Wernicke's Aphasia

	Thrombosis	Embolism	Intracerebral Hemorrhage	Subarachnoid Hemorrhage	Total
With Wernicke's aphasia	0 (0%)	5 (100%)	0 (0%)	0 (0%)	5
Without Wernicke's aphasia	16 (41%)	15 (38%)	1 (3%)	7 (18%)	39

From Mohr JP, Caplan LR, Melski JW, et al: The Harvard Cooperative Stroke Registry: A prospective registry. Neurology 1978;28:754-762.

specifically like our patient: This patient had no motor weakness. I search again the group with Wernicke's aphasia but now stipulate the absence of motor weakness, so the findings might be more useful. I then look at patients with Wernicke's aphasia with no motor weakness, comparing patients who have Wernicke's aphasia but no weakness with patients who have no Wernicke's aphasia and no weakness (see Table 3-12). Now the figures are more impressive because the registry does not contain a single example of thrombosis with Wernicke's aphasia and no weakness. There are, however, a significant number of patients with ICH. From these data, the major differential diagnosis using the past experience of the HSR would be embolus versus ICH.

I now think harder and ask whether there is any other factor that could be added that would differentiate these two conditions: This patient had no history of hypertension and was not hypertensive in the hospital. Hypertension is, of course, common in ICH. If no hypertension is added to the list of search criteria (see Table 3-13), only five patients remain who have Wernicke's aphasia, no weakness, and no hypertension, and all had brain embolism. Using the past experience of the HSR, this patient probably has a cerebral embolus. Of course, the odds would be much higher if the number of patients with Wernicke's aphasia, no weakness, and no hypertension were 100 rather than five, but the computer has allowed quick and precise comparison of this patient with the experience of the registry.

References

1. Caplan LR, Hollander J: The Effective Clinical Neurologist, 2nd ed. Boston: Butterworth-Heinemann, 2001.
2. Caplan LR, Kelly JJ: Consultations in Neurology. Toronto: BC Decker, 1988.
3. Bayes T: An essay towards solving a problem in the doctrine of chances. Philos Trans R Soc Lond 1763;53:270-418. Reprinted in Biometrika 1935;45:296-315.
4. Winkler RL: Introduction to Bayesian Inference and Decision. New York: Holt, Rinehart and Winston, 1972.
5. Aring C, Merritt H: Differential diagnosis between cerebral hemorrhage and cerebral thrombosis. Arch Intern Med 1935;56:435-456.
6. Dalsgaard-Nielsen T: Survey of 1000 cases of apoplexia cerebri. Acta Psychiatr Neurol Scand 1955;30:169-185.
7. Mohr JP, Caplan LR, Melski JW, et al: The Harvard Cooperative Stroke Registry: A prospective registry. Neurology 1978;28:754-762.
8. Whisnant J, Fitzgibbons J, Kurland L, et al: Natural history of stroke in Rochester, Minnesota, 1945-1954. Stroke 1971;2:11-22.
9. Matsumoto N, Whisnant J, Kurland L, et al: Natural history of stroke in Rochester, Minnesota, 1955-1969. Stroke 1973;4:20-29.
10. Caplan LR, Hier DB, D'Cruz I: Cerebral embolism in the Michael Reese Stroke Registry. Stroke 1983;14:530-536.
11. Chambers BR, Donnan GA, Bladin PF: Patterns of stroke: An analysis of the first 700 consecutive admissions to the Austin Hospital Stroke Unit. Aust N Z J Med 1983;13:57-64.
12. Foulkes MA, Wolf PA, Price TR, et al: The Stroke Data Bank: Design, methods, and baseline characteristics. Stroke 1988;19:547-554.
13. Bogousslavsky J, Mille GV, Regli F: The Lausanne Stroke Registry: An analysis of 1,000 consecutive patients with first stroke. Stroke 1988;19:1083-1092.
14. Moulin T, Tatu L, Crepin-Leblond T, et al: The Besancon Stroke Registry: An acute stroke registry of 2,500 consecutive patients. Eur Neurol 1997;38(1):10-20.
15. Heuschmann PU, Kolominsky-Rabas PL, Misselwitz B, et al: Predictors of in-hospital mortality and attributable risks of death after ischemic stroke: The German Stroke Registers Study Group. Arch Intern Med 2004;164:1761-1768.
16. Vemmos KN, Takis CE, Georgilis K, et al: The Athens stroke registry: Results of a five-year hospital-based study. Cerebrovasc Dis 2000;10:133-141.

17. Gross CR, Kase CS, Mohr JP, et al: Stroke in south Alabama: Incidence and diagnostic features—A population based study. Stroke 1984;15:249-255.

18. Oxfordshire Community Stroke Project: Incidence of stroke in Oxfordshire: First year's experience of a community stroke registry. BMJ 1983;287:713-717.

19. Bamford J, Sandercock P, Dennis M, et al: A prospective study of acute cerebrovascular disease in the community: The Oxfordshire Community Stroke Project: 1981-1986. J Neurol Neurosurg Psychiatry 1990;53:16-22.

20. Alter M, Sobel E, McCoy RC, et al: Stroke in the Lehigh Valley: Incidence based on a community-wide hospital registry. Neuroepidemiology 1985;4:1-15.

21. Friday G, Lai SM, Alter M, et al: Stroke in the Lehigh Valley: Racial/ethnic difference. Neurology 1989;39:1165-1168.

22. Yip P-K, Jeng JS, Lee T-K, et al: Subtypes of ischemic stroke in hospital-based stroke registry in Taiwan. Stroke 1997;28:2507-2512.

23. Coull BM, Brockschmidt JK, Howard G, et al: Community hospital-based stroke programs in North Carolina, Oregon and New York. IV. Stroke diagnosis and its relation to demographics, risk factors, and clinical status after stroke. Stroke 1990;21:867-873.

24. Gorelick PB, Hier DB, Caplan LR, et al: Headache in acute cerebrovascular disease. Neurology 1986;36:1445-1450.

25. Gorelick PB, Caplan LR, Hier DB, et al: Racial differences in the distribution of anterior circulation occlusive disease. Neurology 1984;34:54-59.

26. Kieffer S, Takeya Y, Resch J, et al: Racial differences in cerebrovascular disease: Angiographic evaluation of Japanese and American populations. AJR Am J Roentgenol 1967;101:94-99.

27. Heyman A, Fields WS, Keating RD: Joint study of extracranial arterial occlusion. VI. Racial differences in hospitalized patients with ischemic stroke. JAMA 1972;222:285-289.

28. Russo LS: Carotid system transient ischemic attacks, clinical, racial, and angiographic correlations. Stroke 1981;12:470-473.

29. Heyden S, Heyman A, Goree J: Nonembolic occlusion of the middle cerebral and carotid arteries: A comparison of predisposing factors. Stroke 1970;1:363-369.

30. Barnett HJM: The International Collaborative Study of Superficial Temporal Artery-Middle Cerebral Artery Anastomosis. In FC Rose (ed): Advances in Stroke Therapy. New York: Raven Press, 1982, pp 179-182.

31. Huang CY, Chan FL, Yu YL, et al: Cerebrovascular disease in Hong Kong Chinese. Stroke 1990;21:230-235.

32. Feldmann E, Daneault N, Kwan E, et al: Chinese–white differences in the distribution of occlusive cerebrovascular disease. Neurology 1990;40:1541-1545.

33. Caplan LR, Gorelick PB, Hier DB: Race, sex, and occlusive vascular disease: A review. Stroke 1986;17:648-655.

34. Caplan LR: Cerebral ischemia and infarction in blacks. Clinical, autopsy, and angiographic studies. In Gillum RF, Gorelick PB, Cooper ES (eds): Stroke in blacks. Basel: Karger, 1999, pp 7-18.

35. Johnston SC, Gress DR, Browner WS, Sidney S: Short-term prognosis after emergency department diagnosis of TIA. JAMA 2000;284:2901-2906.

36. Daffertshofer M, Mielke O, Pullwitt A, et al: Transient ischemic attacks are more than "ministrokes." Stroke 2004;35:2453-2458.

37. Kleindorfer D, Pangos P, Pancoli A, et al: Incidence and short-term prognosis of transient ischemic attack in a population-based study. Stroke 2005;36:720-724.

38. Hill MD, Yiannakoulias N, Jeerakathil T, et al: The high risk of stroke immediately after transient ischemic attack. A population-based study. Neurology 2004;62:2015-2020.

39. Rothwell PM, Warlow CP: Timing of TIAs preceding stroke. Time window for prevention is very short. Neurology 2005;64:817-820.

40. Touze E, Varenne O, Chatellier G, et al: Risk of myocardial infarction and vascular death after transient ischemic attack and ischemic stroke. Stroke 2005;36:2748-2755.

41. Nguyen-Huynh MN, Johnston SC: Transient ischemic attack: A neurologic emergency. Curr Neurol Neurosci Rep 2005;5:13-20.

42. A classification and outline of cerebrovascular diseases: A report by an ad hoc committee established by the Advisory Council for the National Institute of Neurological Diseases and Blindness, Public Health Service. Neurology 1958;8:395-434.

43. Albers GW, Caplan LR, Easton JD, et al: Transient ischemic attack—Proposal for a new definition. N Engl J Med 2002;347:1713-1716.

44. Marler J, Price TR, Clark GL, et al: Morning increase in onset of ischemic stroke. Stroke 1989;20:473-476.

45. Sloan M, Price TR, Foukes MA, et al: Circadian rhythmicity of stroke onset: Intracerebral and subarachnoid hemorrhage. Ann Neurol 1990;28:226-227.

46. Caplan LR: Course-of-illness graphs. Hosp Pract 1985;20:125-136.

47. Baker R, Rosenbaum A, Caplan LR: Subclavian steal syndrome. Contemp Surg 1974;4:96-104.

48. Caplan LR: Posterior circulation disease. Boston: Blackwell Science, 1996.

49. Reed C, Toole J: Clinical technique for identification of external carotid bruits. Neurology 1981;31:744-746.

50. Fisher CM: Facial pulses in internal carotid artery occlusion. Neurology 1970;20:476-478.

51. Caplan LR: The frontal artery sign: A bedside indicator of internal carotid occlusive disease. N Engl J Med 1973;288:1008-1009.

52. Caplan LR: Transient ischemia and brain and ocular infarction. In Albert DM, Jakobiec FA (eds):

Principles and Practice of Opthalmology, vol 4. Philadelphia: WB Saunders, 1994, pp 2653-2669.

53. Wray SH: Visual aspects of extracranial internal carotid artery disease. In Bernstein EF (ed): Amaurosis Fugax. New York, Springer-Verlag, 1988, pp 72-80.

54. Fisher CM: Observations of the fundus oculi in transient monocular blindness. Neurology 1959;9:333-347.

55. Kearns T, Hollenhorst R: Venous stasis retinopathy of occlusive disease of the carotid artery. Mayo Clin Proc 1963;38:304-312.

56. Carter JE: Chronic ocular ischemia and carotid vascular disease. In EF Bernstein (ed): Amaurosis Fugax. New York: Springer, 1988, pp 118-134.

57. Fisher CM: Dilated pupil in carotid occlusion. Trans Am Neurol Assoc 1966;91:230-231.

58. Prisco D, Marcucci R: Retinal vein thrombosis: Risk factors, pathogenesis and therapeutic approach. Pathophysiol Haemost Thromb 2002;32:308-311.

59. Lahey JM, Kearney JJ, Tunc M: Hypercoagulable states and central retinal vein occlusion. Curr Opin Pulm Med 2003;9:385-392.

60. Caplan LR: The neurological examination. In Fisher M, J Bogousslavsky J (eds): Textbook of Neurology. Boston: Butterworth-Heinemann, 1998, pp 3-18.

61. Heir D, Mondlock J, Caplan L: Behavioral deficits after right hemisphere stroke. Neurology 1983;33:337-344.

62. Caplan LR, Bogousslavsky J: Abnormalities of the right cerebral hemisphere. In Bogousslavsky J, Caplan LR(eds): Stroke Syndromes. Cambridge: Cambridge University Press, 1995, pp 162-168.

63. Caplan LR: The patient with reduced consciousness or coma. In Skillman J (ed): Intensive Care. Boston: Little, Brown, 1975, pp 559-567.

64. Plum F, Posner J: Diagnosis of Stupor and Coma, 3rd ed. Philadelphia: Davis, 1980.

65. Young GB, Ropper AH, Bolton CFB: Coma and Impaired Consciousness: A Clinical Perspective. New York: McGraw-Hill, 1998.

66. Fisher CM: The neurologic examination of the comatose patient. Acta Neurol Scand 1969;45(suppl 36):1-56.

67. Mohr J, Rubinstein L, Kase C, et al: Gaze palsy in hemispheral stroke: The NINCDS Stroke Data Bank. Neurology 1984;34:199.

68. Savitz S, Caplan LR: Current concepts: Vertebrobasilar disease. N Engl J Med 2005; 352:2618-2626.

69. Caplan LR, Schmahmann JD, Kase CS, et al: Caudate infarcts. Arch Neurol 1990;47:133-143.

70. Mendez MF, Adams NL, Skoog-Lewandowski K: Neurobehavioral changes associated with caudate lesions. Neurology 1989;39:349-354.

71. Caplan LR: Caudate infarct. In Donnan G, Norrving B, Bamford J, Bogousslavsky J (eds): Subcortical Stroke, 2nd ed. Oxford: Oxford University Press, 2002, pp 209-223.

72. Graff-Radford NR, Eslinger PJ, Damasio AR, et al: Nonhemorrhage infarction of the thalamus: Behavioral, anatomic and physiologic correlates. Neurology 1984;34:14-23.

73. Bogousslavsky J, Regli F, Uske A: Thalamic infarcts: Clinical syndromes, etiology, and prognosis. Neurology 1988;38:837-848.

74. Barth A, Bogousslavsky J, Caplan LR: Thalamic infarcts and hemorrhages. In Donnan G, Norrving B, Bamford J, Bogousslavsky J (eds): Stroke Syndromes, 2nd ed. Cambridge: Cambridge University Press, 2001, pp 461-468.

75. Eslinger PJ, Reichwein RK: Frontal lobe stroke syndromes. In Donnan G, Norrving B, Bamford J, Bogousslavsky J (eds): Stroke Syndromes, 2nd ed. Cambridge: Cambridge University Press, 2001, pp 232-241.

76. Fisher CM: Abulia minor vs agitated behavior. In Clinical Neurosurgery. Baltimore: Williams & Wilkins, 1983, pp 9-31.

Imaging and Laboratory Diagnosis

4

Having reviewed the basic elements on which diagnosis is based and the preliminary diagnostic impressions from the clinical encounter, I now turn to imaging and laboratory testing. These investigations should be planned to test, confirm, and elaborate on the hypotheses of stroke mechanism and anatomic localization generated from the clinical encounter. A shotgun approach to testing is discouraged. Instead, an individualized and eclectic program of tests should be tailored to the individual patient's problems. Whenever possible, tests should be selected and interpreted sequentially. Results of the initial investigations should be used to help determine the next steps in testing.

In this chapter, I consider various tests in relation to the following series of questions, which clinicians should ask sequentially:

1. Is the brain lesion(s) caused by ischemia or hemorrhage, or is it related to a nonvascular stroke mimic?
2. Where is the brain lesion(s)? What is its size, shape, and extent?
3. What are the nature, site, and severity of the vascular lesion(s), and how do the vascular lesion(s) and brain perfusion abnormalities relate to the brain lesion(s)?
4. Are abnormalities of blood constituents causing or contributing to brain ischemia or hemorrhage?
5. Is the patient with stroke or transient neurologic deficits having seizures?

With these questions in mind, I continue to follow JH, the 36-year-old patient with left hemiparesis introduced in Chapter 3, as he proceeds through the diagnostic laboratory tests.

QUESTION 1: IS THE BRAIN LESION CAUSED BY ISCHEMIA OR HEMORRHAGE, OR IS IT RELATED TO A NONVASCULAR STROKE MIMIC?

Computed Tomography

In JH, the most likely stroke mechanism diagnoses after the clinical encounter are large-artery occlusive disease and cardiogenic brain embolism, with

infarction of the frontal and central regions of the right cerebral hemisphere. Hemorrhage from an unusual cause and even nonstroke etiologies are much less likely but possible causes. The next step is a brain-imaging procedure that allows the clinician to distinguish among these possibilities. A CT scan in this patient (Fig. 4-1A) shows a large, hypodense lesion in the right cerebral hemisphere. This clearly identifies the process as ischemic. A nonvascular lesion such as a brain tumor or abscess or demyelinating lesion large enough to cause a hemiplegia should be readily visible on CT. The lesion shown conforms well to the middle cerebral artery (MCA) territory and involves the surface and depth in a triangular configuration quite typical for infarction. CT scans taken at a later time after brain infarction show more clearly demarcated hypodensity and surrounding edema and mass effect if the infarcts are large (see Fig. 4-1B).

CT is readily available in most hospitals and can reliably show intracerebral hemorrhage (ICH). Immediately after the onset of bleeding, intracerebral hematomas are seen on CT as well-circumscribed areas of high density with smooth borders.[1] Sequential scans in some patients have shown continued bleeding with enlargement of the hematomas in later scans. Occasionally, a blood-fluid level is seen within acute hematomas. Edema develops within the first days and is seen as a dark rim around the white hematoma. As absorption of blood proceeds, the white image becomes more irregular and hypodense, and edema subsides. Ring enhancement of the outer dark zone may occur and may remain evident for weeks after the bleeding. In patients with low hematocrits, or those scanned initially weeks after stroke onset, hematomas can appear as solely hypodense lesions.

When the mechanism is ischemic, CT may show infarction as a low-density lesion or may initially remain normal. The signs of infarction on CT scans can be quite subtle in patients who are imaged within several hours of the onset of symptoms.[1-3] Table 4-1 lists the key diagnostic signs. Newer-generation helical CT scanners yield images in a very short time and provide clearer images and are better able to show these early signs than older generation scanners. Viewing the images on a computer with the ability to vary the

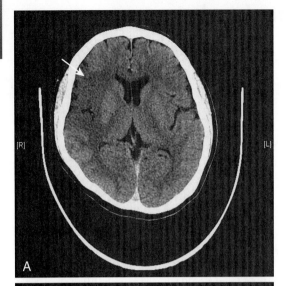

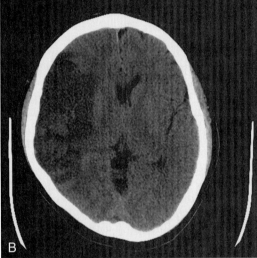

Figure 4-1. Computed tomography nonenhanced scans. (**A**) Recent large infarct *(white arrow)* involving the right middle cerebral-artery territory of the cerebral cortex and underlying white matter. (**B**) Very well-demarcated infarct shown on CT scan taken 36 hours after onset. There is edema surrounding the infarct and mass effect on the ipsilateral lateral ventricle.

Table 4-1.	CT Signs in Patients with Acute Brain Ischemia

Loss of distinction between gray and white matter
Obscuring of basal ganglia density
Loss of definition of the insular cortex
Hypodensity within the infarcted zone
Hyperdense arteries indicating thrombosis or slow flow
Calcific emboli within arteries

contrast also helps identify subtle abnormalities and asymmetries.

Subarachnoid hemorrhage (SAH) is not as reliably diagnosed by CT, especially if the bleeding is minor or has occurred days previously. Increased density is in the cerebrospinal fluid (CSF) adjacent to bone. Visualization depends more on the hematocrit (Hct) in the CSF than on the iron content.[4] Because contrast infusions make this meningeal area bright on CT, SAH is particularly difficult to diagnose if there has not been an unenhanced scan. In those circumstances when SAH is suspected from the clinical findings of headache and restlessness, lumbar puncture (LP) is needed to confirm or exclude SAH.[5,6]

Magnetic Resonance Imaging

MRI shows tomographic sections in multiple planes of proton distribution modified by spin-lattice (T1) and spin-spin (T2) relaxation time.[7,8] Inversion recovery pulse sequences exploit tissue T1 variations to provide contrast, while T2 information is obtained from spin-echo sequences. Ischemia alters water content in the cells (cytotoxic edema), changing their response to a magnetic field. Infarction prolongs the T1 and T2 relaxation constants and appears as a dark, hypointensive image on T1-weighted sequences and as a bright, hyperintensive lesion on T2-weighted films.[7,8] T1-weighted MRI images performed during the first day show infarcts as a loss of gray-white contrast and decreased image intensity (darkness). T2-weighted sequences show hyperintensive bright foci of ischemia. During the next days, lesions become darker on T1-weighted and brighter on T2-weighted images. Increased signal on T2-weighted images may be evident years after the stroke.

MRI is more sensitive than CT in detecting early ischemic changes. Diffusion-weighted images (DWIs)[9-12] and fluid-attenuated inversion recovery (FLAIR)[13] images are especially sensitive for detection of acute brain infarcts. Infarcted areas are shown as bright on DWI and dark on apparent diffusion coefficient (ADC) images. DWI is quite accurate at showing acute infarction even within the first hours after onset of brain ischemia. DWI is effective in both the anterior and posterior circulations.[9-13] Acute, small dot-like white matter, basal ganglionic, and cerebral cortical and cerebellar infarcts are readily shown on DWI images that are not detected on CT scans. The location, pattern, and multiplicity of DWI ischemic lesions can help in suggesting the causative stroke mechanism.[14-16] DWI positivity wanes during the first 7 to 10 days after stroke onset. Lesions seen on DWI images (and confirmed by ADC) usually but not always correspond to areas of infarction. Occasionally these regions or a portion of these DWI+ regions represent reversible ischemia.[17-19] T2-weighted scans show established infarcts as bright. Since DWI images contain some T2 weighting, infarcts that appear bright on T2-weighted images also look bright on DWI images. Care must be taken that the lesions on DWI do not represent the same lesions seen on T2-weighted scans—so-called T2 shine-through. In that circumstance, ADC images do not show a dark region concordant with the DWI+ area and the clinician can conclude that the lesions are not hyperacute.

MRI can also accurately show ICH, especially when echo-planar and gradient-echo susceptibility-weighted images (T2*) are performed.[20-24] These T2*-weighted (susceptibility) images can also show thrombi within intracranial arteries and dural sinuses and veins.[25] The appearances of ICH are quite different from ischemia; they are complex, depend on the duration of time since the bleed, and the choice of MRI technique.[7,8,20-24,26]

Hemoglobin derivatives have paramagnetic effects. The imaging appearance depends on the nature of the compound, oxyhemoglobin, methemoglobin, hemosiderin, or ferritin. The appearance on MRI is also dependent on whether the hemoglobin-derived substances are present inside cells or in the interstitial extracellular spaces. During the first 12 hours after intracerebral bleeding, hematomas contain mostly oxyhemoglobin, which is not paramagnetic. The hematoma appearance during that time reflects mostly protein and water content. On T1-weighted images, the acute hematoma appears as isointense or slightly hypointense (dark), with a surrounding hypointense darker rim. T2-weighted images are often hyperintense (bright), reflecting water content. Between 12 and 48 hours after the onset of hemorrhage, deoxyhemoglobin is formed within extravascular red blood cells (RBCs), especially within the depth of the hematoma. Figure 4-2 shows various MRI sequences of an acute ICH. During the next week, oxidation to methemoglobin occurs, beginning at the periphery of the lesion. By day 5 or 6, T1-weighted images show a central area of bright signal due to short T1, and a darker signal around the hematoma due to edema. On T2-weighted images, the center often becomes dark and is surrounded by bright images. Chronic bleeds contain hemosiderin within macrophages and tissues and show as bright, intense areas on T2-weighted images.[26] Table 4-2 reviews the MRI findings in patients with hematomas at various times after bleeding.

In summary, MRI shows intracerebral hemorrhage less dramatically than CT and requires careful scrutiny of serial images using different acquisition techniques by experienced observers. The presence of mass effects and the location and shape of the lesion can help in the differentiation of hemorrhage from ischemia on MRI. Figure 4-3 show a left thalamic hematoma imaged by CT and MRI.

Patients with SAH are not easy to study by MRI. Restless, ill patients often have difficulty holding still for the time required to produce high-quality images. The relaxation times of blood admixed with CSF approximate the signal from normal brain parenchyma, especially in T1-weighted images. T2 images often do show a bright signal. FLAIR images can often show subarachnoid hemorrhages as a bright signal adjacent to the nulled, low-signal-intensity CSF.[23,27]

Computed Tomography versus Magnetic Resonance Imaging

Brain imaging has become an absolutely integral part of the evaluation of all patients with cerebrovascular disease. Stroke is such a potentially devastating disease that clinicians need all of the objective data available to prognosticate, diagnose, and treat individual stroke patients. CT and MRI are noninvasive and safe, and new-generation scanners produce an enormous amount of clinically useful information. With improvement in technology, MR has, for the most part, replaced CT in most instances. There are, however, still some advantages of CT. I believe that either a CT or an MRI scan should be performed at least once during the course of stroke in each patient. Table 4-3 lists the advantages of CT scanning while Table 4-4 lists the disadvantages.

CT and MRI results depend on the time of the scan in relation to the clinical event. In patients with ischemia, early CT scans are often normal or contain only subtle abnormalities. Contrast enhancement, in my experience, has not been helpful. During the first days after stroke onset, infarcts are usually round or oval and have poorly defined margins. Later, infarcts become more hypodense and dark, and are more wedge-like and circumscribed. Some infarcts that had been hypodense become isodense during weeks 2 and 3 after stroke onset. This so-called fogging effect may obscure the lesion for some time.[1,28] Later, infarcts become hypodense again. Edema also begins to develop within the first days in patients with large infarcts. Edema is manifested by low

4

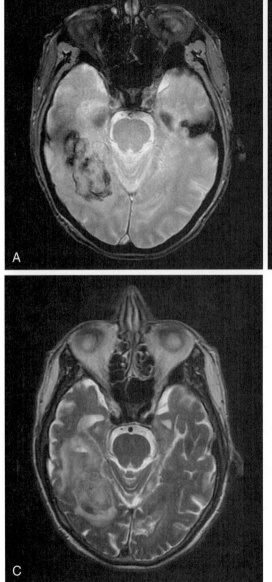

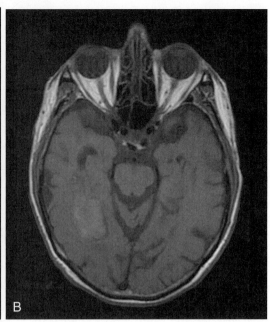

Figure 4-2. MRI scans of a patient with an acute right temporal lobe hemorrhage. (**A**) Gradient-recalled echo (T2*-weighted) scan, (**B**) T1-weighted scan, and (**C**) T2-weighted scan.

Table 4-2.	**Imaging Findings in Patients with Intracerebral Hemorrhage at Various Stages**			
Stage	**CT**	**T2***	**T1**	**T2**
Hyperacute	Bright	Dark	If detectable, dark	If detectable, bright with dark rim
Acute	Bright	Dark	Isodense	Dark
Subacute	Isodense	Dark	Bright	Dark (early) Bright (late)
Chronic	Dark	Dark	Dark	Dark

Note: Dark refers to low signal, and bright to high signal.

Adapted from Bui JD, Caplan LR: Magnetic resonance imaging in intracerebral hemorrhage. Semin Cerebrovasc Dis Stroke 2005;5:172-177.

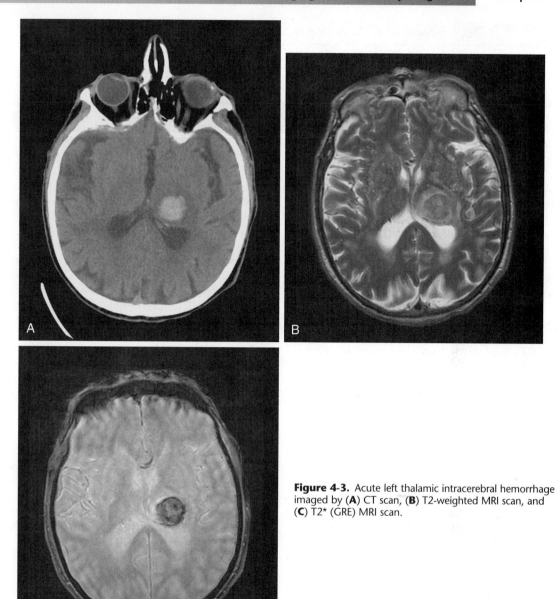

Figure 4-3. Acute left thalamic intracerebral hemorrhage imaged by (**A**) CT scan, (**B**) T2-weighted MRI scan, and (**C**) T2* (GRE) MRI scan.

Table 4-3.   **Advantages of CT Scanning in Stroke Patients**

At present, CT is more readily available. It is generally easier to obtain an acute CT scan in most hospitals than an urgent MRI.

CT is less expensive than MRI.

CT imaging and its interpretation are much less dependent than MRI on selection of technique and filming planes. More experience with CT interpretation makes these scans easier to read by most clinicians who are not stroke neurologists or neuroradiologists.

CT scans of ICH are easier to interpret than MRI scans and, in most circumstances, yield adequate data for clinical decision making without the need for MRI scanning.

CT images subarachnoid blood as well as MRI, and the shorter scanning time of CT is important in restless patients whom you do not want to heavily sedate.

4

Table 4-4. **Disadvantages of CT Scanning in Stroke Patients**

CT is not as sensitive as MRI in detecting and imaging acute brain infarcts.

CT is not accurate in delineating lesions adjacent to bony surfaces (e.g., in the orbital, frontal poles, and temporal lobes). CT is quite inferior to MRI in imaging brainstem and cerebellar infarcts.

CT is mostly a one-plane technique for routine examinations; multiple planes require longer imaging time for reconstruction. MR, by using multiple planes (horizontal, transaxial, coronal, sagittal), shows the three-dimensional location of lesions far better than CT reconstructions.

CT is not useful in detecting and delineating spinal cord infarcts.

density surrounding the lesion and mass effect with displacement of adjacent structures.

FLAIR and diffusion-weighted MRI images show infarcts as bright signals even during the first hours after symptom onset. Despite the fact that a patient clinically has had a transient ischemic attack (TIA) and has no residual symptoms or signs at the time of brain imaging, scans often shows a brain infarct. Nicolaides and colleagues studied 149 patients with hemispheral TIAs and found that 48% had an infarct on CT, most often in the symptomatic hemisphere.[29] MRI is clearly more sensitive than CT in detecting infarcts in patients with TIAs. Inatomi and colleagues studied 129 consecutive TIA patients.[30] The mean time from TIA to MRI was 4.7 plus/minus 2.6 days. Fifty-seven patients (44%) had DWI lesions appropriate to the TIA symptoms. TIA duration of more than 30 minutes and a higher cortical function abnormality during the TIA predicted the presence of DWI lesions.[30] Winbeck et al analyzed signal intensity on DWI and hypodensity on ADC maps to separate TIAs that showed positivity on DWI and strokes.[31] Stroke patients had an increased signal on b-1000 DWI images and a reduced intensity on ADC maps compared with DWI-positive TIA patients.[31]

Lamy and colleagues analyzed how often DWI abnormalities found in TIA patients resolved, and how often they represented brain infarction.[32] They showed that 76% of 59 brain ischemic lesions identified in patients who had clinical transient ischemic attacks represented regions of brain infarction.[32] They confirmed that the TIA-related ADC decrease was moderate when compared to stroke patients, and that ADC values measured in the core of the lesion were quite predictive of long-term brain tissue outcome.[32] Other newer MRI techniques also may help separate transient from persistent ischemia. Bykowski, Latour, and Warach showed that cerebrospinal fluid suppressed DWI imaging and analysis of the concurrent ADC maps helped separate reversible DWI lesions better than standard DWI and ADC images.[33]

When brain infarcts in an appropriate location to explain symptoms are found on DWI in patients who have clinical TIAs, the frequency of recurrent brain ischemia is higher than if no infarcts are shown.[33a,b,c,d] Infarcts on DWI of different ages are particularly indicative of a high risk of recurrent brain ischemia.[33c,d] If the infarcts are in different vascular territories than brain embolism from a central (cardiac or aortic) source is the likely mechanism. When various infarcts of different ages are in the same vascular territory, a proximal large-artery occlusive lesion is likely.

Two other considerations heavily affect the choice of CT versus MR brain imaging—whether the patient is a candidate for thrombolysis, and whether vascular imaging will also be performed acutely. If the patient is a potential candidate for thrombolysis, time is crucial. The availability of emergent CT or MRI will decide which to choose. In the great majority of stroke patients, a study that shows the cervicocranial arteries should be performed concurrent with brain imaging. The need, availability, and feasibility of vascular imaging should also guide the choice of CT versus MRI. Magnetic resonance angiography (MRA) images are readily obtainable at the same time as MRI brain imaging. MRA does not require contrast infusion. Computed tomography angiography (CTA) requires intravenous contrast that can be a problem in patients with allergy to the contrast and in those with abnormal kidney function. Interpretation of the CTA films is aided by software that quickly reformats the images, but if this software is not available, the cross-sections are not easy to read especially if the clinician has not had extensive experience in their interpretation. I believe that all candidates for thrombolysis should have vascular imaging unless the brain image shows a typical hypertensive brain hemorrhage.

In JH, by the time that the patient was seen, 5 hours had elapsed since symptom onset and the severity of his deficit indicated to me that he was unlikely to be a candidate for thrombolysis. MR scanning was not readily available and there were no contraindications to CTA. CT showed the infarct quite well and had indicated without a doubt that the lesion was ischemic. The size of the infarct and the time that had already elapsed indicted that he was not a candidate for thrombolysis.

Lumbar Puncture

Lumbar puncture (LP), introduced into clinical medicine by Quincke in 1891, is still an important diagnostic test. LP is especially important in the diagnosis and management of patients with SAH, and in patients in whom an infectious cause of stroke is suspected. CT and MRI are not particularly sensitive tests for the detection of SAH, especially if bleeding is minor in degree and occurred days before scanning. The accuracy of CT in documenting subarachnoid blood diminishes after 24 hours.[6,34] Large SAHs are often preceded by small warning leaks that are easily overlooked by CT but readily diagnosed by LP. By definition, subarachnoid blood rapidly disseminates and is present in the lumbar theca within minutes. The absence of blood on LP excludes the diagnosis of SAH. When blood is present, the quantity of blood and the pressure of CSF can also be measured and followed by later spinal taps.

Counting the number of erythrocytes in the first and third or fourth tubes of CSF, measurement of the CSF hematocrit, and spectrophotometric analysis of the CSF give an accurate quantitative database. When RBCs lyse, oxyhemoglobin is released into the CSF, reaches a maximum level in approximately 36 hours, and gradually disappears between days 7 and 10.[35-38] Bilirubin is first detectable approximately 10 hours after SAH, reaches a maximum at 48 hours, and persists for approximately 2 to 4 weeks after large hemorrhages. Oxyhemoglobin and methemoglobin are detected at maximal light-absorption peaks at 415 μm on spectrophotometry. The bilirubin peak is approximately 460 μm.[37,38] Sequential LPs with measurement of CSF pressure, quantity of blood, and relative quantities of oxyhemoglobin and bilirubin help to determine the time since the last bleeding and can show evidence of fresh bleeding.

The presence of xanthochromia in the CSF can also be helpful.[37] The CSF collected in a test tube should be spun down quickly in a centrifuge and the supernatant held up against a white piece of paper for comparison to determine if there is a yellowish tint to the fluid. It takes a few hours for the CSF to become xanthochromic after a bleed. A very high CSF protein level can also render the CSF xanthochromic. In the absence of a very high protein content, the presence of xanthochromia indicates that there is a substantial number of RBCs within the subarachnoid space—either due to a subarachnoid hemorrhage or a traumatic spinal tap.

QUESTION 2: WHAT ARE THE NATURE, LOCATION, AND MORPHOLOGY OF THE BRAIN LESION?

The next important questions that the clinician must ask concern the characteristics of the brain lesion found. Where is the lesion? How large is it? What is its extent? What is the effect of the lesion on intracranial structures? Does the location and characteristics of this lesion correlate well with the clinical findings and explain the patient's symptoms and signs? Are there other lesions, and if so, do they have similar or different characteristics from the symptomatic lesion?

Having differentiated ischemia from hemorrhage, the clinician needs to know more about the lesion to predict the most likely stroke mechanism, localize the underlying vessels involved, prognosticate the probable future course, and select optimal treatment. The laboratory answers to the delineation of the morphology of the brain process usually come from neuroimaging with CT or MRI or both. FLAIR and diffusion-weighted MRI scans are especially helpful when patients are tested soon after stroke onset. Tests of brain function, metabolism, and blood flow, such as positron emission tomography (PET), single photon emission CT (SPECT), xenon-enhanced CT (XeCT), can be helpful in localization of the fundamental abnormality in the brain in some patients in whom the results of standard CT and MRI scans are normal or equivocal. Clinicians are fortunate to have available clinical data from the neurologic examination before brain imaging. Having already made hypotheses about lesion localization, clinicians can match these hypotheses with the imaging results. Does the location of the lesion(s) on CT or MRI explain the clinical signs? Could the lesion(s) be asymptomatic, incidental findings not related to the recent event? Are the clinical signs more severe than would be expected from the imaging studies? A discrepancy might indicate that some tissue, although not morphologically damaged enough to show on scans, is not functioning normally. Davalos and colleagues have dubbed this discrepancy a clinical-imaging mismatch.[39]

What if the Lesion Is an Infarct?

Brain ischemia occurs in 80% of stroke patients. In these patients, CT or MRI does not show a hematoma. Hemorrhagic stippling (hemorrhagic infarction) may be present. Lumbar puncture does not show the findings of SAH. Analysis of the neuroimaging findings should allow useful information about the lesion location and morphology. In JH, the lesion shown on CT scan was clearly a brain infarct (see Fig. 4-1).

What Vascular Territory Is Involved?

Identification of the arteries and or veins supplying an area of symptomatic infarction is the first step toward identifying the causative vascular lesion. Ultrasound and vascular imaging tests can then be planned to show the vascular structures involved. Once a plumber has pinpointed a blocked sink, the plumber can examine the water tank, the pump, and the pipes that lead to that blocked region, knowing that mischief must be located within the water delivery system. In 36-year-old JH with left hemiparesis, CT has shown an infarct that involves the deep and superficial territory of the right MCA. Infarction is present above and below the sylvian fissure. The responsible vascular lesion must involve the vascular tree proximal to the origin of the lenticulostriate arteries, which supply the deep territory that is infarcted. These vessels branch from the mainstem of the MCA. The vascular process probably involves the proximal right MCA. Possibilities from viewing only the imaging data include (1) in situ occlusive disease of the right MCA; (2) cardiogenic embolism to the MCA; (3) an intra-arterial embolus from the aorta, right common carotid artery, or right internal carotid artery (ICA); and (4) propagation of clot or embolism from the intracranial portion of the right ICA.

Suppose that the infarct had involved the paramedian frontal lobe cortex in the supply region of the anterior cerebral artery (ACA), in addition to the MCA territory. Clearly, the vascular process would then have had to originate proximal to the ICA intracranial bifurcation into the ACA and MCA. Similarly, within the posterior circulation, the location of infarction yields important clues to the location of the vascular process. In a patient with quadriparesis, MRI shows an infarct in the paramedian basis pontis bilaterally. Careful scrutiny of the films also shows a small infarct in the right cerebellum in the territory of the anterior inferior cerebellar artery, which originates from the lower to midportion of the basilar artery. The lesion must involve the basilar artery proximal to the anterior inferior cerebellar artery branches. The vascular process could be an in situ occlusive lesion within the basilar artery or an embolus to this region arising from the heart, the aorta, the innominate or subclavian arteries, or the cervical or intracranial portion of one of the vertebral arteries. If the cerebellar lesion had involved the posterior inferior cerebellar

artery territory, the clinician would know that the vascular lesion must have affected the intracranial vertebral artery from which the posterior inferior cerebellar artery branches. Knowledge of vascular distribution and supply is essential to localizing the vascular abnormality. Chapter 2 includes diagrams and descriptions of the vascular territories and examples of anterior circulation infarct distributions (see Figs. 2-11 to 2-17, 2-35, and 2-36).

How Large Is the Infarct?

The size of the lesion is helpful in prognosis. Although the severity of the clinical deficit is not always directly proportional to infarct size, larger lesions in the same anatomic area cause more severe deficits than small lesions in the same location. The infarct size, as shown on CT or MRI, should be matched in the clinician's mind with the size of the vascular territory involved. The noninfarcted tissue (entire vascular territory minus the infarct) represents the tissue at risk for further ischemia. To determine the at-risk tissue, the vascular lesion must be known. For example, a small infarct in the territorial supply of a lenticulostriate branch might represent the entire supply of that small penetrating branch. If the vascular lesion were in the MCA proximal to that lenticulostriate branch, a large area of brain tissue would still be at risk for spread of the ischemic damage. Diffusion-weighted and perfusion MRI studies and perfusion CT scanning can give more direct information about the brain tissue at risk for infarction by a given vascular lesion. When the perfusion defect is larger than the diffusion-weighted zone of infarction, the remainder of the brain showing the perfusion deficit is at imminent risk if blood flow to that zone is not improved. Large lesions often exert mass effect and displace normal intracranial contents, especially if edema develops. Large lesions are also more often accompanied by a reduced level of alertness. Mass effect and stupor often dictate treatment strategies aimed at these problems. Large infarcts also represent a relative contraindication for anticoagulant treatment because brain hemorrhages develop much more often in large infarcts than in small ones.

Does the Location and Extent of the Infarct Correlate with the Clinical Findings? Are Other Ischemic Lesions Present?

Clinicians should decide if the lesion found on brain imaging is appropriate to the patient's clinical symptoms and signs. In JH, the right cerebral hemisphere lesion explains quite well his left hemiplegia. A lesion in the left cerebral hemisphere or cerebellum would not have correlated with the clinical findings. In the case of JH, the clinicians could be quite confident that the symptomatic lesion was identified. In some other patients—especially those with TIAs or minor clinical symptoms and signs, and those patients with minor or equivocal brain-imaging findings—it may be more difficult to determine if a brain-imaging lesion relates to the clinical findings. It is also useful to match the extent of the infarct with the severity of the neurologic deficit. When the clinical findings outweigh the brain-imaging lesion, there may be considerable brain tissue that is not functioning normally but is not yet infarcted. This "stunned" brain often retains the ability to return to normal when reperfused.

Many patients have brain infarcts that do not relate to their symptoms. These so-called silent infarcts are common[40]; in these patients, clinical manifestations were absent, minor, or forgotten. The presence of silent and symptomatic infarcts can yield clues as to the mechanism of the present symptomatic infarction. Guilt by association—identification by the company it keeps—is an important, but by no means an infallible, strategy. For example, suppose that a patient is admitted with a pure motor hemiparesis involving his left limbs. CT and MRI do not show a lesion involving the right descending corticospinal system, but five small lacunes in other regions are noted. The likelihood is high that the symptomatic vascular process is also lacunar infarction. Data from the Lausanne Stroke Registry indicates that 62% of recurrent strokes have the same stroke mechanism as the first stroke.[41] If CT or MRI shows multiple scattered cortical infarcts in different vascular territories, then cardiogenic embolism, multiple large-artery occlusive disease, and a hypercoagulable state are the most likely stroke mechanisms.

Are Edema or Mass Effect Present?

Edema can develop around infarcts and may even be potentiated by reperfusion of a blocked artery.[42] Sometimes the zone of actual infarction is quite small, but the surrounding edema zone is large. In young patients, edema may be more threatening than in geriatric patients in whom brain atrophy might allow room for brain expansion. Displacement of midline structures,[43,44] effacement of gyri, encroachment on cisternal spaces, and brainstem displacement can often be judged well on diagnostic-quality CT and MRI scans.

What Is the Age of the Infarct?

There are some general rules for identifying the age of an ischemic lesion. In the beginning of this chapter, I noted some sequential changes that occur in brain infarcts. On CT, well-defined borders, severe hypodensity, and shrinkage of the infarcted brain region all suggest a chronic infarct that is months old. Poor definition from the surrounding brain, edema, mass effect, and contrast enhancement all suggest an acute process. In practice, however, these rules are not often as helpful as clinicians would like them to be. Diffusion-weighted images usually only show bright signal in infarcts that are less than 1 week old. The age of brain infarcts can be estimated by analyzing the lesion characteristics using DWI, apparent diffusion coefficient (ADC), and FLAIR MRI sequences.[33c,44a]

Usually, the history gives the clinician a relatively accurate time of reference. Surprisingly, some acute lesions quickly become well delineated and defined and appear to be older than they actually are. Also, lesions that are months old are not appreciably different on imaging than those that are years old.

What if the Imaging Lesion Represents an Intracerebral Hemorrhage?

Does the Location Provide a Clue as to Etiology of the Hemorrhage?

In Chapter 2, I described and illustrated (Fig. 2-33) the usual loci of hypertensive brain hemorrhages. These are usually deep and are most often located in the lateral ganglionic region, subcortex, thalamus, caudate nucleus, pons, and cerebellum. In a hypertensive patient with a hematoma confined to one of these regions, the likelihood of an etiology other than hypertension is quite low. Angiography in patients with hypertension and deep hematomas has a low yield for showing aneurysms, arteriovenous malformations (AVMs), or other vascular lesions.[45] Hematomas resulting from aneurysms, so-called meningocerebral bleeds, are invariably contiguous to the aneurysms at the brain base or surface. In amyloid angiopathy, hemorrhages are lobar, often multiple, and can be accompanied by small infarcts.[46,47] Anticoagulant-related ICHs are most often lobar or cerebellar, evolve gradually, and enlarge.[48,49] AVMs may be located anywhere in the brain, especially in subependymal locations. Calcifications and heterogeneity within the hematoma raise suspicion of an underlying AVM.

4

How Large Is the Hematoma?

Is there mass effect? By definition, a hematoma represents an extra volume of material in the cranium. Mass effect is more common and more serious in hematomas than in brain infarction. Large size correlates with poor outcome in hematomas at any location. Both mass effect and displacement of adjacent structures are readily analyzed on CT and MRI images. Figure 4-4 is an MRI scan that shows a large ICH with mass effect.

Does the Hematoma Drain into the Cerebrospinal Fluid Pathways?

Is the hemorrhage causing hydrocephalus? Hematomas decompress themselves by draining into the CSF on the surface of the brain and into the ventricular system. In the past, ventricular drainage was considered an ominous sign, but now it is recognized that ventricular drainage is not always bad. The alternative to drainage is an increase in the mass of blood within the brain parenchyma. Nature might have already accomplished decompression of the lesion—a goal that the surgeon hopes to gain by operative drainage.

The mass effect produced by the hematoma and blood within the ventricular system can obstruct the flow of CSF. Blockage of the ventricular system is most common at the foramen of Munro (putaminal bleeds) and at the level of the third (thalamic hemorrhage) and fourth ventricle (cerebellar hemorrhage). Dilatation of

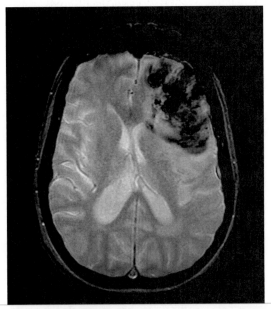

Figure 4-4. T2* (GRE) MRI scan showing a large left frontal hemorrhage with surrounding edema and mass effect.

the ventricular system (hydrocephalus) augments the mass effect of the hematoma and is often amenable to surgical decompression by temporary drainage or permanent shunting of CSF.

What if Imaging Studies Show Subarachnoid Hemorrhage?

Where Is the Blood?

Where is the blood located? Blood may accumulate around a bleeding aneurysm or in the adjacent subarachnoid spaces and cisterns, thus yielding a clue as to the site of bleeding. Blood in the suprasellar cisterns and frontal interhemispheric fissure predicts an anterior communicating artery aneurysm.[50,51] Blood localized predominantly in one sylvian fissure suggests an MCA bifurcation aneurysm on that side.[50,51] Thick blood in the pontine and cerebellopontine angle cisterns predicts a posterior fossa aneurysm. Since the early 1980s, van Gijn and colleagues have identified a pattern of perimesencephalic hemorrhage that does not seem to reflect aneurysmal rupture and has a benign prognosis.[52-54]

How Much Bleeding Has Occurred Generally or Locally?

The thickness of blood on CT or MRI correlates roughly with the degree of bleeding. Figure 4-5A shows a CT scan with thick blood in the subarachnoid cisterns. Figure 4-5B is a CT scan that shows more focal subarachnoid bleeding after trauma. Large subarachnoid bleeds are more often complicated by hydrocephalus and delayed cerebral infarction owing to vasoconstriction than are smaller leaks. Vertical layers of blood clot more than 1 mm thick, or local clots larger than 5 mm in size are often associated with angiographically documented vasoconstriction.[55,56] Repeated LPs, washing away of the blood at the time of aneurysm surgery, and installation of thrombolytic agents such as recombinant tissue plasminogen activator (rt-PA), are strategies that have been used to deal with large subarachnoid bleeds.

In Addition to the Bleeding, Do Regions of Infarction Exist?

SAH is often complicated by vasoconstriction and delayed ischemic damage. Infarction is most often localized to the territory supplied by the artery harboring the aneurysm, but can be located elsewhere. The presence of acute ischemia clearly suggests that vasoconstriction is present. Vasoconstriction can also produce a pattern of

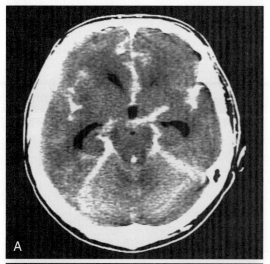

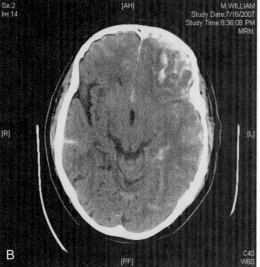

Figure 4-5. CT scans showing subarachnoid blood: (**A**) diffuse white staining of the cisterns and subarachnoid space in a patient with subarachnoid hemorrhage from a ruptured aneurysm, and (**B**) a left frontal contusion after trauma with prominent subarachnoid spread of blood especially seen in the left sulci.

generalized brain ischemia without focal infarction. In brain imaging, this often has the appearance of diffuse brain edema.

Is Hydrocephalus Present?

Blood within the subarachnoid space can diminish the absorptive capability of the arachnoid granulations. Communicating hydrocephalus develops because CSF production exceeds absorption. In Figure 4-5A, the temporal horns of the lateral ventricles are dilated indicating early hydrocephalus. This complication can be managed by repeated LPs to remove CSF or by temporary or permanent CSF drainage or shunting.

What if CT and MRI Show No Acute Brain Lesions?

Normal neuroimaging is common in patients with transient ischemia and early after ischemia develops. FLAIR, diffusion-weighted, and ADC MRI scans are often helpful in those patients who later show infarcts on T2-weighted MRI scans.[9-13,33c,44a] In patients who have only transient ischemia, or persistent ischemia without infarction, the clinical symptoms and signs provide some clues as to localization. EEG, PET, SPECT, and XeCT also help generally to localize the lesion, but they give information about brain electrical and metabolic function and blood flow rather than morphology. Detection of a potentially causative vascular lesion by vascular imaging that corresponds to the clinical localization is very strong evidence that the process is ischemic.

QUESTION 3: WHAT ARE THE NATURE, SITE, AND SEVERITY OF THE VASCULAR LESION(S), AND HOW DO THE VASCULAR LESION(S) AND BRAIN PERFUSION ABNORMALITIES RELATE TO THE BRAIN LESION(S)?

Having localized, characterized, and quantified the process in the brain, the clinician is now ready to identify the vascular lesion(s). The clinical findings and brain imaging results have usually narrowed down the vascular region of interest in the individual stroke patient. In patient JH, it is known that the vascular process must be within the right carotid artery system or lie more proximally in the heart, aorta, or innominate artery.

What if the Stroke Mechanism Is Ischemia?

Ultrasound

Although Christian Doppler discovered the principal idea that underlies ultrasound in 1842, the first clinically applicable devices used to study blood flow were not introduced until the early 1960s. During the 1970s, amplitude modulation and brightness-modulation (B-mode), pulse echo ultrasound were introduced into clinical examinations of the extracranial arteries to detect atherosclerotic changes. The duplex scanner that produced a B-mode image of the extracranial artery being insonated, combined with a pulsed Doppler spectrum analysis, was first introduced in 1979. During the 1980s, duplex scanning became widely used in clinics throughout the world as a means of detecting and quantifying disease of the carotid arteries. Since the early 1980s, major advances in computer technology and electronics have made ultrasound an important tool for identifying occlusive vascular lesions within the neck and basal intracranial cerebral arteries. Ultrasound energy is used to detect interfaces among structures of different densities and to detect moving targets such as RBCs. The ultrasonic information is received through a probe or transducer held over the artery being studied, and the information is converted into electrical energy, either for developing an image or for generating Doppler curves of blood-flow velocity.

Brightness-Modulation Imaging

High-resolution B-mode ultrasound scanning of the neck provides images in several planes of the neck arteries. Figure 4-6 is a B-mode image of a carotid artery plaque. Figure 4-7 shows the usual location of atherosclerotic plaques that develop at the carotid bifurcation in the neck. Figure 4-8 shows transverse sections through various types of carotid artery plaques.

Advances in technology can show these lesions in different planes and allow three-dimensional reconstruction of the arterial lesions (see Fig. 4-7). B-mode scanning is quite accurate at the carotid bifurcation in the neck and at the origin of the vertebral artery (VA) from the subclavian artery. Lesions higher in the neck and more proximally located are technically harder to image well. Figure 4-9 shows a B-mode image of an occluded vertebral artery.

B-mode is quite accurate in assessing the degree of luminal narrowing, in the identification of ulcerations and intraplaque hemorrhages, and for delineating the gross surface-wall characteristics of the carotid arteries.[57,58] When compared with angiography and pathologic study of the arteries at endarterectomy, B-mode generally has good sensitivity and specificity (80%) for detection of significant occlusive lesions.[59-62] Figure 4-10 is a composite B-mode ultrasound image that shows the great potential of the technique for imaging all of the major proximal cervical arteries. However, B-mode performed by itself has limitations. The large size of the ultrasound probe and sharp angulation of the arteries sometimes prevents adequate display of the vessels, especially at the VA origin. Calcifications and clots are not imaged. Soft, irregular, ulcerated plaques and firm, fibrous, or calcified plaques can often be characterized well. Echolucent plaques are usually rich in cholesterol[63] and are susceptible to reduction in size as well as progression. Calcified, hard

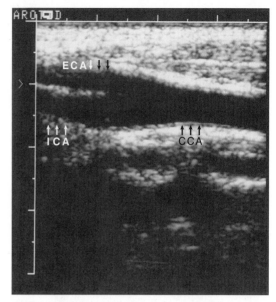

Figure 4-6. B-mode ultrasound of carotid artery bifurcation region. On the left is a small plaque near the origin of the internal carotid artery *(white arrow)*. There is also a thin plaque in the common carotid artery *(black arrows)*. ECA, external carotid artery; ICA, internal carotid artery.

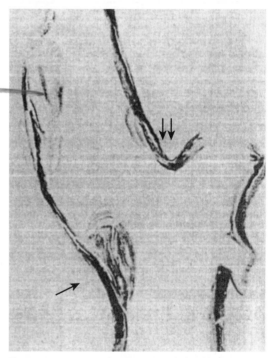

Figure 4-7. Picture of a stained carotid artery specimen: The two *arrows* point to the flow divider between the internal carotid artery on the left and the external carotid artery on the right. The *single arrow* points to a plaque in the characteristic location along the posterior wall of the internal carotid artery opposite the flow divider. (From Hennerici M, Steinke W: Durchblutungsstorungen des Gehirns—neue diagnostische Moglichkeiten. Gütersloh: Verlag Bertelsmann Stiftung, 1987, with permission.)

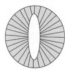

Figure 4-8. Transverse sections through various types of plaques. The plaque on the upper right has had an intramural hemorrhage. (From Hennerici M, Steinke W: Durchblutungsstorungen des Gehirns—neue diagnostische Moglichkeiten. Güterslo h: Verlag Bertelsmann Stiftung, 1987, with permission.)

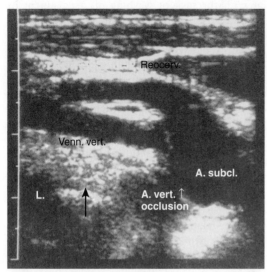

Figure 4-9. B-mode ultrasound figure that shows the subclavian artery on the right and the origin and proximal portion of the right vertebral artery that courses from right to left on the figure. The left vertebral artery is occluded. The vascular structures above the occluded artery are the vertebral vein and the thyrocervical artery. (From LR Caplan: Posterior Circulation Disease: Clinical Findings, Diagnosis, and Management. Reproduced with permission of Blackwell Publishing Ltd.)

echodense plaques in contrast usually do not change much with time.[63] Echolucent plaques with an irregular surface are more likely than echogenic plaques to progress and cause brain infarction.[60,62,64]

Thrombi within the arterial lumen can usually be detected using a combination of the Doppler flow spectra and B-mode ultrasound images. B-mode is quite accurate at separating normal arteries and those with minor plaques from those arteries with severe stenosing lesions (>70% narrowed). More difficult is the separation of arteries with severe pre-occlusive stenosis from those in whom the artery is occluded. Analysis of B-mode images also requires experience and familiarity with the vascular anatomy. Arteries can be misidentified, especially from analyzing only one view. Experience has shown that B-mode imaging is enhanced by the addition of multigated, pulsed-Doppler apparatus. The combined B-mode and Doppler diagnostic systems are called duplex systems. The pulsed-Doppler in this duplex system helps identify the arteries and orientation of B-mode images. The analysis of flow-velocity patterns by Doppler, recorded from different positions within the arterial lumen, provides qualitative

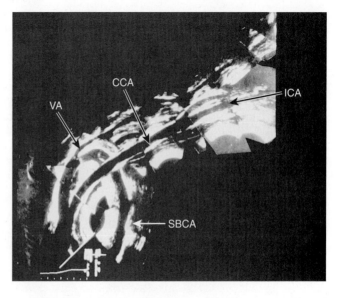

Figure 4-10. Composite B-mode ultrasound image shows the innominate artery and its subclavian, carotid, and vertebral artery branches in the neck. (Courtesy of Burt Eikelboom, MD, and Rob Ackerstaff, MD.) CCA, common carotid artery; ICA, internal carotid artery; SBCA, subclavian artery; VA, vertebral artery. (From Caplan LR: Posterior Circulation Disease: Clinical Findings, Diagnosis, and Management. Reproduced with permission of Blackwell Publishing Ltd.)

and quantitative information about hemodynamic changes. The B-mode images help show the location of the velocity changes. The duplex system offers advantages over either B-mode scanning or Doppler analysis alone. Figure 4-11 shows a duplex scan of a normal VA.

B-mode ultrasound can also be effective in measuring the diameters of the various components of the arterial wall. The intima-media thickness (IMT) can be accurately quantified and followed during sequential ultrasound examinations.[60,62] Thickening of the wall of the carotid artery has been shown to be a marker for systemic atherosclerosis.[60,62,65-67] Finding an increased IMT diameter might stimulate measures to better control atherosclerotic risk factors such as hypertension, smoking, diabetes, and hypercholesterolemia. B-mode imaging can also be performed by using a special probe applied to the posterior pharyngeal wall.[67a,b] This transoral approach is useful in showing the pharyngeal carotid artery and diagnosing and monitoring carotid artery dissections. [67a,b]

Doppler Sonography Systems

CONTINUOUS-WAVE AND PULSED-DOPPLER SYSTEMS

There are two main Doppler systems: continuous-wave (CW) Doppler measures an average velocity for blood moving through an artery or vein beneath the probe; pulsed-Doppler is range gated to measure the velocity of blood in small volumes at specific selected sites within the vessel lumen.[60,62] The CW Doppler device can readily determine mean-flow velocities of the periorbital arteries, the carotid arteries in the neck, and the VAs at their origins and at the cervical region near the skull base (C1 and C2). Moving the Doppler probe along the course of the carotid and

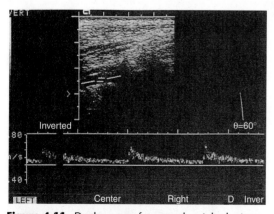

Figure 4-11. Duplex scan of a normal vertebral artery (VA). Top panel shows a brightness modulationof the VA (white lines mark the lumen). Bottom panel shows the Doppler spectrum from this artery.

vertebral arteries allows identification of the bifurcation of the carotid arteries and major changes in audible blood-flow signals. Doppler curves can be analyzed using fast Fourier transform spectral analysis to detect peak frequencies and broadening of the spectrum.[60,68,69]

Figure 4-12 shows Doppler spectra in a patient with carotid artery stenosis in the neck. The severity of stenosis is estimated by the increase in peak systolic frequency, the presence and severity of poststenotic turbulence, and an increase in diastolic blood-flow velocity. Most readers are familiar with the task of washing off a pavement by using a hose. Turning the adjustable end of the hose changes the diameter of the lumen of the nozzle. When the nozzle is tightened, the jet stream of the water is under higher velocity and is more effective in washing the surface. If the nozzle is tightened too much, however, the stream dribbles out or stops altogether. Similarly, in regions of luminal narrowing, blood velocity increases in an inverse proportion to the size of the lumen until a critical reduction in lumen size severely limits flow.

In patients with suspected occlusive disease of the subclavian and innominate arteries, a variety of noninvasive tests can measure blood flow in the arm. The relative velocity of pulsed-wave propagation in the two arms then can be compared. Forearm blood flow can also be studied by oscillography and venous occlusive plethysmography.

COLOR DOPPLER FLOW IMAGING, POWER DOPPLER, AND COMPOUNDED IMAGING

Color Doppler flow imaging (CDFI) improves analysis of arterial plaque surface and configuration. In this technique, the spatial and temporal distribution of color-coded Doppler signals are visualized in real time and displayed as color images superimposed on gray-scale images of the surrounding tissues.[60,68-72] Figure 4-13 shows a CDFI in a patient with near occlusion of an ICA. This technique is especially good for showing changes in blood-flow patterns near small plaques. This technique has an extremely high sensitivity and accuracy for detecting minor, moderate, and severe degrees of carotid artery stenosis.[69-72] CDFI improves evaluation of the extent of carotid artery plaques by the simultaneous two-dimensional display of tissue structure and flow-velocity profile. Real-time images are easier to see and interpret than are curves of velocity. The technology also helps differentiate smooth from irregular surfaces and from ulcerative niches. Severe stenosis cannot always be differentiated from complete occlusion by CDFI.[71] This technique also helps visualization of VA lesions in the neck.

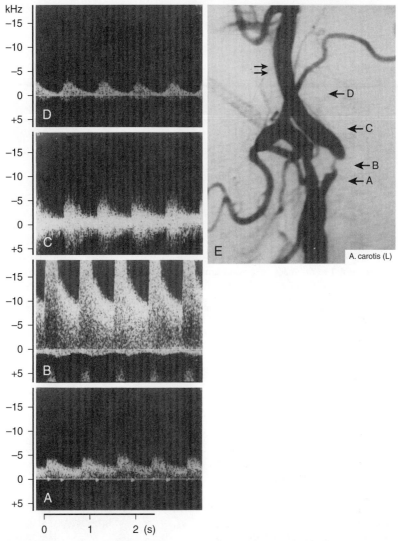

Figure 4-12. Doppler spectra taken from various sites from a patient with the arteriogram shown on the right. At (**A**), the maximal systolic frequency is reduced to 5 kHz; at (**B**), there is increased velocity at the region of stenosis to a maximum of 20 kHz, with an endiastolic velocity of 10 kHz; (**C**) and (**D**) show velocities within the distal artery. The spectra are broadened and show decreased antegrade velocities. (From von Reutern G, Budingen HJ: Ultraschalldiagnostik der hirnversorgenden Arterien. Stuttgart: Georg Thieme Verlag, 1989, with permission.)

Power Doppler is a system based on the display of the integrated power of the Doppler signal obtained from an insonated artery.[60,73,74] This technique is able to remove some of the artifacts and improve some limitations of CDFI. The color display on power Doppler imaging is independent of the angle of insonation. The intravascular surface is better shown using power Doppler. Calcification within plaques can also be visualized with this system. Power Doppler improves the assessment of the severity of carotid artery stenosis and plaque morphology compared with CDFI.[73]

Real-time compounded imaging is a new technique that can enhance visualization and characterization of arterial plaques. The technique uses ultrasound beams that are steered off-axis from the orthogonal beams used in conventional B-mode ultrasound.[57,60] The frames acquired from different angles are then averaged to reduce speckle and improve tissue differentiation. Compound B-mode imaging can suppress edge shadowing and provides better contrast resolution than standard B-mode imaging.[57,60] Plaque motion can also be studied using compound imaging techniques.[74a] Plaque movement in relation to the arterial wall can result in potential "hammering" of the plaque promoting plaque rupture and fissuring and increasing the

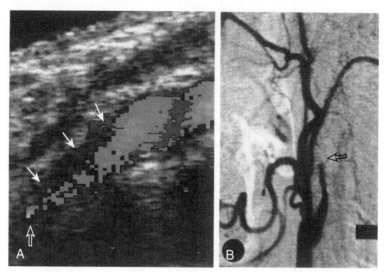

Figure 4-13. An image is shown from a color-flow Dopplar study of an internal carotid artery. **A.** Blood flows from right-to-left. Blood flow in the original image was red and is now displayed in homogenous grey. The lumen is severely narrowed and flow is diminished (*white arrows*) by an extensive atherosclerotic plaque (dark zone above the region of diminished flow). The image in **B** is a cerebral angiogram in the same patient that seems to show a complete occlusion of the artery (*open arrow*).

likelihood of an arterial stenotic lesion becoming symptomatic.[74a]

TRANSCRANIAL DOPPLER ULTRASOUND.

One of the major advances in the field of analysis of vascular lesions has been the introduction of the transcranial Doppler (TCD) system, which permits study of the intracranial arteries. Extracranial ultrasound examinations use pulse frequencies ranging from 3 to 10 MHz. These ultrasound frequencies cannot penetrate bone sufficiently to reflect signals from the intracranial arteries. Aaslid and colleagues showed that signals could be obtained from the MCA and ACA, using a 2-MHz probe directed intracranially from the temporal bone just above the zygomatic arch.[75] Three separate windows are customarily used for probe placement, taking advantage of natural skull foramina or soft-tissue regions.[75-77] The temporal window is used for insonating the MCA and its major branches, the proximal ACA, and the ICA bifurcation as well as the posterior cerebral arteries. A transorbital probe is placed near the eye and is used for studying blood velocities in the ICA siphon and ophthalmic arteries. A suboccipital window through the foramen magnum allows recording of frequencies from the intracranial VAs and the proximal portion of the basilar artery.[78,79] Figure 4-14 shows these ultrasonic windows. From the suboccipital window imaging of the distal VA in the neck and the intracranial VA can be performed (Fig. 4-15).

Early studies using TCD confirmed normal values and techniques and showed that the

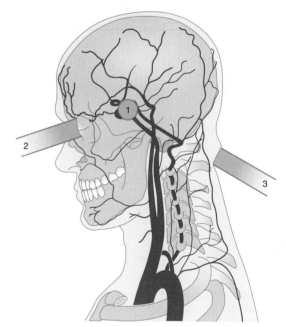

Figure 4-14. Diagram shows locations for transcranial Doppler probes: (**1**) temporal window, (**2**) orbital window, (**3**) suboccipital foramen magnum window. (From von Reutern G, Budingen HJ: Ultraschalldiagnostik der hirnversorgenden Arterien. Stuttgart: Georg Thieme Verlag, 1989, with permission.)

technology was useful in detecting severe stenosis or occlusion of basal cerebral arteries, and for yielding information about the impact of extracranial occlusive disease on flow in intracranial arteries.[78-85] A microprocessor-controlled, directional

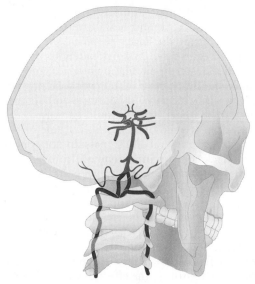

Figure 4-15. The suboccipital window is shown along with the location of the distal vertebral arteries in the neck and the intracranial vertebral and basilar arteries. (Adapted from von Reutern G, Budingen HJ: Ultraschalldiagnostik der hirnversorgenden Arterien. Stuttgart: Georg Thieme Verlag, 1989.)

pulsed-wave adjustable probe is placed at one of the windows and moved until maximal signals are obtained; velocities are then recorded at different depths along the arteries. The introduction of three-dimensional display vascular maps helps orient the insonation to the location of the artery being studied. Specially designed helmets and headbands can be used to hold the probes in place, facilitating monitoring of arteries over time. These improvements allowed the introduction of duplex scanning of intracranial arteries. Power Doppler technology has also been applied to transcranial duplex scanning.[74,86,87] B-mode images of the intra-

cranial arteries can be produced and color coded scans can be obtained from intracranial arteries during transcranial sonography.[70,86,87] Solutions that contain microbubbles can be injected intravenously to obtain contrast-enhancement of the transcranial ultrasound signals. In European countries, the commonest ultrasound contrast agent used is the galactose-palmitic, acid-based agent called "levovist."[86] Contrast enhancement improves the diagnostic capability of transcranial ultrasound scans.[86-90] Newer ultrasonic contrast-enhancing agents are being investigated.[91] Unfortunately, until now microbubble contrast enhancers have not been approved for use in the United States. Interpretation of the results of TCD depends on integrating information from extracranial and transcranial ultrasound and from study of all of the major intracranial arteries at various depths.

TCD has improved the ability of clinicians to study stroke patients at the bedside.[91a] TCD can accurately detect important atherostenotic lesions within the major basal cerebral arteries-the intracranial ICAs, MCAs, intracranial vertebral arteries, and the proximal and middle portions of the basilar artery.[76-78,83-85,91a,b,c] TCD is also helpful in showing the hemodynamic effects of extracranial occlusive lesions on velocities in the intracranial branches. The combination of continuous-wave Doppler, color-flow Doppler, and TCD is effective in screening for major occlusive lesions within the extracranial and intracranial arteries within the posterior circulation as well as in the anterior circulation.[70,92,93] Vascular narrowing due to vasoconstriction and augmented flow through collateral channels and through AVMs all increase blood-flow velocity. TCD can be used to monitor vasoconstriction in patients with SAH.[68,86,94,95] Figure 4-16 shows TCD velocity curves in a patient with an intracranial VA stenosis.

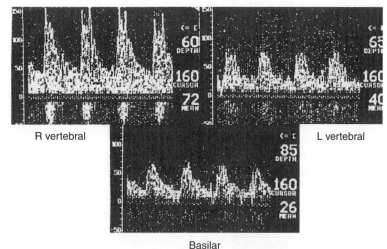

R vertebral   L vertebral

Basilar

Figure 4-16. Transcranial Doppler spectra: The velocities in the right intracranial vertebral artery (VA) are much higher than in the left VA and the basilar artery. Arteriography showed a region of severe stenosis in the intracranial right VA.

4

TCD is also useful in studying collateral circulation in patients with large-artery occlusive lesions. In patients with carotid territory occlusions, blood flow to the ischemic hemisphere through the posterior communicating artery from the vertebrobasilar arterial system and from the contralateral cerebral hemisphere through the anterior communicating artery can be analyzed and quantified.[96-98] Reserve capacity for augmenting blood flow in patients with arterial occlusions can also be studied using TCD and vasodilator stimuli.[99-101] The most common techniques involve either injection of acetazolamide or inhalation of a gas mixture containing CO_2. These promote vasodilatation in normal arteries. Blood flow velocities are monitored using TCD. In normal patients and those with good "vasomotor reactivity," cerebral blood flow increases. When collateral vessels are already maximally dilated, they fail to further augment flow when acetazolamide is injected or when their pCO_2 level is increased. Reduced cerebrovascular reserve capability has been correlated with an increased stroke risk in patients with severe occlusive carotid artery disease.[102] The reduced blood flow reserve capacity reflects a tenuous circulation which is at risk if further vascular stenosis or occlusion develops.

EMBOLUS DETECTION AND MONITORING USING TCD

So far I have discussed the ability of TCD techniques to analyze the presence of arterial occlusions and the effect of occlusions on blood flow. The other very important capability of TCD relates to its use in patients suspected of having brain embolism. Emboli of all kinds can be detected as sudden alterations in flow, with characteristic sound signals.[77,91a,103-109] In this technique TCD probes are positioned over brain arteries, most often the middle and posterior cerebral arteries on each side. When particles pass through the arteries being monitored, they produce an audible chirping noise and high-intensity transient signals (HITS) visible on an oscilloscope. Figure 4-17 shows a microembolic signal (HIT).

The signal characteristics depend on the nature of the particles (gas, thrombus, calcium, cholesterol crystal, etc.), particle size, and particle transit time. Monitoring probes can be placed on the neck and brain arteries. Emboli that arise from the heart or aorta should go equally to each side, proportionately to the anterior and posterior circulation arteries, and the signals should appear in the neck before appearing intracranially. In contrast, emboli that originate in a neck artery should go only to the intracranial arterial branches on the side of the donor artery and embolic signals do not appear in the neck. For example, emboli from the left internal carotid artery (ICA) generate embolic signals detectable in the left middle cerebral artery and not in the neck, posterior cerebral or right-sided arteries. This technique now allows better identification of the nature of embolic materials and their sources and also allows some quantification of the emboli load and a means of monitoring the effect of various therapies on lessening that load.

Emboli monitoring can serve several functions. In patients with TIAs or acute strokes, monitoring might suggest the source of emboli and the quantity of microembolic signals. Monitoring is also useful in patients with known sources of emboli in the heart, aorta, or large arteries. The presence of microemboli in patients with known cardiac lesions may help predict the risk of embolic stroke and also be useful in assessing the effectiveness of various prophylactic regimens in reducing the microembolic load.[106] Monitoring is also helpful in patients with carotid artery disease in the neck.[110,111] Microemboli in patients with severe carotid occlusive disease are often detected after TIAs and minor strokes. The microembolus load decreases soon after carotid occlusion. TCD embolus detection is also useful in patients with known intracranial arterial occlusive disease.[112-114] Long-term ambulatory monitoring is also possible.[115] TCD monitoring has also been used during procedures such as cardiac surgery, carotid artery surgery, and carotid artery stenting. Emboli monitoring is discussed again in the chapter on brain embolism.

TCD can also be used to detect potential right-to-left circulatory system shunts and paradoxical embolism.[77,116-121,121a] Bubbles are injected into an arm vein while the TCD probe is held over a temporal window. In patients without cardiac shunts,

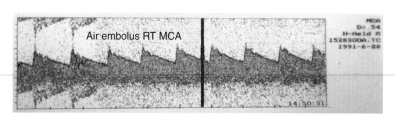

Figure 4-17. Transcranial Doppler ultrasound monitoring of a middle cerebral artery showing a high intensity transient signal (sharp spike) representing a microembolus.

no change is noted over the probe. In the presence of cardiac defects with shunting or pulmonary arteriovenous shunts, air emboli are heard and can be recorded. Figure 4-18 shows air microembolic signals in an MCA during testing for a venous to arterial circulatory shunt. Table 4-5 includes the suggested protocol and reporting.

> In patient JH, ultrasound examinations were quite helpful. Duplex scanning of the ICAs in the neck suggested an occlusion of the right ICA at its origin. The left ICA had only minor disease. TCD showed an inability to detect blood flow in the right MCA. Collateral flow was detected through the right ACA and posterior communicating-cerebral artery (PCA). There was also some damping of flow in the ICA siphon, presumably due to the proximal ICA obstruction in the neck. The left MCA showed normal velocities.

TCD of Cranial Venous Structures

TCD technology has also occasionally been used to study cerebral veins and dural sinuses.[122-126] The major problem is visualizing the location of the veins. Some venous structures such as the superior sagittal sinus are far away from the usual insonating windows. Power-based and color-coded duplex sonography have been most effective in showing the major veins and dural sinuses especially after bubble ultrasound contrast injections.[122] In normal individuals, the deep cerebral veins especially the basal vein of Rosenthal and the vein of Galen can usually be visualized.[123] The dural sinuses are more difficult to image. The straight sinus and transverse sinus can be imaged in more than 50% of individuals but sagittal sinus visualization is poor. Dural sinus occlusion can be suspected by failure to visualize a sinus,[124] by reversal of normal flow direction in a draining vein, and by increased blood flow velocities in the venous structures.[122-126] The patency of the jugular veins can also be assessed. To date, Doppler sonography is probably not an effective screening technique for diagnosis of cerebral venous thrombosis, but may prove useful as a bedside noninvasive method of following changes in the venous

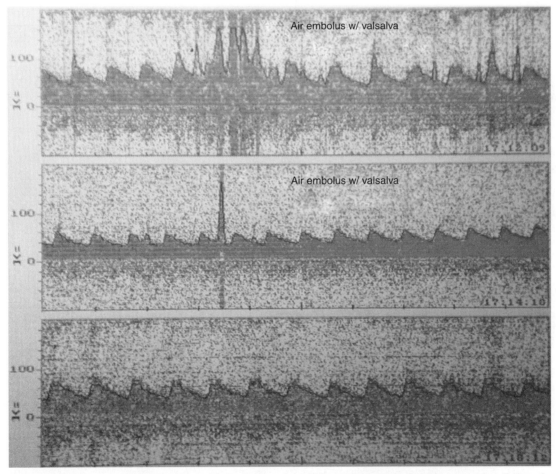

Figure 4-18. Transcranial Doppler ultrasound monitoring of a middle cerebral artery after intravenous installation of air in a patient with a patent foramen ovale.

Table 4-5.   Protocol for TCD Detection and Reporting of Right-to-Left Circulatory Shunts

Performance

1. The patient is in supine position, and an 18-gauge needle is inserted into a cubital vein.
2. A three-way stop-cock connector with two 10-mL syringes is connected to IV access.
3. 9 mL of isotonic (preferably bacteriostatic) saline is forcefully mixed with 1 mL of air.
4. Less than 1 mL of patient blood may be suctioned into syringe for better bubble formation with agitation.
5. At least one MCA is monitored with TCD.
6. The first bolus injection of agitated saline is made with the patient breathing normally.
7. A second bolus injection of similarly prepared agitated saline is made with 10-second Valsalva maneuver initiated 5 seconds after beginning of saline injection.
8. If negative, TCD monitoring is extended up to 1 minute in order to detect potentially late-arriving bubbles suggesting a pulmonary arteriovenous shunt.

Interpretation

1. At times, a so-called curtain of almost continuous signals develops. A four-level categorization is proposed by the International Consensus criteria.[121]
2. No microembolic signals were detected (negative "bubble" test).
3. 1 to 10 MES detected (positive "bubble" test).
4. >10 MES detected with no curtain.
5. A curtain indicates the presence of a large and functional shunt.

From Molina CA, Alexandrov AV: Transcranial Doppler ultrasound. In Caplan LR, Manning WJ (eds): Brain Embolism. New York: Informa Healthcare, 2006, pp 113-128, with permission.

system in patients with venous thrombosis identified by MR venography, CT venography, or catheter cerebral angiography.

Computed Tomography and Magnetic Resonance Imaging

Some information about the neck and brain vessels can often be gleaned from careful scrutiny of CT and MRI scans, especially after contrast enhancement. On plain CT, an acutely thrombosed artery can sometimes be seen as a hyperdense image that has the shape and distribution of an artery or vein.[127] The MCA is the most frequently involved artery.[127-129] Sometimes the intracranial ICA and both the anterior cerebral and middle cerebral artery branches are hyperdense, indicating a top-of-the-carotid-artery occlusion. The hyperdense MCA sign (Fig. 4-19) is virtually diagnostic of the presence of a clot within the MCA. Occasionally, the basilar artery and the PCAs can show similar hyperdensity on unenhanced scans indicating thromboembolic occlusion of these arteries. Calcific particle emboli arising from calcific material in heart valves or a calcified atherostenotic plaque can also sometimes be identified within brain arteries on plain CT scans. Figure 4-20 shows a calcific embolus in an intracranial ICA shown on a CT scan.

Occasionally an intracranial artery can image as a dark linear hypodense structure indicating fat embolism to that artery.[130] Contrast enhancement

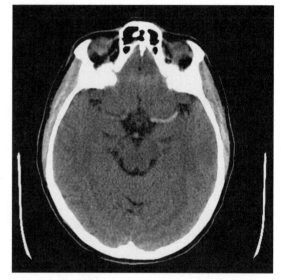

Figure 4-19. CT scan showing a very prominent hyperdense left middle cerebral artery. A cerebral angiogram showed a completely occluded middle cerebral artery and a long thrombus was later extracted from this vessel.

can show large berry aneurysms and dolichoectatic fusiform aneurysms; absence of opacification of an artery can indicate the high probability of occlusion of that vessel. CT can also suggest dural sinus thrombosis by showing thrombosed serpiginous cortical veins, the superior sagittal, or other sinuses as high-density clots on plain CT scans. After contrast enhancement, CT may show a filling defect, representing a clot within the sagittal

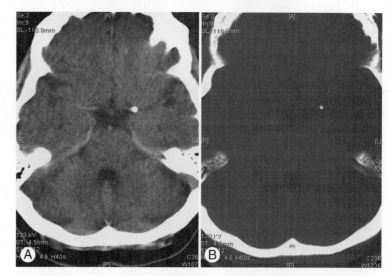

Figure 4-20. (A) CT scan with contrast shows a bright white calcium particle in the right internal carotid artery. **(B)** A bone density film showing that the particle has the same density as bone. (Courtesy of Steven Tanabe, MD, New England Medical Center, Boston.)

sinus, the so-called empty delta sign. Serial cross-sectional CT images of the neck after contrast infusion can also yield information about carotid artery plaques, occlusions, and plaque hemorrhages. High-resolution spiral CT scanning has begun to show plaque characteristics in patients with atherosclerotic lesions in neck arteries.[131] CT of the neck can also show spontaneous and traumatic arterial dissections.

High-resolution MRI is now being used in some centers to characterize atherosclerotic plaques. First used in the heart to show vulnerable coronary artery plaques,[132] the technology has now been explored in imaging atherosclerotic carotid arteries in the neck.[133-137b] Using a surface coil, and high-resolution 1.5-tesla MR scanners, the fibrous caps of atherosclerotic plaques image as a low signal band just outside of the lumen. Rupture of a region within the fibrous cap can also sometimes be imaged. Intraplaque hemorrhages show high signal intensities indicating the presence of a complicated plaque. Researchers are exploring the use of fibrin-specific contrast agents for imaging thrombi within neck arteries; this technique has already been applied to the coronary arteries with success.[138,139] Cross-section views of arterial dissections often show intramural hematomas and luminal encroachment. Fat-saturated images show dissections best. The characteristic finding is a dark small circular or elliptical-shaped flow void representing the compressed lumen surrounded by a bright hyperintense crescent or donut-shaped zone that represents bleeding within the wall of the artery. Figure 4-21 shows a vertebral artery dissection confirmed by MRI.

Flow within brain arteries can also be studied with MRI. Vessels with high-velocity flow appear

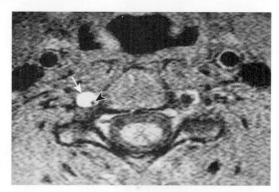

Figure 4-21. MRI with fat-saturation technique showing a dissection within the vertebral artery on the left of the picture *(white arrow)*. The black flow voids in the contralateral vertebral artery and the carotid arteries are well seen in contrast to the tiny flow void in the dissected artery.

black (signal void) on MRI images, whereas arteries with slower flow may show as white hyperintensities. Occlusions can be inferred when a flow void is not seen on images that show cross-section views of arteries. Aneurysms and dissections can also frequently be identified and followed by MRI scanning. High-resolution MRI scanning has also recently been used to characterize intracranial arterial plaques. MRI performed using a 1.5-tesla scanner, eight-channel brain array coils, and a multicontrast imaging technique can show plaques within intracranial arteries.[140] Plaques within the basilar[141] and middle cerebral arteries[142,143] have been imaged using this technique. Figure 4-22 shows a cross-section image of a stenosing plaque in a middle cerebral artery obtained by this MRI technique.

T2*-weighted (also called susceptibility) images can show thrombi within intracranial arteries and veins. Gradient echo images that contain dark

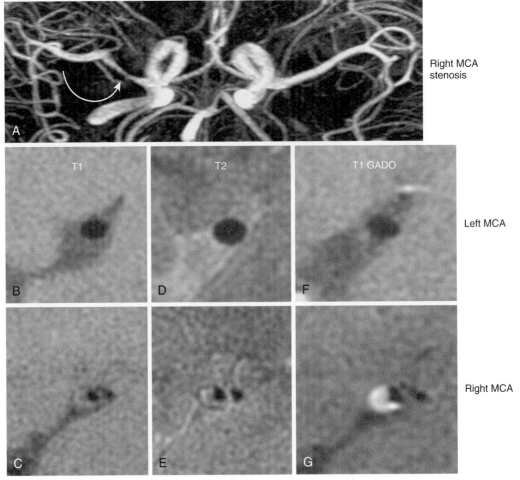

Figure 4-22. The image above shows a stenosis in the middle cerebral artery on the left of the picture *(arrow)*. The images below are cross-sections through the normal middle cerebral artery *(top* images) and the stenosed middle cerebral artery *(lower* images). (Courtesy of Isabelle Klein, MD, Phillippa Lavallee, MD, and Pierre Amarenco, MD, Bichat Hospital, Paris, France.)

hypodense regions that take the shape of intracranial arteries are the MR equivalent of the hyperdense MCA sign seen on CT brain imaging.[144-149] This finding is most common after cardiac and intra-arterial embolic stroke but also may occur in thrombosis engrafted upon intrinsic atherostenotic intracranial lesions. Diffusion-weighted MR images can also show thrombi within veins as hyperdense regions.[150,151]

Enhancement of arteries can be seen after intravenous injection of gadopentetate dimeglumine-diethylenetriaminepenta-acetic acid in patients with brain ischemia and infarction.[152,153] Enhancement best correlates with slow flow and is often found in collateral arteries in patients with brain infarction and proximal vascular occlusions. Fluid-attenuated inversion recovery (FLAIR) images after gadolinium may show delayed enhancement of cerebrospinal fluid spaces especially on the side of brain infarction. This finding indicates breakdown

in the blood-brain barrier and was termed hyperintense acute reperfusion marker (HARM) by Warach and colleagues.[154-156] HARM indicates a high risk of hemorrhagic transformation, increased brain edema, and poor outcome after reperfusion. Another MRI technique, referred to as T2*-permeability imaging can also be used to predict the likelihood of hemorrhagic complications after brain infarction especially after thrombolysis.[156a]

Magnetic Resonance Angiography

MRA offers many advantages over other noninvasive methods of vascular imaging. MRA films can be acquired with and immediately after MRI. MRA examinations are noninvasive and quite safe. High-quality MRAs of the extracranial and intracranial arteries can be achieved by using gradient-echo techniques and short echo times.[157-160] In some scanners, not all of the neck and intracranial arteries can be imaged at the same time. The arch and extracranial arteries require a different technique and different views than the intracranial arteries. Knowledge of the likely location of the vascular lesions helps the examiner focus on particular regions, improving the yield of the examination. Veins can also be studied; the imaging of veins is referred to as MR venography. MRA can be performed using a variety of different techniques, including two-dimensional and three-dimensional time-of-flight and phase-contrast imaging.[158]

MRA is a functional process that creates an image of flow in blood vessels. Unlike standard contrast injection angiograms, the images do not show anatomy. When flow is reduced in an artery, the vessel may appear narrowed or absent even when the artery is normal by contrast angiography; for example, when both intracranial vertebral arteries are severely stenosed or occluded, the basilar artery may not opacify and yet be widely patent. In some patients with severe dolichoectasia, MRA may fail to image the artery because to and fro flow cancel each other and there is insufficient antegrade flow to provide opacity in the artery. At times, contrast infusion of Gadolinium solutions are needed to obtain better images of the arterial circulation.[161-163] To obtain diagnostic-quality images, patients must be cooperative and be able to hold still during the examinations. Patient positioning is critical.

Within the anterior circulation, the ICA origins are usually well visualized, but at times MRA overestimates the severity of luminal narrowing.[164,165] MRA is quite accurate in patients with complete ICA occlusions and has similar sensitivity and specificity to duplex ultrasound in screening for the presence of severe ICA stenotic lesions.[164] Gadolinium enhancement often improves the images in patients with severe arterial narrowing of the carotid artery in the neck.[163] The changing angles and curvature of the ICA in the siphon often makes interpretation of this region more difficult than the straight portions of the artery. The intracranial anterior circulation large arteries are well seen but distal branch arteries are not well imaged.[166-168] The horizontal segment of the MCA and the proximal portions of the superior and inferior divisions of the MCA are usually well shown.

MRA of the vertebral artery origins from the subclavian arteries is often suboptimal because of the overlapping of arteries. Superimposition of arteries sometimes make images difficult to interpret, a problem most older clinicians are aware of in interpreting arch-contrast angiography. Special

views often must be taken to see the origins of the VAs. Filming of the aortic arch and its branches after gadolinium infusion often provides better images of the proximal portions of the innominate, subclavian, and vertebral arteries. The second portion of the VA within the intervertebral foramina is well shown on MRA. The third portion of the VA, that section of the artery that curves around the rostral cervical vertebrae, is often not well seen on MRA because of the sharp angulation and curvature of the artery. The intracranial vertebral arteries and the basilar artery are usually well shown on intracranial MRA, especially the rostral bifurcation of the basilar artery into the PCAs. Quereshi and colleagues evaluated the ability of MRA to detect significant occlusive lesions among 118 patients with brain infarcts.[159] Among the 176 large arteries visualized by both MRA and conventional angiography, angiography confirmed 9 out of 10 (90%) extracranial and 32 out of 40 (80%) intracranial abnormalities shown by MRA. There were few false-negative or false-positive abnormalities.[159] MRA has proven to be an excellent screening technique for occlusive disease. CT or catheter contrast angiography may still be needed in some patients to better delineate the vascular lesions. In some patients who are studied with time-of-flight MRA images of the neck, the jugular vein is also shown. This means that there is reversed flow in the vein, suggesting a proximal stenosis or occlusion of the innominate vein on that side.[169] Figure 4-23 shows a normal MRA taken after gadolinium infusion. Figure 4-24 is an MRA image that shows a stenosing plaque in an internal carotid artery. Figure 4-25 shows an intracranial mRA in a

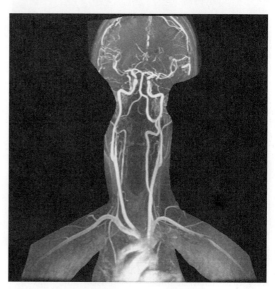

Figure 4-23. Magnetic resonance angiography of the head and neck after gadolinium infusion.

4

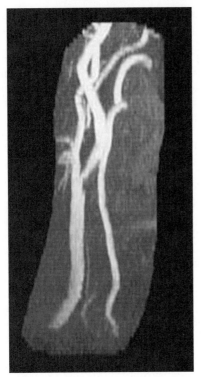

Figure 4-24. Magnetic resonance angiography of the neck showing a stenosing plaque in an internal carotid artery.

patient with an irregular basilar artery. In patient JH, MRA confirmed a right ICA occlusion in the neck. Intracranial views also showed occlusion of the proximal MCA.

Computed Tomography Angiography

Development of more rapid spiral (helical) computed tomography scanners has enabled the development of computed tomography angiography (CTA).[170] This technique involves intravenous injection of a bolus of dye followed by helical scanning. Volumetric data acquisition and improved computerized image manipulation have improved the CTA image display into three-dimensional reformations. CTA is based on anatomic imaging, and when blood flow is severely reduced, CTA has theoretical advantages over MRA, which is a functional imaging technique. The ICAs are well shown in the neck and the results of CTA for quantification of carotid stenosis are comparable to those obtained with MRA.[170-173a] Figure 4-26 shows a CTA of a normal extracranial vertebral artery. Figure 4-27 shows lesions in the neck in a vertebral artery (see Fig. 4-27B) and a carotid artery (see Fig. 4-27A). Compared with conventional angiography there are few false-positive and false-negative results.[170-173]

CTA also provides useful images of intracranial arteries and can show regions of intracranial stenosis, dolichoectasia, and aneurysms.[166,170,174-176,176a] Figure 4-28 shows reconstruction images of CTAs that show intracranial MRA lesions. Bash and

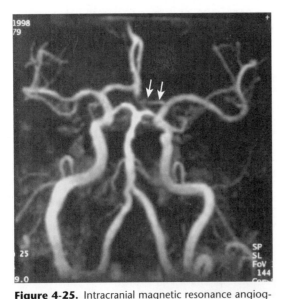

Figure 4-25. Intracranial magnetic resonance angiography. The carotid arteries and their intracranial branches and the vertebral and basilar arteries are well seen. The left A1 segment of the internal carotid artery is hypoplastic *(white arrows)*. The basilar artery has irregularities due to plaques but there are no important stenosing lesions.

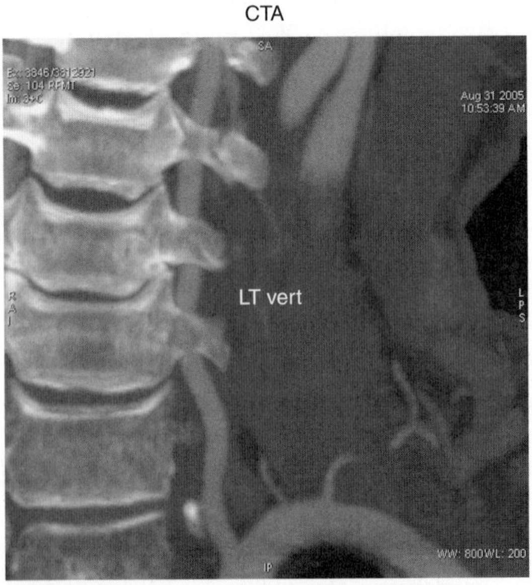

CTA

Figure 4-26. A computed tomography angiograph showing a normal origin of the left vertebral artery in the neck. The artery can be seen to enter the intervertebral foramina and course rostrally.

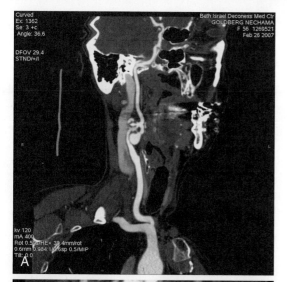

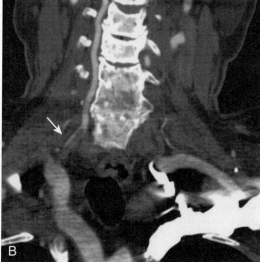

Figure 4-27. Neck computed tomography angiographs. (**A**) An aneurysm is arising from the internal carotid artery. (**B**) A thrombus is seen within the proximal portion of a vertebral artery *(white arrow)*.

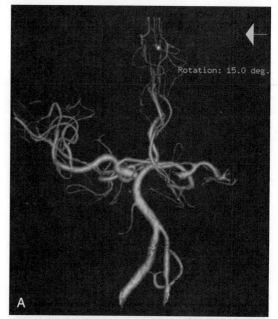

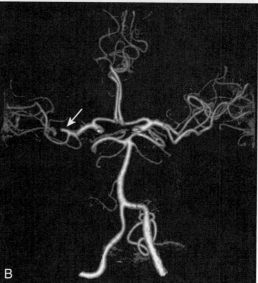

Figure 4-28. Intracranial computed tomography angiographs—maximal intensity projections (MIPS). (**A**) Occlusion of the left mainstem middle cerebral artery on the right of the figure. (**B**) Occlusion of the superior division of the right middle cerebral artery *(white arrow)*.

colleagues compared CTA, MRA, and digital subtraction catheter angiography in 28 patients who had \115 diseased intracranial vascular segments.[166] CTA had a higher sensitivity for intracranial artery stenosis than MRA (98% vs 70%) and for occlusion (100% vs 87%). CTA was superior to MRA especially in patients with low flow states in the posterior circulation.[166] CTA reliably detects aneurysms larger than 3 mm in size,[176] and can be used effectively as the primary vascular diagnostic technique in patients who present with SAH.[176b]

CTA has also been used to predict enlargement and progression of intracerebral hemorrhages.[176c] Tiny enhancing foci within hematomas ("spot sign") shown by CTA indicates active bleeding and correlates with hematoma progression.[176c]

Multimodal Imaging of Brain, Blood Vessels, and Brain Perfusion Using MRI and CT in Acute Ischemic Stroke

The advent of thrombolysis in 1996 made it important for medical centers evaluating patients with acute brain ischemia to obtain anatomical and functional information quickly and safely. New technology and improvements in older techniques now provide clinicians with a menu

4

of different strategies for brain and vascular studies in patients with ischemia. Treating clinicians want to know how much brain is already infarcted, whether large brain-supplying arteries are occluded and where, and the location and portion of the brain that is still at risk for further infarction. Protocols were devised that showed the brain and vascular structures but also included perfusion data able to estimate the regions of brain that were underperfused but not yet infarcted (the so-called ischemic penumbra). This could yield an estimate of the brain tissue still at risk. I have already discussed brain and vascular imaging in the preceding paragraphs. All of the investigations—MRI, FLAIR images, MRA, susceptibility, diffusion and perfusion MRI—can be performed using MR technology within a few minutes. Alternatively, if MR is not readily available or cannot be used, spiral CT can be used to create brain images and CTA of the cervicocranial arteries. Extracranial and transcranial ultrasound can be used as the diagnostic vascular tests in patients who have only had brain imaging or can be used to corroborate and quantify the blood-flow effects of vascular lesions found by CTA and MRA. Ultrasound is also used effectively to monitor the progression and regression of vascular occlusive lesions once they are identified.

MRI Multimodal Protocols

Modern MRI protocols include diffusion and perfusion-weighted imaging along with T2 and T2*-weighted images and MRA. Brain perfusion can be imaged using dynamic contrast-enhanced MR scans.[177-182] Ultrafast imaging after Gd-DTPA injection is used to calculate regional cerebral blood volume (rCBV) and regional cerebral blood flow (rCBF) to produce so-called perfusion-weighted images.[177-186] These images show regions of reduced blood flow when compared to comparable portions of the brain. Perfusion is however quite complex. There are multiple possible measurements such as the relative mean transit time (rMTT) that analyzes the rate of passage of the bolus of gadolinium through the ischemic region, the time to peak, that is the time it takes for the maximum perfusion, and the relative cerebral blood flow and cerebral blood volumes in the ischemic area.[187,187a] The various blood flow measurements sometimes vary; some may be abnormal while other measurements are within the normal range.[186] Within an ischemic zone, perfusion may be quite heterogeneous showing severe hypoperfusion in one area and minor hypoperfusion in another region.[185-187a]

In some centers, it takes additional time to calculate and display perfusion scans, delaying

comparison of the diffusion-weighted scan abnormalities with the perfusion scan. Perhaps just as useful information can be gleaned from the diffusion-weighted scan and the MRA since in most patients, prediction of the hypoperfused region can be estimated by the severity and location of the occluded artery and the clinical neurologic signs (clinical-imaging mismatch[39]).

Researchers and clinicians are now exploring a means of imaging perfusion without the need for contrast infusion. The technique is referred to as arterial spin labeling.[188-191] A radiofrequency pulse is given to the arterial blood column in the neck giving the blood a magnetic label. Continuous arterial spin labeling perfusion magnetic resonance imaging (CASL-pMRI) uses magnetically labeled arterial blood water as a tracer to obtain quantifiable measurements of cerebral blood flow (CBF).[188-191]

Comparison of the region of probable infarction on diffusion-weighted scans with the region of reduced perfusion (either from perfusion-weighted scans or estimated by the MRA results) gives an indication of the part of the brain that is underperfused but not yet infarcted (the presumed ischemic penumbra).[181,182] When the region of reduced perfusion matches the zone of infarction, progression of infarction and progression of neurologic signs are rare. When this information is supplemented by vascular imaging, usually MRA that is acquired at the same time as the diffusion-weighted and perfusion MRI scans, the treating physician has all the useful information needed to assess brain perfusion and to allow a logical decision about the likely utility of acute treatments such as thrombolysis. The cartoon in Figure 4-29 illustrates the components of a multimodal MRI examination emphasizing perfusion/diffusion mismatch. The information gained from the MRI protocols often used to evaluate acute stroke patients. A patient with an occluded MCA shown by MRA who has a large zone of reduced perfusion within the MCA territory shown by perfusion MRI, and a relatively small region of infarction shown by diffusion-weighted MRI represents the ideal candidate for thrombolysis. On the other hand, a large zone of infarction on diffusion-weighted MRI, open ICA and MCA on MRA, and perfusion deficits that match or are less than the zone of infarction on diffusion-weighted scans are characteristics of candidates in whom thrombolysis has little likely utility. In patients who show a large perfusion/diffusion mismatch in whom MRA shows that the artery supplying the ischemia zone is occluded, the infarct invariably enlarges if the artery is not

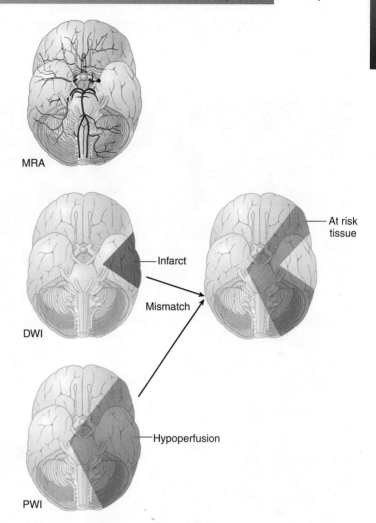

MRA

At risk tissue

Infarct

Mismatch

DWI

Hypoperfusion

Figure 4-29. Cartoon showing a multi-modal MRI protocol emphasizing a perfusion/diffusion mismatch.

PWI

opened quickly.[184] When MRA shows patency of the intracranial artery leading to an ischemic zone, usually no added infarction occurs.[184] The presence of a large-artery occlusion is the main predictor of subsequent acute vascular events in patients with TIAs[191a] and strokes, so that vascular imaging is crucial in patients with cerebrovascular ischemia.

Guidelines for thrombolysis emphasize time; a 3-hour window is usually cited. Modern multimodal MR imaging, however, often shows that important diffusion/perfusion mismatch can still be present long after the 3 hour window. One study showed that among 42 patients in whom MR imaging was performed more than 48 hours after neurologic symptom onset, 15 (36%) still showed a mismatch pattern indicating brain still at risk for further infarction.[192]

All of the clinically relevant data can be acquired rapidly without risk on a single machine, making modern MRI imaging using the new technology far and away the best method of studying acute stroke patients. Figure 4-30A and B shows results of acute MRI stroke protocols in patients with posterior circulation occlusive disease. Although most studies and literature emphasize the utility of multimodal MRI in patients with anterior circulation strokes, the technique can be just as useful in the posterior circulation.[192a]

Figure 4-31 shows MRI studies before and after tPA thrombolysis in a patient with an acute embolic occlusion of the MCA. The use of MRI and other imaging technology for decision making about thrombolysis and other potential therapies will be discussed further in Chapter 5.

COMPUTED TOMOGRAPHY PERFUSION
AND COMPUTED TOMOGRAPHY PROTOCOLS

Brain perfusion can also be studied using contrast-enhanced CT techniques.[193-197a] CT perfusion involves continuous CT acquisition using

4

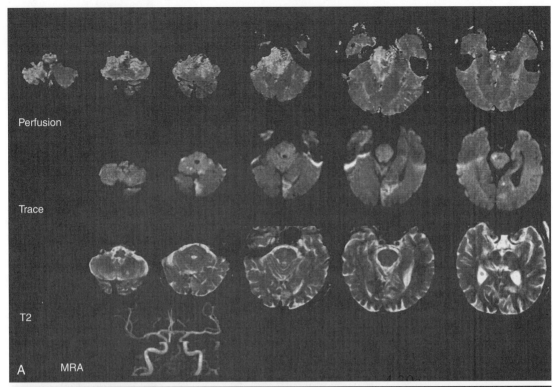

Perfusion

Trace

T2

A   MRA

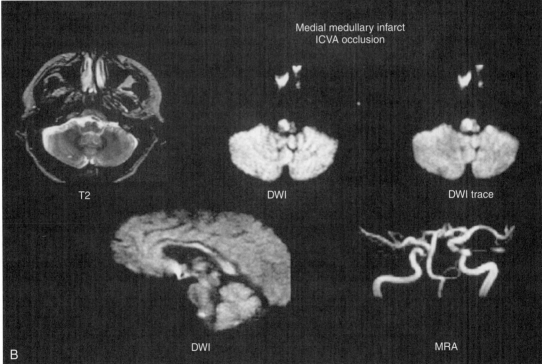

Medial medullary infarct
ICVA occlusion

T2   DWI   DWI trace

B   DWI   MRA

Figure 4-30. Multimodal MRI protocol of patients with severe posterior circulation occlusive disease. (**A**) A patient with bilateral occlusive lesions involving the intracranial vertebral arteries. The perfusion images at the top of the figure show marked reduction in perfusion in the medulla and pons and the right cerebellum. The diffusion images (labeled *Trace*) show a small infarct in the right pons and left occipital lobe. The T2-weighted images show no definite infarction. The MRA shows very poor opacification of the intracranial vertebral arteries. A part of the midbasilar artery is shown. The perfusion abnormality far exceeds the dffusion abnormality in this patient. (**B**) Multimodal MRI protocol in a patient with a right medial medullary infarct. The T2-weighted image is normal. The diffusion images show a well-defined infarct in the right medial medulla spreading a bit beyond the midline. The MRA shows an occlusion of the right intracranial vertebral artery.

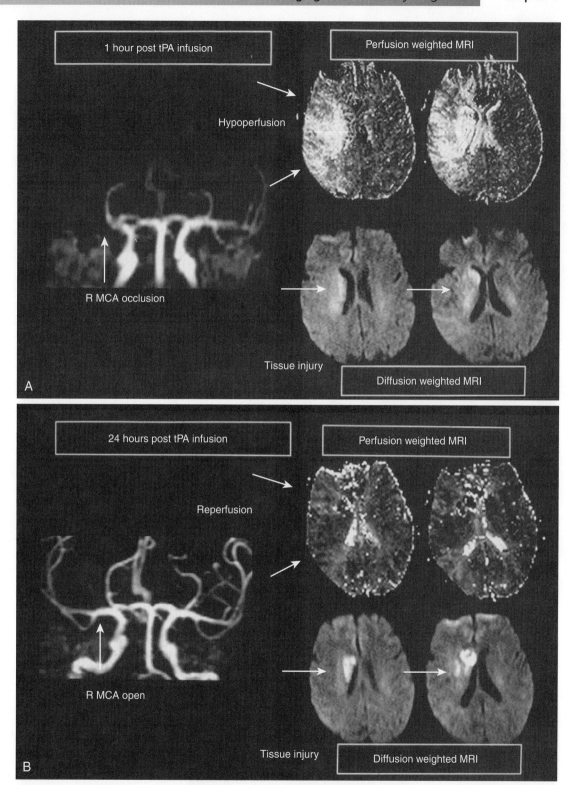

Figure 4-31. MRI protocols in relation to thrombolysis. (**A**) The MRI images were taken 1 hour after tPA infusion was begun. The right middle cerebral artery is occluded on the MRA image *(white arrow)*. The perfusion-weighted images show markedly reduced perfusion in the entire right-middle cerebral artery territory. The diffusion-weighted images show an area of reduced diffusion adjacent to the right lateral ventricle. (**B**) The same MRI protocol taken 24 hours after tPA infusion. The right MCA has now reopened *(white arrow)*. The perfusion has returned to normal and the diffusion-weighted images show only a minimal increase in the area of reduced diffusion compared to the prior DWI images in **A.**

4

a helical scanner during the administration of iodinated dye. The dye increases the intensity in brain regions that are normally perfused but is not as visible in regions that are underperfused. Transit times, cerebral blood flow, and cerebral blood volumes can be calculated using dedicated software. The contrast enhancement in each pixel is compared to the contralateral mirror cerebral region. The values for MTT, rCBF, and rCBV are compared to normal values and known ischemic thresholds and are used to characterize hypoperfused brain regions as being in the core of an infarct and penumbra. Within an established infarct (usually the core of an infarct) both rCBF and rCBV are reduced; within penumbral zones vascular dilatation usually leads to an increase in rCBV so that rCBF is decreased but rCBV is increased.[194] These measurements are more quantitative than now obtainable with contrast-enhanced perfusion-weighted MRI.[197]

When perfusion CT is combined with CT angiography and non-contrast CT scans, comparable information to MRI protocols can be obtained.[191-197] Figure 4-32 shows studies of a patient with a MCA occlusion studied by a multimodal CT protocol. The major difference between acute CT and MRI protocols are that CT does not show the acute area of infarction as well as diffusion-weighted MRI, and a limited number of CT sections can be shown so that some underperfused regions not included in the sections taken are missed while MRI is able to show a much larger area of the brain. Posterior circulation thromboembolism is presently not well studied by CT perfusion protocols.

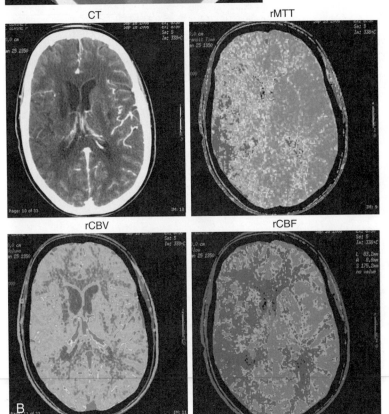

Figure 4-32. Multimodal CT protocol in a 56-year-old woman presenting with acute onset of a left hemiparesis. (**A**) CT scan after contrast infusion shows very poor flow through the right middle cerebral artery *(white arrow)*. (**B**) Head CT shows a right basal ganglia infarct. Perfusion images show a prolonged relative mean transit time (rMTT), slightly decreased relative cerebral blood volume (rCBV) and decreased relative cerebral blood flow (rCBF) involving most of the right MCA territory. (Courtesy of Claudia Chaves, MD, Neurology Department, Lahey Clinic, Burlington, Mass.)

Another method using CT and dye infusion has become popular in Korea. Injection of contrast followed by sequential imaging at specific time intervals ("triphasic perfusion computed tomography") using helical CT can yield rapid information about regions of brain ischemia and blockage of intracranial arteries.[198-200] The technique involves giving a bolus injection using a power injector of contrast into an antecubital vein after a noncontrast CT has been performed. Early, middle, and late phase images are obtained 18, 30, and 80 seconds after the contrast has been injected. Occlusion of the MCA or its branches can be detected from the images even without reformation, allowing rapid decision about thrombolysis. However, only limited CT scan cuts, usually taken along the plane of the MCAs, are imaged. The contrast dye infusion also enhances the brain CT images, yielding a perfusion CT scan that is somewhat comparable to a perfusion image MR scan. Regions of underperfusion do not contain as much of the infused contrast as the uninvolved side. Figure 4-33 is an example of a triphasic CT perfusion study in a patient with a right MCA occlusion.

Multimodal techniques using MRI or CT that include brain, vascular and perfusion imaging are effective in studying patients with acute ischemic stroke for the feasibility of reperfusion.[200a,b,c] CT has the advantage of ready accessibility but the disadvantage of requiring dye infusion and, at present, providing only limited cuts of the brain and vasculature. MRI using DWI and ADC imaging more accurately and effectively shows regions of acute ischemia that will go on to infarction than CT techniques.[200c]

Other Techniques for Studying Perfusion and Vascular Disease

Inhalation of xenon, an inert gas that is not metabolized, has been used for decades to study cerebral blood flow. The development of xenon inhalation combined with CT scanning (XeCT) has allowed imaging of rCBF changes on sequential standard CT slices.[201-203] Xenon enhances or modifies the images, allowing visualization of relative rCBF in regions of interest. This technique facilitates comparison of the zone of infarction on CT with regions of reduced CBF.

Single-photon-emission computed tomography (SPECT) uses ordinary radionuclear camera equipment and does not require a cyclotron to

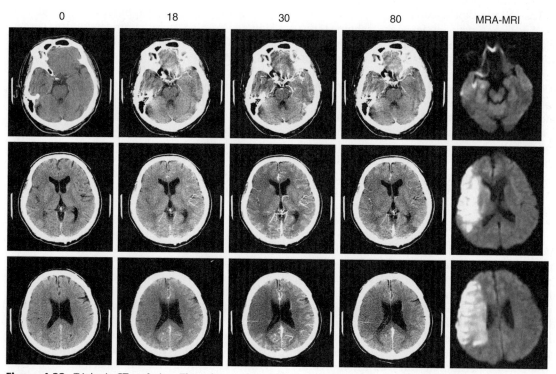

Figure 4-33. Triphasic CT perfusion. The columns show CT scans taken at various sections through the cerebral hemispheres before and 18, 30, and 80 seconds after a contrast infusion. In the upper row, the MCA on the left of the figures is occluded. The MCA territory on the side of the occlusion has much less blood vessel and tissue opacification indicating infarction. The comparable MRA-MRI figures are shown in the far right column. (Courtesy of SJ Lee, MD, Samsung Medical Center, Seoul, Korea.)

4

generate radionuclides. The most common radio-isotopes used now are Technetium-99M-labeled hexamethylpropylene amineoxime (HMPAO) and technetium-99m-labeled ethyl cysteinate dimer (Tc ECD).[204-208] Regional radiotracer uptake can be imaged in three planes. The isotopes measure rCBF rather than metabolic activity. SPECT and XeCT contain no important metabolic information.

A major advantage of SPECT scanning is that imaging does not have to be performed immediately after injection of the radionuclide. The findings on SPECT imaging represent those that were present at the time of injection. Acute treatment could be instituted immediately after injection even before the scans are performed. SPECT does not show the region of infarction but can be used with CT and can be helpful in the diagnosis and management of stroke patients, when the proper questions are asked.[203] Wintermark and colleagues have compared perfusion imaging using MRI, CT, XeCT, and SPECT.[209]

In the past, positron-emission tomography (PET scanning) was used extensively in research centers to quantify cerebral blood flow and metabolism. But PET uses rapidly metabolized radioisotopes and proved to be not practical in the management of patients with acute stroke. MRI has virtually replaced PET in clinical practice but PET is still used for research.

PET is a functional imaging technique that makes it possible to measure in vivo chemical reactions in body organs. Only a small number of suitable positron-emitting radionuclides are available that are integral to most organic biological compounds. These radionuclides have short half-lives, and so a dedicated medical cyclotron is required on site for synthesis, thereby making the equipment and its maintenance quite expensive. Research physicists and chemists are also often needed.

The positron-emitting radionuclides are tagged to physiologically active compounds and given to the patient at acceptably low radiation doses. CT or MRI studies of the distribution of these radionuclides allow for images of brain physiology and metabolism during life. PET scanning allows for quantification and imaging of CBF, the metabolic rate of oxygen, the metabolic rate of glucose, and the oxygen extraction function. These measurements give useful information about blood flow, the metabolic activity, and avidity for oxygen in the local regions studied.[210-214] Reduced regional cerebral blood flow (rCBF) in the range of 10 to 20 mL/100 g per minute can lead to brain stunning (not functioning normal but not irreversibly damaged), a state characterized by decreased electrical activity and reduced cerebral metabolism but increased extraction of oxygen.

In the normal situation, blood flow and metabolism are coupled; however, flow and metabolism are often different in the core of infarcts, as compared with the peripheral zone (penumbra). When oxygen metabolism is markedly depressed, either in association with low rCBF or out of proportion to rCBF, the likelihood of useful return of function in the tissue is small. If oxygen metabolism is preserved and there is a relatively high oxygen extraction function, then the outlook for recovery is better. Baron dubbed the situation of avidity of the local tissue for oxygen in the presence of poor perfusion the misery perfusion syndrome.[212,214] In chronic infarcts, CT regions of hypodensity and PET images of rCBF and the metabolic rate of oxygen are essentially congruous, showing dead tissue with little flow and little metabolism. During some phases of a stroke, rCBF may be increased relative to metabolism, a phenomenon dubbed luxury perfusion. Figure 4-34 illustrates the data generated from PET examinations in a patient with a MCA territory infarct.

Metabolic depression can also occur at sites distant from the zones of infarction. This finding has sometimes been called diaschisis. The recognized regions of reduced metabolism at a distant from brain infarcts and hemorrhages are noted in Table 4-6. These regions that show distant effects provide insight into brain pathways and help guide physiologic approaches to rehabilitation. They also help in understanding previously confusing rCBF results associated with xenon inhalation.

PET can also be used to study changes in flow and metabolism after various types of stimulation. Visual stimuli augment activity in the lateral geniculate body and striate regions. Auditory stimuli activate the medial geniculate body and various temporal and parietal regions, depending on whether music, language, or other auditory stimuli are used and the content of the sound. Speaking and right-limb movement activate parasylvian and frontal regions, predominantly in the left cerebral hemisphere. These studies give important insights into how the brain functions. Also, in some circumstances, rCBF and metabolism might be adequate for baseline function but may not be able to augment satisfactorily after stimulation. These functional studies also have the potential of telling how the damaged brain functions with sensory stimuli and how patterns of metabolism and flow change with recovery. Insight into reparative and adaptive mechanisms could ensue. Without question, PET has opened up large vistas with potential insights into brain function. The expense of the equipment, the length of time required for testing, and the importance of ancillary physicists and chemists limit the applicability of

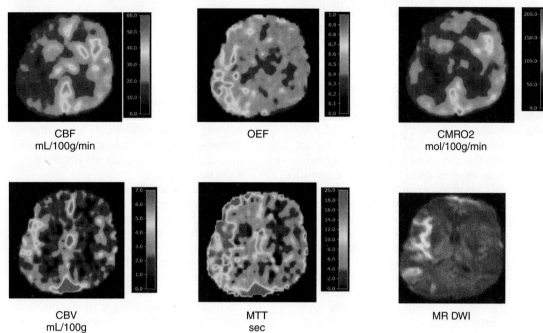

Figure 4-34. PET parametric maps of cerebral blood flow (CBF), oxygen extraction fraction (OEF), oxygen consumption (CMRO₂), cerebral blood volume (CBV) and mean transit time (MTT), as well as the diffusion-weighted (DWI) scan, obtained in a 51-year-old man, 7 to 9 hrs after acute-onset right-sided hemiparesis, homonymous hemianopia and neglect, and global dysphasia. One axial plane is shown for illustration. Images are shown in neurological orientation (i.e., right is shown on the right side). Quantitative grey-white intensity scales are shown to the right of each PET image for interpretation. There is extensive hypoperfusion over the entire left MCA territory, with CBF below the penumbra threshold of 20 mL/100 g/minute in large parts of the affected cortex. The CMRO₂ is also reduced in the entire MCA territory, but less so than predicted by the CBF with massively increased OEF ("misery perfusion"). The CMRO₂ lies above the threshold for irreversible damage (around 39 μmol/100 g/minute) throughout except around the posterior insula and surrounding white matter. The CBV and the MTT are also increased throughout, indicating overridden autoregulation from low perfusion pressure. The DWI lesion is heterogeneous and extensive but smaller than the area of hypoperfusion ("mismatch"); although it is partly congruent with the areas of very low CMRO₂ indicating irreversible damage, it also straddles areas of penumbra, characterized by CBF <20 mL/100 g/minute, high OEF, and CMRO₂ above the irreversibility threshold. (Courtesy of J-C Baron, JV Guadagno, M Takasawa, EA Warburton, et al, University of Cambridge, UK.)

Table 4-6.	Regions of Diaschisis (Reduced Metabolism) Distant from Brain Infarcts and Hemorrhages

Thalamus ipsilateral to a cerebral infarct
Cerebral cortex ipsilateral to thalamic lesion
Cerebral hemisphere contralateral to supratentorial infarct of the opposite hemisphere
Cerebellar hemisphere contralateral to cerebral lesion
Cerebellar hemisphere ipsilateral to pontine infarct

the PET technique to large research centers funded for their studies. Functional MRI studies have begun to develop the capability of demonstrating brain function and activity without the need for a cyclotron. Furthermore, functional MRI can be performed on the same equipment used for brain and vascular imaging.

Recently PET has been used to diagnose cerebral amyloid angiopathy and Alzheimer disease.[214a,b] Radionuclides with an affinity for amyloid (Pittsburgh compound B and fluoroethyl methyl amino-2-naphthyl ethylidene malonitrile) are used during PET scanning to show the quantity and distribution of amyloid within the brain and within brain blood vessels.[214a,b]

Catheter-Contrast Cerebral Angiography

MRA and CTA have the advantage of being able to be performed at the same time as brain imaging and are noninvasive. The advent of

4

high-quality CTA, MRA, and cervical and transcranial ultrasonography have led to a marked decrease in the indications for catheter contrast angiography. Catheter angiography is now performed almost solely using a digital subtraction technique that allows for less dye injection than was used in the past. Digital subtraction cerebral angiography is indicated when the preliminary testing does not satisfactorily clarify the nature of the vascular lesions and when treatment depends on the nature and severity of those vascular lesions. For example, angiography is used in patients in whom carotid artery stenosis has been shown by MRA and duplex sonography, but these two tests give conflicting estimates of the severity of stenosis. Angiography is often required to better define cerebral aneurysms and vascular malformations. Catheter angiography is used as a prelude to intravascular interventions such as intra-arterial thrombolysis and angioplasty because the treatment is given directly within the artery. In experienced hands, angiography gives valuable information and has a relatively low incidence of serious complications. The commonest factors that relate to complications are noted in Table 4-7.

Angiography should be tailored to the clinical question and therapeutic alternatives. Brain and noninvasive vascular imaging (CT or MRI) or ultrasonography, or both, usually should precede angiography. These tests help the angiographer focus on the particular regions of interest. Screening of other arterial regions by noninvasive techniques allows the angiographer to limit the angiographic procedure, thus helping reduce morbidity, time, and expense. The clinician and the angiographer should decide together on the important data clinically needed, considering the clinical context of the study.

I use and teach the following critical angiography "rules"[215]:

1. Tailor angiography to the patient and the individual problem. Avoid extra injections, catheterization, and dye because they increase the risk of the procedure.

2. Follow Sutton's law. Sutton robbed banks because that is where the money is—go after the highest-yield information first. I have seen angiographers, after a catheter had flipped unexpectedly into a vessel that was not the primary focus of attention, take several films "while they were there," believing that the films might be necessary anyway. Too often, a complication or other unforeseen exigency curtails the procedure before the important data are obtained. First things first.

3. The clinician responsible for the patient and the angiographer should plan and discuss the procedure together. Ideally, the procedure should be performed with both present, choosing together the next shot as the data accumulate. Because of time constraints and other commitments, this is not always possible. Telephone contact at critical decision points often is an acceptable substitute. If a clinician cannot be reached during the procedure, discussion of the plan of attack and treatment choices with the angiographer is a minimum requirement. In some circumstances, the relationship between angiographer and clinician is so well oiled by shared past experiences that the angiographer learns how the clinician approaches most common situations. In that case, consultation during the procedure would occur only if unexpected or unusual findings were uncovered. Ideally, if the responsible clinician is not the surgeon who will perform an operative procedure, the surgeon also should be contacted when findings are uncovered that would dictate an operation. Surgeons may have their own demands for studies before surgery, and this is best accomplished during the angiography. Communication between clinicians and neuroradiologists is also important for the performance and interpretation of MRA and CTA protocols, because neuroradiologists should monitor the studies as they are

Table 4-7.	**Factors Related to Complications of Cerebral Angiography**

Equipment, dye, and catheters used
Method, quantity, and rate of dye infusion
Number of injections
Training and experience of angiographer
Whether a large volume of contrast is injected into aortic arch
General medical and psychological state of the patient
Adequacy of hydration
Kidney function
Nature and severity of the occlusive cervicocranial vascular disease

performed to be sure that the information derived answers the queries raised by the clinicians caring for the patient.

4. Avoid an aortic arch injection whenever possible. The yield of arch opacification studies is low. Akers and colleagues reviewed the results of 1000 consecutive patients who had arch angiography, followed by selective catheterization of both carotid and vertebral arteries.[216] Only six (0.6%) had intrathoracic vascular pathology that was hemodynamically important, including four lesions at the common carotid artery origin and two at the innominate artery origin. Three of these lesions (two common carotid arteries and one innominate) would have been discovered if only selective catheterization were performed. Inability to selectively catheterize these arteries and fluoroscopy identify most cases requiring arch injection. The absence of a significant lesion in the head or neck should alert the angiographer to opacify the origin of the artery on the way out. Arch injections usually require 40 to 50 mL of contrast material injected under pressure, so cardiac overload and renal toxicity do occur. A large bolus of dye used for filming the arch limits the amount of dye that should be used during selective catheterization. Arch films are also not easy to read because of overlapping of vessels. In my opinion, there is no reason to perform routine arch angiography. Only the major arteries of interest should be studied using the Seldinger technique of selective catheterization. In addition, intra-arterial digital subtraction filming techniques allow use of less dye while retaining high-quality films.

5. Use the least amount of dye and injections to arrive at a therapeutic decision. Often, the initial opacification provides enough information so that other injections are not needed.

6. Talk to and examine the patient at least briefly after each dye injection, to detect any complication that might dictate stopping the procedure. The neurologic examination depends on the vessels studied. For example, after posterior circulation opacification, check vision and memory; after carotid artery injection, check speech and arm movement.

In JH, I did not perform contrast angiography. The concordance of the MRA, ultrasound data, and the unlikelihood of a treatable lesion persuaded me not to pursue angiography. His clinical deficit was also severe and not reversible.

Cardiac Evaluation

Cardioembolic mechanisms of ischemic stroke are common. The proportion of ischemic strokes generally considered to have originated from cardioembolic sources has increased dramatically with the development of sophisticated technology that has the capability of defining cardiac and vascular lesions. A wide variety of different cardiac lesions are now known to be potential sources of embolism, while in the remote past, only acute myocardial infarction and rheumatic mitral stenosis with atrial fibrillation were generally accepted cardiac sources.

Cardiac emboli arise from a varied assortment of diseases that affect the heart valves, heart rhythm, endocardial surface, and myocardium.[217] Pump failure can cause general cerebral hypoperfusion. In addition, many patients with brain ischemia caused by neck and intracranial atherosclerosis have coexisting coronary artery atherosclerosis. Late deaths in series of patients with ischemic stroke are most often caused by coronary artery disease and myocardial infarction rather than to cerebrovascular disease. These facts should direct the physician's attention to the stroke patient's heart, as well as to the brain and its vascular supply.

The question is not whether to look at the heart but how thoroughly to do so. What is the yield of intensive cardiac investigation? Is it worth the cost? Most clinicians agree that it is important to take a careful cardiac history, particularly seeking symptoms of arrhythmia, congestive heart failure, angina pectoris, and prior myocardial infarctions. The heart should be carefully examined, noting heart size, quality of sounds, rhythm, and presence of gallops, in addition to seeking and characterizing murmurs. An electrocardiogram and chest x-ray should also be obtained routinely because of their high screening value, safety, and low cost.

Table 4-8 lists the demographic features and history features in ischemic stroke patients that indicate the need for echocardiography. Table 4-9 lists the situations recognizable after the preliminary investigations in which echocardiography has a high yield. In these circumstances, intensive cardiac testing is essential. Transthoracic echocardiography (TTE) is usually performed first, and the results may be definitive, and thus transesophageal echocardiography (TEE) would not be required. Because the left atrium is directly anterior to the esophagus, atrial lesions, occult valvular disorders, and ulcerative lesions of the proximal aorta, often missed by transthoracic echocardiography, are detected by the TEE approach. TEE shows many abnormalities not revealed by

Table 4-8.   Situations in Which Echocardiography Has a High Yield in Ischemic Stroke Patients

Known prior heart disease.
Clinical course suggestive of brain embolism—that is, sudden onset of neurological deficit, while active, without prior TIAs.
A history of peripheral embolism in the limbs or abdominal viscera.
Young age with no atherosclerotic risk factors. (Young patients who have no known risk factors for atherosclerosis often harbor unexpected cardiac sources, such as cardiac tumors, intra-atrial defects, or cardiomyopathy.)

Table 4-9.   Preliminary Investigation Results Leading to Important Yield of Echocardiography in Ischemic Stroke Patients

Absence of extracranial and intracranial vascular disease on noninvasive testing
Superficial infarct on CT or MRI in the distribution of a peripheral branch of the MCA or PCA or cerebellar arteries
Hemorrhagic transformation of a brain infarct in one vascular territory
CT or MRI showing infarcts in multiple vascular territories
Normal CTA, MRA, or contrast arteriography in a patient whose clinical deficit and brain imaging are not compatible with lacunar infarction
Angiography (CTA, MRA, or standard catheter) that shows distal cutoff of a brain artery branch or a luminal filling defect without severe proximal arterial stenosis

TTE. The use of TEE in patients with strokes and TIAs has been extensively reviewed.[217-222] TEE is more accurate than TTE in showing atrial and ventricular thrombi, in detecting and quantifying intracardiac shunts, and more often shows spontaneous echo contrast than TTE. Figure 4-35 shows an atrial thrombus and Figure 4-36 shows vegetation on the mitral valve identified on echocardiography in patients with cardiogenic brain embolism.

TEE may not be able to identify a potential cardiac source of emboli. Some thromboemboli are too small to be detected. An embolus that is 1 or 2 mm in size can produce a devastating neurologic deficit, and this size particle is often beyond the resolution of echocardiography.[217,223,224] The other major reason for failure of echocardiography to show a thrombus is that thrombosis and embolism are dynamic processes. When a thrombus leaves the heart to go to the brain, echocardiography may not show a residual thrombus within the heart if performed soon after the clinical event.[223,224] The thrombus may re-form later.

TEE also yields important information about the proximal aorta, a region not imaged by TTE.[225] Figure 4-37 shows different types of

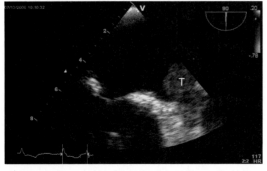

Figure 4-35. Transesophageal echocardiography image at the midesophageal level at 90-degree transducer orientations. A large thrombus (T) is seen along the lateral wall of the left atrium (LA) and filling the left atrial appendage. (Courtesy of Warren Manning, MD, Beth Israel Deaconess Medical Center and Harvard Medical School, Boston, Mass.)

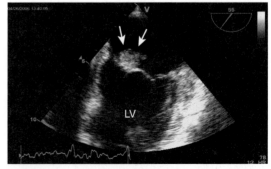

Figure 4-36. Transesophageal image of large vegetation (white arrows) on the anterior mitral valve leaflet. (Courtesy of Susan Yeon, MD, Beth Israel Deaconess Medical Center and Harvard Medical School, Boston, Mass.)

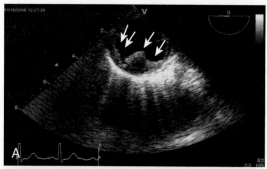

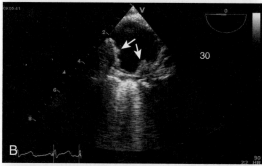

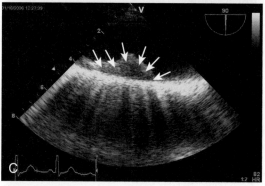

Figure 4-37. (**A**) Transesophageal long-axis (90 degrees) view of thoracic aorta with complex plaque *(white arrows)*. (**B**) Transesophageal echocardiography image at the mid-esophageal level in the horizontal (0 degree) transducer orientation. Two atherosclerotic plaques *(white arrows)* are visible and invaginate into the aortic lumen. (**C**) Transesophageal long-axis (90 degrees) view of thoracic aorta with complex plaque *(white arrows)*. (Courtesy of Susan Yeon, MD, and Warren Manning, MD, Beth Israel Deaconess Medical Center and Harvard Medical School, Boston, Mass.)

aortic plaques detected by TEE. TEE is important in all patients in whom TTE suggests, but does not adequately define, the cardiac pathology, and in all patients in whom other studies (cerebrovascular, hematologic, and other cardiac investigations) do not satisfactorily show the cause of brain embolism and brain ischemia.[220,223] Radionuclide testing, including gated blood pool imaging (multigated acquisition scans), also may be helpful in selected patients as might other cardiac imaging techniques.[226]

The aorta is an important potential source of embolism, especially during angiography and cardiac surgery.[225] Presently, TEE is the most effective method of imaging the aorta for plaques and thrombi. The ascending aorta can also be insonated using a Duplex ultrasound probe placed in the right supraclavicular fossa. The arch and proximal descending thoracic aorta can be imaged using a left supraclavicular probe.[227] The results so far are preliminary but promising. Most plaques are located in the curvature of the arch from the distal ascending aorta to the proximal descending aorta, regions shown by B-mode ultrasound.[227]

When clinical suspicion is high and echocardiography is not diagnostic, CT,[228] MRI, or ultrafast CT[229] of the heart might image cardiac clots. Platelet scintigraphy using radionuclides[230] might also indicate pooling of platelets on the surface of a mural thrombus or other cardiac lesion. Remember also that documentation of a potential cardioembolic source—such as mitral valve prolapse, mitral annulus calcification, or akinetic zones—does not mean per se that the patient has brain embolism. Coexistent atherosclerotic disease may be the cause.

Many patients with atherosclerosis of the carotid and vertebral arteries in the neck have coexistent peripheral vascular occlusive disease and coronary artery disease. Because coronary artery disease, even when silent, can be life-threatening, screening of these patients for silent myocardial ischemia is important, especially if surgery is considered.[231] A variety of different exercise[232,233] and radionuclide techniques[234,235] can detect regions of poor myocardial perfusion. Imaging of the heart after the patient has been given dipyridamole (dipyridamole-thallium myocardial imaging) and some exercise often shows regions of silent ischemia. In one study, among 38 patients with severe cerebrovascular occlusive disease, 60% had reversible or fixed myocardial perfusion deficits using this radionuclide scintigraphic test.[234] Treadmill or supine exercise testing with electrocardiographic monitoring is another commonly used screening technique. Radionuclide angiography can also be helpful in assessing left ventricular function, perfusion at rest, and with exercise. If severe coronary artery disease is suggested by screening tests, coronary angiography may be needed to localize and quantify the coronary artery disease to guide treatment.

The use of routine ambulatory monitoring for cardiac rhythm disturbances is not clear. In patients suspected of brain embolism, the yield is probably high enough to dictate the use of monitoring. However, a review of published results of cardiac rhythm monitoring in patients with acute

4

ischemic stroke estimated that only about one in 20 patients show atrial fibrillation or other embologenic cardiac arrythmias.[235a] In patients with lacunar infarcts and those with a well-defined atherosclerotic extracranial vascular cause for their stroke, the yield is probably low. Cardiac rhythm monitoring should probably be done in any patient whose initial EEG suggests a cardiac rhythm abnormality.

Other Investigations

A wide variety of other tests have been used in the past to study arterial flow in the brain vessels. Most of these investigations have been superseded by newer ultrasound technology and neuroimaging techniques. These include oculoplethysmography and ophthalmodynamometry, techniques that were described in the first two editions of this book but have now been superseded by TCD. A new ultrasound technology, color Doppler imaging of the vessels that supply the eye, has become available and can accurately image and define vascular lesions that involve the ophthalmic and central retinal arteries.[236,237]

The tests described so far help localize and quantify morphologic structural abnormalities in the brain and the brain-supplying arteries.

Two other advances, MR spectroscopy (MRS) and functional MRI, have added new dimensions to the study of stroke and brain ischemia. During MRS, regions of interest as identified by MRI can be analyzed for the relative volumes and localization of various chemical constituents such as choline, creatine, N-acetyl aspartate, lactate, and glutamate.[238-241] Elevated lactate is found soon after infarction; decreased N-acetyl aspartate, creatine, and choline are characteristic of the MRS spectrum in the region of brain infarction. MRS analysis may be useful in the future in distinguishing tissue that is destined to become infarcted from tissue that is reversibly ischemic. MRS may also prove useful in studying patients with various stroke-related metabolic problems, such as mitochondrial disorders that alter brain metabolism.[240]

When certain MRI techniques are used during perceptual, cognitive, and motor tasks, small changes in signal intensity show alterations in local blood flow related to increased brain activity and function during these tasks.[242-244] Functional MRI can yield insights into which parts of the brain are being used to perform various brain functions. This information is probably most relevant to the study of recovery from stroke and may give important insights into spontaneous recovery and the potential of various rehabilitative therapies. Figures 4-38, 4-39, and 4-40 show fMRI scans in some patients with strokes.

What if Brain Imaging Shows an Intracerebral Hemorrhage?

The most common cause of ICH is hypertension, either acute or chronic. When the blood pressure is high and CT or MRI shows a hematoma in a typical location for hypertensive ICH (putamen, caudate nucleus, thalamus, pons, cerebellum), a search for AVMs or aneurysms has a very low yield. In young patients with no hypertension or with intraventricular or lobar hematomas, however, studies of the intracerebral arteries often

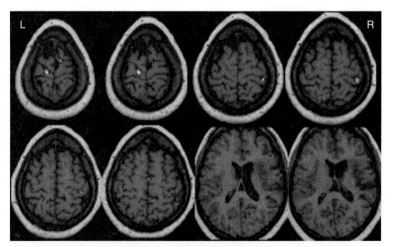

Figure 4-38. Functional MRI scans (fMRI) of a patient with a right cerebral infarct (best seen on the image at the bottom right). When he is asked to try and move his left hand, both the right and left motor regions are activated as shown by spots. (Courtesy of Gottfried Schlaug, MD, Beth Israel Deaconess Medical Center and Harvard Medical School, Boston, Mass.)

Normal   Stroke

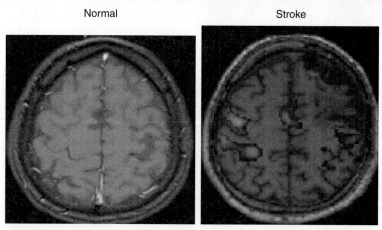

Figure 4-39. Functional MRI scans. On the left is a scan after a normal patient is asked to move the left hand. In the scan on the right, a patient with a right cerebral infarct is asked to move the left hand. The activation in this patient is bilateral but mostly in the nonaffected hemisphere. (Courtesy of Alvaro Pascual-Leone, MD, Beth Israel Deaconess Medical Center and Harvard Medical School, Boston, Mass.)

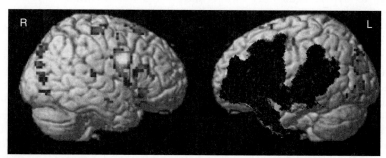

Figure 4-40. fMRI scans in a patient with a large left cerebral infarct that rendered him aphasic. The infarct is shaded black on the figure at the right. Activation is predominantly in the right cerebral hemisphere contralateral to the infarct. (Courtesy of Alvaro Pascual-Leone, MD, Beth Israel Deaconess Medical Center and Harvard Medical School, Boston, Mass.)

show vascular lesions. Patients with ICH after use of cocaine, especially the hydrochloride form, have a relatively high incidence of underlying vascular malformations.[245,246]

MRI can often show AVMs and cavernous angiomas. Vascular channels, serpiginous arteries, mixed-density heterogeneous signals, and the presence of old bleeds containing hemosiderin are clues to the presence of vascular malformations. Contrast-enhanced CT and MRI, plain or enhanced with gadopentetate dimeglumine-diethylenetriaminepenta-acetic acid, can show large aneurysms if they are in the plane of the sections taken. CTA and MRA effectively show AVMs and aneurysms. In some patients, angiography using selective arterial catheterization by the Seldinger technique, with opacification of the arteries supplying the ICH, is needed for definitive exclusion of small AVMs and aneurysms larger than 3 mm. Cavernous and venous angiomas are usually not detected by cerebral angiography.

What if Brain Imaging or Lumbar Puncture Show Subarachnoid Hemorrhage?

Cerebral angiography is still often required for the study of patients with SAH not explainable by trauma or a known bleeding diathesis. Aneurysmal rerupture is such a potentially lethal event that clinicians must be sure an aneurysm is not present in patients with SAH. MRA and CTA[176,247] are useful in screening for aneurysms, but at present, these techniques are probably not definitive enough in many patients for surgical exploration, and dye opacification is still often required. MRI is helpful in detecting small vascular malformations near the ependymal and pial surfaces. MRA and CTA may be useful in following patients after surgical or endovascular treatment of aneurysms and AVMs, and in following unruptured aneurysms and AVMs not treated surgically. TCD is helpful in following patients with aneurysmal SAH in detecting and monitoring vasoconstriction in the basal intracranial arteries.[68,248,249]

QUESTION 4: ARE ABNORMALITIES IN THE BLOOD CAUSING OR ADDING TO BRAIN ISCHEMIA OR HEMORRHAGE?

Once the clinician has determined the nature, site, and severity of the vascular lesion, it is important to find out whether abnormalities of blood constituents are causing or contributing to brain ischemia or hemorrhage. Clinicians must not forget the blood. Abnormalities of the clotting system can lead to hypercoagulability and thrombosis. Even in patients with lesions known to predispose to thromboembolism and brain ischemia, the acute event is often precipitated by a change in the blood and its coagulability. Infections, cancer, and inflammatory bowel disease are examples of conditions that are associated with release of acute-phase reactants that may alter coagulability sufficiently to promote thromboembolism—especially if there is a preexisting lesion that affects an endothelial surface. Bleeding diatheses often cause intracranial bleeding. Abnormalities of the viscosity of blood can alter blood flow, especially in small arterioles and capillaries of the brain, and in patients with occlusive lesions. Increased viscosity can cause or contribute to regional decreases in CBF and potentiate ischemia. Autoimmunity, which can be detected and monitored by blood tests, can lead to occlusive cerebrovascular disease.

What if the Problem Is Ischemia?

The formed cellular elements of the blood—erythrocytes, leukocytes, and platelets—should always be studied. Screening tests of coagulation functions should also be a part of the routine evaluation of patients with brain ischemia. In addition, other blood components may be analyzed, such as serum proteins, coagulation factors, antiphospholipid antibodies, and blood viscosity.

Erythrocytes

Quantitative and qualitative RBC abnormalities can affect blood flow and clotting. The level of the hematocrit clearly affects whole blood viscosity and the rheologic properties of blood. Physicians have long been aware that high Hct levels, such as 60% or more, can cause clotting in normal young adults. In older patients with preexisting atherosclerosis and small-vessel disease, high Hcts that are still within the normal range can compound the vascular disease and limit perfusion. Studies in animals[250] and humans[251-253] confirm that the Hct level can affect blood flow and prognosis even when Hct levels are not frankly polycythemic. The Hct level also has a heavy impact on blood viscosity.[254,255] Lowering the Hct from 45 to 32 results in doubling of CBF.[256] High Hct levels are a factor in reducing reperfusion of ischemic brain and are associated with larger brain infarcts.[257]

Sickle cell disease and other hemoglobinopathies can lead to altered flow and hypercoagulability. Sickle cell disease and spherocytosis are associated with multifocal brain infarcts. TCD documents abnormalities of flow velocities even in young patients with sickle cell disease. These abnormalities correlate well with regions of arterial narrowing and with the occurrence of strokes[258-260] and help select patients for prophylactic blood transfusions.[261,262]

Hemoglobin and Hct certainly should be measured in every patient with stroke. Hemodilution has been advocated as a measure to augment blood flow during acute ischemia. Lowering of relatively high Hct levels by blood donations has been advocated as a measure to prophylactically reduce the risk of stroke in stroke-prone individuals. Hemoglobin electrophoresis is important in those with racial and genetic predispositions to hemoglobinopathies, especially if anemia is present. Careful examination of a stained blood smear for the morphology of RBCs can suggest the possibility of a hemoglobinopathy. Severe anemia also can compound brain ischemia, but low Hct levels are not common in stroke patients.

Leukocytes

The white blood cell (WBC) count is often elevated in patients with myocardial infarction and is also often slightly elevated in patients with brain infarcts. Some have correlated a high WBC count with the severity of carotid atherosclerosis[263] and carotid[264] and aortic arch plaque[265] thickness but interpretation of this finding is clouded by the fact that cigarette smoking is one cause of a high WBC count. Patients with elevated WBC counts also seem to have reduced endothelial reactivity.[266] A relatively elevated WBC is also a marker predicting the likelihood of developing a first stroke.[267] A high WBC count is also a marker of inflammatory activity in the body and inflammation is an important cause of blood vessel damage.[268]

Leukemia with high WBC counts can cause packing of capillaries and small arterioles with aggregates of large WBCs, causing multiple small infarcts and hemorrhages. This is suggested, obviously, by a high leukocrit in the capillary tube used to measure Hct. Measurement of WBC count is usually a routine part of a complete blood cell count, which should be ordered on each stroke patient.

Platelets

Platelets are critical structures active in the initiation of blood coagulation. Evidence of the central importance of platelets in cerebrovascular disease is the enthusiasm clinicians have had for platelet inhibition as a major treatment for patients who have or are at risk of developing brain ischemia. Quantitative and qualitative platelet abnormalities can cause hypercoagulability and bleeding.[268a, 268b,269,270] Thrombocytosis, especially with platelet counts greater than 1 million, can cause hypercoagulability and vascular occlusion and brain infarction.[271-273] Platelet counts should be a routine part of the initial evaluation of patients with ischemic stroke because thrombocytosis can potentiate thrombosis. Low platelet counts can suggest the presence of other disorders, such as the antiphospholipid antibody syndrome, heparin-induced thrombocytopenia, consumptive coagulopathies, lupus erythematosus, and thrombotic thrombocytopenic purpura—all of which are often complicated by brain ischemia. Platelet counts can fall during the course of illness (e.g., after use of heparin),[274,275] so that a baseline count before treatment is useful for later comparison.

Some patients with platelet counts in the normal range have increased platelet aggregation and secretion, or qualitative abnormalities of platelet morphology and function. In vitro platelet function tests are usually performed in hematologic research laboratories, and even experts disagree on their applicability to the in vivo state. Platelet aggregation is usually measured after the addition of various agents known to increase aggregation, such as arachidonic acid, adenosine diphosphate, epinephrine, and collagen.[269,270,276] The extent of platelet activation can also be studied by measuring the levels of beta-thromboglobulin in the blood.[270,276-278] Beta-thromboglobulin is secreted during platelet-release reactions, and, when optimal venipuncture technique is used, the levels are good markers of

in vivo platelet activation and secretion. Simultaneous measurement of platelet factor 4, which has a short half-life, can help control in vitro platelet changes.[277,278] Heparin-induced thrombocytopenia is characterized by elevated anti-heparin/platelet factor 4 antibody titers and these can be measured in patients on heparin.[274,275,280]

Platelet production of thromboxane B2 can be performed by radioimmunoassays and von Willebrand factor antigen can also be quantified.[281-283] Polymorphisms in the platelet glycoprotein II/III fibrinogen receptor have been described; these may also predispose to hypercoagulability and brain and myocardial ischemia.[284]

Fibrinogen, Albumin and Globulins, Blood Viscosity, and Lipids

Fibrinogen is an important part of the coagulation system because fibrinogen is converted to fibrin monomers by the action of thrombin. Fibrin is an essential component of red and white thrombi. Fibrinogen also contributes to blood viscosity because high levels of fibrinogen can increase blood viscosity. Under ordinary circumstances, the Hct and fibrinogen levels are the two most important single predictors of whole-blood viscosity.[252,253]

Normal fibrinogen levels usually range from 250 to 400 mg/dL. High levels of fibrinogen have been shown to be risk factors for stroke in many studies.[285-291] Fibrinogen levels can also rise as acute-phase reactants in the early period after stroke. Ancrod (a defibrogenating enzyme of Malayan pit-viper venom), has been used to lower fibrinogen levels and to decrease fibrin formation, potentially lyse thrombi, and increase blood flow.[292,293] High fibrinogen levels decrease the likelihood of effective reperfusion after thrombolysis.[294]

Omega 3 fish oil preparations containing eicosapentaenoic acid may also act to decrease fibrinogen content.[295] Fibrinogen can also be mechanically removed from the blood. Heparin-mediated extracorporeal low-density lipoprotein precipitation is a system studied by Austrian physicians that removes fibrinogen as well as low-density lipoproteins from the blood and has the capability of quickly and significantly reducing fibrinogen blood levels.[296]

Patients with a predisposition to stroke recurrence have a slightly lower serum albumin level and albumin to globulin ratio than those without recurrence.[286,287] Abnormally high levels of immunoglobulins (Ig) A, IgG, and IgM can indicate autoimmune disease and can be a clue to diagnosis in patients with unexplained

4

brain ischemia. Macroglobulins found in Waldenström's macroglobulinemia and multiple myeloma also can increase blood viscosity and cause or potentiate multiple loci of ischemia. At present, immunoglobulin measurements are not a part of the routine evaluation of stroke patients because of their low yield. In selected patients with clinical and ophthalmoscopic suggestions of hyperviscosity, however, and in those with a high serum globulin level, serum immunoelectrophoresis can be helpful. Another unusual cause of hyperviscosity is a very high titer of lipoproteins. High levels of triglycerides, chylomicra, low-density and very-low-density lipoprotein cholesterol fractions can increase whole blood viscosity.[297,298] Measurement of blood lipids should be performed in every patient with brain ischemia and those with a family history of hyperlipidemia.

Studies have also shown that elevated levels of Lipoprotein (a) {Lp(a)} are an independent risk factor for stroke and other important cardiovascular conditions.[299-301] In a large study among 5888 community-dwelling individuals aged more than 65 years, men in the highest quintile of Lp(a) had three times the risk of stroke and three times the risk of vascular disease–related death compared to the lowest quintile.[299] High Lp(a) levels also have been correlated with the extent of symptomatic intracranial atherosclerosis.[301]

Studies of Coagulation Factors and Coagulation

The prothrombin time (PT) and the activated partial thromboplastin time (aPTT) are excellent screening tests of coagulation function and are routinely available in nearly all hospital laboratories. Measurement of the PT and the aPTT should be a part of the evaluation of all stroke patients. Indications for sometimes ordering other tests of coagulation are noted in Table 4-10.

Some serum proteins—such as antithrombin III, protein C, and protein S—are natural inhibitors of coagulation. A decrease in the level of these substances because of a familial inherited condition or an acquired disease can cause hypercoagulability. An inherited coagulation deficit,

usually referred to as resistance to activated protein C, has been described by Dutch investigators from Leiden.[302-305] In most instances, resistance to activated protein C is caused by a point mutation in the gene that encodes for coagulation factor V.[303] The presence of this mutation, called factor V Leiden, is accompanied by a threefold to fivefold increase in the frequency of venous thromboembolism in the lower extremities[305] and an increased frequency of cerebral venous thrombosis. Factor V Leiden is the most common recognized genetic disorder that leads to hypercoagulability. The second most common genetic mutation that leads to a prothrombotic state is a mutation in the gene encoding prothrombin.[304,306] This mutation involves a transition from guanine to adenine at position 20210 in the sequence of the 3' untranslated region of the prothrombin gene.[304,306] The frequency of cerebral and peripheral venous thrombosis is greatly increased in carriers of the prothrombin gene mutation, especially if they also take oral contraceptive pills.[307] Genetic analysis is warranted in patients with unexplained hypercoagulability, especially those with cerebral venous thrombosis and recurrent peripheral venous thromboembolism.

The level of coagulation factors VII, VIII, IX, and X can be measured in most hematologic laboratories but have not been well studied in large groups of stroke patients. Abnormal levels of factor VIII can cause hypercoagulability and recurrent strokes.[308-310] Factor VIII elevation can be chronic, precede and predispose to stroke, increase as an acute-phase reactant in systemic illnesses such as ulcerative colitis, and can increase secondary to thrombosis. In the latter case, it is a marker and not the cause of the thrombosis.[308-310] High levels of factor VIII activity have been correlated with carotid and coronary atherosclerosis.[311] Levels of other factors have been explored and may be utilized more in the future. High levels of plasma von Willebrand factor increase the risk of stroke and other vascular events in patients with atrial fibrillation,[312] and is a risk factor for first ischemic strokes.[313]

Hemostatic markers of coagulation activity have been used to detect and monitor hypercoagulability.[314] Thrombin acts as a catalyst of

---

Table 4-10.   Potential Reasons to Order Coagulation Testing for Ischemic Stroke Patients

Hypercoagulable state is suspected by acceleration of PT or aPTT.
Multiple vascular occlusions are present and no cardiac source of embolism has been detected.
Occlusion of veins in the upper or lower extremities and the presence of an ischemic stroke.
Dural sinus and/or cerebral venous occlusions.
A past history of recurrent thrombophlebitis or miscarriages.
Known neoplastic, collagen vascular, rheumatologic, or inflammatory diseases are present.

the proteolysis of fibrinogen to fibrin. During this reaction, fibrinopeptide A is generated. The level of fibrin D-dimer is also an index of fibrin generation. The level of the prothrombin activation fragment F1.2 is a measure of in vivo thrombin generation. Increasing intensity of anticoagulation is accompanied by decreasing thrombin generation as measured by the F1.2 levels.[315] Fibrinolysis involves the dissolution of fibrin by endogenous fibrinolytic mechanisms. Fibrinolytic activity can be estimated by the levels of fibrinopeptide B-beta 1-42 and of tissue plasminogen activator and its inhibitor. Thrombosis is favored when thrombin proteolysis of fibrinogen (increased fibrinopeptide A and D-dimer levels) exceeds plasmin proteolysis (increased fibrinopeptide B-beta 1-42 and tissue plasminogen activator to its inhibitor ratio).[278,316-319] Several studies have monitored the levels of these substances in acute stroke patients and during follow-up.[275,314,319] D-dimer testing has been used to monitor the continued need for anticoagulation in patients with venous thromboembolism.[320]

Antiphospholipid Antibodies

Antiphospholipid antibodies (APLAs) are usually IgG or IgM antibodies that bind to negatively charged phospholipids. Phospholipids are important constituents of vascular endothelium, heart proteins, platelets, and other cells.[321-323] Laboratory studies show that sera from patients with APLAs have increased immunoglobulin binding to cerebral endothelium.[323] The two most commonly measured APLAs are anticardiolipin antibody and the so-called lupus anticoagulant (LA). LAs are acquired immunoglobulins that are associated clinically with thrombosis, not bleeding; most patients with LA do not have systemic lupus erythematosus. The laboratory hallmark of LA is a prolonged aPTT that does not correct when normal plasma is added. This indicates the presence of an inhibitor of clotting rather than a deficiency of a necessary coagulation factor.

LA can be sought using a sensitive phospholipid reagent, the kaolin clotting time, or the Russell viper venom time.[321,322] Anticardiolipin antibodies of the IgG or IgM types can be measured as well as more specific antibodies to beta-2-glycoprotein 1. IgG antibody levels, especially those greater than 40 GPL (IgG phospholipid) units, correlate with a relatively high risk of stroke and recurrent stroke.[325] Antiphospholipid antibodies are actually antibodies to a protein, most often beta-2-glycoprotein 1, that is usually bound to a phospholipid.[326] Measurement of beta-2-glycoprotein 1 antibodies is often useful in defining autoimmune activity. Two other antibodies, antiphosphatidyl serine[327] and antiphosphatylinositol,[328] show a high correlation with ischemic stroke especially in the young and in those without another determined cause.[329] The screening tests for syphilis—the VDRL and Reiter protein reaction—depend on the activity of APLAs. False-positive serologic tests for syphilis are often found in patients with APLAs, and thrombocytopenia is present in a third of APLA-positive patients. The clinical syndrome consists of frequent venous and arterial thrombotic events, such as thrombophlebitis, pulmonary embolism, TIAs, strokes, myocardial infarctions, and recurrent fetal loss in women.[321-323] It is likely that the mechanism of recurrent brain ischemia is excessive clotting. APLAs may be directed against the endothelium or platelet membranes and may alter coagulability and vascular functions. APLAs should be measured in situations in which the usual risk factors for ischemic stroke are not present, and certainly in patients with livedo reticularis and strokes (Sneddon's syndrome), and those patients with clinical features matching the primary APLA syndrome.[321-329] Table 4-11 suggests a screening battery in patients suspected of having ischemic strokes related to hypercoagulability.

Table 4-11. Suggested Hypercoagulability Screening Battery

Genetic test for factor V Leiden mutation or coagulation assay for activated protein C resistance
  (if abnormal confirm genetically)
Genetic test for prothrombin G20210A mutation
Functional assay of antithrombin
Functional assay of protein C
Functional assay of protein S and measurements of total and free protein S antigen
Homocysteine
Factor VIII level
Lupus anticoagulant, cardiolipin antibodies, beta-2 glycoprotein 1 antibodies

Note: Ken Bauer, MD, Hematology-Coagulation Department, Harvard Medical School, assisted with the preparation of this table.

Other Blood Measurements

After the demonstration that sugar administration could worsen experimentally induced brain ischemia,[330,331] Plum and colleagues[332,333] noted a poorer prognosis in stroke patients with elevated blood sugar levels. Because blood sugar is a critical metabolite for the brain, there is no doubt that abnormally low levels can be deleterious to patients with stroke. Elevated levels of blood sugar are also often associated with an increased risk of brain damage in patients with brain ischemia and hemorrhage. Blood sugar elevation can be triggered by tissue damage with release of catecholamines and mobilization of sugar. Large infarcts and hemorrhages are often associated with elevations in the blood sugar level.

Patients with hypercalcemia due to hyperparathyroidism also have a higher frequency of stroke, probably due to the vascular and platelet effects of calcium.[334-337] Low serum magnesium can have a similar effect to hypercalcemia. Dehydration diminishes blood volume, thus potentially decreasing blood flow. Measurements of blood urea nitrogen and electrolytes are useful in determining the presence and degree of dehydration and would show important electrolyte imbalance. Blood lipids, including total cholesterol and fractionation into high-density lipoprotein and low-density lipoprotein components, should be measured in each patient with brain ischemia. Markedly increased levels of triglycerides, low-density lipoproteins, and chylomicra can increase blood viscosity. These levels are useful to analyze in patients with known familial hyperlipidemia, premature atherosclerosis, and patients who have clinical hyperviscosity syndromes. A clue to the presence of chylomicra is the presence of milky, lipemic serum, especially after a meal.

> Patient JH had an Hct of 41 and normal WBC and platelet counts. The PT and aPTT were also normal. Renal function and electrolytes were normal. Blood sugar on admission was 145, but levels returned to normal after a few days. HDL cholesterol level was 40 and LDL cholesterol 185.

Other Blood Testing That Reflects Risk Factors

Some measurements are useful in assessing risk factors for stroke and other cardiovascular diseases especially in patients seen in an outpatient setting. In some patients primary stroke prevention is considered, others have already had one or more strokes and secondary prevention of another stroke is the consideration. Since prevention has been shown to be most effective when patients are studied in the hospital and preventive measures are begun at discharge,[338,339] I find it useful to measure these risk factors in the hospital, recognizing that sometimes some elevations may represent acute-phase reactions and not persist later. In that case the measurements should be repeated when the patients are seen as ambulatory patients in follow-up.

An elevated erythrocyte sedimentation rate can be an important clue to the presence of a systemic inflammatory disease or unsuspected vasculitis. It should be ordered in patients with suspected temporal arteritis and in young and elderly patients with unexplained strokes. Studies now also show that elevated C-reactive protein (CRP) and fibrinogen levels as well as homocysteine are risk factors for coronary heart disease, peripheral arterial disease, and stroke.

Elevated homocysteine levels have convincingly been shown to correlate with the risk of ischemic stroke and with large-artery atherosclerosis.[340-345] Homocysteine is a sulfur containing amino acid derived from the metabolism of methionine that circulates bound to plasma proteins. Folic acid, pyridoxine, and B_{12} intake and metabolism are important determinants of homocysteine blood levels. A deficiency in methylenetetrahydrofolate reductase (MTHFR) caused by a polymorphism in the A677V MTHFR gene is a common and important cause of a high homocysteine level.[344] Vegetarians and those with low serum vitamin levels are especially likely to have high serum homocysteine levels. Homocysteine has been associated with hypercoagulability—especially dural sinus thrombosis and with endothelial injury.[305] I have seen a number of patients with very high serum homocysteine levels (>40 μmol/L) who had multiple lacunar-like infarcts in the absence of other risk factors. Homocysteine serum levels are worth measuring, although it is unclear whether vitamin treatment alters the course of vascular disease except in patients with very low B_{12} levels.

Studies now show convincingly that elevated high-sensitivity CRP levels correlate with a risk of stroke, cardiovascular disease, and carotid and intracranial large-artery atherosclerosis.[339,346-349a] CRP is an acute-phase protein discovered in the 1930s that was named for its reaction with the C-polysaccharide cell wall of *Streptococcus pneumoniae*. It is produced in the liver and is a final common pathway of cytokine activation and is produced in response to a variety of infectious and inflammatory stimuli. Some patients with significant atherosclerotic lesions have normal lipids, but high CRP levels, indicating the likely importance of inflammation in contributing to their vascular disease.[340] C-reactive protein levels are also an important measure of activity in patients with temporal arteritis and Takayasu's arteritis.[350]

Measurement of the ESR, fibrinogen level, HDL and LDL cholesterol, high-sensitivity CRP, and homocysteine are useful in suggesting and quantifying the risk of vascular disease and hopefully contributing to preventive measures. I believe they are important to study in patients suspected of having cerebrovascular disease. Table 4-12 notes my suggestions for laboratory testing in patients with ischemic strokes, TIAs, and known cervicocranial arterial lesions.

What if the Patient Has Intracerebral Hemorrhage or Subarachnoid Hemorrhage?

Bleeding diatheses are important causes of intracranial bleeding. Probably the most common bleeding disorders are now iatrogenic, including the use of heparins, warfarin compounds, rt-PA and other fibrinolytic compounds, and possibly the use of aspirin and other antiplatelet substances. Usually, these clinical situations are known and are not diagnostic dilemmas. Hereditary bleeding disorders such as hemophilia are usually well known to both patients and physicians and most patients have had prior systemic hemorrhages before intracranial bleeding events. Thrombocytopenia is another important cause of intracranial bleeding. More recently attention has been focused on an acquired hemorrhagic condition dubbed "hemophilia A," a severe autoimmune bleeding disorder resulting from the presence of autoantibodies directed against clotting factor VIII.[351,352]

A history of prior bleeding episodes (vaginal, dental, postoperative, and so forth) and the presence of systemic purpura or active gum, urine, or bowel bleeding are the best clues to the presence of a bleeding diathesis.

Measurement of PT and partial thromboplastin time (PTT) are usually sufficient to screen for these disorders. Platelet counts detect thrombocytopenia, and the bleeding time is a useful screening procedure measuring platelet function, among other conditions. Hemophilia and other lifelong bleeding diatheses are usually known before the intracranial bleed occurs. Measurement of antihemophilic globulin, antibodies to factor VIII, and other coagulation factors is helpful in patients with previously uncharacterized bleeding disorders.

QUESTION 5: IS THE PATIENT WITH STROKE OR TRANSIENT NEUROLOGIC DEFICITS HAVING SEIZURES?

Electrical Tests of Brain Function

Electroencephalography (EEG) is the oldest available noninvasive test of brain function. Experience has shown that the use of EEG in stroke diagnosis and management is very limited. There are, however, occasional circumstances in which EEG is quite helpful. Seizures and postictal neurologic signs can mimic TIAs. In some patients with stroke or other central nervous system lesions, worsening of a neurologic deficit is caused by clinically unapparent or subtle seizure activity, which is usually dramatically captured by EEG. Some patients with recent-onset strokes, especially those caused by subcortical ICHs or cerebral embolism, have seizures. Patients with acute pontine ischemia or hemorrhage can have unusual limb movements that are easily confused with seizures by those inexperienced with brainstem strokes.[353,354]

In patients in whom the differential diagnosis is between seizures and other transient neurologic conditions EEG can document seizure discharges

Table 4-12. **Suggestions for Blood Testing in All Patients with Ischemic Stroke or TIA**
Hemoglobin
Hematocrit
WBC count (and differential if abnormally high or low)
Platelet count
Activated partial thromboplastin time (APTT)
Prothrombin time (PT)—International Normalized ratio
Serum fibrinogen level
Blood sugar
Serum calcium
Total cholesterol and high-density lipoprotein (HDL) and low-density lipoprotein (LDL) cholesterol
Blood urea nitrogen
Electrolytes (sodium, chloride, potassium, and carbon dioxide)
Homocysteine
C-reactive protein
Erythrocyte sedimentation rate (ESR)

4

or show an EEG suggestive of a seizure disorder. In patients with strokes and known seizures or in less than fully alert patients in whom seizures are a potential cause of decreased alertness, sequential EEGs can document and quantify seizure discharge and thereby guide anticonvulsant management. EEG monitoring of acute stroke patients shows a previously unexpected frequency of seizure activity.[355] Seizures are also quite common in the days, months, and few years after stroke and EEGs can be quite helpful in these patients.[355]

EEGs can also be recorded during somatosensory, visual, and auditory stimuli, and while the patient is performing various cognitive tasks. Computers then subtract the baseline electrical activity and generate a printout of that part of the electrical activity directly attributable to the stimulus and the task-related evoked potentials. Evoked potentials can also be studied via topographic mapping techniques to better localize the abnormalities. These techniques are particularly useful in unresponsive patients, especially after cardiac arrest, when it is impossible to clinically assess cognitive and sensory functions, and in patients under anesthesia.[357-359] In patients with brainstem disease, both brainstem auditory evoked responses and quantified testing of the blink and masseter reflexes can help localize the functional abnormality to particular portions of the brainstem.[360]

These electrical tests are most helpful in answering the following questions: Is the patient having seizures? How much residual electrical activity is present in this comatose patient's cerebrum, and what is the prognosis for long-term outcome? Is this anesthetized patient now having cerebrovascular surgery undergoing damage during the procedure? Are there functional changes in the brain or brainstem not shown by brain-imaging techniques?

> In JH, I did not perform functional imaging or electrical testing. His clinical deficit was severe, and morphologic studies (CT) had shown an extensive infarct. Moreover, his vascular lesion was not treatable. Newer MR technologies were not available at the time he was treated.

QUESTION 6: ARE THERE GENETIC ABNORMALITIES THAT MIGHT CLARIFY THE ETIOLOGY OF THE CEREBROVASCULAR DISEASE AND POTENTIALLY GUIDE TREATMENT OF THE PATIENT AND PREVENTION OR MANAGEMENT OF RELATIVES?

During the last quarter-century, there has been a revolution in molecular biology and genetics. Genetic influences clearly play a large influence in determining who will develop strokes and which subtypes of stroke.[361-363,363a,b] A stimulus to further genetic research was the finding by deCODE genetics that polymorphisms of the phosphodiesterase 4D, camp-specific (PDE4D) gene were prevalent in patients with stroke.[364-366] Genetic analysis of mutations has become instrumental in the diagnosis and understanding of some specific and genetic and mitochondrial diseases.[367-369] A number of genetic disorders have been shown to cause abnormal bleeding and hypercoagulability. Further advances are likely in coming years. The availability of high-density microarrays that allow rapid screening of genome-wide sets that range from 100,000 to more than a million single-nucleotide polymorphisms (SNPs), shows promise of revealing important genetic associations with stroke and stroke risk factors. Pinpointing the genetic etiology and influences on cerebrovascular disease can help the patient's relatives and progeny as well as the patient. I have not included a discussion of molecular biology and genetics in this fourth edition because I personally know little about this field that is developing very quickly. I discuss some specific genetic disorders in Chapter 11 on nonatherosclerotic causes of brain ischemia.

References

1. Eckert B, Zeumer H: Brain computed tomography. In Ginsberg MD, Bogousslavsky J (eds): Cerebrovascular Disease: Pathophysiology, Diagnosis, and Management, vol 2. Boston: Blackwell Science, 1998, pp 1241-1264.
2. von Kummer R, Nolte PN, Schnittger H, et al: Detectability of cerebral hemisphere ischaemic infarcts by CT within 6 hours of stroke. Neuroradiology 1996;38:31-33.
3. Moulin T, Cattin F, Crepin-Leblond T, et al: Early CT signs in acute middle cerebral artery infarction: Predictive value for subsequent infarct location and outcome. Neurology 1996;47:366-375.
4. Norman D, Price D, Boyd D, et al: Quantitative aspects of computed tomography of the blood and cerebrospinal fluid. Radiology 1977;7:223-228.
5. Caplan LR, Flamm ES, Mohr JP, et al: Lumbar puncture and stroke: A statement for physicians by a committee of the Stroke Council of the American Heart Association. Stroke 1987;18:540A-544A.
6. Edlow JA, Caplan LR: Primary care: Avoiding pitfalls in the diagnosis of subarachnoid hemorrhage. N Engl J Med 2000;341:29-36.
7. Beauchamp NJ, Bryan RN: Neuroimaging of Stroke. In Welch KMA, Caplan LR, Reis DJ, Siesjo BK, Weir B (eds): Primer on Cerebrovascular Diseases. San Diego: Academic Press, 1997, pp 599-611.
8. Baird AE, Warach S: Magnetic resonance imaging of acute stroke. J Cereb Blood Flow Metab 1998;18:583-609.

9. Warach S, Chien D, Li W, et al: Fast magnetic resonance diffusion-weighted imaging of acute human stroke. Neurology 1992;42:1717-1723.

10. Warach S, Gaa J, Siewert B, et al: Acute human stroke studied by whole brain echo planar diffusion-weighted magnetic resonance imaging. Ann Neurol 1995;37:231-141.

11. Lansberg MG, Norbash AM, Marks MP, et al: Advantages of adding diffusion-weighted magnetic resonance imaging to conventional imaging for evaluating acute stroke. Arch Neurol 2000;57:1311-1316.

12. Engelter ST, Wetzel SG, Radue EW, et al: The clinical significance of diffusion-weighted imaging in infratentorial strokes. Neurology 2004;62:574-580.

13. Brant-Zawadski M, Atkinson D, Detrick M, et al: Fluid-attenuated inversion recovery (FLAIR) for assessment of cerebral infarction: Initial clinical experience in 50 patients. Stroke 1996;27:1187-1191.

14. Kang DW, Chalela JA, Ezzeddline MA, Warach S: Association of ischemic lesion patterns on early diffusion-weighted imaging with TOAST stroke subtypes. Arch Neurol 2003;60:1730-1734.

15. Bonati LH, Lyrer PA, Wetzel SG, et al: Diffusion-weighted imaging, apparent diffusion coefficient maps and stroke etiology. J Neurol 2005;252:1387-1393.

16. Bonati LH, Kessel-Schaefer A, Linka AZ, et al: Diffusion-weighted imaging in stroke attributable to patent foramen ovale. Stroke 2006;37:20:2030-2034.

17. Kidwell CS, Alger JR, Di Salle F, et al: Diffusion MRI in patients with transient ischemic attacks. Stroke 1999;30:1174-1180.

18. Lecouvet FE, Duprez TP, Raymackers JM, et al: Resolution of early diffusion-weighted and FLAIR MRI abnormalities in a patient with TIA. Neurology 1999;52:1085-1087.

19. Neumann-Haefelin T, Wittsack HJ, Wenserki F, et al: Diffusion- and perfusion-weighted MRI in a patient with prolonged reversible ischaemic neurological deficit. Neuroradiology 2000;42:444-447.

20. Patel MR, Edelman RR, Warach S: Detection of hyperacute primary intraparenchymal hemorrhage by magnetic resonance imaging. Stroke 1996;27:2321-2324.

21. Linfante I, Llinas RH, Caplan LR, Warach S: MRI features of intracerebral hemorrhage within 2 hours from symptom onset. Stroke 2002;30:2263-2267.

22. Chalela JA, Latour LL, Jeffries N, et al: Hemorrhage and early MRI evaluation from the emergency room (HEME-ER): A prospective single center comparison of MRI to CT for the emergency diagnosis of intracranial hemorrhage in patients with suspected acute cerebrovascular disease. Stroke 2003;34:239-240.

23. Schellinger PD, Fiebach JB, Mohr A, et al: The role of stroke MRI in intracranial and subarachnoid hemorrhage. Nervenarzt 2001;72:907-917.

24. Schellinger PD, Jansen O, Fiebach JB, et al: A standardized MRI protocol comparison with CT in hyperacute intracerebral hemorrhage. Stroke 1999;30:765-768.

25. Assouline E, Benziane K, Reizine D, et al: Intra-arterial thrombus visualized on T2 gradient echo imaging in acute ischemic stroke. Cerebrovasc Dis 2005;20:6-11.

26. Dul K, Drayer BP: CT and MR imaging of intracerebral hemorrhage. In Kase CS, Caplan LR (eds): Intracerebral Hemorrhage. Boston: Butterworth-Heinemann, 1994, pp 73-93.

27. Rumboldt Z, Kalousek M, Castillo M: Hyperacute subarachnoid hemorrhage on T2-weighted MR images. AJNR Am J Neuroradiol 2003;24:472-475.

28. Becker H, Desch H, Hacker H, et al: CT fogging effect with ischemic cerebral infarcts. Neuroradiol 1978;18:185-192.

29. Nicolaides AN, Kalodiki E, Ramaswami G, et al: The significance of cerebral infarcts on CT scans in patients with transient ischemic attacks. In Bernstein EF, Callow AD, Nicolaides AN, Shifrin EG (eds): Cerebral Revascularisation. London, Med-Orion, 1993, pp 159-178.

30. Inatomi Y, Kimura K, Yonehara T, et al: DWI abnormlities and clinical characteristics in TIA patients. Neurology 2004;62:376-380.

31. Winbeck K, Bruckmaier K, Etgen T, et al: Transient ischemic attack and stroke can be differentiated by analyzing early diffusion-weighted imaging signal intensity changes. Stroke 2004;35:1095-1099.

32. Lamy C, Oppenheim C, Calvet D, et al: Diffusion-weighted MR imaging in transient ischaemic attacks. Eur Radiol 2006;16:1090-1095.

33. Bykowski J, Latour LL, Warach S: More accurate identification of reversible ischemic injury in human stroke by cerebrospinal fluid suppressed diffusion-weighted imaging. Stroke 2004;35:1100-1106.

33a. Prabhakaran S, Chong JY, Sacco RL: Impact of abnormal diffusion-weighted imaging results on short-term outcome following transient ischemic attack. Arch Neurol 2007;64:1105-1109.

33b. Redgrave JNE, Coutts SB, Schulz UG, et al: Systematic review of associations between the presence of acute ischemic lesions on diffusion-weighted imaging and clinical predictors of early stroke risk after transient ischemic attack. Stroke 2007;38:1482-1488.

33c. Sylaja PN, Coutts SB, Subramaniam S, et al: Acute ischemic lesions of varying ages predict risk of ischemic events in stroke/TIA patients. Neurology 2007;68:415-419.

33d. Caplan LR: Transient ischemic attack with abnormal diffusion-weighted imaging results. What's in a name? Arch Neurol 2007;64:1080-1082.

34. Adams Jr HP, Kassell NF, Turner JC, et al: CT and clinical correlations in recent aneurysmal subarachnoid hemorrhage: A preliminary report of the Cooperative Aneurysm Study. Neurology 1983;33:981-988.

35. Fishman RA: Cerebrospinal fluid in cerebrovascular disorders. In Barnett HJM, Mohr JP, Stein BM, Yatsu FJ (eds): Stroke: Pathophysiology, Diagnosis, and Management. New York: Churchill Livingstone, 1986, pp 109-117.

36. Schluep M, Bogousslavsky J: Cerebrospinal fluid in cerebrovascular disease. In Ginsberg MD, Bogousslavsky J (eds): Cerebrovascular Disease: Pathophysiology, Diagnosis, and Management, vol 2. Boston: Blackwell Science, 1998, pp 1221-1226.

37. Van der Meulen JP: Cerebrospinal fluid xanthrochromia: An objective index. Neurology 1966;16:170-178.

38. Soderstrom CE: Diagnostic significance of CSF spectrophotometry and computer tomography in cerebrovascular disease: A comparative study in 231 cases. Stroke 1977;8:606-612.

39. Davalos A, Blanco M, Pedraza S, et al: The clinical-DWI mismatch: A new diagnostic approach to the brain tissue at risk of infarction. Neurology. 2004;62:2187-2192.

40. Caplan LR: Significance of unexpected (silent) brain infarcts. In Caplan LR, Shifrin EG, Nicolaides AN, Moore WS (eds): Cerebrovascular Ischaemia: Investigation and Management. London: Med-Orion, 1996, pp 423-433.

41. Yamamoto H, Bogousslavsky J: Mechanisms of second and further strokes. J Neurol Neurosurg Psychiatry 1998;64:771-776.

42. Caplan LR: Reperfusion of ischemic brain: Why and why not? In Hacke W, del Zoppo G, Hirschberg M (eds): Thrombolytic Therapy in Acute Stroke. Berlin: Springer, 1991, pp 36-45.

43. Ropper AH: Lateral displacement of the brain and level of consciousness in patients with an acute hemispheral mass. N Engl J Med 1986;314:953-958.

44. Ropper AH: A preliminary MRI study of the geometry of brain displacement and level of consciousness with acute intracranial masses. Neurology 1989;39:622-627.

44a. Lansberg MG, Thijs VN, O'Brien MW, et al: Evolution of apparent diffusion coefficient, diffusion-weighted, and T2-weighted signal intensity of acute stroke. AJNR Am J Neuroradiol 2001;22:637-644.

45. Weisberg LA, Stazio A, Shamsnia M, et al: Non-traumatic parenchymal brain hemorrhages. Medicine (Baltimore) 1990;69:277-295.

46. Kase CS: Cerebral amyloid angiopathy. In Kase CS, Caplan LR (eds): Intracerebral Hemorrhage. Boston: Butterworth-Heinemann, 1994, pp 179-200.

47. Hauw J-J, Seilhean D, Duyckaerts CH: Cerebral amyloid angiopathy. In Ginsberg MD, Bogousslavsky J (eds): Cerebrovascular Disease: Pathophysiology, Diagnosis, and Management. Boston: Blackwell, 1998, pp 1772-1794.

48. Kase C, Robinson R, Stein R, et al: Anticoagulant-related intracerebral hemorrhages. Neurology 1985;35:943-948.

49. Kase CS: Bleeding disorders. In Kase CS, Caplan LR (eds): Intracerebral Hemorrhage. Boston: Butterworth-Heinemann, 1994, pp 117-151.

50. Weisberg L: Computed tomography in aneurysmal subarachnoid hemorrhage. Neurology 1979;29:802-808.

51. Adams H, Kassell N, Torner J, et al: CT and clinical correlations in recent aneurysmal subarachnoid hemorrhage: A preliminary report of the cooperative aneurysm study. Neurology 1983;33:981-988.

52. van Gijn J, van Dongen K: Computerized tomography in subarachnoid hemorrhage: Difference between patients with and without an aneurysm on angiography. Neurology 1980;30:538-539.

53. van Gijn J, van Dongen KJ, Vermeulen M, et al: Perimesencephalic hemorrhage: A non-aneurysmal and benign form of subarachnoid hemorrhage. Neurology 1985;35:493-497.

54. Rinkel GJ, Wijdicks EF, Vermeulen M, et al: Outcome in perimesencephalic (non-aneurysmal) subarachnoid hemorrhage: A follow-up study in 37 patients. Neurology 1990;40:1130-1132.

55. Kistler JP, Crowell R, Davis K, et al: The relation of cerebral vasospasm to the extent and location of subarachnoid blood visualized by CT scan: A prospective study. Neurology 1983;33:424-437.

56. Mohsen F, Pominis S, Illingworth R: Prediction of delayed cerebral ischemia after subarachnoid hemorrhage by computed tomography. J Neurol Neurosurg Psychiatry 1984;47:1197-1202.

57. Kern R, Szabo K, Hennerici M, Meairs S: Characterization of carotid artery plaques using real-time compound B-mode ultrasound. Stroke 2004;35:870-875.

58. Landry A, Spence JD, Fenster A: Measurement of carotid plaque volume by 3-dimensional ultrasound. Stroke 2004;35:864-869.

59. O'Donnell TF, Erdoes L, Mackey W, et al: Correlation of B-mode ultrasound imaging and arteriography with pathologic findings at carotid endarterectomy. Arch Surg 1985;120:443-449.

60. Hennerici M, Baezner H, Daffertshofer M: Ultrasound of cervical arteries. In Caplan LR, Manning WJ (eds): Brain Embolism. New York: Informa Healthcare, 2006, pp 223-242.

61. Schenk EA, Bond G, Aretz T, et al: Multicenter validation study of real-time ultrasonography, arteriography and pathology: Pathologic evaluation of carotid endarterectomy specimens. Stroke 1988;19:289-296.

62. Hennerici M, Meairs S: Imaging arterial wall disease. Cerebrovasc Dis 2000;10(Suppl 5):9-20.

63. Gronholdt M-LM, Nordestgaard BG, Nielsen TG, Sillesen H: Echolucent carotid artery plaques are associated with elevated levels of fasting and postprandial triglyceride-rich lipoproteins. Stroke 1996;27:2166-2172.

64. Geroulakos G, Hobson RW, Nicolaides AW: Ultrasonic carotid plaque morphology. In Caplan LR, Shifrin EG, Nicolaides AN, Moore WS (eds): Cerebrovascular Ischaemia: Investigation and Management. London: Med-Orion, 1996, pp 25-32.

65. O'Leary DH, Polka JF, Kronmal RA, et al: Thickening of the carotid wall: A marker for atherosclerosis in the elderly? Stroke 1996;27:224-231.

66. Bots ML, Hoes AW, Koudstaal PJ, et al: Common carotid intima-media thickness and risk of stroke and myocardial infarction: The Rotterdam Study. Circulation 1997;96:1432-1437.

67. O'Leary DH, Polak JF, Kronmal RA, et al: Carotid artery intima and media thickness as a risk factor for myocardial infarction and stroke risk in older adults. N Engl J Med 1999;340:14-22.

67a. Yakushiji Y, Yasaka M, Takada T, Minematsu K: Serial transoral carotid ultrasonographic findings in extracranial internal carotid artery dissection. J Ultrasound Med 2005;24:877-880.

67b. Yakushijji Y, Takase Y, Kosugi M, et al: Transoral carotid ultrasonography is useful for detection and follow-up of extracranial internal carotid artery dissecting aneurysm. Cerebrovasc Dis 2007;24:144-146.

68. Forteza A, Krejza J, Koch S, Babikian V: Ultrasound imaging of cerebrovascular disease. In Babikian VL, Wechsler LR, Higashida RT (eds): Imaging Cerebrovascular Disease. Philadelphia: Butterworth-Heinemann, 2003, pp 3-35.

69. von Reutern GM, von Budingen HJ: Ultrasound diagnosis of cerebrovascular disease. New York: Georg Thieme, 1993.

70. Bartels E: Color-Coded Duplex Ultrasonography of the Cerebral Vessels. Stuttgart: Schattauer, 1998.

71. Steinke W, Kloetzsch C, Hennerici M: Carotid artery disease assessed by color Doppler flow imaging: correlation with standard Doppler sonography and angiography. AJNR Am J Neuroradiol 1990;11:259-266.

72. Steinke W, Hennerici M, Rautenberg W, Mohr JP: Symptomatic and asymptomatic high-grade carotid stenosis in Doppler color-flow imaging. Neurology 1992;42;131-138.

73. Steinke W, Ries S, Artemis N, et al: Power Doppler imaging of carotid artery stenosis. Comparison with color Doppler flow imaging and angiography. Stroke 1997;28:1981-1987.

74. Griewing B, Doherty C, Kessler CH: Power Doppler ultrasound examination of the intracerebral and extracerebral vasculature. J Neuroimaging 1996;6:32-35.

74a. Lenzi GL, Vicenzini E: The ruler is dead: An analysis of carotid plaque motion. Cerebrovasc Dis 2007;23:121-125.

75. Aaslid R: Transcranial Doppler Sonography. New York: Springer, 1986.

76. Alexandrov AV (ed): Cerebrovascular Ultrasound in Stroke Prevention and Treatment. New York: Futura Blackwell Publishing, 2003.

77. Molina CA, Alexandrov AV: Transcranial Doppler ultrasound. In Caplan LR, Manning WJ (eds): Brain Embolism. New York: Informa Healthcare, 2006, pp 113-128.

78. Babikian VL, Wechsler LR (eds): Transcranial Doppler Ultrasonography, 2nd ed. Boston: Butterworth-Heinemann, 1999.

79. Otis SM, Ringelstein EB: The transcranial Doppler examination: Principles and applications of transcranial doppler sonography. In Tegeler CH, Babikian VL, Gomez CR (eds): Neurosonology. St Louis: Mosby, 1996, pp 113-128.

80. Gomez CR, Brass LM, Tegeler CH, et al: The transcranial Doppler standardization project. Phase 1 results. The TCD Study Group, American Society of Neuroimaging. J Neuroimaging 1993;3:190-192.

81. Caplan LR, Brass LM, DeWitt LD, et al: Transcranial Doppler ultrasound: Present status. Neurology 1990;40:696-700.

82. Hennerici M, Rautenberg W, Sitzer G, et al: Transcranial Doppler ultrasound for the assessment of intracranial arterial flow velocity. Surg Neurol 1987;27:439-448.

83. Hennerici M, Rautenberg W, Schwartz A: Transcranial Doppler ultrasound for the assessment of intracranial arterial flow velocity. II. Evaluation of intracranial arterial disease. Surg Neurol 1987;27:523-532.

84. Demchuk A, Christou I, Wein T, et al: Accuracy and criteria for localizing arterial occlusion with transcranial Doppler. J Neuroimaging 2000;10:1-12.

85. Demchuk AM, Christou I, Wein T, et al: Specific transcranial Doppler flow findings related to the presence and site of arterial occlusion. Stroke 2000;31:140-146.

86. Baumgartner RW: Transcranial color duplex sonography in cerebrovascular disease: A systematic review. Cerebrovasc Dis 2003;16:4-13.

87. Krejza J, Baumagartner RW: Clinical applications of transcranial color-coded duplex sonography. J Neuroimaging 2004;14:215-225.

88. Burns PN: Overview of echo-enhanced vascular ultrasound imaging for clinical diagnosis in neurosonology. J Neuroimaging 1997;7(Suppl 1): S2-S14.

89. Bogdahn U, Becker G, Schlief R, et al: Contrast-enhanced transcranial color-coded real-time sonography. Stroke 1993;24:676-684.

90. Delcker A, Turowski B: Diagnostic value of three-dimensional transcranial contrast duplex sonography. J Neuroimaging 1997;7:139-144.

91. Stolz E, Kaps M: New techniques in ultrasound. In Babikian VL, Wechsler LR, Higashida RT (eds): Imaging Cerebrovascular Disease. Philadelphia: Butterworth-Heinemann, 2003, pp 383-401.

91a. Sharma VK, Tsivgoulis G, Lao AY, Alexandrov AV: Role of transcranial Doppler ultrasonography in evaluation of patients with cerebrovascular disease. Curr Neurol Neurosci Rep 2007;7:8-20.

91b. Tsivgoulis G, Sharma VK, Lao AY, et al: Validation of transcranial Doppler with computed tomography angiography in acute cerebral ischemia. Stroke 2007;38:1245-1249.

91c. Sharma VK, Tsivgoulis G, Lao AY, et al: Noninvasive detection of diffuse intracranaial disease. Stroke 2007;38:3175-3181.

92. Caplan LR: Posterior Circulation Disease: Clinical Findings, Diagnosis, and Management. Boston: Blackwell, 1996.

4

93. Sliwka U, Rautenberg W: Multimodal ultrasound versus angiography for imaging the vertebrobasilar circulation. J Neuroimaging 1998;8:182.

94. Seiler RW, Grolimund P, Asaslid R, et al: Cerebral vasospasm evaluated by transcranial ultrasound correlated with clinical grade and CT-visualized subarachnoid hemorrhage. J Neurosurg 1986;64:594-600.

95. Becker G, Greiner K, Kaune B, et al: Diagnosis and monitoring of subarachnoid hemorrhage by transcranial color-coded real time sonography. Neurosurgery 1991;28:814-820.

96. Chaudhuri R, Padayachee TS, Lewis RR, et al: Non-invasive assessment of the circle of Willis using transcranial pulsed Doppler ultrasound with angiographic correlation. Clin Radiol 1992;46:193-197.

97. Anzola GP, Gasparotti R, Magoni M, Prandini F: Transcranial Doppler sonography and magnetic resonance angiography in the assessment of collateral hemispheric flow in patients with carotid artery disease. Stroke 1995;26:214-217.

98. Klotzsch C, Popescu O, Berlit P: Assessment of the posterior communicating artery by transcranial color-coded duplex sonography. Stroke 1996;27:486-489.

99. Piepgras A, Schmiedek P, Leinsinger G, et al: A simple test to assess cerebrovascular reserve capacity using transcranial Doppler sonography and acetazolamide. Stroke 1990;21:1306-1311.

100. Dahl A, Russell D, Rootwelt K, et al: Cerebral vasoreactivity assesses with transcranial Doppler and regional cerebral blood flow measurements. Dose, concentration, and time of the response to acetazolamide. Stroke 1995;26:2302-2306.

101. Valdueza JM, Draganski B, Hoffman O, et al: Analysis of CO_2 Vasomotor reactivity and vessel diameter changes by simultaneous venous and arterial Doppler recordings. Stroke 1999;30:81-86.

102. Yonas H, Smith HA, Durham SR, et al: Increased stroke risk predicted by compromised cerebral blood flow reactivity. J Neurosurg 1993;79:483-489.

103. Markus HS: Transcranial Doppler detection of circulating cerebral emboli: A review. Stroke 1993;24:1246-1250.

104. Markus HS, Harrison MJ: Microembolic signal detection using ultrasound. Stroke 1995;26:1517-1519.

105. Tong DC, Albers GW: Transcranial Doppler-detected microemboli in patients with acute stroke. Stroke 1995;26:1588-1592.

106. Sliwka U, Job F-P, Wissuwa D, et al: Occurrence of transcranial Doppler high-intensity transient signals in patients with potential cardiac sources of embolism: A prospective study. Stroke 1995;26:2067-2070.

107. Daffertshofer M, Ries S, Schminke U, Hennerici M: High-intensity transient signals in patients with cerebral ischemia. Stroke 1996;27:1844-1849.

108. Sliwka U, Lingnau A, Stohlmann W-D, et al: Prevalence and time course of microembolic signals in patients with acute strokes: A prospective study. Stroke 1997;28:358-363.

109. Ringelstein EB, Droste DW, Babikian VL, et al: Consensus on microembolus detection by TCD. International Consensus Group on Microembolus Detection. Stroke 1998;29:725-729.

110. Siebler M, Nachtmann A, Sitzer M, et al: Cerebral microembolism and the risk of ischemia in asymptomatic high-grade internal carotid artery stenosis. Stroke 1995;26:2184-2186.

111. Molloy J, Markus HS: Asymptomatic embolization predicts stroke and TIA risk in patients with carotid artery stenosis. Stroke 1999;30:1440-1443.

112. Segura T, Serena J, Molins A, Davalos A: Clusters of microembolic signals: A new form of cerebral microembolism presentation in a patient with middle cerebral artery stenosis. Stroke 1998;29:722-724.

113. Wong KS, Li H, Chan YL, et al: Use of transcranial Doppler to predict outcome in patients with intracranial large-artery occlusive disease. Stroke 2003;31:2641-2647.

114. Gao S, Wong KS, Hansberg T, et al: Microembolic signal predicts recurrent cerebral ischemic events in acute stroke patients with middle cerebral artery stenosis. Stroke 2004;35:2832-2836.

115. Mackinnon AD, Aaslid R, Markus HS: Long-term ambulatory monitoring for cerebral emboli using transcranial Doppler ultrasound. Stroke 2004;35:73-78.

116. Teague SM, Sharma MK: Detection of paradoxical cerebral echo contrast embolization by transcranial Doppler ultrasound. Stroke 1991;22:740-745.

117. Chimowitz MI, Nemec JJ, Marwick TH, et al: Transcranial Doppler ultrasound identifies patients with right-to-left cardiac or pulmonary shunts. Neurology 1991;41:1902-1904.

118. Albert A, Muller HR, Hetzel A: Optimized transcranial Doppler technique for the diagnosis of cardiac right-to-left shunts. J Neuroimaging 1997;7:159-163.

119. Di Tullio M, Sacco RL, Venketasubramanian N, et al: Comparison of diagnostic techniques for the detection of a patent foramen ovale in stroke patients. Stroke 1993;24:1020-1024.

120. Klotzsch C, Janzen G, Berlit P: Transesophageal echocardiography and contrast-TCD in the detection of a patent foramen ovale. Experiences with 111 patients. Neurology 1994;44:1603-1606.

121. Jauss M, Zanette E: Detection of right-to-left shunt with ultrasound contrast agent and transcranial Doppler sonography. Cerebrovasc Dis 2000;10:490-496.

121a. Sastry S, Daly K, Chengodu T, McCollum C: Is transcranial Doppler for the detection of venous-to-arterial circulation shunts reproducible? Cerebrovasc Dis 2007;23:424-429.

122. Baumgartner RW, Gonner F, Arnold M, Muri R: Transtemporal power- and frequency-based color-coded duplex sonography of cerebral veins and sinuses. AJNR Am J Neuroradiol 1997;18:1771-1781.

123. Stolz E, Kaps M, Dorndorf W: Assessment of intracranial venous hemodynamics in normal individuals and patients with cerebral venous thrombosis. Stroke 1999;30:70-75.

124. Ries S, Steinke W, Neff KW, Hennerici M: Echo-contrast enhanced transcranial color-coded sonography for the diagnosis of transverse sinus thrombosis. Stroke 1997;28:696-700.

125. Valdueza JM, Hoffmann O, Weih M, et al: Monitoring of venous hemodynamics in patients with cerebral venous thrombosis by transcranial Doppler ultrasound. Arch Neurol 1999;56:229-234.

126. Becker G, Bogdahn U, Gehlberg C, et al: Transcranial color-coded real-time sonography of intracranial veins. J Neuroimaging 1995;5: 87-94.

127. Pressman BD, Tourje EJ, Thompson JR: An early sign of ischemic infarction: Increased density in a cerebral artery. AJNR Am J Neuroradiol 1987;8:645-648.

128. Lays D, Pruvo JP, Godefroy O, et al: Prevalence and significance of hyperdense middle cerebral artery in acute stroke. Stroke 1992;23:317-324.

129. Tomsick T, Brott T, Barsan W, et al: Prognostic value of the hyperdense middle cerebral artery sign and stroke scale score before ultraearly thrombolytic therapy. AJNR Am J Neuroradiol 1996;17:79-85.

130. Lee TC, Bartlett E, Fox AJ, Symons SP: The hypodense artery sign. AJNR Am J Neuroradiol 2005;26:2027-2029.

131. Grunholdt ML: B-mode ultrasound and spiral CT for the assessment of carotid athero-sclerosis. Neuroimaging Clin N Am 2002;12: 421-435.

132. Frank H: Characterization of atherosclerotic plaque by magnetic resonance imaging. Am Heart J 2001;141(Suppl 2):S45-S48.

133. Yuan C, Mitsumori LM, Beach KW, Maravilla KR: Carotid atherosclerotic plaque: Noninvasive MR characterization and identification of vulnerable lesions. Radiology 2001;221: 285-299.

134. Adams GJ, Greene J, Vick 3rd GW, et al: Tracking regression and progression of atherosclerosis in human carotid arteries using high-resolution magnetic resonance imaging. Magn Reson Imaging 2004;22:1249-1258.

135. Honda M, Kitagawa N, Tsutsumi K, et al: High-resolution magnetic resonance imaging for detection of carotid plaques. Neurosurgery 2006;58:338-346.

136. Hatsukami TS, Ross R, Polissar NL, Yuan C: Visualization of fibrous cap thickness and rupture in human atherosclerotic carotid plaque in vivo with high-resolution magnetic resonance imaging. Circulation 2000;102:959-964.

137. Moody AR, Murphy RE, Morgan PS, et al: Characterization of complicated carotid plaque with magnetic resonance direct thrombus imaging in patients with cerebral ischemia. Circulation 2003;107:3047-3052.

137a. Saloner D, Acevedo-Bolton G, Wintermark M, Rapp JH: MRI of geometric and compositional features of vulnerable carotid plaque. Stroke 2007;38(part 2):637-641.

137b. Touzé E, Toussaint J-F, Coste J, et al for the High-Resolution Magnetic Resonanace Imaging in Atherosclerotic Stenosis of the Carotid Artery (HIRISC) Study Group: Reproducibility of high-resolution MRI for the identification and the quantification of carotid atherosclerotic plaque components. Stroke 2007;38:1812-1819.

138. Yuan C, Mitsumori LM, Ferguson MS, et al: In vivo accuracy of multispectral magnetic resonance imaging for identifying lipid-rich necrotic cores and intraplaque hemorrhage in advanced human carotid plaques. Circulation 2001;104:2051-2056.

139. Botnar RM, Buecker A, Wiethoff AJ, et al: In vivo magnetic resonance imaging of coronary thrombosis using a fibrin-binding molecular magnetic resonance contrast agent. Circulation 2004;110:1463-1466.

140. Sirol M, Fuster V, Badimon JJ, et al: Chronic thrombus detection with in vivo magnetic resonance imaging and a fibrin-targeted contrast agent. Circulation 2005;112:1594-1600.

141. Klein IF, Lavallee PC, Schouman-Claeys E, Amaraenco P: High-resolution MRI identifies basilar artery plaques in paramedian pontine infarct. Neurology 2005;64:551-552.

142. Klein IF, Lavallee PC, Touboul P-J, et al: In vivo middle cerebral artery plaque imaging by high-resolution MRI. Neurology 2006;67:327-329.

143. Lam WW, Wong KS, So NM, et al: Plaque volume measurement by magnetic resonance imaging as an index of remodeling of middle cerebral artery: Correlation with transcranial color Doppler and magnetic resonance angiography. Cerebrovasc Dis 2004;17:166-169.

144. Chalela JA, Haaymore JB, Ezzeddine MA, et al: The hypointense MCA sign. Neurology 2002;58:1470.

145. Cho K-H, Kim JS, Kwon SU, et al: Significance of susceptibility vessel sign on T2*-weighted gradient echo imaging for identification of stroke subtypes. Stroke 2005;36:2379-2383.

146. Hermier M, Nighoghossian N: Contribution of susceptibility-weighted imaging to acute stroke assessment. Stroke 2004;35:1989-1994.

147. Assouline E, Benziane K, Reizine D, et al: Intra-arterial thrombus visualized on T2* gradient echo imaging in acute ischemic stroke. Cerebrovasc Dis 2005;20:6-11.

148. Idbaih A, Boukobza M, Crassard I, et al: MRI of clot in cerebral venous thrombosis: high diagnostic value of susceptibility-weighted images. Stroke 2006;37:991-995.

149. Selim M, Fink J, Linfante I, et al: Diagnosis of cerebral venous thrombosis with echo-planar T2*-weighted magnetic resonance imaging. Arch Neurol 2002;59:1021-1026.

150. Lovblad KO, Bassetti C, Schneider J, et al: Diffusion-weighted MR in cerebral venous thrombosis. Cerebrovasc Dis 2001;11:169-176.

151. Favrole P, Guichard JP, Crassard I, et al: Diffusion-weighted imaging of intravascular clots in cerebral venous thrombosis. Stroke 2004;35:99-103.

152. Essig M, von Kummer R, Egelhof T, et al: Vascular MR contrast enhancement in cerebrovascular disease. AJNR Am J Neuroradiol 1996;17:887-894.

153. Lazar EB, Russell EJ, Cohen BA, et al: Contrast-enhanced MR of cerebral arteritis: Intravascular enhancement related to flow stasis within areas of focal arterial ectasia. AJNR Am J Neuroradiol 1992;13:271-276.

154. Warach S, Latour LI: Evidence of reperfusion injury, exacerbated by thrombolytic therapy, in human focal brain ischemia using a novel imaging marker of early blood–brain barrier disruption. Stroke 2004;35(Suppl 1):2659-2661.

155. Latour LL, Kang DW, Ezzeddine MA, et al: Early blood-brain barrier disruption in human focal brain ischemia. Ann Neurol 2004;56:468-477.

156. Schellinger PD, Chalela JA, Kang DW, et al: Diagnostic and prognostic value of early MR Imaging vessel signs in hyperacute stroke patients imaged <3 hours and treated with recombinant tissue plasminogen activator. AJNR Am J Neuroradiol 2005;26:618-624.

156a. Bang OY, Buck BH, Saver JL, et al: Prediction of hemorrhagic transformation after recanalization therapy using T2*-permeability magnetic resonance imaging. Ann Neurol 2007;62:170-176.

157. Edelman RR, Mattle HP, Atkinson DJ, et al: MR angiography. AJR Am J Roentgenol 1990;154:937-946.

158. Bradley WG: Magnetic resonance angiography. In Babikian VL, Wechsler LR, Higashida RT (eds): Imaging Cerebrovascular Disease. Philadelphia: Butterworth-Heinemann, 2003, pp 37-50.

159. Quereshi A, Isa A, Cinnamon J, et al: Magnetic resonance angiography in patients with brain infarction. J Neuroimaging 1998;8:65-70.

160. Gillard JH, Oliverio PJ, Barker PB, et al: MR angiography in acute cerebral ischemia of the anterior circulation: A preliminary report. AJNR Am J Neuroradiol 1997;18:343-350.

161. Yano T, Kodama T, Suzuki Y, Watanabe K: Gadolinium-enhanced 3D time-of-flight MR angiography. Acta Radiol 1997;38:47-54.

162. Leclerc X, Martinat P, Godefroy O, et al: Contrast-enhanced three-dimensional fast imaging with steady-state precession (FISP) MR angiography of supraaortic vessels: Preliminary results. AJNR Am J Neuroradiol 1998;19:1405-1413.

163. U-King-Im J, Trivedi R, Graves M, et al: Contrast-enhanced MR angiography for carotid disease: Diagnostic and potential clinical impact. Neurology 2004;62:1282-1290.

164. Mitti RL, Broderick M, Carpenter JP, et al: Blinded-reader comparison of magnetic resonance angiography and Duplex ultrasonography for carotid artery bifurcation stenosis. Stroke 1994;25:4-10.

165. Levi CR, Mitchell A, Fitt G, Donnan GA: The accuracy of magnetic resonance angiography in the assessment of extracranial carotid artery occlusive disease. Cerebrovasc Dis 1996;6:231-236.

166. Bash S, Villablanca JP, Duckwiler G, et al: Intracranial vascular stenosis and occlusive disease. Evaluation with CT angiography, MR angiography, and digital subtraction angiography. AJNR Am J Neuroradiol 2005;26:1012-1021.

167. Uehara T, Mori E, Tabuchi M, et al: Detection of occlusive lesions in intracranial arteries by three-dimensional time-of-flight magnetic resonance angiography. Cerebrovasc Dis 1994;4:365-370.

168. Johnson BA, Heiserman JE, Drayer BP, Keller PJ: Intracranial MR angiography: Its role in the integrated approach to brain infarction. AJNR Am J Neuroradiol 1994;15:901-908.

169. Ko SB, Kim D-E, Kim SH, Roh J-K: Visualization of venous system by time-of-flight magnetic resonance angiography. J Neuroimaging 2006;16:353-356.

170. Roberts HC, Lee TJ, Dillon WP: Computed tomography angiography. In Babikian VL, Wechsler LR, Higashida RT (eds): Imaging Cerebrovascular Disease. Philadelphia: Butterworth-Heinemann, 2003, pp 51-71.

171. Leclerc X, Godefroy O, Pruvo JP, Leys D: Computed tomographic angiography for the evaluation of carotid artery stenosis. Stroke 1995;26:1577-1581.

172. Josephson S, Bryant S, Mak H, et al: Evaluation of carotid stenosis using CT angiography in the initial evaluation of stroke and TIA. Neurology 2004;63:457-460.

173. Feasby T, Findlay J: CT angiography for the assessment of carotid stenosis. Neurology 2004;63:412-413.

173a. Bartlett ES, Walters TD, Symons SP, Fox AJ: Carotid stenosis index revisitied with direct CT angiography measurement of carotid arteries to quantify carotid stenosis. Stroke 2007;38:286-291.

174. Wong KS, Liang EY, Lam WWM, et al: Spiral computed tomography angiography in the assessment of middle cerebral artery occlusive disease. J Neurol Neurosurg Psychiatry 1995;59:537-539.

175. Skutta B, Furst G, Eilers J, et al: Intracranial stenoocclusive disease: Double detector helical CTA versus digital subtraction angiography. AJNR Am J Neuroradiol 1999;20:791-799.

176. Brisman J, Song JK, Newell DW: Cerebral aneurysms. N Engl J Med 2006;355:928-939.

176a. Nguyen-Huynh MN, Wintermark M, English J, et al: How accurate is CT angiography in evaluating intracranial atherosclerotic disease? Stroke 2008;39:1184-1188.

176b. Nijjar S, Patel B, McGinn G, West M: Computed tomographic angiography as the primary diagnostic study in spontaneous subarachnoid hemorrhage. J Neuroimaging 2007;17:295-299.

176c. Wada R, Aviv RI, Fox AJ, et al: CT angiography "spot sign" predicts hematoma expansion in acute intracerebral hemorrhage. Stroke 2007;38:1257-1262.

177. Warach S, Li W, Ronthal M, Edelman R: Acute cerebral ischemia: evaluation with dynamic contrast-enhanced MR imaging and MR angiography. Radiology 1992;182:41-47.

178. Fisher M, Prichard JW, Warach S. New magnetic resonance techniques for acute ischemic stroke. JAMA 1995;274:908-911.

179. Rother J, Guckel F, Neff W, et al: Assessment of regional cerebral blood flow volume in acute human stroke by use of a single-slice dynamic susceptibility contrast-enhanced magnetic resonance imaging. Stroke 1996;27:1088-1093.

180. Sorensen AG, Buonanno F, Gonzalez RG, et al: Hyperacute stroke: evaluation with combined multisection diffusion-weighted and hemodynamically weighted echo-planar MR imaging. Radiology 1996;199:391-401.

181. Schlaug G, Benfield A, Baird AE, et al: The ischemic penumbra operationally defined by diffusion and perfusion MRI. Neurology 1999;53:1528-1537.

182. Schellinger PD, Fiebach JB, Jansen O, et al: Stroke magnetic resonance imaging within 6 hours after onset of hyperacute cerebral ischemia. Ann Neurol 2001;49:460-469.

183. Chaves C, Silver B, Staroselskaya I, et al: Relation of perfusion-weighted magnetic resonance imaging (MRI) and clinical outcome in patients with ischemic stroke. Cerebrovasc Dis 1999;9(Suppl 1):56.

184. Staroselskaya I, Chaves C, Silver B, et al: Relationship between magnetic resonance arterial patency and perfusion–diffusion mismatch in acute ischemic stroke and its potential clinical use. Arch Neurol 2001;58:1069-1074.

185. Neumann-Haefelin T, Moseley ME, Albers GW: New magnetic resonance imaging methods for cerebrovascular disease: emerging clinical applications. Ann Neurol 2000;47:559-570.

186. Ostergaard L, Sorensen AG, Chesler DA, et al: Combined diffusion-weighted and perfusion-weighted flow heterogeneity magnetic resonance imaging in acute stroke. Stroke 2000;31:1097-1103.

187. Chaves CJ, Staroselskaya I, Linfante I, Llinas R, et al: Patterns of perfusion-weighted imaging in patients with carotid artery occlusive disease. Arch Neurol 2003;60:237-242.

187a. Kane I, Carpenter T, Chappell F, et al: Comparison of 10 different magnetic resonance perfusion imaging processing methods in acute ischemic stroke. Stroke 2007;38:3158-3164.

188. Wong EC: Quantifying CBF with pulsed ASL: Technical and pulse sequence factors. J Magn Reson Imaging 2005;22:727-731.

189. Wang Z, Wang J, Connick TJ, et al: Continuous ASL (CASL) perfusion MRI with an array coil and parallel imaging at 3T. Magn Reson Med 2005;54:732-737.

190. Fernandez-Seara MA, Wang Z, Wang J, et al: Continuous arterial spin labeling perfusion measurements using single shot 3D GRASE at 3 T. Magn Reson Med 2005;54:1241-1247.

191. Ances BM, McGarvey ML, Abrahams JM, et al: Continuous arterial spin labeled perfusion magnetic resonance imaging in patients before and after carotid endarterectomy. J Neuroimaging 2004;14:133-138.

191a. Park K-Y, Youn YC, Chung C-S, et al: Large-artery stenosis predicts subsequent vascular events in patients with transient ischemic attack. J Clin Neurol 2007;3:169-174.

192. Perez A, Restepo L, Kleinman J, et al: Patients with diffusion–perfusion mismatch on magnetic resonance imaging 48 hours or more after stroke symptom onset: Clinical and imaging features. J Neuroimaging 2006;16:329-333.

192a. Linfante I, Llinas RH, Schlaug G, et al: Diffusion-weighted imaging and National Institutes of Health Stroke Scale in the acute phase of posterior-circulation stroke. Arch Neurol 2001;58:621-628.

193. von Kummer R, Weber J: Brain and vascular imaging in acute ischemic stroke: The potential of computed tomography. Neurology 1997;49(Suppl 4):S52-S55.

194. Nabavi DG, Kloska SP, Nam E-M, et al: MOSAIC: Multimodal stroke assessment using computed tomography. Novel diagnostic approach for the prediction of infarction size and clinical outcome. Stroke 2002;33:2819-2826.

195. Koroshetz W: Contrast computed tomography scan in acute stroke: "You can't always get what you want but ... you get what you need." Ann Neurol 2002;51:415-416.

196. Wintermark M, Reichhart M, Thiran J-P, et al: Prognostic accuracy of cerebral blood flow measurement by perfusion computed tomography, at the time of emergency room admission, in acute stroke patients. Ann Neurol 2002;51:417-432.

197. Wintermark M, Reichart M, Cuisenaire O, et al: Comparison of admission perfusion computed tomography and qualitative diffusion- and perfusion-weighted magnetic resonance imaging in acute stroke patients. Stroke 2002;33:2025-2031.

197a. Parsons MW, Pepper EM, Bateman GA, et al: Identification of the penumbra and infarct core on hyperacute noncontrast and perfusion CT. Neurology 2007;68:730-736.

198. Na DG, Byun HS, Lee KH, et al: Acute occlusion of the middle cerebral artery: early evaluation with triphasic helical CT—Preliminary results. Radiology 1998;207:113-122.

199. Lee KH, Cho S-J, Byun HS, et al: Triphasic perfusion computed tomography in acute middle cerebral artery stroke. Arch Neurol 2000;57:990-999.

200. Lee KH, Lee S-J, Cho S-J, et al: Usefulness of triphasic perfusion computed tomography for intravenous thrombolysis with tissue-type plasminogen activator in acute ischemic stroke. Arch Neurol 2000;57:1000-1008.

200a. Kohrmann M, Juttler E, Huttner HB, et al: Acute stroke imaging for thrombolytic therapy—An update. Cerebrovasc Dis 2007;24:161-169.

200b. Wintermark M, Meuli R, Browaeys P, et al: Comparison of CT perfusion and angiography and MRI in selecting stroke patients for acute treatment. Neurology 2007;68:694-697.

200c. Chalela JA, Kidwell CS, Nentwich LM, et al: Magnetic resonance imaging and computed tomography in emergency assessment of patients with suspected acute stroke: A prospective comparison. Lancet 2007;369:293-298.

201. Yonas H, Wolfson SK, Gur D, et al: Clinical experience with the use of xenon-enhanced CT blood flow mapping in cerebral vascular disease. Stroke 1984;15:443-450.

202. Yonas H, Darby JM, Marks EC, et al: CBF measured by Xe-CT: Approach to analysis and normal values. J Cereb Blood Flow Metab 1991;11: 716-725.

203. Hilman J, Sturnegk P, Yonas H, et al: Bedside monitoring of CBF with xenon-CT and a mobile scanner: A novel method in neurointensive care. Br J Neurosurg 2005;19:395-401.

204. Fayad P, Brass LM: Single photon emission computed tomography in cerebrovascular disease. Stroke 1991;22:950-954.

205. Caplan LR: Question-driven technology assessment: SPECT as an example. Neurology 1991;41:187-191.

206. Masdeu JC, Brass LM: SPECT imaging of stroke. J Neuroimaging 1995;5:514-522.

207. Therapeutics and Technology Subcommittee of the American Academy of Neurology: Assessment of Brain SPECT. Neurology 1996;46:278-285.

208. Masdeu JC: Imaging of stroke with single-photon emission computed tomography. In Babikian VL, Wechsler LR, Higashida RT (eds): Imaging Cerebrovascular Disease. Philadelphia: Butterworth-Heinemann, 2003, pp 131-143.

209. Wintermark M, Sesay M, Barbier E, et al: Comparative overview of brain perfusion imaging techniques. JNR J Neuroradiol 2005;32:294-314.

210. Frackowiak R: PET CBF investigations of stroke. In Welch KMA, Caplan LR, Reis DJ, Siesjo B, Weir B (eds): Primer on Cerebrovascular Diseases. San Diego: Academic Press, 1997, pp 636-640.

211. Phelps M, Mazziotta J, Huang S: Study of cerebral function with positron computed tomography. J Cereb Blood Flow Metab 1982;2:113-162.

212. Baron JC, Bousser M, Rey A, et al: Reversal of focal misery-perfusion syndrome by extra-intracranial arterial bypass in hemodynamic cerebral ischemia. Stroke 1981;12:454-459.

213. Marchal G, Furlan M, Beaudouin V, et al: Early spontaneous hyperperfusion after stroke: A marker of favorable tissue outcome. Brain 1996;119:409-419.

214. Baron J-C: Positron emission tomography. In Babikian VL, Wechsler LR, Higashida RT (eds): Imaging Cerebrovascular Disease. Philadelphia: Butterworth-Heinemann, 2003, pp 115-130.

214a. Johnson KA, Gregas M, Becker JA, et al: Imaging of amyloid burden and distribution in cerebral amyloid angiopathy. Ann Neurol 2007;62:229-234.

214b. Vinters HV: Imaging cerebral microvascular amyloid. Ann Neurol 2007;62:209-212.

215. Caplan LR, Wolpert SM: Angiography in patients with occlusive cerebrovascular disease: A stroke neurologist and neuroradiologist's views. AJNR Am J Neuroradiol 1991;12:593-601.

216. Akers DL, Markowitz IA, Kerstein MD: The value of aortic arch study in the evaluation of cerebrovascular insufficiency. Am J Surg 1987;154:230-232.

217. Caplan LR, Manning WJ: Cardiac sources of embolism: The usual suspects. In Caplan LR, Manning WJ (eds): Brain Embolism. New York: Informa Healthcare, 2006, pp 129-159.

218. DeRook FA, Comess KA, Albers GW, Popp RL: Transesophageal echocardiography in the evaluation of stroke. Ann Intern Med 1992;117:922-932.

219. Grullon C, Alam M, Rosman HS, et al: Transesophageal echocardiography in unselected patients with focal cerebral ischemia: When is it useful? Cerebrovasc Dis 1994;4:139-145.

220. Daniel WG, Mugge A: Transesophageal echocardiography. N Engl J Med 1995;332:1268-1279.

221. Horowitz DR, Tuhrim S, Weinberger J, et al: Transesophageal echocardiography: Diagnostic and clinical applications in the evaluation of the stroke patient. J Stroke Cerebrovasc Dis 1997;6:332-336.

222. Manning WJ: Cardiac sources of embolism: Pathophysiology and identification. In Caplan LR, Manning WJ (eds): Brain Embolism. New York: Informa Healthcare, 2006, pp 161-186.

223. Caplan LR: Of birds and nests and cerebral emboli. Rev Neurol 1991;147:265-273.

224. Caplan LR: Brain embolism. In Caplan LR, Chimowitz M, Hurst JW (eds): Practical Clinical Neurocardiology. New York: Marcel Dekker, 1999, pp 35-185.

225. Caplan LR: The aorta as a donor source of brain embolism. In Caplan LR, Manning WJ (eds): Brain Embolism. New York: Informa Healthcare, 2006, pp 187-201.

226. Johnson LL, Pohost GM: Nuclear cardiology. In Schlant RC, Alexander RW (eds): Hurst's The Heart, 8th ed. New York: McGraw-Hill, 1994, pp 2281-2323.

227. Weinberger J, Azhar S, Danisi F, et al: A new noninvasive technique for imaging atherosclerotic plaque in the aortic arch of stroke patients by transcutaneous real-time B-mode ultrasonography. Stroke 1998;29:673-676.

228. Lockwood K, Sherman D, Gerza C, et al: Detection of left atrial thrombi by cardiac CT. Neurology 1984;34:205.

229. Helgason C, Chomka E, Louie E, et al: The potential role for ultrafast cardiac computed tomography in patients with stroke. Stroke 1989;20:465-472.

230. Ezekowitz M, Wilson D, Smith E, et al: Comparison of indium 111 platelet scintigraphy and two-dimensional echocardiography in the diagnosis of left ventricular thrombi. N Engl J Med 1982;306:1509-1513.

231. Rokey R, Rolak LA, Harati Y, et al: Coronary artery disease in patients with cerebrovascular disease: A prospective study. Ann Neurol 1985;16:50-53.

232. Gibbons RJ, Zinsmeister AR, Miller TD: Supine exercise electrocardiography compared with exercise radionuclide angiography in non-invasive identification of severe coronary artery diseases. Ann Intern Med 1990;112:743-749.

233. Engel G, Froelicher VF: ECG exercise testing. In Fuster V, Alexander RW, O'Rourke RA (eds): Hurst's The Heart, 11th ed. New York: Mcgraw-Hill, 2004, pp 467-480.

234. DiPasquale G, Andreoli A, Carini G, et al: Non-invasive screening for silent ischemic heart disease in patients with cerebral ischemia: use of dipyridamole-thallium myocardial imaging. Cerebrovasc Dis 1991;1:31-37.

235. Berman DS, Hachamovitch R, Shaw LJ, et al: Nuclear cardiology. In Fuster V, Alexander RW, O'Rourke RA (eds): Hurst's The Heart, 11th ed. New York: McGraw-Hill, 2004, pp 563-598.

235a. Liao J, Khalid Z, Scallan C, et al: Noninvasive cardiac monitoring for detecting paroxysmal atrial fibrillation or flutter after acute ischemic stroke: A systematic review. Stroke 2007;38:2935-2940.

236. Lieb WE, Flaharty PM, Sergott RC, et al: Color Doppler imaging provides accurate assessment of orbital blood flow in occlusive carotid artery disease. Opthalmology 1991;98:548-552.

237. Hedges TR. Ocular Ischemia. In Caplan LR (ed): Brain Ischemia: Basic Concepts and Clinical Relevance. London: Springer, 1995, pp 61-73.

238. Duijn JH, Matson GB, Maudsley AA, et al: Human brain infarction: Proton MR spectroscopy. Radiology 1992;183:711-718.

239. Castillo M, Kwock L, Mukherij SK: Clinical applications of proton MR spectroscopy. AJNR Am J Neuroradiol 1996;17:1-15.

240. Pavlakis SG, Kingsley PB, Kaplan GP, et al: Magnetic resonance spectroscopy: Use in monitoring MELAS treatment. Arch Neurol 1998;55:849-852.

241. Koroshetz WJ: New techniques in computed tomography, magnetic resonance imaging, and optical imaging in cerebrovascular disease. In Babikian VL, Wechsler LR, Higashida RT (eds): Imaging Cerebrovascular Disease. Philadelphia: Butterworth-Heinemann, 2003, pp 403-412.

242. Belliveau JW, Cohen MS, Weisskoff R, et al: Functional studies of the human brain using high-speed magnetic resonance imaging. J Neuroimaging 1991;1:36-41.

243. Humberstone MR, Sawle GV: Functional magnetic resonance imaging in clinical neurology. Eur Neurol 1996;36:117-124.

244. Love T, Haist F, Nicol J, Swinney D: A functional neuroimaging investigation of the roles of structural complexity and task-demand during auditory sentence processing. Cortex 2006;42:577-590.

245. Levine SR, Brust JCM, Futrell N, et al: A comparative study of the cerebrovascular complications of cocaine-alkaloidal versus hydrochloride-a review. Neurology 1991;41:1173-1177.

246. Caplan LR: Drugs. In Kase CS, Caplan LR (eds): Intracerebral Hemorrhage. Boston: Butterworth-Heinemann, 1994, pp 201-220.

247. Alberico RA, Patel M, Casey S, et al: Evaluation of the circle of Willis with three-dimensional CT angiography in patients with suspected intracranial aneurysms. AJNR Am J Neuroradiol 1995;16:1571-1578.

248. Sekhar L, Wechsler L, Yonas H, et al: Value of transcranial Doppler examination in the diagnosis of cerebral vasospasm after subarachnoid hemorrhage. Neurosurgery 1988;22:813-821.

249. Sloan MA, Haley EC, Kassell NF, et al: Sensitivity and specificity of transcranial Doppler ultrasonography in the diagnosis of vasospasm following subarachnoid hemorrhage. Neurology 1989;39:1514-1518.

250. Pollock S, Tsitsopoulas P, Harrison M: The effect of hematocrit on cerebral perfusion and clinical status following occlusion in the gerbil. Stroke 1982;13:167-170.

251. Harrison M, Pollock S, Kindoll B, et al: Effect of hematocrit on carotid stenosis and cerebral infarction. Lancet 1981;2:114-115.

252. Thomas D, duBoulay G, Marshall J, et al: Effect of hematocrit on cerebral blood flow in man. Lancet 1977;2:941-943.

253. Tohgi H, Yamanouchi H, Murakami M, et al: Importance of the hematocrit as a risk factor in cerebral infarction. Stroke 1978;9:369-374.

254. Grotta J, Ackerman R, Correia J, et al: Whole-blood viscosity parameters and cerebral blood flow. Stroke 1982;13:296-298.

255. Thomas D: Whole blood viscosity and cerebral blood flow. Stroke 1982;13:285-287.

256. Kee Jr DB, Wood JH: Influence of blood rheology on cerebral circulation. In Wood JH (ed): Cerebral Blood Flow: Physiological and Clinical Aspects. New York: McGraw-Hill, 1987, pp 173-185.

257. Allport LE, Parsons MW, Butcher KS, et al: Elevated hematocrit is associated with reduced reperfusion and tissue survival in acute stroke. Neurology 2005;65:1382-1387.

258. Adams RJ, Nichols FT, Figueroa R, et al: Transcranial Doppler correlation with cerebral angiography in sickle cell disease. Stroke 1992;23:1073-1077.

259. Switzer JA, Hess DC, Nichols FT, Adams RJ: Pathophysiology and treatment of stroke in sickle-cell disease: Present and future. Lancet Neurol 2006;5:501-512.

260. Adams RJ: TCD in sickle cell disease: An important and useful test. Pediatr Radiol 2005;35:229-234.

261. Adams RJ, McKie VC, Hsu L, et al: Prevention of a first stroke by transfusions in children with sickle cell anemia and abnormal results on transcranial Doppler ultrasonography. N Engl J Med 1998;339:5-11.

262. Adams RJ, Brambilla D: Optimizing Primary Stroke Prevention in Sickle Cell Anemia (STOP 2) Trial Investigators: Discontinuing prophylactic transfusions used to prevent stroke in sickle cell disease. N Engl J Med 2005;353:2769-2778.

263. Mercuri M, Bond MG, Evans G, et al: Leukocyte count and carotid atherosclerosis. Stroke 1991;22:134.

264. Elkind MS, Cheng I, Boden-Albala B, et al: Elevated white blood cell count and carotid plaque thickness: The Northern Manhattan Stroke Study. Stroke 2001;32:842-849.

265. Elkind MS, Sciacca R, Boden-Albala B, et al: Leukocyte count is associated with aortic arch plaque thickness. Stroke 2002;33: 2587-2592.

266. Elkind MS, Sciacca RR, Boden-Albala B, et al: Leukocyte count is associated with reduced endothelial reactivity. Atherosclerosis 2005; 181:329-338.

267. Elkind MS, Sciacca RR, Boden-Albala B, et al: Relative elevation in baseline leukocyte count predicts first cerebral infarction. Neurology 2005;64:2121-2125.

268. Elkind MS: Inflammation, atherosclerosis, and stroke. Neurologist 2006;12:140-148.

268a. Bennett JS, Kolodziej MA: Disorders of platelet function. Dis Month 1992;38:557-563.

268b. Anderson IR, Feinberg WM: Primary platelet disorders. In Welch KMA, Caplan LR, Reis DJ, Siesjo BK, Weir B (eds): Primer on Cerebrovascular Diseases. San Diego, Academic Press, 1997, pp 401-405.

269. Wu K: Platelet hyperaggregability and thrombosis in patients with thrombocythemia. Ann Intern Med 1978;88:7-11.

270. Arboix A, Besses C, Acin P, et al: Ischemic stroke as first manifestation of essential thrombocythemia: Report of six cases. Stroke 1995; 26:1463-1466.

271. Ogata J, Yonemura K, Kimura K, et al: Cerebral infarction associated with essential thrombocythemia: An autopsy case study. Cerebrovasc Dis 2005;19:201-205.

272. Atkinson JLD, Sundt TM, Kazmier FJ, et al: Heparin-induced thrombocytopenia and thrombosis in ischemic stroke. Mayo Clin Proc 1988;63:353-361.

273. Arepally GM, Ortel TL: Clinical practice. Heparin-induced thrombocytopenia. N Engl J Med 2006;355:809-817.

274. Uchyama S, Takeuchi M, Osawa M, et al: Platelet function tests in thrombotic cerebrovascular disorders. Stroke 1983;14:511-517.

275. Ludlam CA: Evidence for the platelet specificity of beta-thromboglobulin and studies on its plasma concentration in healthy individuals. Br J Haematol 1979;41:271-278.

276. Fisher M, Francis R: Altered coagulation in cerebral ischemia: Platelet, thrombin, and plasmin activity. Arch Neurol 1990;47:1075-1079.

277. Helgason CH, Bolin KM, Hoff JA, et al: Development of aspirin resistance in persons with previous ischemic stroke. Stroke 1994;25: 2331-2336.

278. Yeh RW, Everett BM, Foo SY, et al: Predictors for the development of elevated anti-heparin/ platelet factor 4 antibody titers in patients undergoing cardiac catheterization. Am J Cardiol 2006;98:419-421.

279. Qizilbash N, Duffy S, Prentice CRM, et al: von Willebrand factor and risk of ischemic stroke. Neurology 1997;49:1552-1556.

280. Blann AD: Plasma von Willebrand factor, thrombosis, and the endothelium: The first 30 years. Thromb Haemost 2006;95:49-55.

281. Bowen DJ, Collins PW: Insights into von Willebrand factor proteolysis: Clinical implications. Br J Haematol 2006;133:457-467.

282. Weiss EJ, Bray PF, Tayback M, et al: A polymorphism of a platelet glycoprotein receptor as an inherited risk factor for coronary thrombosis. N Engl J Med 1996;334:1090-1094.

283. Kannel WB, Wolf PA, Castelli WP, et al: Fibrinogen and risk of cardiovascular disease. JAMA 1987;258:1183-1186.

284. Coull BM, Beamer NB, deGarmo PL, et al: Chronic blood hyperviscosity in subjects with acute stroke, transient ischemic attack, and risk factors for stroke. Stroke 1991;22:162-168.

285. Beamer N, Coull BM, Sexton G, et al: Fibrinogen and the albumin-globulin ratio in recurrent stroke. Stroke 1993;24:1133-1139.

286. Ernst E, Resch KL: Fibrinogen as a cardiovascular risk factor: A meta-analysis and review of the literature. Ann Intern Med 1993;118:956-963.

287. Danesh J, Lewington S, Thompson SG, et al: Plasma fibrinogen level and the risk of major cardiovascular diseases and nonvascular mortality: An individual participant meta-analysis. JAMA 2005;294:1799-1809.

288. Rothwell PM, Howard SC, Power DA, et al: Fibrinogen concentration and risk of ischemic stroke and acute coronary events in 5113 patients with transient ischemic attack and minor ischemic stroke. Stroke 2004;35:2300-2305.

289. Mora S, Rifai N, Buring JE, Ridker PM: Additive value of immunoassay-measured fibrinogen and high-sensitivity C-reactive protein levels for predicting incident cardiovascular events. Circulation 2006;114:381-387.

290. The Ancrod Stroke Study Investigators: Ancrod for the treatment of acute ischemic brain infarction. Stroke 1994;25:1755-1759.

291. Atkinson RP: Ancrod in the treatment of acute ischemic stroke. a review of clinical data. Cerebrovasc Dis 1998;8(Suppl 1):23-28.

292. Gonzales-Conejero R, Fernandez-Cadenas I, Iniesta JA, et al: Role of fibrinogen levels and factor XIII V34L polymorphism in thrombolytic therapy in stroke patients. Stroke 2006;37: 2288-2293.

293. Radack K, Deck C, Huster G: Dietary supplementation with low-dose fish oils lowers fibrinogen levels: A randomized double-blind controlled study. Ann Intern Med 1989;111: 757-758.

294. Lechner H, Walzl M, Walzl B, et al: H. E. L. P. application in cerebrovascular disease. In Ernst E, Koenig W, Lowe GDO, Meade TW (eds): Fibrinogen: A New Cardiovascular Risk Factor. Vienna: Blackwell, 1992, pp 408-412.

295. Dashe J: Hyperviscosity and stroke. In Bogousslavsky J, Caplan LR (eds): Uncommon Causes of Stroke. Cambridge: Cambridge University Press, 2001, pp 100-109.

296. Rosenson RS, Lowe GD: Effects of lipids and lipoproteins on thrombosis and rheology. Atherosclerosis 1998;140:271-280.

297. Ariyo A, Thach C, Tracy R for the Cardiovascular Health Study Investigators: Lp (a) lipoprotein, vascular disease, and mortality in the elderly. N Engl J Med 2003;349:2108-2115.

298. Ohira T, Schreiner P, Morrisett JD, et al: Lipoprotein (a) and incident ischemic stroke. The Atherosclerosis Risk in Communities (ARIC) Study. Stroke 2006;37:1407-1412.

299. Arenillas JF, Molina CA, Chacon P, et al: High lipoprotein (a), diabetes, and the extent of symptomatic intracranial atherosclerosis. Neurology 2004;63:27-32.

300. Dahlback B, Carlsson M, Svensson PJ: Familial thrombophilia due to a previously unrecognized mechanism characterized by poor anticoagulant response to activated protein C: Prediction of a cofactor to activated protein C. Proc Natl Acad Sci U S A 1993;90:1004-1008.

301. Zoller B, Dahlback B: Linkage between inherited resistance to activated protein C and factor V gene mutation in venous thrombosis. Lancet 1994;343:1536-1538.

302. Coull BM, Skaff PT: Disorders of coagulation. In Bogousslavsky J, Caplan LR (eds): Uncommon Causes of Stroke. Cambridge: Cambridge University Press, 2001, pp 86-95.

303. Ridker PM, Miletich JP, Stampfer MJ, et al: Factor V Leiden and risks of recurrent idiopathic venous thromboembolism. Circulation 1997;95:1777-1782.

304. Poort SR, Rosendaal FR, Reitsma PH, et al: A common genetic variation in the 3' untranslated region of the prothrombin gene is associated with elevated prothrombin levels and an increase in venous thrombosis. Blood 1996;88: 3698-3703.

305. Martinelli I, Sacchi E, Landi G, et al: High risk of cerebral-vein thrombosis in carriers of a prothrombin-gene mutation and in users of oral contraceptives. N Engl J Med 1998;338: 1793-1797.

306. Kosik KS, Furie B: Thrombotic stroke associated with elevated plasma factor VIII. Arch Neurol 1980;8:435-437.

307. Bhopale GM, Nanda RK: Blood coagulation factor VIII: An overview. J Biosci 2003;28:783-789.

308. Estol C, Pessin MS, DeWitt LD, et al: Stroke and increased factor VIII activity. Neurology 1989;39:225.

309. Pan W-H, Bai C-H, Chen J-R, Chiu H-C: Associations between carotid atherosclerosis and high factor VIII activity, dyslipidemia, and hypertension. Stroke 1997;28:88-94.

310. Lip GYH, Lane D, Van Walraven C, Hart RG: Additive role of plasma von Willebrand factor levels to clinical factors for risk stratification of patients with atrial fibrillation. Stroke 2006;37:2294-2300.

311. Markus HS, Hambley H: Neurology and the blood: haematological abnormalities in ischaemic stroke. J Neurol Neurosurg Psychiatry 1998;64:150-159.

312. Feinberg WM, Cornell ES, Nightingale SD, et al: Relationship between prothrombin activation fragment F1.2 and International Normalized Ratio in patients with atrial fibrillation. Stroke 1997;28:1101-1106.

313. Bongers TN, de Maat MP, van Goor ML, et al: High von Willebrand factor levels increase the risk of first ischemic stroke: Influence of ADAMTS13, inflammation, and genetic variability. Stroke 2006;37:2672-2677.

314. Feinberg WM, Bruck DC, Ring ME, et al: Hemostatic markers in acute stroke. Stroke 1989;20:592-597.

315. Toghi H, Kawashima M, Tamura K, et al: Coagulation-fibrinolysis abnormalities in acute and chronic phases of cerebral thrombosis and embolism. Stroke 1990;21:1663-1667.

316. Jeppeson LL, Jorgensen HS, Nakayama H, et al: Tissue plasminogen activator is elevated in women with ischemic stroke. J Stroke Cerebrovasc Dis 1998;7:187-191.

317. Feinberg WM: Coagulation. In Caplan LR (ed): Brain Ischemia: Basic Concepts and Clinical Relevance. London: Springer, 1995, pp 85-96.

318. Stallworth C, Brey R: Antiphospholipid antibody syndrome. In Bogousslavsky J, Caplan LR (eds): Uncommon Causes of Stroke. Cambridge: Cambridge University Press, 2001, pp 63-77.

319. Coull BM, Goodnight SH: Antiphospholipid antibodies, prothrombotic states, and stroke. Stroke 1990;21:1370-1374.

320. Palareti G, Cosmi B, Legnani C, et al: D-dimer testing to determine the duration of anticoagulant therapy. N Engl J Med 2006;355:1780-1789.

321. Levine SR, Welch KMA: The spectrum of neurologic disease associated with antiphospholipid antibodies: Lupus anticoagulants, and anticardiolipin antibodies. Arch Neurol 1987;44: 876-883.

322. Hess DC, Sheppard S, Adams RJ: Increased immunoglobulin binding to cerebral endothelium in patients with antiphospholipid antibodies. Stroke 1993;24:994-999.

323. Levine SR, Salowich-Palm L, Sawaya K, et al: IgG anticardiolipin antibody titer >40GPL and the risk of subsequent thrombo-occlusive events and death. A prospective cohort study. Stroke 1997;28:1660-1665.

324. Ortel TL: The antiphospholipid syndrome: What are we really measuring? How do we measure it? And how do we treat it? J Thromb Thrombolysis 2006;21:79-83.

325. Tuhrim S, Rand JH, Horowitz DR, et al: Antiphosphatidyl serine antibodies are independently associated with ischemic stroke. Neurology 1999;53:1523-1527.

326. Toschi V, Motta A, Castelli C, et al: High prevalence of antiphosphatidylinositol antibodies in young patients with cerebral ischemia of undetermined cause. Stroke 1998;29:1759-1764.

327. Tanne D, Triplett D, Levine SR: Antiphospholipid-protein antibodies and ischemic stroke: Not just cardiolipin anymore. Stroke 1998;29:1755-1758.

328. Myers R, Yamaguchi S: Nervous system effects of cardiac arrest in monkeys. Arch Neurol 1977;34:65-74.

329. Pulsinelli W, Waldman S, Rawlinson D, et al: Hyperglycemia converts ischemic neuronal damage into brain infarction. Neurology 1982;32:1239-1246.

330. Plum F: What causes infarction in ischemic brain? Neurology 1983;33:222-233.

331. Pulsinelli W, Levy D, Sigsbel B, et al: Increased damage after ischemic stroke in patients with hyperglycemia with or without established diabetes mellitus. Am J Med 1983;74:540-544.

332. Walker G, Williamson P, Ravich R, et al: Hypercalcemia associated with cerebral vasospasm causing infarction. J Neurol Neurosurg Psychiatry 1980;43:464-467.

333. Gorelick PB, Caplan LR: Calcium, hypercalcemia, and stroke. Current concepts of cerebrovascular disease. Stroke 1985;20:13-17.

334. Siesjo B, Kristian T: Cell calcium homeostasis and calcium-related ischemic damage. In Welch KMA, Caplan LR, Reis DJ, et al (eds): Primer on Cerebrovascular Diseases. San Diego: Academic Press, 1997, pp 172-178.

335. Henderson GV, Caplan LR: Calcium, hypercalcemia, magnesium, and brain ischemia. In Bogousslavsky J, Caplan LR (eds): Uncommon Causes of Stroke. Cambridge: Cambridge University Press, 2001, pp 110-113.

336. Ovbiagele B, Saver J, Fredieu A, et al: In-hospital initiation of secondary stroke prevention therapies yields high rates of adherence at follow-up. Stroke 2004;35:2879-2883.

337. Ovbiagele B, Saver J, Fredieu A, et al: PROTECT. A coordinated stroke treatment program to prevent recurrent thromboembolic events. Neurology 2004;63:1217-1222.

338. Ridker PM, Stampfer MJ, Rifai N: Novel risk factors for systemic atherosclerosis: A comparison of C-reactive protein, fibrinogen, homcysteine, lipoprotein (a), and standard cholesterol screening as predictors of peripheral arterial disease. JAMA 2001;285:2481-2485.

339. Sacco RL, Anand K, Lee H-S, et al: Homocysteine and the risk of ischemic stroke in a triethnic cohort. The Northern Manhattan Study. Stroke 2004;35:2263-2269.

340. Tanne D, Haim M, Goldbourt U, et al: Prospective study of serum homocysteine and risk of ischemic stroke among patients with preexisting coronary heart disease. Stroke 2003;34:632-636.

341. Eikelboom JW, Hankey GJ, Anand SS, et al: Association between high homocyst(e)ine and ischemic stroke due to large and small-artery disease but not other etiologic subtypes of ischemic stroke. Stroke 2000;31:1069-1075.

342. Bova I, Chapman J, Sylantiev C, et al: The A677V methylenetetrahydrofolate reductase gene polymorphism and carotid atherosclerosis. Stroke 1999;30:2180-2182.

343. Selhub J, Jacques PF, Rosenberg IH, et al: Serum total homocysteine concentrations in the Third National Health and Nutrition Examination Survey (1991-1994): Population reference ranges and contribution of vitamin status to high serum concentrations. Ann Intern Med 1999;331-339.

344. Ridker PM, Rifai N, Rose L, et al: Comparison of C-reactive protein and low-density lipoprotein cholesterol levels in the prediction of first cardiovascular events. N Engl J Med 2002;347:1557-1565.

345. Eikelboom JW, Hankey GJ, Baker RI, et al: C-reactive protein in ischemic stroke and its etiologic subtypes. J Stroke Cerebrovasc Dis 2003;12:74-81.

346. Arenillas JF, Alvarez-Sabin J, Molina CA, et al: C-reactive protein predicts further ischemic events in first-ever transient ischemic attack or stroke patients with intracranial large-artery occlusive disease. Stroke 2003;34:2463-2470.

347. Wakugawa Y, Kiyohara Y, Tanizaki Y, et al: C-reactive protein and risk of first-ever ischemic and hemorrhagic stroke in general Japanese population. The Hisayama Study. Stroke 2006;37:27-32.

348. Salvarani C, Canini F, Boiardi L, Hunder GG: Laboratory investigations useful in giant cell arteritis and Takayasu's arteritis. Clin Exp Rheumatol 2003;21(Suppl 32):523-528.

349. Lavigne-Lissalde G, Schved JF, Granier C, Villard S: Anti-factor VIII antibodies: A 2005 update. Thromb Haemost 2005;94:760-769.

349a. Schlager O, Exner M, Miekusch W, et al: C-reactive protein predicts future cardiovascular events in patients with carotid stenosis. Stroke 2007;38:1263-1268.

350. Franchini M: Acquired hemophilia A. Hematology 2006;11:119-125.

351. Saposnik G, Caplan LR: Convulsive-like movements in brainstem stroke. Arch Neurol 2001;54:654-657.

352. Ropper AH: "Convulsions" in basilar artery occlusions. Neurology 1988;38:1500-1501.

353. Carrera E, Michel P, Despland PA, et al: Continuous assessment of electrical epileptic activity in acute stroke. Neurology 2006 11;67:99-104.

354. Bladin CF, Alexandrov A, Bellavance A, et al: Seizures after stroke: A prospective multicenter study. Arch Neurol 2000;57:1617-1622.

355. Wilber DJ, Garan H, Finkelstein D, et al: Out-of-hospital cardiac arrest: Use of electrophysiologic testing in the prediction of long-term outcome. N Engl J Med 1988;318-324.

356. Madl C, Kramer L, Domanovits H, et al: Improved outcome prediction in unconscious cardiac arrest survivors with sensory evoked potentials compared with clinical assessment. Crit Care Med 2000;28:721-726.

357. Wijdicks EF, Hijdra A, Young GB, et al: For the Quality Standards Subcommittee of the American Academy of Neurology Practice parameter: Prediction of outcome in comatose survivors after cardiopulmonary resuscitation (an evidence-based review). Report of the Quality Standards Subcommittee of the American Academy of Neurology. Neurology 2006;67:203-210.

358. Tettenborn B, Caplan LR, Krämer G, Hopf H: Electrophysiology in posterior circulation disease. In Berguer R, Caplan LR (eds): Vertebrobasilar Arterial Disease. St Louis: Quality Medical, 1991, pp 124-129.

359. Natowicz M, Kelley RI: Mendelian etiologies of stroke. Ann Neurol 1987;22:175-192.

360. Alberts MJ: Genetics of cerebrovascular disease. Stroke 2004;35:342-344.

361. Meschia JF, Worrall BB: New advances in identifying genetic anomalies in stroke-prone probands. Curr Neurol Neurosci Rep 2004;4:420-426.

362. Gretarsdottir S, Thorleifsson G, Reynisdottir ST, et al: The gene encoding phosphodiesterase 4D confers risk of ischemic stroke. Nat Genet 2003;35:131-138.

363. Yee RYL, Brophy VH, Cheng S, et al: Polymorphisms of the phosphodiesterase 4D, camp-specific (PDE4D) gene and risk of ischemic stroke: A prospective, nested case–control evaluation. Stroke 2006;37:2012-2017.

363a. Dichgans M, Hegele RA: Update on the genetics of stroke and cerebrovascular disease—2006. Stroke 2007;38:216-218.

363b. Dichgans M: Genetics of ischaemic stroke. Lancet Neurol 2007;6:149-161.

364. Worrall BB, Mychaleckyj JC: PDE4D and stroke. A real advance or a case of the emperor's new clothes? Stroke 2006;37:1955-1957.

365. Joutel A, Corpechot C, Ducros A, et al: Notch 3 mutations in CADASIL, a hereditary adult-onset condition causing stroke and dementia. Nature 1996;383:707-710.

366. Ruchoux MM, Domenga V, Brulin P, et al: Transgenic mice expressing mutant Notch3 develop vascular alterations characteristic of cerebral dominant arteriopathy with subcortical infarcts and leukoencephalopathy. Am J Pathol 2003;162:329-342.

367. Penn AMW, Lee JWK, Thuiller P, et al: MELAS syndrome with mitochondrial tRNA Leu(UUR) mutation: Correlation of clinical state, nerve conduction, and muscle 31P magnetic resonance spectroscopy during treatment with nicotinamide and riboflavin. Neurology 1992;42:2147-2152.

368. Ruigrok YM, Rinkel GJE, Wijmenga C: Genetics of intracranial aneurysms. Lancet Neurol 2005;4:179-189.

369. Ruigrok YM, Rinkel GJ, Wijmenga C: The Versican gene and the risk of intracranial aneurysms. Stroke 2006;37:2372-2374.

5 *Treatment*

*Some men see things as they are and say Why? I
dream things that never were and say Why not?*
— GEORGE BERNARD SHAW

The last quarter of the 20th century and first
decade of the 21st can legitimately be considered a time when neurologic and stroke therapeutics reached center stage. Advances in diagnostic technology made it possible to quickly
and safely determine the cause of most strokes.
The methodology of randomized therapeutic
trials progressed as researchers and physicians
began to systematically study various treatments. In this chapter, I introduce the general
underlying principles of treatment of patients
who have acute strokes and outline the types of
therapy available. I will devote the most space
to angioplasty and stenting and thrombolysis
since these treatments have expanded dramatically since the third edition of this monograph.
Prophylactic treatments and stroke prevention
strategies will be discussed in Chapter 17,
avoidance and management of complications in
Chapter 18 and strategies to enhance recovery
and rehabilitation in Chapter 19.

Factors that influence treatment and various
therapeutic strategies are also discussed. The
emphasis of all treatments is on the anatomy,
pathology, and pathophysiology of the cerebrovascular process and on the patient in all
of their socio-psycho-economic-environmental
complexity. Clinicians must use all information
available to make difficult treatment decisions
for individual patient situations. Specific treatments for patients with individual vascular
pathologies and mechanisms (e.g., stenosis of
an internal carotid artery [ICA], cardiac-origin
embolism, and cerebral venous sinus thrombosis) are considered in Part II of this book.

RANDOMIZED TRIALS AND SO-CALLED EVIDENCE-BASED MEDICINE

Randomized trials are important, but they have
limitations.[1] Trials are expensive, time consum-
ing, and require enormous resources. To provide statistically valid results, randomized trials
must contain large numbers of patients with
enough endpoints to analyze. Sufficient endpoints must be reached in a relatively short
period. Many cerebrovascular conditions are
unsuitable for trials. The issue of numbers versus specificity limits trials. For randomized trials to yield statistically valid results, many
patients must be included in the study. If the
results are to be useful, the data must be specifically applicable to individual patients. To
achieve an adequate number of patients, the
condition studied must be common and a
"lumping" strategy must predominate over
"splitting." Patients who are too ill, old, young,
and of childbearing age are often excluded from
trials. Those incapable of giving informed con-
sent or who have too complex or multiple
illnesses are also frequently left out of trials.
These are just the types of stroke patients that
doctors care for every day.

The results of many randomized trials cannot
be applied directly to individual patients. The
term *evidence based* must be used cautiously
when applied to a particular circumstance if that
circumstance has not been specifically studied.
Information from trials must be weighed according to the context of specific treatment decisions.
Conducting trials is different from caring for sick
patients. In trials, the same treatments are given
to all eligible patients depending only on randomization. Departure from the specified treatment makes the results difficult to interpret.
In the clinic, doctors treat individual patients.
George Thibault said it well[2]:

> We then need to decide which approach in our large
> therapeutic armamentarium will be most appropri-
> ate in a particular patient, with a particular stage
> of disease and particular coexisting conditions, and
> at a particular age. Even when randomized clinical
> trials have been performed (which is true for only a
> small number of clinical problems), they will often
> not answer this question specifically for the patient
> sitting in front of us in the office or lying in the
> hospital bed.

First, find out what is wrong with each patient
in as much detail as possible. This includes the
anatomy, pathology, and pathophysiology of the
brain and vascular lesions. The methodology
of diagnosis has been considered in Chapters 3

and 4. If there is clear therapeutic guidance from randomized trials that apply to the patient at hand, then follow those guidelines. If not, use all information from what you know about the condition, what you know about the person, what has been written from published observations, case series, and reports, and what is known about potential treatments to make rational considered treatment decisions.

WHAT FACTORS SHOULD THE CLINICIAN CONSIDER WHEN PLANNING TREATMENT FOR THE INDIVIDUAL STROKE PATIENT?

Socioeconomic and Psychological Factors

Socioeconomic and psychological factors may influence treatment for some patients and their families. A previously unreliable and noncompliant patient cannot be depended on to take anticoagulants. Some patients do not have the economic resources for particular therapies. In other cases, lack of caring family members or friends limits subsequent follow-up and treatment. One person might be disabled by fear of impending disability when informed of the presence of carotid artery disease and a threat of stroke, whereas another individual with a similar condition may weigh the alternatives more dispassionately.

Other Medical Conditions

The presence of preexistent and coexistent medical problems and conditions affects and often limits available treatments. Physicians are more conservative when suggesting surgery for stroke patients who have severe heart disease or advanced cancer. Particular concurrent conditions contraindicate some treatments. An active peptic ulcer or severe uncontrolled arterial hypertension makes anticoagulation unwise. Other conditions, such as severe heart or lung disease, increase the risks of anesthesia and surgery.

The patient's premorbid function and intellect are also critical. A hopelessly demented nursing home resident with a new stroke should be treated humanely but certainly not aggressively. An older widow, depressed and lonely for many years after the passing of her husband and friends, would be managed differently from a happy and pleasant but slightly demented grandmother who draws joy from her family and surroundings. Age is never an absolute contraindication to stroke treatment. Elderly patients cannot tolerate medical and surgical treatments as well as younger patients, nor do they share the same ability to rebound from strokes. The elderly should be handled cautiously. The same diagnostic and therapeutic strategies that apply to younger individuals, however, should be considered for geriatric patients.

NATURE OF THE STROKE

Vascular Lesion

Stroke is a *cerebrovascular disease*. The nature of the causative cerebrovascular process is certainly one of the very most important determinants of potential treatments. Management of ICA occlusion is different from severe ICA stenosis or carotid plaque disease without stenosis. These extracranial large-artery lesions differ greatly from lipohyalinosis of intracranial penetrating arteries caused by hypertension. These intrinsic vascular lesions differ from cardiogenic embolism and hypercoagulability as causes of vascular occlusion. Venous and dural sinus occlusions present very different issues from arterial occlusive disease. The nature, location, and severity of the vascular lesions are key factors in selecting possible and optimal therapeutic strategies.

The Blood

Does the patient have a high hematocrit (Hct) or platelet count? What is the blood viscosity? Are the platelets activated or sticky? Is there a bleeding diathesis? Abnormalities of blood constituents and coagulation functions might suggest some therapeutic strategies and contraindicate other treatments.

In a small number of patients, the hematologic disorder is the primary condition that leads to vascular thrombosis or hemorrhage. In many patients, the coagulation disorder contributes to vascular occlusion. Many acute medical conditions, including infections, systemic vascular occlusions (e.g., myocardial infarction), cancers, and inflammatory diseases such as regional enteritis and ulcerative colitis, are accompanied by platelet activation and an increase in acute-phase reactants that increase blood coagulability. In patients with preexisting cardiac and vascular lesions (e.g., atrial fibrillation, congestive heart failure, and arterial stenosis or ulceration), the increase in coagulability and platelet activation incites the formation of white thrombi, red thrombi, or both at the site of the preexisting condition.

5 Mechanisms and Pathophysiology of Stroke

Was the ischemia caused by local vascular thrombosis, embolism, or circulatory failure? (For example, was the brain ischemia caused by reduced perfusion, or artery-to-artery embolism, or a combination of hypoperfusion and embolism in a patient with severe ICA stenosis?)

Nature, Location, Extent, and Reversibility of the Brain Lesions

If the entire middle cerebral artery (MCA) territory is destroyed, there is little point in reperfusing the MCA territory because only dead brain would be irrigated. Reperfusion might even be harmful.[3,4] In the DEFUSE trial, reperfusion of patients with large infarcts worsened outcomes.[5] If, however, the MCA territory ischemia is reversible and the neurons are stunned and dysfunctional but not yet infarcted, the argument for augmenting MCA blood flow is substantially greater. Imaging using modern CT or MR can define the state of the brain as discussed in Chapter 4. Imaging results can show if feeding arteries are still occluded and the potential reversibility of the ischemia.

The cause of the ischemia and the severity and location of the cardiocerebrovascular lesion is also important in determining the risk for further ischemia. Even if the entire MCA territory in one cerebral hemisphere is irreversibly damaged by cardiac-origin embolism, the opposite cerebral hemisphere and the territory supplied by the posterior circulation is still at risk for further damage.

The size of the lesion, severity of the neurologic deficit, and length of time since the last worsening have traditionally been used to decide if a stroke is "completed."[6] The term *completed stroke* is variously defined and applied and should be discarded. Short of an infallible crystal ball or direct guidance from a deity, doctors cannot predict the future. The fact that a patient is stable today does not predict whether he or she will worsen tomorrow. Patients with so-called completed stroke have as high a frequency of further brain ischemia as those with a transient ischemic attack (TIA) or reversible ischemic neurologic deficit (RIND).[6,7] If, however, the vascular mechanism and pathology are known, the tissue at risk can be estimated. In a patient with penetrating artery disease, a 5-mm basal-ganglionic lacune may represent infarction of the entire territory of that artery. If the same patient with a small basal-ganglia infarct had severe stenosis of the MCA causing reduced flow in the lenticulostriate territory, the potential for further extensive damage is much greater.

Stroke in evolution is a nonspecific term. Almost 30% of stroke patients worsen after entering the hospital. These worsening deficits are related to numerous factors listed in Table 5-1. Knowledge that a patient is worsening should stimulate action. The nature of the therapeutic action, however, depends on the pathophysiology of the patient's particular problem that is causing the worsening.

Pace of Stroke

I have already emphasized that tempo of the illness should not be used as the only criterion for treatment. This does not mean, however, that it should not be considered at all. In fact, the pace of progression dictates the urgency and speed of evaluation and treatment. A patient with a TIA this morning has a greater probability of stroke tomorrow than a patient with a single TIA 3 months ago. The patient with a single TIA a week ago differs from the patient with a flurry of 5 to 10 TIAs yesterday and today. Patients worsening under immediate supervision require more urgent management than patients stable for the past week. An improving patient makes the physician pause before deciding to tamper with natural forces that seem to be at least temporarily succeeding.

The goal of treatment is to prevent brain damage whenever possible. The major determinant of treatment is the nature of the causative cardiocerebrovascular lesion. Ideally, treatments indicated because of the lesion's nature should begin before the patient develops any neurologic worsening.

Personnel and Technology Available for a Given Treatment or Evaluation

Complications and success rates vary widely among hospitals and even within the same medical center depending on the personnel involved. There is striking variability in morbidity and

Table 5-1.	Explanations for Worsening Among Acute Stroke Patients

Failure of collateral circulation
Systemic hypotension
Hypovolemia
Cardiac arrhythmias
Embolization or propagation of thrombus
Progressive occlusion of the arterial lumen
Depression
Intercurrent infections, especially pneumonia and urinary tract infection
Seizures
Pulmonary embolism

mortality for the same surgical procedure—carotid endarterectomy.[8,9] The risk-to-benefit ratio of carotid endarterectomy when the complication rate is 2% is quite different from the situation when it is 10%. The use and complication rate for diagnostic tests, such as cerebral angiography, also vary with the skill, training, and experience of the angiographer and the equipment available. Especially in this era of limited resources, not all medical centers are economically able to specialize equally in all fields.

Physicians owe patients the best available care. Responsibility to the patient must outweigh loyalty to one's colleagues and institution if physicians are to continue to deserve the respect of the community. If a physician or hospital has limited training, experience, interest, and capability in stroke management and the patient's condition and socioeconomic status make it feasible for the patient to go elsewhere, then the physician should send the patient to where the best care is available. The Golden Rule—do unto others what you would want for yourself—is the most important guide to treatment.

Some therapeutic strategies are general and apply to all stroke patients, whereas other strategies depend on the specific problems in the individual patient. Examples of specific problems include (1) focal brain ischemia caused by low flow in a patient with a documented occlusive vascular lesion, (2) increased intracranial pressure (ICP) caused by the mass effect of a hematoma and its surrounding brain edema, (3) a threatened second embolism in a patient with a known cardiac source of embolism, and (4) a threatened recurrence of subarachnoid hemorrhage in a patient with a cerebral aneurysm. The key treatment strategies are listed in Table 5-2.

Table 5-2.	**General Strategies of Stroke Treatment**

Control stroke risk factors to prevent further strokes and vascular disease

Prevent stroke complications (e.g., decubitus ulcers, urinary infections, phlebothrombosis, and pulmonary embolism)

Treat specific pathologies and pathophysiologies (e.g., draining a brain hematoma, reperfusion of an occlusive vascular lesion, managing increased intracranial pressure, reducing coagulability to prevent thrombus formation) in patients with atrial fibrillation

Facilitate recovery

Improve neurologic function

GENERAL CARE

Important general care goals for physicians are to limit suffering, give comfort, and prevent complications. Patients deserve excellent nursing and general care even when no specific therapy seems warranted because of the severity of the deficit, type of stroke, or severe comorbidities. Stroke patients are often at least partially immobilized and may not be able to care for their bodily needs. Key goals are (1) maintenance of adequate nutrition; (2) prevention of contractures or painful, stiff, or frozen joints; (3) prevention of decubiti and of pressure-related peripheral nerve palsies; and (4) prevention of thromboembolic, pulmonary, genitourinary, and skin complications. Table 5-3 lists some stroke complications and general types of treatment for their prevention. Complications are discussed in detail in Chapter 18. Perhaps just as important as these physical problems is maintenance of a positive but realistic outlook for patients, their families, and significant others. Depression is common after stroke, so measures should be instituted early to prevent discouragement.[10] Depression should be recognized and treated when it occurs.

Patients' visits to doctors gives physicians important opportunities to view the whole person and his or her environment. In the hurry to diagnose and treat acute stroke problems, preventive measures are often overlooked. The stroke patient of today, irrespective of cause, is at risk for future strokes and vascular disease in other important organs. Prevention strategies should begin as early as possible. Patients receive wrong messages when some factors are neglected (e.g., food trays rich in red meats, cheese, and ice cream tell the patient with hypercholesterolemia that diet is not important). Nurses or aides who help the patient smoke also convey approbation. While the specific stroke mechanism is investigated and treated, explore general health practices and stroke risk factors and deal with them early in the course. Table 5-4 lists some of these risk factors. These are explored in more detail in Chapter 17.

While exploring diagnosis and treatment of acute stroke, begin to develop rehabilitation strategies. Restorative or rehabilitation therapy depends on the type of handicap and disability, not on the stroke etiology or mechanism. Limb weakness, gait abnormalities, language disturbances, dysphagia, neglect of the left side of space, and hemianopia are different problems that require different rehabilitation and therapy strategies. To be maximally effective, rehabilitation should focus on the individual patient, taking past capabilities, activities, and future needs into consideration. Recovery and rehabilitation are discussed in greater detail in Chapter 19.

Table 5-3.   General Problems and Treatments in Patients with Stroke

Problems	Treatments
Nutritional maintenance (especially if dysphagia is present)	Balanced diet that conforms to suggested calories and content (e.g., low cholesterol and low salt), vitamins when indicated, intravenous feeding, nasogastric tubes, gastronomy
Pulmonary complications (aspiration, pneumonia atelectasis, pulmonary emboli)	Care or avoidance in oral feeding; in dysphagics, study of swallowing before oral feeding; respiratory therapy; early antibiotic treatment of infection; no smoking; anticoagulants (miniheparin or heparinoids); use of special leg boots to prevent phlebothrombosis
Immobility (body or one or more limbs)	Frequent full range-of-motion exercises, frequent turning, prevention of pressure palsies and joint dislocations by slings, and careful limb positioning
Urinary-tract complications (bladder distension, urinary retention, infection)	Catheterization using sterile technique when needed; avoidance when possible of indwelling catheters; early antibiotic treatment; urinary acidification
Skin (decubiti)	Careful, frequent turning; pillows and pads to protect pressure areas; water beds; skin surveillance
Psychological (apathy and depression)	Positive outlook; entire medical care personnel functioning as a team; antidepressants

Adapted from Caplan LR: A general therapeutic perspective on stroke treatment. In: Dunkel R, Schmidley R (eds): Stroke in the Elderly: New Issues in Diagnosis, Treatment and Rehabilitation. New York: Springer Publishing, 1987, pp 60-69, with permission.

Rehabilitation involves an educational process, training patients and their caregivers to understand their handicaps, and devising strategies to overcome them. Recall that the word *doctor* is derived from the Latin word *docere*, which means "to teach" or "to lead." Sometimes well-learned routine tasks, such as walking, eating, or getting on and off a toilet seat, must be performed in a different way. Patients must be instructed and trained to use new approaches. To be successful, the rehabilitation and education process must be shared with the family and others who live with and help the patient. They must carry on and amplify the gains made in the hospital after the patient returns home. If friends and family know the nature of the patient's disabilities, they understand when the patient cannot perform particular tasks and thus modify the patient's environment to make things easier. A kind, understanding, and unhurried approach by all personnel involved is needed. Rehabilitation, like prevention, should start early during the acute stroke period. Passive range-of-movement exercises, speech therapy, and explanation of the neurologic dysfunction can begin during the first days after the stroke.

In many medical centers and physician practices, the locations and personnel involved in stroke prevention, acute treatment, and rehabilitation are different. Primary care physicians have the most opportunity to encourage stroke prevention practices when they see patients in their offices. Neurologists, hospitalists, and other acute-care specialists treat acute strokes in acute-care facilities, sometimes in special stroke or intensive care units. Neurologists do not usually see patients until they already have had a stroke or other cerebrovascular

Table 5-4.   Risk Factors and Potentially Unhealthy Practices

Smoking
Heart disease
Hypertension
Illicit drug use (especially cocaine and amphetamines)
Prescription drugs and their overuse
Overuse of alcohol
Abnormal blood lipids
Oral contraceptives
Sedentary lifestyle, lack of regular exercise
Diabetes
Highly stressful work and home situations
Being overweight
Low fluid intake

event. Other specialists, such as physiatrists, often manage the patient during the recuperative period in rehabilitation hospitals. All phases of care should be a continuum. Ideally, the three types of practitioners should be involved during the acute-care phase. Rehabilitation personnel must be aware of the preventive and acute treatment strategies used during rehabilitation. After being urged to refrain from smoking and watch their diet in the acute-care hospital, what message do patients receive if they are allowed to smoke and eat as they please in the rehabilitation hospital?

Stroke Units and Services

One of the most important therapeutic advances during the last decades of the 20th century in the treatment of patients with acute stroke was the development of stroke services, stroke nurses, stroke specialists, and stroke units. Technological advances in diagnosis and treatment of stroke patients and the complexity of stroke prevention, acute care, and rehabilitation led to the development of specialized stroke services and units in many academic hospitals in the United States, Europe, and Australasia. The advent of thrombolysis and potentially effective care of acute stroke patients gave a boost to this movement and made it clear that efficient rapid throughput of stroke patients by experienced physicians and nurses was essential and advantageous to segregate stroke patients in ICUs and specialized stroke units.

These specialized units were composed of nurses with experience and training in stroke, internists, and stroke neurologists. These stroke units are able to deliver specialized nursing care; attention to management of blood pressure, fluid volumes, and other physiological and biochemical factors; protocols and practices to facilitate rapid and thorough evaluation and treatment, monitor treatment, carry out randomized therapeutic trials, and prevent complications; and education to patients and their families and caregivers about stroke and its prevention and treatment.[11-18] Stroke units also promote an optimistic view of stroke recovery in contrast to the situation previously common on medical wards where stroke patients were often considered undesirable patients with hopeless outcomes.

Once these units began to proliferate, especially in Europe, it became clear that they were a very important major advance. Dedicated stroke units have been convincingly shown to decrease mortality, limit stroke morbidity, and allow more patients to retain their independence and to return home after stroke.[11-18] The milieu and patient care in dedicated stroke units leads to better outcomes. Mortality is reduced. More patients return home, and fewer are transferred to chronic hospitals and nursing homes. Short-term and long-term functional outcomes are also improved. There is no longer any doubt that stroke units work.

ISCHEMIC STROKE

Although mechanisms of ischemia vary, particular themes are applicable to all patients with brain ischemia. Ischemia means inadequate delivery of blood containing required nutrients. Maximizing blood flow to ischemic zones is clearly important. Can areas of vascular blockage in large arteries be opened or circumvented by medical or surgical treatments? Can local perfusion through the microcirculation supplying the ischemic zone be improved? Occlusive thrombosis and thromboembolism are important in most patients with ischemic stroke. Can the coagulation system be altered to diminish the development of white-platelet–fibrin clots and red thrombin-dependent clots? Metabolic changes within the ischemic zone are important in causing cell death. Can the brain be made more resistant to ischemia by manipulating its chemical environment? Edema and raised ICP can promote nerve cell damage. Can they be controlled? I discuss these issues separately.

Maximizing Blood Flow

Different medical and surgical strategies are available to try to improve circulation to an ischemic region distal to a vascular occlusive lesion.

Controlling Position and Activity

In some patients, sitting, standing, and even elevating the head of the bed increase ischemic symptoms.[19,20] The minor reduction in cephalad flow accompanying postural change decreases blood flow through the stenotic vessel or collateral channels just enough to decompensate a fragile equilibrium. Patients may improve when they are treated in a supine or head-down position.[21] Physicians should note if patients are sensitive to postural changes. Initially after the acute stroke, patients should be observed when first sitting or standing, to ensure that blood pressure does not drop excessively or postural symptoms appear. Patients with progressive symptoms caused by ischemia should be nursed in a supine position, sometimes with the feet slightly or moderately elevated.

5

Managing Blood Pressure, Blood Volume, and Cardiac Output

Cerebral blood flow (CBF) increases with rising blood pressure until the pressure becomes high, approaching the malignant range. For this reason, surgeons often administer intravenous agents, such as phenylephrine, to raise blood pressure just before clamping the ICA during an endarterectomy. During the acute period of ischemic stroke, it is unwise to lower the systemic pressure unless it is extremely high (e.g., above 200/120 mm Hg). In some emergency rooms or intensive care units, however, exposing physicians to an elevated blood pressure is like waving a red flag before a bull; they want to move all of the patient's numbers into the normal range, including blood pressure. Remember that physicians treat patients not numbers. The patient's symptoms, signs, and neurologic function are better guides to the appropriateness of a treatment than the measured blood pressure.

In some patients with arterial occlusive lesions, giving medications such as phenylephrine to raise the blood pressure can lead to improved neurologic function.[22-25] Improvement in function is especially likely when there is an arterial occlusion and MRI studies show a diffusion-perfusion mismatch indicating the presence of considerable viable brain tissue.

Blood volume also affects perfusion pressure and blood flow. Some patients who are not able to eat normally become dehydrated and relatively hemoconcentrated. Other factors (i.e., vomiting, eating restrictions because of concern for aspiration, or simply the rush of diagnostic testing occupying patients at mealtimes) contribute to reduced fluid intake during the early hours and days after stroke onset. In general, it is wise to keep blood volume, especially plasma volume, high. Fluids must often be given intravenously or by nasogastric tube. Care, however, must be taken to avoid fluid overload and the complications of cardiac failure and brain edema. Careful monitoring of cardiac and brain function should accompany any therapeutic attempt to augment fluid volume.

Some patients have anoxic-ischemic brain damage caused by cardiac malfunction; in others, a strong pump helps maximize CBF. Attention to cardiac rhythm and pump function is important, especially during the acute, fragile period of brain ischemia. Cardiac output can sometimes be improved by (1) use of digitalis, vasodilators, pacemakers, or medications to treat slow rhythms and heart block; (2) adjustment of already prescribed drugs such as digitalis and diuretics; (3) correction of abnormal serum K^+ and Ca^{++} levels; and (4) control of tachyrhythmias. Cardiac-ejection fractions and output can be monitored noninvasively by echocardiography.

Reperfusion strategies

Table 5-5 lists the various strategies that can be used to effect reperfusion of ischemic zones. Often more than one strategy can be used.

Surgical Endarterectomy or Local Reconstruction

Endarterectomy has been the most common method of unblocking a vessel by direct surgery. This strategy differs from other techniques that augment flow because endarterectomy of a tightly stenotic vessel produces a suddenly large increase in flow. Capillaries, small arterioles, and neurons are often damaged during ischemia. When flooded with blood under high pressure, these abnormal vessels can then bleed. The carotid sinus is also damaged during endarterectomy, leading to failure of the carotid sinus reflex and accelerated hypertension in the hours and days after carotid endarterectomy.[26-28] Elevated blood pressure and flooding of damaged vessels can lead to brain edema and ICH after carotid endarterectomy.[28,29] Care must be taken in the timing of endarterectomy. Blood pressure of patients undergoing carotid endarterectomy must be carefully monitored during the postoperative period. Usually, completely occluded arteries do not lend themselves to direct repair because clots form and propagate distally beyond the site of surgical access in the presence of low flow.

Carotid endarterectomy has been shown to be clearly more effective than medical therapy in patients with neurologically symptomatic, severe (70% luminal narrowing) carotid artery stenosis.[30-32] Endarterectomy not only removes the obstructing lesion dramatically augmenting flow but also removes the source of intra-arterial emboli. Endarterectomy has also been shown to

Table 5-5.	Strategies Used to Effect Reperfusion of Ischemic Brain Regions
Direct arterial surgery—endarterectomy	
Angioplasty	
Stenting	
Thrombolysis	
Mechanical clot retrieval	
Vasodilator treatment of vasoconstriction	
Surgically bypassing an obstructed artery	
Augmenting collateral circulation	

be somewhat effective in selected patients with luminal stenosis in the 50% to 69% range.[33,34] However, patients must be carefully chosen because neurologic and cardiac morbidity and mortality are significant risks.

Vertebral artery surgery can also be performed successfully with low morbidity and mortality when performed by surgeons with extensive experience with the procedure.[35-37] The most common method of vertebral artery reconstruction is to anastamose the vertebral artery to the carotid artery. Vertebral artery endarterectomy can also be performed.

Several randomized trials showed that carotid endarterectomy in carefully selected patients who had severe carotid artery stenosis but no recent symptoms considered related to the carotid disease was more effective than medical treatment in preventing strokes.[38-40] The selected patients had no symptoms of retinal or brain ischemia, severe cardiac disease, or other serious comorbidities and were operated on by selected surgeons who had low surgical complication rates. Women and those over 65 years of age in the European Asymptomatic Carotid Surgery trial (ACST) did not fare as well as men and younger individuals.[40] Endarterectomy has also occasionally been performed successfully in stenosing lesions of the intracranial vertebral arteries.[41,42] Insufficient cases have been studied to determine the indications and effectiveness of surgery versus medical therapy in patients with vertebral artery lesions. Emboli have also been removed directly from the MCA but the procedure did not reduce stroke severity.[43]

Angioplasty and Stenting

Since the 1980s, interventional radiology techniques have become an important therapeutic alternative for many cerebrovascular conditions. At first, interventional techniques using coils, catheters, balloons, glues, and other devices were applied mostly to treatment of patients with intracranial aneurysms and vascular malformations. Transluminal angioplasty, sometimes with insertion of vascular stents, is often performed in patients with coronary artery and peripheral vascular occlusive disease of the limbs. Mechanical vascular dilation has been used to treat fibromuscular dysplasia.

Although coronary artery angioplasty began much earlier, Kerber et al published the first report of endovascular treatment of carotid artery disease with balloon angioplasty in 1980.[44-46] A second small series was reported in 1983[47] and in 1987. Theron and colleagues published a larger series that consisted of 48 patients in whom the

technical success rate was 94% with a major stroke morbidity of 4.1%.[48] By 1995, a review of worldwide experience among 523 patients claimed favorable results: 96.2% technical success, 2.1% morbidity, 6.3% transient minor complications, and no deaths.[49] Operator experience was important in determining the technical success and treatment outcomes: centers with limited experience (<50 cases) reported nearly twice the rate of complications (5.9% vs 2.6%) than those with more substantial experience.[44,45,50,51]

In a larger series, a Spanish neurologist, Gil-Peralta reported the results among 85 carotid artery angioplasties that he performed in patients with severe (>70%) symptomatic carotid stenosis measuring more than 70%.[52] Technical success was achieved in 92% (defined as residual stenosis of <50%), with a 30-day morbidity of 4.9%, and no deaths. The rate of recurrent stenosis was 6.7% at a mean follow-up of 18.7 months, nearly all restenosis developed within 6 months of treatment.[52] Rates of recurrent stenosis in other large series ranged from 0% to 16%.[45,53-56] Early experience showed that angioplasty to treat atherosclerotic disease generated embolic debris composed of atheromatous plaque, cholesterol crystals, thrombus, and platelet aggregates.[57-60]

The development of stenting in conjunction with balloon angioplasty for carotid stenosis was based on reports that showed improved outcomes during coronary interventions when stents were used. These coronary artery studies reported greater event-free survival at 1 year with a lower rate of repeat angioplasty for recurrent stenosis after stenting as compared with angioplasty alone. Stents seemed to reduce the risk of plaque dislodgement, significant intimal dissection, elastic recoil of the vessel wall, and both early and late restenosis. Figure 5-1 is an example of stenting of a very stenotic ICA.

Between 1996 and 1999, there were 11 carotid stent series published in which the total number of patients was 1311.[45] Comparing these reports is difficult due to differences among the patients studied, lesion characteristics, endovascular techniques, and outcome information. The overall reported rate of technical success was more than 95%; procedure-related mortality rates (including cardiac deaths) were 0.6% to 4.5%; major stroke rates were 0% to 4.5%; minor stroke rates were 0% to 6.5%; and the 6-month restenosis rate was less than 5%. Other series that included very high-risk cohorts reported less favorable results.[45]

In the Carotid and Vertebral Transluminal Angioplasty Study (CAVATAS), a large, prospective, randomized, multicenter trial that compared carotid endarterectomy to carotid angioplasty

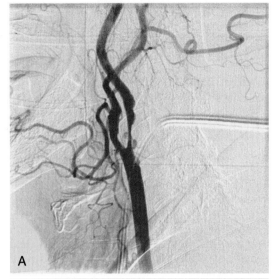

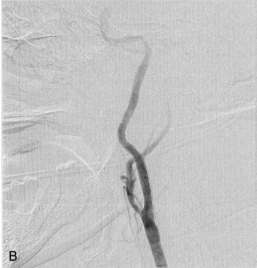

Figure 5-1. (A) Lateral view of catheter-contrast angiogram showing a long, very irregular atherosclerotic lesion that begins in the distal common carotid artery and extends several centimeters into the internal carotid artery. **(B)** Angiographic film after successful placement of a stent across the lesion. (Courtesy of Ajith Thomas, MD, Neurosurgery, Beth Israel Deaconess Medical Center, Boston, Mass.)

surgical and angioplasty groups, and the rate of disabling stroke or death within 30 days of first treatment was 6% in both groups. Preliminary analysis of long-term survival showed no difference in the rate of ipsilateral stroke or any disabling stroke in patients up to 3 years after randomization. The rate of restenosis in the endovascular group was twice that in the surgical cohort, 18% versus 9%, respectively.[62]

The Stenting and Angioplasty with Protection in Patients at High Risk for Endarterectomy (SAPPHIRE) compared carotid stenting using an embolic protection device to endarterectomy in surgically "high-risk" patients with specific comorbidities.[64] A total of 747 patients with more than 50% symptomatic stenosis, or with more than 80% asymptomatic stenosis, were enrolled. Clinical equipoise (stent or surgery) was required for randomization. Primary endpoints were a composite of death, stroke, or myocardial infarction at 30 days and ipsilateral stroke or death within 1 year. The authors concluded that stenting with distal embolic protection was not inferior to endarterectomy ($P = .004$). Moreover, the results narrowly missed the mark for statistical superiority of stenting ($P = .053$). Overall, the risk of stroke, death or MI was 39% lower with stenting at 30 days. The risk of ipsilateral stroke or death was 7.9% lower with stenting at 1 year. Fewer stented patients required reoperation than those who had endarterectomy.

SAPPHIRE was the first trial to show the efficacy of distal embolic filtration protection during stent-supported angioplasty in a high-risk population. Limits to the SAPPHIRE study included the fact that 55% of patients were excluded from randomization as poor surgical candidates, a number that appears high to many surgeons. Additionally, more than 20% of patients in each group had recurrent stenosis following a prior endarterectomy, a condition that potentially favors endovascular treatment. Lastly, inclusion of myocardial infarction in the composite endpoint obscures the effects of stroke and death which were primary endpoints in the large endarterectomy trials.

The Stent-protected Angioplasty versus Carotid Endarterectomy (SPACE) trial included 1183 German, Austrian, and Swiss patients with symptomatic eye or brain ischemia and a severe (>50% luminal narrowing by North American Symptomatic Carotid Endarterectomy Trial [NASCET] criteria) ipsilateral carotid artery stenosis who were allocated to carotid surgery (599) or carotid artery stenting (584).[65] Choice of protection devices, predilatation, balloon size, and stents was left up to the interventionalists. Only 27% of stented patients had protection devices, but there were no differences in endpoints among those treated with

patients with a symptomatic stenosis of 70% or more were randomized to angioplasty or surgery.[61-63] Patients unsuitable for endarterectomy were randomized to percutaneous transluminal angioplasty with or without stenting or to best medical treatment. Among the 504 patients randomized between surgery and angioplasty during 5 years, no significant difference in the risk of stroke or death related to either procedure was found. The rate of any stroke lasting more than 7 days or death within 30 days of first treatment was approximately 10% to 12% in both the and without protective devices. The rate of death or ipsilateral ischemic stroke at 30 days was 6.34% with surgery and 6.84% with stenting, an insignificant difference. Older patients and women tended to do worse with either treatment.[65]

Hoffman and colleagues reviewed the risk scores for peri-interventional complications of carotid artery stenting derived from a prospective registry of 606 consecutive patients treated at a "secondary care hospital" in Austria.[66] The acute stroke rate was 3% (including 13 minor and 5 major periprocedural nonfatal strokes) and 1.3% deaths including four fatal strokes. Diabetes with inadequate glycemic control, age more than 80 years, ulceration of the carotid artery, and a severe contralateral carotid artery stenosis were the major risk factors for periprocedural complications. Patients treated with distal protection devices fared better than those who did not have protection devices.[66]

In a French trial of carotid endarterectomy versus stenting (EVA-3S), the rates of stroke and death were higher in the stent group than the surgical group.[67] The frequency of stroke or death at 30 days was 3.9% in the endarterectomy group and 9.6% in the stented group.[67] Five different stents and seven different protection devices were used; in about 20% of instances (mostly at the beginning of the trial) protection devices were not deployed. The requirements for prior experience of the interventionalists who performed the stenting was less restrictive than in other trials.[68]

The results of the SAPPHIRE trial and other experience showed that distal protection was generally effective and worthwhile. There were, however, potential problems in some patients in deploying the protection devices. When stenotic lesions were very severe, expansion of the lumen by balloon stretching was needed in order to advance the device past the stenotic area. This added risk to the procedure. The protective devices could also irritate or denude the intima above the ultimate stent placement making it a potential nidus for thrombus formation in the hours and days after the procedure. Interventionalists continue to explore different modes of protection and different devices. Flow reversal after common carotid clamping is one strategy now being pursued in some centers.[69] Trials are now being pursued in the United States and Europe to compare interventional treatment (usually using stents and distal protection devices) with endarterectomy. Perhaps it is naive to think one of the two treatments would always be superior. Patients with long lesions, smooth lesions, and very high bifurcations, especially those with coronary artery disease might better be treated using interventional techniques. Patients with focal irregular ulcerated lesions might better be treated surgically. Surgeons are learning both direct surgical and interventional techniques so that they could fit the preferred technique in the individual case to the lesion and the patient.

Angioplasty and stenting has also been used to treat occlusive lesions in other neck arteries. Studies of balloon angioplasty and/or stenting for treatment of subclavian stenosis report excellent patency rates and more favorable results than surgery with amelioration of presenting symptoms in 72% to 100%, technical success in 90% to 100%, periprocedural complications in 0% to 10%, with stroke and death in 0% to 4%.[70-77] Henry et al reported on 113 patients treated for subclavian stenosis or occlusion with either angioplasty alone ($n = 57$) or angioplasty/stenting ($n = 46$) with 91% technical success and a 2.6% complication rate.[73] Procedural failures occurred mostly in occluded vessels. During 4.3 years of average follow-up, restenosis occurred in 16%, the majority of which had been treated with angioplasty only.[73] Schillinger et al reported a higher rate of initial technical success in 115 patients treated for subclavian stenosis with stents: 95% of stented vessels remained patent at 1 year versus 76% treated with angioplasty; however, by 4 years, only 59% of stented vessels remained patent compared with 68% for angioplasty alone.[78]

There are relatively little data on the results of stenting for vertebral artery stenosis near the origin of the artery. The vertebral artery is smaller in diameter than the carotid artery and takes off at an almost 90 degree angle from the subclavian artery making stenting more difficult than in the carotid artery. Although restenosis rates of 9% to 10% within 1 year have been reported,[79-82] 6 of 14 (43%) extracranial vertebral arteries treated with stenting developed restenosis greater than 50% at the 6-month follow-up in the Stenting of Symptomatic Atherosclerotic Lesions in the Vertebral or Intracranial Arteries (SSYLVIA) trial.[82]

The first balloon angioplasties for intracranial occlusive disease were reported in the mid-1980s.[44,83,84] The introduction of improved microballoon catheters and smaller balloon-expandable stents led to a dramatic increase in intracranial interventions. There are many reports of anecdotal experience but only one trial to date. Most reports claim good technical success but the complication rate has been significant.[84] Gress et al reported the results among 25 patients with intracranial vertebrobasilar occlusive disease unresponsive to medical therapies.[85] Angioplasty reduced the stenosis by greater than 40% in all treated vessels.[85] Marks and colleagues reported a 91% success rate in decreasing the severity of stenosis among 23 patients with intracranial arterial stenosis.[86] There was one periprocedural death. During follow-up that averaged 35 weeks, the annual stroke rate in territories fed by angioplastied arteries was 3.2%.[86] Connors and Wojak noted that their experience led to a change in technique during a 9-year period during which they had treated 70 patients with intracranial occlusive disease.[87] They had learned to use slow inflation of an undersized balloon and aimed at moderate reduction of the luminal stenosis rather than normalization.[87] Takis et al[88] and others reported complications that included arterial dissections, arterial thrombi requiring thrombolysis, and procedure-related brain infarcts.

Following the experience in the coronary and carotid arteries, intracranial stents began to be used. Gomez et al[89] and Yu et al[90] reported their experience with 12 and 18 patients, respectively, in whom they stented a severely stenotic basilar artery. Gomez et al reported no periprocedural complications and no new stroke or deaths during a half-year follow-up.[89] Yu et al reported 11% neurologic complications and 28% of patients had several minor episodes of ischemia.[90] After a mean of 2 years, 83% of patients had excellent functional outcome and 56% were considered asymptomatic in relation to their cerebrovascular disease.[90] Kessler et al reported their results in 16 patients with basilar artery (12) and intracranial vertebral artery (4) stenosis who were treated with stents.[91] Stenoses were reduced from a median of 84% (67% to 98%) to a median of 12% (2% to 20%).[91] Narrowing of the stents was found on follow-up angiography in all cases, with restenosis ranging from 10% to 32% luminal narrowing. Vascular perforations occurred in one patient.[91]

Long-term results were reported by Marks et al among 37 intracranial angioplasties[92] and by Wojak et al in among their 84 procedures (62 angioplasties and 22 stents).[93] There were two periprocedural deaths and one minor stroke in the series of Markus et al.[59] The average stenosis decreased from 84% to 43%. The annual stroke rate in the territory of the treated lesions was 3.4% but was 4.5% in patients with more than 50% residual stenosis.[92] In the Wojak et al series, the periprocedural stroke or death rate was 4.8%.[93] During a mean of 4.6 months, angiographic restenosis developed in 23 patients, 13 of whom were retreated without recognized complications.[93]

The SSYLVIA trial was a multicenter, nonrandomized, prospective feasibility study, which evaluated the Neurolink intracranial stent system for treatment of patients with single target vertebral or intracranial artery stenosis greater than 50%.[82] Among 61 patients enrolled, 43 (70.5%) had an intracranial stenosis and 18 (29.5%) had an extracranial vertebral artery stenosis. During the first 30 days, 6.6% of patients had strokes but no deaths. Successful stent placement was achieved in 58/61 (95%) of procedures. Although restenosis occurred in 35% of patients, 61% were asymptomatic.[82]

The Wingspan stent technique represented a new concept in cerebral artery revascularization by use of balloon angioplasty followed by placement of a self-expanding nitinol microstent across the atherosclerotic lesion in the brain. In a prospective multicenter study among 45 patients, enrolled from 12 European sites, with symptomatic intracranial atherosclerosis (>50% stenosis), revascularization using the Wingspan stent was performed.[94,95] Among these patients, 95% had strokes, and 29% had TIAs. Technical success was achieved in 98% (44/45) of cases. The composite 30-day death or ipsilateral stroke rate was 4.5% (2/44), and the 6-month death or ipsilateral stroke rate was 7.1% (3/42), with the all-cause stroke rate of 9.5% (4/42).[95]

Further experience with the Wingspan stent is now accumulating. One report described the results among U.S. centers of Wingspan stent deployment in 78 patients with 82 intracranial atherostenotic lesions.[96] Two thirds of the lesions showed greater than 70% stenosis. All but one of the lesions was successfully stented during the first procedure session. There were five (6.1%) major procedural neurologic complications, four of which proved fatal within 30 days after the procedure.[96] Figure 5-2 is an example of a lesion in the proximal portion of a MCA treated with a Wingspan stent.

Drug-eluting stents have been used in the coronary circulation to attempt to reduce restenosis rates. These stents may require longer-term, more aggressive antiplatelet therapy to reduce the risk of white-platelet thrombi formation on the stents than on bare stents. Drug-eluting stents are now also being used to treat both extracranial and intracranial arterial stenoses but their relative long-term safety and efficacy are as yet uncertain.[97,98] Further studies are needed to determine whether drug elution provides an important benefit.

Thrombolysis

Rationale and Early Studies

Clots can also be lysed chemically. In the body, thrombus formation stimulates an endogenous fibrinolytic mechanism for thrombolysis. Factor XII, the release of tissue plasminogen activator, and other substances promote conversion of plasminogen to plasmin, the active fibrinolytic

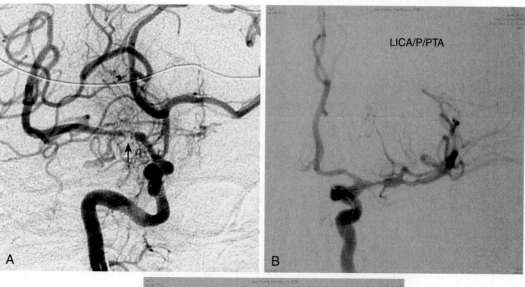

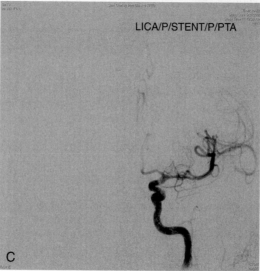

Figure 5-2. Left carotid angiograms in a patient with acute left cerebral ischemia. **A,** The initial angiogram shows a severe stenosis of the left MCA beginning near the origin of the artery. There is poststenotic dilatation. **B,** Angiogram after angioplasty before stent placement. **C,** Angiogram after placement of neuroform stent. (Courtesy of Ajith Thomas, MD, Neurosurgery, Beth Israel Deaconess Medical Center, Boston, Mass.)

enzyme.[99-101] Plasmin activity is concentrated at the sites of fibrin deposition. Fibrinolytic drugs degrade the fibrin network mesh of red erythrocyte-fibrin clots. They do not lyse white platelet-fibrin thrombi but instead may activate platelets.[101] Endogenous formation of plasmin is probably responsible for some examples of spontaneous recanalization of thrombosed arteries. The ideal thromolytic agent would adhere specifically to fibrin in clots and would not cause systemic fibrinogenolysis. Lowering fibrinogen levels excessively can promote bleeding.

Physicians began to explore the use of thrombolytic agents during the 1950s for a variety of systemic thromboembolic conditions. Early attempts used bovine or human thrombolysins or streptokinase. During the early 1960s, Meyer and colleagues randomized 73 patients with worsening strokes to receive streptokinase intravenously and/or concomitant anticoagulants within 3 days of stroke onset.[102,103] Clots lysis was successful in some patients, but 10 patients died, and some had brain hemorrhages. After these studies, streptokinase was thought to be too dangerous to use. Use of streptokinase for systemic and cardiac thromboembolism was considered contraindicated in the presence of brain lesions or past strokes.

5

Observational Studies of Intravenous and Intra-Arterial Thrombolysis in Patients with Known Arterial Lesions before NINDS Study

During the 1980s, stimulated by success in treating coronary artery thrombosis, clinicians turned again to "clot busters" to treat cerebrovascular thromboembolism. My colleagues and I at the New England Medical Center in Boston were involved in some of the early studies with American, German, and Japanese colleagues. Streptokinase, urokinase, and rt-PA were the most common agents used. In these early studies, acute stroke patients were screened clinically and by CT, and then angiography was performed. If an intracranial arterial occlusion was shown, thrombolytic drugs were given either intra-arterially (IA) into the clots, or intravenously (IV). Follow-up angiography was performed after treatment to assess recanalization. Both anterior and posterior circulation thromboembolism were treated. These studies were observational only since controls were seldom used and patients were not randomized but successive patients meeting protocol requirements were treated.[104-107]

The results of these early studies were not included in the publications of the results of the later randomized trials. In all of these early angiographic studies, and in angiographically controlled trials since release of rt-PA, recanalization heavily correlated with outcome. As far as is known, thrombolytic agents act only by lysing clots. If arteries are not opened the drugs do not facilitate recovery. Knowing the recanalization rate of agents given IV and IA in patients with various occlusive arterial lesions is extremely helpful in choosing appropriate therapy.

Among patients treated using IA thrombolytic agents under angiographic control, the agents were given within 24 hours.[104-107] The presence and extent of reperfusion depended mostly on the location of the occluded artery and the mechanism of the stroke. Among 449 patients treated in 17 studies, 64% had effective recanalization after therapy. Mainstem and divisional middle cerebral artery (MCA) occlusions responded best, while ICA occlusions responded poorly. Distal MCA branch occlusions did not respond as well as more proximal MCA lesions, probably because the blockage was beyond the reach of interventional catheters. Basilar artery occlusions were recanalized in 69% of patients. Thrombolysis of occlusions of the intracranial carotid artery (ICA) bifurcation (the carotid "T" portion) was almost invariably unsuccessful. Embolic occlusions were more successfully recanalized than thrombosis engrafted upon in-situ atherosclerosis. Reocclusions did occur and

transluminal angioplasty was sometimes used after thrombolysis to keep occluded arteries open. Recanalization was helped by mechanical clot disruption. Intracranial hemorrhagic complications occurred in 18.5% of patients and 42% of treated patients had good outcomes as judged by the authors of the reports.[104-107]

In other clinical studies, the vascular lesions were defined by angiography but thrombolytic drugs were given IV.[104-107] Only two of these studies had control patients who were not given a thrombolytic drug. In six series, rt-PA was given within 6 hours and one study had an 8-hour window. Among 370 patients treated with IV rt-PA, one third of the arteries treated showed significant recanalization compared to only 5% of 58 control arteries. MCA branch occlusions recanalized best followed by occlusions of the superior and inferior divisions of the MCA. Mainstem MCA occlusions recanalized less often than branch and division MCA lesions. ICA occlusions recanalized seldom and there were no recanalizations when both the ICA and MCA were occluded. Very few patients with documented basilar artery occlusions were given intravenous rt-PA and only one sixth recanalized. In one study, Grond et al reported favorable results of treatment in 10 of 12 patients with acute vertebrobasilar territory ischemia given IV rt-PA followed by heparin, but the occlusive vascular lesions were not documented before treatment.[108] Embolic occlusions recanalized more often than in-situ thrombosis of atherostenotic arteries. Recanalization was better when there was angiographic evidence of good collateral circulation prior to administration of rt-PA. Both hemorrhagic infarction and hematomas were more common with IV than with IA treatment possibly because of the larger dose used in IV treatment.[104-107]

Randomized Trials of Intravenous (NINDS and ECASS I, II, and III) and Intra-Arterial Therapy (PROACT I and II)

None of the IV randomized trials recommended or reported vascular testing before treatment, and all used clinical findings and CT as entry requirements. The single randomized trial of IA treatment required catheter cerebral angiography before treatment.

The first reported large multicenter randomized trial of IV thrombolysis was the European Cooperative Acute Stroke Study (ECASS I), which included 620 patients with acute hemispheral strokes among 75 hospitals in 14 European countries.[109,110] A total of 313 patients were randomized to receive rt-PA (1.1 mg/kg) and 307 patients were randomized to placebo. Treatment was given within 6 hours of the onset of symptoms of brain ischemia. Patients who had major early infarct signs (diffuse hemispheral swelling, parenchymal hypodensity, effacement of cerebral sulci in more than one third of the MCA territory) and hemorrhage on initial CT scans, which were read at the local site, were excluded. An independent blinded CT scan reading panel later retrospectively reviewed the CT scans and determined protocol violations of the CT scan entry criteria. Many patients (109, including 66 patients in the rt-PA group and 43 in the placebo-treated group) had protocol deviations, mostly because of failure at local centers to recognize CT abnormalities that should have excluded patients. Considering the entire group of patients treated, the study was considered negative. There was a bimodal result—more patients treated with rt-PA had good outcomes but more patients did poorly and more patients died.[109,110]

In ECASS I, among rt-PA treated patients in the target population (those patients who had no protocol violations) there was a significantly better outcome and hospital stay was significantly shorter. Intracerebral hemorrhages and death were more common in rt-PA treated patients, but these differences were not statistically significant. Large parenchymal hematomas were more often found in rt-PA treated patients. Patients treated with rt-PA within 3 hours did better than controls and those treated with rt-PA between 3 and 6 hours.[111]

The ECASS I study showed that treatment of patients with early infarct signs on CT scan could be hazardous. Reading of the CT scans at the local hospitals was often unreliable. Some hemorrhages and many early infarcts were missed by local physicians. The mortality and brain hemorrhage rate among patients with protocol violations treated with rt-PA was extremely high, 33.3% and 40%, respectively. Among 52 patients included in the study despite major early infarct signs, 40% died.[109-111]

The next study reported was the National Institute of Neurological Disorders and Stroke (NINDS) study.[112] The major study differences compared to ECASS were lower rt-PA dose, earlier treatment (302 patients were treated within 90 minutes and 322 between 90 and 180 minutes), and no exclusion of patients because of brain ischemia on entry CT scans. Patients who received intravenous rt-PA were at least 30% more likely to have minor or no disability at 3 months. Symptomatic intracerebral hemorrhages were more common in the rt-PA–treated patients (6.4% vs 0.6%) and more often developed in patients who had more severe neurologic deficits at entry and in patients 75 years or older. The mortality at 3 months was 17% in the rt-PA group versus 21% in the placebo group.[112] There seemed to be no important difference in outcome in the groups with varying etiologies, but the quick entry and absence of vascular and cardiac imaging made the clinical diagnosis of stroke etiology and mechanism tentative at best. A committee that reviewed the NINDS results reported that the stroke subtype results were not valid.[113]

In the European Cooperative Acute Stroke Study (ECASS II) trial, investigators treated 800 patients from Europe, Australia, and New Zealand with rt-PA or placebo within 6 hours of stroke onset.[114] They administered the rt-PA dose used in the NINDS trial rather than the higher dose used in ECASS I. Patients with major infarcts on CT scan were excluded but vascular imaging was not performed before treatment. Guidelines for control of hypertension were more explicit than in ECASS I or the NINDS trial. In ECASS II, 36.6% of placebo-treated patients had favorable outcomes—a better result than thrombolysed patients in the ECASS I and NINDS trials. Among the rt-PA–treated group, 40.3% had favorable outcomes; this was not a statistically significant difference from the placebo-treated group. Treatment results and frequency of hemorrhages were similar in the 0- to 3-hour and 3- to 6-hour treatment groups.[114] In the interval between the two ECASS trials, stroke centers had developed widely in Europe and were manned by experienced stroke neurologists, internists, and nurses. The results in the placebo and thrombolysis groups reflect better medical care delivered in dedicated stroke centers.

The ATANTIS study used a protocol similar to the NINDS trial to study patients treated with rt-PA in a 3- to 5-hour window.[115] This study failed to show effectiveness according to its preset criteria. Analysis of the pooled data from six rt-PA trials shows that the earlier patients are treated the more the likelihood of a favorable outcome. Treatment after 3 hours, especially between 3 to 4.5 hours, was also effective but not as effective as earlier treatment[116,117] (Table 5-6). The ECASS III trial showed that rt-PA was effective in patients treated between 3 and 4.5 hours after stroke symptom onset.[117a]

Three randomized trials of IV streptokinase in patients without identification of vascular lesions were launched; all were stopped prematurely because of a high rate of brain hemorrhages in patients treated with streptokinase.[118]

The Prolyse in Acute Cerebral Thromboembolism (PROACT) trials studied the effectiveness of intra-arterially administered pro-urokinase (r-proUK) in patients who had angiographically documented MCA occlusions.[119-121] PROACT I

Table 5-6.　Pooled Analysis of the NINDS, ECASS, and ATLANTIS Trials: Odds Ratio for Favorable Outcome at 3 Months after Brain Infarct

Time Range	Odds Ratio	Confidence Interval	rt-PA Treated	Placebo
0-90 min	2.81	1.75-4.5	161	150
91-180 min	1.55	1.12-2.15	302	315
181-270 min	1.40	1.05-1.85	390	411
270-360 min	1.15	0.90-1.47	538	508

From Clark WM, Wissman S, Albers GW, (eds): Recombinant tissue-type plasminogen activator (altepase) for ischemic stroke 3 to 5 hours after symptom onset. The ATLANTIS study: A randomized controlled trial. Altepase Thrombolysis for Acute Non-interventional Therapy in Acute Stroke. JAMA 1999 282:2019-2026, with permission.

compared the recanalization rate of locally injected, IA r-proUK versus heparin within 6 hours of onset in patients with a radiographically proven MCA occlusion.[119] The interventionalist was not permitted to mechanically disturb the clot (contrary to the usual practice in the community) and was to inject r-proUK at the proximal end of the thrombus. There was successful recanalization in 15/26 (58%) of patients treated with medication while 2/14 (14%) recanalized with heparin alone.

PROACT II was more extensive.[120] Although it was an open-label study, the follow-up was blinded to medication versus placebo. About one fifth of patients thought clinically by their doctors to have MCA occlusions had no occlusive arterial lesions at angiography. Forty percent of patients in the treatment group had slight or no neurologic disability at day 90 compared with 25% of the control group (P = .04). The mortality rates were similar—25% in the treatment group versus 27% in the placebo group. The symptomatic hemorrhage rate was 10% in the treatment group versus 2% in the placebo group (P = .04). The study showed favorable recanalization rates in the treatment group (66%) versus 18% in the control group (P < .001).[120] Patients overall benefited from IA thrombolysis despite the excess hemorrhage rate and there was no excess mortality.[120,121] Although IA thrombolytic treatment was effective and met the pretrial guidelines discussed with the FDA, the drug was not approved.

A randomized trial of intra-arterial urokinase in patients with angiographically confirmed occlusions of the M1 or M2 portions of one of the MCAs was performed in Japan.[122,123] Intravenous heparin was given and angiograms performed. In patients with MCA occlusions intra-arterial urokinase was given and disruption of clot by guidewire was allowed. Patients (114, 57 in the urokinase group and 57 controls) were treated within 6 hours. Favorable outcome (Rankin 0 to 2 at 90 days) was present in 49% of the urokinase group and 39% of the control group and excellent outcome (Rankin 0 to 1 at 90 days) occurred in 42% of the urokinase group and 23% of controls.[122] Intracerebral hemorrhage during the first day occurred in 9% after IA urokinase and in 2% of controls. The death rate was 5% in the fibrinolytic group and 3.5% in the control group. The study was prematurely stopped when IV rTPA was approved in Japan. Although the results did not show a statistically significant advantage of IA urokinase, the results look promising if a sufficient number of patients had been enrolled.[122]

Results of Thrombolytic Drug Use after FDA Approval of rt-PA in United States

Release of the results of the NINDS trial gave momentum to a movement in the United States to quickly (much too quickly in my opinion) introduce IV thrombolysis widely into the community. During the summer of 1996, about 6 months after the publication of the NINDS trial, the FDA approved the use of rt-PA for the treatment of stroke patients when the drug was given within the first 3 hours. The American Heart Association[124] and American Academy of Neurology[125] published treatment recommendations that exactly followed the inclusion and exclusions and the treatment protocols of the NINDS trial. The recommendations suggest that a CT scan done before thrombolysis should not show major infarction, mass effect, edema, or hemorrhage. The guidelines do not require or suggest MRI or vascular tests before treatment. American Heart Association/American Stroke Association guidelines published in 2007 concerning early management of adults with ischemic stroke do not substantially alter the original guidelines concerning IV tPA administration.[126]

Postmarketing experience was extensive. It has been estimated that only about 1% to 2% of stroke patients in the United States receive rt-PA.

An analysis of data contained in U.S. national hospital discharge surveys for 1999 to 2001, showed that among 1,796,513 admissions for ischemic stroke, 11,283 (0.6%) had IV thrombolysis and 1314 (0.07%) had IA thrombolysis.[127] Results of studies that attempted to follow published guidelines have varied widely. One study that included experienced investigators active in the ATLANTIS 3- to 5-hour window study (Standard Treatment with Alteplase Study {STARS}) collected further experience with thrombolysis during the first 3 hours.[128] At 30 days, 35% had very favorable outcomes; the symptomatic hemorrhage rate was 3.3%, and asymptomatic hemorrhages were found in 8.2%.[128] These results mimicked those of the NINDS trial. In experienced hands, the NINDS results could be duplicated in academic and community centers.

Results of a survey that included 1205 patients treated in Canada, United States, and Germany showed that 33% of patients had a good outcome and the symptomatic hemorrhage rate was 6%.[129] Unfortunately the experience has not all been good. In Cleveland only, 70/3948 (1.8%) acute stroke patients seen during 1 year received tPA.[130] Fully half had protocol violations. Eleven patients (15.7%) had symptomatic hemorrhages of which six were fatal.[130] Fortunately, later results from Cleveland had improved.[131]

Intravenous thrombolysis with rt-PA was approved in Germany in August 2000 for use within 3 hours after onset of focal brain ischemia. Eleven neurology departments that had acute stroke units participated in the German Stroke Study Collaboration before and after approval and consecutively registered all patients admitted within 24 hours after acute ischemic strokes.[132] The frequency of intravenous thrombolysis in the patients increased from 4.8% before approval to 7.9% after approval; more older patients were treated and the delay between symptom onset and imaging was significantly shorter during the second study period.[132] In Germany over a 1-year period, 384/13,440 (3%) of acute stroke patients received tPA.[133] In-hospital mortality was significantly higher for patients treated with tPA (11.7%) than those not treated (4.5%) (P < .0001). Patients treated in hospitals with fewer than five instances of thrombolysis per year had a 3.3 odds ratio of higher in-hospital mortality. Patients treated after 3 hours fared worse than those treated within 3 hours.[133] A large single center cohort of 450 patients was given IV tPA in Cologne, Germany.[134] Heparin was allowed 1 hour after tPA in patients considered at high risk for recurring thrombosis, and was administered to 184/450 (41%) acute stroke patients. The efficacy and safety results were comparable to those in the NINDS study.[134] In the NINDS trial and later guidelines, heparin is recommended to be held for at least 24 hrs after IV thrombolysis.

In Europe, approval of rt-PA for acute stroke came much later than in the United States. The European Medicines Evaluation Agency (EMEA) conditionally approved alteplase (rt-PA) in September 2002 for treatment of ischemic stroke by experienced clinicians within 3 hours of symptom onset. One of the conditions required by the European Union regulatory authorities for the definitive approval of thrombolytic therapy was that treatment safety would be monitored during a 3-year period by entering all treated patients in a Web register. Since that time, physicians performing thrombolysis in Europe have been urged to enter all of their cases in the SITS Monitoring Study–SITS-MOST Registry.[135] In this registry, during a 4-year period, data from 6483 patients from 285 centers in 14 countries were entered.[136] At 24 hours, 1.7% of patients had symptomatic intracerebral hemorrhages compared with 8.6% in the previously reported pooled randomized controlled trials. The mortality rate at 3 months in SITS-MOST was 11.3% compared with 17.3% in the pooled randomized controlled trials. The investigators concluded that intravenous alteplase use was safe and effective in routine clinical practice when given within 3 hours of stroke onset, even at medical centers with little previous experience of thrombolytic therapy for acute stroke.[136]

In summary, when experienced stroke centers followed published guidelines for IV thrombolysis, the results mirrored the NINDS results. Inexperience and protocol violations greatly worsened the results.

IA thrombolysis has also been pursued in the community and in academic centers after PROACT II. Interventionalists customarily manipulate occlusive thrombi with their catheters and inject thrombolytic drug directly into the clots, a practice not permitted in the PROACT trials. IA thrombolysis has been performed widely in centers that have the needed technology, capability, and experience.[121,137-141] Much experience is available that allows prediction of the safety and effectiveness of IA treatment in patients with various stroke severities, various vascular occlusive lesions, treated at various times after symptom onset.[138,139]

Evaluating the Present Practice of Thrombolysis—2008

Clearly, if an unbiased committee were to write a report card on the status of thrombolysis to date, they would find much good and much to be desired. Finally there was a drug that all agreed

5

was an effective stroke treatment. Before tissue type plasminogen activator (tPA) therapeutic nihilism prevailed. Approval of tPA was a wake-up call. *Stroke can and should be treated.* Stroke patients must be hustled quickly into medical centers, and doctors and hospitals must become prepared and able to treat them. Doctors and the media, politicians, and authorities called the attention of the public and of doctors to stroke.

But unfortunately, doctors and medical centers have been slow to heed the call. Only about 1% to 2% of acute stroke patients are now treated with thrombolytics. About 4% to 5% of patients who arrive at medical centers and are eligible for thrombolysis under present guidelines actually receive it. Many hospitals, doctors, ambulance services, and emergency room units are still not adequately prepared to treat acute stroke patients. Some physicians, especially emergency room doctors remain unconvinced about thrombolysis and are unwilling to give thrombolytic drugs for stroke patients. The guidelines for treatment are hopelessly outdated and do not take into consideration advances made since the randomized NINDS and ECASS trials. There are not enough doctors sufficiently trained and experienced to handle acute stroke patients. There is still much that is not known about thrombolysis (and is not likely to be learned unless the present guidelines are updated).

A Look Ahead: Recent Technology and Therapeutic Developments

EARLIER TREATMENT

Spurred by the availability of a proven treatment for acute ischemic stroke, researchers and clinicians have explored a number of new strategies for rapid treatment and reperfusion.[142] The most important new strategies are listed in Table 5-7.

The most expeditious way to begin treatment of patients would be to begin treatment in the field when the ambulance personnel arrive. Physicians are exploring the feasibility of prehospital administration of drugs, especially neuroprotective agents.[143-145] Theoretically, increasing the brain's resistance to ischemia would provide a longer time window for thrombolysis. In a pilot study (FAST-MAG), University of California-Los Angeles investigators showed the feasibility of administering a loading dose of magnesium sulfate in the field.[145] Among 20 patients with a mean age 74, the magnesium infusion began a median of 100 minutes after symptom onset and 70% were infused within 2 hours of onset. The interval from paramedic arrival on the scene to the time of starting administration of the study agent was field initiated, 26 minutes (range 15 to 64) versus in-hospital initiated (historic controls), 139 minutes.[145]

Table 5-7. New Thrombolytic Strategies
Faster treatment, even before the hospital
Lengthening the time window for treatment and improving selection of candidates by using more advanced CT, MRI, and ultrasound technologies including vascular imaging
Telemedicine communications with stroke centers
Newer thrombolytics
Bridging strategies—IV and then selective IA thrombolysis
Enhancing thrombolysis by using TCD-related techniques
Multiple reperfusion and neuroprotection combinations
Mechanical recanalization as an assist to thrombolysis

Better clinical and technological diagnosis in the field would also accelerate early treatment. Researchers are exploring portable CT equipment that could be carried in an ambulance (a "stroke-mobile") that would allow CT brain and vascular imaging in the field. Computer transmission of the images to a stroke center experienced clinician might allow that individual to direct administration of a thrombolytic and/or other agents before hospital arrival.

Clearly the earliest steps are also important: educating patients and the public about calling 911 in case of suspected stroke, training those who answer the calls to recognize an acute neurologic problem and to dispatch an ambulance as an emergency that is appropriately equipped with experienced personnel and technology, and training ambulance personnel in recognition of strokes and in their emergency management.

DEVELOPMENT OF COMPETENT MEDICAL CENTERS AND STROKE PATIENT DELIVERY TO SUCH CENTERS

Not all hospitals are equally suited to manage acute brain ischemia patients (Table 5-8). An important goal is to develop regional stroke centers with advanced capabilities in stroke management. Many large U.S. and European cities now have such centers. Also needed are community-based centers that have adequate personnel and technology that can efficiently and safely administer thrombolytics and other treatments. Since many self-designated centers are not adequately equipped, criteria and evaluation strategies must be developed for accrediting competent centers. Listed in Table 5-9 are

Table 5-8.	**Alternatives for Hospitals That Receive Acute Stroke Patients**

If your medical center intends to treat acute stroke patients, develop systems and protocols for rapid delivery, efficient evaluation, and rapid throughput of patients with suspected acute strokes and TIAs. Be sure that physicians managing the patients are experienced in stroke care and the technology available is adequate.

Choose not to accept patients suspected of having acute stroke and divert them to a nearby stroke center if such is available.

Upgrade the facility to meet standards and then accept patients.

If it is not feasible to divert to a nearby facility, consider connecting with such a facility by telemedicine or consultative arrangements to facilitate care.

---

alternatives for hospitals that receive acute stroke patients. Telemedicine has been used effectively in Paris, Germany, and parts of the United States.[146-148] This allows doctors at stroke centers to help with the acute care of stroke patients at distant sites and will become even more important in the future. The use of telemedicine will likely increase the frequency and appropriateness of stroke thrombolysis.[148]

SELECTION OF CANDIDATES FOR THROMBOLYSIS USING MODERN UP-TO-DATE TECHNOLOGY

When the ECASS and NINDS studies were planned, available technology was limited. Since then there has been a dramatic upgrade in MRI, CT, and ultrasound technology. I have discussed at length in Chapter 4 the capability of this technology to yield information about the presence, location, and amount of infarcted

Table 5-9.	**Data Needed to Logically Choose Treatment for Patients with Acute Ischemic Stroke**

Location, nature, and severity of any arterial occlusions

Mechanism of the brain ischemia—hypoperfusion or embolism

Composition and coagulability of blood

Extent of brain injury and brain at risk for further infarction. How much brain is already irreversibly damaged, how much is ischemic and not functioning but reversible (stunned), and how much is functioning, yet underperfused, and thus threatened?

---

brain and arterial and venous occlusions. Most authorities agree that thrombolysis can be effective if given within 3 hours following present guidelines, but are the present guidelines optimal? Could thrombolytic treatment be improved? Are there patients now excluded such as those who awaken with neurologic symptoms, those who have minor deficits or have improved substantially, and those treatable only after 3 hours who could respond to treatment? Are there some patients now treated under the guidelines who should not be treated because of little likelihood of success and high risk of hemorrhage or edema?

Knowledge gained from modern brain and vascular imaging can help select for treatment some patients now included and excluded under present guidelines. The present guidelines: use a firm 3-hour window; do not suggest or even mention vascular imaging; and exclude patients who awaken with deficits, have mild or improving signs, or have seizures.

Some patients' brains are at risk for further ischemia hours after the present 3-hour deadline. Early and recent studies document many instances of improvement and recanalization after the 3-hour window.[105-107,149-153] The pooled analysis of the ECSS, NINDS, and ATLANTIS data[121] (Table 5-6) shows an advantage of thrombolysis during the 3- to 4.5-hour window and possibly in the 4.5- to 6-hour time interval.

Patients who awaken with neurologic symptoms often have brain and vascular imaging that shows treatable vascular occlusion patterns and no or small infarcts and are excellent candidates for thrombolysis.[154]

Many patients who enter with slight deficits or improving signs later develop severe strokes. Improving or slight deficits are one of the most common reasons for present exclusion from thrombolysis. Several series show that a substantial number of patients who later deteriorate have occlusive vascular lesions that are amenable to thrombolytic treatment.[155-157]

Many patients already have large infarcts and little recoverable brain when brain imaging is performed within 3 hours. These patients can be harmed by thrombolysis.[5,109]

Seizures at or near onset do occur in some acute ischemic stroke patients, especially those with embolic strokes.[158] The occurrence of a seizure should not exclude an otherwise appropriate candidate for thrombolysis from being treated.

Knowing whether there is an arterial occlusion and its location and the extent of infarction already present might lead clinicians to choose no thrombolysis, IV treatment, or to consider IA treatment, or combined IV and then IA treatment. The site of arterial occlusion clearly strongly effects the likelihood of reperfusion after IV and IA thrombolysis.[105,107,149,150] The more one knows about the patient, the more logically the clinician can choose acute and more chronic treatment. The present guidelines desperately need revision to account for information gained since the NINDS trial was published.

Modern MRI and CT protocols along with clinical data are now being used in the attempt to better select patients likely to benefit from thrombolysis and those at most risk of hemorrhage and other complications.[159-176] A selection system based on pathology and pathophysiology is preferred over selection by a clock. Trials (EPITHET,[169] DIAS,[170] and DEFUSE[5]) and extensive experience[174] have established the feasibility of using modern brain and vascular imaging to optimally choose patients for thrombolysis.

The Desmoteplase in Acute Ischemic Stroke (DIAS) trial was a placebo-controlled, double-blind, randomized dose-finding phase II trial of Desmoteplase.[170] Desmoteplase is derived from vampire bat saliva and is a plasminogen activator fibrinolytic enzyme with high-fibrin selectivity and a long terminal half-life.[177] Fibrin-selectivity is important since the agent tends to bind at the site of the thrombus and not cause systemic fibrinogenolysis. In DIAS, patients were selected for fibrinolysis if they had a diffusion/perfusion mismatch on MRI and were treated within a 3- to 9-hour window. The patients treated with desmoteplase had a higher rate of reperfusion and better clinical outcomes than placebo-treated controls.[170]

The Diffusion and Perfusion Imaging Evaluation for Understanding Stroke Evolution (DEFUSE) trial studied whether MRI criteria helped determine responders to IV tPA in patients treated between 3 to 6 hours after stroke symptom onset.[5] A diffusion/perfusion mismatch occurred in 54% of patients with interpretable PWI scans and in this group early reperfusion was associated with a favorable response in 56% of patients compared to only 19% of patients with no mismatch. In addition, those with large DWI lesions fared worse with a very low rate of good clinical response and a high rate of hemorrhage when reperfusion occurred.[5] MRA showed that 44/68 (65%) of patients had a symptomatic arterial occlusion before treatment. Complete early recanalization occurred in 27% and partial recanalization in 16% as determined by follow-up MRA. Patients with early recanalization had a 74% reduction in PWI volume compared with 16% with no recanalization.[5] Symptomatic intracerebral bleeding occurred in 9.5% of patients, especially in those with a large DWI volume infarct before thrombolysis.[175]

DIAS and DEFUSE showed that MRI and MRA could be used effectively to select patients for thrombolysis even within the 3- to 9-hour window. Modern CT profiles that include CTA and perfusion CT should also be able to select patients with arterial occlusions with no or small infarcts and larger perfusion defects that would be amenable to thrombolysis irrespective of time.[161-163]

Table 5-9 lists the data needed for optimal treatment of patients with acute brain ischemia.

Combined IV and Selective IA Thrombolysis

Recognizing that IV thrombolysis was very often ineffective but that primary IA treatment took time to initiate, investigators began to study the feasibility of giving IV tPA and following that treatment with IA thrombolysis in selected patients.[178-183] This strategy was dubbed *bridging* by the investigators.[178-181] Intravenous rt-PA was given within 3 hours at a dose of 0.6 mg/kg maximum with a 15% bolus and the rest infused over 30 minutes. Angiography was then performed and if thrombus was shown rt-PA was infused intra-arterially up to a total of 22 mg. An IV bolus of heparin was given when thrombus was identified by angiography and heparin flush solution was given until the catheter was removed.[178-181] The 80 patients treated had a mean baseline NIHSS score of 18. Mean time to IV rt-PA was 140 minutes. The rate of symptomatic intracranial hemorrhage was 6.3% (comparable to the 6.6% in the NINDS trial) and the treated patients had better 3-month outcomes than the NINDS placebo-treated patients (odds ratio >2).[180,181] Among the 77 patients who had angiography 28 had major occlusions or severe stenosis of the ICA as well as tandem MCA or MCA branch occlusions. Among 62 patients who received IA rt-PA, 11% had complete recanalization and partial or complete recanalization developed in 56%.[180] Those who were reperfused had relatively good outcomes as in other studies.

Other investigators used transcranial Doppler (TCD) to select patients for IA thrombolysis.[182] TCD was used to monitor the effectiveness of IV thrombolysis; if TCD showed effective, recanalization IV treatment was continued. If the insonated occluded artery did not recanalize, IA treatment was given.[183] Keris et al treated patients who had no major infarct signs on CT scan with IA rt-PA if they had arterial occlusions; the IA dose was then followed by an IV infusion.[184]

These studies all showed the feasibility of combining IV and IA treatment using arterial occlusions as detected by angiography or TCD as a guide to select patients for IA treatment.

Non–rt-PA Thrombolytics

STREPTOKINASE

Streptokinase has been used widely in patients with coronary ischemia, although patients with past strokes were excluded from most streptokinase cardiac trials. There were three randomized trials of IV streptokinase in patients with acute ischemic strokes; all were stopped prematurely because of a high rate of brain hemorrhages in patients treated with streptokinase.[118] No vascular studies were reported and inclusion depended on CT scan results. Researchers and clinicians speculated that the dose of streptokinase may have been excessive in these trials, but there has been no further enthusiasm for further streptokinase use or trials.

UROKINASES

Intravenous and intra-arterial urokinase (UK) was used often in early pre-NINDS observational studies and continues to be given in some medical centers.[185-189] Pro-urokinase was used in the successful PROACT trials,[119-121] but has not been approved to be marketed and is not presently available. Australian investigators performed a pilot randomized controlled trial of intra-arterial urokinase within 24 hours of symptom onset in 16 patients with stroke and angiographic evidence of posterior circulation vascular occlusions.[187] Four of the 8 treated with IA UK did well compared to one of eight in the control group.

Intra-arterial urokinase (IA-UK) thrombolysis is often given in Japan to selected patients with acute cerebral artery occlusions. Japanese investigators performed a case-control retrospective analysis using data from Japan's Multicenter Stroke Investigator's Collaboration (J-MUSIC that included 16,922 acute ischemic stroke patients.[188] They compared outcomes among 91 patients who received IA-UK for cardioembolic stroke with 182 controls. A favorable outcome (Rankin 0-2) and mean Rankin score at discharge were better in the UK-treated group.[188] A review of IA-UK treated patients analyzed factors related to complications of that treatment. Investigators in Taiwan performed a preliminary dose-finding, safety, and efficacy trial of human tissue urokinase-type plasminogen activator (HTUPA) given intravenously to 33 patients with acute ischemic strokes.[190] They concluded that IV HTUPA, given at 0.3 mg/kg as a bolus injection within 5 hours after symptom onset, had an acceptable safety and efficacious profile in patients with acute ischemic stroke; further trials of this agent are planned.[190]

ANCROD

Ancrod, a purified venom extract from the Malaysian pit viper induces rapid systemic defibrinogenation.[191-193] It has been used in Canada and Europe since the 1970s in patients with peripheral limb vascular disease, deep-vein thrombosis, and central retinal artery thrombosis to induce reperfusion.[193] Two preliminary studies in the 1980s involving, respectively, 20 and 30 ischemic stroke patients indicated that ancrod was possibly safe and effective.[194,195]

A randomized, placebo-controlled trial was performed in the United States of ancrod in ischemic stroke patients ($n = 132$) treated within 6 hours of symptom onset.[191] Neurologic function as measured by the Scandinavian Stroke Scale was significantly better in the ancrod-treated patients ($P = .04$), and there were no recognized symptomatic intracranial hemorrhages. No vascular studies were reported so that the mechanism of improvement was not clear. Did the lowering of fibrinogen lyse occlusive clots? Did lowering of fibrinogen effectively reduce blood viscosity so that blood flow was increased in collateral vessels?

A second study, the Stroke Treatment with Ancrod Trial (STAT), was performed in the United States and Canada.[192] A total of 500 patients with acute or progressing ischemic deficits were treated with a continuous 72-hour infusion of ancrod ($n = 248$) or placebo ($n = 252$) followed by 1-hour infusions at 96 and 120 hours. The aim was to reduce fibrinogen levels to below 200. More patients treated with ancrod achieved favorable functional status than those treated with placebo (42.2% vs 34.4%, $P = .04$). There were more symptomatic and asymptomatic intracranial hemorrhages in the ancrod-treated group. No data about vascular lesions were included in the report of the trial.[192] The European Stroke Treatment with Ancrod trial (ESTAT) was performed and enrolled 1222 patients.[196] Patients were treated within 6 hours in contrast to the 3-hour window in the STAT trial. Functional outcome at 3 months was the same in the ancrod- and placebo-treated groups. There were more hemorrhages and more deaths in the ancrod-treated group.[196] No further trials of ancrod are being pursued or planned, as far as I know.

TENECTEPLASE

Tenecteplase (TNK) is a biogenetic variant of wildtype rtPA that may be given as a single bolus injection.[191] It is posited to have an eightfold higher affinity for fibrin and a longer half-life

5

than rtPA. In a trial of 17,000 patients with myocardial infarction, TNK was compared with rtPA in reference to bleeding; fewer patients treated with TNK had major systemic bleeding but intracranial bleeding and mortality were similar.[197] A preliminary exploratory trial of 75 patients showed promising results and a dose-finding trial of TNK is in progress in the United States but has not been reported.[191]

Researchers and clinicians have continued to search for fibrinolytic agents that might prove superior to rt-PA.[191]

Reperfusion Using Mechanical Devices

Mechanical clot removal strategies are now being tested, especially in patients in whom thrombolysis would pose a high risk. Multiple strategies have and continue to be explored. The most common are techniques that directly lyse or retrieve thrombi from arteries. Direct angioplasty or stenting of thrombosed arteries has also been performed. Mechanical reperfusion has been performed instead of thrombolysis, with thrombolysis, and after thrombolysis.[198,199] Theoretically, mechanical clot dissolution poses less risk of bleeding during and after reperfusion. Most reports are anecdotal series of few cases.

One mechanical clot retrieval device has been studied in therapeutic trials.[200-203] This device looks like a corkscrew (Fig. 5-3). The device is delivered thru a catheter to the clot and the device is directed into the clot. The clot is then pulled back through the catheter and is delivered out of the vascular system. The Mechanical Embolus Removal in Cerebral Ischemia (MERCI) I study was a phase-I trial designed to evaluate the safety and efficacy of this mechanical embolectomy device.[200] Twenty-eight patients were treated in seven U.S. centers. Included were patients with NIHSS scores equal to or higher than 10 who were treated within 8 hours from symptoms onset who

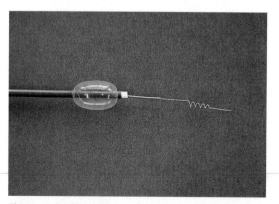

Figure 5-3. The MERCI retriever device.

had a contra-indication to intravenous thrombolysis and had occlusion of a major cerebral artery on angiography and no large hypodensity on a CT scan. The median NIHSS was 22. Successful recanalization with mechanical embolectomy only was achieved in 12 (43%) patients, and with additional intra-arterial tissue plasminogen activator in 18 (64%) patients. Twelve asymptomatic and no symptomatic intracranial hemorrhages occurred. At 1 month, 9 of 30 revascularized patients and 0 of 10 nonrevascularized patients had achieved significant recovery.[200]

A larger prospective, nonrandomized, multicenter trial of the MERCI retriever enrolled 151 patients who were ineligible for intravenous tPA.[201] Recanalization was achieved in 48% (68/141) of patients in whom the device was deployed. Clinically important procedural complications occurred in 10 (7.1%) patients. Symptomatic intracranial hemorrhages developed in 11 of 141 (7.8%) patients. Good neurologic outcomes (modified Rankin score ≤2) were more frequent at 90 days in patients with successful recanalization compared with patients with unsuccessful recanalization (46% vs 10%) and mortality was less (32% vs 54%, $P = .01$). As a result of this trial, the MERCI retriever was approved by the device division of the U.S. FDA for use in patients with intracranial occlusions.

The Multi MERCI trial is an ongoing international, multicenter, prospective, single-arm trial of patients treated within 8 hours of symptom onset who had received IV tPA but did not recanalize or who were ineligible for IV tPA.[202] Primary outcome was vascular recanalization and safety. Among 111 patients in whom the thrombectomy procedure was performed, 30 (27%) had received IV tPA before intervention. Treatment with the retriever alone resulted in successful recanalization in 60 of 111 (54%) treatable arteries and in 77 of 111 (69%) after adjunctive therapy (IA tPA, mechanical manipulation). Symptomatic intracranial hemorrhage occurred in 10 (9.0%) patients, 2 of 30 (6.7%) in patients pretreated with IV tPA, and 8 of 81 (9.9%) in those without. Clinically significant procedural complications occurred in 5 (4.5%) patients.[202] A pooled analysis of outcomes in patients with intracranial ICA occlusions ($n = 80$) in the MERCI and Multi MERCI Part I trials, showed that mechanical reperfusion had a high rate of successful recanalization and improved outcome over those patients who did not recanalize.[203]

The NINDS-funded MR and recanalization of stroke clots using embolectomy (MR-RESCUE) trial is now enrolling patients who present within 8 hours after symptom onset who are selected using MR perfusion and diffusion studies criteria to either have thrombectomy using a modified MERCI retriever system or medical management.[191]

A number of other mechanical instrument techniques have been used instead of chemical thrombolysis or as an adjunct to thrombolysis. Qureshi and colleagues reported their experience with treatment of 19 patients who had arterial occlusions but were considered poor candidates for full-dose chemical thrombolysis with what they dubbed "aggressive mechanical clot disruption" and low-dose IA tPA.[204] They used snare manipulation for distal clots and angioplasty for proximal occlusions and treated patients within 9 hours after symptom onset. Noser et al used aggressive mechanical clot disruption in 32 patients with ICA and/or MCA occlusions.[205] They first infused IV rtPA if patients were treated within 3 hours or primary IA rtPA if they presented later. If angiography showed persistent occlusion 60 to 90 minutes after repeated tPA infusions, they used balloon angioplasty, stents, or a snare instrument to recanalize the occluded artery. They advanced the snare device through a microcatheter into the clot matrix and made multiple passes through the thrombus using the fully extended loop of the snare to fragment or capture the clot.[205] Others have used mechanical thrombectomy with various devices or stenting along with thrombolysis to successfully recanalize MCA[206,207] and basilar artery occlusions.[208,209] Exploration of laser-thrombolysis and other mechanical devices continues at a rapid pace. Interventionalists will in the future have a wide array of potential chemical and mechanical tools capable of opening occluded arteries.

Multiple Neuroprotective and Thrombolytic Combinations

The history of acute stroke treatment reflects the limited effectiveness of any single treatment. Reperfusion of occluded arteries is considered by all to be the single most important goal of treatment. Reperfusion is strongly associated with improved clinical outcome.[210] The faster that thromboemboli are lysed, the better the outcome.[211] Even late reperfusion is associated with better outcomes than failure to reperfuse.[212,213] Unfortunately thrombolysis is underutilized mostly because appropriate candidates for thrombolysis do not reach stroke centers equipped to manage them in sufficient time to be treated effectively. Even in patients who are treated "in time," the present thrombolytics do not recanalize the occluded artery. Researchers and clinicians have begun to explore multiple

sequential or concurrent treatments—a "cocktail" approach.[214] The two most commonly used strategies follow: (1) giving a neuroprotective drug before thrombolysis in an attempt to lengthen the time window available for thrombolysis. Increasing the brain's resistance to ischemia could lengthen the time that reperfusion might save neurons, and (2) augmenting the effect of the presently used thrombolytic agents by using antiplatelet or anticoagulant drugs concurrently or after thrombolysis to open arteries and to keep arteries open.

Clinicians continue to search for effective neuroprotective agents. Unfortunately, the search has been mostly unsuccessful. I discuss neuroprotection in some detail later in this chapter. I mentioned the FAST-MAG trial earlier.[145] The idea behind the trial is to give a magnesium sulfate infusion in the field as a potential neuroprotectant before hospital evaluation for thrombolysis. Others are exploring the potential for citicoline to be used in combination with thrombolysis.[215] Citicoline has been studied in clinical trials in acute ischemic stroke patients that showed the substance was very safe and there were some suggestions of effectiveness.[216,217] Citicoline was effective in a rat model of acute embolic stroke when combined with thrombolysis.[218] NXY-059 proved safe and effective in the SAINT I trial,[219-221] but was not effective in the SAINT II trial.[222] Theoretically, the concurrent use of a safe and an effective neuroprotectant might help resuscitate ischemic neurons, protect against reperfusion injury, as well as lengthen the time window for reperfusion.[223]

In many patients, IV and IA thrombolytic agents are ineffective in lysing clots and in effecting important reperfusion. In other patients thrombolysis is initially effective but the artery reoccludes.[224] Alexandrov and Grotta found that reocclusion after initial recanalization developed in about a third of their patients who had initially recanalized after IV rtPA.[224] Clinicians have explored the use of glycoprotein IIb/IIIa inhibitors as an adjunct to thrombolysis and other reperfusion strategies. The GpIIb/IIIa inhibitors abciximab,[225,226] tirofiban,[227-229] and eptifibatide[229] have all been administered in preliminary studies along with thrombolytics. Hemorrhage was a major concern in the AbESTT trials of abciximide for acute ischemic stroke[226,230] and was a problem when abciximide was combined with neurointerventional procedures and thrombolysis.[225] Tirofiban has been used: with heparin before IA urokinase and mechanical devices,[227] concurrent with IV rtPA,[228] and after IV rtPA.[229] The dose of thrombolytics was usually reduced. Preliminary results were suggestive of an added

5

effect and hemorrhage was not a major problem in these preliminary explorations with tirofiban. Eptifibatide was used as a part of multimodal reperfusion strategies among 168 patients treated with IA tPA or urokinase and/or mechanical devices.[229] Eptifibatide was given concurrent with or after the thrombolytic agent and seemed to enhance recanalization in a retrospective review.[229]

Standard anticoagulants and antiplatelet agents have also been used as adjuncts to thrombolytic drugs. Heparin has been variously used immediately after IV and IA thrombolysis, although its use was prohibited for 24 hours in the NINDS and PROACT trials. In one study, the use of heparin just after thrombolysis did not increase the rate of symptomatic hemorrhagic complications.[231] In another study, among 300 consecutive acute stroke patients treated with IV rtPA, 92 were pretreated with aspirin (100 to 500 mg), and with low-dose ($n = 122$) or high-dose ($n = 153$) heparin.[232] The authors concluded that pretreatment with aspirin in this group of patients did not increase the rate of symptomatic hemorrhage even in those also given heparin.[232] An ongoing study, the Argatroban tPA Stroke Study is exploring the safety and efficacy of giving argatroban after IV rtPA.[233] At this time, it is not clear which agents if any should be given (routinely or selectively) before, during, or after thrombolysis or mechanical reperfusion.

The Use of Ultrasound as an Adjunct to Enhance Thrombolysis

Transcranial Doppler ultrasound (TCD) has been used effectively to diagnose and localize intracranial arterial occlusions and to monitor whether spontaneous or treatment-related recanalization has occurred.[224,234] Preliminary small studies suggested that continuous monitoring of the middle cerebral artery using TCD ultrasound during thrombolysis might augment the lytic effect of the thrombolytic agent.[235,236] In a randomized trial, CLOTBUST patients were randomly assigned to receive continuous 2-MHz TCD (the target group, $n = 63$) or placebo (the control group, $n = 63$).[237] The primary combined endpoint was complete recanalization as assessed by TCD or dramatic clinical recovery. Symptomatic intracerebral hemorrhage occurred in 3 patients in the target group and in 3 in the control group. Complete recanalization or dramatic clinical recovery within 2 hours after the administration of a tPA bolus occurred in 31 patients in the target group (49%), compared with 19 patients in the control group (30%; $P = .03$). Twenty-four hours after treatment, 24 patients in the target group (44%) and 21 in the control group (40%) had a

dramatic clinical recovery ($P = .7$). At 3 months, 22/53 (42%) patients in the target group and 14/49 in the control group (29%) had favorable outcomes (as indicated by a score of 0 to 1 on the modified Rankin scale) ($P = .20$). The results of this trial suggested further that continuous transcranial Doppler might augment t-PA–induced arterial recanalization.[237]

Ultrasound has the potential to physically loosen fibrin bridges within red blood clots, allowing erythrocytes to escape and the clot to dissolve.[238] In one preliminary study, 15 patients who were ineligible for thrombolysis were randomized to have or not have continuous TCD monitoring.[239] The group that had TCD monitoring more often recanalized and showed more neurologic improvement than those patients not monitored but the numbers were very small.[239] In another preliminary study, TCD monitoring of thrombolysis was compared with no monitoring, and with monitoring combined with three doses of 2.5 g (400 mg/mL) of a galactose-based microbubble solution. There was a suggestion that the microbubble infusion potentiated and accelerated the effect of ultrasound on thrombolysis.[240] There are many reasons to recommend TCD monitoring during and shortly after thrombolysis in centers that have the capability.

Thrombolytic treatment has brought much excitement and enthusiasm to the care of patients with acute ischemic stroke. As one can readily see from the length and complexity of this review, the field is ever changing and new agents, devices, and means of evaluation are being explored and studied in observation studies and trials. Table 5-10 lists my present recommendations for thrombolysis. Key factors for these decisions are knowledge of the presence, location, and nature of arterial occlusion, time since symptom onset if known, presence and amount of infarction and threatened brain, availability of other potentially effective treatments, and the wishes of patients informed about the risks and benefits of the recommendations.

Surgically Bypassing Blockage Regions

A surgical bypass can be created connecting one vessel to another beyond an obstruction in the neck (e.g., a common carotid artery to vertebral artery connection) or intracranially creating an artificial conduit between extracranial branches and intracranial arteries. One artery can be directly sewn to another, or a venous conduit can be interposed. When the vessel to be bypassed is stenotic but still patent, creation of a distal shunt has been shown to further reduce flow through the region of stenosis and promote thrombotic

Table 5-10.	**Caplan's Present Recommendations for Thrombolysis at Stroke Centers That Have Experienced Stroke Clinicians and Modern Technology**

1. If the patient is seen within 3 hours and the cause is clear clinically (e.g., atrial fibrillation) and the CT does not show a large region of hypodensity, it is reasonable to give tPA using the guidelines without further study.
2. If the cause is not obvious and/or the patient does not meet guidelines (stroke on awakening, uncertain onset time, .3 hours of symptoms, minor or improving deficit, or usual exclusion), then further brain and vascular imaging are suggested. This could be MRI with T2*, DWI, MRA, or CT with CTA, or CT or MR with neck and transcranial Doppler.
3. Transcranial Doppler monitoring before, during, and shortly after thrombolysis is optimal if available. This allows recognition of recanalization and reocclusions.

After brain and vascular evaluation

Situations in which I do not recommend thrombolysis:
• Large infarct already present and little at-risk tissue
• No occlusion and lacunar syndrome
Situations in which I recommend IV thrombolysis (followed by IA if recanalization does not occur):
• Occluded intracranial artery (MCA or branch or ICVA) especially if the mechanism is embolic and no or small infarct and considerable at-risk tissue
• Occluded ICA in the neck seen within 3 hours (although treatment is often unsuccessful)
Situation in which I usually recommend angiography with consideration of IA thrombolysis with or without mechanical clot retrieval and/or angioplasty/stenting:
• Basilar artery occlusions
• Carotid T occlusions with considerable at risk tissue
• >6 hours after symptom onset
• Some patients with ICA neck occlusions
• Some patients whose clinical pictures (demography and recurrent TIAs) suggest in-situ atherothrombotic intracranial occlusive disease especially after IV treatment does not produce effective recanalization

occlusion of the previously stenotic artery.[241,242] Clots that form at the site of occlusion might embolize distally, causing new ischemic damage.

Many anecdotal reports noted the effectiveness of extracranial to intracranial artery bypass using the superficial temporal artery as the donor artery and an MCA branch as the recipient artery. A large, randomized study of the effectiveness of such extracranial-intracranial bypasses, however, proved beyond reasonable doubt that the surgery as it was customarily performed at the time had no benefit.[243] In some circumstances, operated patients fared worse than patients treated medically.[243] The patients in this series had surgery approximately 6 weeks or more after the last symptomatic episode of brain ischemia or stroke to prevent reperfusion hemorrhage in regions where the capillaries and arterioles might be ischemic and vulnerable to leakage. Following the report of this study, surgeons and stroke clinicians asked the following questions[244]:

1. Would bypass procedures earlier in the course (although more risky) be more effective?
2. Would a larger recipient artery (e.g., intracranial ICA, mainstem MCA, or a large conduit

such as an interposed vein or larger artery improve results?
3. Might there be some small well-selected groups of patients (e.g., those with severe persistent hypoperfusion confirmed by modern technology) who could benefit?[245]

Since the publication of the international EC/IC bypass trial a number of new technological advances and techniques have been introduced. Surgeons have created higher volume bypasses by using the intracranial ICA or MCA or major branches as the recipient artery instead of distal branches of the superior or inferior divisions as was the former practice.[246,247] Tulleken and colleagues introduced a technique that uses excimer laser equipment to help create a high flow shunt connecting a large venous or arterial interposed graft between the superficial temporal artery and the intracranial ICA or proximal MCA.[248,249] After sewing the donor artery directly into a ring placed on the surface of the recipient large artery, the excimer laser makes an opening through the recipient artery that opens the anastomosis. The theoretical advantage is that no clipping or stoppage of blood flow occurs during the bypass procedure.[248,249]

5

Studies have shown that patients who continue to have ischemic symptoms after ICA occlusions, those with increased oxygen extraction fractions as determined by positron emission tomography (PET) scanning, and those with reduced cerebrovascular reserve have a relatively high risk of new brain infarction. The Carotid Occlusion Study showed that ipsilateral increased O_2 extraction fraction (OEF) as measured by PET is a powerful independent risk factor for subsequent stroke in patients with symptomatic complete carotid artery occlusion. The ipsilateral ischemic stroke rate at 2 years was 5.3% in 42 patients with normal OEF and 26.5% in 39 patients with increased OEF ($P = .004$). In patients in whom hemispheric symptoms developed within 120 days, the 2-year ipsilateral stroke rates were 12% in 27 patients with normal OEF and 50% in 18 patients with increased OEF. PET studies show that anastomosis of the superficial temporal artery (STA) to a middle cerebral artery (MCA) cortical branch can restore OEF to normal. Investigators have shown conclusively that reduced cerebrovascular reserve (as measured in a variety of ways) in the cerebral hemisphere supplied by an occluded carotid artery predicts a relatively high risk of brain infarction compared to patients with normal reserve.[250-254]

These studies have given an impetus to examine the utility of EC/IC bypass in selected patients in new trials.[255-257] The Carotid Occlusion Surgery Study (COSS) is recruiting patients with recently symptomatic ICA occlusion and increased ipsilateral OEF for a randomized study testing the utility of surgical bypass.[255,256] Other studies will use reduced cerebrovascular reserve in patients who have symptomatic carotid artery occlusions as an inclusion criteria.[256]

Bypass surgery has also been used in patients with moya moya syndrome. The most common indication for attempts to augment intracranial blood flow has been brain ischemia and brain infarction. A variety of different structures have been placed over the ischemic brain including omentum, gracilis muscle, temporalis muscle with its blood supply, superficial temporal artery with attached galea, and a vascular portion of the dura mater and arachnoid.[258] These procedures are often considered effective in children with moya moya although they have not been studied definitively in randomized trials.[259] Superficial temporal artery to middle cerebral artery anastomoses have also been performed, but in young individuals the arteries are rather small. Adult patients with moya moya often present with hemorrhages from deep penetrating arteries that are overloaded in attempting to deliver adequate collateral blood supply. A multicenter, prospective randomized trial (Japan Adult Moya Moya trial) to test the utility of extracranial-intracranial (EC-IC) bypass for treating adult patients with moya moya disease who had episodes of intracranial bleeding is now being performed in Japan.[260] Treatment of moya moya will be discussed in more detail in Chapter 11.

Bypass operations have also been performed in the past for vertebrobasilar ischemia.[247] These procedures have now been almost entirely superceded by intracranial angioplasty and stenting.

Increasing Blood Flow in the Collateral Circulation and Perfusion in the Ischemic-Zone Capillary Bed

Vasodilating agents have long been prescribed to increase blood flow. Carbon dioxide (CO_2) is the oldest known vasodilator. Physicians have attempted to dilate brain arteries by asking patients to breathe air with high CO_2 content. Other agents include cyclandelate, isoxsuprine, hydergine, papaverine, and nicotinic acid. A woeful lack of information exists regarding the effect and use of vasodilating agents on CBF in patients with TIAs or ischemic strokes.[261] Abnormal or even paradoxical responses of the cerebral circulation in stroke patients might theoretically render vasodilator treatment ineffective or even harmful.[261] Cerebral arteries have relatively few elastic fibers in the media and are less responsive than systemic vessels to vasodilator stimuli. Vasodilator agents produce more systemic than cerebral vasodilation and could thus lead to hypotension or globally decreased CBF. Arteries within nonischemic regions should retain the ability to vasodilate, whereas arteries within ischemic zones could be sufficiently damaged by ischemia and so lose their ability to dilate. In that circumstance, vasodilating drugs could result in an increased flow into nonischemic areas creating a type of "steal away" from the ischemic areas.

Some pharmaceutical agents have vasoconstrictive effects in some arteries and vasodilator effects in others. Even individual drugs sometimes have different effects on the same circulation depending on dose and other factors. Serotonin has been shown to dilate normal coronary arteries but constrict coronary arteries when the endothelium is diseased.[262] None of the available agents have been thoroughly studied in individuals with cerebrovascular disease. Technology to study regional cerebral blood flow (rCBF) and flow in the brain arteries is now available allowing more definitive analysis of the effect of various agents on blood flow, symptoms, and outcomes.

In situations such as SAH or migraine, in which there is known vasospasm, agents that decrease vasoconstriction may have beneficial effects. Acetazolamide (Diamox) has been used as a provocative agent to acutely dilate brain arteries to test the brain's vascular reserve capability to further augment blood flow. Flow is measured in basal intracranial arteries by transcranial Doppler before and after acetazolamide is given intravenously.[263] In one study of patients with occlusive disease of intracranial or extracranial arteries, intravenous acetazolamide did increase rCBF but mostly on the nonobstructed side.[264] Acetazolamide is taken orally and could be administered to out-patients with occlusive disease in an attempt to augment blood flow but this strategy has not been extensively studied as a treatment in ischemic stroke patients.

Calcium channel-blocking agents have been tested since 1987 to determine if they improve function in patients with ischemic stroke and SAH. Calcium has a number of actions that can influence the outcome of ischemia.[265] These include promoting vasoconstriction by effects on vascular smooth muscle, altering coagulation (some of the coagulation reactions require Ca^{++}), killing cells when extracellular Ca^{++} passes through cell membranes into the intracellular compartment, and lowering systemic blood pressure.[265,266]

A preliminary study of nimodipine in patients with SAH suggested some beneficial effects on cerebral vasospasm.[267] Later studies also showed some beneficial effects on morbidity, mortality, and on prevention of delayed ischemic infarction in patients with SAH. It was not clear in these studies whether or not nimodipine successfully increased blood flow or decreased the arterial vasoconstriction.[268-270] Trials of the effectiveness of nimodipine in patients with ischemic stroke, however, have had disappointing results,[271] although nimodipine may help in the most severe cases if given early enough.[272] Therapeutic benefits probably result more from blockage of extracellular to intracellular movement of Ca^{++} than from reversal of vasoconstriction.

Newer calcium channel blockers might have more selective cerebral vasodilating effects. Newer technology allows monitoring of blood flow acutely, chronically, focally, and globally. Newer drugs and some untested, older agents can be studied in the laboratory and clinic.

Volume expansion is another method used to attempt to augment cerebral blood flow and increase perfusion within the microcirculation of the brain. Physicians have attempted to increase blood volume by simply increasing fluid intake or by using various volume expanders. Albumin, plasma, and solutions of colloids and crystalloids have been used.[273] Albumin has been extensively studied in experimental models of brain ischemia and does increase local cerebral blood flow in ischemic zones.[274] In the ALIAS pilot trial 82 patients with acute ischemic stroke with a NIHSS of 6 or higher received a 25% albumin solution beginning within 16 hours of stroke onset.[275,276] Six successive dose tiers were assessed (range, 0.34 to 2.05 g/kg). Forty-two patients also received standard-of-care intravenous tPA. After adjusting for the tPA effect, the probability of good outcome (defined as modified Rankin Scale 0 to 1 or NIH Stroke Scale 0 to 1 at 3 months) at the highest three albumin doses was 81% greater than in the lower-dose tiers (relative risk, 1.81; 95% confidence interval, 1.11 to 2.94) and was 95% greater than in the comparable NINDS rt-PA Stroke Study cohort (relative risk, 1.95; 95% confidence interval, 1.47 to 2.57). The tPA-treated subjects who received higher-dose albumin (ALB) were three times more likely to achieve a good outcome than subjects receiving lower-dose albumin, suggesting a positive synergistic effect between albumin and tPA.[276] The investigators posited that albumin might have a neuroprotective effect in addition to expansion of blood volume and augmentation of blood flow. An ALIAS Phase III trial is planned.[274-276]

Mannitol, most often used to treat brain edema in patients with edematous brain infarcts and brain hemorrhages, may also temporarily expand intravascular volume and increase microcirculatory blood flow. Most often, the expansion of blood volume related to use of osmotic agents is in serum volume, thus effectively diluting the more viscous erythrocyte portion of the blood. This is referred to as hemodilution. The two major determinants of blood viscosity within brain vessels are fibrinogen and Hct. Lowering the Hct by hemodilution may reduce whole blood viscosity and increase blood flow.[277,278] The optimal Hct for blood flow and preservation of oxygen transport is approximately 33%.[279]

Rapid hemodilution with reduction of the Hct theoretically could significantly improve blood flow to ischemic zones. Hemodilution may be isovolemic (i.e., blood replaced with equivalent fluid volume) or replacement may be more (hypervolemic) or less (hypovolemic) than the original blood volume. Plasma, Ringer's lactate solution, albumin, or colloid solutions such as dextran 40 or hydroxyethyl starch are often used for fluid replacement. Volume is important to maintain during hemodilution because either hypovolemia with excessively reduced volume, hypervolemia with potential cardiac overload, and brain edema can be harmful. Centers using hemodilution therapy must have experience in this technique. The most frequently used colloidal solutions are dextrans and starches. Dextrans are polysaccharide molecules made by the action of bacteria on sucrose. The most commonly used solution (10% dextran solution in normal saline or 5% dextrose) is called dextran 40 and contains molecules ranging from a molecular weight of 10,000 to 80,000 (average 40,000). Infusion causes rapid volume expansion but rapid urinary excretion of the dextran molecules of less than 50,000 molecular weight leads to an osmotic diuresis with reduction in plasma volume. Dextran also coats red blood cells, platelets, and endothelium and this capability is posited to decrease blood viscosity and prevent cellular aggregation to improve microcirculatory flow. Dextran has a potential antithrombotic action by its hemodiluting effect, erythrocyte coating, and decreased platelet aggregation. Another frequently used colloidal solution is hydroxyethyl starch. Dextran and hydroxyethyl starch solutions have been used to treat stroke, usually as part of hemodilution protocols, but these agents have not been shown to improve outcome in clinical trials.[277,280-283] Plasma and Ringer's lactate solution have also been used but have not been well studied in therapeutic trials.

Another means of reducing viscosity and also potentially altering blood coagulability is the use of substances that reduce fibrinogen levels. Fibrinogen contributes significantly to whole blood viscosity[284] and high fibrinogen levels have been noted to predict stroke recurrence in high-risk patients.[285-288] Ancrod, an agent discussed earlier in this chapter under thrombolysis, selectively acts on fibrinogen and inhibits formation of cross-linked fibrin.[288] Ancrod can reduce fibrinogen levels to approximately 100 mg/dL. In one study at onset, the mean plasma fibrinogen level was 385 mg/dL.[288] After intravenous infusions of ancrod, D-dimer levels rose, indicating clot lysis. Fibrinogen levels fell to a mean of 116 mg/dL at 6 hours and 52 mg/dL at 24 hours after beginning treatment.[289] Liu and colleagues analyzed the data from trials of fibrinogen-depleting agents and concluded that more information is needed.[290]

Another method of rapidly reducing blood fibrinogen levels and whole blood viscosity is to use plasmaphoresis techniques. Investigators in Austria developed a technique that they named *heparin-induced, extracorporeal low-density lipoprotein precipitation* (HELP).[291,292] In this system, blood is removed from a cubital vein and passed through a filter that separates the cellular components from the plasma. Isovolemic acetate buffer and heparin are added to the plasma. Fibrinogen, low-density lipoprotein (LDL) cholesterol, and

triglycerides are removed by this process. The blood is then reinfused into the cubital vein on the opposite side. HELP treatment reduces fibrinogen levels, lowers whole-blood viscosity at high and low shear rates, lowers plasma viscosity, and reduces red cell transit time.[291-293] This pharesis technique has been used for decades in the United States and Europe to treat patients with familial hypercholesterolemia.[293] It is quite effective in preventing premature atherosclerosis. Fibrinogen depletion after treatment is dramatic but temporary, lasting less than 2 weeks. Pharesis also lowers C-reactive protein quite effectively.[294] This treatment has been used acutely to augment cerebral blood flow and can also be used repeatedly in patients with microvascular occlusive disease with vascular dementia who have high fibrinogen levels. The effectiveness of the fibrinogen depletion (acutely or chronically) in preventing stroke or limiting the extent of brain infarction has not been studied well in patients who have normal cholesterol levels.

Omega-3 fatty acids, especially eicosopentanoic acid, can also lower blood fibrinogen levels, although the effect is quite variable.[295-297] In a preliminary study, eicosopentanoic acid also reduced blood viscosity, especially in those patients with high baseline viscosities.[295] Eicosopentanoic acid and omega-3 fatty acids, plentiful in various fish oils, have the potential to reduce platelet aggregability in addition to their effects on fibrinogen and viscosity. The low frequency of atherosclerosis in Eskimos has been posited to be related to diets rich in fish and omega-3 fatty acids. These substances have not been tested in stroke prevention or treatment. Atromid, ticlopidine, and pentoxyphilline also have some fibrinogen-lowering effects.

Another strategy that has been used experimentally to improve microcirculatory flow and oxygen delivery is the use of perfluorochemicals. Perfluorochemicals are relatively small molecules, much smaller than erythrocytes. They can carry and release oxygen yet are not metabolized, remain chemically inert, and have low surface tension.[298] When patients or laboratory animals breathe 100% oxygen, these small molecules become saturated with oxygen. Perfluorochemicals have been used mostly as so-called white blood given to patients who are severely anemic but refuse blood transfusions for religious reasons.[299,300] Theoretically, small molecules can squeeze through vascular passages that block erythrocytes and thereby succeed in delivering needed oxygen to the ischemic stunned penumbral brain tissue. In clinical studies, however, investigators have not been able to attain concentrations of perfluorochemicals ("fluocrits") high enough to provide useful oxygen-carrying capabilities.[300] In experimental stroke models, perfusion of the ventricular and subarachnoid fluid spaces with highly oxygenated fluorocarbons decreases the extent of brain infarction.[301,302] The concept of delivering oxygen to tissues by using fluorocarbon emulsions shows promise.

In patients with low flow, stagnation causes clot formation and embolization. Measures to prevent embolization, discussed in the following section, are also applicable to many low-flow situations.

Prevention of Clot Formation, Propagation, and Embolism

The formation of a thrombus depends on a number of interrelated factors that include local vascular injury or roughening, the number of platelets and their activation, and the presence of serum coagulant and anticoagulant substances. Thrombi can be divided into red erythrocyte-fibrin clots and white platelet-fibrin clots. Red clots are treated with thrombolytic drugs and heparins, warfarin, factor Xa inhibitors, and direct thrombin inhibitors.[303] In contrast, white clot formation is prevented by so-called antiplatelet agents (aspirin, clopidogrel, dipyridamole, cilostazol, and others).[303-305] In general, red clots, erythrocyte-fibrin thrombi, tend to form in regions where there is low flow or stagnation, whereas smaller, so-called white platelet clots adhere to roughened places in faster-moving streams of blood.

Red thrombi are most apt to develop when flow is reduced. Dilated cardiac atria especially those with inefficient contractility as found with atrial fibrillation, regions of hypokinesia of the cardiac ventricles, and frank ventricular aneurysms often harbor red clots. Red thrombi are also often formed in heart chambers when ejection fractions are low. Red thrombi tend to form on the surface of myocardial infarcts. Thrombi formed in the leg and pelvic veins that pass through defects in the cardiac atrial and ventricular septa or pass through arteriovenous fistulae in the lungs are nearly always red thrombi. Both red and white thrombi often form along damaged heart valves especially those made of prosthetic materials.

Red thrombi are composed mostly of red blood cells and fibrin. They tend to form in areas of slowed blood flow. Their formation does not require an abnormal vessel wall or tissue thromboplastin. Red clots are formed by activation of circulating coagulation factors. The final step in the coagulation cascade is the conversion of the soluble protein fibrinogen into insoluble polymers called fibrin. Fibrin strands form a network of fibers that entangle the formed blood elements (platelets, erythrocytes, and leukocytes) into a clot. Fibrin is quite adhesive and is capable of contracting. The fibrinogen-fibrin reaction occurs when factor II, prothrombin is converted to thrombin. The amounts of circulating fibrinogen and prothrombin are important in these reactions.

Prothrombin is activated in two different ways. In the so-called extrinsic system of coagulation, a tissue or endothelial injury releases thromboplastic substances, tissue factors, which in turn cause both platelet activation and activation of blood serine protease coagulation factors, especially factors V, VII, and X. Activation of factor X catalyzes the reaction of prothrombin to thrombin. Activation of platelets causes them to agglutinate, to adhere to the injured vessel wall, and to release various intracellular substances, which in turn also activate the coagulation system.[303,306,307]

The complementary intrinsic coagulation system refers to blood-coagulation factors that circulate in inactive forms (factors V, VIII [antihemophilic globulin], IX, X, XI, XII) and are intrinsic to the blood. Activation of factor XII from an inert precursor form to an activated form triggers a series of reactions, the coagulation cascade, in which the various blood-clotting factors are sequentially converted to their active enzymatic forms. Ultimately, these reactions lead to activation of factor X, which catalyzes the prothrombin–thrombin reaction.

White clots are composed of platelets and fibrin and do not contain red blood cells. White clots form almost exclusively in areas in which the endothelial surface is abnormal, characteristically in fast-moving bloodstreams. Irregular valvular and endothelial surfaces predispose to platelet-fibrin thrombi forming in areas of irregularities. In many patients thrombosis involves first the deposition of white clots on denuded or abnormal endothelium. Platelets adhere to the abnormal endothelium and aggregate forming a white clot. Platelet activation also stimulates thrombin generation which in turn can lead to the deposition of red thrombi superimposed upon the white thrombi.[308] An analysis of thrombi retrieved from cerebral arteries of patients with acute ischemic stroke most often showed a pattern of mixed white and red clots.[309]

Standard "anticoagulants", including heparin (and low-molecular-weight heparin and heparinoids), warfarin, factor Xa inhibitors, and direct thrombin inhibitors argatroban, ximelagatran, and dabigitran, theoretically should be more useful in preventing red clots, whereas antiplatelet agglutinating agents should be better at preventing white platelet plugs.[282] Heparin and warfarin and direct thrombin inhibitors should work best in occlusive disease of veins and large arteries and in cardiac disorders that predispose to cardiac-origin thromboembolism, whereas agents that decrease platelet aggregation might have an advantage in arterial plaque disease without severe stenosis. Thrombolytic agents lyse red clots but are not thought to lyse white clots. In fact they may stimulate platelet activation instead.

Polycythemia and thrombocytosis increase the probability of clot formation. Frequent blood donations, removal of causes of secondary erythremia such as cigarette smoking, and specific antineoplastic treatment of polycythemia vera are therapeutic alternatives for reduction of the hematocrit. In the acute situation, hemodilution decreases the hematocrit reducing viscosity and thrombotic tendencies. Thrombocytosis can also cause a clotting tendency and usually accompanies hematologic proliferative disorders that require specific therapy. Severe anemia also may promote thrombosis.

Anticoagulants

Heparin and Heparins

Heparin, a biological substance derived from tissues of various animals (most often bovine lungs and porcine intestines), has been used clinically since the 1940s. Heparin derives its name from the original description of it as an aqueous extract of liver (hepar) that showed anticoagulant activity in vitro.[310] Heparin decreases hyperlipemia and has a variety of different anticoagulant effects. The anticoagulant properties of heparin are due to the ability of components of the compound to bind to antithrombin III (AT III). AT III slowly binds to thrombin and the serine proteases factors VIIa, IXa, Xa, XIa, and XIIa and neutralizes these compounds. Heparin binds to AT III and dramatically accelerates the complex formation of AT III with thrombin and also with coagulation factors Xa and XIa.[311,312] Heparin also antagonizes thromboplastin and prevents thrombi from reacting with fibrinogen to form fibrin. Heparin is a heterogeneous mixture of sulfated mucopolysaccharides containing at least 21 compounds ranging in size from 3000 to 37,500 daltons.[313]

Heparin has been used most often during the acute phase of thrombosis or embolism. The necessity of giving the drug parenterally has limited its long-term use. Heparin has also been used during pregnancy in patients who require anticoagulation because of the potential adverse effects of warfarin on the fetus. Heparin can be given as an intravenous bolus, a continuous-drip infusion, or, less effectively, subcutaneously. Dosage is usually adjusted to keep the activated partial thromboplastin time (aPTT) at 1.5 to 2.5 times the mean of the normal control values.[310,314,315]

Heparin has usually been given acutely to maintain anticoagulation until warfarin therapy reaches therapeutic levels. There are two main reasons behind this practice. Heparin works very quickly while warfarin takes days to reach therapeutic levels. The other reason relates to prevention of hypercoagulability that occasionally develops with the initiation of warfarin without preceding heparin. Warfarin-induced skin necrosis mostly occurs in patients with hereditary protein C deficiency. It is a rare occurrence and almost invariably develops in the setting of acute thrombosis when there is inflammation and cytokine elaboration. There is no need in ambulatory patients with atrial fibrillation without thrombosis to give heparin along with warfarin or to test such individuals for protein C deficiency. The only exception would be a patient with known protein C deficiency in whom it would be wise to build up the warfarin dose slowly starting from a dose of 2 mg.

Some patients treated with heparin develop a drop in their platelet count (thrombocytopenia) and new ischemic events.[316-319] There are two varieties of heparin-induced thrombocytopenia (HITS). The most common variety involves a slight degree of thrombocytopenia usually beginning 1 to 5 days after the start of heparin owing to heparin-induced platelet aggregation. Ischemia does not result and platelet counts return to normal despite continuation of heparin. In the more severe form of heparin-induced thrombocytopenia, antibodies of the IgG and IgM groups become bound to platelets and platelet counts fall, usually during the second week of treatment. Often, thrombocytopenia is severe (10,000 mm^3) and thromboembolic and hemorrhagic complications may develop owing to consumption of coagulation factors and platelets. Blockage of small arteries by white platelet-fibrin clots can cause regions of skin and visceral organ necrosis, termed the *white clot syndrome*. Occasionally, thrombosis seems to be precipitated by heparin without thrombocytopenia.[320]

The anticoagulant activities of various commercial preparations of heparin vary among sources and even within batches from the same source.[311-314] These variations lead to variability in clinical effectiveness and unexpected bleeding. Unfractionated heparin has begun to be replaced by low-molecular-weight heparins and heparinoids. Crude commercial preparations of heparin can be separated into low- and high-molecular-weight fractions. Low-molecular-weight heparins are fragments of standard heparin with molecular weights of 4000 to 6000.[321,322] Heparinoids are heparin analogues, natural or semisynthetic sulfated glycosaminoglycans, prepared by tissue extraction or by blending various components.[322,323] They are related structurally to heparin and have similar biological functions, especially anticoagulant effects. Heparins, low-molecular-weight heparins, and heparinoids act as anticoagulants by binding to plasma antithrombin III. This interaction induces a conformational change in antithrombin III that increases its ability to inactivate coagulation enzymes, including thrombin and activated factor X (factor Xa).

Low-molecular-weight heparins are thought to have more favorable bioavailability and pharmacokinetics than standard heparin. Their plasma half-lives are two to four times that of heparin.[321] Low-molecular weight heparins are posited to cause fewer hemorrhagic complications than standard heparin because they have less pronounced effect on platelet function and vascular permeability.[321,322] Some evidence suggests that low-molecular-weight heparin has more anticoagulant effect than unfractionated heparin and does not activate platelets.[311,323] Heparin's bleeding complications most likely relate to effects on platelets, especially inhibition of platelet aggregation which is mostly an action of the high-molecular-weight components in heparin.[323] Low-molecular-weight heparins also cause less heparin-related thrombocytopenia, heparin-related skin necrosis, and white clot syndromes. While heparin is monitored closely using the PTT, low-molecular-weight heparins and heparinoids can be monitored by measuring anti–factor Xa activity. However not all laboratories have high-quality reliably reproducible analyses of anti-factor Xa. Heparinoids and low-molecular-weight heparins are more convenient to use than standard heparin and are often used in patients outside of acute-care hospital settings. Although low-molecular-weight heparins have been well studied in patients with lower extremity phlebothrombosis and pulmonary embolism, there are few studies in stroke patients.

The effectiveness of heparins and anticoagulants in ischemic stroke has not been well studied except in regard to atrial fibrillation. Heparin followed by warfarin has often been used in patients with cardiogenic embolism who are at high risk for early re-embolization. Recent studies also suggest that heparin is effective in patients with cerebral dural sinus thrombosis and in patients with extracranial dissections and in selected patients with large-artery occlusive disease. Because the indications for anticoagulation (except for timing) relate to both heparin and warfarin, I will review them after discussing warfarin.

Warfarin

Warfarin is a water-soluble derivative of coumaric acid that is absorbed by the small intestine and transported in the blood loosely bound to albumin. Its therapeutic effect is to inhibit the action of vitamin K necessary for the biological synthesis of factors II (prothrombin), VII, IX, and X.[324] By depressing these procoagulant factors, warfarin affects the so-called intrinsic cascade and the extrinsic coagulation pathway.[324,325] Warfarin works quite differently from heparin. In some patients who have continued transient spells or progressive ischemic symptoms despite warfarin anticoagulation, symptoms may almost miraculously stop when heparin is substituted for warfarin. In the past, prothrombin times were usually maintained at 2.0-2.5 times the control value. This therapeutic range was selected as that level slightly below that at which bleeding occurred.[324,325] Wessler and Gitel provide data that persuasively show that the dosage at which warfarin protects against thrombosis is probably far below that needed to cause bleeding.[324] In one study of 96 patients with venous thromboses treated with various intensities of oral anticoagulation, higher intensity therapy measured by more prolonged prothrombin times caused more bleeding. Less intense therapy was equally effective in preventing recurrent thromboembolism.[326] Others have also corroborated the safety and effectiveness of less intense warfarin anticoagulation.[327,328]

Because of the wide variation in thromboplastin reagents used, the World Health Organization designated a single batch of human brain thromboplastin as an international standard.[329] Manufacturers calibrate their reagent against the international standard and calculate an International Sensitivity Index that relates their reagent to the international standard. Using the International Sensitivity Index and the prothrombin times, the International Normalized Ratio (INR) can be readily calculated. Various expert groups have published recommendations for intensity of anticoagulation based on the international system.[329,330] Generally, two intensities of anticoagulation have been recommended: a less intense range (INR 2.0-3.0) and a more intense range (INR 3.0-4.5).[329] The higher intensity range clearly has more risk of bleeding. Stroke Prevention in Reversible Ischemia Trial (SPIRIT), a large Dutch trial that compared the effectiveness of aspirin versus oral anticoagulation (INR target range, 3.0 to 4.5) was prematurely stopped after an interim analysis showed an unacceptable rate of hemorrhage in the anticoagulant-treated group.[331] In another analysis, the frequency of bleeding increased by a factor of 1.43 for each 0.5 unit increase in the INR.[327]

5

Genetic analysis can identify some individuals who are more sensitive to warfarin compounds. Various alleles in the Genes CYP2C9 and VKORCI render patients more susceptible to bleeding during warfarin administration.[332] VKORCI variants are especially common in patients of Asian origin. Genetic analysis can be useful in guiding the dose of warfarins.[333,334] Pharmacogenetic biomarkers may also become important in the use of direct thrombin inhibitors, other types of anticoagulants, and anticonvulsants.[335]

The Atrial Fibrillation Investigators analyzed the results of five trials of anticoagulation in patients with atrial fibrillation (INR target range, 1.4 to 4.2) and recommended a target range of 2.0-3.0 as having the best benefit and risk results.[336,337] Hylek and colleagues also analyzed the results of anticoagulation in atrial fibrillation trials and found that the rate of stroke increased when the INR fell below 2.0. Optimal protection occurred in patients with INRs between 2.0 and 3.0.[338] No further protection was attributable to INRs above 3.0.[338] In most patients, I aim at an INR between 2.0 and 3.0. In patients older than 75 years, I use an INR target of 2.0 to 2.5.

Indications and Timing of Anticoagulants

Cardiac-Origin Embolism

Until the 1990s, the effectiveness of warfarin had not been tested in modern randomized trials in patients with known pathologies. Early observational studies showed the effectiveness of warfarin in patients with rheumatic mitral stenosis who had brain embolism.[339-342] Trials of stroke prophylaxis in patients with atrial fibrillation who did not have valvular heart disease have now documented a dramatic benefit of warfarin treatment.[342-351] All trials showed a consistent and considerable risk reduction for stroke in patients treated with warfarin. Warfarin is approximately 50% more effective than aspirin in reducing the rate of stroke in patients with atrial fibrillation who do not have valvular disease.[350] The rate of intracranial hemorrhages and major bleeding episodes was low in all groups in all trials except in warfarin-treated patients older than 75 years in the Stroke Prevention in Atrial Fibrillation (SPAF II) study.[347,348] In that study, 7 of 197 warfarin-treated older patients had intracranial hemorrhages that were most often fatal. Caution must be used in prescribing warfarin to patients older than 75 years. Other characteristics found on echocardiography should help select those in most need of anticoagulation. Favoring anticoagulation are: atrial and ventricular thrombi, spontaneous echo contrast, atrial enlargement, valvular disease, ventricular regions of aneurismal dilatation akinesis or hypokinesis, and low cardiac ejection fraction.

The various cardiac sources that are potential indications for anticoagulation are listed in Table 5-11. In many the relative value of anticoagulants versus other treatments such as platelet inhibitors has not been well studied. Although clinicians often eclectically choose which atrial fibrillation patients who have not had a stroke to anticoagulate, nearly all agree that anticoagulants are indicated in atrial fibrillation patients who have had a cardiac-origin embolic brain infarct.

Controversy still exists about how soon to anticoagulate. Early anticoagulation of patients with atrial fibrillation-related strokes can be safe and effective.[352,353] In a nonrandomized, noncontrolled observational study, Chamorro et al treated all patients with atrial fibrillation who had presumed cardioembolic strokes with either intravenous or subcutaneously administered unfractionated heparin as soon as a CT scan had excluded brain hemorrhage.[354] In 74 patients heparin was given within 6 hours, while heparin was begun between 6 and 48 hours after symptom onset in 157 other patients. Comparing the early-treated and late-treated groups, those treated within

Table 5-11.	Cardiac Sources of Emboli and Anticoagulation

Anticoagulants indicated

Atrial fibrillation
Thrombus found in heart on echocardiography
Ventricular aneurysm
Hypokinetic ventricle
Acute myocardial infarction
Very low ejection fraction
Mitral stenosis with large left atrium
Spontaneous echo contrast and large left atrium
Prosthetic mechanical valves

Antibiotics indicated

Bacterial endocarditis

Antiplatelets indicated

Libman Sacks endocarditis
Fibrotic valve disease in antiphospholipid antibody syndrome
Nonthrombotic (marantic) endocarditis
Fibrous strands

Anticoagulants sometimes used

Mitral valve prolapse (with thrombi)
Mitral annulus calcification (with thrombi)
Patent foramen ovale especially with atrial septal aneurysm
Calcific aortic stenosis

6 hours had more functional recovery at hospital discharge. Treatment with intravenous heparin more often led to therapeutic and excessive levels of anticoagulation than subcutaneously administered heparin. The rate of serious brain hemorrhage was low. Patients with recurrent strokes had lower mean APTT ratios than those without recurrence, and patients with hemorrhage had higher mean APTT ratios than those without hemorrhage, especially when APTT ratios were compared on the day of hemorrhage.[354] Clinicians could conclude from this study that, in patients with atrial fibrillation who have cardioembolic strokes, (1) early heparin treatment is relatively safe, (2) patients treated early seem to do better than those treated later, and (3) therapeutic and excessive APTT ratios are more often achieved with intravenous compared to subcutaneously administered heparin.

How should a clinician decide on when to treat an individual patient with cardiogenic brain embolism? The Cerebral Embolism Task Force published two reviews that analyzed published reports to determine the frequency and timing of stroke recurrence in patients with brain embolism due to a variety of different cardiac lesions and also analyzed the frequency of hemorrhagic complications of heparin treatment.[355,356] They concluded that stroke recurrence during the first 2 weeks after cardiac-origin brain embolism was uncommon especially in patients with nonrheumatic atrial fibrillation, and hemorrhagic complications were relatively common and related to size of infarction, intensity of anticoagulation, and the presence of hemorrhagic changes on CT scans.[355] Considering these findings they recommended delaying CT scanning and anticoagulation. They recommended treatment for individual patients by applying aggregate data from large groups of patients to all individuals.

The Cerebral Embolism Study Group conducted a randomized trial of immediate versus delayed anticoagulation in patients with cardiogenic brain embolism and reviewed 30 cases of hemorrhagic infarction or parenchymatous hematomas developing in patients with cardiogenic emblism.[357] These studies led them to conclude that brain hemorrhage in embolic strokes was most common in large infarcts and that early CT might not accurately estimate infarct size.[357] In contrast, Furlan et al studied 54 consecutive patients with acute, nonseptic embolic brain infarcts, and showed that hemorrhagic complications were rare even in patients with large infarcts and that recurrent strokes were related to inadequate intensity of anticoagulation. They recommended early anticoagulation for all patients with nonseptic cardioembolic brain infarcts.[358] Pessin

et al showed that patients with hemorrhagic infarction on CT scan seemed to have no adverse effects when heparin was continued despite the CT findings.[359] Internists have always anticoagulated patients with pulmonary embolism despite the presence of hemoptysis and hemorrhagic pulmonary infarcts. Chamorro and colleagues performed a retrospective analysis of the safety of heparin anticoagulation among 83 patients with presumed embolic brain infarcts treated within 72 hours and found that severity of stroke and infarct size did not predict hemorrhagic changes or clinical worsening.[360]

I urge weighing the benefits versus the risks of any given treatment in the individual patient. Regarding the timing of anticoagulation in patients with cardiac-origin embolism, the risk of early recurrence if not anticoagulated should be weighed against the risk of early anticoagulation. The probability of early recurrence in atrial fibrillation patients depends on the number of prior embolic events, the presence of valve abnormalities, atrial size, the presence of atrial or auricular appendage thrombi, the presence of ventricular lesions, ventricular function, ejection fraction, and blood and coagulation factors. The risk of hemorrhage with heparin relates to the patient's blood pressure, coagulation factors, use of a bolus starting dose, and the route and intensity of anticoagulation. The data are conflicting about the relevance of the size of infarction and the severity of the neurologic deficit, and the presence of hemorrhagic infarction on CT scans. Echocardiography can help decide on the risk of early recurrence.

Anticoagulants are not routinely used as prophylaxis in patients with mitral valve prolapse (MVP), mitral annulus calcification (MAC), calcific aortic stenosis, and those with fibrotic valve lesions (Libman-Sacks endocarditis in patients with lupus erythematosis, the antiphospholipid antibody syndrome and nonthrombotic (marantic) endocarditis), cardiac myxomas, and bacterial endocarditis. Anticoagulants are continued in patients with bacterial endocarditis if there was a preexisting indication such as atrial fibrillation, and prosthetic heart valves. Some patients with MVP and MAC have thrombi attached to their mitral valves and so anticoagulants are then used.

The data regarding optimal prophylaxis in patients with atrial septal defects or patent foramen ovale (PFO) are to date not conclusive and also should be eclectic and depend on individual circumstances. The data from echocardiographic studies show that there is a strong association between atrial septal aneurysms and interatrial shunts, and that the presence of either atrial septal aneurysms and/or PFOs is strongly associated with the presence of cryptogenic stroke especially among young stroke patients.[361-364] The mechanism by which atrial septal aneurysms contribute to brain embolism has not been satisfactorily clarified but these lesions can harbor thrombi. Thrombus was seen within an atrial septal aneurysm in one patient,[365] and has been found within the base of atrial septal aneurysms at necropsy.[366]

The recurrence rate of stroke in patients with PFOs and the effect of various treatments on recurrence has occasionally been studied.[364,367-370] Bogousslavsky et al studied stroke recurrence among 140 consecutive patients who had PFOs and brain ischemic events, one fourth of whom also had atrial septal aneurysms.[367] During a mean follow-up period of 3 years, the stroke or death rate was 2.4% per year; 8 patients had a recurrent brain infarct. Ninety-two (66%) took aspirin at a dose of 250 mg per day, while 37 (26%) were given anticoagulants and 11 (8%) had surgical closure of the PFO within 12 weeks of the stroke after anticoagulant treatment. There was no significant difference in the effect of any of the treatments on recurrence. The relatively low rate of recurrence contrasted with the severity of the initial stroke which left disabling effects in half the patients.[367] In a French multicenter study, 132 patients with PFOs and/or atrial septal aneurysms and cryptogenic stroke were followed for an average of 22.6 months.[368] The recurrence rate was approximately 2% to 3% at 2 years and was higher in patients with both PFOs and atrial septal aneurysms. Recurrences occurred in four patients who were taking antiplatelet agents and in one treated with anticoagulants.[368] Bridges and colleagues reported the results of transcatheter closure of PFOs among 36 patients with PFOs of whom half had multiple ischemic events.[369] In 28 (78%) the closure was complete and another 5 had nearly complete closure. No patient had a recurrent stroke during 8.4 months of follow-up, but 4 had transient ischemic events.[369]

The Patent Foramen Ovale in Cryptogenic Stroke Study (PICSS)[370] was a substudy of the Warfarin Aspirin Recurrent Stroke Study (WARSS).[371] All patients in WARSS who had TEEs were eligible; In PICSS 312 stroke patients were treated with warfarin and 318 received aspirin. Large PFOs were much more common in patients with cryptogenic strokes. Among the cryptogenic stroke patients, warfarin treatment was slightly but not significantly better than aspirin in regard to annual rate of stroke or death (4.75% vs 8.95%; relative risk, 0.53; confidence interval, 0.18 to 1.58) because the numbers were small and the confidence intervals were wide.[370]

The available data regarding optimal treatment of PFO-related strokes are inconclusive. The presence of both a PFO and an atrial septal aneurysm substantially increases the risk of stroke occurrence. Large defect, spontaneous right to left shunting, and large number of bubbles shunted may indicate a higher risk of paradoxical embolism. Warfarin and surgical or transcatheter closure are posited to be more effective than drugs that effect platelet functions but studies have not definitively shown their superiority.

Dural Sinus and Cerebral Venous Thrombosis

Occlusions of the venous structures that drain the brain are due to red erythrocyte-fibrin thrombi. Since standard anticoagulants are effective in preventing peripheral phlebothrombosis and pulmonary embolism, it is logical to posit that anticoagulation would be effective in patients with venous occlusions involving nervous system structures. Case reports and reviews showed that patients do not worsen or develop new hemorrhages after heparin anticoagulation.[372-379] In one study, among 82 heparin-treated patients, there were no deaths and 77% of patients recovered completely.[373] In another study, among 79 patients given anticoagulants, 94% improved and survived while only half of 157 patients not given anticoagulants survived.[374] Meta-analysis of two trials showed an absolute risk reduction in mortality of 14% and a relative risk reduction of 70% in heparin-treated patients.[375,376] Among 102 patients with cerebral venous thromboses, (43 of whom had intracerebral hemorrhages), those not treated with heparin fared worse and had higher mortality.[376] In a double-blind, placebo-controlled multicenter trial, cerebral venous thrombosis (CVT) patients treated with low-molecular-weight heparin had better outcomes than those given placebo.[377] No new symptomatic brain hemorrhages occurred. Prevention of pulmonary embolism is another reason to administer anticoagulants to patients with dural sinus thrombosis.[379] Most clinicians now agree that heparin and anticoagulants are indicated in patients with CVT. The duration of anticoagulation has not been well studied.

Large-Artery Thrombosis and Arterial Dissections

The use of anticoagulants in the treatment of stroke patients with noncardioembolic strokes continues to be controversial.[380,381] Many neurologists use heparin during the acute phase of stroke and continue with warfarin, while others do not use heparin and believe strongly that it should not be used at all and seldom use warfarin.

Heparin should not be indiscriminately used in all brain ischemia patients. Bleeding complications will outweigh therapeutic benefit. Heparins should theoretically be useful in patients with fresh red erythrocyte-fibrin thrombi within large arteries to prevent the development of fresh clots and intra-arterial embolism. Warfarin is posited to be effective in preventing red clot development in patients with severe large-artery stenosis. Warfarin might be useful in preventing fresh clot from forming during the first 3 to 6 weeks after an arterial occlusion.

Unfortunately randomized trials have not adequately studied anticoagulants in patients with conditions likely to respond to treatment. Reported trials lumped patients with brain ischemia together without diagnostic investigations that defined stroke etiology, stroke subtypes, or vascular lesions.

Worsening and development of new neurologic deficits can occur when thrombi form, propagate, and embolize. Stroke worsening, even when thrombi are present, occurs in only about 20% to 33% of ischemic strokes.[382] Worsening in patients with atherothrombotic large-artery occlusive disease is due to perfusion failure and propagation and embolization of occlusive thrombi. Randomized trials in patients with noncardioembolic brain ischemia to effectively determine anticoagulant utility must be (1) eclectic and include only patients in whom brain and cardiac and vascular imaging show high-risk, artery-to-artery embolic brain infarcts in patients with documented severe extracranial or intracranial large-artery occlusive disease; (2) powered to account for clinical worsening and/or new brain infarcts in less than one third of patients; and (3) anticoagulant activity must be closely and effectively monitored to ensure infrequent bleeding. No available trials even remotely meet these criteria. In the International Stroke Trial (IST), the largest heparin trial, vascular and cardiac imaging were not reported, some patients had no brain imaging before treatment, heparin was given subcutaneously while elsewhere heparins are usually given intravenously, and levels of anticoagulation were not always closely monitored.[383] Heparin effectively prevented pulmonary embolism.[383]

The results of two trials suggest that anticoagulation might be effective in patients with acute ischemic stroke caused by large-artery thromboembolism.[384-386] In a trial performed in Hong Kong among 312 patients with acute ischemic stroke, low-molecular-weight heparin was more effective than placebo.[384] This study found a significant dose-dependent reduction in the risk of death or dependency among patients treated with low-molecular-weight heparin. Although vascular studies were not mandated, most patients with ischemic stroke in Hong Kong have intracranial artery occlusive disease. Patients with cardiac lesions that required anticoagulation were not included in this study. However another study of low-molecular-weight heparin in Asian patients with large-artery occlusive disease (mostly intracranial) did not show a benefit of nadroparin over aspirin.[387]

In the Trial of ORG 10172 in Acute Stroke Treatment (TOAST), the low-molecular-weight heparinoid ORG 10172 was given within 24 hours of the onset of symptoms of an acute ischemic stroke.[385] This heparinoid was then given by continuous intravenous infusion for 7 days with the dose adjusted after 24 hours to maintain the anti-Xa factor activity at 0.6 to 0.8 antifactor Xa units per milliliter. ORG 10172 (Danaparoid) is a mixture of glycosaminoglycans with a mean molecular weight of 5500 isolated from porcine intestinal mucosa. The antifactor Xa activity of Danaparoid is attributed to its heparin sulfate component which has a high affinity for antithrombin III. Although Danaparoid treatment was not effective in terms of the entire group of patients with ischemic stroke, there was effectiveness in the group of patients that were diagnosed as having large-artery atherosclerosis.[386] In this group, heparinoid reduced the number of recurrences of stroke during the 7 days of infusion, and the rates of favorable and very favorable outcomes were significantly higher in patients given heparinoid when compared with placebo. Sixty-eight percent of patients with large-artery atherosclerosis treated with Danaparoid had favorable outcome versus 54.7% treated with placebo ($P = .04$); 43% of patients with large-artery atherosclerosis treated with Danaparoid had very favorable outcomes versus 29.1% treated with placebo ($P = .02$). Recurrent strokes developed in 6% of Danaparoid-treated patients with large-artery atherosclerosis versus 11% of those treated with placebo. Because of the small numbers the figures for recurrent strokes did not meet statistical significance.[386]

In the WARRS trial, coumadin and aspirin were equally effective in preventing new strokes.[371] The drugs were given within a month of stroke onset, not always acutely, and secondary prevention of new strokes was studied. The number of patients with documented large-artery disease was small and vascular studies were not required or reported. Some patients received heparin acutely and then aspirin. Some patients did not receive heparin but were given coumadin within a month. The data do not relate well to the use of heparin/warfarin during the acute stroke.

In the Warfarin-Aspirin for Symptomatic Intracranial Disease (WASID) trial of patients with severe intracranial atherosclerosis, there was no significant difference in the prevention of new strokes between aspirin and warfarin.[388] Again the study drugs were initiated often weeks after the last ischemic event. Warfarin was difficult to control. In those patients who were maintained within the target therapeutic INR range, warfarin performed better than 1300 mg of aspirin per day. In those who were below the target range more infarcts developed, and more hemorrhages developed in those above the target INR range.[388,389]

I administer heparin to patients with acute arterial dissections. Unfortunately, there are no data from trials about the effectiveness of heparin or any other treatment in patients with arterial dissections. Therapeutics in patients with dissection has not been studied in trials, although most stroke clinicians use anticoagulants when the diagnosis of extracranial arterial dissection is made. Although transient ocular and brain ischemia may develop when a dissection causes a complete or near complete arterial occlusion, the great majority of strokes are caused by embolization of thrombi formed in the region of the dissection. Thrombus is often present within the lumen, either as a result of communication of the intramural hematoma with the lumen or because of stasis of blood flow caused by luminal compromise. Perturbation of the endothelium leads to the release of tissue factors that promote thrombosis. The luminal clot is usually loosely adherent to the intima and can readily embolize distally. In the weeks and months after dissection, the intramural blood is absorbed and the narrowed lumen usually returns to its normal size; if the artery becomes completely occluded, it remains occluded in about 75% of patients. Anecdotally many neurologists use heparin and follow with warfarin in this situation and believe it effective, although initially there was much concern that it could enlarge the intramural clot. The duration of anticoagulation in patients with arterial dissections has not been studied.

Clearly, more trials are needed in patients with documented cardiac and cardiovascular lesions. Until the results of such trials are available, I use and recommend the use of anticoagulants in patients who have or are at risk of developing red clots. In some, after preliminary use of heparin, warfarin is given for a period of 3 to 6 weeks until clots become organized and adhere to the vascular wall. In other patients, mostly those with cardiac thrombi, arrhythmias, cardiac lesions promoting thrombus formation, or severe stenosis of large arteries, warfarin is given indefinitely until the risk of thrombosis diminishes or anticoagulants become contraindicated. My present practice is to monitor vascular occlusive lesions by ultrasound or vascular imaging (CTA or MRA). I stop warfarin

approximately 1 month after stenotic lesions are shown to have become occluded or after dissected or atherostenotic occluded arteries recanalize. Warfarin is also used for some patients with congenital or acquired hypercoagulable states.

Warfarin has proven to be a difficult drug to use. Studies in nonacademic community settings[390] (Fig. 5-4) and even in anticoagulation clinics (Fig. 5-5)[391] has shown that many patients remain under or over anticoagulated even in the

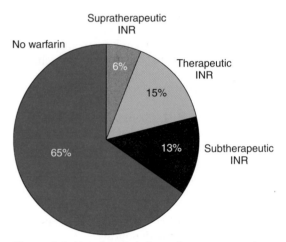

Figure 5-4. Use of warfarin in a primary care population. All patients analyzed were judged to be appropriate candidates for warfarin according to guidelines. There were no contraindications to warfarin treatment. (Data from Samsa GP, Matchar DB, Goldstein LB, et al: Quality of anticoagulation management among patients with atrial fibrillation. Results of a review of medical records from 2 communities. Arch Intern Med 2000;160:967-973.)

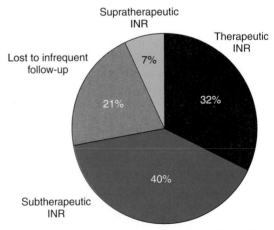

Figure 5-5. Adequacy of warfarin control achieved in an anticoagulation clinic. Distribution of INR values based on a target range of 2 to 3. (Data from Chiquette E, Amato MG, Bussey HL: Comparison of an anticoagulation clinic with usual medical care: Anticoagulation control, patient outcomes, and health care costs. Arch Intern Med 1998;158:1641-1647.)

best of situations. Warfarin anticoagulation is difficult to control because of individual variance in dose and the effect of a variety of foods and pharmaceutical agents on vitamin k, prothrombin and liver functions. Especially worrisome is the observation that important INR changes may develop just before major hemorrhages. One study showed that when INRs were plotted in relation to the time before the onset of bleeding, a marked increase in the patients' INRs was observed only shortly before the bleeding began.[392]

The adequacy of anticoagulation is important. In the WASID study of the prevention of recurrent stroke in patients with intracranial occlusive vascular disease, although there were no differences in stroke recurrence in patients treated with warfarin versus aspirin, those in the target anticoagulation range had less strokes and less bleeding than those patients treated with aspirin and those outside of the INR range chosen.[388,389] Although warfarin anticoagulation has been definitively shown to be effective in a number of conditions including atrial fibrillation, many primary care physicians and internists are reluctant to prescribe it because of the perceived difficulty in keeping the INR in target range, the seriousness of complications, and medico-legal implications of adverse events.

Newer Anticoagulants: Factor Xa and Thrombin Inhibitors

Red thrombi are composed mostly of red blood cells and fibrin. They are formed by activation of circulating coagulation factors; their formation does not require an abnormal vessel wall or tissue thromboplastin. The final step in the coagulation cascade is the conversion of the soluble protein fibrinogen into insoluble polymers called fibrin. Fibrin strands form a network of fibers that entangle the formed blood elements (platelets, erythrocytes, and leukocytes) into a clot. Fibrin is quite adhesive and is capable of contracting. Activation of factor X to Xa catalyzes the conversion of prothrombin (factor II) to thrombin. Thrombin in turn catalyzes the fibrinogen to fibrin conversion.

Several key components in the coagulation system—prothrombin, factor Xa, and thrombin—are targets for pharmacological anticoagulation. New drugs are now being developed by a number of pharmaceutical companies and tested in trials. It is important for neurologists dealing with stroke patients and stroke prevention to understand the present anticoagulants and newer agents that will likely be soon become available.

The new anticoagulant agents mostly target inhibition of factor Xa or thrombin. Direct inhibitors of thrombin offer many potential advantages.[393] Argabatran is an intravenous agent used often in Asia instead of heparin.[394] It has also been used in the United States and Europe mostly in patients with heparin-induced thrombocytopenia.[395] One trial showed that it could be effective in patients with acute ischemic stroke.[396] Its safety record and control are comparable or better than heparins. Ximelagatran is an oral direct thrombin inhibitor that was studied in trials and approved in Europe, but was not approved in the United States. In studies of patients with deep-vein thrombosis[397] and atrial fibrillation,[398-400] ximelagatran was as effective or more effective than warfarin and caused less bleeding. Ximelagatran acts quickly so that heparins are not needed. The dose is constant and does not require monitoring by either APTT or INR determinations. There is no important effect of foods or other drugs. Ximelagatran is given twice per day. The Food and Drug Administration (FDA) in the United States failed to authorize release of ximelagatran in the United States because of liver enzyme abnormalities. Unfortunately, there is no antidote to reverse the activity of ximelagatran or other direct thrombin inhibitors if bleeding develops. Other orally administered direct thrombin inhibitors such as dabigitran are now undergoing trials.

Factor Xa inhibition is also a viable form of anticoagulation.[401] Several indirect inhibitors of factor Xa have been made and have undergone trials. Fondaparinux is a pentasaccharide given subcutaneously that causes less bleeding than heparins and does not cause thrombocytopenia. It has been very effective in trials to prevent phlebothrombosis and pulmonary emboli in patients who have had recent surgery[402] and in medical hospitalized patients.[403] Fondaparinux has been more effective than low-molecular-weight heparin in patients with acute coronary syndromes.[404-406] Fondaparinux is excreted through the kidneys and accumulates in patients with renal impairment. There is no antidote. Fondaparinux seems not to inhibit catheter thrombosis in patients who undergo interventional radiology procedures. Other indirect and direct inhibitors of factor Xa are being synthesized and prepared for trials in humans.

Factor Xa has been referred to as the "gatekeeper" of the coagulation cascade.[406] It mediates the entry of the extrinsic (tissue factor) and intrinsic coagulation pathways to the conversion of prothrombin to thrombin. On the other hand direct thrombin inhibitors directly inhibit thrombin generation. In the future it is likely that either

5

direct thrombin inhibitors and/or factor Xa inhibitors will likely replace heparins and warfarin for rapid, safe, and effective anticoagulation. Neurologists need to be alert to this research.[407]

Drugs That Modify Platelet Functions

Aspirin

The first clinical observations on aspirin as an anticoagulant was probably made by a practitioner named Craven.[407] Craven, observing that dental patients bled more if they had used aspirin, urged friends and his patients to take one or two aspirin tablets per day. He later published the effectiveness of this strategy in preventing coronary and cerebral thrombosis among 8000 men in articles in the *Mississippi Valley Medical Journal*, not a periodical on many neurologists' bookshelf.[408,409] Twenty years later, case reports from the United States and Britain on the effectiveness of aspirin in preventing attacks of transient monocular blindness brought more attention to the subject.[410,411] The American[412] and Canadian[413] aspirin trials soon ensued in the late 1970s.

Aspirin and other nonsteroidal anti-inflammatory drugs, such as indomethacin, phenylbutazone, and ibuprofen, inhibit platelet release reactions secondary to adenosine diphosphate-induced platelet aggregation and platelet adhesion to collagen when tested in vitro.[414] Aspirin inhibits platelet aggregation and secretion by preventing the synthesis of prostaglandins and thromboxane A2. This action is achieved by inhibiting the cyclo-oxygenase enzyme that converts arachidonic acid to prostaglandin G2, the precursor of thromboxane A2.[415] Aspirin, however, also inhibits the production of prostacyclin by endothelial cells. Prostacyclin has a potent platelet antiaggregant and vasodilator effect.[416]

The optimal therapeutic dosage of aspirin is still controversial. The American,[412] Canadian,[413] and WASID[388] trials used four 5-grain aspirin tablets (about 1300 mg) each day. Some investigators posit that smaller doses produce the desired inhibition of platelet functions and do not inhibit production of prostacyclin by endothelial cells.[417,418] In vitro studies of the effects of small- and larger-dose aspirin on prostaglandin and prostacyclin formation have used normal, young animal vessels; however, in patients with extracranial vascular disease, the endothelium is frequently damaged and might no longer be able to synthesize prostacyclin. In the British UK-TIA trial, one 300-mg dose of aspirin per day was as effective as higher doses.[419] In the Swedish Aspirin Low-Dose trial, 75 mg of aspirin per day

resulted in a statistically significant 18% reduction in stroke and death,[420] while in the Dutch TIA trial, even 30 mg was as effective and better tolerated than 300 mg of aspirin per day.[421]

Patients who are given aspirin do not all have the same effect on platelet functions as measured in vitro.[422-427] Helgason and colleagues studied the effectiveness of aspirin on platelet function measured in vitro.[424] Among 107 patients who received 325 mg of aspirin per day, inhibition of platelet aggregation was complete in 85 (79%) and partial in 22 (20.5%). Among nine patients who did not respond to 325 mg of aspirin, escalating the dose to 650 mg per day resulted in complete platelet inhibition in 5 (56%). An increase to 975 mg caused complete inhibition in 1 of the 4 patients who did not respond to 650 mg. The 3 patients who did not respond to 975 mg had only partial inhibition at a 1300-mg dose of aspirin.[424] Others have also shown a variability of response on platelet aggregation tested in vitro according to the dose of aspirin.[425] Genetic factors clearly play a role in aspirin effects and those of virtually all other drugs. Some patients require more aspirin than others. Platelets interact with the endothelium and arterial wall, so platelet function is only one of the factors that relates to the deposition of platelet-fibrin and erythrocyte-fibrin thrombi. The presence and importance of "aspirin resistance" continues to be debated.[425] Most neurologists now use aspirin doses that vary from 50 to 325 mg of aspirin per day. Gastrointestinal bleeding and gastritis are important and common side effects of aspirin. The frequency of these side effects is dose related.

Dipyridamole

Dipyridamole is a pyramidopyrimidine compound that, acting as a phosphodiesterase inhibitor, modestly reduces platelet function.[428,429] Dipyridamole also has important endothelial activity and acts as a vasodilator.[428] Dipyridamole inhibits the attachment of platelets to the endothelium. In rabbits, a combination of aspirin and dipyridamole protected against thrombosis induced by combined chemical and electrical stimuli when neither drug did so separately.[430] In a study reported in 1971, Sullivan and colleagues showed a beneficial effect of adding dipyridamole in a dose of 400 mg per day to warfarin anticoagulation to effectively prevent brain embolic strokes in patients who had prosthetic heart valves.[431] Two trials reported during the early 1980s showed no benefit of dipyridamole even when added to aspirin.[432,433] In the Canadian-American trial, dipyridamole in doses of 300 mg per day had no significant therapeutic effect when added to 1300 mg per day aspirin in patients with TIA or minor stroke.[432] In a French trial, 225 mg of dipyridamole used with 1000 mg of aspirin was not better than aspirin alone.[433]

Dipyridamole in the form given in these two trials had variable gastrointestinal absorption related to gastric acidity, and required four times per day dosing because of its pharmacokinetics. The dose of dipyridamole was relatively low and likely did not produce adequate sustained blood levels. An extended release form of dipyridamole has longer activity and much improved absorption. Two trials—European Stroke Prevention Studies (ESPS I and ESPS II) reported a beneficial effect on stroke prevention of extended release dipyridamole when used with aspirin.[434-437] In ESPS I, dipyridamole 75 mg three times per day plus aspirin 330 mg three times per day given for 2 years showed a 38% reduction in stroke compared to placebo in patients with ischemic strokes or TIAs.[434] In the ESPS II trial, 6602 patients took either placebo, aspirin (25 mg twice per day), dipyridamole in a modified-release form at 200 mg twice per day, or aspirin and dipyridamole 25 mg of aspirin plus 200 mg of modified-release dipyridamole twice per day.[435] The relative risk reduction for the combined endpoints of stroke and death were 13.2% for aspirin, 15.4% for dipyridamole, and 24.4% for the combination of aspirin and dipyridamole. The combined therapy reduced the stroke risk 23.1% over aspirin alone and 24.7% over dipyridamole alone.[434-437]

A more recent trial, carried out in the Netherlands, also studied the effectiveness of dipyridamole in stroke prevention of patients who had recent transient ischemic attacks or minor strokes.[438] Several features distinguish this trial (ESPRIT) from the ESPS trials: varied dose of aspirin (30 to 325 mg, median dose 75 mg), 17% of patients assigned to dipyridamole did not receive the extended-release form; and the trial was not initiated or funded by a pharmaceutical company. The primary outcome studied was the composite of death from all vascular causes, nonfatal stroke, nonfatal myocardial infarction, and major bleeding. These outcomes occurred in 13% of patients assigned to aspirin-dipyridamole versus 16% of those in the aspirin group. Ischemic stroke developed in 7% of those assigned to aspirin-dipyridamole versus 8.4% of those assigned to aspirin. Cardiac events were also more common in those on aspirin.[438] A recent meta-analysis concluded that "the combination of aspirin and dipyridamole was more effective than aspirin alone in preventing stroke and other serious vascular events in patients with minor strokes and TIAs."[439]

Thienopyridines: Clopidogrel and Ticlopidine

Ticlopidine hydrochloride was the first thienopyridine derivate studied in trials and introduced into practice. The thienopyridines inhibit the adenosine diphosphate pathway of platelet aggregation; unlike aspirin they do not inhibit the cyclooxygenase pathway.[440,441] In the Ticlopidine-Aspirin Stroke Study (TASS), a large, randomized trial, ticlopidine showed a relative risk reduction of approximately 30% in minimizing the rate of stroke, myocardial infarction, and vascular death in men and women who had a previous minor stroke.[442] In the Canadian-American Ticlopidine Study (CATS), ticlopidine (500 mg daily) was slightly more effective than aspirin (1300 mg daily) in reducing the rate of stroke in patients with TIAs or minor strokes.[443] In the clinical trials, ticlopidine had a relatively high rate of side effects, especially diarrhea and skin rash. Neutropenia, sometimes severe, was a serious but infrequent complication of ticlopidine (approximately 1% of patients).[442,443] Patients taking ticlopidine had a slightly elevated cholesterol level.[442] Bennett et al reported 60 patients with thrombotic thrombocytopenic purpura after using ticlopidine,[444] and thrombocytopenia has been noted by others as a ticlopidine side effect.[441] Ticlopidine was introduced into stroke prophylaxis in the early 1990s but recognition of serious side effects and the introduction of clopidogrel (a thienopyridine with a closely related chemical structure that differs from ticlopidine by the addition of a carboxymethyl side group) an agent that had similar effectiveness but fewer severe side effects led to the gradual disappearance of ticlopidine as a newly prescribed antiplatelet agent.

The Clopidogrel versus Aspirin in Patients at Risk of Ischemic Events (CAPRIE) trial was a randomized, double-blinded trial of clopidogrel (75 mg/day) versus aspirin (325 mg/day) in preventing ischemic events (ischemic stroke, myocardial infarction, and vascular death).[445] During 3 years, 19,185 patients were entered, including 6421 ischemic stroke patients, 6302 patients with myocardial infarcts, and 6452 patients who had atherosclerotic peripheral vascular occlusive disease. Clopidogrel had a relative risk reduction over aspirin of 8.7%, considering all endpoints. The frequency of stroke was 405 out of 17,636 (2.30%) for clopidogrel versus 430 out of 17,519 (2.45%) for aspirin. The frequency of myocardial infarction was more effectively reduced by clopidogrel than the frequency of stroke.[445] Clopidogrel had an excellent safety record in this large trial; the frequency of neutropenia and thrombocytopenia in patients using clopidogrel were no different than for aspirin,[445] but clopidogrel was later reported to be associated with thrombotic thrombocytopenic purpura in another report.[446]

Reasoning that decreasing platelet activities by two different mechanisms might prove superior to single agents alone, the MATCH trial tested aspirin (75 mg/day) plus clopidogrel (75 mg/day) against clopidogrel (75 mg/day) alone in patients with brain ischemia.[447,448] The combination was not superior in decreasing the primary outcome measure (reduction in ischemic stroke, myocardial infarction, vascular death, and rehospitalization for acute ischemic events) and caused more life-threatening bleeding, often intracranial.[447,448]

The Clopidogrel and Aspirin versus Aspirin Alone for the Prevention of Atherothrombotic Events (CHARISMA) trial studied the effectiveness of adding clopidogrel to aspirin for stroke prevention.[449] The trial included 15,063 patients with either clinically evident cardiovascular disease (coronary, cerebrovascular, or peripheral vascular) or multiple risk factors. Overall clopidogrel plus aspirin was not more effective than aspirin alone in reducing the rate of myocardial infarction, stroke, or death from cardiovascular causes. Moderate and severe bleeding were more common in those taking both clopidogrel and aspirin.[449]

The combination of clopidogrel and aspirin causes more bleeding than either agent alone, and is probably not more effective in preventing stroke. Clopidogrel and aspirin are effective in preventing thrombi in patients who have had interventional procedures involving angioplasty and stenting, and in patients with acute coronary syndromes and myocardial infarction.[449-453]

Among 20,332 stroke patients treated in the Prevention Regimen for Effectively Avoiding Second Strokes (PRoFESS) trial, there were similar rates of recurrent stroke in patients treated with aspirin plus extended-release dipyridamole (916 patients [9.0%]) and clopidogrel (898 patients [8.8%]).[454] There were more major hemorrhagic events attributable to aspirin plus extended-release dipyridamole. In PRoFESS, treatment with telmisartan, an angiotensin-receptor blocker, initiated soon after ischemic strokes and continued for 2.5 years did not significantly reduce the rate of recurrent stroke, major cardiovascular events, or diabetes.[454a] Another thienopyridine, prasugrel is now under investigation for treatment of patients with coronary and cerebrovascular disease.[455]

Cilostazol

Cilostazol is a phosphodiesterase inhibitor that, like dipyridamole, has both antiplatelet and vasodilator effects.[456,457] In a trial in Japan that included more than 1000 patients with brain infarcts acquired 1 to 6 months before entry,

cilostazol 100 mg twice daily showed a 42.3% relative risk reduction (CI, 10.3% to 62.9%, $P = .013$) in reducing the frequency of recurrent brain infarction in an intention-to-treat analysis.[458] In a study of Korean patients with intracranial arterial stenosis, 200 mg of cilostazol plus 100 mg of aspirin was more effective than 100 mg of aspirin alone in reducing the frequency of progression and increasing the frequency of regression of stenotic lesions ($P = .008$).[459] Cilostazol has been shown to increase cerebral blood flow in patients with atherosclerotic risk factors.[460] Cilostazol is often used in patients with peripheral vascular occlusive disease. To date its effect on stroke prevention has been mainly studied in Asians, and the patients studied have had a high frequency of penetrating artery disease (lacunar strokes) and intracranial large-artery disease. Its effect in Caucasian patients in the United States and Europe has not been studied in any depth.

GP IIb/IIIa antagonists

The advent of drugs that are antagonists of the glycoprotein platelet IIb/IIIa complex gives promise of even more effective inhibition of platelet functions. The platelet glycoprotein IIb/IIIa complex is the site of binding to adhesive proteins including fibrinogen. Binding to fibrinogen activates platelet aggregation and adhesion to blood vessels. Abciximab is a humanized monoclonal antibody that binds to the GP IIb/IIIa complex on platelets.[461,462] Abciximab has been used mostly intravenously and acutely in patients after invasive coronary and cerebral revascularization procedures.[461,463,464] This agent causes a profound impairment of the function of platelets similar to a temporary thrombasthenia so that the rate of bleeding is potentially high.[461] The use of abciximab during the first 24 hours after stroke proved safe in a preliminary study.[465] The Abciximab in Emergent Stroke Treatment Trial II (AbESTT-II), a double-blind, randomized phase III trial designed to compare abciximab with placebo for the treatment of acute ischemic stroke patients, did not show efficacy and was terminated prematurely for safety reasons—excessive bleeding.[230]

Some patients develop a veritable carpet of white platelet-fibrin thrombi after vascular surgery and interventional vascular treatments. In that setting abciximab may prove very useful. Abciximab has also been used during interventional procedures to accomplish reperfusion in acute stroke patients as an adjunct to thrombolytic agents.[466-468] Cardiologists often use abciximab or other GP IIb/IIIa antagonists along with thrombolytics, other antiplatelets, and anticoagulants as a potent intravenous "cocktail" in patients with acute coronary-related cardiac ischemia.[469,470]

Other parenteral small molecule, nonantibody GP IIb/IIIa antagonists, tirofiban and eptifbatide have shorter duration of antiplatelet activity and have been shown to improve outcomes after coronary procedures and have less bleeding complications than abciximab.[461,471] GP IIb/IIIa inhibiting agents that can be used orally and chronically are now being tested but to-date have been associated with excess bleeding and have not been introduced into clinical practice. Lotrifiban, an orally administered GP IIb/IIIa inhibitor, was studied in a trial (BRAVO) that included 9190 patients admitted with coronary or cerebrovascular disease.[472] Lotrifiban was given 30 or 50 mg twice per day or placebo was given with aspirin. Lotrifiban administration was associated with a significantly higher death rate due to vascular disease and more serious bleeding. Lotrifiban use was not associated with a significant decrease in the composite endpoint of all-cause mortality, myocardial infarction, recurrent ischemia requiring hospitalization or urgent revascularization.[472]

Natural Food Substances

There is considerable interest in the potential effects of natural substances such as eicosopentanoic acid (EPA)—a substance found in high concentration in fish and in omega-3-oils—as agents that affect platelet functions and are contained in natural foods.[473] EPA reduces fibrinogen levels and decreases whole blood viscosity,[295,296] as well as inhibiting platelet functions and decreasing thrombin generation.[297] Black tree fungus, a common component of Chinese foods, is also purported to have platelet-inhibiting functions. A Japanese traditional herbal medicine called Orengedokuto given in a clinically relevant dose has been shown to decrease platelet activation and aggregation.[474] These and other natural food substances that have antiplatelet properties may become popular among patients that seek natural alternative remedies rather than prescription drugs.

The Antiplatelet Trialists Collaboration,[475,476] the Antithrombotic Trialists' Collaboration,[477] and Cochrane[478] and other reviews[479,480] analyzed the relative effects of antiplatelet drugs on stroke prevention and other vascular events in detail. None of the published studies mandated rigorous evaluation of the heart, aorta, and craniocerebral arteries or technology-assisted diagnosis of stroke mechanisms. None of the studies showed which drugs were effective for which vascular lesions. More studies are needed comparing antiplatelet drugs with other strategies in patients with well-defined vascular lesions.

Some investigators and clinicians have used a combination of warfarin anticoagulants and platelet antiaggregants, usually aspirin, in patients with severe atherosclerosis who did not respond to more conventional treatments.[481] This combination was effective but resulted in a higher bleeding-complication rate.[481,482] I have also used this strategy in patients in whom warfarin was indicated but was ineffective when used alone.

A useful strategy may be to use platelet antiaggregants when there is no obstruction to flow and ischemia is most likely due to the process of platelet plugs and small white (or white and red) clots. Heparin (or low-molecular-weight heparin or heparinoids) and warfarin are reserved for situations of tight stenosis or clots within the heart. These standard anticoagulants are also used for 3 to 4 weeks in patients with a recent in situ occlusion within a large artery. Results of the use of these strategies to date are anecdotal and have not been tested scientifically. Table 5-12 reviews my present recommendations for the use of platelet antiaggregants and anticoagulants.

Increasing the Brain's Resistance to Ischemia ("Neuroprotection")

Theoretically, there might be substances or strategies that make the brain relatively resistant, at least for some time, to the deleterious effect of lack of oxygen and energy delivery, that is, keeping brain cells alive despite poor perfusion. I have discussed some of these so-called neuroprotection strategies that have been used in combination with thrombolysis earlier in this chapter. Trials of putative neuroprotectants, when used alone without adjunctive measures to enhance reperfusion, have all resulted in failure as of this writing. Many failed because agents that were effective in experimental animal models of acute ischemia simply had no or little benefit in humans with brain ischemia. Many failures are likely due to suboptimal trial design and testing.

Neuronal death depends on multiple factors,[483] including (1) level of activity (the more work that goes on, the more fuel is needed), (2) presence of local metabolites such as lactic acid[484,485] and oxygen-free radicals,[486-489] (3) temperature of the system (at low temperatures there is less metabolism and less need for fuel),[489-491] (4) integrity of the neuronal cell membranes, and (5) influx of calcium into cells and the extracellular-to-intracellular gradient for calcium.[492-494]

Experimental evidence from global ischemia experiments in young animals indicates that hyperglycemia makes the brain more vulnerable to ischemia.[485] Sugar increases metabolism and leads

Table 5-12.	**Present Recommended Use of Platelet Aggregants and Anticoagulants**

Heparin (standard intravenous dose, short term: 2 to 4 weeks)—Usually given by constant IV infusion keeping aPTT between 60 and 100 seconds (1.5 to 2, control aPTT)
1. Immediate therapy of definite cardiac-origin brain embolism. (*Note:* Large cerebral infarct, hypertension, bacterial endocarditis, or sepsis would delay or contraindicate this use.)
2. For patients with severe stenosis or occlusion of the ICA origin, ICA siphon, MCA, VA, or basilar artery, with less than a severe clinical deficit, treatment then could be shifted to warfarin or surgery.
3. Heparin (subcutaneous minidose) for prophylaxis of deep-vein occlusion in patients immobilized by stroke (unless contraindicated).

Warfarin—Usually overlapped with heparin, keeping INR between 2.0 and 3.0
1. Long term (>3 months) in patients with cardiogenic brain embolization and rheumatic heart disease, atrial fibrillation with large atria or prior cerebral embolism, prosthetic valves, and some hypercoagulable states.
2. Long term (>3 months) in patients with severe stenosis of the ICA origin, ICA siphon, MCA stem, VA, basilar artery. Used until studies show artery has been occluded for at least 3 weeks.
3. Shorter term (3 to 6 weeks) in patients with recent occlusion of the ICA, MCA, VA, or basilar arteries.

Platelet antiaggregants (aspirin, clopidogrel, combined aspirin-dipyridamole, cilostazol)
1. For patients with plaque disease of the extracranial and intracranial arteries without severe stenosis.
2. For patients with polycythemia or thrombocytosis and related ischemic attacks.

APTT, activated partial thromboplastin time; ICA, internal carotid artery; INR, International Normalized Ratio; MCA, middle cerebral artery; VA, vertebral artery.

to the production of lactic acid. Acidosis can be destructive to brain tissue.[495] Hyperglycemia is known to be associated with poor outcomes in patients with brain ischemia and brain hemorrhage.[496-499] A high concentration of extracellular calcium can also contribute to final neuronal death. Lowering of blood sugars and reducing calcium influx into cells has been one posited means of protecting neurons from cell death.

Neurotransmitters, especially glutamate, released at sites of ischemia might overexcite neurons and cause toxic damage, thereby increasing the effects of the initial ischemia.[500-503] This theory, often referred to as the excitotoxin hypothesis, has stimulated much research concerning neurotransmitters and ischemia and attempts to counter the harmful effects of excess neurotransmitter release. The excitotoxin hypothesis was introduced by Olney and colleagues to describe the mechanism by which glutamate and some other acidic amino acids caused neuronal lesions in periventricular structures when given systemically to mice.[500-503] Electrophysiologic studies showed that these compounds functioned as neuronal excitants and damaged the periventricular structures studied. Hypothetically, hypoxia and ischemia caused energy depletion and release of glutamate into the tissues. Glutamate then was taken up by receptors and excited the cells already depleted of blood supply, ultimately leading to neuronal death. Putative neurotoxins include glutamate, kainic acid, N-methyl-D-aspartate

(NMDA), and homocysteic acid. By far, glutamate has been the most studied. These compounds have various receptor types, usually referred to as NMDA and non-NMDA receptors, including quisqualate and kainate receptors.

Experimental evidence supports the role of excitotoxins in potentiating ischemia. When kainic acid is injected into the hippocampus of experimental animals, it causes a pattern of cell death similar to hypoxic-ischemic damage.[503] The concentration of glutamate in the extracellular compartment in ischemic brain is increased. Deafferentation of specific intrahippocampal excitatory pathways seems to protect against ischemic damage. Finally, drugs that block excitatory neurotransmission are sometimes protective when given to animals early after experimentally induced ischemia.

Glutamate opens membrane sodium conductance, allowing a large influx of sodium to enter cells. Chloride ion and water follow the sodium, causing cytotoxic edema. Transmembrane influx of calcium into cells leads to a toxic increase in cytosolic free calcium that can kills cells.[492,493] Experimentally, a number of competitive and noncompetitive NMDA receptor antagonists have been used, including MK 801, dextrorphan, dextromethorphan, ketamine, magnesium, memantine, selfotel, aptiganel, felbamate, and phencyclidine.[504-506] Although the vast bulk of the work on excitatory neurotransmitters has been in laboratory animals, preliminary studies have been carried out in human stroke patients.[504-506] Many of the agents used have had prominent central nervous system or cardiovascular toxicity. Agitation, confusion, sedation, hallucinations, catatonia, and psychotic behavior occur during therapy with many of the NMDA channel antagonists. Unfortunately the agents used have been associated with unacceptable frequencies of side effects especially psychosis.

Some investigators posit that free radicals found during hypoxic injury may lead to further neuronal damage.[486-488] A free radical is an atom, group of atoms, or molecule having one or more unpaired electrons in its outermost orbit. Covalent chemical bonds usually have paired electrons; free radicals are molecules with an open bond, which accounts for their extreme reactivity. The free radicals of importance in brain ischemia are superoxide and hydroxyl radicals. Hydrogen peroxide can generate hydroxyl radicals in reaction with superoxide. Xanthine oxidase is the major enzyme that generates superoxide radicals. Free radicals can react with and damage proteins, nucleic acids, lipids, and other molecules and can initiate destructive chain reactions.[486-488] Oxygen radicals can also damage blood vessels and cause vasodilation, increased permeability, endothelial and smooth muscle injury, and increased platelet aggregation.[488]

Strategies to prevent and neutralize oxygen free radicals have been attempted mostly in experimental animals. The agents used are often referred to as free radical scavengers. Unfortunately, none have proved effective in man in preliminary trials. The most recent free radical scavenger to be tested in human trials was NXY-059. This agent proved safe and effective in the SAINT I trial[219-221] but was not effective in the SAINT II trial,[222] and the pharmaceutical company that produced and studied the drug has said that it will not pursue its use for stroke neuroprotection.

One cytoprotective strategy is to give a substrate that might help injured neurons to recover. Citicoline (cytidine-5-diphosphocholine) is the agent in this category that has been used most often in experimental animals and humans. Citicoline is an intermediary in the biosynthesis of the membrane phospholipid phosphatidylcholine and is used to enhance the synthesis of this lipid in the brain. Citicoline has been used alone and in combination with thrombolysis.[215] Citicoline has been studied in clinical trials in acute ischemic stroke patients that showed the substance was very safe and there were some suggestions of effectiveness.[216,217] Citicoline was effective in a rat model of acute embolic stroke when combined with thrombolysis.[218]

The most important substrates used by nerve cells are oxygen and sugar. I have already noted the problems with administration of sugar. Hyperglycemia increases lactate production and likely has adverse rather than protective effects.[495-499] Administration of oxygen was thought to potentially induce vasoconstriction in arteries feeding ischemic brain tissue so that only recently has its use been explored in patients with acute brain ischemia. Because hyperbaric oxygen therapy was known to be effective in divers who developed bends—a disorder in which gas was introduced into blood vessels during pressure changes during diving—it seemed worth trying in patients with brain ischemia. Unfortunately preliminary trials of hyperbaric oxygen in acute stroke patients showed no benefit and the pressure chamber could cause harm by reducing arterial input flow.[507,508] Preliminary studies of bedside inhaled oxygen show promise in widening the window during which spontaneous or induced reperfusion could save neurons from damage.[509,510]

Another neuroprotective strategy has been to reduce the metabolic needs of brain tissue, thus allowing survival despite less energy delivery. This strategy also hopes to enlarge the time window during which reperfusion would be effective. The two most common strategies in this category are to induce hypothermia[511-518] and to use barbiturates at or near anesthesia levels.[519,520] These interventions reduce cerebral energy and metabolism and thereby reduce the brain's requirements for fuel, oxygen, and blood. However, each can lead to circulatory changes and can complicate the examination and management of stroke patients. Hypothermia has been used effectively in reducing brain injury in patients after cardiac arrest, and this has been its most commonly used clinical application.[512,513] Preliminary trials show some suggestion of effectiveness in patients with large brain infarcts.[514-516] In these observational studies, hypothermia has been used alone[514,515] or with hemicraniectomy decompression.[516] Newer techniques of administering hypothermia have made its use more promising,[517] and trials of hypothermia in acute ischemic stroke are being pursued.[518] Cooling to effective hypothermic levels is not simple. Shivering and discomfort usually requires rather heavy sedation, and changes in electrolytes are common, as is potential cardiac arrhythmias. Hypothermia should not be used as a neuroprotective strategy except in medical centers that have considerable experience with its use. Barbiturate use also involves practical problems in managing patients with induced coma and has not been pursued clinically in acute stroke patients.

5

As of this writing, no neuroprotective strategy has proved effective in man. Armchair ideas and theories abound and far outweigh the data, but this field of investigation still may prove fruitful in the future. Trials in human stroke patients have not always been well designed to show an effect of the various therapies. They have customarily been given to all patients with acute stroke, and in the vast majority of trials and studies full brain and vascular imaging have not been mandated at entry or follow-up.

Among all patients with acute brain ischemia:

- Many would already have large infarcts. These could be identified by DWI MRI scans or full CT protocols. Dead brain would likely not respond to neuroprotection.
- In many the blood vessels supplying the ischemic brain would be occluded. The neuroprotective agents might not reach the ischemic neurons because the roads are blocked. Administering the agents to patients who have open arteries or are undergoing thrombolysis or other reperfusion techniques would be most effective.
- White matter infarcts especially lacunes might not respond to neuroprotective agents that are cytoprotective since the white matter consists of tracts and not neurons.

If a neuroprotective agent proves effective among patients who are studied thoroughly using modern neuroimaging who have small or no brain infarcts, open arteries (or are undergoing reperfusion), and nonlacunar mechanisms, and the agent is safe, it will become widely used. The presently pursued strategy of treating all acute stroke patients provides a very difficult barrier for any neuroprotective agent to hurdle. Meetings of stroke researchers and clinicians and pharmaceutical companies have engendered guidelines (STAIRS) for studying neuroprotective agents.[521-523]

Statins (HMG-CoA Reductase Inhibitors)

Because of their pleotrophic effects in stroke and vascular disease prevention and their potential in neuroprotection, statins are worth separate consideration in this chapter. The 3-hydroxy-3-methylglutaryl coenzyme A reductase inhibitors (statins) were initially prescribed because of their potent affect in lowering serum cholesterol, especially the low-density lipoprotein component. Early trials showed that statin drugs not only reduced cholesterol levels but also were effective in reducing coronary artery disease-related events and mortality, even in patients with average levels

of cholesterol.[524-526] Analysis of randomized trials of statins also shows a clear and rather dramatic reduction in the incidence of stroke.[527-529] Use of statin drugs slows progression of coronary artery lesions[530] and carotid artery atherosclerotic plaques.[531-533] Aggressive therapy with high doses of statins (equivalent of 80 mg of atorvastatin) has been shown to be more effective than lower doses in patients with coronary artery disease[530] and in preventing strokes in those patients who had TIAs or strokes.[534,535] In a review of over 8800 patients who had a history of cerebrovascular disease and were treated with statins, there was a reduction in subsequent ischemic strokes and total strokes but an increase in hemorrhagic strokes.[536] Other studies that contained fewer patients who had cerebrovascular disease did not show an increase in hemorrhagic strokes.[536]

Preliminary studies suggest that statins may also have potent neuroprotective effects.[535,537-540] Large doses of statins increase cerebral blood flow at the ischemic core and penumbra. One mechanism of this increase in blood flow is related to an increase in endothelium-derived nitric oxide synthase (eNOS).[540-542] The beneficial effects of the statins on nearly all aspects of atherosclerotic disease morbidity and mortality are not entirely explained by reduction in serum lipid levels. Basic research indicates some other important salutary effects of the statins including (1) normalization of the vascular endothelium, (2) anti-inflammatory effects reduce CRP as well as LDL cholesterol[530] and high CRP levels are strong predictors of the occurrence of coronary and cerebrovascular events,[543-545] (3) depletion and stabilization of the lipid core content of plaques, (4) strengthening of the fibrous cap of plaques, (5) decrease in formation of platelet-fibrin thrombi and decreased deposition of white clots on endothelial surfaces, (6) reduction in the thrombogenicity of plaque elements,[546] and (7) increase in cerebrovascular reactivity, which might prove effective in reducing vasospasm after subarachnoid hemorrhage[547] and improving blood flow in patients with lacunar infarction due to penetrating artery disease.[548] There are many potential indications for statin use in patients with stroke and many types of cerebrovascular disease.[535,540,549]

High-dose statins have proved very safe with less than 1% of serious complications.[534] Furthermore discontinuation of statin administration in patients with coronary or cerebrovascular events can promote the development of myocardial and brain damage.[550-552] In one trial that included 215 patients in whom statins were not given for the first 3 days after an acute ischemic stroke, statin withdrawal was associated with increased infarct volumes, higher Rankin scores, and an increased risk of death or dependency at 3 months.[552] Neuromuscular symptoms and findings include asymptomatic creatine kinase (CK) elevations, cramps, stiffness, exercise intolerance, proximal muscle weakness, and rhabdomyolysis.[553,554] Severe myopathy is rare. Hydrophilic statins (pravastatin and atorvastatin), when used at high doses are associated with elevated transaminases but not CK, while lipophilic statins (simvastatin, lovasatatin) in high doses are associated with high CK levels and not transaminase.[553]

INCREASED INTRACRANIAL PRESSURE AND BRAIN EDEMA AND THEIR CONTROL

Large ischemic and hemorrhagic strokes often increase the volume and pressure inside the cranium. Herniations, shifts in intracranial contents, and generalized increase in intracranial pressure (ICP) are all common causes of death in patients with large strokes. Treatment of these patients often includes strategies to control changes in ICP. Subarachnoid hemorrhage is also accompanied by increased blood within the cranium, often complicated by decreased drainage of cerebrospinal fluid. Patients with subarachnoid hemorrhage almost always have increased ICP.

The cranium can be thought of as an almost completely closed structure within a rigid container. The brain and its interstitial fluid account for approximately 80% of the intracranial volume, whereas cerebrospinal fluid (CSF) and blood within vessels each account for approximately 10% of the volume.[555] When ICP rises, adaptation occurs mostly by altering the CSF and vascular compartments. Less CSF can be produced or more can be absorbed. Blood volume inside the cranium can also be reduced. Most blood is contained in the low-pressure venous system, and this volume can be reduced.[555] ICP has a major effect on pressure and flow in brain blood vessels. To maintain viability of brain tissue, there must be adequate cerebral perfusion pressure. In supine patients, cerebral perfusion pressure is approximately equal to the mean systemic arterial blood pressure minus the mean ICP.[555] Either an increase in ICP or a decrease in systemic blood pressure can further compromise rCBF to brain regions that are already ischemic. For practical purposes, there are only a few mechanisms of ICP elevation in stroke patients. These include (1) introduction of new contents into the cranium, such as a hematoma within the brain or subarachnoid hemorrhage; (2) edema in and around infarcts and hemorrhages; (3) obstruction of the ventricular system leading to hydrocephalus; and (4) decreased absorption of CSF caused by subarachnoid bleeding or inflammation. Each of these problems dictates different treatment strategies.

REDUCING OR LIMITING THE SIZE OF AN INTRACEREBRAL HEMORRHAGE

Unlike brain infarction, a hemorrhage always introduces extra volume into the closed cranial cavity. The larger the hemorrhage, the more the intracranial volume is expanded. In addition, the local blood collection induces surrounding edema, which further increases the volume of extra matter within the brain. Serial brain imaging studies have confirmed that hematomas often expand during the first hours after symptom onset.[556-558] About 35% to 40% of hematomas expand within a 3- to 6-hour period after onset. Expansion of hematoma volume is an important factor that increases morbidity and mortality in patients with intracerebral hemorrhages.[559] Edema usually develops around the hematoma beginning within the first 48 hours and often increases during the first week. Larger hematomas have more surrounding edema than smaller ones. Hemoglobin products and thrombin may promote edema formation. The volume of perihematomal edema also correlates with outcome.[560] ICP is generally elevated, especially in the region of the hematoma; the pressure changes can lead to a shift of midline structures and herniation into other dural compartments. The aim of therapy is to limit the size of the hemorrhage. This can be accomplished by limiting the bleeding, treating the accompanying edema, or draining the hematoma. In the case of hemorrhage caused by a vascular malformation or aneurysm, removing the offending vascular lesion also prevents recurrent hemorrhage.

The most important method to stop the bleeding is to reduce arterial tension. When I was a stroke fellow, before the advent of CT scanning, Dr Miller Fisher would sometimes transiently occlude with his finger the ipsilateral carotid artery in a patient with a clinical hypertensive basal ganglionic hemorrhage in order to diminish blood flow and stop the bleeding. The strategy is similar to the placement of a tourniquet on a limb proximal to bleeding. Overzealous blood pressure reduction, however, can be harmful because the elevated blood pressure helps perfuse brain tissue remote from the hemorrhage. The increased ICP is transmitted passively to the cerebral veins and dural sinuses increasing the pressures in those structures. The arterial pressure

5

must rise to produce an effective arteriovenous pressure differential to perfuse the brain. Excessive reduction in blood pressure could decrease brain perfusion. The patient's alertness and neurologic findings must be carefully monitored as the blood pressure is lowered.

When hemorrhage is caused by a bleeding diathesis, correction of the coagulopathy is critical in containing the hemorrhage. Use of antihemophilic globulin in hemophiliacs and reversal of warfarin-induced hypoprothrombinemia by fresh frozen plasma or vitamin K or activated factor VII are examples of such therapeutic interventions.

Recently, clinicians and investigators have attempted to limit hematoma expansion even in patients without coagulopathies by administering recombinant activated factor VII (rFVIIa) to patients early in the course of intracerebral hemorrhages.[561-563] A randomized trial of rFVIIa showed some effectiveness but also some risk related to the induced hypercoagulability. In this trial 399 patients with CT confirmed intracerebral hematomas were randomly assigned within 3 hours after onset to receive placebo (96 patients) or 40 μg of rFVIIa per kilogram (108 patients), 80 μg/kg (92 patients), or 160 μg/kg (103 patients) within 1 hour after the initial CT scan. The primary outcome measure was the percent change in the volume of the intracerebral hemorrhage measured at 24 hours. Hematoma volume increased more in the placebo group than in the rFVIIa groups. The mean increase was 29% in the placebo group, contrasted with 16%, 14%, and 11% in those given 40 μg, 80 μg, and 160 μg of rFVIIa/kg, respectively ($P = .01$ for the comparison of the three rFVIIa groups with the placebo group). Growth in the volume of intracerebral hemorrhage was reduced by 3.3 mL, 4.5 mL, and 5.8 mL in the three treatment groups, compared with the placebo group ($P = .01$). Sixty-nine percent of placebo-treated patients died or were severely disabled compared with 55%, 49%, and 54% of patients given 40, 80, and 160 μg of rFVIIa, respectively ($P = .004$ for the comparison of the three rFVIIa groups with the placebo group). Mortality at 90 days was 29% for patients who received placebo, as compared with 18% in the 3 rFVIIa groups combined ($P = .02$). Serious thromboembolic adverse events, mainly myocardial or cerebral infarction, occurred in 7% of rFVIIa-treated patients, compared with 2% of those given placebo ($P = .12$).[562] In a second trial, 841 patients with intracerebral hemorrhage were randomized to placebo (268 patients), 20 microg of rFVIIa per kilogram of body weight (276 patients), or 80 microg of rFVIIa per kilogram (297 patients) within 4 hours after stroke onset.[563a] Hemostatic therapy with rFVIIa reduced growth of the hematoma but did not improve survival or functional outcome. In another report elevated

troponin occurred in 20% and myocardial infarction in 10% of 20 ICH patients treated with rFVIIa compared with troponin elevation in 3% and myocardial infarction in 1% of 110 ICH patients who received standard medical management.[564] In patients with preexisting severe vascular occlusive disease involving the coronary or peripheral arteries, or past venous thromboembolism, the administration of rFVIIa poses a risk of myocardial infarction or venous occlusion with pulmonary embolism.

Drainage of hematomas can provide rapid decompression. Some patients may decompress their own lesions through spontaneous dissection of the hematoma that drains into the ventricle or the subarachnoid space. Ease of surgical drainage will depend on the location of the lesion and its proximity to the surface. Lobar, putaminal, and cerebellar hemorrhages are easiest to drain surgically; thalamic and pontine hemorrhages are difficult to drain effectively.[565,566] The purpose of drainage is to reduce critical volume expansion that threatens life. Drainage of the hematoma leaves a residual cavity that disconnects brain pathways. Although allowing survival, drainage probably does not reduce the final neurologic deficit. In comparable-sized infarcts, the cortex is invariably destroyed, whereas hematomas usually spare the cortex. For this reason, recovery from hemorrhages is usually better than from infarcts of equal size.

Open surgical drainage of intracerebral hematomas remains controversial. Unfortunately clinical series and trials have not settled the issues concerning surgical drainage of intracerebral hematomas.[567] A meta-analysis[568] and a Cochrane review[569] conclude that there was insufficient evidence regarding surgical treatment. Case series lump patients with different location hemorrhages, of different sizes, operated on by different surgeons, using different surgical techniques, at different times. No wonder conclusions are difficult. The prevailing opinion of most neurologists has been that patients with very large hematomas who have reduced consciousness are not helped by drainage since the outcome is so bleak with or without surgical decompression. Similarly there is little use in draining very small hematomas since patients recover well without drainage. Patients with moderate-sized lobar and cerebellar hemorrhages, especially when associated with hematoma enlargement, mass effect, and clinical worsening, are those most likely to respond to decompressive surgery.

The largest randomized trial to date, the STICH trial, failed to show a definite superiority of either medical or surgical treatment.[567,570] In STICH, 1033 patients from 83 centers in 27 countries were randomized to surgery within 24 hours of randomization or initial conservative treatment.

Among those randomized to early surgery, 26% had a favorable outcome compared with 24% randomized to initial conservative treatment (odds ratio, 0.89; 95% confidence interval, 0.66 to 1.19; $P = .414$). In this analysis deep and lobar hemorrhages were considered together. Among the 530 patients randomized to initial conservative treatment, 140 crossed over and had surgery, complicating the analysis and interpretation of the results.[571] The investigators concluded that overall "patients with spontaneous supratentorial intracerebral hemorrhage in neurosurgical units show no overall benefit from early surgery when compared with initial conservative treatment."[570] The STICH trial did show that the presence of intraventricular bleeding and hydrocephalus adversely affected outcomes.[572]

The timing of decompressive surgery is clearly important. Initially the intracerebral blood is liquid. Later the blood coagulates and solidifies and is more difficult to remove. Much later the intracerebral clot again becomes softer and more liquid. Unfortunately the present CT and MRI technologies do not reliably reflect the liquidity unless there is a fluid level within the hematoma. Clinicians posited that very early surgery, within 4 hours after symptom onset, might allow drainage of liquid blood and lead to better outcomes than surgery after 12 hours.[573] A planned study to test this hypothesis was stopped prematurely after 11 patients in the 4-hour arm had surgery.[573] Median time to surgery was 180 minutes; median hematoma volume was 40 mL; median baseline NIH Stroke Scale score was 19. Postoperative rebleeding occurred in four patients, three of whom died. Rebleeding occurred in 40% of the patients treated within 4 hours, compared with 12% of the patients treated within 12 hours. A relationship between postoperative rebleeding and mortality was apparent.[572] Clearly, too early surgery often led to rebleeding, which adversely affected outcome. The ideal time to operate is unknown.

Two advances in treatment raise hopes of improving drainage of hematomas—stereotactic drainage with or without thrombolytic softening of intracerebral clots. Stereotactic surgery has been performed for ICH for nearly two decades.[574-578] It has been used more often in Asian countries than in the West. Drainage is performed through a small burr hole and no cortisectomy is involved. Stereotactic surgery has been preformed with and without a stereotactic frame and with and without administration of a thrombolytic agent directly into the intracerebral clot. The results show promise and are likely to prove superior in the hands of experienced surgeons to direct surgical drainage. Endoscopic drainage of blood is another promising technique.[578] Drainage of subacute hemorrhages, by reducing intracranial pressure can improve alertness and reduce the frequency and severity of medical complications that often develop in stuporous patients.[576]

Since intraventricular blood, especially a large amount, adversely affects outcome, clinicians have posited that more aggressive drainage of the ventricular blood might improve outcomes in patients with brain hemorrhages that included the cerebral ventricles.[579] A preliminary trial showed that intraventricular thrombolysis with urokinase was able to speed the resolution of intraventricular blood clots, compared with treatment with ventricular drainage alone.[579]

I believe that, in the foreseeable future, more aggressive drainage of hematomas using advanced stereotactic and endoscopic techniques and thrombolytic agents to liquefy clots will result in improved outcomes for patients with intracerebral hematomas. Brain edema surrounding the hematomas can be treated with agents discussed in the next section.

Treatment of Brain Edema and Increased Intracranial Pressure

Brain infarcts, hemorrhages, and subarachnoid bleeding can cause secondary effects that lead to swelling of the brain. The resulting increase in ICP contributes to reduction in consciousness and increases the likelihood of a bad outcome. The three major processes that swell the brain are vascular congestion, so-called vasogenic brain edema, and cytotoxic edema. The potential volume of distended brain capillaries is great. When consciousness is reduced, patients may hypoventilate, thus raising the partial pressure of arterial carbon dioxide. Carbon dioxide is a potent vasodilator. The potential importance of vascular congestion can be shown by the use of mechanical hyperventilation in rapidly reducing elevated ICP.[555,580] Hyperventilation causes an almost immediate decrease in ICP but the peak decrement occurs approximately 30 minutes after the carbon dioxide partial pressure (Pco_2) is reduced.[555,580] The initial acute reduction in PCO_2 of 5 to 10 mm Hg often reduces ICP by 25% to 30%.[555] The PCO_2 should be kept between 25 and 35 mm Hg. Blood gases should be monitored using capillary oximetry in patients with reduced consciousness. The ICP-reducing effect of hyperventilation is temporary and lasts only 1 to 2 days.[581] In many patients, it may be necessary to use sedation and a curare-like drug to adequately control mechanical hyperventilation. Reducing the volume of blood in the head reduces ICP irrespective of the cause. Even

5

when there is no important vascular dilation or congestion, decreasing the amount of venous blood volume in the cranium allows acute decompression of intracranial contents.

Infarcts and hematomas are often accompanied by considerable edema during the acute period. The two basic types of brain edema are customarily classified as vasogenic and cytotoxic.[582] Water in the interstitial or extracellular compartment has been traditionally called vasogenic edema after Klatzo.[583] This type of edema responds to osmotic diuretics, such as mannitol and glycerol. Glycerol is an effective osmotic dehydrating agent that reduces ICP and can be given either orally or intravenously.[584-586] When given intravenously, glycerol should be infused every 2 hours but can be given every 4 to 6 hours orally.[555] Glycerol is a purified preparation of glycerine. Glycerine is readily obtained over the counter in most pharmacies and the impurities are not absorbed and are excreted in the feces. Glycerine is a very useful agent in out-patients who continue to have brain edema after hospital discharge.

A 20% to 25% solution of Mannitol has been the most common osmotic agent used to reduce ICP. Although dosage varies, the typical initial dose of mannitol is 0.75 to 1 g/kg followed by 0.25 to 0.5 g/kg every 3 to 5 hours depending on the ICP.[555] Small doses of 0.25 g/kg may decrease ICP as well as higher doses, but the effect of small doses lasts a shorter time.[555,587] Mannitol may also improve microcirculatory perfusion in the regions directly surrounding hematomas. More recently many neurology intensivists have begun to use hypertonic saline (about 23% solution) to reduce brain edema. This strategy has been effective in reversing brain herniation symptoms and has been well tolerated.[588,589] Elevated head position and barbiturate sedation also reduce ICP. Patients with intracerebral hematomas and increased ICP should be nursed in a sitting position.

The effect of corticosteroids is controversial, but most studies show no benefit of steroids in patients with brain hemorrhages and infarcts.[555] Vasogenic edema commonly surrounds hematomas. Many clinicians use mannitol in patients with large hematomas. There is theoretical concern, however, that hypertonic agents could diffuse into the hematoma during continued bleeding and increase the volume of the hematoma.

The second type of brain edema, so-called cytotoxic edema, is caused by swelling of the cells so that the water is intracellular.[582] Most of the edema in patients with ischemia is intracellular and does not respond to corticosteroids. Cytotoxic edema is said to account for the positivity of brain images seen on DWI-MRI scans in patients with acute brain infarcts. Ischemia can also produce some vasogenic edema. This develops later, however, when brain cell necrosis has released substances that compromise the blood-brain barrier and lead to extracellular edema.

Both vasogenic and cytotoxic edema may be potentiated by reperfusion of brain tissue.[582,590] When the arterial supply to a brain region is blocked, the capillaries and small blood vessels may be damaged by the resulting ischemia. When this region is reperfused, the damaged capillaries leak fluid because of injury to the endothelium and basement membranes. Increased brain edema and brain hemorrhage are potential complications of reperfusion after thrombolytic treatment. The reperfused blood may also carry or promote circulation of substances to the region, such as excitotoxins and Ca^{++} ions that might enhance cell damage leading to more cytotoxic edema.[3,591]

Clinical trials have not shown a general beneficial effect from corticosteroids in ischemic stroke or primary supratentorial intracerebral hemorrhage.[555,581-593] Most authorities do not recommend their use in patients with brain infarcts. In most infarct patients, edema is not clinically important except when there is massive infarction and the prognosis is already poor. Dramatic edema does develop in certain younger patients, however, despite seemingly limited infarction. In this circumstance, osmotic agents and steroids are probably helpful. I have also seen extensive brain edema develop in young patients with subdural hematomas. In that circumstance, steroids have been effective in my experience.

Recently, physicians working in intensive care units have begun to prefer hypertonic saline to mannitol infusions.[555,594] Solutions of IV fluid that contain 1.25% to 3% saline can be used to produce a slow but hopefully sustained rise in osmolality. Alternatively bolus infusions of varying amounts of saline (e.g., 23.4% or 10%) saline can be used instead of mannitol.[595-598] Phlebitis is a problem with hypertonic saline infusions unless a central catheter is used. Congestive heart failure can also develop as a complication of expansion of the intravascular fluid volume.[596,598] Intravenous albumin infusions have also been used in experimental animal models and in a preliminary trial in humans.[274-276,490] Albumin is posited to be a potential neuroprotective agent as well as potentially improving brain edema. Pulmonary edema is a known complication of albumin infusion.

Occasionally, surgical decompression with removal of infarcted and edematous brain has been performed in patients with herniations or increased ICP. Most often, the infarction has involved the cerebellum with resultant compression of the brainstem and fourth ventricle.[599-600] The infarcted cerebellum acts much like a hematoma causing critical mass effect in the posterior cranial fossa, a relatively small, enclosed compartment. Hemicraniectomy has been increasingly used to treat patients with large cerebral infarcts.[516,602-607] Decompressive hemicraniectomy involves removing a large bone flap of approximately 12 cm that usually includes the frontal, parietal, and temporal bones and part of the occipital squama.[604] The dura mater is opened and a dural patch is used for closure. At first, the surgery was limited to patients with large right cerebral hemisphere infarcts because it was thought that survivors with large left hemisphere infarcts would remain hopelessly disabled by aphasia and right hemiplegia.[602] Initially, surgery was only performed after a major shift in brain contents had occurred and the patient became stuporous. Some studies, however, show surprisingly good results even in patients with large left hemisphere infarcts.[516,603,604] The prognosis of patients with large middle cerebral artery territory infarcts is so poor[608] that aggressive therapy is warranted, especially in young, previously healthy individuals. Occasional patients, even those with uncal herniation, do respond and survive after the use of acute hyperventilation followed by mannitol.[609] Survival from massive cerebral infarction is better when hemicraniectomy is performed early before herniation occurs.[602-607]

Hydrocephalus can be caused by ventricular drainage system blockage, most commonly at the level of the aqueduct or fourth ventricle, or by failure of CSF absorption caused by plugging of the meninges by blood and blood products. In SAH, the ventricles may enlarge early in the course, and some patients develop persistent hydrocephalus.[610] Ventricular shunting is needed in only a minority of patients with SAH because, in many patients, the hydrocephalus is temporary. Most other patients respond to repeated lumbar punctures and the use of acetazolamide to decrease CSF production. Large cerebellar infarcts and hemorrhages distort the fourth ventricle, leading to obstructive hydrocephalus.[599,611] Insertion of a ventricular drain or shunt can be life-saving in that situation and can allow recovery in some patients, without the need for direct surgery on the posterior fossa lesion.[611] The decision whether to treat patients with large cerebellar infarcts with ventricular drainage or removal of a large portion of the infarct depends on the clinical and neuroimaging findings in the individual patient.[612,613]

PROMOTING RECOVERY

The previous sections discussed prevention and minimization of ischemic brain damage. What if damage has already occurred and an infarct or hemorrhage is already present? The incidence of stroke is projected to increase considerably during the next few decades because of the rapidly increasing number of individuals over 70 in the population.[614,615] Stroke is predicted to account for 6.2% of the total burden of illness by the year 2020.[615] Even with optimal treatment of patients with acute brain ischemia and hemorrhages, many will have residual brain damage. Are there agents or strategies that might improve function or accelerate and promote maximum recovery? The study of recovery from brain injuries has been greatly facilitated by new technologies such as functional MRI (fMRI) and transcranial magnetic stimulation (TMS). Stem cell research has kindled a reawakening of research on the plasticity of the nervous system and regeneration. These advances in research and technology have stimulated research and clinical interest in neurologic recovery.[616] I will briefly mention herein various strategies for facilitating recovery but will cover this topic in more detail in Chapter 19. I will not discuss standard physical or occupational therapy in this chapter but will limit the discussion to novel strategies now being pursued and studied.

The most dramatic new research in promoting recovery relates to transplantation of primitive stem cells into patients with stroke.[617,618] Early transplantation experiments in animals showed that grafted neurons survive and remain viable only if they are immature before they have elaborated axonal connections. Preliminary studies in man, using postmitotic human neuron-like cells (NT2N) derived originally from a human testicular germ cell tumor, have shown the feasibility of implanting these cells into humans after striato-capsular infarcts and hemorrhages.[617-620] Cyclosporine immunosuppression was given to the transplanted patients. Some patients seemed to improve.[619,620] There were no major safety issues. Transplantation of fetal porcine cells derived from the lateral ganglionic eminence have also been transplanted into 5 patients with basal ganglionic infarct cavities.[617,621] To prevent rejection in this study, the cells were pretreated with an anti-MHC1 antibody and no immunosuppressive drugs were given to the patients.[621]

Stem cell research in stroke patients is clearly very preliminary. When primitive embryonal cells are used, the transplants often also contain abundant growth factors that could stimulate endogenous proliferation of neural elements. Researchers are exploring the potential for using bone marrow stromal cells.[617,618,622-624] and blood from the human umbilical cord[618,623,625] as potential donor sources of cells and accompanying growth factors. Many questions arise[617]:

1. When to transplant? If too early, ischemia may reduce the potential for the implants to take and cytokines and leukocytes could impair implantation. Also prognosis is often less evident during the acute period making it less likely that patients and physicians would opt for an experimental procedure soon after stroke onset. Transplantation weeks or months after the stroke may not be very effective and may be too late.

2. Which cells to use as a donor source and how many?

3. Which strokes? Should only patients with infarcts limited to one area (e.g., the putamen) be chosen? Would transplants be effective if a number of divergent neuronal cells are infarcted (cortical, putaminal, hippocampal, etc.)? What about size? What if the infarction is predominantly white matter or involves important white matter tracts such as those that travel in the internal capsule?

4. Which site to implant? Directly into the infarct or in the presumed penumbra? Multiple site injections or one large implant? Hopefully, ongoing research will answer these queries if not curtailed by political and religious authorities.

Another strategy to promote recovery is a derivation of the old saying, "Use it or lose it." Stimulating the brain region damaged by the stroke might promote plasticity and encourage assumption of the functions of the damaged areas by other brain regions. Researchers have explored the effectiveness of forcing use of a hemiparetic arm by constraining the good arm.[626-628] Preliminary studies investigated the effect of therapeutic interventions for the arm in the acute phase after stroke, with follow-ups at a maximum of 12 months.[626,628] A relatively small study of forced use of the upper extremity in chronic stroke patients reported in 1999, suggested some benefit.[626] A much larger multisite randomized clinical trial conducted at 7 United States academic centers between January 2001 and January 2003 entitled the Extremity Constraint Induced Therapy Evaluation (EXCITE) trial, enrolled 222 patients with predominantly ischemic stroke.[628] Participants were assigned to receive either constraint-induced movement therapy wearing a restraining mitt on the less-affected hand while engaging in therapy on the weak arm and hand ($n = 106$) or usual and customary care that ranged from no treatment after formal acute stroke rehabilitation to pharmacologic or physiotherapeutic interventions ($n = 116$). Among patients who had a stroke within the previous 3 to 9 months, restraint and physical therapy on the affected hand produced statistically significant and clinically relevant improvements in arm motor function that persisted for at least 1 year.[628]

Others have examined the effect of sensory and sensory motor stimulation of paretic limbs. One study examined the effect of repetitive sensorimotor training of the arm after stroke.[629] One hundred consecutive stroke patients were randomly assigned either to an experimental group that received daily additional sensorimotor stimulation of the arm or to a control group. The treatment period was 6 weeks. Assessments of the patients were made before and after treatment and at 6 and 12 months after stroke, and 62 patients at 5 years after stroke. At the 5-year follow-up, there was a statistically significant difference in function tests favoring the treatment group that received early, repetitive, and targeted stimulation of the paretic arm. Extra stimulation of the arm during the acute phase after a stroke resulted in a clinically meaningful and long-lasting salutary effect on motor function.[629] Another study showed that 100-Hz current applied to finger surfaces in patients with chronic poststroke deficits improved the use of utensils with the involved hand.[630,631] Many different types of sensory input—optokinetic, neck proprioceptive, vestibular, and somatosensory—show improvement in neglect in stroke patients.[631,632]

Another way to attempt to facilitate functional recovery is to directly stimulate the brain.[633-637] Repetitive transcranial magnetic stimulation (rTMS) has potential long-term effects on cerebral cortex excitability. Researchers have begun to explore the potential of rTMS in facilitating recovery. Both inhibitory and facilitatory effects can result from rTMS depending on the frequency range of the stimulation. When applied to the primary motor cortex M1, low-frequency (1 Hz) stimulation inhibits excitability while high-frequency (5 to 20 Hz) stimulation increases cortical excitability. Two studies showed that low-frequency rTMS applied to the motor cortex on the side opposite a brain infarct improved function in the hand that was weakened by the stroke.[633,634] The authors posited that inhibition of activity contralateral to the infarct facilitated activity in the hemisphere harboring the brain infarct.[633,634] Other studies showed that rTMS (applied at a frequency of 3 Hz[635] and 10 Hz[637]) to the motor cortex on the side of a brain infarct improved function of the contralateral weak hand. Often rTMS was applied along with routine standard physical and occupational therapy.

Pharmacological interventions have also been explored. Stroke-related injury to nerve cells affects their ability to secrete or respond to neurotransmitters. One popular strategy is to attempt to restore function by replacing neurotransmitters known to be active in damaged regions. Results to date of this approach are mostly anecdotal experiences or small trials. L-Dopa is given to patients with Parkinson's disease to replace depleted dopamine because of nigrostriatal degeneration. Acetylcholine-like drugs have been tried in an attempt to treat the hypothesized cholinergic deficit in Alzheimer's disease. After this lead, a few clinicians have tried neurotransmitters in stroke patients. In one patient with bilateral paramedian thalamic infarcts who was apathetic and habitually assumed sleeping postures, bromocriptine, a dopamine agonist, led to improvement in spontaneity and less time in bed.[638,639] In a patient who had been aphasic since a left frontal-lobe hemorrhage 3.5 years before study, bromocriptine led to an improvement in speech fluency and a reduction in hesitancy when talking.[640] Several small studies suggested that bromocriptine using an average dose of 30 mg alone or with carbidopa/levadopa preparations can improve speech fluency in some patients with Broca's and transcortical motor aphasia.[640,641] Bromocriptine was also effective in a patient with neglect of the left side of space owing to a right frontoparietal and striatal infarct.[642] Neglect and lack of attention were improved while taking bromocriptine and worsened after the drug was withdrawn. Bromocriptine and lisuride have been used effectively to treat abulia in four patients with degenerative diseases and strokes.[643] In all of these circumstances, bromocriptine presumably had no healing effect on the damaged tissues; it merely improved functional capacity.

Amphetamines have also been given to promote recovery and enhance function. After the animal experiments of Feeney and colleagues,[643,644] who found that amphetamines coupled with motor activity accelerated recovery of beam-walking ability in rats, some investigators began to try amphetamines in stroke patients.[631,645-648] In rats, neither saline (if the rats had low blood volumes, also used as a control) nor amphetamine alone facilitated recovery after sensorimotor-cortex lesions. A single 2-mg/kg injection of amphetamines and continued experience walking on the beam were needed.[645,646] In contrast, animals given haloperidol performed far worse than controls.[644] Amphetamines were also effective in promoting recovery of function in animals with experimental sensorimotor-cortex lesions.[647] In a preliminary human study, 10 mg of D-amphetamine sulfate and physical therapy led to accelerated recovery when compared with patients given placebo and therapy.[645] Amphetamine had to be given early to be effective. A single 10-mg dose of

D-amphetamine followed by training improved hand function capabilities in some normal individuals when training alone had not done so.[649] In another study that used normal young volunteers, a single dose of a selective norepinephrine reuptake inhibitor enhanced motor skill acquisition and corticomotor excitability as studied by TMS.[650] From the available studies, it is not clear whether amphetamine has a specific effect in promoting recovery or merely a general stimulatory function when combined with physical activity. Amphetamine administration might lead to long-term potentiation of cell function or merely promote nonspecific stimulation of less-than-normal cells.

Some pharmacological agents have the potential of retarding recovery. Haloperidol has a definite negative effect on recovery.[643-645] Similarly, drugs that enhance gamma-aminobutyric acid transmission, such as diazepam, might increase inhibition of function and also delay recovery.[651] Stroke patients are often exposed to polypharmacy.[652,653] Some drugs have been prescribed before the stroke and others are given after the stroke to treat various symptoms and general medical conditions. In general, the acute and chronic effects of concurrent drugs on recovery have been poorly studied but are clearly important.[654,655] Sedatives, anticonvulsants, haloperidol, and opiates should be avoided when possible.

CONCLUDING COMMENTS AND RULES

Stroke is a complex disease. Care should include (1) stroke and atherosclerosis risk assessment and stroke prevention strategies, (2) rapid clinical evaluation and diagnosis, (3) rapid complete brain and vascular imaging studies and blood tests, (4) management of blood pressure and fluid balance, (5) medical or surgical treatment (or both) of the process causing the acute stroke, (6) early use of rehabilitation techniques, (7) surveillance and treatment to prevent common stroke complications (e.g., aspiration, phlebothrombosis, urinary and pulmonary infections, and bed sores), and (8) education for patients and their families regarding their specific problems and stroke in general.

Because patients with strokes often develop second and third strokes that are different in etiology from the initial stroke,[656] all patients should be fully investigated for conditions that may cause future strokes. Consideration should be given to prophylaxis of all of the risks found.[657]

The field of stroke treatment is changing so quickly that I have included much armchair theorizing and investigational strategies. I suggest the following rules for clinicians to use when approaching treatment in their patients with strokes and cerebrovascular disease:

1. Begin preventive strategies early. Educate patients and families about stroke risk factors and their control early during hospitalization.
2. Treatment of the acute stroke, prevention of the next stroke, and rehabilitation should be concurrent themes throughout hospitalization and recovery.
3. Avoid common stroke complications, such as deep-vein thrombosis, aspiration, hypovolemia, pressure sores, contractures, and urinary tract infections. These problems are easier to prevent than treat.
4. Plan treatment of the acute stroke by analyzing the mechanism and pathophysiology in the individual patient. The time course of the symptoms should never be the sole guide to treatment.
5. The clinician should determine the location and severity of the vascular lesion, the blood constituents and coagulation functions, and the state of the brain (e.g., normal, stunned, or irreversibly damaged).
6. Determine precisely what is wrong with every stroke patient. Stroke is a cerebrovascular disease and diagnosis involves finding the cardiac-cerebrovascular-hematologic cause. Precise diagnosis has great intrinsic value. It allows better estimates of prognosis and guides logical treatment.
7. Unblocking occlusive arterial lesions with endarterectomy or thrombolysis should be considered when there is no brain damage or when ischemia is recent and possibly reversible.
8. Prevention of thrombus formation, propagation, and embolization is often possible by using drugs that modify platelet aggregation and adhesion and by using anticoagulants of the heparin, heparinoid, and warfarin groups. I suggest using antiplatelet aggregants (e.g., aspirin) to prevent white clots and heparin and warfarin to counteract red clots.
9. When an artery is acutely occluded, anticoagulants are used for 3 to 6 weeks until the occlusive thrombus has organized and become adherent to the artery. In contrast, longer-term anticoagulants are warranted for severe stenosis in large arteries and for continued potential for embolism (e.g., in chronic cardiac lesions that represent a risk for cardiogenic embolism).
10. Try to maximize blood flow to ischemic regions during the acute stroke. Avoid excessive reduction of blood pressure and hypovolemia during the acute stage of infarction.
11. Cardiac disease and mortality are high in most stroke patients. Always consider the heart and its blood supply in addition to the brain.

Discussion of these general treatments and strategies is expanded in Part II (Stroke Syndromes) and III (Prevention, Complications, and Rehabilitation) of this book.

References

1. Caplan LR: Evidence-based medicine. Concerns of a clinical neurologist. J Neurol Neurosurg Psychiatry 2001;71:569-576.
2. Thibault GE: Clinical problem solving: Too old for what? N Engl J Med 1993;328:946-950.
3. Caplan LR: Reperfusion of ischemic brain: Why and why not? In Hacke W, DelZoppo G, Hirschberg M (eds): Thrombolytic Therapy in Acute Ischemic Stroke. Berlin: Springer, 1991, pp 36-45.
4. Babbs C: Reperfusion injury of postischemic tissues. Ann Emerg Med 1988;17:1148-1157.
5. Albers GW, Thijs VN, Wechsler L, et al: MRI profiles predict clinical response to early reperfusion: The Diffusion and Perfusion Imaging Evaluation for Understanding Stroke Evolution (DEFUSE) Study. Ann Neurol 2006;60:508-517.
6. Caplan LR: Are terms such as completed stroke or RIND of continued usefulness? Stroke 1983;14:431-433.
7. Caplan LR: TIAs—We need to return to the question, what is wrong with Mr. Jones? Neurology 1988;38:791-793.
8. Cebul RD, Snow RJ, Pine R, et al: Indications, outcomes, and provider volumes for carotid endarterectomy. JAMA 1998;279:1282-1287.
9. Wennberg DE, Lucas FL, Birkmeyer JD, et al: Variation in carotid endarterectomy mortality in the medicare population. Trial hospitals, volume, and patient characteristics. JAMA 1998;279:1278-1281.
10. Robinson RG, Lipsey JR, Price TR: Diagnosis and clinical management of post-stroke depression. Psychosomatics 1985;26:769-778.
11. Indredavik B, Bakke F, Solberg R, et al: Benefit of a stroke unit: A randomized controlled trial. Stroke 1991;22:1026-1031.
12. Indredavik B, Slordahl SA, Bakke F, et al: Stroke unit treatment. Long term effects. Stroke 1997;28:1861-1866.
13. Diez-Tejedor E, Fuentes B: Acute care in stroke: Do stroke units make the difference? Cerebrovasc Dis 2001;11(suppl 1):31-39.
14. Birbeck GL, Zingmond DS, Cui X, Vickrey BG: Multispecialty stroke services in California

hospitals are associated with reduced mortality. Neurology 2006;66:1527-1532.

15. Stroke Unit Trialists' Collaboration: Collaborative systematic review of the randomized trials of organised in-patient (stroke unit) care after stroke. BMJ 1997;314:1151-1159.

16. Stroke Unit Trialists' Collaboration: How do stroke units improve patient outcomes? A collaborative systematic review of the randomized trials. Stroke 1997;28:2139-2144.

17. Leys D, Ringelstein EB, Kaste M, Hacke W: The main components of stroke unit care: Results of a European expert survey. European Stroke Initiative Committee. Cerebrovasc Dis 2007;23:344-352.

18. Candelise L, Gattinoni M, Bersano A, et al: Stroke unit care for acute stroke patients: An observational follow-up study. PROSIT Study Group. Lancet 2007;369:299-305.

19. Caplan LR, Sergay S: Positional cerebral ischemia. J Neurol Neurosurg Psychiatry 1976;39:385-391.

20. Toole J: Effects of change of head, limb, and body position on cephalic circulation. N Engl J Med 1968;279:307-311.

21. Wojner-Alexander AW, Garami Z, Chernyshev OY, Alexandrov AV: Heads down: Flat positioning improves blood flow velocity in acute ischemic stroke. Neurology 2005;64;1354-1357.

22. Rordorf G, Cramer SC, Efird JT, Schwamm LH, Buonanno F:Koroshetz WJ: Pharmacological elevation of blood pressure in acute stroke. Clinical effects and safety. Stroke 1997;28:2133-2138.

23. Hillis AE, Ulatowski JA, Barker PB, et al: A pilot randomized trial of induced blood pressure elevation: Effects on function and focal perfusion in acute and subacute stroke. Cerebrovasc Dis 2003;16(3):236-246.

24. Chalela JA, Dunn B, Todd JW, Warach S: Induced hypertension improves cerebral blood flow in acute ischemic stroke. Neurology 2005;64:1979.

25. Hillis AE, Kane A, Tufflash E, et al: Reperfusion of specific brain regions by raising blood pressure restores selective language functions in subacute stroke. Brain Lang 2001;79:495-510.

26. Lehv M, Salzman E, Silen W: Hypertension complicating carotid endarterectomy. Stroke 1970;1:307-313.

27. Holton P, Wood J: The effects of bilateral removal of the carotid bodies and denervation of the carotid sinus in two human subjects. J Physiol 1965;181:365-378.

28. Breen JC, Caplan LR, DeWitt LD, et al: Brain edema after carotid surgery. Neurology 1996;46:175-181.

29. Caplan LR, Skillman J, Ojemann R, et al: Intracerebral hemorrhage following carotid endarterectomy: A hypertensive complication. Stroke 1978;9:457-460.

30. North American Symptomatic Carotid Endarterectomy Trial Collaborators: Beneficial effect of carotid endarterectomy in symptomatic patients with high-grade carotid stenosis. N Engl J Med 1991;325:445-453.

31. MRC European Carotid Surgery Trial: Interim results for symptomatic patients with severe (70-99%) or with mild (0-29%) carotid stenosis. Lancet 1991;337:1235-1243.

32. Biller J, Feinberg WM, Castaldo JE, et al: Guidelines for carotid endarterectomy. A statement for healthcare professionals from a special writing group of the Stroke Council, American Heart Association. Stroke 1998;29:554-562.

33. Barnett HJM, Taylor DW, Eliasziw M, et al: Benefit of carotid endarterectomy in patients with symptomatic moderate or severe stenosis. North American Symptomatic Carotid Endarterectomy Trial Collaborators. N Engl J Med 1998;339: 1415-1425.

34. European Carotid Surgery Trialists' Collaborative Group: Randomised trial of endarterectomy for recently symptomatic carotid stenosis: Final results of the MRC European Carotid Surgery Trial (ECST). Lancet 1998;351: 1379-1387.

35. Spetzler RF, Hadley MN, Martin NA, et al: Vertebrobasilar insufficiency: I: Microsurgical treatment of extracranial vertebrobasilar disease. J Neurosurg 1987;66:648-661.

36. Kieffer E, Koskas F, Bahnini A, et al: Long-term results after reconstruction of the cervical vertebral artery. In Caplan LR, Shifrin EG, Nicolaides AN, Moore WS (eds): Cerebrovascular Ischaemia—Investigation and Management. London: Med-Orion, 1996, pp 617-625.

37. Berguer R, Flynn LM, Kline RA, Caplan LR: Surgical reconstruction of the extracranial vertebral artery: Management and outcome. J Vasc Surg 2000;31:9-18.

38. Executive Committee for the Asymptomatic Carotid Atherosclerosis Study: Endarterectomy for symptomatic carotid artery stenosis. JAMA 1995;273:1421-1428.

39. Halliday AW, Thomas D, Mansfield A: The Asymptomatic Carotid Surgery Trial (ACST). Rationale and design. Steering Committee. Eur J Vasc Surg 1994;8:703-710.

40. Halliday A, Mansfield A, Marro J, et al: Prevention of disabling and fatal strokes by successful carotid endarterectomy in patients without recent neurological symptoms: Randomised controlled trial. Lancet 2004;363:1491-1502.

41. Hopkins LN, Martin NA, Hadley MN, et al: Vertebrobasilar insufficiency: II: Microsurgical treatment of intracranial vertebrobasilar disease. J Neurosurg 1987;66:662-674.

42. Ausman JI, Diaz FG, Pearce JE, et al: Endarterectomy of the vertebral artery from C2 to posterior inferior cerebellar artery intracranially. Surg Neurol 1982;18:400-404.

43. Meyer FB, Piepgras DG, Sundt TM, et al: Emergency embolectomy for acute occlusion of the middle cerebral artery. J Neurosurg 1985;62: 639-647.

44. Caplan LR, Meyers PM, Schumacher HC: Angioplasty and stenting to treat occlusive vascular disease. Rev Neurol Dis 2006;3(1):8-18.

45. Meyers PM, Schumacher C, Higashida RT, et al: Use of stents to treat extracranial cerebro-vascular disease. Ann Rev Med 2006;57:437-454.

46. Kerber CW, Cromwell LD, Loehden OL: Catheter dilatation of proximal carotid stenosis during distal bifurcation endarterectomy. AJNR Am J Neuroradiol 1980;1:348-349.

47. Bockenheimer SA, Mathias K: Percutaneous transluminal angioplasty in arteriosclerotic internal carotid artery stenosis. AJNR Am J Neuroradiol 1983;4:791-792.

48. Theron J, Raymond J, Casasco A, Courtheoux F: Percutaneous angioplasty of atherosclerotic and postsurgical stenosis of carotid arteries. AJNR Am J Neuroradiol 1987;8:495-500.

49. Kachel R: Results of balloon angioplasty in the carotid arteries. J Endovasc Surg 1996;3:22-30.

50. Wholey MH, Wholey M, Mathias K, et al: Global experience in cervical carotid artery stent place-ment. Catheter Cardiovasc Interv 2000;50: 160-167.

51. Roubin GS, New G, Iyer SS, et al: Immediate and late clinical outcomes of carotid artery stenting in patients with symptomatic and asymptomatic carotid artery stenosis: A 5-year prospective analysis. Circulation 2001;103:532-537.

52. Gil-Peralta A, Mayol A, Marcos JR, et al: Percutane-ous transluminal angioplasty of the symptomatic atherosclerotic carotid arteries. Results, complications, and follow-up. Stroke 1996;27: 2271-2273.

53. Munari LM, Belloni G, Perretti A, et al: Carotid percutaneous angioplasty. Neurol Res 1992;14: 156-158.

54. Eckert B, Zanella FE, Thie A, et al: Angioplasty of the internal carotid artery: Results, complications and follow-up in 6 cases. Cerebrovas Dis 1996;27:2271-2273.

55. Higashida R, Tsai F, Halbach V, et al: Transluminal angioplasty, thrombolysis, and stenting for extra-cranial and intracranial cerebral vascular disease. J Intervent Cardiol 1996;9:245-255.

56. Theron JG, Payelle GG, Coskun O, et al: Carotid artery stenosis: Treatment with protected balloon angioplasty and stent placement. Radiology 1996;201:627-636.

57. Crawley F, Clifton A, Buckenham T, et al: Com-parison of hemodynamic cerebral ischemia and microembolic signals detected during carotid endarterectomy and carotid angioplasty. Stroke 1997;28:2460-2464.

58. Eckert B, Thie A, Valdueza J, et al: Transcranial Doppler sonographic monitoring during percutaneous transluminal angioplasty of the internal carotid artery. Neuroradiology 1997;39:229-234.

59. Markus HS, Clifton A, Buckenham T, Brown MM: Carotid angioplasty. Detection of embolic signals during and after the procedure. Stroke 1994;25: 2403-2406.

60. McCleary AJ, Nelson M, Dearden NM, et al: Cerebral haemodynamics and embolization during carotid angioplasty in high-risk patients. Br J Surg 1998;85:771-774.

61. Endovascular versus surgical treatment in patients with carotid stenosis in the Carotid and Vertebral Artery Transluminal Angioplasty Study (CAVATAS): A randomised trial. Lancet 2001;357:1729-1737.

62. Brown MM: Vascular surgical society of Great Britain and Ireland: Results of the carotid and vertebral artery transluminal angioplasty study. Br J Surg 1999;86:710-711.

63. Coward LJ, McCabe DJH, Ederle J, et al: Long-term outcome after angioplasty and stenting for symptomatic vertebral artery stenosis compared with medical treatment in the Carotid and Verte-bral Artery Transluminal Angioplasty Study (CAVATAS). A randomized trial. CAVATAS Investigators. Stroke 2007;38:1526-1530.

64. Yadav J, Wholey M, Kuntz KM, et al: Protected carotid-artery stenting versus endarterectomy in high-risk patients. N Engl J Med 2004;351: 1493-1501.

65. SPACE Collaborative Group: 30 day results from the SPACE trial of stent-protected angioplasty versus carotid endarterectomy in symptomatic patients: A randomized non-inferiority trial. Lancet 2006;368:1239-1247.

66. Hoffman R, Niessner K, Kypta A, et al: Risk score for peri-interventional complications of carotid artery stenting. Stroke 2006;37:2557-2561.

67. Mas J-L, Chatellier G, Beyssen B, et al: Endarterectomy versus stenting in patients with symptomatic severe carotid stenosis. N Engl J Med 2006;355:1660-1671.

68. Qureshi A: Carotid angioplasty and stent placement after EVA-3S trial. Stroke 2007;38:1993-1996.

69. Ribo M, Molina C, Alvarez B, et al: Transcranial Doppler monitoring of transcervical carotid stenting with flow reversal protection. Stroke 2006;37:2846-2849.

70. Hadjipetrou P, Cox S, Piemonte T, Eisenhauer A: Percutaneous revascularization of atherosclerotic obstruction of aortic arch vessels. J Am Coll Cardiol 1999;33:1238-1245.

71. Dorros G, Lewin RF, Jamnadas P, Mathiak LM: Peripheral transluminal angioplasty of the subcla-vian and innominate arteries utilizing the bra-chial approach: Acute outcome and follow-up. Catheter Cardiovasc Diagn 1990;19:71-76.

72. Hebrang A, Maskovic J, Tomac B: Percutaneous transluminal angioplasty of the subclavian arter-ies: Long-term results in 52 patients. AJR Am J Roentgenol 1991;156:1091-1094.

73. Henry M, Amor M, Henry I, et al: Percutaneous transluminal angioplasty of the subclavian arteries. J Endovasc Surg 199;6:33-41.

74. Millaire A, Trinca M, Marache P, et al: Subcla-vian angioplasty: Immediate and late results in 50 patients. Catheter Cardiovasc Diagn 1993;29:8-17.

75. Motarjeme A: Percutaneous transluminal angioplasty of supra-aortic vessels. J Endovasc Surg 1996;3:171-181.

76. Motarjeme A, Keifer JW, Zuska AJ, Nabawi P: Percutaneous transluminal angioplasty for treat-ment of subclavian steal. Radiology 1985;155:611-613.

77. Vitek JJ: 1989. Subclavian artery angioplasty and the origin of the vertebral artery. Radiology 1989;170:407-409.

78. Schillinger M, Haumer M, Schillinger S, et al: Risk stratification for subclavian artery angioplasty: Is there an increased rate of restenosis after stent implantation? J Endovasc Ther 2001;8:550-557.

79. Chastain HD 2nd, Campbell MS, Iyer S, et al: Extracranial vertebral artery stent placement: In-hospital and follow-up results. J Neurosurg 1999;91:547-552.

80. Piotin M, Spelle L, Martin JB, et al: Percutaneous transluminal angioplasty and stenting of the proximal vertebral artery for symptomatic stenosis. AJNR Am J Neuroradiol 2000;21:727-731.

81. Higashida R, Tsai F, Halbach V, et al: Transluminal angioplasty, thrombolysis, and stenting for extracranial and intracranial cerebral vascular disease. J Intervent Cardiol 1996;9:245-255.

82. SSYLVIA Study Investigators: Stenting of Symptomatic Atherosclerotic Lesions in the Vertebral or Intracranial Arteries (SSYLVIA): Study results. Stroke 2004;35:1388-1392.

83. Meyers PM, Schumacher HC, Tanji K, et al: Use of stents to treat intracranial cerebrovascular disease. Ann Rev Med 2007;58:107-122.

84. Higashida RT, Meyers PM, Connors 3rd JJ, et al: Intracranial angioplasty and stenting for cerebral atherosclerosis: A position statement of the American Society of Interventional and Therapeutic Neuroradiology, Society of Interventional Radiology, and the American Society of Neuroradiology. AJNR Am J Neuroradiol 2005;26:2323-2327.

85. Gress DR, Smith WS, Dowd CF, et al: Angioplasty for intracranial symptomatic vertebrobasilar ischemia. Neurosurgery 2002;51:23-27.

86. Marks MP, Marcellus M, Norbash AM, et al: Outcome of angioplasty for atherosclerotic intracranial stenosis. Stroke 1999;30:1065-1069.

87. Connors 3rd JJ, Wojak JC: Percutaneous transluminal angioplasty for intracranial atherosclerotic lesions: Evolution of technique and short-term results. J Neurosurg 1999;91:415-423.

88. Takis C, Kwan ES, Pessin MS, et al: Intracranial angioplasty: Experience and complications. AJNR Am J Neuroradiol 1997;18:1661-1668.

89. Gomez CR, Misra VK, Liu MW, et al: Elective stenting of symptomatic basilar artery stenosis. Stroke 2000;31:95-99.

90. Yu W, Smith WS, Singh V, et al: Long-term outcome of endovascular stenting for symptomatic basilar artery stenosis. Neurology 2005;64:1055-1057.

91. Kessler IM, Mounayer C, Piotin M, et al: The use of balloon-expandable stents in the treatment of intracranial arterial diseases: A 5-year single-center experience. AJNR Am J Neuroradiol 2005;26:2342-2348.

92. Marks MP, Marcellus ML, Do HM, et al: Intracranial angioplasty without stenting for symptomatic atherosclerotic stenosis: Long-term follow-up. AJNR Am J Neuroradiol 2005;26:525-530.

93. Wojak JC, Dunlap DC, Hargrave KR, et al: Intracranial angioplasty and stenting: Long-term results from a single center. AJNR Am J Neuroradiol 2006;27:1882-1892.

94. Henkes H, Miloslavaski E, Lowens S, et al: Treatment of intracranial atherosclerotic stenoses with balloon dilatation and self-expanding stent deployment (WingSpan). Neuroradiology 2005;47:222-228.

95. Bose A, Hartmann M, Henkes H, et al: A novel, self-expanding nitinol stent in medically refractory intracranial atherosclerotic stenoses. The Wingspan Study. Stroke 2007;38:1531-1537.

96. Fiorella D, Levy EI, Turk AS, et al: US multicenter experience with the Wingspan stent system for the treatment of intracranial atheromatous disease. Periprocedural results. Stroke 2007;38:881-887.

97. Gupta R, Al-Ali F, Thomas AJ, et al: Safety, feasibility, and short-term follow-up of drug-eluting stent placement in the intracranial and extracranial circulation. Stroke 2006;37:2562-2566.

98. Schuchhman M: Trading retenosis for thrombosis? New questions about drug-eluting stents. N Engl J Med 2006;355:1949-1952.

99. Collen D: On the regulation and control of fibrinolysis: Edward Kowalsky Memorial Lecture. Throm Haemost 1980;43:77-89.

100. Sloan MA: Thrombolysis and stroke, past and future. Arch Neurol 1987;44:748-768.

101. del Zoppo GJ, Hosomi N: Mechanisms of thrombolysis. In Lyden PD (ed): Thrombolytic Therapy for Acute Stroke. Totowa, NJ: Humana Press, 2005, pp 3-27.

102. Meyer JS, Gilroy J, Barnhart ME, et al: Anticoagulants plus streptokinase therapy in progressive stroke. JAMA 1964;189:373.

103. Meyer JS, Gilroy J, Barnhart ME, Johnson JF: Therapeutic Thrombolysis, in Cerebral Thromboembolism: Randomized Evaluation of Streptokinase. In Millikan C, Siekert R, Whisnant JP (eds): Cerebral Vascular Disease, 4th Princeton Conference. New York: Grune & Stratton, 1965, pp 200-213.

104. del Zoppo GJ: Thrombolytic therapy in cerebrovascular disease. Stroke 1988;19:1174-1179.

105. Pessin MS, del Zoppo GJ, Furlan AJ: Thrombolytic treatment in acute stroke: Review and Update of Selected Topics. In Cerebrovascular Diseases, 19th Princeton Conference, 1994. Boston: Butterworth-Heinemann, 1995, pp 409-418.

106. Caplan LR: Caplan's Stroke: A Clinical Approach, 3rd ed. Boston: Butterworth-Heinemann, 2000.

107. Caplan LR: Thrombolysis 2004: The good, the bad, and the ugly. Rev Neurol Dis 2004;1:16-26.

108. Grond M, Rudolf J, Schmulling S, et al: Early intravenous thrombolysis with recombinant tissue-type plasminogen activator in vertebrobasilar ischemic stroke. Arch Neurol 1998;55:466-469.

109. Hacke W, Kaste M, Fieschi C, et al: Intravenous thrombolysis with recombinant tissue plasminogen activator for acute hemispheric stroke. The European Cooperative Acute Stroke Study (ECASS). JAMA 1995;274:1017-1025.

110. Fisher M, Pessin MS, Furlan AJ: ECASS: Lessons for future thrombolytic stroke trials. JAMA 1995;274:1058-1059.

111. Steiner T, Bluhmki E, Kaste M, et al: The ECASS 3-hour cohort. Secondary analysis of ECASS data by time stratification. Cerebrovasc Dis 1998;8:198-203.

112. National Institute of Neurological Disorders and Stroke rt-PA Study Group. Tissue plasminogen activator for acute ischemic stroke. N Engl J Med 1995;333:1581-1587.

113. Ingall TJ, O'Fallon WM, Asplund K, et al: Findings from the reanalysis of the NINDS tissue plasminogen activator for acute ischemic stroke treatment trial. Stroke 2004;35:2418-2424.

114. Hacke W, Kaste M, Fieschi C, et al: Randomised double-blind placebo-controlled trial of thrombolytic therapy with intravenous alteplase in acute ischaemic stroke (ECASS II). Lancet 1998;352:1245-1251.

115. Clark WM, Wissman S, Albers GW, et al: Recombinant tissue-type plasminogen activator (Altepase) for ischemic stroke 3 to 5 hours after symptom onset. The ATLANTIS study: A randomized controlled trial. Altepase Thrombolysis for Acute Non-interventional Therapy in Acute Stroke. JAMA 1999;282: 2019-2026.

116. ATLANTIS, ECASS, and NINDS rt-PA Study Group Investigators: Association of outcome with early stroke treatment. Pooled analysis of the ATLANTIS, ECASS, and NINDS stroke trials. Lancet 2004;363:768-774.

117. Flaherty ML, Jauch EC, Kothari RU, Broderick JP: Intravenous thrombolytic therapy for acute ischemic stroke: Results of large, randomized clinical trials. In Lyden PD (ed): Thrombolytic Therapy for Acute Stroke, 2nd ed. Totowa, NJ, Humana Press, 2005, pp 111-127.

117a. Hacke W, Kaste M, Bluhmki E, et al for the ECASS Investigators: Thrombolysis with alteplase 3 to 4.5 hours at the acute ischemic stroke. N Engl J Med 2008;359:1317-1329.

118. Donnan GA, Davis SM, Chambers BR, et al: Trials of streptokinase in severe acute ischemic stroke. Lancet 1995;345:578-579.

119. del Zoppo GJ, Higashida RT, Furlan AJ, et al: PROACT: A phase II randomized trial of recombinant pro-urokinase by direct arterial delivery in acute middle cerebral artery stroke. PROACT Investigators. Prolyse in Acute Cerebral Thromboembolism. Stroke 1998;29:4-11.

120. Furlan AJ, Higashida RT, Wechsler L, et al: PROACT II. Intra-arterial pro-urokinase for acute ischemic stroke. A randomized controlled trial. JAMA 1999;282:2003-2011.

121. Furlan AJ, Higashida R, Katzan I, et al: Intra-arterial thrombolysis in acute ischemic stroke. In Lyden PD (ed): Thrombolytic Therapy for Acute Stroke, 2nd ed. Totowa, NJ: Humana Press, 2005, pp 159-184.

122. Ogawa A, Mori E, Minematsu K, et al: Randomized trial of intraarterial infusion of urokinase within 6 hours of middle cerebral artery stroke. The Middle Cerebral Artery Embolism Local Fibrinolytic Intervention Trial (MELT) Japan. Stroke 2007;38:2633-2639.

123. Saver JL: Intra-arterial fibrinolysis for acute ischemic stroke. The message of MELT. Stroke 2007;38:2627-2628.

124. Adams HP, Brott TG, Furlan AJ, et al: Use of thrombolytic drugs. A supplement to the guidelines for the management of patients with acute ischemic stroke. A statement for health care professionals from a special writing group of the Stroke Council American Heart Association. Stroke 1996;27:1711-1718.

125. Quality Standards Subcommittee of the American Academy of Neurology: Practice advisory: Thrombolytic therapy for acute ischemic stroke-summary statement. Neurology 1996;47:835-839.

126. Adams HP, del Zoppo G, Alberts MJ, et al: Guidelines for the early management of adults with ischemic stroke. A guideline from the American Heart Association/American Stroke Association. Stroke 2007;38:1655-1711.

127. Qureshi AI, Suri MF, Nasar A, et al: Thrombolysis for ischemic stroke in the United States: Data from National Hospital Discharge Survey 1999-2001. Neurosurgery 2005;57:647-654.

128. Albers CW, Bates VE, Clark WM, et al: Intravenous tissue-type plasminogen activator for treatment of acute stroke: The Standard Treatment with Altepase to Reverse Stroke (STARS) Study. JAMA 2000;283:1145-1150.

129. Demchuk AM, Tanne D, Hill MD, et al: Predictors of good outcome after intravenous tPA for acute ischemic stroke. Neurology 2001;57:474-480.

130. Katzan IL, Furlan AJ, Lloyd LE, et al: Use of tissue-type plasminogen activator for acute ischemic stroke. The Cleveland experience. JAMA 2000;283:1151-1158.

131. Katzan IL, Hammer MD, Furlan AJ, et al: Quality improvement and tissue-type plasminogen activator for acute ischemic stroke: A Cleveland update. Stroke 2003;34:799-800.

132. Weimar C, Kraywinkel K, Maschke M, Diener HC: Intravenous thrombolysis in german stroke units before and after regulatory approval of recombinant tissue plasminogen activator. Cerebrovasc Dis 2006;22:429-431.

133. Heuschmann PU, Berger K, Misselwitz B, et al: Frequency of thrombolytic therapy in patients with acute ischemic stroke and the risk of in-hospital mortality. The German Stroke Registers Study Group. Stroke 2003;34:1106-1113.

134. Sobesky J, Frackowiak M, Weber OZ, et al: The Cologne stroke experience: Safety and outcome in 450 patients treated with IV thrombolysis. Cerebrovasc Dis 2007;24:56-65.

135. Toni D, Lorenzano S, Puca E, Prencipe M: The SITS-MOST registry. Neurol Sci 2006;27(suppl 3): S260-S262.

136. Wahlgren N, Ahmed N, Dávalos A, et al: Thrombolysis with alteplase for acute ischaemic stroke in the Safe Implementation of Thrombolysis in Stroke-Monitoring Study (SITS-MOST): An observational study. Lancet 2007;369(9558):275-282.

137. Edwards MT, Murphy MM, Geraghty JJ, et al: Intra-arterial cerebral thrombolysis for acute ischemic stroke in a community hospital. AJNR Am J Neuroradiol 1999;20:1682-1687.

138. Suarez JI, Sunshine JL, Tarr R, et al: Predictors of clinical improvement, angiographic recanalization, and intracranial hemorrhage after intra-arterial thrombolysis for acute ischemic stroke. Stroke 1999;30:2094-2100.

139. Lisboa RC, Jovanovic BD, Alberts MJ: Analysis of the safety and efficacy of intra-arterial thrombolytic therapy of ischemic stroke. Stroke 2002;33:2866-2871.

140. Quereshi AI, Ali Z, Suri MFK, et al: Intra-arterial third generation recombinant tissue plasminogen activator (reteplase) for acute ischemic stroke. Neurosurgery 2001;49:41-50.

141. Arnold M, Schroth G, Nedeltchev K, et al: Intra-arterial thrombolysis in 100 patients with acute stroke due to middle cerebral artery occlusion. Stroke 2002;33:1828-1833.

142. Molina C, Saver JL: Extending reperfusion therapy for acute ischemic stroke: Emerging pharmacological, mechanical, and imaging strategies. Stroke 2005;36:2311-2320.

143. Rajajee V, Saver J: Prehospital care of the acute stroke patient. Tech Vasc Interv Radiol 2005;8:74-80.

144. Crocco T, Gullett T, Davis SM, et al: Feasibility of neuroprotective agent administration by prehospital personnel in an urban setting. Stroke 2003;34:1918-1922.

145. Saver JL, Kidwell C, Eckstein M, et al: Prehospital neuroprotective therapy for acute stroke: Results of the Field Administration of Stroke Therapy-Magnesium (FAST-MAG) pilot trial. Stroke 2004;35:e106-108.

146. LaMonte MP, Bahouth MN, Hu P, et al: Telemedicine for acute stroke: Triumphs and pitfalls. Stroke 2003;34:725-728.

147. Audebert HJ, Kukla C, Clarmann von Claranau S: Telemedicine for safe and extended use of thrombolysis in stroke: The Telemedic Pilot Project for Integrative Stroke Care (TEMPiS) in Bavaria. Stroke 2005;36:287-291.

148. Audebert HJ, Kukla C, Vatankhah B, et al: Comparison of tissue plasminogen activator administration management between Telestroke Network hospitals and academic stroke centers: The Telemedical Pilot Project for Integrative Stroke Care in Bavaria/Germany. Stroke 2006;37:1822-1827.

149. del Zoppo GJ, Poeck K, Pessin MS, et al: Recombinant tissue plasminogen activator in acute thrombotic and embolic stroke. Ann Neurol 1992;32:78-86.

150. Wolpert SM, Bruckmann H, Greenlee R, et al: Neuroradiologic evaluation of patients with acute stroke treated with recombinant tissue plasminogen activator. The rt-PA Acute Stroke Study Group. AJNR Am J Neuroradiol 1993;14:3-13.

151. Grond M, Rudolf J, Schmulling S, et al: Early intravenous thrombolysis with recombinant tissue-type plasminogen activator in vertebro-basilar ischemic stroke. Arch Neurol 1998;55:466-469.

152. Montavont A, Nighoghossian N, Derex L, et al: Intravenous r-tPA in vertebrobasilar acute infarcts. Neurology 2004;62:1854-1856.

153. Lindsberg PI, Soinne L, Tatlisumak T, et al: Long-term outcome after intravenous thrombolysis of basilar artery occlusion. JAMA 2004;292:1883-1885.

154. Fink JN, Kumar S, Horkan C, et al: The stroke patient who woke up; clinical and radiological features, including diffusion and perfusion MRI. Stroke 2002;33:988-993.

155. Barber PA, Zhang J, Demchuk AM, et al: Why are stroke patients excluded from tPA therapy? An analysis of patient eligibility. Neurology 2001;56:1015-1020.

156. Smith EE, Abdullah AR, Petkovska I, et al: Poor outcomes in patients who do not receive intravenous tissue plasminogen activator because of mild or improving ischemic stroke. Stroke 2005;36:2497-2499.

157. Rajajee V, Kidwell C, Starkman S, et al: Early MRI and outcomes of untreated patients with mild or improving ischemic stroke. Neurology 2006;67:980-984.

158. Selim M, Kumar S, Fink J, et al: Seizure at stroke onset: Should it be an absolute contraindication to thrombolysis. Cerebrovasc Dis 2002;14:54-57.

159. Schellinger PD, Fiebach JB, Jansen O, et al: Stroke magnetic resonance imaging within 6 hours after onset of hyperacute cerebral ischemia. Ann Neurol 2001;49:460-469.

160. Neumann-Haefelin T, Moseley ME, Albers GW: New magnetic resonance imaging methods for cerebrovascular disease: Emerging clinical applications. Ann Neurol 2000;47:559-570.

161. Koroshetz W: Contrast computed tomography scan in acute stroke: "You can't always get what you want but ... you get what you need." Ann Neurol 2002;51:415-416.

162. Wintermark M, Reichhart M, Thiran J-P, et al: Prognostic accuracy of cerebral blood flow measurement by perfusion computed tomography, at the time of emergency room admission, in acute stroke patients. Ann Neurol 2002;51:417-432.

163. Wintermark M, Reichart M, Cuisenaire O, et al: Comparison of admission perfusion computed tomography and qualitative diffusion- and perfusion-weighted magnetic resonance imaging in acute stroke patients. Stroke 2002;33:2025-2031.

164. Sanak D, Nosal V, Horak D, et al: Impact of diffusion-weighted MRI-measured initial cerebral infarction volume on clinical outcome in acute stroke patients with middle cerebral artery

occlusion treated by thrombolysis. Neuroradiology 2006;48:632-639.

165. Kohrmann M, Juttler E, Fiebach JB, et al: MRI versus CT-based thrombolysis treatment within and beyond the 3 h time window after stroke onset: A cohort study. Lancet Neurol 2006;5: 661-667.

166. Davis SM, Donnan GA, Butcher KS, Parsons MW: Selection of thrombolytic therapy beyond 3 hours using MRI. Curr Opin Neurol 2005;18:47-52.

167. Butcher KS, Parsons MW, Donnan GA, Davis SM: Refining the perfusion-diffusion mismatch hypothesis. Stroke 2005;36:1153-1159.

168. Prosser J, Butcher KS, Allport LE, et al: Clinical-diffusion mismatch predicts the putative penumbra with high specificity. Stroke 2005;36: 1700-1704.

169. Butcher KS, Parsons M, MacGregor L, et al: Refining the perfusion-diffusion mismatch hypothesis. EPITHET Investigators. Stroke 2005;36:1153-1159.

170. Hacke W, Albers G, Al-Rawi Y, et al: The Desmoteplase in Acute Ischemic Stroke Trial (DIAS). Stroke 2005;36:66-73.

171. Schellinger PD, Fiebach JB, Hacke W: Imaging-based decision making in thrombolytic therapy for ischemic stroke. Present status. Stroke 2003;34:575-583.

172. Hjort N, Butcher K, Davis SM, et al: E Magnetic resonance imaging criteria for thrombolysis in acute cerebral infarct. Stroke 2005;36:388-397.

173. Kohrmann M, Juttler E, Fiebach JB, et al: MRI versus CT-based thrombolysis treatment within and beyond the 3 h time window after stroke onset: A cohort study. Lancet Neurol 2006;5: 661-667.

174. Schellinger PD, Thomalla G, Fiehler J, et al: MRI-based and CT-based thrombolytic therapy in acute stroke within and beyond established time windows. An analysis of 1210 patients. Stroke 2007;38:2640-2645.

175. Lansberg MG, Thijs VN, Bammer R, et al: Risk factors of symptomatic intracerebral hemorrhage after tPA therapy for acute stroke. DEFUSE Investigators. Stroke 2007;38:2275-2278.

176. Fiehler J, Albers GW, Boulanger J-M, et al: Bleeding Risk Analysis in Stroke Imaging Before ThromboLysis (BRASIL). Pooled analysis of T2*-weighted magnetic resonance imaging data from 570 patients. MR STROKE Group. Stroke 2007;38:2738-2744.

177. Liberatore GT, Samson A, Bladin C, et al: Vampire bat salivary plasminogen activator (desmoteplase): A unique fibrinolytic enzyme that does not promote neurodegeneration. Stroke 2003;34:537-543.

178. Lewandowski CA, Frankel M, Tomsick TA, et al: Combined intravenous and intra-arterial r-TPA versus intra-arterial therapy of acute ischemic stroke. Emergency Management of Stroke (EMS) Bridging Trial. Stroke 1999;30: 2598-2605.

179. Ernst R, Panicoli A, Tomsick T, et al: Combined intravenous and intraarterial recombinant tissue plasminogen activator in acute ischemic stroke. Stroke 2000;31:2552-2557.

180. IMS Investigators: Combined intravenous and intra-arterial recanalization for acute ischemic stroke: The Interventional Management of Stroke study. Stroke 2004;35:904-911.

181. IMS Study Investigators: Hemorrhage in the Interventional Management of Stroke Study. Stroke 2006;37:847-851.

182. Sekoranja L, Loulidi J, Yilmaz H, et al: Intravenous versus combined (intravenous and intra-arterial) thrombolysis in acute ischemic stroke. A transcranial color-coded duplex sonography-guided pilot study. Stroke 2006;37:1805-1809.

183. IMS II Investigators: The Interventional Management of Stroke (IMS) II study. Stroke 2007;38: 2127-2135.

184. Keris V, Rudnicka S, Vorona V, et al: Combined intraarterial/intravenous thrombolysis for acute ischemic stroke. AJNR Am J Neuroradiol 2001;22:352-358.

185. Ducrocq X, Bracard S, Taillandier L, et al: Comparison of intravenous and intra-arterial urokinase thrombolysis for acute ischaemic stroke. J Neuroradiol 2005;32:26-32.

186. Sugg RM, Noser EA, Shaltoni HM, et al: Intra-arterial reteplase compared to urokinase for thrombolytic recanalization in acute ischemic stroke. AJNR Am J Neuroradiol 2006;27:769-773.

187. Macleod MR, Davis SM, Mitchell PI, et al: Results of a multicentre, randomised controlled trial of intra-arterial urokinase in the treatment of acute posterior circulation ischaemic stroke. Cerebrovasc Dis 2005;20:12-17.

188. Inoue T, Kimura K, Minematsu K, et al: A case–control analysis of intra-arterial urokinase thrombolysis in acute cardioembolic stroke. Japan Multicenter Stroke Investigators Collaborators. Cerebrovasc Dis 2005;19:225-228.

189. Titschwell DL, Coplin WM, Becker KJ, et al: Intra-arterial urokinase for acute ischemic stroke: Factors associated with complications. Neurology 2001;57:1100-1103.

190. Hu HH, Teng MM, Hsu LC, et al: A pilot study of a new thrombolytic agent for acute ischemic stroke in Taiwan within a five-hour window. Stroke 2006;37:918-919.

191. Fanale CV, Lyden PD: Thrombolytic therapy for acute ischemic stroke. In Bhardwaj A, Alkayed NJ, Kirsch JR, Traystman RJ (eds): Acute Stroke, Bench to Bedside. New York: Informa Healthcare 2007, pp 217-228.

192. Ancrod Stroke Study Investigators: Ancrod for the treatment of acute ischemic brain infarction. Stroke 1994;25:1755-1759.

193. Sherman DG, Atkinson RP, Chippendale T, et al: Intravenous ancrod for treatment for acute ischemic stroke. JAMA 2000;283:2395-2403.

194. Hossman V, Heiss W-D, Bewermeyer H, Wiedemann G: Controlled trial of ancrod in ischemic stroke. Arch Neurol 1983;40:803-808.

195. Olinger CP, Brott TG, Barsan WG, et al: Use of ancrod in acute progressing ischemic cerebral infarction. Ann Emerg Med 1988;17:1208-1209.

196. Hennerici M, Kay R, Bogousslavsky J, et al: Intravenous ancrod for acute ischaemic stroke in the European Stroke Treatment with Ancrod Trial: A randomized controlled trial. Lancet 2006;368:1871-1878.

197. Van de Werf F, Adgey J, Ardissino D, et al: Single-bolus tenecteplase compared with front-loaded alteplase in acute myocardial infarction: The Assent-2 double-blind randomized trial. Lancet 1999;354:716-722.

198. Fussell D, Schumacher C, Meyers PM, Higashida RT: Mechanical interventions to treat acute stroke. Curr Neurol Neurosci Reports 2007;7:21-27.

199. Qureshi A, Janjua N, Kirmani J, et al: Mechanical disruption of thrombus following intravenous tissue plasminogen activator for ischemic stroke. J Neuroimag 2007;17:124-130.

200. Gobin YP, Starkman S, Duckwiler GR, et al: MERCI 1: A phase 1 study of mechanical embolus removal in cerebral ischemia. Stroke 2004;35:2848-2854.

201. Smith WS, Sung G, Starkman S, et al: Safety and efficacy of mechanical embolectomy in acute ischemic stroke: Results of the MERCI trial. Stroke 2005;36:1432-1438.

202. Smith WS: Safety of mechanical thrombectomy and intravenous tissue plasminogen activator in acute ischemic stroke. Results of the Multi Mechanical Embolus Removal in Cerebral Ischemia (MERCI) trial, part I. AJNR Am J Neuroradiol 2006;27:1177-1182.

203. Flint A, Duckwiler GR, Budzik RF, et al: Mechanical thrombectomy of intracranial internal carotid occlusion. Pooled results of the MERCI and Multi MERCI part I trials. Stroke 2007;38:1274-1280.

204. Qureshi AI, Siddiqui AM, Suri MF, et al: Aggressive mechanical clot disruption and low-dose intra-arterial third-generation thrombolytic agent for ischemic stroke: A prospective study. Neurosurgery 2002;51:1319-1327.

205. Noser EA, Shaltoni HM, Hall CE, et al: Aggressive mechanical clot disruption. A safe adjunct to thrombolytic therapy in acute stroke? Stroke 2005;36:292-296.

206. Lansberg MG, Fields JD, Albers GW, et al: Mechanical thrombectomy following intravenous thrombolysis in the treatment of acute stroke. Arch Neurol 2005;62:1763-1765.

207. Gupta R, Jovin TG, Tayal A, Horowitz MB: Urgent stenting of the M2 (superior) division of the middle cerebral artery after systemic thrombolysis in acute stroke. AJNR Am J Neuroradiol 2006;27:521-523.

208. Lin DD, Gailloud P, Beauchamp NJ, et al: Combined stent placement and thrombolysis in acute vertebrobasilar ischemic stroke. AJNR Am J Neuroradiol 2003;24:1827-1833.

209. Bergui M, Stura D, Daniele D, et al: Mechanical thrombolysis in ischemic stroke attributable to basilar artery occlusion as first-line treatment. Stroke 2006;37:145-150.

210. Rha J-H, Saver JL: The impact of recanalization on ischemic stroke outcome. A meta-analysis. Stroke 2007;38:967-973.

211. Delgado-Mederos R, Rovira A, Alvaraez-Sabin J, et al: Speed of tPA-induced clot lysis predicts DWI lesion evolution in acute stroke. Stroke 2007;38:955-960.

212. Wunderlich MT, Goertler M, Postert T, et al: Recanalization after intravenous thrombolysis. Does a recanalization time window exist? Neurology 2007;68:1364-1368.

213. Uchino K, Anderson DC: Better late than never. The story of arterial recanalization in acute ischemic stroke. Neurology 2007;68:1335-1336.

214. Sacco RL, Chong J, Prabhakaran S, Elkind MSV: Experimental treatments for acute ischaemic stroke. Lancet 2007;369:331-341.

215. Overgaard K, Meden P: Citicoline—the first effective neuroprotectant to be combined with thrombolysis in acute ischemic stroke. J Neurol Sci 2006;247:119-120.

216. Clark WM, Wechsler LR, Sabounjian LA, et al: A phase III randomized efficacy trial of 2000 mg citicoline in acute ischemic stroke patients. Neurology 2001;57:1595-1602.

217. Warach S, Pettigrew LC, Dashe JF, et al: Effect of citicoline on ischemic lesions as measured by diffusion-weighted magnetic resonance imaging. Citicoline 010 Investigators. Ann Neurol 2000;48:713-722.

218. Alonso de Lecinana M, Gutierrez M, Roda JM, et al: Effect of combined therapy with thrombolysis and citicoline in a rat model of embolic stroke. J Neurol Sci 2006;247:121-129.

219. Lees KR, Zivin JA, Ashwood T, et al: NXY-059 for acute ischemic stroke. Stroke Acute Ischemic NXY Treatment (SAINT I) Investigators. N Engl J Med 2006;354:588-600.

220. Hess DC: NXY-059. A hopeful sign in the treatment of stroke. Stroke 2006;37:2649-2650.

221. Fisher M: NXY-059 for acute ischemic stroke. The promise of neuroprotection is finally realized. Stroke 2006;37:2651-2652.

222. Shuaib A, Lees KR, Lyden P, et al: NXY-059 for the treatment of acute ischemic stroke. SAINT II Trial Investigators. N Engl J Med 2007;357:562-571.

223. Steiner T, Hacke W: Combination therapy with neuroprotectants an thrombolytics in acute ischemic stroke. Eur Neurol 1998;40:1-8.

224. Alexandrov AV, Grotta JC: Arterial reocclusion in stroke patients treated with intravenous tissue plasminogen activator. Neurology 2002;59:862-867.

225. Quereshi AL, Saad M, Zaidat OO, et al: Intracerebral hemorrhages associated with neurointerventional procedures using a combination of antithrombotic agents including abciximab. Stroke 2002;33:1916-1919.

226. Abciximab Emergent Stroke Treatment Trial (AbESTT) Investigators: Emergency administration of abciximab for treatment of patients with

5

acute ischemic stroke: Results of a randomized phase 2 trial. Stroke 2005;36:880-890.

227. Mangiafico S, Cellerini M, Nencini P, et al: Intravenous glycoprotein IIb/IIIa inhibitor (Tirofiban) followed by intra-arterial urokinase and mechanical thrombolysis in stroke. AJNR Am J Neuroradiol 2005;26:2595-2601.

228. Straub S, Junghans U, Jovanovic V, et al: Systemic thrombolysis with recombinant tissue plasminogen activator and tirofiban in acute middle cerebral artery occlusion. Stroke 2004;35:705-709.

229. Seitz RJ, Meisel S, Moll M, et al: The effect of combined thrombolysis with rtPA and tirofiban on ischemic brain lesions. Neurology 2004;62:2110-2112.

230. Adams HP, Effron MB, Torner J, et al: Emergency administration of abciximab for treatment of patients with acute ischemic stroke: Results of an international phase III trial. Abciximab in Emergency Treatment of Stroke trial (AbESTT-II). Stroke 2008;39:87-99.

231. Grond M, Rudolf J, Neveling M, et al: Risk of immediate heparin after rt-PA therapy in acute ischemic stroke. Cerebrovasc Dis 1997;318-323.

232. Schmulling S, Rudolf J, Strotmann-Tack T, et al: Acetylsalicylic acid pretreatment, concomitant heparin therapy and the risk of early intracranial hemorrhage following systemic thrombolysis for acute ischemic stroke. Cerebrovasc Dis 2003;16: 183-190.

233. Sugg R, Pary JF, Uchino K, et al: Argatroban tPA Stroke Study. Study design and results in the first treatment cohort. Arch Neurol 2006;63: 1057-1062.

234. Alexandrov AV, Demchuk AM, Felberg RA, et al: Intracranial clot dissolution is associated with embolic signals on transcranial Doppler. J Neuroimag 2000;10:27-32.

235. Alexandrov AV, Demchuk AM, Felberg RA, et al: High rate of complete recanalization and dramatic clinical recovery during tPA infusion when continuously monitored with 2-Mhz transcranial Doppler monitoring. Stroke 2000;31: 610-614.

236. Eggers J, Koch B, Meyer K, et al: Effect of ultrasound on thrombosis of middle cerebral artery occlusion. Ann Neurol 2003;53:797-800.

237. Alexandrov AV, Molina CA, Grotta JC, et al: Ultrasound-enhanced systemic thrombolysis for acute ischemic stroke. N Engl J Med 2004;351:2170-2178.

238. Polak JF: Ultrasound energy and the dissolution of thrombus. N Engl J Med 2004;351:2154-2155.

239. Eggers J, Seidel G, Koch B, Konig I: Sonothrombolysis in acute ischemic stroke for patients ineligible for rt-PA. Neurology 2005;64:1052-1054.

240. Molina C, Ribo M, Rubiera M, et al: Microbubble administration accelerates clot lysis during continuous 2-Mhz ultrasound monitoring in stroke patients treated with intravenous tissue plasminogen activator. Stroke 2006;37: 425-429.

241. Furlan A, Little J, Dohn D: Arterial occlusion following anastomosis of the superficial temporal artery to middle cerebral artery. Stroke 1980;11:91-95.

242. Gumerlock M, Ono H, Neurvelt E: Can a patent extracranial-intracranial bypass provoke the conversion of an intracranial arterial stenosis to a symptomatic occlusion? Neurosurgery 1983;12:391-400.

243. EC-IC Bypass Study Group: Failure of the extracranial-intracranial arterial bypass to reduce the risk of ischemic stroke. N Engl J Med 1985;313:1191-1200.

244. Caplan LR, Piepgras DG, Quest DO, et al: EC-IC bypass 10 years later: Is it valuable? Surg Neurol 1996;46:416-423.

245. Przybylski GJ, Yonas H, Smith HA: Reduced stroke risk in patients with compromised cerebral blood flow reactivity treated with superficial temporal artery to distal middle cerebral artery bypass surgery. J Stroke Cerebrovasc Dis 1998;7:302-309.

246. Diaz FG, Umansky F, Mehta B, et al: Cerebral revascularization to a main limb of the middle cerebral artery in the sylvian fissure, an alternative to conventional anastamosis. J Neurosurg 1985;63:21-29.

247. Diaz FG: Technique for extracranial-intracranial bypass grafting. In Moore WS (ed): Surgery for Cerebrovascular Disease, 2nd ed. Philadelphia: WB Saunders, 1996, pp 638-654.

248. Tulleken CAF, Verdaasdonk RM, Mansvelt Beck RJ, Mali WPM: The modified excimer laser-assisted high flow bypass operation. Surg Neurol 1996;46:424-429.

249. Klijn CJM, Kappelle LJ, van der Zwan A, et al: Excimer laser-assisted high-flow extracranial/intracranial bypass in patients with symptomatic carotid artery occlusion at high risk of recurrent cerebral ischemia. Safety and long-term outcome. Stroke 2002;33:2451-2458.

250. Grubb Jr RL, Powers WJ, Derdeyn CP, et al: The Carotid Occlusion Surgery Study. Neurosurg Focus 2003;14:e9

251. Derdeyn CP, Grubb Jr RL, Powers WJ: Cerebral hemodynamic impairment: Methods of measurement and association with stroke risk. Neurology 1999;53:251-259.

252. Grubb Jr RL, Derdeyn CP, Fritsch SM, et al: The importance of hemodynamic factors in the prognosis of symptomatic carotid occlusion. JAMA 1998;280:1055–1060.

253. Powers WJ: Cerebral hemodynamics in ischemic cerebrovascular disease. Ann Neurol 1991;29: 231-240.

254. Yokota C, Hasegawa Y, Minematsu K, Yamaguchi T: Effect of acetazolamide reactivity and long-term outcome in patients with major cerebral artery occlusive disease. Stroke 1998;29:640-644.

255. Vernieri F, Pasqualetti P, Passarelli F, et al: Outcome of carotid artery occlusion is predicted by cerebrovascular reactivity. Stroke 1999;30: 593-598.

256. Grubb Jr RL: Extracranial-intracranial arterial bypass for treatment of occlusion of the internal carotid artery. Curr Neurol Neurosci Rep 2004;4:23-30.

257. Adams Jr HP, Powers WJ, Grubb Jr RL, et al: Preview of a new trial of extracranial-to-intracranial arterial anastomosis: The carotid occlusion surgery study. Neurosurg Clin North Am 2001;12:613-624.

258. Garg BP, Bruno A, Biller J: Moyamoya disease and cerebral ischemia. In Batjer HH, Caplan LR, Friberg L, Greenlee RG Jr, Kopitnik TA Jr, Young WL (eds): Cerebrovascular Disease. Philadelphia: Lippincott-Raven, 1997, pp 489-499.

259. Scott RM, Smith JL, Robertson RL, et al: Long-term outcome in children with moyamoya syndrome after cranial revascularization by pial synangiosis. J Neurosurg 2004;100(2 suppl Pediatrics):142-149.

260. Miyamoto S: Study design for a prospective randomized trial of extracranial-intracranial bypass surgery for adults with moyamoya disease and hemorrhagic onset—The Japan Adult Moyamoya Trial Group. Neurol Med Chir (Tokyo) 2004;44:218-219.

261. Caplan LR: Use of vasodilating drugs for cerebral symptomatology. In Miller R, Greenblatt D (eds): Drug Therapy Reviews. Amsterdam: Elsevier, 1979, pp 305-317.

262. Golino P, Pisclone F, Willerson JT, et al: Divergent effects of serotonin in coronary-artery dimensions and blood flow in patients with coronary atherosclerosis and control patients. N Engl J Med 1991;324:641-648.

263. Piepgras A, Schmiedek P, Leinsinger G, et al: A simple test to assess cerebrovascular reserve capacity using transcranial Doppler sonography and acetazolamide. Stroke 1990;21:1306-1311.

264. Hojer-Pedusen E: Effect of acetazolamide on cerebral blood flow in subacute and chronic cerebrovascular disease. Stroke 1987;18:887-891.

265. Braunwald E: Mechanism of action of calcium-channel blocking agents. N Engl J Med 1982;307:1618-1627.

266. Gorelick PB, Caplan LR: Calcium, hypercalcemia and stroke. Current concepts of cerebrovascular disease. Stroke 1985;20:13-17.

267. Allen G, Ahn H, Preziosi T, et al: Cerebral arterial spasm: A controlled trial of nimodipine in patients with subarachnoid hemorrhage. N Engl J Med 1983;308:619-624.

268. Phillipon J, Grob R, Dagreou F, et al: Prevention of vasospasm in subarachnoid hemorrhage: A controlled study with nimodipine. Acta Neurochir (Wien) 1986;82:110-114.

269. Jan M, Buchheit F, Tremoulet M: Therapeutic trial of intravenous nimodipine in patients with established cerebral vasospasm after rupture of intracranial aneurysms. Neurosurg 1988;23:154-157.

270. Pickard JD, Murray GD, Illingworth R, et al: Effect of oral nimodipine on cerebral infarction and outcome after subarachnoid hemorrhage: British Aneurysm Nimodipine Trial. BMJ 1989;298:636-642.

271. TRUST Study Group: Randomized, double-blind placebo-controlled trial of nimodipine in acute stroke. Lancet 1990;336:1205-1209.

272. American Nimodipine Study Group: Clinical trial of nimodipine in acute ischemic stroke. Stroke 1992;23:3-8.

273. Heros RC, Korosue K: Hemodilution for cerebral ischemia. Stroke 1989;20:423-427.

274. Huh PW, Belayev L, Zhao W, et al: The effect of high-dose albumin therapy on local cerebral perfusion after transient focal cerebral ischemia in rats. Brain Res 1998;804:105-113.

275. Ginsberg MD, Hill MD, Palesch YY, et al: The ALIAS Pilot Trial: A dose-escalation and safety study of albumin therapy for acute ischemic stroke—I: Physiological responses and safety results. Stroke 2006;37:2100-2106.

276. Palesch YY, Hill MD, Ryckborst KJ, et al: The ALIAS Pilot Trial: A dose-escalation and safety study of albumin therapy for acute ischemic stroke—II: Neurologic outcome and efficacy analysis. Stroke 2006;37:2107-2114.

277. Thomas DJ: Hemodilution in acute stroke. Stroke 1985;16:763-764.

278. Thomas DJ, duBoulay GH, Marshall J, et al: Effect of haemotocrit on cerebral blood flow in man. Lancet 1977;2:941-943.

279. Wood JH, Kee DB: Hemorrheology of the cerebral circulation in stroke. Stroke 1985;16:765-772.

280. Strand T, Asplund K, Eriksson S, et al: A randomized controlled trial of hemodilution therapy in acute stroke. Stroke 1984;15:980-989.

281. Staedt U, Schlierf G, Oster P, et al: Hypervolemic hemodilution with 10% HES 200/0.5 and 10% dextran 40 in patients with ischemic stroke. In Hartmann A, Kuschinsky E (eds): Cerebral Ischemia and Hemorrheology. New York: Springer, 1987, pp 429-435.

282. Scandinavian Stroke Study Group: Multicenter trial of hemodilution in acute ischemic stroke: Results of subgroup analyses. Stroke 1988;19:464-471.

283. Aichner FT, Fazekas F, Brainin M, et al: Hypervolemic hemodilution in acute ischemic stroke. The Multicenter Austrian Hemodilution Stroke Trial (MAHST). Stroke 1998;29:743-749.

284. Grotta J, Ackerman R, Correia J, et al: Whole-blood viscosity parameters and cerebral blood flow. Stroke 1982;13:296-298.

285. Coull BM, Beamer NB, deGarmo PL, et al: Chronic blood hyperviscosity in subjects with acute stroke, transient ischemic attacks, and risk factors for stroke. Stroke 1991;22:162-168.

286. Beamer N, Coull BM, Sexton G, et al: Fibrinogen and the albumin-globulin ratio in recurrent stroke. Stroke 1993;24:1133-1139.

287. Ernst E, Resch KL: Fibrinogen as a cardiovascular risk factor: A meta-analysis and review of the literature. Ann Intern Med 1993;118:956-963.

288. Rothwell PM, Howard SC, Power DA, et al: Fibrinogen concentration and risk of ischemic stroke and acute coronary events in 5113 patients with transient ischemic attack and minor ischemic stroke. Stroke 2004;35:2300-2305.

289. Olinger CP, Brott TG, Barsan TG, et al: Use of ancrod in acute or progressing ischemic cerebral infarction. Ann Emerg Med 1988;17:1208-1209.

290. Liu M, Counsell C, Wardlaw J, Sandercock P: A systematic review of randomized evidence for fibrinogen-depleting agents in acute ischemic stroke. J Stroke Cerebrovasc Dis 1998;7:63-69.

291. Schuff-Werner P, Schutz E, Seyde WC, et al: Improved haemorheology associated with a reduction in plasma fibrinogen and LDL in patients being treated by heparin-induced extracorporeal LDL precipitation (HELP). Eur J Clin Invest 1989;19:30-37.

292. Walzl M, Lechner H, Walzl B, Schied G: Improved neurological recovery of cerebral infarctions after plasmapheretic reduction of lipids and fibrinogen. Stroke 1993;24:1447-1451.

293. Bambauer R, Schiel R, Latza R: Low-density lipoprotein apheresis: An overview. Ther Apher Dial 2003;7:382-390.

294. Wieland E, Schettler V, Armstrong VW: Highly effective reduction of C-reactive protein in patients with coronary heart disease by extracorporeal low density lipoprotein apheresis. Atherosclerosis 2002;162:187-191.

295. Radack K, Deck C, Huster G: Dietary supplementation with low-dose fish oils lowers fibrinogen levels: A randomized double-blind controlled study. Ann Intern Med 1989;111:757-758.

296. Kobayashi S, Hirai A, Terano T, et al: Reduction in blood viscosity by eicosopentaenoic acid. Lancet 1981;2:197.

297. Vanschoonbeek K, Feijge MA, Paquay M, et al: Variable hypocoagulant effect of fish oil intake in humans: Modulation of fibrinogen level and thrombin generation. Arterioscler Thromb Vasc Biol 2004;24:1734-1740.

298. Geyer RP: Oxygen transport in vivo by means of perfluorochemical preparations. N Engl J Med 1982;307:304-306.

299. Tremper KK, Friedman AE, Levine EM, et al: The preoperative treatment of severely anemic patients with a perfluorochemical oxygen-transport fluid, Fluosol-DA. N Engl J Med 1982;307:277-283.

300. Gould SA, Rosen AL, Sehgal L, et al: Fluosol-DA as a red-cell substitute in acute anemia. N Engl J Med 1986;314:1653-1656.

301. Bose B, Osterholm JL, Triolo A: Focal cerebral ischemia: Reduction in size of infarcts by ventriculo-subarachnoid perfusion with fluorocarbon emulsions. Brain Res 1985;328:223-231.

302. Bell RD, Frazer GD, Osterholm JL, Duckett SW: A novel treatment for ischemic intracranial hypertension in cats. Stroke 1991;22:80-83.

303. del Zoppo GJ: Vascular hemostasis and brain embolism. In Caplan LR, Manning WJ (eds): Brain Embolism. New York, Informa Healthcare, 2006, pp 243-258.

304. Weksler B: Antithrombotic therapies in the management of cerebral ischemia. In Plum F, Pulsinelli W (eds): Cerebrovascular Diseases: Proceedings of the Fourteenth Princeton Conference. New York: Raven Press, 1985, pp 211-223.

305. Caplan LR: Antiplatelet therapy in stroke: Present and future. Cerebrovasc Dis 2006;21(suppl 1):1-6.

306. Bloom AL, Thomas DP: Haemostasis and Thrombosis. Edinburgh: Churchill-Livingstone, 1987.

307. Deykin D: Thrombogenesis. N Engl J Med 1967;276:622-628.

308. Hemker HC, Lindhout T: Interaction of platelet activation and coagulation. In Fuster V, Topol EJ, Nabel EG (eds): Atherothrombosis and Coronary Artery Disease, 2nd ed. Philadelphia: Lippincott-Williams & Wilkins, 2005, pp 569-581.

309. Marder VJ, Chute DJ, Starkman S, et al: Analysis of thrombi retrieved from cerebral arteries of patients with acute ischemic stroke. Stroke 2006;37:2086-2093.

310. Francis CW, Kaplan KL: Principles of antithrombotic therapy. In Lichtman MA, Kipps TJ, Kaushansky K, et al (eds): Williams Hematology, 7th ed. New York: McGraw-Hill, 2006, pp 283-300.

311. Caplan LR: Review: Anticoagulation for cerebral ischemia. Clin Neuropharm 1986;9:399-414.

312. Damus P, Hicks M, Rosenberg R: Anticoagulant action of heparin. Nature 1973;246:355-357.

313. Wu K: New pharmacologic approaches to thromboembolic disorders. Hosp Pract 1985;20:101-120.

314. Hirsh J: Heparin. N Engl J Med 1991;324:1565-1574.

315. Salzman E, Deykin D, Shapiro R, et al: Management of heparin therapy. N Engl J Med 1975;292:1046-1050.

316. Warkentin TE, Levine MN, Hirsh J, et al: Heparin-induced thrombocytopenia in patients treated with low-molecular-weight heparin or unfractionated heparin. N Engl J Med 1995;332:1330-1335.

317. Becker PS, Miller VT: Heparin-induced thrombocytopenia. Stroke 1989;20:1449-1459.

318. Arepally GM, Ortel TL: Clinical practice. Heparin-induced thrombocytopenia. N Engl J Med 2006;24:355:809-817.

319. Das P, Ziada K, Steinhubl SR, et al: Heparin-induced thrombocytopenia and cardiovascular diseases. Am Heart J 2006;152:19-26.

320. Phelan BK: Heparin-associated thrombosis without thrombocytopenia. Ann Intern Med 1983;99:637-638.

321. Weitz JI: Low-molecular-weight heparins. N Engl J Med 1997;337:688-698.

322. Gordon DL, Linhardt R, Adams HP: Low-molecular-weight heparins and heparinoids and

their use in acute or progressing ischemic stroke. Clin Neuropharmacol 1990;13:522-543.

323. Rosenberg R, Lam L: Correlation between structure and function of heparin. Proc Nat Acad Sci U S A 1979;76:3198-3202.

324. Wessler S, Gitel S: Warfarin: From bedside to bench. N Engl J Med 1984;311:645-652.

325. Deykin D: Warfarin therapy. N Engl J Med 1970;283:691-694.

326. Hull R, Hirsch J, Jay R, et al: Different intensities of oral anticoagulant therapy in the treatment of proximal-vein thrombosis. N Engl J Med 1982;307:1676-1681.

327. Taberner D, Poller L, Burslem R, et al: Oral anticoagulants controlled by the British cooperative: Thromboplastin versus low dose heparin in prophylaxis of deep vein thromboses. BMJ 1977;1:272-274.

328. Frances CW, Marder VJ, Evan CM, et al: Two-step warfarin therapy: Prevention of post-operative venous thrombosis without excessive bleeding. JAMA 1983;249:374-378.

329. Hirsh J, Poller L, Deykin D, et al: Optimal therapeutic range for oral anticoagulants. Chest 1989;95(suppl):S5-S11.

330. Poller L: The effect of low-dose warfarin on the risk of stroke in patients with nonrheumatic atrial fibrillation. N Engl J Med 1991;325:129-130.

331. Sconce EA, Khan TI, Wynne HA, et al: The impact of CYP2C9 and VKORC1 genetic polymorphism and patient characteristics upon warfarin dose requirements: Proposal for a new dosing regimen. Blood 2005;106: 2329-2333.

332. Rieder MJ, Reiner AP, Gage BF, et al: Effect of VKORC1 haplotypes on transcriptional regulation and warfarin dose. N Engl J Med 2005;352: 2285-2293.

333. Yin T, Miyata T:Warfarin dose and the pharmacogenomics of CYP2C9 and VKORC1—rationale and perspectives. Thromb Res 2007; 120(1):1-10.

334. Ingelman-Sundberg M: Pharmacogenetic biomarkers for prediction of adverse drug reactions. N Engl J Med 208;358:637-639.

335. Stroke Prevention in Reversible Ischemia Trial (SPIRIT) Study Group: A randomized trial of anticoagulants versus aspirin after cerebral ischemia of presumed arterial origin. Ann Neurol 1997;42:857-865.

336. Atrial Fibrillation Investigators: Risk factors for stroke and efficacy of antithrombotic therapy in atrial fibrillation: Analysis of pooled data from 5 randomized clinical trials. Arch Intern Med 1994;154:1949-1957.

337. Hart RG: Oral anticoagulation for secondary prevention of stroke. Cerebrovasc Dis 1997;7(suppl 6):24-29.

338. Hylek EM, Skates SJ, Sheehan MA, Singer DE: An analysis of the lowest effective intensity of prophylactic anticoagulation for patients with nonrheumatic atrial fibrillation. N Engl J Med 1996;335:540-546.

339. Fleming HA, Bailey SM: Mitral valve disease, systemic embolism and anticoagulants. Postgrad Med J 1971;47:599-604.

340. Adams GF, Merrett JD, Hutchinson WM, Pollock AM: Cerebral embolism and mitral stenosis: Survival with and without anticoagulants. J Neurol Neurosurg Psychiatry 1974;37:378-383.

341. Carter AB: Prognosis of cerebral embolism. Lancet 1965;2:514-519.

342. Caplan LR: Brain embolism. In Caplan LR, Chimowitz MI, Hurst JW. Clinical Neurocardiology. New York: Marcel Dekker, 1999, pp 35-185.

343. Boston Area Anticoagulation Trial for Atrial Fibrillation Investigators: The effect of low-dose warfarin on the risk of stroke in patients with nonrheumatic atrial fibrillation. N Engl J Med 1990;323:1505-1511.

344. EAFT (European Atrial Fibrillation Trial) Study Group: Silent brain infarction in nonrheumatic atrial fibrillation. Neurology 1996;46:159-165.

345. EAFT (European Atrial Fibrillation Trial) Study Group: Secondary prevention in non-rheumatic atrial fibrillation after transient ischaemic attack or minor stroke. Lancet 1993;342:1255-1262.

346. Petersen P, Godtfredsen J, Boysen G, et al: Placebo-controlled, randomized trial of warfarin and aspirin for prevention of thromboembolic complications in chronic atrial fibrillation: The Copenhagen AFASAK study. Lancet 1989;1: 175-179.

347. Stroke Prevention in Atrial Fibrillation Investigators: The stroke prevention in atrial fibrillation study: Final results. Circulation 1991;84: 527-539.

348. Stroke Prevention in Atrial Fibrillation Investigators: Warfarin versus aspirin for prevention of thromboembolism in atrial fibrillation: Stroke Prevention in Atrial Fibrillation II Study. Lancet 1994;343:687-691.

349. Stroke Prevention in Atrial Fibrillation Investigators: Adjusted-dose warfarin versus low-intensity, fixed-dose warfarin plus aspirin for high-risk patients with atrial fibrillation: Stroke Prevention in Atrial Fibrillation III randomised clinical trial. Lancet 1996;348:633-638.

350. Albers G: Atrial fibrillation and stroke. Three new studies, three remaining questions. Arch Intern Med 1994;154:1443-1448.

351. Manning WJ: Cardiac source of embolism: Treatment. In Caplan LR, Manning WJ (eds): Brain Embolism. New York: Informa Healthcare, 2006, pp 289-318.

352. Cerebral Embolism Study Group: Immediate anticoagulation of embolic stroke: A randomized trial. Stroke 1983;14:668-676.

353. Chamorro A, Vila N, Saiz A, et al: Early anticoagulation after large cerebral embolic infarction. Neurology 1995;45:861-865.

354. Chamorro A, Vila N, Ascaso C, Blanc R: Heparin in acute stroke with atrial fibrillation. Clinical relevance of early treatment. Arch Neurol 1999;56:1098-1102.

355. Cerebral Embolism Task Force: Cardiogenic brain embolism. Arch Neurol 1986;43:71-84.

356. Cerebral Embolism Task Force: Cardiogenic brain embolism. The second report of the Cerebral Embolism Task Force. Arch Neurol 1989;46:727-743.

357. Cerebral Embolism Study Group: Immediate anticoagulation of embolic stroke: Brain hemorrhage and management options. Stroke 1984;15:779-789.

358. Furlan AJ, Cavalier S, Hobbs RE, et al: Hemorrhage and anticoagulation after nonseptic embolic brain infarction. Neurology 1982;32:280-282.

359. Pessin MS, Estol C, Lafranchise F, Caplan LR: Safety of anticoagulation after hemorrhagic infarction. Neurology 1993;43:1298-1303.

360. Chamorro A, Vila N, Saiz A, et al: Early anticoagulation after large cerebral embolic infarction. Neurology 1995;45:861-865.

361. Nater B, Bogousslavsky J, Regli F, Stauffer J-C: Stroke patterns with atrial septal aneurysms. Cerebrovasc Dis 1992;2:342-346.

362. Belkin RN, Hurwitz BJ, Kisslo J: Atrial septal aneurysm: Association with cerebrovascular and peripheral embolic events. Stroke 1987;18:856-862.

363. Cabanes L, Mas JL, Cohen A, et al: Atrial septal aneurysm and patent foramen ovale as risk factors for cryptogenic stroke in patients less than 55 years of age. A study using transesophageal echocardiography. Stroke 1993;24:1865-1873.

364. Mas JL, Arquizan C, Lamy C, et al: Recurrent cerebrovascular events associated with patent foramen ovale, atrial septal aneurysm, or both. N Engl J Med 2001;345:1740-1746.

365. Grosgogeat Y, Lhermitte F, Carpenter A, et al: Aneurysme de la cloison interauriculaire revele par une embolie cerebrale. Arch Mal Coeur 1973;66:169-177.

366. Silver MD, Dorsey JS: Aneurysms of the septum primum in adults. Arch Pathol Lab Med 1978;102:62-65.

367. Bogousslavsky J, Garazi S, Jeanrenaud X, et al: Stroke recurrence in patients with patent foramen ovale: The Lausanne study. Neurology 1996;46:1301-1305.

368. French Study Group on Patent Foramen Ovale and Atrial Septal Aneurysm: Recurrent cerebrovascular events in patients with patent foramen ovale or atrial septal aneurysms and cryptogenic stroke or TIA. Am Heart J 1995;130:1083-1088.

369. Bridges ND, Hellensbrand W, Catson L, et al: Transcatheter closure of patent foramen ovale after presumed paradoxical embolism. Circulation 1982;86:1902-1908.

370. Homma S, Sacco RL, Di Tullio MR, et al: Effect of medical treatment in stroke patients with patent foramen ovale: Patent Foramen Ovale in Cryptogenic Stroke Study. Circulation 2002;105:893-898.

371. Mohr JP, Thompson JLP, Lazar RM, et al: A comparison of warfarin and aspirin for the prevention of recurrent ischemic stroke.

372. Bousser M-G, Ross Russell R: Cerebral venous thrombosis. London: WB Saunders, 1997.

373. Ameri A, Bousser M-G: Cerebral venous thrombosis. Neurol Clin 1992;10:87-111.

374. Jacewicz M, Plum F: Aseptic cerebral venous thrombosis. In Einhaupl K, Kempski O, Baethmann A (eds): Cerebral Sinus Thrombosis: Experimental and Clinical Aspects. New York: Plenum, 1990, pp 157-170.

375. Einhaupl KM, Villringer A, Meister W, et al: Heparin treatment in sinus venous thrombosis. Lancet 1991;338:597-600.

376. Meister W, Einhaupl K, Villringer A, et al: Treatment of patients with cerebral sinus and vein thrombosis with heparin. In Einhaupl K, Kempski O, Baethmann A (eds): Cerebral Sinus Thrombosis. Experimental and Clinical Aspects. New York: Plenum, 1990, pp 225-230.

377. De Bruijn SF, Stam J: Randomized, placebo-controlled trial of anticoagulant treatment with low-molecular-weight heparin for cerebral venous thrombosis. Stroke 1999;30:484-488.

378. Caplan LR: Venous and dural sinus thrombosis. In Caplan LR: Posterior Circulation Disease. Clinical Findings, Diagnosis, and Management. Boston: Blackwell Science, 1996, pp 569-592.

379. Diaz JM, Schiffman JS, Urban ES: Superior sagittal sinus thrombosis and pulmonary embolism: A syndrome rediscovered. Acta Neurol Scand 1992;86:390-396.

380. Caplan LR: Resolved: Heparin may be useful in selected patients with brain ischemia. Stroke 2003;34:230-231.

381. Caplan LR: Anticoagulants to prevent stroke occurrence and worsening. Israel Med Assoc J: 2006;8:773-778.

382. Caplan LR: Worsening in ischemic stroke patients: Is it time for a new strategy? Stroke 2002;33:1443-1445.

383. International Stroke Trial Collaboration Group: The International Stroke Trial (IST): A randomised trial of aspirin, subcutaneous heparin, both, or neither among 19,435 patients with acute stroke. Lancet 1997;349:1569-1581.

384. Kay R, Wong KS, Yu YL, et al: Low-molecular-weight heparin for the treatment of acute ischemic stroke. N Engl J Med 1995;333:1588-1593.

385. Publications Committee for the Trial of ORG 10172 in Acute Stroke Treatment (TOAST) Investigators: Low molecular weight heparinoid, ORG 10172 (Danaparoid), and outcome after acute ischemic stroke. A randomized controlled trial. JAMA 1998;279:1265-1272.

386. Adams HP, Bendixen BH, Leira EC, et al: Antithrombotic treatment of ischemic stroke among patients with occlusion or severe stenosis of the internal carotid artery: A report of the Trial of Org 10172 in Acute Stroke Treatment (TOAST). Neurology 1999;53:122-125.

387. Wong KS, Chen C, Ng PW, et al: Low-molecular-weight heparin compared with

Warfarin-Aspirin Recurrent Stroke Study Group. N Engl J Med 2001;345:1444-1451.

aspirin for the treatment of acute ischaemic stroke in Asian patients with large artery occlusive disease: A randomized study. FISS-tris Study Investigators. Lancet Neurol 2007; 6:407-413.

388. Chimowitz MI, Lynn MJ, Howlett-Smith H, et al: Comparison of warfarin and aspirin for symptomatic intracranial arterial stenosis. N Engl J Med 2005;352:1305-1316.

389. Koroshetz W: Warfarin, aspirin, and intracranial vascular disease. N Engl J Med 2005;352: 1368-1370.

390. Samsa GP, Matchar DB, Goldstein LB, et al: Quality of anticoagulation management among patients with atrial fibrillation. Results of a review of medical records from 2 communities. Arch Intern Med 2000;160:967-973.

391. Chiquette E, Amato MG, Bussey HL: Comparison of an anticoagulation clinic with usual medical care: Anticoagulation control, patient outcomes, and health care costs. Arch Intern Med 1998;158:1641-1647.

392. Kucher N, Connolly S, Beckman JA, et al: International normalized ratio increase before warfarin-associated hemorrhage: Brief and subtle. Arch Intern Med 2004:164:2176-2179.

393. Di Nisio M, Middledorp S, Buller H: Direct thrombin inhibitors. N Eng J Med 2005;353:1028-1040.

394. Kobayashi W, Tazaki Y: Effect of the thrombin inhibitor argabatran in acute cerebral thrombosis. Semin Thromb Hemost 1997;23:531-534.

395. Lewis BE, Wallis DE, Leya F, et al: Argabatran anticoagulation in patients with heparin-induced thrombocytopenia. Arch Intern Med 2003;163:1849-1856.

396. LaMonte MP, Nash ML, Wang DZ, et al: Argabatran anticoagulation in patients with acute ischemic stroke (ARGIS-1). Stroke 2004;35:1677-1682.

397. Fiessinger J-N, Huisman MV, Davidson BL, et al: Ximelagatran vs low-molecular-weight heparin and warfarin for the treatment of deep vein thrombosis: A randomized trial. THRIVE Treatment Study Investigators. JAMA 2005;293:681-689.

398. Olsson SB: Executive Steering Committee on Behalf of SPORTIF III Investigators. Stroke prevention with the oral direct thrombin inhibitor ximelagatran compared with warfarin in patients with non-valvular atrial fibrillation (SPORTIF III): Randomized controlled trial. Lancet 2003;362:1691-1698.

399. Albers GW, Diener HC, Frison L, et al: Ximelagatran vs warfarin for stroke prevention in patients with nonvalvular atrial fibrillation: A randomized trial. SPORTIF Executive Steering Committee for the SPORTIF V Investigators. JAMA 2005;293:690-698.

400. Akins PT, Feldman HA, Zoble RG, et al: Secondary stroke prevention with ximelagatran versus warfarin in patients with atrial fibrillation.

Pooled anaysis of SPORTIF III and V clinical trials. Stroke 2007;38:874-880.

401. Bauer KA: New anticoagulants: Anti IIa vs anti Xa—Is one better? J Thromb Thrombolysis 2006;21:67-72.

402. Turpie AG, Bauer KA, Eriksson BI, Lassen MR: Postoperative Fondaparinux vs enoxaparin for the prevention of venous thromboembolism in major orthopedic surgery: A meta-analysis of 4 randomized double-blind studies. Arch Intern Med 2002;162:1833-1840.

403. Cohen AT, Davidson BL, Gallus AS, et al: Efficacy and safety of fondaparinux for the prevention of venous thromboembolism in older acute medical patients: Randomised placebo controlled trial. ARTEMIS Investigators. BMJ 2006;332:325-329.

404. Yusuf S, Mehta SR, Chrolavicius S, et al: Comparison of fondaparinux and enoxaparin in acute coronary syndromes. Fifth Organization to Assess Strategies in Acute Ischemic Syndromes Investigators. N Engl J Med 2006;354:1464-1476.

405. OASIS-6 Trial Group: Effects of fondaparinux on mortality and reinfarction in patients with acute ST-segment elevation myocardial infarction. The OASIS-6 randomized trial. JAMA 2006;295: 1519-1530.

406. Rajagopal V, Bhatt DL: Factor Xa inhibitors in acute coronary syndromes: Moving from mythology to reality. J Thromb Haemostasis 2005;3: 436-438.

407. Fields WS, Lemak NA: A history of stroke: Its recognition and treatment. New York: Oxford University Press, 1989, pp 115-119.

408. Craven LL: Experiences with aspirin (acetylsalicylic acid) in the nonspecific prophylaxis of coronary thrombosis. Mississippi Valley Med J 1953;75:38-44.

409. Craven LL: Prevention of coronary and cerebral thrombosis. Mississippi Valley Med J 1956;78:213-215.

410. Mundall J, Quintero P, von Kaulla K, et al: Transient monocular blindness and increased platelet aggregability treated with aspirin—a case report. Neurology 1971;21:402.

411. Harrison MJG, Marshall J, Meadows JC, et al: Effect of aspirin in amaurosis fugax. Lancet 1971;2:743-744.

412. Fields WS, Lemak N, Frankowski R, et al: Controlled trial of aspirin in cerebral ischemia. Stroke 1977;8:301-306.

413. Barnett HJM: The Canadian Cooperative Study: A randomial trial of aspirin and sulfinpyrazone in threatened stroke. N Engl J Med 1978;299:53-59.

414. Moncada S, Vane J: Arachidonic acid metabolites and the interactions between platelets and blood vessel walls. N Engl J Med 1979; 300:1142-1147.

415. Nurden AT: Platelet function and pharmacology of antiplatelet drugs. Cerebrovasc Dis 1997;7 (suppl 6):2-9.

416. Moncada C: Biologic and therapeutic potential of prostacyclin. Stroke 1983;14:157-168.

417. Preston F, Whipps S, Jackson C, et al: Inhibition of prostacyclin and platelet thromboxane A2 after low dose aspirin. N Engl J Med 1981;304:76-79.

418. Weksler B, Pelt S, Alonso D, et al: Differential inhibition by aspirin of vascular and platelet prostaglandin synthesis in atherosclerotic patients. N Engl J Med 1983;308:800-805.

419. UK-TIA Study Group: The UK-TIA Aspirin Trial: The interim results. BMJ 1988;296:316-320.

420. SALT Collaborative Group: Swedish Aspirin Low-Dose Trial (SALT) of 75 mg aspirin as secondary prophylaxis after cerebrovascular ischemic events. Lancet 1991;338:1345-1349.

421. Dutch TIA Trial Study Group: A comparison of two doses of aspirin (30 mg vs 283 mg a day) in patients after a transient ischemic attack or minor stroke. N Engl J Med 1991;325:1261-1266.

422. Schwartz KA: Aspirin resistance: A review of diagnostic methodology, mechanisms, and clinical utility. Adv Clin Chem 2006;42:81-110.

423. Helgason CM, Hoff JA, Kondos GT, Brace LD: Platelet aggregation in patients with atrial fibrillation taking aspirin or warfarin. Stroke 1993;24:1458-1461.

424. Helgason CM, Tortorice L, Winkler S, et al: Aspirin response and failure in cerebral infarction. Stroke 1993;24:345-350.

425. Dalen JE: Aspirin resistance: Is it real? Is it clinically significant? Am J Med 2007;120:1-4.

426. Chen W-H, Cheng X, Lee P-Y, et al: Aspirin resistance and adverse clinical events in patients with coronary artery disease. Am J Med 2007;120:631-635.

427. Hohlfeld T, Weber A-A, Junghans U, et al: Variable platelet response to aspirin in patients with ischemic stroke. Cerebrovasc Dis 2007; 24:43-50.

428. Caplan LR: Antiplatelet therapy in stroke prevention: Present and future. Cerbrovasc Dis 2006;21(suppl 1);1-6.

429. Fitzgerald GA: Dipyridamole. N Engl J Med 1987;316:1247-1257.

430. Honour A, Hochaday T, Mann J: The synergistic effect of aspirin and dipyridamole upon platelet thrombi in living blood vessels. Br J Exp Path 1977;58:268-272.

431. Sullivan J, Harken D, Gorlin R: Pharmacologic control of thromboembolic complications of aortic valve replacement. N Engl J Med 1971; 284:1391-1394.

432. Fields WS, Yatsu F, Conomy J, et al: Persantine-aspirin trial in cerebral ischemia: The American-Canadian Cooperative Study group. Stroke 1983;14:97-103.

433. Bousser MG, Eschwege E, Hagenah M, et al: AICLA controlled trial of aspirin and dipyridamole in the secondary prevention of athero-thrombotic cerebral ischemia. Stroke 1983;14:5-14.

434. ESPS Group: European Stroke Prevention Study (ESPS): Principal endpoints. Lancet 1987;2: 1351-1354.

435. Diener HC, Cunha L, Forbes C, et al: European Stroke Prevention Study 2. Dipyridamole and acetylsalicylic acid in the secondary prevention of stroke. J Neurol Sci 1996;143:1-13.

436. Leonardi-Bee J, Bath PMW, Bousser M-G, et al: Dipyridamole for preventing recurrent ischemic stroke and other vascular events. A meta-analysis of individual patient data from randomized controlled trials. Stroke 2005;36:162-168.

437. Sacco RL, Sivenius J, Diener H-C: Efficacy of aspirin plus extended-release dipyridamole in preventing recurrent stroke in high-risk populations. Arch Neurol 2005;62:403-408.

438. ESPRIT Study Group: Aspirin plus dipyridamole versus aspirin alone after cerebral ischaemia of arterial origin (ESPRIT): Randomized controlled trial. Lancet 2006;367:1665-1673.

439. Verro P, Gorelick PB, Nguyen D: Aspirin plus dipyridamole versus aspirin for prevention of vascular events after stroke or TIA: A meta-analysis

440. Bousser M-G, Roberts RS, Gent M: Ticlopidine and Clopidogrel in secondary stroke prevention. Cerebrovasc Dis 1997;7(suppl 6):17-23.

441. Sharis PJ, Cannon CP, Loscalzo J: The antiplatelet effects of ticlopidine and clopidogrel. Ann Intern Med 1998;129:394-405.

442. Hass WK, Easton JD, Adams HP, et al: A randomized trial comparing ticlopidine hydrochloride with aspirin for the prevention of stroke in high-risk patients. N Engl J Med 1989;321: 501-507.

443. Gent M, Easton JD, Hachinski V, et al: The Canadian American Ticlopidine Study (CATS) in thromboembolic stroke. Lancet 1989;1: 1215-1220.

444. Bennett CL, Weinberg PD, Rozenberg-Ben-Dror K, et al: Thrombotic thrombocytopenic purpura associated with ticlopidine. A report of 60 cases. Ann Intern Med 1998;128:541-544.

445. CAPRIE Steering Committee: A randomised, blinded, trial of clopidogrel versus aspirin in patients at risk of ischaemic events. Lancet 1996;348:1329-1339.

446. Bennett CL, Connors JM, Carwile JM, et al: Thrombotic thrombocytopenic purpura associated with clopidogrel. N Engl J Med 2000;342:1773-1777.

447. Diener H-C, Bogousslavsky J, Brass LM, et al: Aspirin and clopidogrel vs clopidogrel alone after recent ischemic stroke or transient ischemic attack in high-risk patients (MATCH): Randomized, double-blind, placebo-controlled trial. MATCH Investigators. Lancet 2004;364:331-337.

448. Hankey GJ, Eikelboom JW: Adding aspirin to clopidogrel after TIA and ischemic stroke. Benefits do not match risks. Neurology 2005;64: 1117-1121.

449. Bhatt DL, Fox KAA, Hacke W, et al: Clopidogrel and aspirin versus aspirin alone for the prevention of atherothrombotic events. CHARISMA Investigators. N Engl J Med 2006;354:1706-1717.

450. Steinhubl SR, Berger PB, Mann JT III, et al: Early and sustained dual oral antiplatelet therapy following precutaneous coronary intervention: A randomized controlled trial. JAMA 2002;288:2411-2420.

451. Chaturverdi S, Yadav JS: The role of antiplatelet therapy in carotid stenting for ischemic stroke prevention. Stroke 2006;37:1572-1577.

452. Clopidogrel in Unstable Angina to Prevent Recurrent Events Trial Investigators: Effect of clopidogrel in addition to aspirin in patients with acute coronary syndromes without ST-segment elevation. N Engl J Med 2001;345:494-502.

453. Chen ZM, Jiang LX, Chen YP, et al: Addition of clopidogrel to aspirin in 45,852 patients with acute myocardial infarction: Randomised placebo-controlled trial. Lancet 2005;366:1607-1621.

454. Sacco RL, Diener H-C, Yusuf S, et al for the PRoFESS Study Group: Aspirin and extended-release dipyridamole versus clopidogrel for recurrent stroke. N Engl J Med 2008;359:1238-1251.

454a. Yusuf S, Diener H-C, Sacco RL, et al for the PRoFESS Study Group: Telmisartan to prevent recurrent stroke and cardiovascular events. N Engl J Med 2008;359:1225-1237.

455. Wiviott SD, Braunwald E, McCabe CH, et al: Prasugrel versus clopidogrel in patients with acute coronary syndromes. TRITON-TIMI 38 Investigators. N Engl J Med 2007;357:2001-2015.

456. Ikeda Y, Kikuchi M, Murakami H: Comparison of the inhibitory effects of cilostazol, acetylsalicylic acid, and ticlopidine on platelet function ex vivo: Randomized, double-blind cross-over study. Drug Res 1987;37:563-566.

457. Tanaka K, Ishikawa T, Hagiwara M, et al: Effects of cilostazol, a selective camp phosphodiesterase inhibitor, on the contraction of vascular smooth muscle. Pharmacology 1988;36:313-320.

458. Gotoh F, Tohgi H, Hirai S, et al: Cilostazol Stroke Prevention Study: A placebo-controlled double-blind trial for secondary prevention of cerebral infarction. J Stroke Cerebrovasc Dis 2000;9:147-157.

459. Kwon SU, Cho Y-J, Koo J-S, et al: Cilostazol prevents the progression of the symptomatic intracranial stenosis. The multicenter double-blind placebo-controlled trial of cilostazol in symptomatic intracranial arterial stenosis. Stroke 2005;36:782-786.

460. Ameriso S, Lagos R, Ferreira LM, et al: Cerebrovascular effects of cilostazol in patients with atherosclerotic disease. J Stroke Cerebrovasc Dis 2006;15:273-276.

461. Weksler B: Antiplatelet agents in stroke prevention. Cerebrovasc Dis 2000;10(suppl 5)41-48.

462. Tcheng JE: Differences among the parenteral glycoprotein IIb/IIIa inhibitors and implications for treatment. Am J Cardiol 1999;83:7E-15E:

463. Lefkovits J, Plow EF, Topol EJ: Platelet glycoprotein IIb/IIIa receptors in cardiovascular medicine. N Engl J Med 1995;332:1553-1559.

464. Wallace RC, Furlan AJ, Moliterno DJ, et al: Basilar artery rethrombosis: Successful treatment with platelet glycoprotein IIb/IIIa receptor inhibitor. AJNR Am J Neuroradiol 1997;18:1257-1260.

465. Abciximab in Acute Ischemic Stroke Investigators: Abciximab in acute ischemic stroke: A randomized, double-blind, placebo-controlled dose-escalation study. Stroke 2000;31:601-609.

466. Qureshi AI, Harris-Lane P, Kirmani JF, et al: Intra-arterial reteplase and intravenous abciximab in patients with acute ischemic stroke: An open-label, dose-ranging, phase I study. Neurosurgery 2006;59:789-796.

467. Eckert B, Koch C, Thomalla G, et al: Aggressive therapy with intravenous abciximab and intra-arterial rtPA and additional PTA/stenting improves clinical outcome in acute vertebrobasilar occlusion: Combined local fibrinolysis and intravenous abciximab in acute vertebrobasilar stroke treatment (FAST): Results of a multicenter study. Stroke 2005;36:1160-1165.

468. Velat GJ, Burry MV, Eskioglu E, et al: The use of abciximab in the treatment of acute cerebral thromboembolic events during neuroendovascular procedures. Surg Neurol 2006;65:352-358.

469. Heer T, Zeymer U, Juenger C, et al: Beneficial effects of abciximab in patients with primary percutaneous intervention for acute ST segment elevation myocardial infarction in clinical practice. Acute Coronary Syndromes Registry Investigators. Heart 2006;92:1484-1489.

470. De Luca G, Suryapranata H, Stone GW, et al: Abciximab as adjunctive therapy to reperfusion in acute ST-segment elevation myocardial infarction: A meta-analysis of randomized trials. JAMA 2005;293:1759-1765.

471. Coller BS: Anti GpIIb/IIIa drugs: Current status and future directions. Thromb Haemostast 2001;86:427-443.

472. Topol E, Easton D, Harrington R, et al: Randomized double-blind placebo-controlled international trial of the oral IIb/IIIa antagonist lotrafiban in coronary and cerebrovascular disease. Circulation 2003;108:16-23.

473. Dyerberg J, Bang H, Stofferson E, et al: Eicosopentanoic acid and prevention of thrombosis and atherosclerosis. Lancet 1978;2:117-119.

474. Kimura Y, Shimizu M, Kohara S, et al: Antiplatelet effects of a Kampo medicine, Orengedokuto. J Stroke Cerebrovasc Dis 2006;15:277-282.

475. Antiplatelet Trialists' Collaboration: Secondary prevention of vascular disease by prolonged antiplatelet treatment. BMJ 1988;296:320-331.

476. Antiplatelet Trialists' Collaboration: Collaborative overview of randomised trials of antiplatelet therapy. 1. Prevention of death, myocardial infarction, and stroke by prolonged antiplatelet therapy in various categories of patients. BMJ 1994;308:81-106.

477. Antithrombotic Trialists' Collaboration: Collaborative meta-analysis of randomized trials of

5

antiplatelet therapy for prevention of death, myocardial infarction, and stroke in high risk patients. BMJ 2002;524:71-86.

478. Gubitz G, Sandercock P, Counsell C: Antiplatelet therapy for acute ischaemic stroke. Cochrane Database Syst Rev 2000;(2):CD000029. Cochrane Database Syst Rev 2003;(2):CD000029.

479. Tran H, Anand SS: Oral antiplatelet therapy in cerebrovascular disease, coronary artery disease, and peripheral arterial disease. JAMA 2004;292:1867-1874.

480. Diener H-C: Secondary stroke prevention with antiplatelet drugs: have we reached the ceiling? Int J Stroke 2006;1:4-8.

481. Miller A, Lees R: Simultaneous therapy with antiplatelet and anticoagulant drugs in symptomatic cardiovascular disease. Stroke 1985;16:668-675.

482. Chesebro J, Fuster V, Elveback L, et al: Trial of combined warfarin plus dipyridamole or aspirin therapy in prosthetic heart valve replacement: Danger of aspirin combined with warfarin. Am J Cardiol 1983;51:1537-1541.

483. Garcia J: Mechanisms of cell death in ischemia. In Caplan LR (ed): Brain Ischemia: Basic Concepts and Clinical Relevance. London: Springer, 1995, pp 7-18.

484. Plum F: What causes infarction in ischemic brain? Neurology 1983;33:222-233.

485. Myers R: Lactic acid accumulation as a cause of brain edema and cerebral necrosis resulting from oxygen deprivation. In Korobkin R, Guilleminault C (eds): Advances in Perinatal Neurology. New York: Spectrum, 1979, pp 88-114.

486. McCord JM: Oxygen-derived free radicals in postischemic tissue injury. N Engl J Med 1985;312:159-163.

487. Floyd RA: Production of free radicals. In Welch KMA, Caplan LR, Reis DJ, et al (eds): Primer on Cerebrovascular Diseases. San Diego: Academic, 1997, pp 165-169.

488. Kontos H: Oxygen radicals in cerebral ischemia: The 2001 Willis Lecture. Stroke 2001;32:2712-2716.

489. Ginsberg MD: Adventures in the pathophysiology of brain ischemia: Penumbra, gene expression, neuroprotection: The 2002 Thomas Willis Lecture. Stroke 2003;34:214-223.

490. Busto R, Dietrich WD, Globus MYT, et al: The importance of brain temperature in cerebral ischemic injury. Stroke 1989;20:1113-1114.

491. Dietrich WD, Busto R: Hyperthermia and Brain Ischemia. In Welch KMA, Caplan LR, Reis DJ, et al (eds): Primer on Cerebrovascular Diseases. San Diego: Academic, 1997, pp 165-169.

492. Siesjo BK, Bengtsson F: Calcium fluxes, calcium antagonists, and calcium-related pathology in brain ischemia, hypoglycemia and spreading depression: A unifying hypothesis. J Cereb Blood Flow Metab 1989;9:127-140.

493. Tymianski M, Sattler RG: Is calcium involved in excitotoxic or ischemic neuronal damage? In Welch KMA, Caplan LR, Reis DJ, et al (eds): Primer on Cerebrovascular Diseases. San Diego: Academic, 1997, pp 190-192.

494. Siesjo B: Historical overview: Calcium, ischemia and death of brain cells. Ann N Y Acad Sci 1988; 522:638-661.

495. Siesjo B, Smith M-L: Mechanism of acidosis-related damage. In Welch KMA, Caplan LR, Reis DJ, et al (eds): Primer on Cerebrovascular Diseases. San Diego: Academic, 1997, pp 223-226.

496. Adams HP, Olingrr CP, Marler JR, et al: Comparison of admission serum glucose concentration with neurologic outcome in cerebral infarction. Stroke 1988;19:455-458.

497. Woo E, Lam CW, Kay R: The influence of hyperglycemia and diabetes mellitus on immediate and 3-month morbidity and mortality after acute stroke. Arch Neurol 1990;47:1174-1177.

498. Alvarez-Sabin J, Molina C, Montaner J, et al: Effects of admission hyperglycemia on stroke outcome in reperfused tissue plasminogen activator—treated patients. Stroke 2003;34: 1235-1241.

499. Passero S, Ciacci G, Ulivelli M: The influence of diabetes and hyperglycemia on clinical course after intracerebral hemorrhage. Neurology 2003;61:1351-1356.

500. Choi DW: The Excitotoxic Concept. In Welch KMA, Caplan LR, Reis DJ, et al (eds): Primer on Cerebrovascular Diseases. San Diego: Academic, 1997, pp 187-190.

501. Choi DW: Excitotoxicity and stroke. In Caplan LR (ed): Brain Ischemia: Basic Concepts and Clinical Relevance. London: Springer, 1995, pp 29-36.

502. Olney JW: Brain lesion, obesity, and other disturbances in mice treated with monosodium glutamate. Science 1969;164:719-721.

503. Meldrum B: Excitotoxicity in ischemia: An overview. In Ginsberg MD, Dietrich WD (eds): Cerebrovascular Diseases. New York: Raven Press, 1989, pp 47-60.

504. Small DL, Buchan AM: NMDA and AMPA receptor antagonists in global and focal ischemia. In Welch KMA, Caplan LR, Reis DJ, et al (eds): Primer on Cerebrovascular Diseases. San Diego: Academic, 1997, pp 244-247.

505. Onai MZ, Fisher M: Thrombolytic and cytoprotective therapies for acute ischemic stroke: A clinical overview. Drugs Today 1996;32: 573-592.

506. Lees KR: Cerestat and other NMDA antagonists in ischemic stroke. Neurology 1997;49(suppl 4): S66-S69.

507. Nighoghossian N, Trouillas P, Adeleine P, Salord F: Hyperbaric oxygen in the treatment of acute ischemic stroke. A double-blind pilot study. Stroke 1995;26:1369-1372.

508. Rusyniak DE, Kirk MA, May JD, et al: Hyperbaric oxygen therapy in acute ischemic stroke: Results of the Hyperbaric Oxygen in Acute Ischemic Stroke Trial Pilot Study. Stroke 2003;34:571-574.

509. Kim HY, Singhal AB, Lo EH: Normobaric hyperoxia extends the reperfusion window in focal cerebral ischemia. Ann Neurol 2005;57: 571-575.

510. Singhal AB, Benner T, Roccatagliata L, et al: A pilot study of normobaric oxygen therapy in acute ischemic stroke. Stroke 2005;36: 797-802.

511. Ginsberg MD: Hypothermic neuroprotection in cerebral ischemia. In Welch KMA, Caplan LR, Reis DJ, et al (eds): Primer on Cerebrovascular Diseases. San Diego: Academic, 1997, pp 272-275.

512. Bernard SA, Gray TW, Buist MD, et al: Treatment of comatose survivors of out-of-hospital cardiac arrest with induced hypothermia. N Engl J Med 2002;346:557-563.

513. Mayer SA: Hypothermia for neuroprotection after cardiac arrest. Curr Neurol Neurosci Rep 2002;2:525-526.

514. Schwab S, Schwarz S, Spranger M, et al: Moderate hypothermia in the treatment of patients with severe middle cerebral artery infarction. Stroke 1998;29:2461-2466.

515. Schwab S, Georgiadis D, Berrouschot J, et al: Feasibility and safety of moderate hypothermia after massive hemispheric infarction. Stroke 2001;32:2033-2035.

516. Georgiadis D, Schwarz S, Aschoff A, Schwab S: Hemicraniectomy and moderate hypothermia in patients with severe ischemic stroke. Stroke 2002;33:1584-1588.

517. Abou-Chebl A, DeGeorgia MA, Andrefsky JC, Krieger DW: Technical refinements and drawbacks of a surface cooling technique for the treatment of severe acute ischemic stroke. Neurocrit Care 2004;1:131-143.

518. Krieger DW, De Georgia MA, Abou-Chebl A, et al: Cooling for acute ischemic brain damage (cool aid): An open pilot study of induced hypothermia in acute ischemic stroke. Stroke 2001;32:1847-1854.

519. Safar P: Amelioration of post-ischemic brain damage with barbiturates. Current concepts in cerebrovascular disease. Stroke 1980;15:1-5.

520. Black K, Weidler J, Jallad N, et al: Delayed pentobarbital therapy of acute focal cerebral ischemia. Stroke 1978;9:245-251.

521. Stroke Therapy Academic Industry Roundtable II (STAIR-II): Recommendations for clinical trial evaluation of acute stroke therapies. Stroke 2001;32:1598-1606.

522. Fisher M: Recommendations for advancing development of acute stroke therapies: Stroke Therapy Academic Industry Roundtable 3. Stroke 2003;34:1539-1546.

523. Fisher M, Albers GW, Donnan GA, et al: Enhancing the development and approval of acute stroke therapies: Stroke Therapy Academic Industry Roundtable. Stroke 2005; 36:1808-1813.

524. Shepherd J, Cobbe SM, Ford I, et al: Prevention of coronary heart disease with pravastatin in men with hypercholesterolemia. N Engl J Med 1995;333:1301-1307.

525. Scandinavian Simastatin Survival Study Group: Randomised trial of cholesterol lowering of 444 patients with coronary heart disease: The Scandinavian Simvastatin Survival Study (4S). Lancet 1994;344:1383-1389.

526. Sacks FM, Pfeffer MA, Moye LA, et al: The effect of pravastatin on coronary events after myocardial infarction in patients with average cholesterol levels. N Engl J Med 1996;335:1001-1009.

527. Hebert P, Gaziano JM, Chan KS, Hennekens CH: Cholesterol lowering with statin drugs, risk of stroke, and total mortality. An overview of randomized trials. JAMA 1997;278:313-321.

528. Blauw GJ, Lagaay AM, Smelt AHM, et al: Stroke, statins, and cholesterol. A meta-analysis of randomized placebo-controlled double-blind trials with HMG-CoA reductase inhibitors. Stroke 1997;28:946-950.

529. Bucher HC, Griffith LE, Guyatt GH: Effect of HMGcoA reductase inhibitors on stroke. A meta-analysis of randomized controlled trials. Ann Intern Med 1998;128:89-95.

530. Nissen SE, Tuzcu M, Schoenhagen P: Stain therapy, LDL cholesterol, C-reactive protein, and coronary artery disease. Reversal of Atherosclerosis with Aggressive Lipid Lowering (REVERSAL) Investigators. N Engl J Med 2005;352:29-38.

531. Furberg CD, Adams HP, Applegate WB, et al: Effect of lovostatin on early carotid atherosclerosis and cardiovascular events. The Asymptomatic Carotid Artery Progression Study (ACAPS) Research Group. Circulation 1994;90:1679-1687.

532. Crouse JR, Byington RP, Bond MG, et al: Pravastatin, lipids, and atherosclerosis in the carotid arteries (PLAC II). Am J Cardiol 1995; 75:455-459.

533. Hodis HN, Mack WJ, LaBree L, et al: Reduction in carotid arterial wall thickness using lovastatin and dietary therapy. A randomized controlled clinical trial. Ann Intern Med 1996;124:548-556.

534. Stroke Prevention by Aggressive Reduction in Cholesterol Levels (SPARCL) Investigators: High-dose atorvastatin after stroke or transient ischemic attack. N Engl J Med 2006;355: 549-559.

535. Amarenco P, Goldstein LB, Szarek M, et al: Effects of intense low-density lipoprotein cholesterol reduction in patients with stroke or transient ischemic attack. The Stroke Prevention by Aggressive Reduction in Cholesterol Levels (SPARCL) Trial. Stroke 2007;38:3198-3204.

536. Vergouwen MDI, de Haan RJ, Vermuelen M, Roos YBWEM: Statin treatment and the occurrence of hemorrhagic stroke in patients with a history of cerebrovascular disease. Stroke 2008;39:497-502.

537. Sanossian N, Ovbiagele B: Drug insight: Translating evidence on statin therapy into clinical benefits. Nat Clin Pract Neurol 2008;4:43-49.

538. Schwartz GG, Olsson AG, Ezekowitz MD, et al: Effects of atorvastatin on early recurrent ischemic events in acute coronary syndromes. The MIRACL Study: A randomized controlled trial. JAMA 2001;285:1711-1718.

539. Elkind MS, Flint AC, Sciacca RR, Sacco RL: Lipid-lowering agent used at ischemic stroke

onset is associated with decreased mortality. Neurology 2005;65:253-258.

540. Amarenco P, Moskowitz MA: The dynamics of statins. From event prevention to neuroprotection. Stroke 2006;37:294-296.

541. Endres M, Laufs U, Huang Z, et al: Stroke protection by 3-hydroxy-3-methylglutaryl (HMG)-CoA reductase inhibitors mediated by endothelial nitric oxide synthase. Proc Nat Acad Sci U S A 1998;95:8880-8885.

542. Endres M, Laufs U, Liao JK, Moscowitz MA: Targetting eNOS for stroke protection. Trends Neurosci 2004;27:283-289.

543. Ridker PM, Rifai N, Rose L, et al: Comparison of C-reactive protein and low-density lipoprotein cholesterol levels in the prediction of first cardiovascular events. N Engl J Med 2002;347:1557-1565.

544. Eikelboom JW, Hankey GJ, Baker RI, et al: C-reactive protein in ischemic stroke and its etiologic subtypes. J Stroke Cerebrovasc Dis 2003;12:74-81.

545. Arenillas JF, Alvarez-Sabin J, Molina CA, et al: C-reactive protein predicts further ischemic events in first-ever transient ischemic attack or stroke patients with intracranial large-artery occlusive disease. Stroke 2003;34:2463-2470.

546. Rosenson RS, Tangney CC: Antiatherothrombotic properties of statins. Implications for cardiovascular event reduction. JAMA 1996;279:1643-1650.

547. Carod-Artal FJ: Statins and cerebral vasomotor reactivity. Implications for a new therapy. Stroke 2006;37:2446-2448.

548. Pretnar-Oblak J, Sabovic M, Sebestjen M, et al: The influence of atorvastatin treatment on L-arginine cerebrovascular reactivity and flow-mediated dilatation in patients with lacunar infarction. Stroke 2006;37:2540-2545.

549. Ovbiagele B, Kidwell CS, Saver JL: Expanding indications for statins in cerebral ischemia. A quantitative study. Arch Neurol 2005;62:67-72.

550. Endres M, Laufs U: Discontinuation of statin treatment in stroke patients. Stroke 2006;37:2640-2643.

551. Colivicchi F, Bassi A, Santini M, Caltagirone C: Discontinuation of statin therapy and clinical outcome after ischemic stroke. Stroke 2007;38:2652-2657.

552. Blanco M, Nombela F, Castellanos M, et al: Statin treatment withdrawal in ischemic stroke. A controlled randomized trial. Neurology 2007;69:904-910.

553. Dale KM, White CM, Henyan NN, Kluger J, Coleman CI: Impact of statin dosing intensity on transaminase and creatine kinase. Am J Med 2007;120:706-712.

554. Radcliffe KA, Campbell WW: Statin myopathy. Curr Neurol Neurosci Rep 2008;8:66-72.

555. Ropper AH, Gress DR, Diringer MN, et al: Neurological and Neurosurgical Intensive Care, 3rd ed. New York: Raven Press, 2003.

556. Kazui S, Naritomi H, Yamamoto H, et al: Enlargement of spontaneous intracerebral hemorrhage. Incidence and time course. Stroke 1996;27:1783-1787.

557. Brott T, Broderick J, Kothari R, et al: Early hemorrhage growth in patients with intracerebral hemorrhage. Stroke 1997;28:1-5.

558. Qureshi AI, Tuhrim S, Broderick JP, et al: Spontaneous intracerebral hemorrhage. N Engl J Med 2001;344:1450-1460.

559. Davis SM, Broderick J, Hennerici M, et al: Hematoma growth is a determinant of mortality and poor outcome after intracerebral hemorrhage. Recombinant Activated Factor VII Intracerebral Hemorrhage Trial Investigators. Neurology 2006;66:1175-1181.

560. Gebel Jr JM, Jauch EC, Brott TG, et al: Relative edema volume is a predictor of outcome in patients with hyperacute spontaneous intracerebral hemorrhage. Stroke 2002;33:2636-2641.

561. Mayer SA: Ultra-early hemostatic therapy for intracerebral hemorrhage. Stroke 2003;34:224-229.

562. Mayer SA, Brun NC, Broderick J, et al: Safety and feasibility of recombinant factor VIIa for acute intracerebral hemorrhage. Europe/AustralAsia NovoSeven ICH Trial Investigators. Stroke 2005;36:74-79.

563. Mayer SA, Brun NC, Begtrup K, et al: Recombinant activated factor VII for acute intracerebral hemorrhage. Recombinant Activated Factor VII Intracerebral Hemorrhage Trial Investigators. N Engl J Med 2005;352:777-785.

563a. Mayer SA, Brun NC, Begtrup K, et al for the FAST Trial Investigators: Efficacy and safety of recombinant activated factor VII for acute intracerebral hemorrhage. N Engl J Med 2008;358:2127-2137.

564. Sugg RM, Gonzales NR, Matherne DE, et al: Myocardial injury in patients with intracerebral hemorrhage treated with recombinant factor VIIa. Neurology 2006;67(6):934-935.

565. Kase CS, Crowell RM: Prognosis and treatment of patients with intracerebral hemorrhage. In Kase CS, Caplan LR (eds): Intracerebral Hemorrhage. Boston: Butterworth-Heinemann, 1994, pp 467-489.

566. Kase CS, Caplan LR: Therapy of intracerebral hemorrhage. In Brandt T, Caplan LR, Dichgans J, et al (eds): Neurological Disorders: Course and Treatment. San Diego: Academic, 1996, pp 277-288.

567. Rabinstein AA, Wijdicks EFM: Surgery for intracerebral hematoma: The search for the elusive right candidate. Rev Neurol Dis 2006;3:163-172.

568. Prasad K, Browman G, Srivastava A, Menon G: Surgery in primary supratentorial intracerebral hematoma: A meta-analysis of randomized trials. Acta Neurol Scand 1997;95:103-110.

569. Prasad K, Shrivastava A: Surgery for primary supratentorial intracerebral haemorrhage. Cochrane Database Syst Rev 2000;CD000200.

570. Mendelow AD, Gregson BA, Fernandes HM, et al: Early surgery versus initial conservative treatment in patients with spontaneous supratentorial intracerebral haematomas in the International Surgical Trial in Intracerebral Haemorrhage (STICH): A randomised trial. Lancet 2005;365:387-397.

571. Prasad KS, Gregson BA, Bhattathiri PS, et al: The significance of crossovers after randomization in the STICH trial. Acta Neurochir Suppl 2006; 96:61-64.

572. Bhattathiri PS, Gregson B, Prasad KS, et al: Intraventricular hemorrhage and hydrocephalus after spontaneous intracerebral hemorrhage: Results from the STICH trial. Acta Neurochir Suppl 2006;96:65-68.

573. Morgenstern LB, Demchuk AM, Kim DH, et al: Rebleeding leads to poor outcome in ultra-early craniotomy for intracerebral hemorrhage. Neurology 2001;56:1294-1299.

574. Shields CB, Friedman WA: The role of stereotactic technology in the management of intracerebral hemorrhage. Neurosurg Clin North Am 1992;3:685-702.

575. Niizuma H, Shimizu Y, Yonemitsu T, et al: Results of stereotactic aspiration in 175 cases of putaminal hemorrhage. Neurosurgery 1989; 24:814-819.

576. Marquardt G, Wolff R, Sager A, et al: Subacute stereotactic aspiration of haematomas within the basal ganglia reduces occurrence of complications in the course of haemorrhagic stroke in non-comatose patients. Cerebrovasc Dis 2003;15: 252-257.

577. Thiex R, Rohde V, Rohde I, et al: Frame-based and frameless stereotactic hematoma puncture and subsequent fibrinolytic therapy for the treatment of spontaneous intracerebral hemorrhage. J Neurol 2004;251:1443-1450.

578. Cho DY, Chen CC, Chang CS, et al: Endoscopic surgery for spontaneous basal ganglia hemorrhage: Comparing endoscopic surgery, stereotactic aspiration, and craniotomy in noncomatose patients. Surg Neurol 2006;65:547-556.

579. Naff NJ, Hanley DF, Keyl PM, et al: Intraventricular thrombolysis speeds blood clot resolution: Results of a pilot, prospective, randomized, double-blind, controlled trial. Neurosurgery 2004;54:577-584.

580. Zervas N, Hedley-White J: Successful treatment of cerebral herniation in five patients. N Engl J Med 1973;286:1075-1077.

581. Krieger D, Hacke W: The Intensive Care of the Stroke Patient. In Barnett HJM, et al (eds): Stroke: Pathophysiology, Diagnosis, and Management, 3rd ed. New York: Churchill Livingstone, 1998, pp 1133-1154.

582. O'Brien MD: Ischemic cerebral edema. In Caplan LR (ed): Brain Ischemia: Basic Concepts and Clinical Relevance. London: Springer, 1995, pp 43-50.

583. Klatzo I: Neuropathological aspects of brain edema. J Neuropathol Exp Neurol 1967; 26:1-14.

584. Newkirk T, Tourtellotte W, Reinglass J: Prolonged control of increased intracranial pressure with glycerin. Arch Neurol 1972;27:95-96.

585. Buckell M, Walsh L: Effect of glycerol by mouth on raised intracranial pressure in man. Lancet 1964;1:1151-1152.

586. Frank MS, Nahata MC, Hilty MD: Glycerol: A review of its pharmacology, pharmacokinetics, adverse reactions and clinical use. Pharmacotherapy 1981;1:147-160.

587. Marshall LF, Smith RW, Rauscher LA, et al: Mannitol dose requirements in brain-injured patients. J Neurosurg 1978;48:169-172.

588. Qureshi A, Suarez J: Use of hypertonic saline solutions in treatment of cerebral edema and intracranial hypertension. Crit Care Med 2000; 28:3301-3313.

589. Koenig MA, Bryan M, Lewin JL, et al: Reversal of transtentorial herniation with hypertonic saline. Neurology 2008;70:1023-1029.

590. Kuroiwa M, Shibutani M, Okeda R: Blood-brain barrier disruption and exacerbation of ischemic brain edema after restoration of blood flow in experimental focal cerebral ischemia. Acta Neuropathol 1988;76:62-70.

591. Mulley G, Wilcox R, Mitchell J: Dexamethasone in acute stroke. BMJ 1978;2:994-996.

592. O'Brien MD: Ischemic cerebral edema. A review. Stroke 1979;10:623-628.

593. Poungvarin N, Bhoopat W, Viriyavejakul A, et al: Effects of dexamethasone in primary supratentorial intracerebral hemorrhage. N Engl J Med 1987;316:1229-1233.

594. Bardutzky J, Schwab S: Antiedema therapy in ischemic stroke. Stroke 2007;38:3084-3094.

595. Shackford SR, Bourguignon PR, Wald SL, et al: Hypertonic saline resuscitation of patients with head injury: A prospective, randomized clinical trial. J Trauma 1998;44:50-58.

596. Suarez JI, Qureshi AI, Bhardwaj A, et al: Treatment of refractory intracranial hypertension with 23.4% saline. Crit Care Med 1998;26: 1118-1122.

597. Schwarz S, Georgiadis D, Aschoff A, Scwab S: Effects of hypertonic (10%) saline in patients with raised intracranial pressure after stroke. Stroke 2002;33:136-140.

598. Suarez JI: Hypertonic saline for cerebral edema and elevated intracranial pressure. Cleveland Clin J Med 2004;71(suppl 1):S9-S13.

599. Caplan LR: Cerebellar infarcts. In Caplan LR: Posterior Circulation Disease: Clinical Findings, Diagnosis, and Management. Boston: Blackwell Science, 1996, pp 492-543.

600. Lehrich J, Winkler G, Ojemann R: Cerebellar infarction with brainstem compression: Diagnosis and surgical treatment. Arch Neurol 1970;22: 490-498.

601. Feeley MP: Cerebellar infarction. Neurosurg 1979;4:7-11.

602. Delashaw JB, Broaddus WC, Kassell NF, et al: Treatment of right hemispheric cerebral infarction by hemicraniotomy. Stroke 1990;21:874-881.

603. Schwab S, Rieke K, Aschoff A, et al: Hemicraniotomy in space-occupying hemispheric infarction: useful early intervention or desperate activism. Cerebrovasc Dis 1996;6:325-329.

604. Schwab S, Steiner T, Aschoff A, et al: Early hemicraniectomy in patients with complete middle cerebral artery infarction. Stroke 1998;29:1888-1893.

605. Vahedi K, Vicaut E, Mateo J, et al: Sequential-design, multicenter, randomized, controlled trial of early decompressive craniectomy in malignant middle cerebral artery infarction (DECIMAL Trial). Stroke 2007;38:2506-2517.

606. Vahedi K, Hofmeijer J, Juettler E, et al: Decompressive surgery in malignant infarction of the middle cerebral artery. Lancet Neurol 2007;6: 315-322.

607. Mayer SA: Hemicraniectomy. A second chance on life for patients with space-occupying MCA infarction. Stroke 2007;38:2410-2412.

608. Heinsius T, Bogousslavsky J, Van Melle G: Large infarcts in the middle cerebral artery territory: Etiology and outcome patterns. Neurology 1998;50:341-350.

609. Wijdicks E, Schievink W, McGough PF: Dramatic reversal of the uncal syndrome and brain edema from infarction in the middle cerebral artery territory. Cerebrovasc Dis 1997;7:349-352.

610. Graff-Radford NR, Torner J, Adams Jr HP, Kassell NF: Factors associated with hydrocephalus after subarachnoid hemorrhage. A report of the Co-operative Aneurysm Study. Arch Neurol 1989;46:744-752.

611. Greenberg J, Shubick D, Shenkin H: Acute hydrocephalus in cerebellar infarct and hemorrhage. Neurology 1961;11:697-700.

612. Khan M, Polyzoidis K, Adegbite A, et al: Massive cerebellar infarction: "conservative" management. Stroke 1983;14:745-751.

613. Rieke K, Krieger D, Adams H-P, et al: Therapeutic strategies in space-occupying cerebellar infarction based on clinical, neuroradiological, and neurophysiological data. Cerebrovasc Dis 1993;3:45-55.

614. Meairs S, Wahlgren N, Dirnagl O, et al: Stroke research priorities for the next decade—a representative view of the European Scientific community. Cerebrovasc Dis 2006;22:75-82.

615. Menken M, Munsat TL, Toole JF: The global burden of disease study: Implications for neurology. Arch Neurol 2000;57:418-420.

616. Caplan LR: Treatment of patients with stroke. Arch Neurol 2002;59:703-707.

617. Savitz SI, Rosenbaum DM, Dinsmore JH, et al: Cell transplantation for stroke. Ann Neurol 2002;52:266-275.

618. Kodziolka D, Wechsler L, Goldstein S, et al: Transplantation of cultured human neuronal cells for patients with stroke. Neurology 2000;55:565-569.

619. Bliss T, Guzman R, Daadi M, Steinberg GK: Cell transplantation therapy for stroke. Stroke 2007;38(part 2):817-826.

620. Kondziolka D, Steinberg GK, Wechsler L, et al: Neurotransplantation for patients with subcortical motor stroke: A phase 2 randomized trial. J Neurosurg 2005;103:38-45.

621. Savitz SI, Dinsmore J, Wu J, et al: Neurotransplantation of fetal porcine cells in patients with basal ganglia infarcts: A preliminary safety and feasibility study. Cerebrovasc Dis 2005;20:101-107.

622. Chopp M, Li Y: Transplantation of bone marrow stromal cells for treatment of central nervous system diseases. Adv Exp Med Biol 2006; 585:49-64.

623. Chen J, Chopp M: Neurorestorative treatment of stroke: Cell and pharmacological approaches. NeuroRx 2006;3:466-473.

624. Chen J, Sanberg PR, Li Y, et al: Intravenous administration of human umbilical cord blood reduces behavioral deficits after stroke in rats. Stroke 2001;32:2682-2688.

625. Shen LH, Li Y, Chen J, et al: One-year follow-up after bone marrow stromal cell treatment in middle-aged female rats with stroke. Stroke 2007;38:2150-2156.

626. van der Lee JH, Wagenaar RC, Lankhorst GJ, et al: Forced use of the upper extremity in chronic stroke patients: Results from a single-blind randomized clinical trial. Stroke 1999;30: 2369-2375.

627. Wolf SL, Winstein CJ, Miller JP, et al: Effect of constraint-induced movement therapy on upper extremity function 3 to 9 months after stroke: The EXCITE randomized clinical trial. JAMA 2006;296:2095-2104.

628. Dopkin BH: Interpreting the randomized clinical trial of constraint-induced movement therapy. Arch Neurol 2007;64:336-338.

629. Feys H, De Weerdt, Verbeke G, et al: Early and repetitive stimulation of the arm can substantially improve the long-term outcome after stroke: A 5-year follow-up study of a randomized trial. Stroke 2004;35:924-929.

630. Dannebaum R, Dykes R: Sensory loss in the hand after sensory stroke: Therapeutic rationale. Arch Phys Med Rehabil 1988;69:833-839.

631. Dobkin BH: Stroke. In Dobkin BH: Neurologic Rehabilitation. Philadelphia, FA Davis, 1996, pp 157-217.

632. Teasell RW, Kalra L: What's new in stroke rehabilitation. Stroke 2004;35:383-385.

633. Takeuchi N, Chuma T, Matsuo Y, et al: Repetitive transcranial magnetic stimulation of contralesional primary motor cortex improves hand function after stroke. Stroke 2005;36: 2681-2686.

634. Kobayashi M, Hutchinson S, Theoret H, et al: Repetitive transcranial magnetic stimulation of the motor cortex improves ipsilateral sequential simple finger movements. Neurology 2004; 62:91-98.

635. Khedr EM, Ahmed MA, Fathy N, Rothwell JC: Therapeutic trial of repetitive transcranial magnetic stimulation after acute ischemic stroke. Neurology 2005;65:466-468.

636. Kim Y-H, You SH, Ko M-H, et al: Repetitive transcranial magnetic stimulation-induced corticomotor excitability and associated motor skill acquisition in chronic stroke. Stroke 2006; 37:1471-1476.

637. Kluger BM, Triggs WJ: Use of transcranial magnetic stimulation to influence behavior. Curr Neurol Neurosci Rep 2007;7:491-497.

638. Khedr EM, Ahmed MA, Fathy N, Rothwell JC: Therapeutic trial of repetitive transcranial magnetic stimulation after acute ischemic stroke. Neurology 2005;65:466-468.

639. Catsman-Beirevoets C, Harskamp F: Compulsive pre-sleep behavior and apathy due to bilateral thalamic stroke: Response to bromocriptine. Neurology 1988;38:647-648.

640. Albert ML, Bachman D, Morgan A, et al: Pharmacotherapy for aphasia. Neurology 1988;38: 877-879.

641. Sabe L, Leiguarda R, Sarkstein S: An open-label trial of bromcriptine in nonfluent aphasia. Neurology 1992;42:1637-1638.

642. Fleet WS, Watson RT, Valenstein E, et al: Dopamine agonist therapy for neglect in humans. Neurology 1986;36(suppl):347.

643. Barrett K: Treating organic abulia with bromocriptine and lisuride: Four case studies. J Neurol Neurosurg Psychiatry 1991;54: 718-721.

644. Feeney DM, Gonzalez A, Law WA: Amphetamine, haloperidol and experience interact to affect the rate of recovery after motor cortex injury. Science 1982;217:855-857.

645. Houda DA, Feeney DM: Haldoperidol blocks amphetamine induced recovery of binocular depth perception after bilateral visual cortex abilities in the cat. Proc West Pharmacol Soc 1985;28:209-211.

646. Davis JN, Crisostomo EA, Duncan P, et al: Amphetamine and physical therapy facilitate recovery of function from stroke: Correlative animal and human studies. In Raichle ME, Powers W (eds): Cerebrovascular Diseases. New York: Raven Press, 1987, pp 297-304.

647. Goldstein LB: Amphetamine-facilitated functional recovery after stroke. In Ginsberg MD, Dietrich WD (eds): Cerebrovascular Diseases. New York: Raven Press, 1989, pp 303-308.

648. Hurwitz BE, Dietrich D, McCabe PM, et al: Amphetamine promotes recovery from sensory-motor integration deficit after thrombotic infarction of the primary somatosensory rat cortex. Stroke 1991;22: 648-654.

649. Reding MJ, Solomon B, Borucki S: The effect of dextroamphetamine on motor recovery after stroke. Neurology 1995;45(suppl 4):A222.

650. Sawaki L, Cohen LG, Classen J, et al: Enhancement of use-dependent plasticity by d-amphetamine. Neurology 2002;59:1262-1264.

651. Plewnia C, Hoppe J, Cohen LG, Berloff C: Improved motor skill acquisition after selective stimulation of central norepinephrine. Neurology 2004;62:2124-2126.

652. Hernandez TC, Kiefel J, Barth TM, et al: Disruption and facilitation of recovery of behavioral function: Implication of the gamma-aminobutyric acid/benzodiazepine receptor complex. In Ginsberg MD, Dietrich WD (eds): Cerebrovascular Diseases. New York: Raven Press, 1989, pp 327-334.

653. Goldstein LB, Davis JN: Physician prescribing patterns following hospital admission for ischemic cerebrovascular disease. Neurology 1988;38:1806-1809.

654. Goldstein LB: Potential effects of common drugs on stroke recovery. Arch Neurol 1998;55: 454-456.

655. Goldstein LB: Common drugs may influence motor recovery after stroke. The Sygen in Acute Stroke Study Investigators. Neurology 1995;45: 865-871.

656. Yamamoto H, Bogopusslavsky J: Mechanisms of second and further strokes. J Neurol Neurosurg Psychiatry 1998;64:771-776.

657. Caplan LR: Prevention of strokes and recurrent strokes. J Neurol Neurosurg Psychiatry 1998;64:716.

Stroke Syndromes II

Large Artery Occlusive Disease of the Anterior Circulation

6

Specific clinical and laboratory aspects of occlusive disease of the commonly involved arteries are analyzed in this chapter. Examples of typical patients are included to discuss management and illustrate the most common clinical and imaging findings. The general epidemiologic, etiologic, and pathologic features that relate to large artery occlusive lesions are discussed in Part I of this book.

OCCLUSIVE DISEASE OF THE INTERNAL CAROTID ARTERY

Atherosclerotic Internal Carotid Artery Disease in the Neck

The modern era in ischemic cerebrovascular disease began in 1951 with Miller Fisher's key report that called attention to the clinical findings in patients with occlusion of the internal carotid artery (ICA) in the neck.[1,2] Previously, ischemic strokes in the anterior circulation were invariably attributed to middle cerebral artery (MCA) disease. Fisher called attention to warning episodes in patients with carotid artery disease that preceded strokes. He recognized that attacks of eye and hemispheral ischemic symptoms were diagnostic of carotid artery disease in the neck. He dubbed these episodes transient ischemic attacks (TIAs).[1,3] Fisher commented, "It is even conceivable that some day surgery will find a way to bypass the occluded portion of the artery during the period of ominous fleeting symptoms." At that time, angiography required a surgical cut-down and only single-frame, hand-pulled films were available. During the next decades, the advent of safer and more widespread angiography led to increased recognition of the frequency and importance of ICA disease in the neck. Newer, noninvasive techniques now make possible reliable detection of carotid artery lesions in outpatients.

The first carotid surgical procedures were performed during the early 1950s.[1,4] During the 1960s and 1970s, improved diagnostic capability, safer anesthesia, advanced surgical techniques, and an increase in the number of vascular surgeons caused an explosion in the amount of operative procedures performed on the carotid arteries. In 1985, more than 107,000 endarterectomies were performed in the United States, making it one of the three most common surgical procedures.[4] After 1987, the number of endarterectomies began to decrease in response to widespread concern about the indications, use, and complications of the procedure.[5,6]

In 1991, North American and European controlled trial results[7,8] showed an important therapeutic benefit of endarterectomy in symptomatic patients with high-grade stenosis. These reports gave the procedure more credibility and served as an impetus for more vascular surgery. Subsequent reports from the North American[9] and European[10] carotid surgery trials showed that endarterectomy was beneficial in selected patients who had moderately severe stenosis (50% to 69%) when operated on by surgeons who had documented records of low surgical morbidity and mortality. Trials also showed that selected patients who had severe carotid artery disease without recognized symptoms also could benefit from carotid artery surgery.[11,12] Selection of the surgeon is most important since the frequency of complications, morbidity, and mortality figures still vary widely among surgeons and medical centers, even within the same city.[13,14]

During the last decade interventional procedures to open stenosed carotid arteries—angioplasty and stenting—have increasingly been performed instead of surgery in symptomatic and asymptomatic patients considered appropriate candidates. Angioplasty and stenting are now performed by many different specialists including neuroradiologists, vascular surgeons, cardiologists, neurologists, and neurosurgeons. Trials now attempt to sort out the relative risks and benefits of angioplasty/stenting compared to open surgical repair.[15,16] I return to the important question of treatment after reviewing the epidemiologic, clinical, and laboratory features of ICA occlusive disease in the neck.

A 58-year-old man, HL, awakened with a numb and weak left hand. He had a myocardial infarction 6 years earlier and continued to have angina pectoris on moderate exertion. During the past year, he developed pain in the left calf that abated when he stopped to rest or walked more than two blocks.

The major cause of ICA occlusive disease in the neck is atherosclerotic narrowing of the vessel. The lesion usually begins in the distal common carotid artery (CCA) and extends to the first few proximal centimeters of the ICA and external carotid artery (ECA), almost always more severely narrowing the ICA. The usual site of the lesion is shown in Figure 4-7. This lesion is found more often in whites than in African Americans or Asians, and in men more than women.[17,18] Occlusive disease of the large systemic arteries, especially the coronary, iliac, and femoral arteries, often accompanies carotid atherosclerosis. Coexisting angina pectoris, myocardial infarction, and limb claudication are common.[19] Risk factors for the development of proximal ICA disease are similar to those for coronary artery disease and include hypertension, smoking, diabetes, and hypercholesterolemia. Mortality in patients with ICA disease is usually cardiac. Attention is appropriately focused on the heart and brain, and the brain's circulation.

> Although HL did not volunteer other symptoms, direct questioning revealed several important warning signs. In the months before presentation, he had two brief episodes of transient obscuration of vision in his right eye. A dark shade descended from above, rather quickly blocking vision completely on one occasion, and obscuring only the upper half of vision during the other episode. The attacks were brief and lasted less than a minute each. He also had three episodes of transient neurologic dysfunction. These episodes consisted of stumbling after his left leg gave way during one episode, and slurred speech, and numbness of the left arm, hand, and face in the other two episodes. The initial episode was 3 months earlier, the most recent 3 days earlier. He noted unaccustomed, frequent headaches in the weeks before presentation.

Atherosclerotic plaques most often gradually narrow the ICA lumen. Ulceration, attachment of platelet nidi and clots to crevices in plaques, and hemorrhage into plaques become more common as the arterial lumen becomes increasingly narrowed. Plaques usually contain a lipid core and fibrous cap. When there is a break in the fibrous cap, contact of the lipid core with the contents of the lumen activates platelets and can activate the coagulation cascade, promoting the deposition of white and red thrombi onto the plaque surface. Plugs of platelets and thrombin may detach from the arterial wall and embolize to distal vessels, causing transient or prolonged brain and eye dysfunction. Reduction in blood flow can also lead to periodic insufficiency in distal perfusion. For these reasons, TIAs often occur as the artery narrows and so warn of an impending stroke. Many times when an artery occludes, adequate collateral circulation develops and no permanent neurologic damage ensues.

The single most important clue to an ICA localization of the occlusive process is an attack of transient monocular blindness. Often, the vision loss is described as a dimming, darkening, or obscuration. An apparent shade or curtain usually falls from above, but may move from the side like a theater curtain. After a brief period of seconds or a few minutes, the curtain lifts or recedes. This usually leaves no permanent visual loss. These attacks of transient visual obscuration are caused by decreased blood flow through the ophthalmic artery, the first branch of the ICA. Amaurosis fugax occurs when the lesion affects the ICA proximal to the ophthalmic artery (in the neck or proximal carotid siphon) or involves the ophthalmic artery itself. Diminished flow or pressure in the ophthalmic artery is a clue to the presence of carotid artery disease.

In migraine, the most common differential diagnostic consideration, patients usually describe brightness, glittering, flickering, and movement within the visual field, which lasts 15 to 30 minutes and is seldom monocular. Occasionally, patients with severe ICA occlusive disease report unilateral spells of reduced vision after exposure to bright light, a type of retinal claudication.[20] In some patients with bilateral ICA disease, the transient loss of vision can be bilateral. As in HL, individuals may not volunteer information about temporary visual loss because they consider it completely unrelated to the present problem. The physician must directly and repeatedly ask about specific symptoms of ocular and brain ischemia.

Episodes of hemispheral ischemia are also usually brief. Attacks may be quite varied and include various deficits in different limbs during individual attacks. Sometimes, however, the spells are stereotyped. In some patients with critical stenosis, the attacks are frequent and may be precipitated by suddenly standing or a drop in blood pressure.[21] Frequent, brief, machine-gun—like attacks usually mean low flow caused by proximal severe stenosis. Emboli generally produce longer, less frequent attacks. In disease of larger vessels, such as the ICA, TIAs may occur during a period of months, as compared with a briefer span of hours, days, or a week in patients with lacunar infarction caused by disease of smaller blood vessels. As the ICA narrows, collateral circulation develops, leading to dilation of arteries and the onset of unaccustomed headache. It is unusual, however, for headache to be the only symptom; in my experience, headache is usually accompanied by TIAs. The most common symptoms of ICA disease in the neck are listed in Table 6-1.

Table 6-1.	Symptoms of Internal Carotid Artery Disease

Attacks of transient monocular blindness
Transient ischemic attacks, sometimes variegated, and occurring during a span of weeks or months
Frequent, unaccustomed headache
Commonly associated history of coronary or peripheral vascular disease

Table 6-2.	Signs of Internal Carotid Artery Disease

Neck
High-pitched, focal, long bruit at bifurcation
Face
Increased angular, brow, cheek (ABC) pulses[23]
Frontal artery sign[24]
Increase in superficial temporal artery
Retina
Cholesterol crystals[25]
Platelet plugs[26]
Retinal infarcts
Reduced caliber of arteries
Less severe hypertensive changes
Venous stasis retinopathy[27,28]
Reduced retinal artery pressure

On examination, HL had moderate weakness of the left arm, slight weakness of the left psoas muscle, and severe weakness of the left hand. Position sense was decreased in the left hand and HL could not accurately localize left-limb touch stimuli, nor recognize objects in the left hand. He drew a clock poorly (Fig. 6-1, top) and also copied inaccurately (Figure 6-1, bottom). A soft, high-pitched bruit was audible at the right carotid bifurcation in the neck. A right Horner's syndrome was noted.

Physical examination of the blood vessels and eyes often yields important clues to an ICA location of the lesion (Table 6-2). Palpation of the neck is not helpful unless the CCA is occluded, in which case there is no palpable carotid pulse on that side. Even when the ICA is occluded, the CCA pulse is usually transmitted to the ICA in the neck. The presence of a typical bruit (i.e., a high-pitched, long, focal sound heard loudest over the carotid bifurcation) is virtually diagnostic of localized ICA disease. In some patients with severe ICA occlusive disease, however, flow is so severely diminished that no bruit is audible. When a bruit at the bifurcation is also audible over the ipsilateral eye, the physician can be confident that the bruit is of ICA origin and that the artery is patent. A bruit also can arise from the proximal ECA. In this case, the bruit usually radiates toward the jaw and can be diminished by pressure on ECA branches.[22] When the ICA is occluded or severely stenosed, ECA collaterals may feed into the orbit and may be palpable at the angular, brow, and cheek (ABC) regions (see Fig. 3-5).[23] Blood flow may be found to flow retrograde down the frontal artery into the orbit[24] (see Fig. 3-6).

Ischemia to the iris or retina on the side of the carotid occlusive lesion is another helpful clue. Retinal arteries on the side of the carotid lesion may be reduced in caliber or show fewer hypertensive changes than their counterparts in the opposite retina. White, fluffy exudates or focal retinal atrophy can represent infarction. Small cholesterol crystal emboli are highly refractile bodies that usually lodge at bifurcations of retinal arteries.[25] White platelet plugs can also be transiently seen within retinal arteries.[26] Figures 3-8, 3-9, and 3-10 show examples of retinal vascular changes in patients with severe ICA disease in the neck.

Venous stasis retinopathy is a descriptive term for the ophthalmoscopic appearance found in patients with chronic ICA occlusion, and is characterized by microaneurysms, small-dot retinal hemorrhages, and dilated, dark retinal veins, sometimes of irregular caliber[27,28] (Figs. 3-11 and 6-2) The retina in this condition resembles diabetic

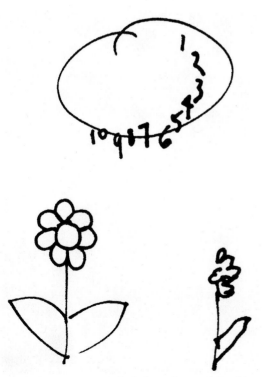

Figure 6-1. At top is a clock drawn by a patient with right parietal lobe lesion. At bottom is the patient's copy *(right)* of a daisy drawn by the examiner *(left)*.

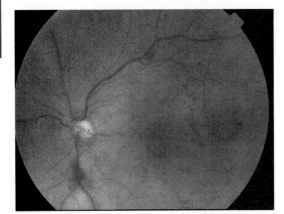

Figure 6-2. A photograph of the optic fundus in a patient with a carotid artery occlusion showing central venous retinopathy. There are dilated veins and many blot and dot hemorrhages mostly in the periphery of the retina. (Courtesy of Thomas Hedges III, MD.)

retinopathy but can usually be distinguished by unilaterality, location in the midportion of the retina, and its association with low retinal arterial pressure as measured by diminished ophthalmic blood-flow velocities by transcranial Doppler (TCD). The presence of venous stasis retinopathy always means that flow reduction in the ophthalmic artery is severe and longstanding.

Neurologic findings are caused by infarction of brain regions within the ICA circulation. Signs in patients with ICA disease are difficult to separate clinically from those in patients with intrinsic lesions of the MCA.[29,30] The most common loci of infarction are within the MCA territory. Weakness is common and usually affects the contralateral hand and face more than the leg. When sensory loss is present, it usually is of the cortical type with loss of position sense, point localization, and stereognosis on the opposite side of the body. Again, the hand and face often show more sensory abnormalities than the trunk and lower extremity. When bilateral simultaneous tactile stimuli are presented to the arms, the stimulus contralateral to the lesion is often not reported by the patient. Neglect of the opposite side of visual space and an attentional hemianopia are also common findings, especially when the infarct is in the right cerebral hemisphere. Poor drawing and copying, impersistence with tasks, diminished emotional responsiveness, and anosognosia (lack of awareness of the deficit) also frequently accompany right ICA-territory infarction.[31,32] Aphasia is a common sequel to left-sided infarction. Occasionally, the infarct is located predominantly in the territory of the anterior cerebral artery (ACA); foot, leg, and shoulder weakness predominate. Rarely, when the posterior cerebral artery (PCA) is supplied

directly by the ICA, an infarct caused by ICA occlusion can lie solely within the PCA territory and can manifest as a hemianopia without other signs.[33,34]

A duplex ultrasound scan was performed. B-mode showed some flat plaques within the distal right CCA and severe atherosclerotic disease at the right ICA origin with near occlusion. The Doppler frequencies also suggested high-grade stenosis of the right ICA. The left carotid artery showed only minor disease. TCD examination revealed lower flow velocities in the right ICA siphon, and the right MCA and ACA. Computed tomography (CT) showed a hypodensity in the cortical parietal lobe affecting the postcentral gyrus and superior parietal lobule. CT angiography (CTA) showed severe, irregular narrowing of the ICA at its origin with a residual lumen of approximately 1 mm (95% luminal narrowing) (Fig. 6-3). The carotid siphon and MCA were normal. Echocardiography and Holter monitoring were normal.

Noninvasive diagnostic tests are discussed in Chapter 4. Figures 4-6, 4-10, 4-12, and 4-13 show ultrasound studies of the ICA in the neck. In this patient, ultrasonography showed a severe flow-reducing lesion at the ICA origin and CTA

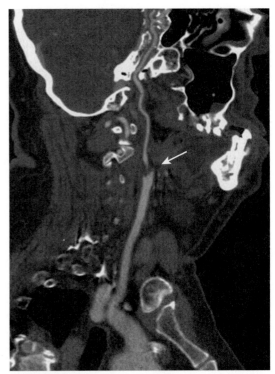

Figure 6-3. Computed tomography angiogram (CTA) of the neck, lateral view showing very severe stenosis at the origin of the internal carotid artery.

confirmed the finding and showed the artery quite well. The concordance of the two vascular tests made it unnecessary to proceed to diagnostic catheter angiography. If angioplasty and/or stenting is performed, angiographic images of the artery would be performed as an adjunct to the therapeutic procedure. MRA is also a useful screening test although the severity of stenosis is sometimes over estimated. Figures 4-24 and 6-4A show stenosing ICA lesions imaged by MRA. Figure 6-4B shows the same lesion shown in Fig. 6-4A studied by catheter contrast-digital angiography.

In patients with ICA atherosclerotic occlusive disease, there are several frequent patterns of disease. When the ICA is occluded, the vessel may be angiographically absent or show a pointed, tapering, or rounded stump.[35] Barnett and colleagues called attention to embolization from the stump of previously occluded carotid arteries.[36] Stenotic lesions can be ulcerated, smooth, or irregular. The lesions may be long and tapered or may slope abruptly like a shelf. B-mode scans and color—Doppler-flow ultrasound imaging (CDFI) studies of the carotid origin can help define the nature of plaques, presence of ulceration, and dynamics of flow. An example of a CDFI study is shown in Fig. 4-13. Calcific, smooth plaques are less often the source of intra-arterial emboli and usually do not show rapid enlargement, whereas irregular, heterogeneous, ulcerated, soft plaques often progress and are frequently the source of emboli. Cross-section images of the carotid artery using advanced MRI and CT techniques can also yield useful information about the nature of plaques. When angiography is complete, it is often possible to detect embolic occlusion of the MCA or its branches, so-called occlusio supra occlusionem.[37]

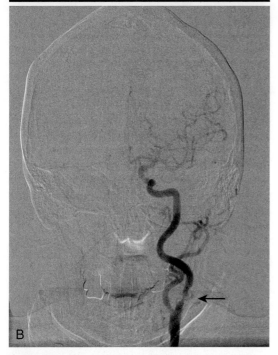

Brain Imaging Findings in Patients with Internal Carotid Artery Disease

CT scans of patients with carotid artery occlusion or severe stenosis show several common patterns of distribution of infarction (Fig. 6-5). These patterns include (1) watershed or borderzone infarction between the territories of the ACA and MCA, and between the MCA and PCA; (2) subcortical white-matter infarcts often referred to as "internal border-zone" infarcts; (3) wedge-shaped, pial-artery territory infarcts; and (4) infarction of the basal ganglia and lentiform nucleus.[37]

The border-zone and subcortical white matter lesions are probably caused by a combination of reduced flow and embolism. TCD monitoring of patients with symptomatic ICA disease often shows frequent microemboli passing through the MCA.[38,39] Most such microemboli are composed of white-platelet-fibrin thrombi. As the ICA narrows, blood flow velocity increases within the center of the artery and flow-separation becomes more prominent. Flow is reduced in some parts of the artery especially on the outer perimeter of the residual lumen. When subtotal or complete occlusion of the ICA develops, the bloodstream flow diminishes because of reduced volume of flow and blood flow

Figure 6-4. (A) Magnetic resonance angiogram (MRA) of the neck showing a severe stenosis at the internal carotid artery origin on the right. (B) Dye-contrast cerebral angiogram in the same patient showing a localized cylindrical region of stenosis in the internal carotid artery.

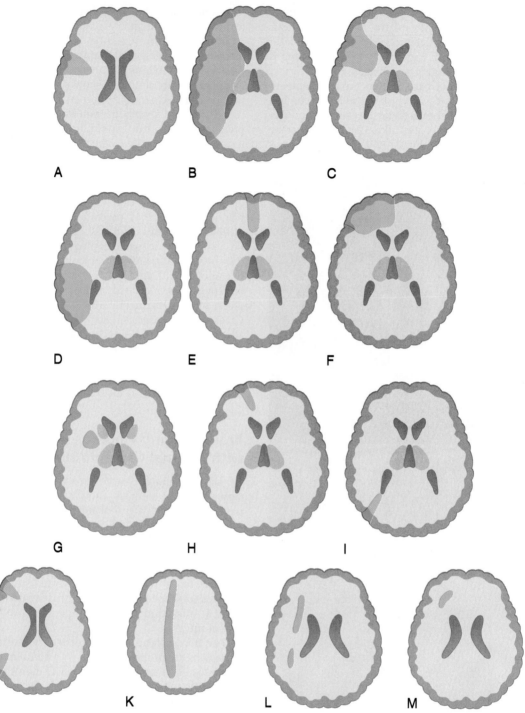

Figure 6-5. Most common CT locations of infarcts in the anterior circulation (infarcts are shown by *hatched gray*): (**A**) wedge-shaped MCA infarct, (**B**) entire MCA territory, (**C**) superior-division MCA, (**D**) inferior division MCA, (**E**) ACA, (**F**) ACA and MCA, (**G**) striatocapsular infarct, (**H**) wedge-shaped anterior watershed infarct, (**I**) wedge-shaped posterior watershed infarct, (**J**) anterior and posterior watershed infarcts, (**K**) linear watershed infarct, (**L**) ovular deep watershed infarct, and (**M**) small white-matter watershed infarct.

velocity also is decreased. Antegrade perfusion becomes less effective. This reduced perfusion and pressure decreases washout and throughput of emboli especially in arterial border zones.[40,41] MRI using DWI may show tiny dot lesions often in the internal and cortical border-zone regions that result from these small emboli. Figure 6-6A and B shows such small dot infarcts. At times these small dot lesions are accompanied by larger infarcts in the center of the MCA

distribution resulting from larger emboli as shown in Figs. 6-7A and B, or as a vertical linear distribution within the internal border zone on the side of the ICA occlusion (Fig. 6-7C).

Larger pial and basal ganglia infarcts are caused by emboli to the mainstem MCA, its superior or inferior division trunks, or penetrating artery branches. These larger emboli most likely contain red clots, sometimes engrafted on white clots. Emboli removed from cerebral arteries by an embolus retrieving technique usually showed mixed elements of white and red clots.[42] In my experience, watershed infarction and large, superficial infarcts in the MCA territory are the most common lesions found on CT and MRI in patients with severe ICA obstructive disease. The mechanism of stroke in patient HL was a small superior parietal-lobe infarct caused by an embolus from the ICA stenosis in the neck. Cardiac testing did not show an alternative embologenic donor source in the heart.

> HL was placed on heparin therapy for 1 week of treatment and was then switched to warfarin. The international normalized ratio (INR) was maintained between 2.0 and 2.5. At 4 weeks, an uncomplicated carotid endarterectomy was performed. Blood pressure was carefully monitored postoperatively, but did not elevate. The patient had minimal residual neurologic signs of clumsiness and slight numbness of his left hand, but was able to return to his former work.

In my present practice, choice of treatment for patients with ICA disease in the neck depends on the following:

1. Severity of the stenosis.
2. Anatomy of the carotid artery and stenosing plaque. A high carotid artery bifurcation and a long stenotic lesion increase the difficulty of surgery and are factors that favor stenting if aggressive treatment of the lesion is warranted.
3. Presence of a recent cerebral infarct as determined by a persistent clinical deficit and an appropriate CT, or magnetic resonance imaging (MRI) lesion.
4. General health of the patient, especially any contraindication to surgery, warfarin anticoagulation, or agents that decrease platelet agglutination.
5. Morbidity and mortality record of the surgeon who would undertake surgery and of the hospital where the surgery would take place.
6. Experience and record of the interventionalist who would perform angioplasty or stenting of the carotid artery lesion.

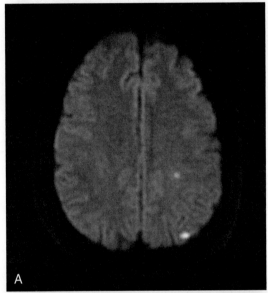

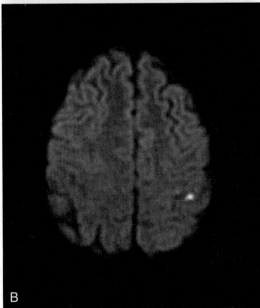

Figure 6-6. Diffusion-weighted MRI scans showing small-dot regions of hyperintensity in patients with unilateral severe carotid artery occlusive lesions. (**A**) Two dot lesions are seen within the posterior border-zone region. (**B**) There is a single dot lesion near the hand area of the cerebral cortex.

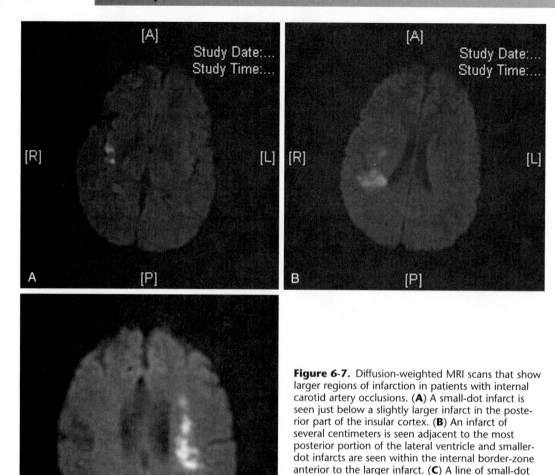

Figure 6-7. Diffusion-weighted MRI scans that show larger regions of infarction in patients with internal carotid artery occlusions. (**A**) A small-dot infarct is seen just below a slightly larger infarct in the posterior part of the insular cortex. (**B**) An infarct of several centimeters is seen adjacent to the most posterior portion of the lateral ventricle and smaller-dot infarcts are seen within the internal border-zone anterior to the larger infarct. (**C**) A line of small-dot hyperintensities is shown within the internal border-zone region.

7. Attitude of the patient and family toward the situation after the alternative courses of action has been discussed.

Physicians and surgeons at the Mayo clinic carefully analyzed the neurologic, medical, and angiographic risks of carotid surgery. I rely heavily on their analysis in patients in whom I consider aggressive repair of the ICA (surgery or angioplasty/stenting).[43] Their categorization of the complications of carotid surgery are listed in Table 6-3. The general topic of carotid artery surgery and stenting, including the results of observational studies and trials, has already been discussed at length in Chapter 5. Management of symptomatic patients with TIAs or small,

nondisabling strokes who have various ICA lesions are considered in the following section.

Complete Occlusion of the Internal Carotid Artery in the Neck

I do not recommend surgery or stenting for complete occlusion of the ICA in the neck. When the ICA occludes, clot quickly propagates high into the neck, often as far as the carotid siphon and beyond. Because there are no ICA branches in the neck, collateral flow patterns promote extension of clot toward the first branch, the ophthalmic artery. It is technically difficult to open completely occluded ICAs, and attempts to suction clots can lead to distal embolization. If it were

Table 6-3.	Risks of Carotid Endarterectomies

Neurologic Risks

Progressive course of brain ischemia
Recent stroke

Vascular Anatomy Risks

High carotid bifurcation

Long Lesion (3 cm distally in internal carotid artery or 5 cm into common carotid artery)

Thrombus within the ICA
Contralateral ICA stenosis or occlusion
Intracranial stenosis or occlusion

Medical Risks

Hypertension
Coronary artery disease
Diabetes
Obesity
Smoking
Chronic obstructive pulmonary disease
Congestive heart failure

Adapted from Sundt TM, Sandok BA, Whisnant JP: Carotid endarterectomy complications and preoperative assessment of risk. Mayo Clin Proc 1975;50:301-306.

known that an occlusion had become complete minutes or a few hours before, as might happen after angiography, or after surgery, exploration of the neck would be reasonable. That circumstance is rare in my experience. Angiography can yield clues as to the extent of the occlusive thrombosis. If opacification of the contralateral ICA shows retrograde filling of the occluded ICA down into the neck, it is more likely that the surgeon might be able to open the ICA surgically or the interventionist to successfully recanalize the artery using thrombolysis and stenting.

When the patient arrives at the hospital soon after the onset of stroke symptoms, and CT or MRI do not show a large region of infarction, thrombolytic therapy can be considered. Intravenous recombinant tissue plasminogen activator has often failed to recanalize occlusions of the ICA in the neck or intracranially.[44,45] Some interventionists have been able to physically manipulate the ICA clot with a catheter and inject urokinase or rt-PA directly into the thrombus. This lyses the clot and allows recanalization.[46,47] When an embolus arising from the ICA has blocked the MCA, the interventionist can manipulate the catheter to the MCA clot and affect thrombolysis by injecting the thrombolytic agent into the intracranial thrombus.[46,47] When neck or intracranial thrombi are superimposed on severe atherostenotic lesions; however,

thrombi almost always reoccur, unless the stenosis is removed by angioplasty shortly after successful thrombolysis. The use of thrombolysis in the setting of ICA thrombosis has never been compared with anticoagulant therapy. I have not had occasion to use this aggressive approach in patients with acute ICA thrombosis.

I treat patients with acute ICA thrombosis with bed rest, keeping the head flat or slightly lower than the feet, to augment blood flow to the head. I try to avoid hypotension and have used agents, such as ephedrine, which raise blood pressure in some patients. I avoid antihypertensive drugs during the first 1 to 2 weeks unless the blood pressure is in the malignant range (e.g., greater than 225/125 mm Hg). If the patient is normotensive and there is no contraindication to the use of anticoagulants, I use intravenous heparin, followed by warfarin for a short period (2 to 6 weeks), to attempt to prevent embolization of fresh clots and discourage clot propagation. After this period, I do not use anticoagulants, but rather aspirin in doses of one 325-mg tablet per day or aspirin 25/modified-release dipyridamole 200 mg twice a day. I sometimes use 75 mg of clopidogrel or cilostazole 200 mg twice a day in patients who are aspirin-intolerant.

Caution must be exercised in the diagnosis of complete ICA occlusion because a severe reduction in flow can lead to collapse of the artery above the high-grade block. Angiography produces a picture that closely resembles occlusion (so called pseudo-occlusion[48]), but late films usually show a trickle of dye ascending anterograde toward the siphon. Color-flow Doppler ultrasound also sometimes visualizes flow through a pseudo-occlusion not seen with standard angiography.[49] Figure 4-13 shows such a circumstance. CT in cross-section of the high neck after contrast can show blood in the ICA, documenting preserved anterograde flow.[50] In pseudo-occlusion, the residual flow, albeit small, makes it possible for the surgeon to open the artery. Patients with pseudo-occlusion are considered to have severe stenosis. Analysis of the data from the North American Symptomatic Carotid Endarterectomy Trial (NASCET) showed that patients with near occlusion do not have an increased risk of acute stroke compared with those with lesser degrees of severe stenosis (70% to 94%), nor do they have a higher rate of surgical complications.[51] In my experience, the course of patients with pseudo-occlusion is identical to that of occlusion and the artery has in fact collapsed. I treat them in the same way that I manage patients with complete occlusions.

6

In patients with ICA occlusion, the deficit usually develops at, or shortly after, the time of occlusion when embolization and low flow are maximal. A chronic low-flow state, so-called misery perfusion,[52] may occur but only rarely persists. Occasionally, patients with known ICA occlusion develop transient symptoms, especially if they become hypotensive from overzealous antihypertensive treatment, or from dehydration or hypovolemia. The most common symptoms are transient obscurations of vision in the ipsilateral eye and/or weakness or numbness of the contralateral limbs. An unusual, but characteristic, sign of hypoperfusion is a so-called limb-shaking TIA.[53,54] Usually when standing or active, the patient develops a flapping flexion-extension tremor with impressive shaking and oscillation of the arm and hand contralateral to the occluded ICA. Occasionally, the lower extremity is involved. The shaking stops when the patient sits or lies down, and is caused by ischemia rather than a seizure.

I have not referred patients with ICA occlusion for ECA-ICA bypass, but would consider doing so if there were persistent, recurrent ischemic attacks or if positron emission tomography (PET), single-photon emission computed tomography (SPECT), or other new technology documented persistent misery perfusion. Sequential TCD studies of blood-flow velocity in the MCA and ACA, especially after acetazolamide infusion, also yield information about distal flow and the reserve capacity of the carotid tributaries to dilate. These laboratory techniques are discussed in Chapter 4. A trial is now underway to test whether superficial temporal artery to MCA bypass is useful in patients with chronic ICA occlusions who have poor cerebrovascular reserve, or PET scan evidence of continued ischemia.[55] Since acetazolamide augments blood flow in some patients with ICA occlusions, I have treated some patients with oral acetazolamide although there are no trial data on this approach.

Severe Stenosis of the Internal Carotid Artery in the Neck

In my opinion, severe stenosis of the ICA in the neck, when symptomatic, requires aggressive treatment (surgery or angioplasty/stenting) unless there is a severe, disabling brain infarct in the territory of the stenotic ICA. The reported results of North American[7,9] and European trials[8,10] support carotid endarterectomy in these patients. Most clinicians apply the same inclusion criteria to interventional treatment. What constitutes a severe stenosis? The two principal criteria are (1) the degree of

anatomic narrowing of the artery and (2) presence of significant reduction in flow velocity and pressure in tributary vessels shown by TCD.[56] A residual lumen of less than 1.5 mm (70% to 99% stenosis) invariably represents severe stenosis and nearly always impedes intracranial blood flow in the ICA branches. When the severely stenotic ICA is examined histologically, compound ulcers are often found.[57,58] Although these lesions may also be found in nonstenosed vessels, they become more frequent as the artery narrows.

When patients have TIAs, but no persistent neurologic deficit, and severe stenosis of the ICA with a residual lumen of less than 1.5 mm (70% to 99% stenosis), I believe that aggressive treatment should be performed urgently. If there is evidence of infarction, persistent abnormal neurologic signs or symptoms, or a new infarct on CT or MRI, I prefer to wait several weeks before opening the ICA because of the possibility of intracerebral hemorrhage (ICH) after opening of the artery.[59,60] Many instances of postendarterectomy ICH are explained by hypertension after manipulation of the carotid receptors in the neck.[61-64] Careful postoperative monitoring of blood pressure and effective treatment of hypertension (if it develops) should prevent ICH. Intracranial hemorrhage is less common after carotid stenting, perhaps because the frequency of severe hypertension after percutaneous manipulation of the ICA is less frequent than after surgery.

Endarterectomy in patients with severe stenosis can also be followed by a "hyperperfusion syndrome."[63,64] Sudden flooding of previously underperfused brain with blood can overwhelm the autoregulatory capacity of the region and lead to headache, seizures, focal neurologic signs, brain edema, and brain hemorrhage.[64] Hypertension, often acute and severe, is also usually present in patients with severe effects of the hyperperfusion syndrome. Recognition of the syndrome and rapid, effective treatment of hypertension usually prevents serious brain edema and hemorrhage. Hyperperfusion may also develop after carotid stenting,[65] but is less common than after surgery.

When there is a persistent neurologic deficit, I prefer to use heparin, then warfarin, to keep the INR between 2.0 and 2.5. As long as the patient remains stable or improves, I wait 4 to 6 weeks. If, however, there are further attacks or worsening during this waiting interval, I suggest opening the ICA without further delay, because in my experience, severe deficits commonly develop if aggressive treatment is not performed in these patients. Also, if patients worsen during observation in the hospital and continue to progress despite heparin therapy, I urge emergency correction of a critical

ICA stenosis. Some patients improve dramatically immediately after arterial opening.

The choice between surgery and interventional treatment is evolving because of the many ongoing trials comparing the two treatments. I have analyzed the existing material in detail in Chapter 5. I believe that in the future angioplasty/stenting will gradually replace surgery in most circumstances. Now the choice depends on (1) the availability and experience, training, and past results of the individual who will perform the surgery or the percutaneous interventional treatment; (2) the nature, location, and severity of the ICA lesion and the presence of other arterial lesions; (3) comorbidities that would preclude surgery or interventional treatment; and (4) the wishes of the patient after information is shared. Patients with long lesions, smooth lesions, and very high carotid bifurcations, especially those with coronary artery disease might better be treated using interventional techniques. Patients with focal irregular ulcerated lesions might better be treated surgically.

In patients with severe ICA stenosis, if surgery and angioplasty/stenting cannot be performed or if the patient refuses these procedures, I choose to anticoagulate with warfarin. I also treat risk factors aggressively and prescribe a 3-hydroxy-3-methylglutaryl coenzyme A reductase inhibitor (statin) in high dose (e.g., 40 to 80 mg atorvastatin) and often an ACE inhibitor. The duration of anticoagulation is uncertain and should be individualized. I use the results of sequential duplex scans to guide the duration of anticoagulation. Arteries with tight stenosis frequently occlude on follow-up scans, often without new symptoms.[66,67] During the 4 to 6 weeks after occlusion, thrombi become organized and adherent, after which embolization is rare. I switch from warfarin to one aspirin, per day, or two capsules of aspirin 25 mg combined with modified release dipyridamole 200 mg, 4 to 6 weeks after scans show complete occlusion. While the lumen remains narrowed but patent, I continue warfarin. In some patients, plaques regress and the lumen may become less narrowed. In these individuals, a switch to antiplatelet therapy also seems logical. No studies have been undertaken to test the strategy that I have outlined.

Plaque Disease of the Internal Carotid Artery in the Neck with Slight or Moderate Stenosis

I suggest prophylactic treatment with 3-hydroxy-3-methylglutaryl coenzyme A reductase inhibitors (statins) and an agent that decreases platelet aggregation for ICA plaque disease in the neck. Recent evidence favors rather high doses of statins.[68] I do not recommend warfarin anticoagulation or aggressive treatment. Although it is true that ulceration can occur in nonstenotic lesions, and that ulcers can be the source of artery-to-artery embolization, this occurs less frequently in patients without severe stenosis. In the presence of a severe stenosing lesion, the physician can be more confident that this is the responsible lesion rather than another plaque. Furthermore, the natural history of plaques has not been well studied. They may reendothelialize and heal. Plaques are ubiquitous in individuals older than 40 years, and current angiographic and noninvasive techniques do not infallibly predict the presence of ulceration on histologic examination. Agents that decrease platelet aggregation are posited to be most effective when there are nonstenosing plaques and high-velocity flow continues.

Antiplatelet agents (aspirin, aspirin combined with modified-release dipyridamole, clopidogrel, and cilostazole) have theoretical advantages over warfarin, an agent that probably works best in slow-moving vascular streams to prevent red thrombi. At present, I prefer aspirin, or aspirin combined with modified-release dipyridamole to other agents. The dose of aspirin is uncertain. I usually prescribe one 325-mg tablet per day. Clopidogrel 75 mg a day, or cilostazol 200 mg twice a day are alternative antiplatelet agents. An accurate, reproducible in vitro test of the effectiveness of the platelet antiaggregants might lead clinicians to titrate the dose in individual patients, and so monitor effectiveness of the drug.

When plaques are shallow, the decision to use platelet antiaggregant agents is clear. As plaques become larger, more irregular, or clearly ulcerated, and luminal narrowing approaches 50% to 70%, the therapeutic decision becomes more difficult and should be individualized. NASCET and the European Carotid Surgery Trials showed modest benefit from surgery in patients with this severity of stenosis. The benefit-to-risk ratio, however, is highly dependent on the individual patient and surgeon characteristics.[9,10] In a young patient with a lesion in this gray zone of near-critical stenosis, who has several TIAs and is a good candidate for aggressive vascular opening, I probably would choose surgery or angioplasty/stenting.

Carotid Artery Clots

Some patients with atherosclerotic plaques in the neck, with or without severe stenosis, have thrombi that are grossly visible on angiography.[69,70] Figures 6-8A and B are angiograms that show filling defects due to clot formation within the ICA, Fig. 2-4 is a carotid artery specimen removed at autopsy that contains a large clot. In some of these patients, free-floating thrombi are attached to plaques and coagulation functions are normal, whereas in others, a hypercoagulable state has promoted the formation of carotid thrombi. Cancer, active inflammatory disease such as Crohn's disease, and ulcerative colitis can increase acute-phase reactants and promote thrombosis

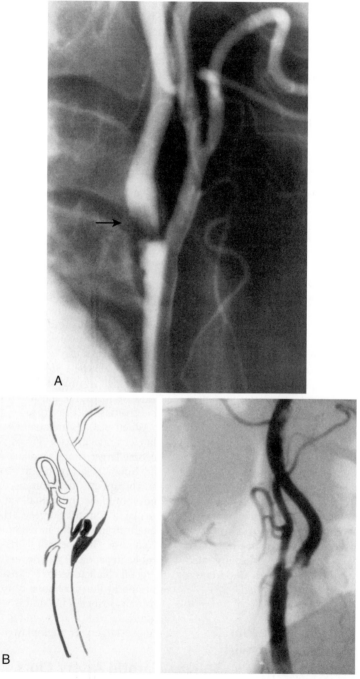

A

B

Figure 6-8. Dye-contrast digital subtraction cerebral angiograms showing thrombi within the internal carotid artery. (**A**) The *black arrow* points to a filling defect caused by a thrombus. (**B**) The angiogram on the right shows a filling defect at the origin of the internal carotid artery. On the left is a cartoon in which the plaque and thrombus are shown in *black*.

on endothelial lesions. These patients should be treated urgently. In a review of prior cases of patients with intraluminal clot, both surgery and warfarin anticoagulation were effective in preventing further stroke.[69] Clot recurred after surgery, however, in patients with coagulopathy.[70] The blood coagulation profiles of these patients should be carefully studied before treatment. Screening for common cancers especially adenocarcinomas is often indicated. In the NASCET study, the presence of ICA thrombi increased the surgical risk.[71]

Asymptomatic Patients with Internal Carotid Artery Disease in the Neck

The preceding discussion of treatment concerned symptomatic patients with TIA or stroke. It now has become commonplace to document ICA disease in the neck in patients who have no apparent central nervous system symptoms. The most common circumstances provoking carotid artery investigation are an audible neck bruit or imminent surgical procedures on the aorta, coronary, or peripheral-limb vessels. Some instances are discovered at angiography for indications other than vascular disease, or when an angiogram shows ICA disease on the asymptomatic side. Should these lesions be repaired before symptoms develop?

I seldom recommend carotid endarterectomy in asymptomatic patients. These patients do not have an unusual risk of stroke during surgery on other major vessels. Furthermore, stroke is unusual without preceding TIAs. In most medical centers, the risk of surgery and angiography (approximately 6% combined morbidity and mortality) or angioplasty/stenting is probably as great as, if not greater than, the risk of stroke without prior TIA. Analysis of a large series of patients followed for years showed that the annual stroke risk is likely less than 2%.[72]

Results of several studies of asymptomatic lesions are important to consider. In one series of 168 prospectively studied patients with known ICA stenosis, 26 patients (15%) had TIAs only; three patients had TIAs but refused surgery and had subsequent strokes; and just one patient developed sudden stroke without warning.[73] In another series of patients with carotid stenosis followed for 2 years among 318 patients, 5% developed TIAs, but only two patients had a stroke without a preceding TIA.[74] Sequential studies show that stenotic arteries often occlude without symptoms.[66,67] In patients undergoing endarterectomy who have bilateral carotid artery

stenosis, subsequent stroke on the unoperated side is uncommon.[74] Even when a bruit is detected before elective noncardiac vascular surgery, the incidence of postoperative stroke is not increased.[75] In patients who must have cardiac surgery, postoperative strokes are usually caused by cardiogenic emboli.

Treatment of asymptomatic patients must be individualized.[76] I do not think surgery or interventional repair of the ICA in asymptomatic patients should be seriously considered unless the stenosis is severe (>80% luminal narrowing). When made aware of a definite risk of stroke, some patients become quite anxious and psychologically tolerate knowledge of that risk poorly. They prefer the small gamble of an intraprocedural complication to the sword that they sense hangs perpetually over them. The situation must be fully discussed with the patient, and the benefits and risks of medical and surgical therapy explained. In patients who do not elect surgery, I teach them about TIAs and urge them to immediately report any attacks. I prescribe statin drugs and antiplatelet aggregants and follow the carotid artery disease with sequential duplex ultrasound examinations. Significant increase in severity of the stenosis does increase the risk of a stroke and there is some evidence favoring aggressive treatment.[77] The occurrence of TIAs puts patients in the symptomatic category and makes them surgical candidates.

The Asymptomatic Carotid Artery Study showed a modest benefit for carotid endarterectomy in men who had more than 60% carotid stenosis, and did not have important cardiac or other comorbidity.[78] Surgeons who participated in this study were carefully selected, and the perioperative surgical morbidity and mortality was low (2.3%). The risk of stroke attributed to angiography was 1.2%.[78] A European study also reported a benefit for surgery, but women and those over 65 years of age did not fare as well as men and younger individuals.[79] The results of these studies and the topic of treatment of patients who have carotid artery stenosis with no symptoms has aroused considerable controversy.[80-82] Many neurologists and vascular surgeons question the need for catheter angiography in these patients and rely on duplex ultrasound and vascular imaging with MRA or CTA. The decision remains an individual one for each patient. Factors that should be considered when deciding between medical or surgical or interventional treatment include the anatomic aspects of the plaque (e.g., location, extent, degree of stenosis, heterogeneity, and echodensity), change in the plaque during conservative medical treatment with statins and platelet antiaggregants, comorbidities, especially

6

the presence of hypertension and coronary artery disease, the experience and results of the surgeon and the interventionalist chosen, and the biases and wishes of the well-informed patient.[76]

Data are now accruing about the results of angioplasty/stenting in patients with asymptomatic ICA atherosclerotic disease. If, with experience and better materials, the morbidity and mortality figures for interventional treatment in patients with severe and moderate stenosis become extremely low, I and many others will have to rethink our approach to these patients.

Extracranial Carotid Artery Dissections

After atherosclerosis, dissection is the next most common lesion that affects the carotid artery in the neck. I discuss dissections in more detail in Chapter 11. Carotid artery dissections usually involve the pharyngeal portion of the artery above the origin but below entry into the skull. Dissections are tears in arteries, almost always involving the medial coat. Dissections are customarily referred to as traumatic or spontaneous in origin. The great majority of dissections, however, probably involve some trauma or mechanical stress. Sudden neck movements and stretching are likely to cause dissection. Some inciting events are trivial, such as lunging for a tennis shot or turning the neck while driving to see other cars to the side and rear. Many patients forget such events or believe them to be too inconsequential to mention. Congenital and acquired abnormalities of the arterial media and elastic tissue, especially fibromuscular dysplasia, make patients more vulnerable to dissection. Most patients with dissection, however, do not have concurrent disorders. Migraine is more common in patients with dissection. The posited explanation for the relationship between migraine and dissection is that edema of the vessel wall during a migraine attack makes the involved artery more vulnerable to tearing.

Arterial dissections probably begin with a tear in the media that then leads to bleeding within the arterial wall. Intramural blood then dissects longitudinally, spreading along the vessel proximally and distally. Dissections can tear through the intima, allowing partially coagulated intramural blood to enter the lumen of the artery. The arterial wall, expanded by intramural blood, also compresses the lumen. Dissections probably begin from the luminal side at the intimal surface in some patients and dissect into the media. Intimal flaps are often present on the intimal surface. At times, the major dissection plane is between the media and the adventitia, causing an aneurysmal outpouching of the arterial wall.

Extracranial dissections cause symptoms primarily by the presence of luminal compromise and luminal clot. Dissections through the adventitia lead to rupture into the surrounding neck, muscles, and fascia, a process that causes neck pain and formation of a pseudoaneurysm, but usually does not further compromise blood flow. Thrombus is present within the lumen because of rupture of intramural clot into the lumen or thrombus formation in situ within the lumen. Narrowing of the lumen by the intramural blood, with alteration in blood flow and irritation of the endothelium causing release of endothelins and tissue factors, and activation of platelets and the coagulation cascade, all contribute to formation of intraluminal thrombus. Brain ischemia can result from hypoperfusion (usually from acute luminal compromise), embolism, or both. Hypoperfusion usually causes transient ischemia, but seldom is prolonged enough to cause infarction. Infarction is more often caused by embolization or propagation of luminal thrombus.

The major symptoms of carotid artery dissection in the neck are (1) neck, head, and face pain; (2) Horner's syndrome; (3) pulsatile tinnitus; (4) transient ipsilateral monocular vision loss; (5) transient hemispheral attacks with contralateral limb numbness or weakness; (6) sudden onset strokes; and (7) palsy of lower cranial nerves (IX-XII).[83-85]

I separate symptoms related to the arterial wall from those related to brain ischemia. The commonest symptoms not indicative of brain ischemia are pain, Horner's syndrome, pulsatile tinnitus, and loss of function of lower cranial nerves. Many patients present with pain and headache as their only symptoms and do not have neurologic findings. The pain is often in the neck, face, or jaw. Headaches may be generalized, but are most often on the side of the dissection. Features of Horner's syndrome are caused by involvement of the sympathetic fibers along the dilated carotid artery segments. Pulsatile tinnitus is explained by the course of the internal carotid artery near the tympanic membrane. I personally have not seen a patient present with nonischemic findings (other then pain and headache) that were present for a week or more who later developed brain ischemia.

Neurologic symptoms related to hypoperfusion are usually multiple, brief TIAs, referred to as carotid allegro by Miller Fisher because of their rapidity. Sudden-onset strokes are usually caused by embolism of clot from the region of dissection. The distended, dilated carotid artery at the skull base can compress the lower cranial nerves (IX to XII) that exit this region. The diagnosis of carotid artery dissection can be suggested by ultrasound when the ultrasonographer explores the neck with the probe from above the carotid bifurcation to the skull base.[86] MRA, CTA, and standard angiography are helpful. Figures 6-9A and B show MRAs of a patient with a carotid dissection. A cross-section of fat-saturated MRI scans of the neck in this patient shows a characteristic change in the signal intensity in the wall of the artery. Figure 6-10 is an angiogram that shows a characteristic aneurysm in the pharyngeal ICA from a patient with a carotid dissection. A montage of angiograms in patients with carotid artery dissections is found in Figure 11-3.

There have been no controlled trials of medical therapy. Table 6-4 lists various treatments given in large series of patients with cervical, mostly carotid artery dissections.[83,85,87,88] Fully 87% of the 572 patients were treated with anticoagulants in these series. Prevention of embolization of thrombus at or shortly after the dissection should prevent stroke. Anticoagulants have not seemed to increase the extent of the dissections, a major theoretical concern.

One report does give some evidence that occasionally anticoagulation can be problematic.[89] I use heparin than warfarin in those patients who have neurologic ischemic symptoms, in those with severe narrowing of the arterial lumen, and those with intracranial embolic occlusions. My reasons for choosing anticoagulants over antiplatelets follow: (1) evidence that red-clot (erythrocyte-fibrin) thromboemboli enter the arterial lumen in dissection patients and anticoagulants are more effective against red clots than antiplatelets, (2) many reports of others that anticoagulants are effective and

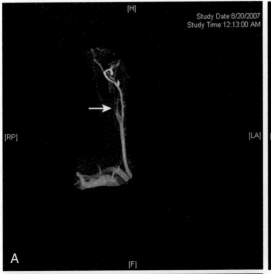
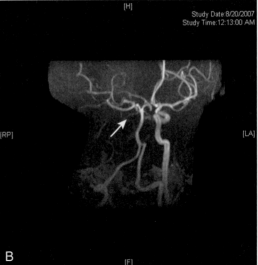
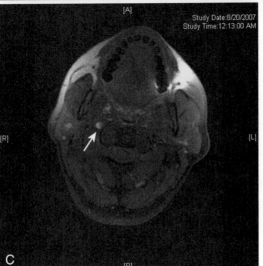

Figure 6-9. Dissection of the internal carotid artery. (**A**) Magnetic resonance angiogram showing narrowing with tapering of the internal carotid artery *(white arrow)* above its origin. (**B**) Magnetic resonance angiogram showing that the distal right internal carotid artery does not opacify. The *white arrow* indicates where the vessel should be visible. (**C**) Fat-saturated MRI image showing a half-moon—shaped hyperintensity *(white arrow)* that represents blood or edema within the dissected right internal carotid artery.

6

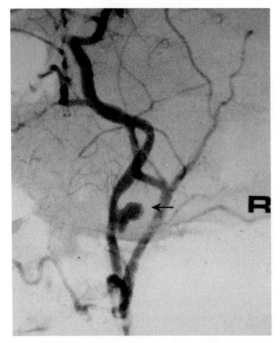

Figure 6-10. Right internal carotid dye-contrast digital subtraction cerebral angiogram showing an aneurysmal outpouching within the pharyngeal portion of the internal carotid artery in a patient with a carotid artery dissection.

platelet function such as aspirin, clopidogrel, or aspirin with modified-release dipyridamole.

Thrombolytics have been given to a few patients with ICA neck dissections. They might be effective in patients with intracranial red clot embolization who do not have obstruction of the pharyngeal ICA who are seen soon after neurologic symptom onset and do not already have large brain infarcts. These circumstances are very unusual in my experience. IV tPA is likely to be ineffective when the ICA is occluded. Stenting is rarely indicated since in patients without occlusions, the arterial lumens usually open well with time and anticoagulants are effective in preventing further thrombi from forming and embolizing. Stenting may be useful in the very rare patient who has tight luminal narrowing and continues to have brain ischemia despite anticoagulants.[90]

Intracranial Internal Carotid Artery Occlusive Disease

Narrowing and thrombotic occlusion of the ICA occur at the siphon far less often than at the ICA origin. The siphon includes the S-shaped portion of the carotid artery from its entry through the carotid foramen into the petrous bone to its exit from the cavernous sinus above the petrous clinoid. The ophthalmic artery originates from the ICA within the siphon. Less is known about the pathology of the artery in its entirely intraosseous course because the bone is seldom removed for study. Calcification of the ICA in the siphon is common.[91] Studies of groups of patients with ICA siphon disease report a high frequency of strokes, frequent coexistent extracranial vascular disease, and a high death rate from coronary artery disease.[92-97]

relatively safe, and (3) personal experience with more than 200 dissection patients treated with anticoagulants. I do, however, favor a randomized trial testing this choice of anticoagulant treatment. Because the risk of embolization is only during the acute period, I use heparin, followed by warfarin, and try to maximize cerebral blood flow (CBF) during the acute period, to augment collateral circulation. Healing of dissections can be monitored using MRI, MRA, CTA, and ultrasound. I stop anticoagulants after 6 weeks in patients with dissected arteries that remain occluded. I continue anticoagulants in patients with widely patent arteries until luminal stenosis improves and blood flow is not importantly obstructed. When arterial blood flow is improved, I switch to drugs that modify

> RY, a 70-year-old African-American man, had an attack of transient weakness of his right leg 1 week before he awakened with weakness of the right face and leg. This was accompanied by an unaccustomed reluctance to speak. He repeated spoken language normally and comprehension

Table 6-4.   Acute Treatment in Patients with Neck Arterial Dissections in Three Series

Series	n	Antiplatelets	Anticoagulants	t-PA	Surgery
Biousse et al[83]	80	15 (19%)	58 (73%)	0	1 (1%)
Engelter et al[87]	33	8 (24%)	25 (76%)	0	0
Touze et al[88]	459	24 (5%)	416 (91%)[a]	2 (0.4%)	0
Totals	572	47 (8%)	499 (87%)	2 (0.3%)	1 (0.2%)

[a]405 heparin and 11 warfarin.

of written and spoken language was good. There was a past history of hypertension, angina pectoris and a high-pitched focal bruit was audible over the right neck.

The epidemiology of carotid siphon disease is probably similar to ICA-origin disease. African Americans, however, have an unexpectedly high incidence of this lesion.[17] Accompanying disease at the ICA and vertebral artery origins is common. In one series of ICA-siphon disease patients, tandem ICA origin and siphon disease occurred in 62% of patients.[92] TIAs are less frequent and fewer in number in patients with siphon disease when compared with ICA-origin disease. The ratio of strokes to TIAs and asymptomatic patients is higher in carotid-siphon disease.

The presence of amaurosis fugax depends on the level of the lesion in the siphon. In my experience, the occlusive lesion is most often distal to the ophthalmic artery origin, so that ICA siphon disease is an uncommon cause of transient monocular visual loss. On examination, there are usually no signs of collateral circulation through the ECA vessels of the face. The ocular and retinal pathologies discussed in ICA-origin disease are uncommon. I have, however, seen a number of patients with angiographically verified thrombotic occlusion of the carotid siphon, who days later developed signs of decreased ophthalmic flow and reduced central retinal artery pressure. The mechanism of delayed ophthalmic ischemia is retrograde extension of the clot below the ophthalmic artery branch, a phenomenon documented at necropsy in patients with stenosis and thrombosis of the ICA siphon.[98] The thrombus can also extend retrograde into the neck and mimic occlusive disease at the ICA origin. Retrograde extension of clot is, however, rare if the siphon occlusion is caused by embolism.[98]

Too few patients have been well studied to allow a comparison of the topography and distribution of cerebral infarcts in patients with ICA-siphon disease, as compared with disease of the ICA origin or the MCA. My impression is that separate infarcts in portions of the ACA and MCA territories are more common in siphon disease. The leg is more often paretic in siphon disease, indicating ACA-territory damage. Sometimes, the lesions affect the center of the ACA and MCA territories, causing weakness of the lower extremity and face with relative sparing of the hand, whereas in ICA-origin disease, upper-extremity weakness is most common.

In RY, a carotid duplex scan showed moderate stenosis (50%) of the right ICA origin. TCD showed increased blood-flow velocities through the orbital window at the left carotid siphon,

and reduced velocities in the left MCA and ACA. Velocities in the right intracranial arteries were normal. Angiography by femoral catheterization revealed severe stenosis of the left ICA just as it entered the siphon, well below the ophthalmic-artery origin (Fig. 6-11). The left ICA origin had a shallow plaque without stenosis. No definite distal-branch artery occlusion was seen. MRI showed small infarcts in the paramedian frontal lobe and in the left posterior parietal lobe.

Ultrasound studies confirmed severe carotid-siphon disease on the side appropriate to the symptoms and the infarcts found on MRI. TCD is effective for detecting and quantifying stenotic lesions of the intracranial ICA.[99,100] MRAs of the carotid siphon

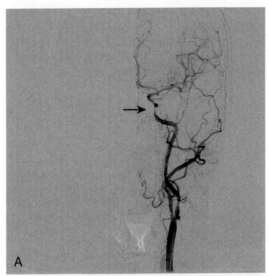

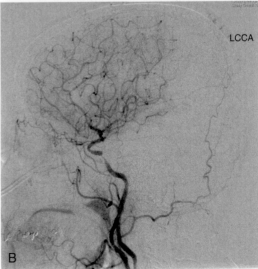

Figure 6-11. Dye contrast digital subtraction left carotid artery cerebral angiogram. (**A**) Anteroposterior view showing a severe area of narrowing of the internal carotid artery as it enters the carotid siphon. (**B**) Lateral view of the lesion. (Courtesy of Ajith Thomas, MD.)

are often difficult to interpret. Tortuosity makes this a common area for artifacts. CTAs are more useful than MRAs in this region. The contralateral ICA-origin lesion was asymptomatic and not severe enough to reduce flow. The clinical signs of leg and foot weakness and transcortical motor aphasia were caused by ACA-territory ischemia. The infarct was caused by either low flow with good MCA collaterals or embolism originating from the irregular siphon stenosis.

> RY was given intravenous heparin. After a slight increase in leg weakness during the first day, he stabilized. Warfarin was begun on day 5. On day 7, heparin was discontinued. The patient was maintained on warfarin therapy for 1 year, at which time he developed a fatal myocardial infarction.

Reviews in the 1980s confirm that ICA-siphon disease has a worse prognosis than ICA-origin disease.[92-97] Intracranial occlusive disease in general carries a worse prognosis than disease in the neck.[101] The closer the obstructing lesion to the brain, the more likely that infarction will occur. At the same time, when infarction is related to localized in-situ atherosclerosis, the infarcts tend to be relatively smaller than those caused by intra-arterial emboli originating in the neck, aorta, or heart.

Late strokes and cardiac death are common. Stenosis of the ICA in the siphon seems to be more stable than other intracranial lesions. Follow-up angiography shows a low rate of progression or regression of stenotic carotid siphon atherosclerotic lesions.[102] Lesions within the siphon cannot be treated surgically. Therapeutic alternatives include thrombolytics for patients who arrive soon after stroke onset, and to prevent worsening and for secondary stroke prevention antiplatelet agglutinating agents, warfarin, angioplasty, and ECA-ICA bypass to MCA branches. There have been no prospective controlled studies to fully document the effectiveness, or lack thereof, of any medical treatment in patients with disease of the carotid siphon, mostly because the number of recognized patients is relatively small. In some series, white men with TIAs relating to siphon disease had a relatively good outcome after warfarin therapy.[93,94] Studies[103] and trials[104-107] that compared antiplatelets and anticoagulants in patients with intracranial disease have contained too few patients with ICA siphon disease to yield meaningful results for this specific group of patients. The tortuous, windy course and calcification within the siphon makes angioplasty or stenting of stenotic lesions difficult and risky. Some balloon angioplasties, however, have been performed without stents.[108-111]

In patients who have occlusion of the ICA siphon and who arrive within 6 hours of neurologic symptom onset, thrombolysis should be considered in those patients who have no or small brain infarcts. There are few reported such cases. Within the first 3 hours, IV treatment should be used. If unsuccessful, IA treatment can then be pursued. Others will choose to begin directly with IA thrombolysis after angiography.

I suggest warfarin for those patients with tight ICA siphon stenosis, and preserved anterograde flow who have no contraindication to anticoagulation. I reserve antiplatelet agglutinating agents, such as aspirin, clopidogrel, cilostazole, and combined low-dose aspirin and dipyridamole for patients who have minor irregularity of the artery without severe impediment to flow. As with disease of the ICA origin, attention should also be directed to the heart because of the high incidence of associated cardiac morbidity (as in the case of RY).

In some patients, there is associated severe disease of the ICA origin in addition to the siphon stenosis. In these patients with tandem lesions, operation on the ICA in the neck is sometimes followed by opening of the siphon lesion on follow-up angiography.[112] This occurrence is explained by preoperative distal collapse or narrowing of the artery as a result of diminished flow. In the face of complete occlusion of the ICA siphon, there is no gain in opening an ICA-origin stenosis. If, however, the ICA stenosis at the siphon is not critical, carotid endarterectomy or stenting of the more proximal ICA-origin lesion might greatly augment flow.

In the presence of severe critical stenosis at both neck and intracranial sites, angioplasty/stenting can be performed at both sites during a single procedure. When tandem ICA occlusive lesions are present along with other occlusive extracranial and/or intracranial lesions, I generally choose anticoagulants and high dose statins rather than aggressive attempts to open the tandem lesions. Aggressive surgery or interventional treatment mandates cessation of anticoagulants before and shortly after interventions and the use of anticoagulants plus antiplatelets after interventional treatment. This scenario carries a relatively high risk of occlusion of other stenotic arteries during the cessation of anticoagulants and/or hemorrhage during the weeks and few months after the interventional procedures. In my estimate, the risks outweigh the benefits in most patients with widespread occlusive disease. I usually choose warfarin therapy for these patients.

Top of the Carotid Artery Occlusions

Occlusions of the intracranial carotid artery bifurcation are predominantly embolic.[113,114] This portion of the ICA is often called the T portion because of its shape. When an embolus blocks the distal intracranial ICA, the result is usually a large infarct that includes the anterior and MCA territory. Death or severe disability often results. Occlusions of the distal intracranial carotid artery have been thought to seldom recanalize with either intravenous or intra-arterial thrombolytic treatment.[114-116] More recent analysis is more optimistic about the potential for carotid T recanalization after thrombolysis.[117]

Prophylactic management of patients with emboli to the carotid T depends on the nature and site of the lesion from which the thromboembolus originated. Severe stenosis and thrombotic occlusion of the supraclinoid carotid artery before its intracranial bifurcation into MCA and ACA branches (top of the carotid) rarely occurs. In my experience, an unusual number of patients with a lesion at this site have had coagulation abnormalities, such as sickle cell disease or circulating lupus anticoagulant.

Intracranial Dissections Involving the Carotid Artery and Its Branches

Intracranial anterior circulation dissections are much less common than those that involve the extracranial—mostly pharyngeal portion—of the ICA. When intracranial dissections do occur they often involve the ICA within or above the carotid siphon. Past reports of intracranial ICA dissections emphasize severe morbidity and mortality. My colleagues and I recently reported 10 patients who had spontaneous intracranial ICA dissections.[118] The ages ranged from 15 to 59 (mean age 28). Severe retroorbital or temporal headache followed by contralateral hemiparesis was the most common initial clinical symptom. No patient had vascular risk factors or a history of neck or head trauma. One patient had only a TIA, but the other nine had brain infarcts, one accompanied by some subarachnoid bleeding. The most common location of the dissection was in the supraclinoid ICA (eight patients) with extension to the middle cerebral artery or anterior cerebral artery in two patients each. Aneurysm formation in the ipsilateral anterior cerebral artery was seen in one patient. Two patients had a total occlusion of the supraclinoid portion of the ICA. All patients did well, with no ($n = 3$), mild ($n = 4$), or moderate ($n = 3$) disability on the Modified Rankin Scale during a 3-month follow-up period.[118] Others have also reported patients, often children and young adults, with intracranial ICA dissections that resulted in relatively good outcomes.[119] Dissections may also begin in the MCAs.

OCCLUSION OR SEVERE STENOSIS OF THE MIDDLE CEREBRAL ARTERY STEM OR ITS MAJOR UPPER AND LOWER TRUNKS

Occlusion of the MCA was a common diagnosis in the era before cerebral angiography. After Fisher and others called attention to the high incidence of extracranial ICA disease[1-3] and angiography became prevalent, most patients formerly diagnosed with MCA occlusion were found instead to have ICA disease in the neck. The vast majority of MCA occlusions are embolic, arising from a proximal ICA plaque or from the heart or aorta. The observations on the rarity of occlusive lesions in the intracranial anterior circulation were generated at hospitals with a predominance of white patients. Studies of African-American[17,18,120,121] and Asian[122-126] patients, however, show a higher frequency of intracranial occlusive disease of the MCA and its major trunk branches than is found in white patients. A recent necropsy study in Paris of the MCAs in 339 predominantly white stroke patients showed that 11% had nonstenotic atherosclerotic plaques, 13% had plaques causing 30% to 74% stenosis, and 6% had 75% to 99% stenosis or in-situ occlusion.[126a] Figure 6-12 shows the most common patterns of infarction in patients with MCA occlusions.

> A 48-year-old Chinese woman, AC, awakened with weakness of the right face and was unable to speak. These symptoms cleared during the day. Three days later, during the morning, she became unable to speak normally and recognized weakness of her right limbs. She had a past history of slight hypertension, but had no history of coronary or peripheral vascular disease. She came to the hospital 10 hours after the symptoms began.

In my experience, patients with MCA occlusive disease, when compared with patients with ICA disease, are more often African American or Asian, young, female, hypertensive, and diabetic.[19,29,125,127] They also have had a lower incidence of hypercholesterolemia and associated coronary and peripheral vascular disease. Patients of Japanese, Chinese, Korean, and Thai descent, as well as diabetics and women taking contraceptive pills, share a propensity for MCA pathology

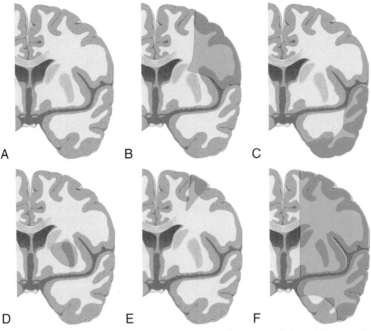

Figure 6-12. Common patterns of infarction with MCA occlusion: (**A**) normal cerebral hemisphere in coronal section, (**B**) occlusion of the upper trunk of the MCA, (**C**) occlusion of the lower trunk of the MCA, (**D**) infarct of the deep basal ganglia, (**E**) wedge infarct in the pial territory, and (**F**) whole MCA occlusion.

with African Americans. As in atherosclerotic neck disease, active lipid-laden plaques and ulcerations predispose to deposition of white and red thrombi and thrombosis of the artery.[127a] The loosely attached thrombi can propagate and embolize distally as well as occlude the orifices of the penetrating lenticulostriate arteries.

Although TIAs do occur in patients with MCA disease, they are probably less frequent than with ICA disease and occur during a shorter time span.[29,123] The frequency of TIAs in patients with MCA disease also seems to vary with race. In four series of predominantly white patients with MCA occlusive disease, TIAs were a more frequent presentation than stroke.[128-131] The TIA to stroke ratios in these studies were 15 to 1,[128] 15 to 6,[129] 13 to 11,[130] and 9 to 4.[131] In contrast, the TIA to stroke ratio in a predominantly African American patient series was 4 to 16.[29] It was 3 to 20 in a series of mostly Chinese-origin patients,[127] and 8 to 28 in a series of Japanese patients.[132] Smoking was an important risk factor in a large study that reported its frequency. Eighty percent of patients with MCA occlusion and 72% of patients with MCA stenosis had a history of cigarette smoking.[126] Because the vascular lesion is intracranial and, of course, beyond the ophthalmic artery supply, transient monocular blindness does not occur.

During the first 3 days in the hospital, AC progressively worsened, gradually developing a complete right hemiplegia, minor tingling of the right limbs, and mutism. Examination revealed no bruits, facial, or limb-pulse abnormalities.

Patients with MCA disease often develop their deficits more gradually than comparable series of patients with ICA disease.[29,127] Patients with MCA disease often note their abnormalities on awakening in the morning or after a nap and often have subsequent fluctuations or progression during the next 1 to 7 days. This gradual onset and progressive course support a low-flow contribution to the ischemia. Deficits begin when flow is most sluggish, and collateral circulation takes time to develop and equilibrate. Recent studies using TCD show that microemboli often originate from regions of MCA stenosis.[133-135] As in the ICA, reduced perfusion results in poor washout of emboli. Production of thromboemboli and reduced clearance both contribute to infarction.[40,41] In contrast, patients with ICA disease more often have sudden-onset deficits while awake and thereafter remain stable (a course better explained by embolism of large white, red, or mixed clots from their ICA lesion than by reduced perfusion alone).

Because the occlusive process is intracranial, there are no important associated signs of extracranial disease. Neurologic findings vary, depending on the location of the vascular occlusion and the brain ischemia. The following sections discuss the most common patterns of neurologic deficits seen in patients with MCA disease. Although these syndromes are discussed under the heading of intrinsic MCA-occlusive disease, the patterns are more commonly caused by embolism to the MCA territory. Figure 6-13 shows the common patterns of MCA occlusion and their anatomic and clinical correlates.

Occlusion or Stenosis of Upper Division of the Middle Cerebral Artery

The superior division of the MCA supplies the frontal and superior parietal lobes. It can be thought of as supplying the MCA territory above the sylvian fissure. Occasionally, when the mainstem MCA is short, the lenticulostriate vessels

arise from the proximal portion of the superior trunk.[29,136,137] In that case, the internal capsule and lateral basal ganglia are also nourished by the superior trunk.

The findings include (1) hemiplegia, more severe in the face, hand, and upper extremity, with relative sparing of the lower extremity; (2) hemisensory loss, usually including decreased pinprick and position sense, sometimes sparing the leg; (3) conjugate eye deviation, with the eyes resting toward the side of the brain lesion; and (4) neglect of the contralateral side of space, especially to visual stimuli. Visual neglect is usually more severe in patients with right hemisphere lesions.

When the lesion is in the left dominant hemisphere, there invariably is an accompanying aphasia. Verbal output is sparse and patients do not do what they are asked to do with either hand. They may follow whole-body commands, however, such as turn over, sit, and stand. They

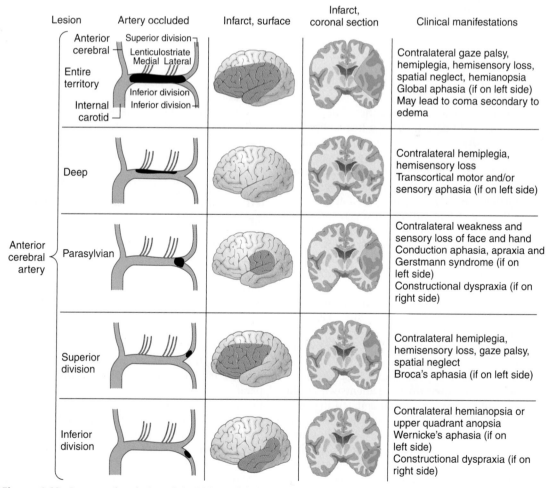

Figure 6-13. Patterns of occlusion of the MCA and their anatomic correlates.

may be able to nod appropriately to yes and no questions, but comprehension of written material is poor. With time, a pattern of Broca's aphasia evolves with sparse, effortful speech, poor pronunciation of syllables, and omission of filler words. Comprehension of spoken language, however, is preserved.

In superior-division MCA infarcts in the right hemisphere, patients often seem unaware of their deficit (anosognosia) and may not admit they are hemiplegic or impaired in any way.[31,32,138] Some patients are also impersistent, performing requested tasks quickly, but fail to persevere and terminate tasks prematurely.[31,32,139] When asked to read, patients with right superior-trunk occlusions often omit the left of the page or paragraph, and do not heed people or objects to their left.

Occlusion of the Inferior Division of the Middle Cerebral Artery

The inferior division of the MCA usually supplies the lateral surface of the temporal lobe and inferior parietal lobule. The supply is mostly inferior and posterior to the sylvian fissure. The anterior, medial, and inferior portions of the temporal lobes are supplied by other arteries.

In contrast to patients with lesions of the superior division, patients with occlusion of the MCA inferior division usually have no elementary motor or sensory abnormalities. They often have a visual field defect, either a hemianopia or an upper quadrantanopia, affecting the contralateral visual field.

When the left hemisphere is involved, patients have a Wernicke-type aphasia. Speech is fluent, and syllables are well pronounced. Patients use wrong or nonexistent words, however, and what is said may make little sense. Comprehension and repetition of spoken language are poor. There may be relative sparing of written comprehension, with the patient preferring that words be written rather than spoken.[140,141] When the right hemisphere is affected, patients draw and copy poorly, and may have difficulty finding their way about or reading a map.

Behavioral abnormalities also frequently accompany temporal-lobe infarctions. Patients with Wernicke's aphasia are sometimes irascible, paranoid, and may become violent. Patients with right temporal infarcts often have an agitated hyperactive state resembling delirium tremens.[142-144] Diagnosis of right inferior-trunk occlusion is sometimes difficult unless patients are examined thoroughly. The key neurologic findings are a left visual-field defect and poor drawing and copying in an agitated person.[144]

Deep Infarction of the Middle Cerebral Artery Territory

Basal ganglia and internal-capsule infarction is usually explained by occlusion of the mainstem MCA before its lenticulostriate branches. Excellent potential exists for collateral circulation over the convexities but poor collateral circulation in the deep basal gray nuclei and the internal capsule. For this reason, some patients with MCA occlusion have selective ischemia of the deep lenticulostriate territory. Collateral circulation, however, is adequate to prevent cortical infarction. On CT or MRI scans, the lesions can be confused with lacunes, but are larger and often extend to the inferior brain surface. Some have called these lesions giant lacunes.[29,145] The preferred term for these deep MCA lenticulostriate-territory lesions, however, is *striatocapsular infarcts*.[113,146,147]

Patients with stratiocapsular infarcts are invariably hemiparetic, but the distribution of weakness in face, arm, and leg is variable. Sensory loss is usually minor because the posterior portion of the internal capsule is spared. When the lesion is in the left hemisphere, after a short period of temporary mutism, speech is sparse and dysarthric, but repetition of spoken language is preserved. Comprehension of spoken and written language depends on the size and anteroposterior extent of the lesion.[148,149] When the right hemisphere is involved, there often is neglect of contralateral visual and tactile stimuli, but this is usually more transient than with parietal cortical infarction.

Mainstem Occlusion with Total Infarction of the Middle Cerebral Artery Territory

Mainstem occlusion with total infarction of the MCA territory is most common in patients with embolism to the proximal MCA (Fig. 6-9). In most patients with intrinsic occlusive disease of the MCA, there is sufficient collateral circulation to spare at least the outer borders of the territory.

These patients are usually devastated. Among 208 patients with large MCA-territory infarcts in one series, the mortality rate was 17%. Fifty percent of patients had severe disability.[150] Severe paralysis, hemisensory loss, attentional hemianopia, and conjugate eye deviation to the opposite side were found. When the left hemisphere is involved, there is a global aphasia. Right hemisphere lesions produce severe neglect, anosognosia, disinterest or poor motivation, apathy, and severe constructional apraxia. Recovery to useful function is unusual.[151]

Brain edema with swelling of the infarcted hemisphere, causing a midline shift and brain herniations, is an important complication in patients with large MCA-territory infarction.[150,152,153] This complication is especially apt to develop in young patients with large embolic MCA-territory infarcts. Coma usually heralds a fatal outcome. Some patients with large MCA-territory infarcts and severe brain edema have been treated with hemicraniectomy with favorable outcomes.[152,153]

Segmental Infarction in the Middle Cerebral Artery Territory

Segmental infarctions in the MCA territory are caused by occlusion of the distal cortical branches of the upper or lower division of the MCA. They are almost invariably embolic and are seldom caused by intrinsic atheromatous occlusion of a convexity branch. The syndromes are quite variable and depend on the branch affected.

Insula of Reil Infarction

Infarction of a portion of the insular cortex is quite common in patients with embolic occlusion of the MCA. One of the clues to MCA infarction, known for some time, is the so-called "insular ribbon" sign on CT scans of patients with acute brain ischemia. Figure 6-14 is an MRI of an infarct involving predominantly a portion of the insular cortex. Among 150 consecutive patients

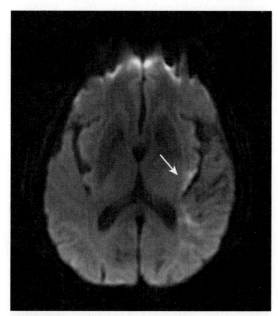

Figure 6-14. MRI-DWI image showing a infarct involving predominantly the inferior portion of the left insular cortex (white arrow).

with acute nonlacunar brain ischemia studied at the Beth Israel Deaconess Medical Center in Boston using modern multimodal MRI, we found that 72 (48%) had insular infarcts on DWI.[154] Major insular lesions were present in 34 (23%) and 38 (25%) had minor lesions. Insula infarcts were associated with lenticulostriate territory infarction, more severe neurologic deficits, and proximal MCA occlusion detected on MRA.[154]

Several patterns were apparent: infarction limited to the anterior portion of the insula, often accompanied by infarcts in the suprasylvian territory of the MCA; infarcts limited to the posterior insula, often accompanied by temporal and inferior parietal lobe infarction in territory supplied by the inferior division of the MCA; and major infarcts involving the anterior and posterior insula, often accompanied by striatocapsular infarcts and/or involvement of cortical and subcortical territories supplied by the superior and/or inferior division of the MCA.[154] The superior division of the MCA supplies the anterior insular cortex, and the inferior division supplies the posterior insular cortex. When the entire insula (or parts of the anterior and posterior insula) are infarcted, the occlusive lesion must have at some time involved the mainstem MCA.

Animal and some human observations indicate that the insular cortex has important autonomic and cardiovascular control functions.[155-159] Oppenheimer and colleagues stimulated the insular cortex of human epileptic patients.[155,156] They found that when they electrically stimulated areas of the left human insular cortex, bradycardia, and blood pressure depression responses resulted, while stimulation of the right insular cortex elicited tachycardia and pressor effects.[155] Stimulation of the left insula decreased protective parasympathetic effects and increased cardiovascular sympathetic effects on the heart rate and blood pressure. This asymmetry of autonomic function was also shown by Yoon and colleagues who studied autonomic function in patients evaluated for epilepsy surgery.[157] They found that the right cerebral hemisphere predominantly modulated sympathetic nervous system activity. Hachinski et al showed that rats with experimentally induced, right-middle cerebral artery occlusions developed an increase in Q-T intervals and had elevated plasma norepinephrine levels, while sham-operated and left-middle cerebral artery occlusion animals had neither of these findings. They concluded that right-cerebral hemisphere infarcts caused more sympathetic nervous system perturbations than comparable left hemisphere infarcts.[158] Other investigators have shown using power spectrum analysis of heart rate variability that stroke patients with middle cerebral artery territory infarcts have

6

a significant sympathetic/parasympathetic imbalance.[159] These cardiovascular changes have usually been predominantly attributed to the insula of Reil in the respective cerebral hemispheres.

> Neck ultrasound in patient AC was normal. Blood-sugar levels were 240 on admission and remained elevated until insulin was begun. DWI-MRI showed a deep striatocapsular infarct. Perfusion MRI showed a large perfusion defect occupying most of the deep and superficial MCA territory. TCD showed an absence of flow velocities in the left MCA with normal ACA ¦and right-sided values. Angiography showed occlusion of the left mainstem MCA after a tapered, irregular origin.

CT patterns of MCA-territory infarction have already been described. The most common patterns are wedge-shaped, pial-territory infarcts, and subcortical, deep basal ganglia, and internal-capsule infarcts.[127] Hyperdensity of the MCA in noncontrast-enhanced CT scans is an important and relatively common finding in patients with acute-onset MCA-territory infarcts (Fig. 4-19). In one series among 55 patients, one third had the hyperdense MCA sign.[160] TCD is a useful technique for showing MCA disease.[99,100,161,162] Stenosis often causes high velocities when insonating at the depth of the lesion. When the MCA is occluded, flow and velocities decline, and often no signal can be obtained. TCD can be used to rapidly diagnose embolic MCA occlusion and monitor recanalization during and after thrombolysis.[162] TCD monitoring sometimes shows microembolic signals in patients with MCA stenosis.[134,135,162,163] This indicates embolism from the MCA lesion, a situation also documented to occur at necropsy in patients with thrombi engrafted on MCA stenotic lesions.[164]

MRA and CTA, with concentration on intracranial views, can also usually document severe MCA occlusive lesions.[165,166] Using standard dye-contrast angiography, MCA occlusion is best seen on the anteroposterior view of a selective ICA injection. At times, the occlusion is near the MCA trifurcation, so oblique views are needed. The area of poorest supply of MCA tributaries is best identified on lateral views. At times, poor opacification of inferior and superior trunk arteries is seen, and it is difficult to identify the precise point of narrowing or occlusion.

AC was treated with heparin. The neurologic deficit, however, progressed. She remained on warfarin for 2 months. Repeat angiography showed good collateral filling of the MCA from ACA and PCA branches. The infarct on a T2-weighted MRI scan at 2 months matched the perfusion defect on the perfusion-weighted MRI performed initially.

Therapy of intrinsic MCA disease is uncertain because there have been few series of patients studied and seldom have the studies included treatment begun during the acute period of ischemia. In patients with acute thrombotic or embolic MCA occlusion, thrombolytic treatment is sometimes effective if given early enough. Thrombolytic therapy is more likely to lead to recanalization in patients with MCA emboli than in those with in-situ thrombosis engrafted on atherostenosis. Intravenous[44,45,167-170] and intra-arterial[115,116,171] thrombolysis have been effective in recanalizing MCA embolic occlusions. In patients with thrombotic disease within the MCA, thrombi often reform within the MCA after thrombolysis unless angioplasty is performed after the clot is lysed.

Angioplasty and stenting have been increasingly performed to dilate occlusive MCA-stenotic lesions.[108-111,172-174] Figure 5-2 contains angiograms of a patient with an irregular MCA mainstem stenosis that was treated successfully with a wingspan stent. Angioplasty can be complicated by occlusion of lenticulostriate branches with resultant striatocapsular infarction.[173] Dissection and vasoconstriction are other complications of angioplasty on the mainstem MCA.[173] The success of angioplasty depends greatly on the location, length, angulation, and morphology of the MCA-occlusive lesion.[174]

Heparin, low-molecular-weight heparin, and heparinoids have been given to patients with acute-thrombotic and embolic-MCA occlusions. Warfarin is then used to attempt to prevent propagation and embolization from the MCA thrombus during a period of 6 weeks to 3 months. During this time, the clot becomes organized and adherent, and collateral circulation maximizes. Warfarin has been also used to prevent total occlusion of a stenosed MCA. In the series of Hinton et al., Caucasian patients often stabilized while taking warfarin.[128] However, in series of black and Asian patients, anticoagulation has been reported to be less successful.[29,95,127] MCA pathology and pathophysiology may differ among whites, blacks, Asians, and others.

In the Warfarin-Aspirin Symptomatic Intracranial Disease Study (WASID) that retrospectively compared outcome in patients with intracranial occlusive disease treated with aspirin or warfarin, warfarin was more effective.[103] In this study, MCA-stenotic lesions were the most common intracranial stenotic lesions studied and the patients were treated acutely usually with heparin followed by warfarin.[103] In the prospective WASID Trial, aspirin (1300 mg/day) was as effective and caused less hemorrhage than warfarin.[105,106] However, this trial was a secondary prevention trial and patients were enrolled after the acute ischemic period. Warfarin was a bit more effective than aspirin, and did not cause excessive bleeding in those patients in whom the INR values remained in the therapeutic range.

I tend to use warfarin anticoagulation in patients with severe MCA stenosis, keeping the INR between 2.0 and 2.5. If ischemic symptoms are not controlled, I pursue angioplasty or stenting in selected patients with lesions amenable to this treatment.

OCCLUSION OR SEVERE STENOSIS OF THE ANTERIOR CEREBRAL ARTERY

Intrinsic occlusive disease of the ACA is unusual. Most ACA-territory infarcts are caused by embolism from the heart or ICA. Many patients with intrinsic disease of the ACA also have extensive ICA and MCA disease, often with multiple infarcts, making clinicopathologic correlation of the ACA lesions difficult.[175] Some ACA-territory infarcts are caused by occlusive disease of the ICA. Others are caused by vasospasm-related ischemia in patients with SAH who have aneurysms of the anterior communicating artery.[176] In one study of cerebral infarcts documented by CT, 13 of 413 (3%) were in the ACA territory.[177] Eight of the 13 patients with ACA-territory ischemia had angiography that showed five ACA occlusions. In three other patients, angiography showed ACA occlusion, but the CT showed no infarction in this territory. Nearly all patients in this series with occlusion of the ACA had severe occlusive disease at the origin of the ICA in the neck or in the carotid siphon on the side of the ACA lesion.[177] The most likely mechanism of ACA-territory infarction in this group of patients was intra-arterial embolism arising from the more proximal ICA lesions. In one patient, the authors postulated that intra-arterial embolic material traveled from an occluded ICA origin to the contralateral ACA, through a widely patent anterior communicating artery.

In the Lausanne Stroke Registry, 27 of 1490 patients (1.8%) with first-ever strokes had infarcts limited to the ACA territory.[178] Ten of the 27 patients had ICA-occlusive lesions and seven had cardiac-origin embolism. Only one patient, a Vietnamese man, had intrinsic ACA-occlusive disease. In the remainder of the patients, the cause of the ACA-territory infarcts was not discovered.[178] Occasionally, dissections may involve the anterior cerebral artery usually in the A2 portions of the artery.[179,180]

My experience and that of others[177,178,181-183] leads me to the following opinions about the mechanisms of ACA-territory infarction: (1) ACA-territory infarction is most often embolic; (2) embolism is most often intra-arterial, arising from proximal ICA occlusive disease; (3) when intrinsic atherostenosis affects the ACA, patients usually have widespread extracranial and intracranial occlusive disease with multiple brain infarcts; (4) patients of Asian extraction often have predominantly intracranial occlusive disease, sometimes involving the ACA; and (5) stenotic lesions of the ACA are not always in the horizontal first portion of the artery, but can involve the pericallosal artery and other branches. Figure 6-15 depicts patterns of ACA occlusion and their anatomic correlates.

The ACA, after its brief horizontal A1 segment, gives off penetrating arteries that supply anteromedial portions of the caudate nucleus, anterior limb of the internal capsule, and the anterior perforated substance.[184-187] One group of these penetrators is usually termed "the artery of Heubner," but analyses of anatomic specimens shows that there are more often a group of relatively parallel Heubner and medial striate arteries rather than a single artery.[185,187] After reaching the midline, the ACA swings posteriorly and divides to form the pericallosal and callosomarginal

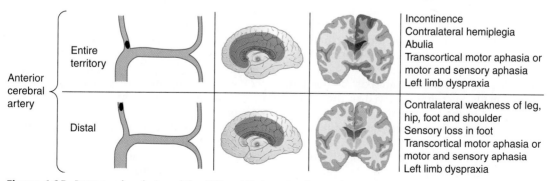

Figure 6-15. Patterns of occlusion of the ACA and their anatomic correlates.

Anterior cerebral artery	Entire territory			Incontinence Contralateral hemiplegia Abulia Transcortical motor aphasia or motor and sensory aphasia Left limb dyspraxia
	Distal			Contralateral weakness of leg, hip, foot and shoulder Sensory loss in foot Transcortical motor aphasia or motor and sensory aphasia Left limb dyspraxia

arteries that supply the paramedian frontal lobe above the corpus callosum. Figures 2-11, 2-12, and 2-15 show the ACA and its usual region of supply. At times, the A1 segment of the ACA on one side may be absent or hypoplastic, so that both ACAs are supplied by one ICA. The extent of infarction after ACA occlusion depends on the location of the obstruction and the pattern of the anterior circle of Willis.

> A 75-year-old man, CF, awakened from a nap with paralysis of his left leg and foot. He also had slight tingling in his left toes. Examination showed complete paralysis of the left lower extremity. When asked to salute, wave goodbye, or pretend to throw a ball, he performed these functions normally with the right arm, but used incorrect movements with the left arm. His arms, however, were not weak or clumsy. The patient was surprised to find that, on occasion, the left hand would grasp the right hand in the midst of an activity and seemed to do things without his will.

The single most important clue to an ACA-territory infarct is the distribution of motor weakness. Paralysis is usually greatest in the foot, but is also severe in the proximal thigh. Shoulder shrug is weak on the involved side, but the hand and face are usually normal if the deep ACA territory is spared. Some patients with anterior or large ACA-territory infarcts have a hemiplegia.[181-183] Some patients with medial frontal infarcts in the ACA territory have prominent motor neglect.[188] These individuals have little voluntary movement on the hemiparetic side. Despite the lack of spontaneous movement, strong prodding induces slow, clumsy arm movements. In these patients, the lower-extremity paralysis is explained by involvement of the precentral gyrus motor cortex. The upper limb motor dysfunction, however, is related to infarction of the premotor cortex anterior to the precentral gyrus.[188] Cortical sensory loss is also present in the weak limbs but is usually slight. The patient may have difficulty touching the spot on his or her lower extremity touched by the examiner, be unable to identify numbers written on his or her foot with a blunt pencil, or extinguish bilateral tactile stimuli on the paralyzed foot and leg. A grasp reflex is often present in the hand contralateral to the infarct.

Another helpful sign is apraxia of the left arm. Normally, speech is received in the posterior portions of the left cerebral hemisphere. To communicate language to regions of the right hemisphere that control the left limbs, the information goes forward toward the left frontal region and then across the corpus callosum to the right frontal region. In ACA-territory infarcts, the corpus callosum or its adjacent white matter is often infarcted. This interrupts the pathway, regardless of whether the right or left ACA territory is infarcted.[189,190] This disconnection can be detected by the following simple bedside tests:

1. Ask the patient to perform spoken commands with the right and left arms. Patients with ACA infarction may be unable to perform the commands correctly using the left hand. The fact that they follow the commands normally with the right hand proves they understand the commands.
2. Ask the patient to write or print first with the right hand, then with the left hand. Some patients with ACA infarction make aphasic errors when they write using the left hand.
3. Ask the patient to name objects placed first in the left hand, then in the right hand. Patients with an ACA infarct may be unable to name objects in their left hand, but can select the same objects by vision or touch and can name them correctly when placed in the right hand.

The topic of left limb apraxia was reviewed by Geschwind and Kaplan,[189,190] and has often been referred to as an *anterior disconnection syndrome*.

When the infarct involves the left ACA territory and supplementary motor cortex, a transcortical motor and sensory aphasia often results.[181,182,191-193] Despite reduced spontaneous speech, the patient can repeat spoken language well. Incontinence that is characterized by inability to control micturition, although the urge to urinate is preserved, may occur especially in patients with bilateral lesions. Patients with unilateral ACA infarcts or bilateral frontal infarcts are often abulic. They are apathetic with decreased spontaneity, slowness in responding to queries or commands, and use terse speech that is limited in amount.[192,193] These patients have difficulty counting quickly from 20 to 1, or in persevering with any protracted task such as crossing off all the letter A's in a paragraph or telling the examiner without prodding each time their finger is moved or touched. In some patients, the decreased activity is intermittent. At one moment patients speak. The next moment they stare blankly and pay no heed to queries or conversation, as if their brain were temporarily shut off.[194]

Another phenomenon found in some patients with frontal-lobe infarction related to ACA disease has been called the alien hand sign.[195-197] CF had noticed that his left hand had a mind of its own, often doing things that he did not will it to do. This sign is most common in the right hand that interferes with willed movements of the left hand. One hand acts against the other or acts involuntarily. Similar findings occur in patients with epilepsy after surgical cutting of the corpus callosum, making it likely that the phenomenon is caused by defective interhemispheric connections. Forced grasping and a heightened grasp reflex found often contralateral to frontal-lobe lesions may also play a role in causing this sign.

> CT showed a moderate-sized, right medial frontal infarct in CF (Figure 6-16), and angiography documented severe stenosis of the right ACA before it formed the callosomarginal artery. After physical therapy, he was able to walk with a brace.

MRI is able to show the topography of ACA-territory infarction quite well. Figure 6-16 is a CT and Figure 6-17 an MRI showing typical paramedian ACA-territory infarct in patients who had paralysis of the contralateral foot, leg, and thigh. Little is known about treatment for intrinsic ACA disease. I elected not to expose this older gentleman with an already sizable infarct to the risk of anticoagulation because little additional damage would ensue, even if the remainder of the right ACA territory were infarcted.

Occasionally, patients have the sudden development of bilateral ACA-territory infarction.[198-200] Figure 6-18 is a CT scan that shows a large, bilateral ACA-territory infarct. Figure 6-19 is a necropsy specimen of a patient with asymmetric large right and left ACA-territory infarcts. Bilateral ACA-territory infarction is most often

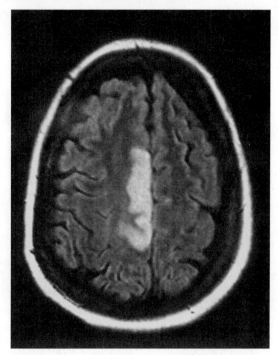

Figure 6-17. MRI FLAIR image showing a typical anterior cerebral artery cortical infarct located along the paramedian cerebral cortex.

explained by hypoplasia or absence of the A1 segment of the ACA on one side. In that circumstance, the territories of the ACA on both sides are supplied by one ACA. On angiography, dye instillation into one ICA produces bilateral ACA opacification. Occlusion of the ICA or ACA supplying both sides leads to bilateral frontal-lobe infarction. The resulting clinical picture is sudden apathy, abulia, and incontinence.[198-200] When the paracentral lobule is involved, weakness on one or both sides occurs. This predominantly affects the lower extremities. The sudden onset of a frontal lobe type of dementia presents a striking clinical picture, especially to those unfamiliar with this rare syndrome.

Caudate Infarcts

One of the major branch territories of the ACA is that of the recurrent arteries of Heubner, which supply the head of the caudate nucleus and the anterior limb of the internal capsule.[184-187] Much of the lateral portion of the caudate nucleus is supplied by the lateral lenticulostriate branches of the MCA. Although older descriptions spoke of a single Heubner's artery, newer dissections show there usually are multiple, parallel penetrating arteries arising from the ACA near the anterior communicating artery junction. In approximately

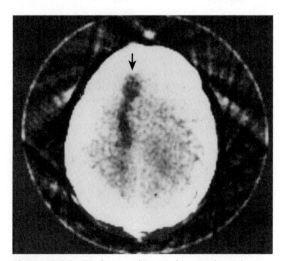

Figure 6-16. CT showing linear infarct in the right ACA territory *(black arrow)*.

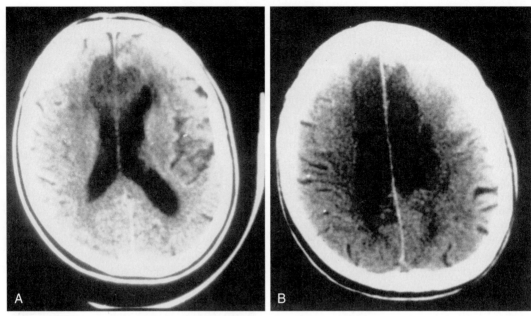

Figure 6-18. CT scan showing large bilateral paramedian ACA territory infarcts in a patient who suddenly developed bilateral lower-limb paralysis and mutism. (**A**) CT showing bilateral infarction involving the corpus callosum and cingulate gyri just anterior to the lateral ventricles. (**B**) Higher CT section showing extensive bilateral paramedian ACA territory infarction. (Courtesy of Noble David, MD.)

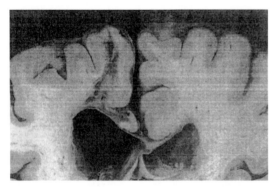

Figure 6-19. Postmortem necropsy coronal slice of brain showing a large ACA-territory infarct above the very enlarged left lateral ventricle. The corpus callosum is necrotic, and the infarct extends toward the right cingulate gyrus.

25% of individuals, there is a single Heubner's artery; often, there are two, three, or even four recurrent arteries.[184,185] Occlusion of one of these penetrating arteries, or of the parent ACA before the origin of the perforators, leads to infarcts in the head of the caudate nucleus. Frequently, the infarction also involves the anterior limb of the internal capsule and the most anterior part of the putamen. Medial and lateral lenticulostriate artery branches of the MCA supply the caudate nucleus, anterior limb of the internal capsule, and the putamen. Figure 6-20 shows a montage of the findings from CT scans from a series of patients with caudate infarcts.[186]

The clinical signs of caudate infarction are quite variable. Motor weakness is not prominent, although many patients have slight, but usually transient, hemiparesis. Among 18 patients in one series, 13 patients (78%) had some weakness in the limbs contralateral to the infarct. In most patients, however, the motor dysfunction was minor and recovered quickly.[186] Dysarthria is a more common finding and was present in 11 of 18 patients (61%) with caudate infarcts in one series,[186] and in 18 of 21 patients (86%) in another series.[201] Occasionally, patients with caudate infarcts have a movement disorder, usually choreoathetosis in the contralateral limbs, as the major clinical manifestation of caudate nucleus infarction.[202]

Most important are changes in behavior.[186,201,203] The most common behavioral change, in my experience, has been abulia.[186,201] Families describe the patients as more apathetic, uninterested, inert, laconic, and inactive than they were before the stroke. Slowness is a frequent theme; each activity takes longer and requires more concentration and effort. Another frequent abnormality, especially in patients with right caudate infarcts, is restlessness and hyperactivity. Some patients speak incessantly, call out, and appear agitated, confused, and delirious, closely resembling patients with right temporal-lobe infarcts.[143,144,186,201] In some patients with caudate infarction, restlessness and agitation alternate with apathy and inertia. Slight aphasia can be found in left caudate infarcts. Some patients with right caudate lesions have left visual neglect.[186,201]

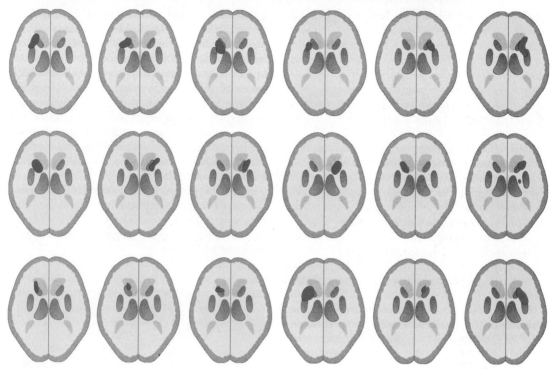

Figure 6-20. Montage of drawings of CT scans showing caudate-nucleus infarcts.

The cognitive and behavioral abnormalities found in patients with caudate infarcts closely resemble the clinical signs found in patients with lesions in the medial thalamus and the frontal and temporal lobes. Anatomic and physiologic studies have shown strong interconnections between the caudate nucleus and various cortical regions, and between the caudate nucleus and the thalamus, globus pallidus, and substantia nigra.[204,205] Caudato-nigro-thalamo-cortical circuits are intimately related to planning, thinking, acting, and other higher cortical functions.[186,204]

The causes of caudate infarction are diverse. The most lateral portion is supplied by the medial and lateral striate penetrators of the MCA. Occlusion of these branches, or of the parent proximal MCA, can lead to striatocapsular infarction, including the caudate nucleus. Occlusion of the ACA, by intrinsic atherosclerosis or more often by embolism, is another important mechanism of caudate infarction. In most patients, the lesions are probably caused by atheromatous branch disease at the origins of these penetrating arteries.[186,206] In a 1990 series of patients with caudate infarcts, risk factors for small artery disease were prevalent.[186] Among the 18 patients, hypertension (77%) and diabetes (33%) were common, five patients had both diabetes and hypertension, and only 3 of 18 patients had neither hypertension nor diabetes. Only 1 of the 18 patients had confirmed large-artery disease (ICA siphon stenosis). One patient had a cardiac source

of embolism (mitral stenosis).[186] These data suggest that most caudate infarcts are caused by atheromatous branch disease. This conclusion, however, must be tentative without more clinical and necropsy data. At present, I suggest screening patients with caudate infarcts with cardiac testing, ultrasound, or CTA or MRA before diagnosing a small artery etiology.

Occlusion of the Anterior Choroidal Artery

Neuroimaging (CT and MRI) often shows infarction limited to the territory of the anterior choroidal artery (AChA). Often AChA territory infarction is accompanied by infarcts in the MCA territory as part of an occlusion of the intracranial ICA. The AChA originates from the ICA after its ophthalmic and posterior communicating branches, and courses posteriorly and laterally to supply the globus pallidus, lateral geniculate body, posterior limb of the internal capsule, and medial temporal lobe.[207,208] There is a small supply to the thalamus. Figure 2-16 shows the AChA and its supply regions. Occasionally, there are anomalies of the AChA.[209] The artery can occasionally arise from the MCA or from the posterior communicating artery. Sometimes, the AChA is a larger-than-normal vessel that supplies the temporo-occipital lobes, the usual territory of the posterior cerebral artery.[209]

Before CT, occlusion of the anterior choroidal artery had seldom been diagnosed during life. Cooper, at first inadvertently and later purposefully, tied this vessel in Parkinsonian patients to stop tremor. The results were variable.[210]

Analyses of various series of patients[211-216] shows that the syndrome of the anterior choroidal artery includes the following:

- Hemiparesis affecting the face, arm, and leg
- Prominent hemisensory loss that is often temporary
- Homonymous hemianopia
- When the lateral geniculate body is infarcted, an unusual hemianopia, with sparing of a beak-shaped tongue of vision, within the center of the hemianopic visual field[217]
- Absence of persistent neglect, aphasia, or other higher cortical-function abnormalities

Hemiparesis is the most consistent finding. Dysarthria and hemisensory abnormalities are present less often and usually do not persist. Hemianopia is the least common sign. Some patients with bilateral AChA-territory capsular infarcts have severe dysarthria and may even become mute.[218]

The diagnosis of AChA territory infarction is verified by CT (Fig. 6-21) or MRI (Fig. 6-22), which shows infarction in the pallidum and lateral geniculate body adjacent to the temporal horn,[211,216,219] and by occlusion of the AChA demonstrated angiographically. Many of the reported patients with AChA-territory infarcts have been diabetic or hypertensive.[211,216,220] Most often, infarction in AChA territory is caused by occlusion of the AChA. The pathology is probably that of intracranial branch atheromatous disease.[206] Carotid artery occlusion, vasospasm in patients with carotid artery aneurysms, and cardiac-origin embolism are occasionally responsible for AChA-territory infarction, often coupled with MCA-territory infarcts.[221,222]

The posterior cerebral artery PCA is occasionally supplied directly through the posterior communicating branch of the ICA. This vessel is considered in Chapter 7 because it usually arises from the basilar artery.

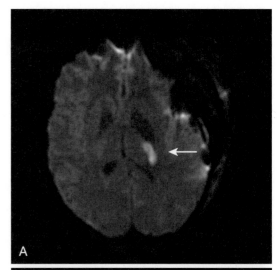

A

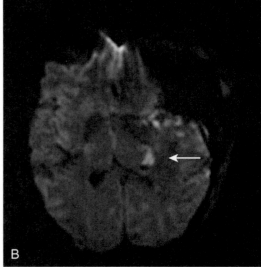

B

Figure 6-22. Diffusion-weighted MRI scans (**A**) and (**B**) showing infarcts in the territory of the anterior choroidal artery (*white arrows*).

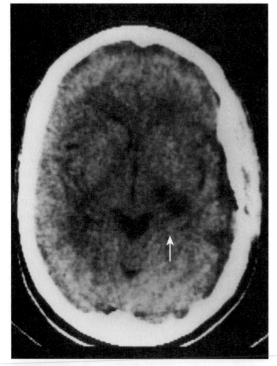

Figure 6-21. CT scan showing an anterior choroidal artery territory infarct (*white arrow*).

References

1. Estol CJ: Dr C Miller Fisher and the history of carotid artery disease. Stroke 1996;27:559-566.
2. Fisher CM: Occlusion of the internal carotid artery. Arch Neurol Psychiatry 1951;65:346-377.
3. Fisher M: Occlusion of the carotid arteries. Arch Neurol Psychiatry 1954;72:187-204.
4. Thompson JE: The evolution of surgery for the treatment and prevention of stroke: The Willis lecture. Stroke 1996;27:1427-1434.
5. Dyken M: Carotid endarterectomy studies: A glimmering of science. Stroke 1986;17:355-358.
6. Barnett HJ, Plum F, Walton J: Carotid endarterectomy-an expression of concern. Stroke 1984;15:941-943.
7. NASCET Collaborators: Beneficial effect of carotid endarterectomy in symptomatic patients with high-grade carotid stenosis. N Engl J Med 1991;325:445-453.
8. European Carotid Surgery Trialists Collaborative Group: Interim results for symptomatic patients with severe (70—99%) or with mild (0—19%) carotid stenosis. Lancet 1991;337:1235-1243.
9. Barnett HJM, Taylor DW, Eliasziw M, et al: Benefit of carotid endarterectomy in patients with symptomatic moderate or severe stenosis. North American Symptomatic Carotid Endarterectomy Trial Collaborators. N Engl J Med 1998;339:1415-1425.
10. European Carotid Surgery Trialists' Collaborative Group: Randomised trial of endarterectomy for recently symptomatic carotid stenosis: Final results of the MRC European Carotid Surgery Trial (ECST). Lancet 1998;351:1379-1387.
11. Executive Committee for the Asymptomatic Carotid Atherosclerosis Study: Endarterectomy for symptomatic carotid artery stenosis. JAMA 1995;273:1421-1428.
12. Halliday A, Mansfield A, Marro J, et al: Prevention of disabling and fatal strokes by successful carotid endarterectomy in patients without recent neurological symptoms: Randomised controlled trial. Lancet 2004;363:1491-1502.
13. Wennberg DE, Lucas FL, Birkmeyer JD, et al: Variation in carotid endarterectomy mortality in the Medicare population. JAMA 1998;279:1278-1281.
14. Kempczinski RF, Brott TG, Labutta RJ: The influence of surgical specialist and caseload on the results of carotid endarterectomy. J Vasc Surg 1986;3:911-916.
15. Meyers PM, Schumacher C, Higashida RT, et al: Use of stents to treat extracranial cerebrovascular disease. Ann Rev Med 2006;57:437-454.
16. Caplan LR, Meyers PM, Schumacher HC: Angioplasty and stenting to treat occlusive vascular disease. Rev Neurol Dis 2006;3:8-18.
17. Gorelick PB, Caplan LR, Hier DB, et al: Racial differences in the distribution of anterior circulation occlusive disease. Neurology 1984;34:54-59.
18. Caplan LR, Gorelick PB, Hier DB: Race, sex, and occlusive cerebrovascular disease: A review. Stroke 1986;17:648-655.
19. Mohr JP, Caplan LR, Melski J, et al: The Harvard Cooperative Stroke Registry: A prospective registry. Neurology 1978;28:752-754.
20. Furlan A, Whisnant J, Kearns T: Unilateral visual loss in bright light. Arch Neurol 1979;36:675-676.
21. Caplan LR, Sergay S: Positional cerebral ischemia. J Neurol Neurosurg Psychiatry 1976;39:385-391.
22. Reed C, Toole J: Clinical technique for identification of external carotid bruits. Neurology 1981;31:744-746.
23. Fisher CM: Facial pulses in internal carotid artery occlusion. Neurology 1970;20:476-478.
24. Caplan LR: The frontal artery sign. N Engl J Med 1973;288:1008-1009.
25. Hollenhorst R: Ocular manifestations of insufficiency or thrombosis of the internal carotid artery. Am J Ophthalmol 1959;47:753-767.
26. Fisher CM: Observations of the fundus oculi in transient monocular blindness. Neurology 1959;9:333-347.
27. Kearns T, Hollenhorst R: Venous stasis retinopathy of occlusive disease of the carotid artery. Mayo Clin Proc 1963;38:304-312.
28. Carter JE: Chronic ocular ischemia and carotid vascular disease. In Bernstein EF (ed): Amaurosis Fugax. New York: Springer, 1988, pp 118-134.
29. Caplan LR, Babikian V, Helgason C, et al: Occlusive disease of the middle cerebral artery. Neurology 1985;35:975-982.
30. Neau J-P, Bogousslavsky J: Superficial middle cerebral artery syndromes. In Bogousslavsky J, Caplan LR (eds): Stroke Syndromes, 2nd ed. Cambridge: Cambridge University Press, 2001, pp 405-427.
31. Caplan LR, Bogousslavsky J: Abnormalities of the right cerebral hemisphere. In Bogousslavsky J, Caplan LR (eds): Stroke Syndromes. Cambridge: Cambridge University Press, 1995, pp 162-168.
32. Hier DB, Mondlock J, Caplan LR: Behavioral abnormalities after right hemisphere stroke. Neurology 1983;33:337-344.
33. Pessin MS, Kwan E, Scott RM, Hedges TR: Occipital infarction with hemianopsia from carotid occlusive disease. Stroke 1989;20:409-411.
34. Linn FH, Chang H-M, Caplan LR: Carotid artery disease: A rare cause of posterior cerebral artery territory infarction. J Neurovasc Dis 1997;2:31-34.
35. Pessin M, Duncan G, Davis K, et al: Angiographic appearance of carotid occlusion in acute stroke. Stroke 1980;11:485-487.
36. Barnett HJM, Peerless S, Kaufmann J: "Stump" of internal carotid artery: A source for further cerebral embolic ischemia. Stroke 1978;9:448-452.
37. Ringelstein E, Zeumer H, Angelou D: The pathogenesis of strokes from internal carotid artery occlusion: Diagnostic and therapeutic implications. Stroke 1983;14:867-875.

38. Orlandi G, Parenti G, Bertolucci A, Murri L: Silent cerebral microembolism in asymptomatic and symptomatic carotid artery stenoses of low and high degree. Eur Neurol 1997;38:39-43.

39. Droste DW, Dittrich R, Kerveny V, et al: Prevalence and frequency of microembolic signals in 105 patients with extracranial carotid artery occlusive disease. J Neurol Neurosurg Psychiatry 1999;67:525-528.

40. Caplan LR, Hennerici M: Impaired clearance of emboli (washout) is an important link between hypoperfusion, embolism, and ischemic stroke. Arch Neurol 1998;55:1475-1482.

41. Caplan LR, Wong K-S, Gao S, et al: Is hypoperfusion an important cause of strokes? If so, how? Cerebrovasc Dis 2006;21:145-153.

42. Marder VJ, Chute DJ, Starkman S, et al: Analysis of thrombi retrieved from cerebral arteries of patients with acute ischemic stroke. Stroke 2006;37:2086-2093.

43. Sundt T, Sandok BA, Whisnant JP: Carotid endarterectomy: Complications and preoperative assessment. Mayo Clin Proc 1975;50:301-306.

44. del Zoppo GJ, Poeck K, Pessin MS, et al: Recombinant tissue plasminogen activator in acute thrombotic and embolic stroke. Ann Neurol 1992;32:78-86.

45. Linfante I, Llinas RH, Selim M, et al: Clinical and vascular outcome in internal carotid artery versus middle cerebral artery occlusions after intravenous tissue plasminogen activator. Stroke 2002;33:2066-2071.

46. Casto L, Caverni L, Canerlingo M, et al: Intraarterial thrombolysis in acute ischaemic stroke: Experience with a superselective catheter embedded in the clot. J Neurol Neurosurg Psychiatry 1996;60:667-670.

47. Barnwell SL, Clark WM, Nguyen TT, et al: Safety and efficacy of delayed intra-arterial urokinase therapy with mechanical clot disruption for thromboembolic stroke. AJNR Am J Neuroradiol 1994;15:1817-1822.

48. Sekhar L, Heros R: Atheromatous pseudo-occlusion of the internal carotid artery. J Neurosurg 1980;52:782-789.

49. Steinke W, Kloetzsch C, Hennerici M: Symptomatic and asymptomatic high-grade carotid stenosis in Doppler color-flow imaging. Neurology 1992;42:131-138.

50. Riles T, Posner M, Cohen W, et al: Rapid sequential CT scanning of the occluded internal carotid artery. Stroke 1982;13:124.

51. Morganstern LB, Fox AJ, Sharpe BL, et al: The risks and benefits of carotid endarterectomy in patients with near occlusion of the carotid artery. Neurology 1997;48:911-915.

52. Baron JC: Stroke research in the modern era: Images versus dogma. Cerebrovasc Dis 2005;20:154-163.

53. Baquis GD, Pessin MS, Scott RM: Limb shaking—A carotid TIA. Stroke 1985;16:444-448.

54. Yanigahara T, Piepgras DG, Klass DW: Repetitive involuntary movement associated with episodic cerebral ischemia. Ann Neurol 1985;18:244-250.

55. Grubb Jr RL, Powers WJ, Derdeyn CP, et al: The Carotid Occlusion Surgery Study. Neurosurg Focus 2003;14:e9

56. Can U, Furie K, Suwanwela N, et al: Transcranial Doppler ultrasound criteria for hemodynamically significant internal carotid artery stenosis based on residual lumen diameter calculated from en bloc endarterectomy specimens. Stroke 1997;28:1966-1971.

57. Fisher CM, Ojemann RG: A clinico-pathological study of carotid endarterectomy plaques. Rev Neurol (Paris) 1986;39:273-299.

58. Fisher M, Paganini-Hill A, Martin A, et al: Carotid plaque pathology: Thrombosis, ulceration, and stroke pathogenesis. Stroke 2005;36:253-257.

59. Caplan LR, Skillman J, Ojemann R, et al: Intracerebral hemorrhage following carotid endarterectomy: A hypertensive complication. Stroke 1978;9:457-460.

60. Piepgras DG, Morgan MK, Sundt TM, et al: Intracerebral hemorrhage after carotid endarterectomy. J Neurosurg 1988;68:532-536.

61. Wade J, Larson C, Hickey R, et al: Effect of carotid endarterectomy on carotid chemoreceptor and baroreceptor function in man. N Engl J Med 1970;282:823-829.

62. Countee R, Sapru H, Vijayanathan T, et al: "Other syndromes" of the carotid bifurcation. In Smith RR (ed): Stroke and the Extracranial Vessels. New York: Raven Press, 1984, pp 345-357.

63. Reigel MM, Hollier LH, Sundt TM, et al: Cerebral hyperperfusion syndrome: A cause of neurologic dysfunction after carotid endarterectomy. J Vasc Surg 1987;5:628-634.

64. Breen JC, Caplan LR, DeWitt LD, et al: Brain edema after carotid surgery. Neurology 1996;46:175-181.

65. Abou-Chebl A, Yadav JS, Reginelli JP, et al: Intracranial hemorrhage and hyperperfusion syndrome following carotid artery stenting: Risk factors, prevention, and treatment. J Am Coll Cardiol 2004;43:1596-1561.

66. Hennerici M, Rautenberg W, Struck R: Spontaneous clinical course of asymptomatic vascular processes of the extracranial cerebral arteries. Klin Wochenschr 1984;62:570-576.

67. Hennerici M, Hulsbower HB, Hefter K, et al: Natural history of asymptomatic extracranial disease: Results of a long-term prospective study. Brain 1987;110:777-791.

68. Stroke Prevention by Aggressive Reduction in Cholesterol Levels (SPARCL) Investigators: High-dose atorvastatin after stroke or transient ischemic attack. N Engl J Med 2006;355:549-559.

69. Caplan LR, Stein R, Patel D, et al: Intraluminal clot of the carotid artery detected angiographically. Neurology 1984;34:1175-1181.

70. Pessin MS, Abbott BF, Prager R, et al: Clinical and angiographic features of carotid circulation thrombus. Neurology 1986;36:518-523.

71. Buchan A, Gates P, Pelz D, Barnett HJM: Intraluminal thrombus in the cerebral circulation. Implications for surgical management. Stroke 1988;19: 681-687.

72. Nadareishvili ZG, Rothwell PM, Beletsky V, et al: Long-term risk of stroke and other vascular events in patients with asymptomatic carotid artery stenosis. Arch Neurol 2002;59:1162-1166.

73. Humphries A, Young J, Santilli P, et al: Unoperated asymptomatic significant carotid artery stenosis: A review of 182 instances. Surgery 1976;80:694-698.

74. Durward Q, Ferguson G, Barr H: The natural history of asymptomatic carotid bifurcation plaques. Stroke 1982;13:459-464.

75. Ropper A, Wechsler L, Wilson L: Carotid bruits and the risk of stroke in elective surgery. N Engl J Med 1982;307:1387-1390.

76. Caplan LR: A 79-year-old musician with asymptomatic carotid artery disease. JAMA 1995; 274:1383-1389.

77. Chambers BR, Norris JW: Outcome in patients with asymptomatic neck bruits. N Engl J Med 1986;315:860-865.

78. Executive Committee for the Asymptomatic Carotid Atherosclerosis Study (ACAS): Endarterectomy for asymptomatic carotid artery stenosis. JAMA 1995;273:1421-1428.

79. Halliday A, Mansfield A, Marro J, et al: Prevention of disabling and fatal strokes by successful carotid endarterectomy in patients without recent neurological symptoms: Randomised controlled trial. Lancet 2004;363:1491-1502.

80. Brott T, Toole J: Medical compared with surgical treatment of asymptomatic carotid artery stenosis. Ann Intern Med 1995;123:720-722.

81. Warlow C: Surgical treatment of asymptomatic carotid stenosis. Cerebrovasc Dis 1996; 6(Suppl 1):7-14.

82. Perry JR, Szalai JP, Norris JW: Consensus against both endarterectomy and routine screening for asymptomatic carotid artery stenosis. Canadian Stroke Consortium. Arch Neurol 1997;54:25-28.

83. Biousse V, D'Anglejan-Chatillon J, Toboul P-J, et al: Time course of symptoms in extracranial carotid artery dissections. A series of 80 patients. Stroke 1995;26:235-239.

84. Bogousslavsky J, Despland PA, Regli F: Spontaneous carotid dissection with acute stroke. Arch Neurol 1987;44:137-140.

85. Baumagartner RW, Bogousslavsky J: Clinical manifestations of carotid dissection. In Baumgartner RW, Bogousslavsky J, Caso V, Paciaroni M (eds): Handbook on Cerebral Artery Dissection. Basel: Karger, 2005, pp 70-76.

86. Sturznegger M: Ultrasound findings in spontaneous carotid artery dissection: The value of Duplex sonography. Arch Neurol 1991;48: 1057-1063.

87. Engelter ST, Lyrer PA, Kirsch EC, Steck AJ: Long-term follow-up after extracranial internal carotid artery dissection. Eur Neurol 2000;44:199-204.

88. Touze E, Gauvrit J-Y, Moulin T, et al: Risk of stroke and recurrent dissection after a cervical artery dissection. A multicenter study. Neurology 2003;61:1347-1351.

89. Dreier JP, Lurtzing F, Kappmeier M, et al: Delayed occlusion after internal carotid artery dissection under heparin. Cerebrovasc Dis 2004;18:296-303.

90. Kadkhodayan Y, Jeck DT, Moran CJ, et al: Angioplasty and stenting in carotid dissection with and without pseudoaneurysm. AJNR Am J Neuroradiol 2005;26:2328-2335.

91. Fisher CM, Gore I, Okabe N, et al: Calcification of the carotid siphon. Circulation 1965;32: 538-548.

92. Marzewski D, Furlan A, St Louis P, et al: Intracranial internal carotid artery stenosis: Long-term prognosis. Stroke 1982;13:821-824.

93. Craig D, Meguro K, Watridge G, et al: Intracranial internal carotid artery stenosis. Stroke 1982;13: 825-828.

94. Wechsler LR, Kistler JP, Davis KR, et al: The prognosis of carotid siphon stenosis. Stroke 1986;17:714-718.

95. Caplan LR: Cerebrovascular disease: Larger artery occlusive disease. In Appel S (ed): Current Neurology, vol 8. Chicago: Yearbook Medical, 1988, pp 179-226.

96. Borozan PG, Schuler JJ, LaRosa MP, et al: The natural history of isolated carotid siphon stenosis. TJ Vasc Surg 1984;1:744-749.

97. Bogousslavsky J: 1987. Prognosis of carotid siphon stenosis. Stroke 1987;18:537.

98. Castaigne P, Lhermitte F, Gautier JC, et al: Internal carotid artery occlusion: A study of 61 instances in 50 patients with postmortem data. Brain 1970;93:231-258.

99. Ley-Pozo J, Ringelstein EB: Noninvasive detection of occlusive disease of the carotid siphon and middle cerebral artery. Ann Neurol 1990;28: 640-647.

100. Sloan MA, Alexandrov AV, Tegeler CH, et al: Assessment: Transcranial Doppler ultrasonography: Report of the Therapeutics and Technology Assessment Subcommittee of the American Academy of Neurology. Neurology 2004;62: 1468-1481.

101. Thijs VN, Albers GW: Symptomatic intracranial atherosclerosis: outcome of patients who fail antithrombotic therapy. Neurology 2000;55:490-497.

102. Akins PT, Pilgram TK, Cross DT, Moran CJ: Natural history of stenosis from intracranial atherosclerosis by serial angiography. Stroke 1998; 29:433-438.

103. Chimowitz MI, Kokkinos J, Strong J, et al: The Warfarin-Aspirin Symptomatic Intracranial Disease Study. Neurology 1995;45:1488-1493.

104. Mohr JP, Thompson JL, Lazar RM, et al: A comparison of warfarin and aspirin for the prevention of recurrent ischemic stroke. N Engl J Med 2001;345:1444-1451.

105. Chimowitz MI, Lynn MJ, Howlett-Smith H, et al: Comparison of warfarin and aspirin for

symptomatic intracranial arterial stenosis.
N Engl J Med 2005;352:1305-1316.

106. Kasner SE, Chimowitz MI, Lynn MJ, et al: Predictors of ischemic stroke in the territory of a symptomatic intracranial arterial stenosis. Warfarin Aspirin Symptomatic Intracranial Disease Trial Investigators. Circulation 2006; 113:555-563.

107. Kasner SE, Lynn MJ, Chimowitz MI, et al: Warfarin vs aspirin for symptomatic intracranial stenosis: Subgroup analyses from WASID. Neurology 2006;67:1275-1278.

108. Callahan III AS, Berger BL: Balloon angioplasty of intracranial arteries for stroke prevention. J Neuroimaging 1997;7:232-235.

109. Marks MP, Marcellus M, Norbash AM, et al: Outcome of angioplasty for atherosclerotic intracranial stenosis. Stroke 1999;30:1065-1069.

110. Connors 3rd JJ, Wojak JC: Percutaneous transluminal angioplasty for intracranial atherosclerotic lesions: Evolution of technique and short-term results. J Neurosurg 1999;91:415-423.

111. Marks MP, Marcellus ML, Do HM, et al: Intracranial angioplasty without stenting for symptomatic atherosclerotic stenosis: Long-term follow-up. AJNR Am J Neuroradiol 2005; 26:525-530.

112. Day A, Rhoton A, Quisling R: Resolving siphon stenosis following endarterectomy. Stroke 1980;11:278-281.

113. Bladin PF, Berkovic SF: Striatocapsular infarction. Neurology 1984;34:1423-1430.

114. Jansen O, von Kummer R, Forsting M, et al: Thrombolytic therapy in acute occlusion of the intracranial internal carotid artery bifurcation. AJNR Am J Neuroradiol 1995;16:1977-1986.

115. Zeumer H, Freitag HJ, Zanella F, et al: Local intra-arterial thrombolytic therapy in patients with stroke: urokinase versus recombinant tissue plasminogen activator (rt-PA). Neuroradiology 1993;35:159-162.

116. Gonner F, Remonda L, Mattle H, et al: Local intra-arterial thrombolysis in acute ischemic stroke. Stroke 1998;29:1894-1900.

117. Zaidat OO, Suarez JI, Santillan C, et al: Response to intra-arterial and combined intravenous and intra-arterial thrombolytic therapy in patients with distal internal carotid artery occlusion. Stroke 2002;33:1821-1827.

118. Chaves C, Estol C, Esnaola MM, et al: Spontaneous intracranial internal carotid artery dissection: Report of 10 patients. Arch Neurol 2002;59: 977-981.

119. Pelkonen O, Tikkakoski T, Leinonen S, et al: Intracranial arterial dissection. Neuroradiology 1998;40:442-447.

120. Russo L: Carotid system transient ischemic attacks: Clinical, racial, and angiographic correlations. Stroke 1981;12:470-473.

121. Bauer R, Sheehan S, Wechsler N, et al: Arteriographic study of sites, incidence, and treatment of arteriosclerotic cerebrovascular lesions. Neurology 1962;12:698-711.

122. Kieffer S, Takeya Y, Resch J, et al: Racial differences in cerebrovascular disease: Angiographic evaluation of Japanese and American populations. AJR Am J Roentgenol 1967;101:94-99.

123. Brust R: Patterns of cerebrovascular disease in Japanese and other population groups in Hawaii: An angiographic study. Stroke 1975;6: 539-542.

124. Kubo H: Transient cerebral ischemic attacks: An arteriographic study. Naika 1968;22:969-978.

125. Feldmann E, Daneault N, Kwan E, et al: Chinese-white differences in the distribution of occlusive cerebrovascular disease. Neurology 1990;40:1541-1545.

126. Bogousslavsky J, Barnett JHM, Fox AJ, et al: Atherosclerotic disease of the middle cerebral artery. EC-IC Bypass Study Group. Stroke 1986;17:1112-1120.

126a. Mazighi M, Labreuche J, Gongora-Rivera F, et al: Autopsy prevalence of intracranaial atherosclerosis in patients with fatal stroke. Stroke 2008;39:1142-1147.

127. Yoo K-M, Shin H-K, Chang H-M, Caplan LR: Middle cerebral artery occlusive disease: The New England Medical Center Stroke registry. J Stroke Cerebrovasc Dis 1998;7:344-351.

127a. Chen XY, Wong KS, Lam WWM, et al: Middle cerebral artery atherosclerosis: histological comparison between plaques associated with and not associated with infarct in a postmortem study. Cerebrovasc Dis 2008;25:74-80.

127b. Ogata J, Yutani C, Otsubo R, et al: Heart and vessel pathology underlying brain infarction in 142 stroke patients. Ann Neurol 2008;63:770-781.

128. Hinton R, Mohr JP, Ackerman R, et al: Symptomatic middle cerebral artery stenosis. Ann Neurol 1979;5:152-157.

129. Corston RN, Kendall BE, Marshall J: Prognosis in middle cerebral artery stenosis. Stroke 1984; 15:237-241.

130. Moulin DE, Lo R, Chiang J, et al: Prognosis in middle cerebral artery occlusion. Stroke 1985; 16:282-284.

131. Feldmeyer JJ, Merendaz C, Regli F: Stenosis symptomatiques de l'artere cerebrale moyenne. Rev Neurol (Paris) 1983;139:725-736.

132. Naritomi H, Sawada T, Kuriyama Y, et al: Effect of chronic middle cerebral artery stenosis on the local cerebral hemodynamics. Stroke 1985; 16:214-219.

133. Segura T, Serena J, Molins A, Davalos A: Clusters of microembolic signals: A new form of cerebral microembolism in a patient with middle cerebral artery stenosis. Stroke 1998;29:722-724.

134. Wong KS, Gao S, Chan YL, et al: Mechanisms of acute cerebral infarctions in patients with middle cerebral artery stenosis: A diffusion-weighted imaging and microemboli monitoring study. Ann Neurol 2002;52:74-81.

135. Gao S, Wong KS, Hansberg T, et al: Microembolic signal predicts recurrent cerebral ischemic events in acute stroke patients with middle cerebral artery stenosis. Stroke 2004;35:2832-2836.

136. Jain K: Some observations on the anatomy of the middle cerebral artery. Can J Surg 1964;7: 134-139.
137. Kaplan H: Anatomy and embryology of the arterial system of the forebrain. In Vinken P, Bruyn G (eds): Handbook of Clinical Neurology, vol 11. Amsterdam: North Holland, 1972, pp 1-23.
138. Hier DB, Gorelick PB, Shindler AG: Topics in Behavioral Neurology and Neuropsychology. Boston: Butterworth, 1987.
139. Fisher CM: Left hemiplegia and motor impersistence. J Nerv Ment Dis 1956;123:201-218.
140. Hier DB, Mohr JP: Incongruous oral and written naming: Evidence for a subdivision of the syndromes of Wernicke's aphasia. Brain Lang 1977;4:115-126.
141. Sevush S, Roeltgen D, Campanella D, et al: Preserved oral reading in Wernicke's aphasia. Neurology 1983;33:916-920.
142. Awada A, Poncet M, Signoret J: Confrontation de la Salpetriere 4 Mai 1983: Troubles des compartement soudains avec agitation chez un homme de 68 ans. Rev Neurol (Paris) 1984; 140:446-451.
143. Schmidley J, Messing R: Agitated confusional states in patients with right hemisphere infarctions. Stroke 1984:15;883-885.
144. Caplan LR, Kelly M, Kase CS, et al: Infarcts of the inferior division of the right middle cerebral artery. Neurology 1986;36:1015-1020.
145. Adams H, Damasio H, Putnam S, et al: Middle cerebral artery occlusion as a cause of isolated subcortical infarction. Stroke 1983;14:948-952.
146. Weiller C, Ringelstein EB, Reiche W, et al: The large striatocapsular infarct: A clinical and pathological entity. Arch Neurol 1990;47:1085-1091.
147. Caplan LR: The large striato-capsular infarct: A clinical and pathophysiologic entity: Critique. Neurol Chronicle 1991;1:12-13.
148. Damasio A, Damasio H, Rizzo M, et al: Aphasia with nonhemorrhagic lesions in the basal ganglia and internal capsule. Arch Neurol 1982;89:15-20.
149. Naesser M, Alexander M, Estabrooks N, et al: Aphasia with predominantly subcortical lesion sites. Arch Neurol 1982;39:2-14.
150. Heinsius T, Bogousslavsky J, van Melle G: Large infarcts in the middle cerebral artery territory. Etiology and outcome patterns. Neurology 1998; 50:341-350.
151. Hier DB, Mondlock J, Caplan LR: Recovery of behavioral abnormalities after right hemisphere stroke. Neurology 1983;33:345-350.
152. Schwab S, Rieke K, Aschoff A, et al: Hemicraniotomy in space-occupying hemisopheric infarction:useful early intervention or desperate activism. Cerebrovasc Dis 1996;6:325-329.
153. Schwab S, Steiner T, Aschoff A, et al: Early hemicraniectomy in patients with complete middle cerebral artery infarction. Stroke 1998;29: 1888-1893.
154. Fink JN, Selim MH, Kumar S, et al: Insular cortex infarction in acute middle cerebral artery territory stroke: Predictor of stroke severity and vascular lesion. Arch Neurol 2005;62: 1081-1085.
155. Oppenheimer SM, Cechetto DF, Hachinski VC: Cerebrogenic cardiac arrythmias: Cerebral ECG influences and their role in sudden death. Arch Neurol 1990;47:513-519.
156. Oppenheimer SM, Wilson JX, Guiraudon C, Cechetto DF: Insular cortex stimulation produces lethal cardiac arrythmias: A mechanism of sudden death. Brain Res 1991;550:115-121.
157. Yoon R-W, Morillo CA, Cechetto DF, Hachinski V: Cerebral hemispheric lateralization in cardiac autonomic control. Arch Neurol 1997;54:741-744.
158. Hachinski VC, Oppenheimer SM, Wilson JX, et al: Assymetry of sympathetic consequences of experimental stroke. Arch Neurol 1992;49: 697-702.
159. Giubilei F, Strano S, Lino S, et al: Autonomic nervous system activity during sleep in middle cerebral artery infarction. Cerebrovasc Dis 1998;8:118-123.
160. Tomsick T, Brott T, Barsan W, et al: Prognostic value of the hyperdense middle cerebral artery sign and stroke scale score before ultraearly thrombolytic therapy. AJNR Am J Neuroradiol 1996;17:79-85.
161. Alexandros AV, Bladin CF, Norris JW: Intracranial blood flow velocities in acute ischemic stroke. Stroke 1994;25:1378-1383.
162. Molina CA, Alexandrov AV: Transcranial Doppler ultrasound. In Caplan LR, Manning WJ (eds): Brain Embolism. New York: Informa Healthcare, 2006, pp 113-128.
163. Segura T, Serena J, Molins A, Davalos A: Clusters of microembolic signals: A new form of cerebral microembolism presentation in a patient with middle cerebral artery stenosis. Stroke 1998;29: 722-724.
164. Masuda J, Yutani C, Miyashita T, Yamaguchi T: Artery-to-artery embolism from a thrombus formed in a stenotic middle cerebral artery. Report of an autopsy case. Stroke 1987;18:680-684.
165. Wong KS, Lam WWM, Liang E, et al: Variability of magnetic resonance angiography and computed tomography angiography in grading middle cerebral artery stenosis. Stroke 1996;27: 1084-1087.
166. Bash S, Villablanca JP, Duckwiler G, et al: Intracranial vascular stenosis and occlusive disease. Evaluation with CT angiography, MR angiography, and digital subtraction angiography. AJNR Am J Neuroradiol 2005;26:1012-1021.
167. Mori E, Yoneda Y, Tabuchi M, et al: Intravenous recombinant tissue plasminogen activator in acute carotid artery territory stroke. Neurology 1992;42:976-982.
168. Trouillas P, Nighogossian N, Getenet J, et al: Open trial of intravenous tissue plasminogen activator in acute carotid territory stroke. Stroke 1996;27:882-890.
169. Wolpert SM, Bruckman H, Greenlee R, et al: Neuroradiologic evaluation of patients with

acute stroke treated with recombinant tissue plasminogen activator. AJNR Am J Neuroradiol 1993;14:3-13.

170. Albers GW, Thijs VN, Wechsler L, et al: MRI profiles predict clinical response to early reperfusion: The Diffusion and Perfusion Imaging Evaluation for Understanding Stroke Evolution (DEFUSE) Study. Ann Neurol 2006;60:508-517.

171. del Zoppo GJ, Higashida R, Furlan AJ, et al: PROACT: A phase II randomized trial of recombinant pro-urokinase by direct arterial delivery in acute middle cerebral artery stroke. Stroke 1998;29:4-11.

172. Meyers PM, Schumacher HC, Tanji K, et al: Use of stents to treat intracranial cerebrovascular disease. Ann Rev Med 2007;58:107-122.

173. Chaturverdi S, Caplan LR: Angioplasty for intracranial atherosclerosis: Is the treatment worse than the disease? Neurology 2003;61:1647-1648.

174. Mori T, Fukuoka M, Kazita K, Mori K: Follow-up study after intracranial percutaneous transluminal cerebral balloon angioplasty. AJNR Am J Neuroradiol 1998;19:1525-1533.

175. Critchley M: The anterior cerebral artery, and its syndromes. Brain 1930;53:120-165.

176. Uihlein A, Thomas R, Cleary J: Aneurysms of the anterior communicating artery complex. Mayo Clin Proc 1967;42:73-87.

177. Gacs G, Fox A, Barnett HJM, et al: Occurrence and mechanisms of occlusion of the anterior cerebral artery. Stroke 1983;14:952-959.

178. Bogousslavsky J, Regli F: Anterior cerebral artery territory infarction in the Lausanne Stroke Registry. Clinical and etiologic patterns. Arch Neurol 1990;47:144-150.

179. Ohkuma H, Suzuki S, Kikkawa T, Shimamura N: Neuroradiologic and clinical features of arterial dissection of the anterior cerebral artery. AJNR Am J Neuroradiol 2003;24:691-699.

180. Koyama S, Kotani A, Sasaki J: Spontaneous dissecting aneurysm of the anterior cerebral artery: Report of two cases. Surg Neurol 1996;46:55-61.

181. Brust JC: Anterior cerebral artery. In Barnett HJM, Mohr JP, Stein B, Yatsu F (eds): Stroke: Pathophysiology, Diagnosis and Management, 3rd ed. New York: Churchill Livingstone, 1998, pp 401-425.

182. Brust JC, Sawada T, Kazui S: Anterior cerebral artery. In Bogousslavsky J, Caplan LR (eds): Stroke Syndromes, 2nd ed. Cambridge: Cambridge University Press, 2001, pp 439-450.

183. Nagaratnam N, Davies D, Chen E: Clinical effects of anterior cerebral artery infarction. J Stroke Cerebrovasc Dis 1998;7:391-397.

184. Rhoton AL, Sacki N, Pearlmutter D, Zeal A: Microsurgical anatomy of common aneurysm sites. Clin Neurosurg 1978;26:248-306.

185. Gorczyca W, Mohr G: Microvascular anatomy of Heubner's recurrent artery. J Neurosurg 1976;44:359-367.

186. Caplan LR, Schmahmann JD, Kase CS, et al: Caudate infarcts. Arch Neurol 1990;47:133-143.

187. Dunker R, Harris A: Surgical anatomy of the proximal anterior cerebral artery. J Neurosurg 1976;44:359-367.

188. Chamarro A, Marshall RS, Valls-Sole J, et al: Motor behavior in stroke patients with isolated medial frontal ischemic infarction. Stroke 1997;28:1755-1760.

189. Geschwind N, Kaplan E: A human cerebral deconnection syndrome. Neurology 1962;12:675-695.

190. Geschwind N: Disconnection syndromes in animals and man. Brain 1965;88:237-294, 585-644.

191. Rubens A: Aphasia with infarction in the territory of the anterior cerebral artery. Cortex 1975;11:239-250.

192. Alexander M, Schmitt M: The aphasia syndrome of stroke in the left anterior cerebral artery territory. Arch Neurol 1980;37:97-100.

192a. Ross E: Left medial parietal lobe and receptive language functions: Mixed transcortical aphasia after left anterior cerebral artery infarction. Neurology 1980;30:144-151.

192b. Fisher CM: Abulia minor versus agitated behavior. Clin Neurosurg 1983;31:9-31.

193. Fesenmeier JT, Kuzniecky R, Garcia J: Akinetic mutism caused by bilateral anterior cerebral tuberculous arteritis. Neurology 1990;40:1005-1006.

194. Fisher CM: Intermittent interruption of behavior. Trans Am Neurol Assoc 1968;93:209-210.

195. Brion S, Jedynak C-P: Trouble du tranfer interhemispherique a propos de trois observations de tumeurs du corps calleux. Le signe de al main etrangere. Rev Neurol (Paris) 1972;126:257-266.

196. Goldberg G, Mayer NH, Toglia JU: Medial frontal cortex infarction and the alien hand sign. Arch Neurol 1981;38:683-686.

197. Geschwind DH, Iacoboni M, Mega MS, et al: Alien hand syndrome: Interhemispheric motor disconnection due to a lesion in the midbody of the corpus callosum. Neurology 1995;45:802-808.

198. Freeman FR: Akinetic mutism and bilateral anterior cerebral artery occlusion. J Neurol Neurosurg Psychiatry 1971;34:693-694.

199. Borggreve F, De Deyn PP, Marien P, et al: Bilateral infarction in the anterior cerebral artery vascular territory due to an unusual anomaly of the circle of Willis. Stroke 1994;25:1279-1281.

200. Ferbert A, Thorn A: Bilateral anterior cerebral territory infarction in the differential diagnosis of basilar artery occlusion. J Neurology 1992;239:162-164.

201. Caplan LR: Caudate infarcts. In Donnan G, Norrving B, Bamford J, Boigousslavsky J (eds): Subcortical Stroke, 2nd ed. Oxford: Oxford University Press, 2002, pp 209-223.

202. Saris S: Chorea caused by caudate infarction. Arch Neurol 1983;40:590-591.

203. Mendez M, Adams N, Lewandowski K: Neurobehavioral changes associated with caudate lesions. Neurology 1989;39:349-354.

204. Alexander GE, DeLong MR, Strick PL: Parallel organization of functionally segregated circuits linking basal ganglia and cortex. Ann Rev Neurosci 1986;9:357-381.

205. Alexander GE, Delong MR: Microstimulation of the primate neostriatum: I: Physiological properties of striatal microexcitable zones. J Neurophysiol 1985;53:1417-1432.

206. Caplan LR: Intracranial branch atheromatous disease. Neurology 1989;39:1246-1250.

207. Rhoton A, Fuji K, Fradd B: Microsurgical anatomy of the anterior choroidal artery. Surg Neurol 1979;12:171-187.

208. Mohr JP, Steinke W, Timsit SG, et al: The anterior choroidal artery does not supply the corona radiata and lateral ventricular wall. Stroke 1991; 22:1502-1507.

209. Takahashi S, Suga T, Kawata Y, Sakamoto K: Anterior choroidal artery:angiographic analysis of variations and anomalies. AJNR Am J Neuroradiol 1990;11:719-729.

210. Cooper I: Surgical occlusions of the anterior choroidal artery in Parkinsonism. Surg Gynecol Obstet 1954;99:207-219.

211. Helgason C, Caplan LR, Goodwin V, et al: Anterior choroidal territory infarction: Case reports and review. Arch Neurol 1986;43:681-686.

212. Vuadens P, Bogousslavsky J: Anterior choroidal artery territory infarcts. In Bogousslavsky J, Caplan LR (eds): Stroke Syndromes, 2nd ed. Cambridge: Cambridge University Press, 2001, pp 451-460.

213. Ward T, Bernat J, Goldstein A: Occlusion of the anterior choroidal artery. J Neurol Neurosurg Psychiatry 1984;47:1046-1049.

214. Masson M, DeCroix JP, Henin D, et al: Syndrome de l'artere choroidienne anterieure: Etude clinique et tomodensitometrique de 4 cas. Rev Neurol (Paris) 1983;139:553-559.

215. Decroix JP, Graveleau PH, Masson M, Cambier J: Infarction in the territory of the anterior choroidal artery: A clinical and computerized tomographic study of 16 cases. Brain 1986;109: 1071-1085.

216. Helgason CM: Anterior choroidal artery territory infarction. In Donnan G, Norrving B, Bamford J, Bogousslavsky J (eds): Lacunar and Other Subcortical Infarctions. Oxford: Oxford University Press, 1995, pp 131-138.

217. Frisen L: Quadruple sector anopia and sectorial optic atrophy: A syndrome of the distal anterior choroidal artery. J Neurol Neurosurg Psychiatry 1979;42:590-594.

218. Helgason C, Wilbur A, Weiss A, et al: Acute pseudobulbar mutism due to discrete bilateral capsular infarction in the territory of the anterior choroidal artery. Brain 1988;111:507-524.

219. Damasio H: A computed tomographic guide to the identification of cerebral vascular territories. Arch Neurol 1983;40:138-142.

220. Bruno A, Graff-Radford NR, Biller J, Adams HP: Anterior choroidal artery territory infarction: A small vessel disease. Stroke 1989;20:616-619.

221. Mayer JM, Lanoe Y, Pedetti L, Fabry B: Anterior choroidal-artery territory infarction and carotid occlusion. Cerebrovasc Dis 1992;2:315-316.

222. Leys D, Mounier-Vehier F, Lavenu I, et al: Anterior choroidal artery territory infarcts. Study of presumed mechanisms. Stroke 1994; 25:837-842.

7

Large Vessel Occlusive Disease of the Posterior Circulation

Following the suggestion of American[1-5] and British[1,6] authors during the late 1950s and early 1960s, physicians lumped posterior circulation ischemia under the catchall terms *vertebrobasilar insufficiency* (VBI) or *vertebrobasilar territory infarction*. Various treatments were tried in groups of patients with VBI.[1,7] As was found in the case of large, heterogeneous groups of patients with anterior and posterior circulation disease lumped under the categories of transient ischemic attack (TIA), progressing, or so-called completed stroke, no single treatment strategy proved helpful for the group as a whole. With the advent of better brain imaging, more angiography, better surgery, and safe, noninvasive diagnostic techniques, physicians and surgeons began to consider treatment of individual patients with anterior circulation disease, depending on the (1) nature, severity, and location of their vascular lesions; (2) degree of infarction; (3) hematologic-coagulation findings; and (4) general health of the patient.

The same strategy should be applied to patients with vertebrobasilar disease because this category is even more heterogeneous than anterior-circulation ischemic disease.[1,2,8,9] This chapter follows this idea and categorizes posterior circulation occlusive disease, depending on the causative vascular lesions. Remember that in the posterior circulation, considerably more tissue is fed by small, penetrating arteries, so the proportion of small-artery to large-artery disease is higher than in the anterior circulation. Lacunes and penetrating branch territory infarcts within the vertebrobasilar system are considered in Chapter 8. A monograph devoted entirely to posterior circulation disease[1] discusses this topic in much more detail than is possible in this chapter.

OCCLUSION OR SEVERE STENOSIS OF THE SUBCLAVIAN AND INNOMINATE ARTERIES

The extracranial vertebral arteries (ECVAs) arise from the proximal subclavian arteries. The subclavian artery arises in the great majority of patients as the last brachiocephalic branch of the aortic arch, while the right subclavian artery originates from the innominate artery. Thus, disease of the subclavian or innominate arteries before the ECVA origins can lead to changes in vertebral artery blood flow. Reivich et al[10] and others[11-13] brought this practical fact to the attention of physicians when they recognized the subclavian steal syndrome. In this syndrome, obstruction to the proximal subclavian artery led to a low-pressure system within the ipsilateral VA and in blood vessels of the ipsilateral upper extremity. Blood from a higher-pressure system, the contralateral vertebral artery and basilar artery, was diverted and flowed retrograde down the ipsilateral vertebral artery into the arm (Fig. 7-1). Figure 7-2 shows an arteriogram from a patient with subclavian steal.

In the nearly 3 decades since the description of this syndrome, knowledge of its natural history, diagnosis, and treatment has greatly expanded. Most often, subclavian artery disease is detected when patients with coronary, carotid, or peripheral vascular occlusive disease in the legs are referred to ultrasound laboratories for noninvasive testing. Most patients with subclavian artery disease are asymptomatic. In those with symptoms, most complaints relate to arm ischemia. Fatigue, aching after exercise, and coolness are described by some patients, especially those that use their arms vigorously during athletics or work. In a large series of patients with subclavian steal, studied in 1988 by Hennerici and colleagues using ultrasound documentation of vertebral artery reversed flow, one third of patients reported pain, numbness, or fatigue in the arm.[14] Only 15 of the 324 patients (4.8%) studied, however, had objective physical signs of brachial ischemia or embolism.[14] Neurologic symptoms are not common unless there is accompanying carotid artery disease. Among 155 patients, 116 patients (74%) with a unilateral subclavian steal shown by ultrasonography had no neurologic symptoms.[14]

JK, a 53-year-old laborer, noted occasional dizziness, sometimes with diplopia and fuzzy vision, when he worked. The attacks were brief, and always went away within seconds when he stopped working. For 6 months, his left hand felt cool and occasionally ached after he exercised.

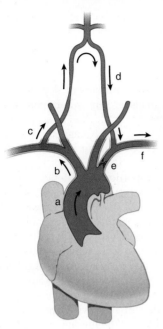

Figure 7-1. Subclavian steal: (**a**) aortic arch, (**b**) innominate artery, (**c**) right VA, (**d**) left VA, (**e**) occlusion of subclavian artery proximal to the left VA, (**f**) subclavian artery. *Arrows* represent direction of flow. VA, vertebral artery.

The most frequent symptoms of subclavian artery disease relate to the ipsilateral arm and hand. Coolness, weakness, and pain on use of the arm are common, but may not be severe enough for the patient to consult a doctor. When there is impairment of vertebral artery flow (decreased antegrade flow or retrograde flow), patients may report spells of dizziness. Dizziness is by far the most common neurologic symptom of subclavian steal syndrome, and usually has a spinning or vertiginous character. Diplopia, decreased vision, oscillopsia, and staggering occur but less frequently, often accompanying the dizziness. The attacks are brief and may occasionally be brought on by exercising the ischemic arm, a diagnostic point that is sometimes useful during examination. In most patients, however, exercise of the ischemic limb does not provoke neurologic symptoms or signs.

On examination of JK, the left radial pulse was smaller in volume and delayed relative to the carotid and right radial pulses. Blood pressure was 160/90 mm Hg in the right arm, and 120/50 mm Hg in the left. The left hand felt cool. There was a loud bruit in the left supraclavicular region that decreased slightly as the

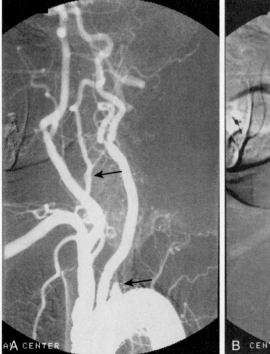
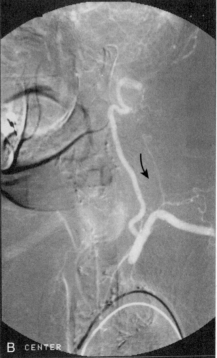

Figure 7-2. Subtraction arch angiograms from a patient with subclavian steal syndrome. **A,** Arch angiogram early phase. The right subclavian artery and right vertebral artery *(large black arrow)* fill normally. The left subclavian artery is occluded just above its origin *(lower, small black arrow).* **B,** Arch angiogram, later films. The left vertebral artery is now opacified after filling from the right ICVA, and blood is flowing retrograde down the left vertebral artery into the left subclavian artery beyond the occlusion *(large curved arrow).* (From Caplan LR: Posterior Circulation Disease: Clinical Findings, Diagnosis, and Management. Boston: Blackwell, 1996, with permission.)

blood pressure cuff on the left arm was inflated to a pressure exceeding 120 mm Hg. There also was a loud, high-pitched focal bruit at the right carotid bifurcation. Neurologic examination was normal.

The diagnosis of subclavian-artery occlusive disease can usually be made by physical examination. Invariably, there is a difference in the wrist and the antecubital pulses in the two arms. The pulse in the affected limb is of smaller volume and is delayed relative to the contralateral arm. The blood pressure is also reduced asymmetrically. In my experience, however, the pulse asymmetry has usually been more obvious than the blood pressure difference. I do not know of a single case of subclavian steal syndrome in which the pulse was symmetric and a blood pressure difference was prominent. I believe that it is more important to carefully feel both wrist pulses simultaneously than it is to routinely measure blood pressure in both arms. A supraclavicular bruit may be present. When the bruit originates from an ECVA stenosis without subclavian narrowing, inflating a blood pressure cuff above systolic pressure may augment the bruit by directing more blood into the ECVA. When the bruit is caused by subclavian or innominate artery stenosis, similarly inflating the cuff reduces flow into the arm, so the bruit becomes softer.

Atherosclerotic subclavian artery stenosis occurs in 0.5% to 2% of patients. The left side is more often affected than the right, and the segment proximal to the vertebral artery more often than the segment distal to the vertebral origin. Atherosclerosis of the proximal subclavian artery is usually associated with occlusive disease in other large arteries, typically the coronary, lower extremity, and other extracranial arteries. In JK, the loud, focal, right carotid bruit indicated important concomitant right internal carotid artery (ICA) disease.

Other diseases, especially temporal arteritis[15] and Takayasu's disease,[16,17] can lead to subclavian stenosis. Temporal arteritis with involvement of aortic arch branches is rare and is limited to geriatric patients. Takayasu's arteritis is most common in young Asian girls and women, and middle-aged men in India. Takayasu's is also known as pulseless disease because of the almost invariable loss of arterial pulses at the wrist. In these patients, arterial blood pressure measurements taken in the usual way are not a reliable reflection of systemic blood pressure.

Baseball pitchers and cricket bowlers are also at risk for developing innominate and subclavian artery disease because of their arm mechanics during throwing. A cervical rib or chronic use of an arm crutch can also lead to stenosis or aneurysmal

dilation of the subclavian artery. Clots can form in the diseased vessel and periodically embolize to individual finger arteries, causing a syndrome that can be confused with unilateral Raynaud's syndrome. When the lesion affects the innominate artery, signs and symptoms of decreased carotid artery flow can also occur. Innominate artery disease is much less common than subclavian artery disease.[18,19] Figure 7-3 is a magnetic resonance angiogram (MRA) of a patient with severe innominate artery stenosis.

A large proportion of patients with innominate artery disease are cigarette smokers. In series of patients with innominate artery disease, women are more often affected than men, in contrast to patients with carotid, subclavian, and peripheral vascular occlusive disease, in which there is a male preponderance.[18] Although right subclavian steal is much less frequent than left, it is more serious and more important to treat. Two early patients, reported by Symonds, had right subclavian-artery occlusion with spread of clot into the innominate and carotid arterial systems.[20] Since then, occasional patients who had recurrent arm and brain ischemia, caused by embolization of floating thrombi within the innominate artery, have been reported.[1,21,22]

An illustrative case report described the events in a well-known professional baseball pitcher.[23] Symptoms began when the pitcher noted his throwing arm suddenly went "dead" and his first

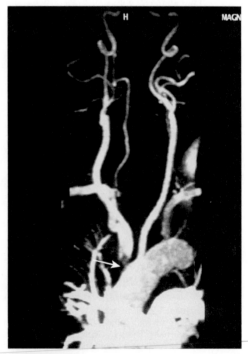

Figure 7-3. Gadolinium-enhanced MRA of the aortic arch region showing a severe stenosis of the proximal innominate artery *(white arrow)*.

three digits felt numb. Angiography showed complete occlusion of the right subclavian artery just proximal to the medial edge of the first rib. Five days later while exercising, he suddenly developed a left hemiplegia and confusion.[23] Subsequent angiography showed that the clot had propagated proximally to block the innominate artery, and had embolized into ICA branches intracranially.[23]

I had a patient who presented with a rather remarkable constellation of symptoms and signs that included (1) transient right monocular visual loss, (2) coldness of the right arm, (3) left upper-extremity weakness, (4) double vision, (5) dizziness, (6) ataxia, and (7) a left homonymous hemianopia. Evaluation, including magnetic resonance imaging (MRI) and angiography, showed a stenosis of the innominate artery with a superimposed thrombus. Infarcts were present within the right MCA territory, right posterior cerebral artery (PCA) territory, and the cerebellar territory supplied by the superior cerebellar artery (SCA). The patient had embolized through the right carotid artery branch of the innominate artery, to the ipsilateral eye and the MCA, and through the ipsilateral subclavian-ECVA to the distal basilar artery and its PCA and SCA branches. The array of ipsilateral arm and eye ischemia, accompanied by anterior and posterior circulation ischemia (or both), is diagnostic of innominate artery disease.

Although frequent attacks of posterior circulation ischemia may occur in patients with subclavian steal, development of a posterior circulation stroke is rare.[1,14,24] There is usually much smoke but little fire. I could find only two documented, reported examples of serious brainstem or cerebellar infarction in patients with subclavian steal, and each followed severe hypotension. Among 407 patients with posterior circulation TIAs and ischemic strokes in the New England Medical Center Posterior Circulation Registry, only two had symptoms (TIAs) attributable to significant subclavian or innominate artery disease.[1,2,25,26]

> Noninvasive testing of JK's arms showed reduced left forearm blood flow measured by oscillography. Duplex ultrasonography showed severe stenosis 2 cm beyond the origin of the left subclavian artery. Continuous wave (CW) Doppler examination at C2 revealed a reversal of flow in the left ECVA. Transcranial Doppler (TCD) blood-flow velocities were normal. MRI was normal. Angiography confirmed a high-grade stenosis of the left subclavian artery, with retrograde flow down the left vertebral artery on delayed films. A moderately severe stenosis (2.5-mm residual lumen) of the right ICA and slight stenosis of the left ICA at their origins were also evident. The intracranial arteries were normal. He was treated with a combination of

25 mg of aspirin and 200 mg of modified-release dipyridamole twice a day and was urged to limit vigorous exercising of the left arm. The episodes of dizziness persisted for 2 months and then stopped. He has been followed for symptoms of anterior circulation ischemia.

Noninvasive testing of flow in the arm should allow the diagnosis of subclavian artery stenosis. Helpful are oscillographic measurements of forearm blood flow, venous occlusive plethysmography of the arm,[27] and analysis of the relative velocities of pulse-wave propagation in the two arms.[28]

Doppler sonography gives an accurate indication of flow in the proximal ECVA system. Hennerici et al studied the accuracy of CW Doppler in detecting innominate and subclavian artery lesions.[19] All 21 patients with Doppler-detected innominate artery stenosis and all 66 patients with subclavian steal had angiography that confirmed the ultrasound findings.[19] In patients with slight or moderate subclavian-artery stenosis, reduction of flow is found in the ECVA during systole. The flow, however, is usually antegrade. With increasingly severe subclavian artery stenosis, blood flow reverses during systole, but remains cephalad in diastole, or blood flow is persistently decreased.[14,29-32] The subclavian arteries are often well shown by duplex sonography and CW Doppler[33] (see Figs. 4-9 and 4-10). The left subclavian artery B-mode images are usually obtained 1 to 4 cm above the subclavian artery origin. Duplex scanning of the right subclavian artery is more problematic because the proximal right subclavian artery makes a posterolateral curve.[33] TCD recordings give information about the intracranial effects of the proximal arterial disease.[14,31,32] Hennerici et al reported the TCD findings in 50 patients with subclavian steal: 47 unilateral and three bilateral.[14] Most patients had normal brachial artery flow velocities and retrograde flow, irrespective of the flow pattern in the proximal ECVA. CTA and MRA can also show the innominate and subclavian arteries as well as the ECVAs, especially when arch films are taken after gadolinium infusions. Figure 4-23 is a gadolinium-enhanced MRA that shows normal subclavian, innominate, and vertebral arteries. Figure 7-3 is a gadolinium-enhanced study that shows severe innominate artery disease. Figure 4-26 is a CTA showing the left subclavian artery and the origin of the vertebral artery.

When angiography is performed, it is especially important to obtain delayed films of ECVA flow; otherwise, the retrograde phase of flow might be missed. It is also important to assess the carotid arteries carefully because often there is associated occlusive disease in other arteries.

Subclavian artery disease is usually relatively benign. The spells of posterior circulation ischemia and the arm symptoms often improve with time, as collateral circulation to the arm develops. Operations on the proximal subclavian or innominate artery, when performed by thoracotomy, are more serious operative procedures than vascular surgery involving only a neck incision. Angioplasty and stenting have recently almost entirely replaced surgery on the innominate and subclavian arteries.

Surgery on the subclavian and innominate arteries is much more difficult than carotid artery surgery and has more frequent complications. In a systematic review of 2496 patients, the average complication rate associated with surgery was 16%, with a stroke rate of 3%, and mortality rate of 2%.[34] Studies of balloon angioplasty and/or stenting for treatment of subclavian stenosis report more favorable results than surgery with improvement or cessation of presenting symptoms in 72% to 100%, technical success in 90% to 100%, periprocedural complications in 0% to 10%, and stroke and death in 0% to 4%.[35-41] Stenting has also been performed in patients with subclavian artery stenosis with very good technical success and patency rates. In one series, Henry et al reported the results among 113 patients treated for subclavian stenosis or occlusion with either angioplasty alone ($n = 57$) or stenting ($n = 46$) with 91% technical success and 2.6% complication rate.[37] Procedural failures were mostly in patients with occluded vessels. Over 4.3 years of average follow-up, restenosis occurred in 16%, the majority of whom had been treated with angioplasty only.[37] In contrast, Schillinger et al found a higher rate of initial technical success in 115 patients in whom stents were applied for subclavian stenosis: 95% of stented vessels remained patent at 1 year versus 76% treated with angioplasty; however, by 4 years, only 59% of stented vessels remained patent compared with 68% for angioplasty alone.[42]

Sometimes, the intriguing radiologic demonstration of reversal of VA flow seduces surgeons into operating on the subclavian artery (by repair of the subclavian artery or ligation of the proximal ECVA) or interventionalist into angioplasty or stenting of the narrowed artery. When the patient is incapacitated by arm ischemia (e.g., if the syndrome occurs in a golfer or a pitcher), repair is indicated. When the disease affects the right innominate or subclavian artery, serious carotid-territory infarction can ensue, so aggressive treatment is often indicated. In most other patients, I suggest watchful waiting. I try to reduce risk factors, such as smoking, hypertension, and hyperlipidemia, and observe the patient for

attacks related to the anterior circulation. I usually prescribe a statin in high doses (equivalent of 80 mg of atorvastatin), a platelet antiaggregant, and often an ACE inhibitor or ACE receptor blocker.

OCCLUSION OR SEVERE STENOSIS OF THE VERTEBRAL ARTERY IN THE NECK

Proximal Atherosclerotic Extracranial Vertebral Artery Disease

The most frequent location for atherosclerotic disease of the ECVAs is at their origin from the subclavian arteries. Atherosclerosis at this site shares epidemiologic features with its close cousin, atherosclerosis of the ICA origin. In fact, the two sites are frequently affected in the same individuals.[43-45] My colleagues and I have found that stenosis at the ECVA origins is found less often in African Americans and Asians than in whites.[1,46] Proximal ECVA stenosis is often accompanied by hypertension, smoking, coronary artery disease, and peripheral vascular occlusive disease. ECVA was the most common site of atherosclerotic narrowing in the New England Medical Center Posterior Circulation Registry series among 407 patients with vertebrobasilar TIAs and strokes.[1,25,26] A total of 131 patients (32%) had significant (>50%) narrowing of the ECVA, 29 bilaterally. Many patients with severe ECVA disease also had severe occlusive disease within the intracranial vertebrobasilar arterial system, sometimes at multiple sites.[25,26] Among patients who had occlusive lesions at only one site, 52 had only proximal ECVA disease (15 bilaterally).[25,26]

> LM, a 63-year-old white man, had repeated attacks of spinning dizziness during the past 2 weeks. In some spells, the only symptom was dizziness. In others, diplopia and staggering occurred. In one attack, his right limbs felt transiently weak. The attacks were brief, lasting 30 seconds to 4 minutes. They tended to occur while he was quietly resting, and never occurred during exertion. He also had occasional left occipital headaches.

The most frequently reported symptom during TIAs caused by ECVA-origin disease is dizziness. The attacks are indistinguishable from those described by patients with subclavian steal, except that ECVA-origin TIAs are not precipitated by effort or by arm exertion. Although dizziness is the most common symptom, it is seldom the only neurologic symptom. Usually, in at least some attacks, dizziness is accompanied by other definite signs of hindbrain ischemia. Diplopia, oscillopsia, weakness of the legs, hemiparesis, or numbness are often mentioned if the patient is closely questioned. Fisher wrote that he had not seen a patient with repeated spells of unaccompanied dizziness occurring during a period of 6 weeks or more that were caused by documented VA disease.[47] In the years since this report, I have also not seen such a patient. However, there are isolated reports of isolated dizziness and vertigo associated with occlusive posterior circulation lesions,[48,49] and, of course, now we do not wait 6 weeks to investigate the cause. Because dizziness is a common neurologic symptom and is in most cases not caused by cerebrovascular disease, I seldom diagnose ECVA disease in patients with repeated, unaccompanied dizziness. True vertigo, present only on rising and retiring, and true positional vertigo are never caused by ECVA-origin disease. In patients with risk factors for stroke and unaccompanied spells of dizziness, I usually order ultrasound or CTA or MRA to detect lesions of the vertebral arteries in the neck or intracranially.

VA atheromas often originate in the subclavian artery and spread to the proximal few centimeters of the ECVA. They may also arise at the origin of the ECVA. Little has been written about the morphology of VA-origin lesions. Although ulceration and plaque hemorrhage are commonly recognized when carotid endarterectomy specimens are examined, ECVA lesions are said to be fibrous and smooth and seldom ulcerate.[50,51] Scant pathologic data about ECVA-origin lesions exist because ECVA surgery is usually performed by using a bypass, so the vessel is not available for pathologic examination. Careful necropsy examinations of the ECVAs have not been reported subsequent to recognition of the importance of plaque ulceration and hemorrhage. ICA- and ECVA-origin lesions cannot be assumed to be morphologically identical. The geometry of the two origins is quite different. The ECVA arises at nearly 90 degrees from the subclavian artery, whereas the ICA is almost a direct 180-degree extension of the common carotid artery (CCA). Caliber and flow disparities between the ICA and ECVA origins also exist. Only a small fraction of subclavian flow goes into each ECVA, a much smaller artery, whereas a high proportion of CCA blood goes into the ICA, a vessel of nearly the same size.

In 1989, Pelouze reported a man with multiple attacks of vertigo and brainstem ischemia, which continued despite prescription of aspirin.[52] Angiography showed irregular stenosis near the ECVA origin and a B-mode ultrasound scan suggested an ulcerated plaque. An ECVA endarterectomy was performed, and the surgical specimen showed an ulcerated, irregular plaque that represented the source of multiple intracranial posterior circulation emboli.[52] The question of the frequency of ECVA-origin plaque ulceration is of great importance, but remains unsolved until more necropsy or surgical specimens are carefully examined. Do small platelet-fibrin and erythrocyte-fibrin emboli arise frequently from the proximal ECVA and embolize to distal arteries in the posterior circulation? Would agents that reduce platelet aggregability or anticoagulants (or both) be effective for patients with ECVA-origin TIAs?

Two important anatomic facts explain why ECVA-origin lesions seldom cause chronic, hemodynamically significant low flow to the vertebrobasilar system:

1. The vertebral arteries are paired vessels that unite to form a single basilar artery; only rarely is there complete atresia of one vertebral artery, although asymmetries are frequent.
2. The ECVA gives off numerous muscular and other branches as it ascends in the neck. In contrast, there are no nuchal branches of the ICA.

In the vertebral artery system, there is much more potential for development of adequate collateral circulation, than when a carotid artery occludes. Figure 7-4 shows collaterals filling the distal ECVA in a patient with ECVA-origin occlusion. Even when there is bilateral occlusion of the ECVAs, some patients do not develop posterior circulation infarcts.[1,25,26,53-58] ECVA-origin disease is more benign than ICA-origin disease from a hemodynamic aspect. Only 13 patients who had ECVA disease among the 407 patients in the New England Medical Center Posterior Circulation Registry had a chronic, recurrent low flow mechanism of brain ischemia.[26] In 12 of these 13, there was severe bilateral, vertebral artery occlusive disease. Six had severe bilateral ECVA disease and 6 had severe intracranial vertebral artery (ICVA) disease contralateral to severe disease of one ECVA. The only patient who did not have bilateral vertebral artery disease, had a unilateral ECVA occlusion and bilateral ICA occlusions. All 13 patients had TIAs. Only two had brain infarcts, one affecting the occipital lobe and the other the temporal lobe and cerebellum. TIAs were multiple and recurred during 1 week to several months. Dizziness, often accompanied by veering to one side and gait ataxia, visual blurring, perioral paresthesias, and diplopia were the commonest TIA symptoms.[26]

Embolization of white platelet-fibrin and red erythrocyte-fibrin thrombi from atherostenotic occlusive lesions is the most important presentation of ECVA-origin disease.[1,2,26,54-58] During one

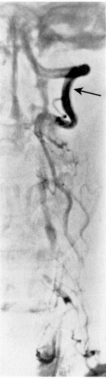

Figure 7-4. Subclavian artery angiogram showing filling of the distal extracranial VA *(black arrow)* from collaterals. (From Caplan LR: Posterior Circulation Disease: Clinical Findings, Diagnosis, and Management. Boston: Blackwell, 1996, with permission.)

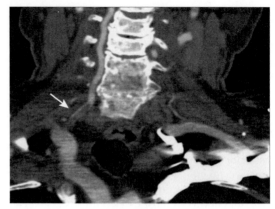

Figure 7-5. CT angiogram showing a filling defect *(white arrow)* representing a thrombus that formed at the origin of the right vertebral artery.

stenosis of the left ECVA origin (Figure 7-6). Intracranial films showed good basilar artery filling. The right VA was normal. He was treated with warfarin and had no further attacks. Six months later, B-mode, CW Doppler, and color Doppler flow imaging (CDFI) suggested complete occlusion of the proximal ECVA with no antegrade flow. Warfarin was stopped a month later without subsequent ischemic spells.

In patients with proximal ECVA disease, a bruit can often be heard over the supraclavicular region. Physicians should auscultate by moving

2-week period, I cared for three patients with intra-arterial posterior circulation embolism arising from an occlusive lesion at the ECVA origin. A similar situation is well known in the anterior circulation. A patient is admitted with a small MCA-territory infarct, and ultrasound or angiography shows an occlusion at the ICA origin. The recently formed occlusive thrombus has fragmented and embolized distally. Among 407 patients in the New England Medical Center Posterior Circulation Registry, 80 patients had very severe preocclusive stenosis or occlusion of the proximal ECVA. In 45 (56%) of these 80 patients, embolization from the VA lesion was the most likely cause of brain ischemia.[54] Figure 7-5 is a CTA that shows a thrombus at the origin of the vertebral artery in the neck. Intra-arterial embolism to the intracranial posterior circulation arteries occurs much more often than is presently recognized.

> Neurologic examination of LM was normal. A high-pitched focal bruit was audible in the left supraclavicular fossa, and a soft bruit was heard over the right posterior mastoid region. The MRI was normal. Noninvasive testing confirmed a reduction of flow in the left ECVA. A catheter digital-subtraction angiogram showed severe

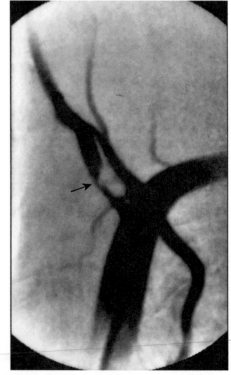

Figure 7-6. Subclavian angiogram showing severe stenosis of the left vertebral artery origin *(arrow)*.

the stethoscope bell to listen over the posterior cervical muscles and mastoid. Sometimes, as in the patient LM, a bruit is heard over the contralateral side because of increased collateral blood flow. B-mode scans can image the proximal VA in the segment between the origin of the artery until its entrance into the foramen transversaria of the cervical vertebrae.[1,31-33] Color flow Doppler imaging (CFDI) is also helpful in showing the origin of the ECVA and distal flow patterns. Figure 7-7 shows a CFDI image of the origin of the ECVA from the subclavian artery. CW Doppler insonation in the low neck and at the C2 region is the most effective means of monitoring ECVA blood flow. In the presence of a severe occlusive lesion at the ECVA origin, blood flow is usually retrograde or to-and-from above the occlusive lesion. CTA has been able to show the vertebral artery origin from the subclavian artery, at times better than using MRA. MRA, especially with gadolinium enhancement and attention to the aortic arch branches, can also most often provide diagnostic quality images of the proximal ECVA.

Data about the natural history of disease of the ECVA origin and the response of patients with this lesion to various treatments are insufficient to warrant firm conclusions as to the best therapy. Moufarrij and colleagues reviewed the Cleveland Clinic experience with VA lesions.[59] Long-term follow-up of their series of more than 80 patients with greater than 75% stenosis of the ECVA origin showed that only two patients had brainstem strokes. These two patients also had basilar artery stenosis.[59]

Vascular surgeons with considerable experience in operating on the ECVA have shown that they can bypass ECVA-origin lesions with low morbidity and mortality.[1,51,52,60-64] Angioplasty and stenting have been performed much less often on the ECVA than on the ICA. Some reports cite a restenosis rates of 9% to 10% within 1 year.[65-69] In the Stenting of Symptomatic Atherosclerotic Lesions in the Vertebral or Intracranial Arteries (SSYLVIA) trial, 6 of 14 (43%) extracranial vertebral arteries treated with stenting developed restenosis more than 50% at 6 months follow-up.[69] This preliminary experience with ECVA angioplasty/stenting has raised concerns that the restenosis rate of interventional treatment of the ECVA may be relatively high.

No data exist about the effectiveness or lack thereof of antiplatelet aggregating agents or warfarin in patients with proximal ECVA disease. In the case of LM, I chose warfarin to prevent thrombosis and subsequent embolization in a vessel with low-antegrade blood flow. If the lesion had been less stenotic, I would have chosen aspirin or aspirin combined with modified-release dipyridamole to prevent fibrin-platelet emboli. In some patients, I have chosen surgical reconstruction. I have not had extensive experience with ECVA angioplasty/ stenting. Clearly, more data are needed regarding the natural history of ECVA-origin disease and its response to medical, surgical, and interventional treatments. The advent of CTA and MRA and wider application of noninvasive techniques to the posterior circulation may provide groups of patients with ECVA-origin disease who can be followed prospectively and studied to determine the relative effectiveness and risks of various potential therapies.

Dissections of the ECVA

Dissections usually involve portions of arteries that are mobile and rarely occur at the origins of arteries. Vertebral artery dissections are also discussed in detail in Chapter 11. The carotid and vertebral arteries are relatively fixed at their origins from the common carotid and subclavian arteries. The ECVAs are anchored at their origin from the subclavian artery and during their course through bone within the intervertebral foramina (V_2 portion), and also by the dura at the point of intracranial penetration. The short movable segments between these anchored regions are most vulnerable to tearing and stretching. Dissections can involve the proximal (V_1) portion of the ECVA usually beginning well above the vessel origin from the subclavian artery, affecting the artery before it enters the intervertebral foramina at C5 or C6. V_1 dissections are almost always unilateral. The distal extracranial portion (V_3) is the most common location for dissection. This segment is relatively mobile and so vulnerable to tearing by sudden motion and stretching as might occur during chiropractic manipulation. Distal

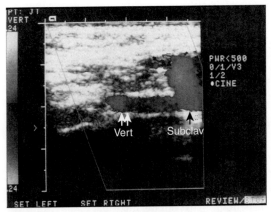

Figure 7-7. An image is shown from a color-flow Doppler study of the vertebral artery of the proximal extracranial vertebral artery. Blood flows from the subclavaian artery *(right)* into the vertebral artery.

ECVA dissections may extend into the ICVA and proximally into the V_2 segment. Distal ECVA dissections are usually bilateral, even though pain and other symptoms may be unilateral.

ECVA dissections were first recognized in patients who had either neck trauma or chiropractic manipulation, but ECVA injuries also have been reported in patients who manipulate their own necks or who have maintained their necks in a fixed position for some time. ECVA dissections also occur after surgery and resuscitation, presumably because of sustained neck positions in patients who are anesthetized or unresponsive. These lesions most often involve the distal ECVA (V_3). Spontaneous ECVA dissections closely mimic those related to trauma. Pain in the posterior neck or occiput is common, as is generalized headache.

Pain often precedes neurologic symptoms by hours, days, and, rarely, weeks.[70-76] Some patients with ECVA dissections have only neck pain and do not develop neurologic symptoms or signs. TIAs most often include dizziness, diplopia, veering, staggering, and dysarthria. TIAs are less common in ECVA dissections than in ICA dissections. Infarcts usually cause signs that begin suddenly. The commonest patterns of ischemic brain damage are cerebellar infarction in PICA cerebellar territory distribution and lateral medullary infarction. As in extracranial ICA dissections, infarcts are invariably explained by embolization of fresh thrombus to the ICVA. Occasionally, dissections extend or begin intracranially. Sometimes, emboli reach the superior cerebellar arteries (SCAs), the main basilar artery, or the posterior cerebral arteries (PCAs). Young age and presentation with pain and no or minor neurologic signs are features predictive of a good prognosis.[76]

ECVA dissections also can cause cervical root pain. Aneurysmal dilatation of the ECVA adjacent to nerve roots causes the radicular pain and can lead to radicular distribution motor, sensory, and reflex abnormalities. Occasionally spinal cord infarction results because of hypoperfusion in the supply zones of arteries from the ECVA that supply the cervical spinal cord. Many patients with ECVA dissections have headache, pain, and TIAs without lasting neurologic deficits.

Duplex scans of the ECVAs can suggest dissection. Typical findings are increased arterial diameter, decreased pulsatility, intravascular abnormal echoes, and hemodynamic evidence of decreased flow. Color Doppler flow imaging can also show the regions of dissection within the neck. Diminished flow in the high neck at the level of the atlas detected by CW Doppler and decreased flow in the ICVA shown by transcranial Doppler (TCD) suggest the presence of distal ECVA dissections. Dye-contrast catheter cerebral angiography is still the optimal method of imaging the extracranial vertebral arteries in patients suspected of having vertebral artery dissections. Figure 11-5 is a montage of angiograms that show vertebral artery dissections.

Intracranial Vertebral Artery Disease

Severe atherosclerotic narrowing is rare in the cervical portions of the vertebral arteries, except at their origins. Plaques are relatively routinely observed opposite osteophytes but rarely narrow the vessel.[1,50] The distal ECVA is vulnerable to trauma,[1] dissections, and fibromuscular dysplasia. The distal cervical ECVA is occasionally severely narrowed in patients with temporal arteritis[77] and in women taking high estrogen-content contraceptive pills.[78]

Atherosclerosis of the intracranial vertebral arteries (ICVAs) is most severe in the distal segment of the arteries, often at the vertebral-basilar junction.[1,79,80] Narrowing often extends into the proximal portion of the basilar artery. Less often, stenosis involves the ICVA just after it penetrates the dura to enter the cranium. In contrast to patients with proximal ECVA disease, there is no single typical patient with ICVA occlusive disease. Therefore, four different patient examples are presented and discussed herein.

Patient 1

A 57-year-old white man, WA, had a transient attack of dizziness and diplopia when he arose from a nap. Awakening the next day, he felt dizzy, as if the room were rocking or wavering like a ship. He felt a series of sharp, painful jabs in his left eye. His left face seemed strangely numb. He veered to the left when he tried to sit or stand. His left arm was clumsy. His voice was hoarse, and he gagged as he tried to swallow water. Vomiting and hiccups developed as the morning progressed, so he went to the hospital. Examination showed diminished pain and temperature sensation on the left face and right body, including the limbs; nystagmus with greater amplitude on looking leftward; diminished left corneal reflex; left ptosis, and a smaller left pupil; clumsiness of the left hand and foot; and decreased palatal motion on the left.

The most frequent findings in patients with ICVA occlusion are related to ischemia of the lateral medulla, the lesion illustrated by this patient.[1] In patients with lateral medullary infarction, the most common vascular lesion is occlusion of the proximal or middle portion of the ICVA.[1,81] Penetrating branches to the lateral medulla arise from the middle and distal two-thirds of the ICVAs and penetrate through the lateral medullary fossa to reach and supply the lateral medullary tegmentum.[1,82,83] The medial branches of the posterior inferior cerebellar arteries (PICAs) supply only a small portion of the dorsal medullary tegmentum.[83] The ICVA occlusive lesions decrease flow in these penetrators. Less often, lateral medullary infarction is caused by occlusion of one of the small medullary branches.

Important symptoms and signs of lateral medullary infarction can be understood best by recalling the anatomic nuclei and tracts in the lateral medulla (Fig. 7-8).

1. Nucleus and descending spinal tract of V. Symptoms include sharp jabs or stabs of pain in the ipsilateral eye and face and a feeling of numbness of the face; examination usually confirms decreased pinprick and temperature sensations on the ipsilateral face, and a reduced corneal reflex.
2. Vestibular nuclei and their connections. Feelings of dizziness or instability of the environment result from dysfunction of the vestibular system and may invoke vomiting; careful examination usually shows nystagmus with coarse rotatory eye movements when looking to the ipsilateral side and small-amplitude, faster nystagmus when looking contralaterally[1]; sometimes, the eyes forcibly deviate to the side of the lesion, known as *ocular lateral pulsion*.[1,84,85]

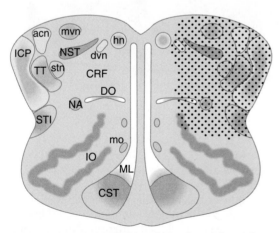

Figure 7-8. Cartoon of a dorsal lateral medullary infarct (Wallenberg's syndrome). acn, accessory cuneate nucleus; CRF, central reticular formation; CST, corticospinal tract; DO, dorsal accessory olivary nucleus; dvn, dorsal vagal nucleus; hn, hypoglossal nucleus; ICP, inferior cerebellar peduncle; IO, inferior olivary nucleus; ML, medial lemniscus; mo, medial accessory olivary nucleus; mvn, medial vestibular nucleus; NA, nucleus ambiguus; NST, nucleus of the solitary tract; STT, spinothalamic tract; stn, spinal trigeminal nucleus; TT, trigeminal tract.

3. Spinothalamic tract. Lesions of this structure usually produce diminished pinprick and temperature sensation in the contralateral limbs and body; this loss of function is seldom spontaneously recognized or reported by patients. Some patients note that they cannot feel hot or cold in the involved limbs. Most individuals only recognize the sensory abnormality during sensory testing when examined neurologically. Occasionally a sensory level is present on the contralateral trunk with pain and temperature loss on the trunk below that level and in the lower extremity.[1,86] At times, the pinprick and temperature loss extends to the contralateral face because of involvement of the crossed quintothalamic tract, which appends itself medially to the spinothalamic tract.[1,86] Rarely, the loss of pain and temperature sensation is totally contralateral and involves the face, arm, trunk, and leg.[1,86] Rarely the clinical findings are dominated by sensory symptoms and signs sometimes with a level on the trunk.[86a,b]
4. Restiform body (inferior cerebellar peduncle). Symptoms include veering or leaning toward the side of the lesion and clumsiness of the ipsilateral limbs; on examination, hypotonia and exaggerated rebound of the ipsilateral arm are common, but frank intention tremor is not; on standing or sitting, patients often lean or tilt to the side of the lesion.
5. Autonomic nervous system nuclei and tracts. The descending sympathetic system traverses the lateral medulla in the lateral reticular formation; dysfunction causes an ipsilateral Horner's syndrome; and the dorsal motor nucleus of the vagus is sometimes affected, leading to tachycardia and a labile increased blood pressure.
6. Nucleus ambiguus: When the infarct extends medially, it often affects this nucleus, causing hoarseness and dysphagia. The pharynx and palate are weak on the side of the lesion, sometimes causing patients to retain food within the piriform recess of the pharynx. A crow-like cough represents an attempt to extricate food from this area. At times, there is also ipsilateral facial weakness, perhaps related to ischemia of the caudal part of the VII-nerve nucleus, just rostral to the nucleus ambiguus, or involvement of corticobulbar fibers going toward the VII-nerve nucleus.[1]
7. Abnormal respiratory control: Initiation and control of respiration are known to involve the lateral pontine and medullary tegmentum. Poliomyelitis and bilateral medullary infarcts are well known to cause decreased respiratory drive.[87] Levin and

Margolis described a single patient with failure of automatic respirations ("Ondine's curse," or sleep-related apnea) caused by a one-sided lateral medullary infarct.[88] Bogousslavsky et al described in detail the clinical and autopsy findings in two patients with one-sided lateral medullopontine infarction who had respiratory failure.[89] Hypoventilation is probably related to involvement of the nucleus of the solitary tract, nucleus ambiguus, nucleus retroambiguus, and nuclei parvocellularis and gigantocellularis.[1,89]

When infarction is limited to the lateral medulla, prognosis for recovery is good,[1,90] although there are three exceptions to this rule[1,91]:

1. Some patients also have infarction in the ipsilateral inferior cerebellum, a region fed by the PICA. When the ICVA occlusion is long and extends to block the orifices of both PICA and the lateral medullary penetrators, both lateral medullary and cerebellar infarction develop. This occurs in about one in six patients with lateral medullary infarction. When the infarct is large, headache, head tilt, and stupor can result. A posterior fossa pressure cone can develop and cause death from medullary compression.[1]

2. Some patients with lateral medullary infarcts die suddenly; although the etiology of sudden death is uncertain, it is most likely caused by an increase in vagal tone (secondary to involvement of the dorsal motor nucleus of the vagus), or to involvement of automatic respiratory centers.

3. Some patients with one-sided lateral medullary infarcts have occlusive lesions in both ICVAs. Development of symptomatic ischemia, in the lateral medulla contralateral to the infarct, has a serious prognosis because of the frequency of autonomic dysfunction and loss of automatic control of respiration. Some patients with bilateral ICVA disease have a poor outcome once symptoms develop.[1,79,80,92]

Because of these important problems, it has been my practice to evaluate patients with lateral medullary infarcts for cerebellar infarction and cerebellar mass effect using MRI, to study the ICVAs noninvasively using MRA, CTA, or TCD, and to monitor respiration early in the course of the illness. Figures 7-9 and 7-10 are MRIs that clearly show lateral medullary infarcts.

In some patients with ICVA occlusion, ischemia of the medial medulla accompanies the lateral medullary infarct. This phenomenon is explained by an ICVA occlusion that blocks the

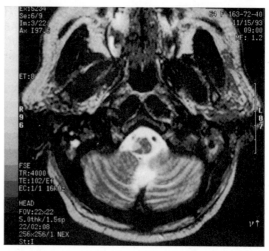

Figure 7-9. T2-weighted MRI scan. A small area of hyperintensity is shown in the left lateral medulla. The flow void in the adjacent left intracranial vertebral artery has been obliterated because of occlusion of that vessel. The right vertebral artery flow void is clearly visible and is normal.

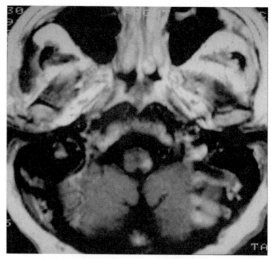

Figure 7-10. T2-weighted MRI scan. A small infarct is seen in the right dorsal lateral medulla.

anterior spinal artery orifices.[93] In addition to the signs already mentioned, a hemiparesis affects the contralateral arm and leg because of ischemia to the medullary pyramid. Ipsilateral weakness of the tongue and contralateral loss of position sense are less frequent findings and are explained by involvement of the hypoglossal nerve and the medial lemniscus.[94-96] The combination of medial and lateral medullary infarcts is often referred to as *hemimedullary infarction* and is caused by a long occlusion of the distal ICVA (that spares the PICA branch). Occlusion of the distal portion of the ICVA that blocks only the orifice of the anterior spinal artery can cause infarction, limited to the medial medulla, without associated lateral medullary infarction.[96] Rarely medial medullary infarction is bilateral and may extend caudally into the rostral spinal cord, causing a syndrome of quadriparesis difficult to separate from basilar artery occlusion with pontine infarction.[96a,b] The MRI in Figure 7-11 shows a bilateral medial medullary infarct.

In WA, B-mode and CW Doppler of the ECVA were normal. TCD showed an increase in blood-flow velocities in the left ICVA. Right ICVA pressures were normal. MRA showed severe stenosis of the left ICVA, just after the artery entered the cranium.

TCD can give accurate indications of occlusive lesions, involving the ICVAs, using insonation through a suboccipital foramen magnum window.[31,32] After the TCD and MRA results, the patient was treated with warfarin. The arterial stenosis is being followed by serial TCD examinations.

Patient 2

A 48-year-old woman, AD, suddenly felt dizzy and unsteady on her feet. She vomited and became unable to walk. When examined, the only positive findings were gait ataxia and slight conjugate gaze paresis to the left. CT was normal. The next morning, she was sleepy and reported severe headache. Her neck was stiff and she preferred to stay stationary in bed. A complete left conjugate gaze paresis to oculocephalic maneuvers was evident, and the left corneal reflex was reduced. Both plantar responses were extensor. CT showed a large area of hypodensity in the left cerebellum. The fourth ventricle was not visible,

and the lateral ventricles were enlarged. MRI confirmed a large PICA-territory cerebellar infarct (Figure 7-12). She became stuporous and difficult to arouse. She was treated with intravenous steroids and mannitol, but did not awaken. Soft, necrotic, cerebellar tissue was removed through a left posterior fossa craniotomy, after which she made an excellent recovery.

The most common vascular lesion found in patients with cerebellar infarction is occlusion or severe stenosis of the ICVA.[1,97-99] Often, the ICVA occlusion is caused by embolism, the thrombus arising from a source in the heart, or proximal vascular system.[1,100,101] The syndrome of cerebellar infarction is often difficult to diagnose. Symptoms

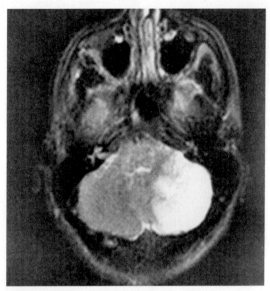

Figure 7-12. MRI T2-weighted axial image showing large PICA-territory infarct.

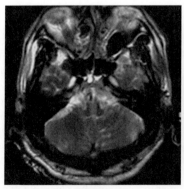
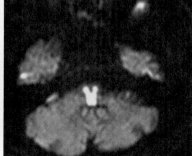

T2WI   DWI

Figure 7-11. MRI scans of a patient with a bilateral medial medullary infarct. The scan on the left is a T2-weighted scan. The hyperintensity in the medial medullar base and tegmentum is visible but is slight. The Diffusion-weighted scan on the right shows the abnormality much more obviously. (Courtesy of Yasumasa Yamamoto, MD, Kyoto, Japan.)

can resemble labyrinthitis and can appear deceptively slight. Gait ataxia and vomiting are often accompanied by dizziness, closely mimicking the findings in patients with cerebellar hemorrhage.[1,101,102] Most often, no signs of lateral medullary ischemia are evident. Initial CT scans may be normal. It is important to make certain that the fourth ventricle is of normal size and is in normal position. In retrospect, this was not done in this patient. Review of the initial films revealed slight rightward deviation and tilting of the fourth ventricle. MRI is more accurate in detecting early cerebellar ischemia. Especially important for localization are T2-weighted sagittal sections. On sagittal films, localization of the vascular territory involved is relatively easy. Lesions above the horizontal fissure are in the SCA territory. Lesions below the fissure are localized to anterior inferior cerebellar artery (AICA) or PICA territories, depending on anterior or posterior localization on the inferior surface of the cerebellum. Figure 7-13 shows a PICA-territory infarct on a T2-weighted sagittal MRI section. Compare this image with Figure 7-14A and B that show superior cerebellar artery (SCA) territory cerebellar infarcts. Figure 7-15 is a sagittal MRI that shows PICA and SCA territory infarcts on the same side.

Swollen cerebellar lesions may compress the cerebellopontine angle, leading to involvement of the ipsilateral fifth, sixth, seventh, and eighth cranial nerves. Compression of the medulla and pons is the probable cause of conjugate-gaze paresis to the ipsilateral side. This finding is especially important because the presence of a conjugate-gaze palsy, without contralateral hemiplegia, is virtually diagnostic of a cerebellar space-taking lesion. With more severe compression, the plantar responses become extensor, systolic pressure rises, diastolic pressure falls, the pulse may slow, and respiration may cease.

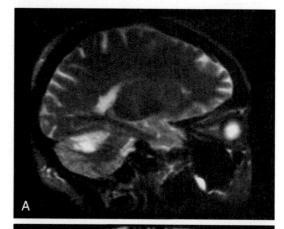

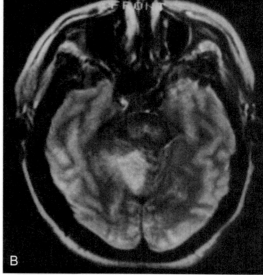

Figure 7-14. T2-weighted MRI scans. **A,** An infarct is seen in the superior portion of the cerebellum in the territory of the superior cerebellar artery. **B,** Axial scan showing an infarct in the superior portion of the cerebellar vermis in the territory of the medial branch of the superior cerebellar artery.

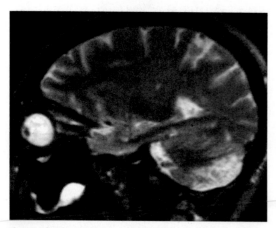

Figure 7-13. MRI T2-weighted sagittal view showing an infarct in the posterior inferior portion of the cerebellum.

As the cerebellum swells, hypodensity usually appears on repeat CT scans. Posterior fossa cisterns are compressed, and the ventricles become enlarged because of compression of the fourth ventricle. On MRI, compression of the contralateral vermis and brainstem are usually evident. Without treatment, death often ensues.[1,103-105] The preferred therapy is decompression of the swollen cerebellum. In some patients, medical decompression using steroids and osmotic agents has been helpful. Success has also been achieved in some patients by placing a ventricular drain in the lateral ventricles.[106,107] It is often difficult to separate brainstem pressure caused by cerebellar infarction, from brainstem ischemia caused by the propagation of clot into the basilar artery. MRI scans are helpful in making this distinction,

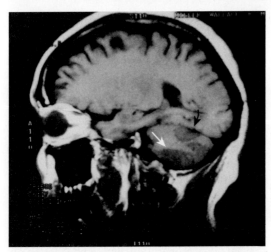

Figure 7-15. T1-weighted MRI scan sagittal projection showing infarcts in the posterior inferior cerebellar artery territory *(white arrow)* and also in the superior cerebellar artery territory *(curved black arrow)* on the same side. (From Caplan LR: Posterior Circulation Disease: Clinical Findings, Diagnosis, and Management. Boston: Blackwell, 1996, with permission.)

but MRA or catheter angiography (or both) are often necessary to visualize the vascular lesions.

Patient 2, AD, is an example of a large cerebellar infarct. In other patients, cerebellar infarcts are quite small and cause little or no abnormal neurologic signs. Infarcts limited to the medial vermis in territory supplied by the medial branch of PICA often present as isolated vertigo.[49] Examination may be normal except for nystagmus and gait ataxia. The most important signs of infarction of the posterior inferior cerebellum are alteration of posture, gait ataxia, and limb hypotonia. Patients topple, lean, or veer to the ipsilateral side when they sit or stand. In many patients, standing or walking is impossible during the acute period and helpers may be needed to support them in maintaining an erect posture. When they become able to walk, patients often feel as if they are being pulled to the side of the lesion. They veer, lean, or weave to the side, especially on turns. The ipsilateral limbs usually do not show a cerebellar type of rhythmic intention tremor. Hypotonia of the ipsilateral arm can best be shown by having the patient quickly lower or raise the outstretched hands together, braking the ascent or descent suddenly. The arm on the ipsilateral side often overshoots and is not as quickly braked. In some patients, the ipsilateral arm also makes a slower ascent or descent to facilitate braking. Some patients have great difficulty in feeding themselves with the ataxic limbs. They overshoot targets and have difficulty pointing accurately to moving targets.

Embolism from the heart or ECVA can cause cerebellar infarction by blocking the ICVA, PICA, or SCA. Cardiac evaluation and MRA or standard angiography can usually delineate the nature of the causative vascular disease.

Patient 3

A 65-year-old man, BE, had transient headache and dizziness on two occasions, 7 and 10 days before admission. On the day of admission, he suddenly became blind and agitated. When examined 5 hours later, he could not recall events of the past 3 weeks. He could form no new memories and had a complete right hemianopia. No other abnormalities of brainstem or central nervous system function were evident. CT revealed infarcts in the left occipital and temporal lobes in the distribution of the left PCA. MRI also showed a small infarct in the left cerebellum, in PICA territory. Angiography revealed occlusion of the left ICVA and embolic amputation of the left PCA. All other vessels were normal or showed only minor atheroma. Cardiac evaluation was normal.

This patient had an ICVA occlusion, followed by an embolus to the distal basilar artery system. In retrospect, the two episodes of dizziness probably represented transient cerebellar or medullary ischemia. When the vertebrobasilar system has been studied at necropsy, embolic occlusions are common in the PCAs.[1,108] These emboli may arise from recent occlusion within the ECVAs or the ICVAs.[1,56,57,109] Koroshetz and Ropper studied 12 patients with PCA infarcts and brainstem symptoms.[109] They found that three patients had intraarterial embolism arising from a donor site in the ICVA. The three other patients had lesions of the ICVAs and the ECVAs. All of the patients had intra-arterial embolism as the cause of PCA infarction.[109] Documentation of artery-to-artery emboli, from freshly occluded vertebral arteries, has led me to prescribe heparin or warfarin for such patients during the time it takes for the clot to solidify and attach to the artery (3 to 4 weeks). Insufficient data exist to determine the risk/benefit ratio of anticoagulants for preventing embolization and progressing infarction in patients with recent ICVA occlusions. Thrombolysis is another potential therapeutic strategy to treat recent ICVA occlusion, although there is no published data.

Patient 4

A 60-year-old hypertensive, diabetic African-American man, EO, noted diplopia and dizziness after arising from a nap. The symptoms were transient. Two days later, he staggered and had double vision. On examination, he had gait ataxia, nystagmus, and slight left facial weakness. When he stood, he became dizzy, felt weak, and his vision dimmed. He was treated

7

with heparin and bed rest. Six days later, he gradually became stuporous and quadriplegic. He died soon after of pneumonia. Necropsy revealed bilateral occlusion of the ICVAs and extensive necrosis of the cerebellar hemispheres, medulla, and pons.

Bilateral ICVA disease is relatively common. Among 430 patients in the New England Medical Center Posterior Circulation Registry, 21% had severe ICVA occlusive disease[79] and 42 patients (10%) had bilateral severe ICVA occlusive disease.[80] The diagnosis of bilateral ICVA occlusion is often difficult.[1,92] Early symptoms may be deceptively mild and are usually referable to the cerebellum and lateral medulla, like those seen in patients 1 (WA) and 2 (AD). Because of a low-flow system, the symptoms are often positionally sensitive, worsening when the patient sits or stands or when blood pressure falls spontaneously or after treatment. Usually, TIAs continue and are multiple and stereotyped.[80] Symptoms and signs may also gradually progress.[92] Heparin is most often ineffective because the progressive ischemia is caused by reduced brainstem perfusion rather than thrombus propagation or embolization. Figure 4-30A is a multimodal MRI in a patient with bilateral ICVA occlusions showing severe perfusion abnormalities in the medulla, pons, and cerebellum. Ataxia and pyramidal signs and symptoms predominate. At times, ischemia of the PCA territories also leads to abnormalities of vision, memory, and behavior. Bilateral ICVA occlusive lesions are most common in hypertensive and diabetic patients.[1,80,92] Death caused by extensive hindbrain ischemia can result.[92]

In the 1970s and 1980s, a preferred treatment for patients with persistent brainstem ischemia related to bilateral ICVA disease was surgical creation of shunts from a variety of different donor arteries—mostly the occipital and superficial temporal arterial branches of the external carotid arteries to various posterior circulation arteries distal to the ICVA obstruction.[110-112] Endarterectomy of a stenotic ICVA was also occasionally performed when the stenotic lesion was proximal in the ICVA.[113] More recently, the preferred treatment has become angioplasty with or without stenting of one of the stenotic ICVAs.[114]

Patients 1 through 4 illustrate serious posterior circulation infarction caused by ICVA disease. In some patients, this vascular lesion is tolerated without symptoms or with only minor TIAs. As a general rule, however, the more distally located a vascular lesion is along the path from the proximal subclavian-vertebral junction to the distal basilar artery, the more likely it is to cause infarction. The more proximal the lesion, the more likely it is to be more benign.

Little is known about optimal treatment of lesions of the ICVA. Allen and others have performed direct endarterectomies on the ICVA, usually in its proximal portion.[113] Interventional radiologists have the capability to perform angioplasties on the ICVA.[115] I have been involved in the treatment of three patients with bilateral ICVA occlusive disease in whom unilateral ICVA angioplasty effectively stopped TIAs.[114] Thrombolytic treatment could also lyse ICVA thrombi if given early enough after occlusion. In the patient examples and discussion, I have emphasized the need for vigilance to detect large cerebellar infarcts and decompress these lesions. I often use short-term heparin or warfarin therapy for patients with ICVA occlusions in an attempt to prevent clot propagation and embolization. In some patients with severe ICVA stenosis, I have used longer-term warfarin (6 months to 1 year), keeping the international normalized ratio (INR) between 2 and 2.5. I follow patients with ICVA stenosis with serial TCD, and MRA examinations for progression of the vascular lesion to complete occlusion or for recanalization with disappearance of critical stenosis. I stop anticoagulants approximately a month after documented occlusion or reestablishment of wide patency. I have no data that support these choices of treatment, but they make good sense to me at the present time. I await careful prospective studies of treatment of patients with ICVA disease.

OCCLUSION OR SEVERE STENOSIS OF THE BASILAR ARTERY

In a landmark report, Kubik and Adams called attention to the clinical and pathologic features of occlusion of the basilar artery.[116] Characterized by quadriparesis and cranial nerve abnormalities, which allowed for accurate diagnosis during life, the disorder was then considered invariably fatal. We now know that the outcome of patients with basilar-artery occlusive disease is quite variable. Some patients die or are left severely disabled, whereas others survive with little or no deficit.[1,117-122] Prognosis depends on the rapidity of the occlusion, location, and extent of the thrombosis, presence of occlusive disease in other posterior circulation arteries, and development of adequate collateral circulation.

A 63-year-old man, OL, was unable to rise from bed because of weakness in both his legs. He had a myocardial infarction 5 years earlier. During the past 2 weeks, he had two transient episodes of diplopia, one accompanied by momentary buckling of the legs. During the past month, he had occasional, severe occipital headaches. For the past 3 days, he had noted weakness of his left leg and diplopia but refused to seek medical care.

Atherosclerosis commonly affects the first few centimeters of the basilar artery. Stenosis can also occur in the middle and distal segments.[1,118,119,121,122] Patients with basilar-artery atherosclerosis have a high frequency of atherosclerosis elsewhere, especially in the coronary, carotid, and iliofemoral arteries. In Kubik and Adams' original report,[116] most patients developed signs abruptly without previous warnings. Their paper preceded recognition of the frequency and importance of TIAs, however, and emanated from the pathology laboratory. Careful questioning of most patients with basilar-artery occlusive disease elicits descriptions of attacks of temporary brainstem dysfunction before their strokes, as in patient OL. The most common symptoms during these TIAs are (1) diplopia; (2) dizziness, most often without true spinning; (3) weakness of both legs; and (4) weakness alternating between different limbs in different attacks. As in occlusive disease of other large extracranial and cranial arteries, some patients develop prominent headache during the weeks before and during development of a critical decrease in blood flow. With basilar-artery occlusive disease, the headache is usually occipital, often spreading to the vertex of the head.

> On examination, OL's limbs were weak, more so on his right side. He could not move his right arm and leg, but could lift the left heel off the bed to a height of 15 cm for 5 seconds before it would fall. He could adduct the left shoulder toward himself by sliding it along the bed, but could not lift the arm or move his fingers. Both plantar responses were extensor. Pinprick and touch perception were normal. He could not look to the right. On gazing to the left, only the left eye moved but with abducting nystagmus. No adduction of the right eye on attempted left gaze occurred. His voice was dysarthric, and secretions pooled in the back of his throat.

The basilar artery forms from the merging of the two ICVAs at the medullopontine junction. The basilar artery ends at the junction of the pons and midbrain. The major territory of supply of the basilar artery is the pons, especially the basis pontis. The tegmentum of the pons has a rich, collateral supply of vessels but depends primarily on the SCAs, vessels that originate from the rostral basilar artery just before it bifurcates. Occlusion of the basilar artery often causes ischemia in the pontine base bilaterally, sometimes extending into the medial tegmentum on one or both sides. Figure 7-16 shows an example of the distribution of ischemia in basilar-artery occlusion, patterned after Kubik and Adams.[116] Note that the medulla and cerebellar hemispheres are usually spared, in contrast to the situation when one or both ICVAs are blocked. Blockage of the midbasilar artery at the orifice of the AICAs often is accompanied by infarction in the anterior inferior cerebellum on one or both sides.[1,101,123,124] Figure 7-17 is a necropsy specimen of the pons in a patient with basilar artery occlusion that shows a pattern similar to that drawn in Figure 7-16.

Visualizing the anatomic regions of damage helps in predicting and understanding the usual neurologic signs and symptoms that accompany basilar-artery occlusion:

1. Paralysis of the limbs. Weakness is usually bilateral but may be asymmetric, as in patient OL's presentation; stiffness, hyperreflexia, and extensor plantar reflexes are found on examination of the weak limbs. Some patients present with a hemiparesis, but also usually have weakness and reflex changes in the limbs contralateral to the hemiparesis on examination.[1] Hemiparesis was more common than quadriparesis in patients with basilar artery occlusion studied in the New England Medical Center Posterior Circulation Registry.[1,118]

2. Bulbar or pseudobulbar paralysis of the cranial musculature. The infarct can directly involve cranial motor nuclei, causing paralysis of the face, palate, pharynx, neck, or tongue on one or both sides. The IX-XII nerve nuclei are located within the medullary tegmentum, which is usually below the level of the infarct. Weakness of the cranial musculature innervated by these nuclei causes dysarthria, dysphonia, hoarseness, dysphagia, and tongue weakness. These are common findings in patients with basilar artery occlusion and pontine infarction. The pontine lesion interrupts corticofugal descending fibers destined for these cranial-nerve nuclei. The resulting weakness is referred to as pseudobulbar because it involves the descending pathways controlling the bulbar nuclei rather than the nuclei themselves. Exaggerated jaw and facial reflexes, increased gag reflex, and easily induced emotional incontinence with excessive laughing and/or crying accompany the weakness. In some cases, the limb and bulbar paralysis is so severe that the patient cannot communicate verbally or by gesture. Such patients have been referred to as locked-in because of their loss of motor function.[1] Eye movement or eye-blinking signals can sometimes be arranged, which clearly prove the patient is alert and intellectually preserved despite the paralysis.

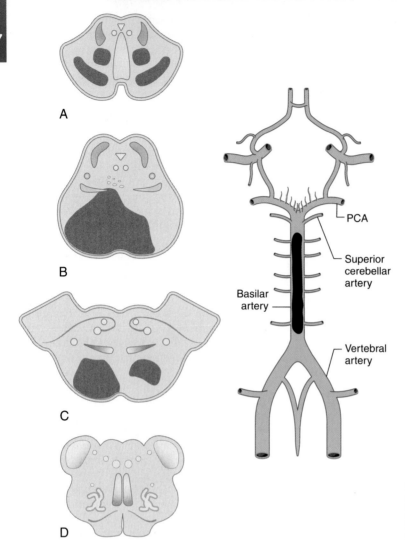

Figure 7-16. Cartoon showing the pons with an infarct caused by occlusion of the basilar artery: (**A**) midbrain, (**B**) upper pons, (**C**) lower pons, and (**D**) medulla.

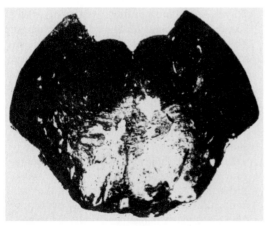

Figure 7-17. Myelin-stained section of the pons showing a large infarct limited to the paramedian portion of the base in a patient with basilar artery occlusion. (From Caplan LR: Posterior Circulation Disease: Clinical Findings, Diagnosis, and Management. Boston: Blackwell, 1996, with permission.)

3. Absence of sensory or cerebellar abnormalities. The infarct usually affects the midline and paramedian structures in the basis pontis. Collateral circulation is generally through the circumferential vessels, which course around the lateral portions of the brainstem, and supply the lateral base, tegmentum, and cerebellum. Figure 7-18A is a cartoon that shows the potential paths of collateral supply when the basilar artery is occluded. And Figure 7-18B is a cerebral angiogram that shows cerebellar artery collaterals filling the upper basilar artery in a patient with proximal basilar artery occlusion. The cerebellar hemispheres are mostly nourished by the PICA, which originates before the basilar artery, and the SCA, which is preserved when the basilar-artery clot does not extend to the distal basilar artery. Infarcts involving the AICA portion of the cerebellum and the basis pontis do occur

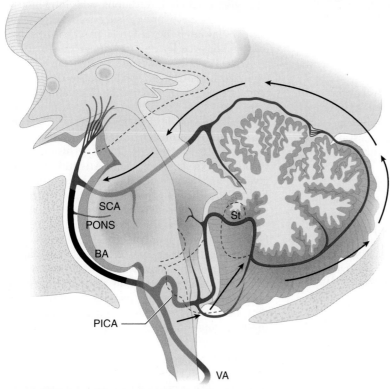

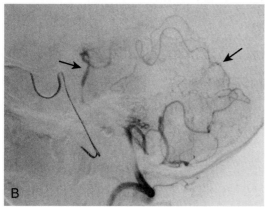

Figure 7-18. A, Drawing of the brainstem and cerebellum in sagittal section. The cerebellar arteries are well shown. When the basilar artery occludes blood can flow from the intracranial vertebral artery (VA) to the posterior inferior cerebellar artery (PICA) over the cerebellum to the superior cerebellar artery (SCA), and from there into the distal basilar artery (BA). **B,** Vertebral angiogram, lateral view: Basilar artery is occluded; rostral basilar artery is filled *(arrow, upper left)* from collaterals going around the cerebellum *(arrow, upper right)* from PICA to SCA branches.

but the usual clinical cerebellar signs are overshadowed by the accompanying paralysis and pyramidal tract abnormalities. The spinothalamic tracts and the cerebellum are often spared from the ischemia.

4. Abnormalities of eye movement. The sixth-nerve nuclei, medial longitudinal fasciculi (MLF), and pontine lateral gaze centers are located in the paramedian pontine tegmentum, and therefore are vulnerable to ischemia in this region. Lesions of the sixth nerve or nucleus cause paralysis of abduction of the eye. An MLF lesion produces a defect in adduction of the ipsilateral eye on gaze directed to the opposite side and nystagmus of the contralateral abducting eye. This syndrome, called an internuclear

ophthalmoplegia, can be bilateral. Lesions of the paramedian pontine tegmentum may also affect the paramedian pontine reticular formation (PPRF), the so-called pontine lateral gaze center that mediates gaze to the same side. A lesion of this region causes an ipsilateral conjugate-gaze paresis. A unilateral lesion can affect both the PPRF and the MLF on the same side. The resulting syndrome was present in patient OL, and has been called the one-and-one-half syndrome by Fisher[1,125] because only one half of gaze (scoring 1 for gaze to each side) is preserved. OL had paralysis of right gaze caused by a lesion of the right PPRF and paralysis of the adducting right eye on gaze to the left caused by involvement of the right MLF.

5. Nystagmus. The vestibular nuclei and their connections are also commonly affected, causing vertical and horizontal nystagmus.

6. Other eye signs. Ptosis, small pupils, and ocular skewing are also often found in patients with basilar-artery occlusion.

7. Coma. If the lesion interrupts function of the medial pontine tegmentum bilaterally, coma may develop.[1,126] Reduced consciousness is a poor prognostic sign, but care must be taken in differentiating reduced alertness from the locked-in state.

CT of OL was normal. MRI on the 1st day showed ischemia in the mid and lower pons bilaterally in the basis pontis. The basilar-artery flow void was absent in the lower pons. Heparin was given intravenously in a continuous-drip infusion. During the first 24 hours, the patient developed increased weakness of the right leg. He remained stable thereafter, and by day 10 he could lift both arms and speak more clearly. MRA on day 2 was technically poor but suggested a basilar artery occlusion. Catheter angiography on day 10 showed slight irregularity without stenosis of the ECVAs at their origins. The basilar artery was occluded just after its origin. An ICA injection opacified the rostral basilar artery through the posterior communicating artery. By day 14, he could sit with help and had no blood pressure drop or increased weakness when he did so. Heparin was stopped after coumadin had achieved an INR of 2.5. He recovered partially during rehabilitation and had no further worsening of signs or symptoms.

CT is not especially sensitive in imaging brainstem infarcts, although this capability has improved with newer-generation scanners. CT is, however, reliable in excluding primary brainstem hemorrhage, one of the differential diagnostic considerations. MRI provides better imaging of brainstem and cerebellar infarcts.[118-120,127] In the patient OL, and in others with bilateral abnormalities of brainstem function, the principal differential diagnosis is between basilar-artery obstruction and obliteration of basilar branch arteries bilaterally, despite a patent basilar artery.[128] This distinction can usually be made by vascular imaging tests, CTA, MRA, and catheter angiography.[118-120,127,129]

When OL presented, the lack of a history of prior stroke and the extensive nature of the bilateral signs made it highly probable that the lesion involved the main basilar artery. He had persistent neurologic signs for more than 72 hours, so he was not a candidate for thrombolysis. If he had presented within 24 hours, I would have considered catheter angiography followed by intra-arterial thrombolysis if his basilar artery were occluded. I would have performed MRA as a screening test as soon as he presented before performing angiography. Both intravenous and intra-arterial thrombolysis have proved successful in patients with basilar artery occlusion even when treatment has been delayed for up to 24 hours.[130,131,131a]

I gave heparin intravenously after the CT scan excluded hemorrhage. I prefer not to do invasive studies early in the course of fluctuating brainstem ischemia, performing angiography only when the diagnosis remains uncertain, or when intra-arterial treatment (thrombolysis, angioplasty, or both) is considered. Reduced perfusion of the brainstem is a major problem. Attention must be given to maximizing blood flow. I keep patients at bed rest with their heads flat. Blood pressure should not be lowered unless it is in the malignant range, and cardiac failure should be treated. Dehydration and hypovolemia should be avoided. During the initial course of the ischemia (up to 2 weeks), patients may develop additional symptoms when they sit, stand, or are merely propped up in bed.[132] I observe patients carefully when they sit or stand, checking their pulse and blood pressure and noting any change in neurologic symptoms and signs. Ambulation should be gradual and carefully supervised. TCD is sometimes not accurate in showing basilar-artery disease because the lesion is often beyond the range of the suboccipital probe. MRI can suggest basilar-artery occlusion by the absence of the usual basilar-artery flow void. CTA and MRA are usually able to define basilar-artery disease.[120,133-135] Figure 7-19 shows an MRA of a patient with basilar artery stenosis and occlusion.

When there is strong clinical suspicion that the vascular lesion affects the main basilar artery, or when the clinical picture is confusing and preliminary vascular imaging studies do not clarify the nature of the vascular lesion, I use angiography to help decide the next therapeutic step. Catheter angiography is usually deferred 2 to 7 days while the patient continues to receive heparin until the clinical course appears stable. If

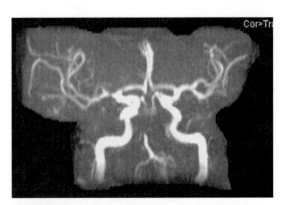

Figure 7-19. Intracranial MRA. The basilar artery stops abruptly.

the patient with ischemia has not stabilized and continues to deteriorate despite heparin, I then suggest angiography earlier. If CTA, MRA, or angiography shows a complete basilar-artery occlusion, I continue heparin, followed by warfarin, for a total of 6 to 8 weeks, and use aspirin or combined aspirin and modified-release dipyridamole thereafter. If there is a severe stenosis of the basilar artery without occlusion, I usually use long-term warfarin treatment in an attempt to prevent occlusion. If there is only minor plaque disease in the major basilar artery, I select agents, such as aspirin or aspirin with dipyridamole, which decrease platelet aggregation and agglutination.

In patients with no obvious intrinsic lesions by angiography, it is important to think of the possibility of embolism and be certain that studies are adequate to exclude a cardiogenic embolus or embolism from the aorta or the proximal innominate, subclavian or vertebral arteries. Angioplasty and stenting has been performed to open basilar-artery stenotic lesions, but this procedure can result in obliteration of paramedian and other arteries that penetrate from the basilar artery.[115]

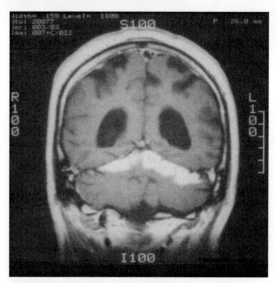

Figure 7-20. T2-weighted MRI scan, coronal view. There is bilateral infarction in the superior portion of the cerebellum in the territory of the bilateral superior cerebellar arteries (SCAs) in a patient with a basilar artery occlusion that blocks the orifices of the SCAs. I have dubbed this appearance icing on a cake.

> A 38-year-old man, PG, was discovered comatose by his son. That morning he had been normal, according to his wife, who recalled no recent signs of ill health in her husband. He had no history of heart or vascular disease. On examination, his pupils were dilated and fixed at 8 mm each. His eyes were deviated down and outward. Lateral motion in each eye was obtained by oculocephalic maneuvers. No abnormal motor signs were evident.

The bilateral III nerve dysfunction and coma suggested a midbrain lesion. This could be caused by a large supratentorial space-taking lesion with midbrain compression or by an intrinsic lesion within the midbrain. Because of the lack of history, absence of stroke risk factors, and limitation of the neurologic examination by coma, I believed it mandatory to order urgent neuroimaging tests.

> The CT in patient PG was normal with and without contrast. MRI could not be performed urgently. The next day, diffusion-weighted and T2-weighted images showed infarction in the paramedian thalamus and midbrain tegmentum. MRA was normal. An echocardiogram showed a left atrial myxoma.

In most patients with basilar artery occlusion, the thrombus is limited to the proximal basilar artery. In some patients, the occlusion extends to the distal basilar-artery segment; in other patients, more often in African Americans, occlusion or severe stenosis can predominantly affect the distal basilar artery.[1,46,121] Figure 7-20 shows a patient with a bilateral superior cerebellar artery territory infarct caused by a localized stenosis that was located at the orifices of the SCAs. SCA territory infarction is accompanied most often by dysarthria and limb dysmetria and intention tremor. Dizziness and gait ataxia are less prominent signs compared to patients with PICA territory cerebellar infarction.

Occlusion of the distal basilar artery is most often caused by embolism from the heart or the proximal vertebral artery system. Emboli small enough to pass through the vertebral arteries do not usually lodge in the proximal basilar artery, a vessel larger than each ICVA, but travel to the distal basilar artery or its terminal branches. The distal basilar artery supplies the midbrain and diencephalon through small vessels that pierce the posterior perforated substance. Signs of dysfunction in this territory include the following[1,136-138]:

1. Pupillary abnormalities. The lesion often interrupts the afferent reflex arc by interfering with fibers going toward the Edinger-Westphal nucleus. The III-nerve nucleus can also be involved, as well as the rostral descending sympathetic system. The pupils are usually abnormal and can be small, midposition, or dilated, depending on the level and extent of the lesion. Decreased pupillary reactivity and eccentricity of the pupil are also found. Sometimes a pupil attains an oval shape.[139]
2. Eye movement abnormalities. Vertical gaze abnormalities are common in patients with rostral brainstem lesions.[140-142] Paralysis of upward or downward gaze is common. The

7

eyes may also be skewed and may be deviated at rest, most often downward and inward. Hyperconvergence, retractory nystagmus, and pseudo VI–nerve paresis are other oculomotor abnormalities.[1,125,136,138] The failure of ocular abduction in patients with pseudo-VI paresis is explained by hyperadduction of the eye. The adduction vector neutralizes the abduction motion and so abduction is incomplete. The lesion is of course far rostral to the VI nerve nucleus or fibers.[1,125,136,138]

3. Altered level of alertness. Hypersomnolence or frank coma can result from bilateral paramedian rostral brainstem dysfunction. After the acute phase, the patient may remain relatively inert and apathetic. Some patients sleep many hours a day unless stimulated or coaxed into activities.

4. Amnesia. Memory loss can accompany thalamic infarction. Patients are unable to form new memories and may not be able to recall events just preceding their stroke. There may be an array of other behavioral abnormalities, including agitation, hallucinations, and abnormalities that mimic lesions of the frontal lobe. Cognitive deficits often persist in patients with left and bilateral paramedian thalamic infarcts.[142a]

In PG, the bilateral III–nerve palsies identified a midbrain lesion that was confirmed by MRI. Because the most frequent cause is embolic, the cardiac and vascular investigations are important. Identification of the left atrial myxoma led to successful removal of the cardiac tumor. The patient awakened on day 4 after his stroke and was left with a bilateral III–nerve palsy as his only important, persistent, neurologic sign. In other patients with top-of-the-basilar emboli, the distribution of infarction varies and may include the midbrain and thalami and the territories of the SCAs and PCAs. Infarction can be limited to one SCA or PCA. Figure 7-21 shows MRI and CTA scans in a patient with a top-of-the-basilar embolus. Infarcts are shown in the midbrain, superior cerebellum, and bilateral posterior cerebral artery territories.

OCCLUSION OR SEVERE STENOSIS OF THE POSTERIOR CEREBRAL ARTERIES

The PCAs are the major terminal branches of the basilar artery. In approximately 30% of patients, one basilar communicating segment is hypoplastic, and the PCA is derived primarily from the ipsilateral ICA through its posterior communicating artery branch. Intrinsic atheromatous disease of the PCA most often affects the origin of the

vessel. Its epidemiology is similar to disease of the proximal MCA. Infarcts in the PCA territory are often caused by emboli to the posterior circulation.[1,56,57,108,109,143-145] Castaigne and colleagues in a necropsy study identified 30 infarcts within PCA territory.[108] The most common mechanism of infarction was embolism from a proximal occlusive lesion within the vertebrobasilar system (15 of 30, 50%). In eight patients, clot propagated from the basilar artery into the PCA. Only three patients had thrombosis of the PCA engrafted on previous atherosclerotic narrowing.[108]

Pessin, myself, and colleagues studied the mechanism of infarction in 35 patients with hemianopia and a unilateral infarct on CT limited to the PCA territory on one side.[143] Figure 7-22 is a montage of the CT lesions from this study. The most frequent mechanism of infarction was embolism. A cardiac source of embolism was present in 10 patients (28.5%), and intra-arterial embolism arising from proximal posterior circulation lesions was found in six patients (17%). In 11 other patients, the clinical and angiographic findings suggested embolism, but no definite donor site was established. Among the 35 patients, 27 (77%) had embolic occlusion of PCA branches.[143] Among 79 patients with PCA-territory infarction in the New England Medical Center Posterior Circulation Registry, embolism was the most likely stroke mechanism in 65 patients (82%).[145] Series of patients with PCA-territory infarcts reported by other centers have shown that embolism is the predominant cause of these infarcts.[1,144,145]

An analogy can be drawn between the two brain circulations. In the anterior circulation, emboli usually lodge in MCA branches, leading to cortical infarcts; in the posterior circulation, emboli traverse the vertebral and basilar arteries and ultimately lodge in PCA branches, producing cortical infarcts. Intrinsic disease of the MCA and PCA does occur, but is far less common than cardiogenic or artery-to-artery embolization. When intrinsic atherosclerosis of the PCA is present, the clinical presentation usually consists of transient hemianopic visual symptoms, sometimes accompanied by transient hemisensory symptoms on the same side.[146]

A 64-year-old African-American woman, MA, awakened and realized she could not see to her left. She was able to read and could clearly identify objects in the room, but found it necessary to turn to the left to "see better." She also noted a dull pain behind her right eye. She was not aware of any difficulty with her limbs, walking, or thinking. During the past few weeks, she had several attacks of diminished vision to her left, each lasting a few minutes. On examination, there was a left homonymous hemianopia with

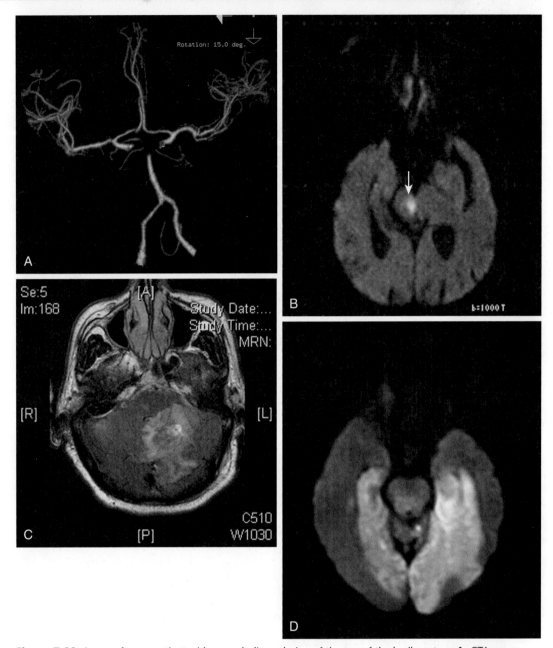

Figure 7-21. Images from a patient with an embolic occlusion of the top of the basilar artery. **A,** CTA reconstructed. The very distal portion of the basilar artery and the left posterior cerebral artery do not opacify. **B,** Diffusion weighted MRI image showing an infarct *(arrow)* in the medial midbrain. **C,** Diffusion-weighted MRI scan showing an infarct involving the left superior cerebellar artery territory of the cerebellum and the left dorsal pontine tegmentum. **D,** Diffusion-weighted MRI scan showing extensive occipital lobe infarction bilaterally in the territory of the posterior cerebral arteries.

slight sparing of the most central portion of the left visual field. She could read, note the color and nature of objects and pictures, draw common objects, copy drawings, and accurately bisect lines scattered on a page. Motor, sensory, and reflex functions and gait were normal.

After giving off penetrating branches to the midbrain and thalamus, the PCA supplies branches to the occipital lobes and supplies the medial and inferior portions of the temporal lobes (Fig. 7-23). Headache in patients with PCA disease is often retro-orbital or above the eye, probably reflecting the fact that the upper surface of the tentorium is innervated by the first division of the fifth nerve. Infarction in the cerebral territories of the PCA most often affects

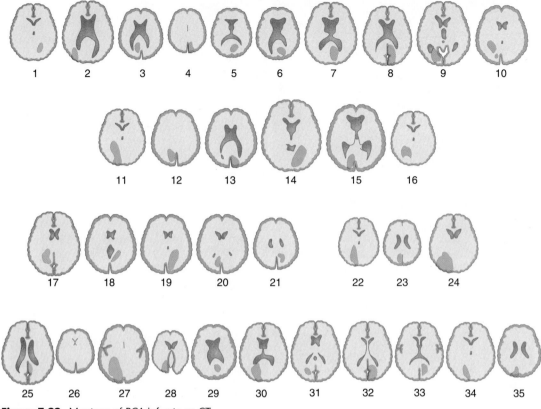

Figure 7-22. Montage of PCA infarcts on CT.

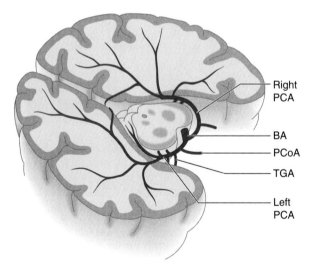

Right
PCA

BA

PCoA

TGA

Left
PCA

Figure 7-23. Cartoon of the posterior cerebral arteries and their branches. BA, basilar artery; PCA, posterior cerebral artery; PCoA, posterior communicating artery; TGA, thalamogeniculate artery pedicle. (Drawn by Laurel Cook-Lhowe.)

vision and somatic sensation, but seldom causes paralysis.[1,143-147]

Visual-Field Abnormalities

The single most common finding in patients with PCA-territory infarction is a hemianopia.[1,143-148] Hemianopia is caused by infarction of the striate visual cortex on the banks of the calcarine fissure, a region supplied by the calcarine branch of the PCA, or it is caused by interruption of the geniculo-calcarine tract as it nears the visual cortex. If just the lower bank of the calcarine fissure is involved, the lingual gyrus, a superior quadrant-field defect results. An inferior quadrantanopia results if the lesion affects the cuneus on the upper bank of the calcarine fissure.

When infarction is restricted to the striate cortex and does not extend into the adjacent parietal cortex, the patient is fully aware of the visual field loss. Usually described as a void, blackness, or limitation of vision to one side, patients usually recognize that they must focus extra attention to the hemianopic field. When given written material or pictures, patients with hemianopia caused by occipital lobe infarction are able to see and interpret the stimuli normally, although it may take them a bit longer to explore the hemianopic visual field. They will often cant the picture obliquely and hold it in the preserved visual field.

Hemianopia and visual neglect are not synonymous, nor is visual neglect merely a more or less severe form of hemianopia. In patients with occipital lobe infarcts, physicians can reliably map out the visual fields by confrontation. At times, the central or medial part of the field is spared, known as *macular sparing*. Optokinetic nystagmus is normal. Some patients, although they accurately report motion or the presence of objects in their hemianopic field, cannot identify the nature, location, or color of that object.[1,148]

In contrast, patients with infarction in the parietal lobe, most often in MCA territory, who have preservation of geniculo-calcarine fibers and the striate cortex, have visual neglect. Their findings are quite different from those in patients with medial occipital infarction. Patients with visual neglect are usually unaware of their visual-field defect. They often (1) ignore objects in the abnormal visual field; (2) do not notice words in their impaired field, often reading only half of a headline or paragraph; (3) miss objects in pictures in the neglected field; and (4) have reduced optokinetic nystagmus to the side of the visual defect.[148] Poor drawing and copying are also often associated with visual neglect. When the parieto-occipital and temporal branches of the PCA are involved, leading to large infarcts in the entire PCA territory, both a hemianopia and visual neglect are present. More often, in isolated infarcts of the striate cortex, patients have a hemianopia without neglect. In my experience, visual neglect without a hemianopia is always caused by infarction within the MCA territory.

Somatosensory Abnormalities

The lateral thalamus is the site of the major somatosensory relay nuclei, the ventroposteromedial and lateral nuclei. Ischemia to these nuclei or white matter tracts carrying fibers from the thalamus to somatosensory cortex (postcentral gyrus and the sensory 2 region in the parietal operculum) produces sensory symptoms and signs, usually without paralysis.[144,145,149] Patients describe paresthesias or numbness in the face, limbs, and trunk. On examination, their touch, pinprick, and position senses are sometimes reduced. In many patients, the sensory symptoms far outweigh abnormalities that can be shown on examination.[150] The combination of hemisensory loss, with hemianopia and without paralysis, is virtually diagnostic of infarction in the PCA territory. The occlusive lesion is within the PCA, before the thalamogeniculate branches to the lateral thalamus.[149,150]

Motor Abnormalities

Rarely, occlusion of the proximal portion of the PCA can cause a hemiplegia.[1,142,144,145,151-153] Penetrating branches from the most proximal portion of the PCA penetrate into the midbrain to supply the cerebral peduncle. PCA-origin occlusions cause hemiplegia related to midbrain peduncular infarction accompanied by a hemisensory loss caused by lateral thalamic infarction and hemianopia caused by occipital lobe infarction. The resultant neurologic deficit is not easily distinguished clinically from MCA or anterior choroidal artery territory infarcts, but separation is made readily by CT and MRI results. Figure 7-24 from Hommel et al[153] shows the proximal branches of the PCA.

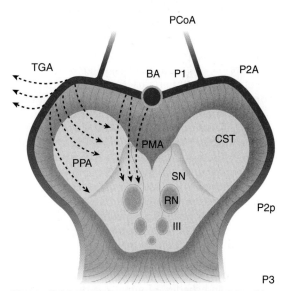

Figure 7-24. Axial diagram of the midbrain arteries. BA, basilar artery; PCoA, posterior communicating artery; P1, proximal segment of the PCA; P2A, anterior segment of the P2 part of the PCA; P2p, posterior segment of the P2 part of the PCA; P3, P3 part of the PCA; TGA, thalamogeniculate arteries; PPA, peduncular perforating arteries; PMA, paramedian arteries; CST, corticospinal tract in cerebral peduncle; SN, substantia nigra; RN, red nucleus; III, oculomotor nucleus.

When the lateral thalamus is infarcted and the midbrain is spared, patients often show a hemiataxia and choreic and dystonic movements on the same side as the hemisensory symptoms. The limb ataxia is likely related to interruption of cerebellofugal fibers from the superior cerebellar peduncle and red nucleus that synapse in the ventrolateral nucleus of the thalamus. The motor abnormalities of choreoathetosis and dystonia probably relate to interruption of extrapyramidal fibers from the ansa lenticularis that are destined for the ventral lateral and ventral anterior thalamic nuclei. In some patients with lateral thalamic infarcts, transient involuntary choreiform and athetotic movements are present during the first days after the stroke.[1,150]

Cognitive and Behavioral Abnormalities

When the left PCA territory is infarcted, several additional findings may occur:

1. Alexia without agraphia. Infarction of the left occipital lobe and splenium of the corpus callosum is associated with a remarkable clinical syndrome—an inability to read despite retained ability to write correctly, first described by Dejerine,[154] and later amplified by Geschwind and Fusillo.[155] Because the left visual cortex is infarcted, patients see with their right occipital lobe and their left visual field. To name what they see, the information must be communicated from the right occipital cortex to the language region in the left temporal and parietal lobes. Infarction of the corpus callosum or adjacent white matter paths interrupts communication between the right occipital cortex and the left hemisphere. Patients have difficulty naming what they see. The most conspicuous abnormality is in reading. Although usually able to name individual letters or numbers, the patient cannot read words or phrases. Because the speech cortex is normal, they retain the ability to speak, repeat speech, write, and spell aloud. Although they are able to write a paragraph, they often cannot read it back moments later. Usually accompanying the dyslexia is a defect in color naming.[1,148,155,156] Patients can match colors and shades, proving that their perception of colors is normal. They can also describe the usual color of familiar objects and can even color correctly when given an array of crayons. Nonetheless, they are unable to give a color its correct name.

2. Anomic or transcortical sensory aphasia.[157] Some patients with left PCA-territory infarction

have difficulty naming objects. Others can repeat, but not understand, spoken language.

3. Gerstmann syndrome. PCA-territory infarction can undercut the angular gyrus, leading to a host of findings, usually lumped together as Gerstmann syndrome.[1] These findings include (1) difficulty telling right from left, (2) difficulty in naming digits on their own or on others' hands, (3) constructional dyspraxia, (4) agraphia, and (5) difficulty in calculating. In any single patient, all features may appear together or one or more may occur in isolation. Gerstmann syndrome also occurs when the angular gyrus region is infarcted during left MCA-territory infarction.

4. Altered memory. A defect in acquisition of new memories is common when both medial temporal lobes are damaged,[1,158-160] but also occurs in lesions limited to the left medial temporal lobe.[1,156,158-162] The memory deficit in unilateral lesions is usually not permanent, but has lasted up to 6 months. Patients cannot recall recent events and when given new information, they cannot recall it moments later. They often repeat statements and questions spoken only minutes before.

5. Associative visual agnosia.[1,148,156,163,164] Some patients with left PCA territory infarction have difficulty understanding the nature and use of objects presented visually. They can trace with their fingers and copy objects, demonstrating that visual perception is preserved. They can often name objects if the objects are presented in their hand and explored by touch or when the objects are described verbally. One patient, when shown a pair of scissors, had no idea what it was. When the instrument was placed in her hand, she was able to name it. When asked to list five objects that might be used for cutting, she included scissors, indicating that the name of the object was available to the patient.[156]

Infarcts of the right PCA territory are often accompanied by prosopagnosia, difficulty in recognizing familiar faces.[1,148,164-166] At times, patients cannot recognize their spouses, children, or even their own images in a mirror. Despite the seeming inability to recognize, match, or identify faces, physiologic tests of autonomic function are consistent with familiarity on a subconscious level.[166] Disorientation to place and an inability to recall routes and read or revisualize the location of places on maps are also common findings in patients with right PCA-territory infarcts.[148,167] Patients with right occipitotemporal infarcts also may have difficulty revisualizing what a given object or person should look like. Dreams may also be devoid of visual imagery. Visual neglect is much more common after lesions of the right PCA territory.

When the PCA territory is infarcted bilaterally, the most common findings are cortical blindness, amnesia, and agitated delirium.[1,136,144,147,168-170] Most often, bilateral PCA-territory infarction is caused by embolism with blockage of the distal basilar artery bifurcation. Figure 7-21D is an MRI that shows bilateral PCA infarcts in a patient rendered blind by an embolus. Cortically blind patients cannot see or identify objects in either visual field, but have preserved pupillary light reflexes.[1,148,168] Some patients with cortical blindness do not volunteer or admit that they cannot see and they seem to avoid barriers in their way. Amnesia caused by bilateral medial temporal-lobe infarction may be permanent and closely resembles Korsakoff's syndrome.[158] In addition, infarcting the hippocampus, fusiform, and lingual gyri, usually bilaterally, leads to an agitated hyperactive state that could be confused with delirium tremens.[1,169,170] When infarction is limited to the lower banks of the calcarine fissures bilaterally, the major findings are prosopagnosia and defective color vision.[1,148,164,171,172] In contrast to patients with alexia without agraphia who cannot name colors, these patients cannot recognize, match, or name colors correctly.[171,172]

> CT showed an infarct in patient MA in the medial occipital lobe on the right. Angiography was not performed. Extracranial Doppler examination at C2 did not show reversed VA flow on either side. TCD showed a focal region of increased blood-flow velocity in the right PCA. MRI showed that the occipital infarct involved striate cortex above and below the calcarine fissure. MRA showed a focal narrowing of the right PCA. Cardiac echo and rhythm monitoring were normal. She was discharged on aspirin therapy. The findings did not change during the ensuing years of follow-up.

CT can accurately reflect the vascular territory involved. In this patient, it confirmed that the lesion was in the territory of the calcarine branch of the right PCA.[1,144,147,173,174] CT also showed that the lesion was ischemic and not caused by intracerebral hemorrhage. MRI is probably better able to image small associated lesions in the thalamus, midbrain, and more proximal brainstem and cerebellum, thus helping to localize the offending vascular lesion. Sagittal T2-weighted MRI sections through the medial occipital lobes can also identify the location of the lesions in relation to the calcarine fissure and the optic radiations, and thereby help prognosticate recovery of visual field defects.

Figure 7-25 contains axial and coronal MRI views of occipital lobe infarcts caused by embolism to the PCA—a montage of MRI lesions in patients with PCA territory infarcts.

The occipital lobe is a site of predilection for amyloid angiopathy. Hemorrhage from amyloid angiopathy often occurs in the absence of hypertension and can mimic an ischemic stroke. Little is known at present about optimum therapy for patients with intrinsic disease of the PCA. When infarction is limited to branches of the PCA, cardiogenic embolism should be considered and appropriate investigations performed to exclude it.

In patient MA, there was no clinical or laboratory evidence to suggest cardiac-origin embolism. Noninvasive studies gave no evidence for an ECVA occlusion in the neck, a potential source of intra-arterial embolism to the PCA. If ECVA occlusion had been suggested by noninvasive tests,

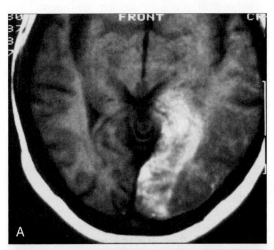

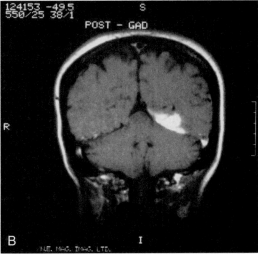

Figure 7-25. T2-weighted MRI scans showing infarction in posterior cerebral artery territory. **A,** Axial view showing large occipital lobe infarct. **B,** Coronal view showing smaller occipital lobe infarct.

7

or if epidemiologic and ecologic factors had favored an ECVA-origin lesion, a gadolinium-enhanced MRA examination of the subclavian ECVA-origin region, or CTA, or catheter angiography would have been ordered. She was African American and had no history of coronary or peripheral vascular disease, and did not have hypercholesterolemia. These factors weighed against the likelihood of a proximal ECVA lesion.[46] The absence of brainstem symptoms and normal ICVA blood-flow velocities on TCD examination argued against an ICVA occlusion. The TCD findings of a focal increase in blood-flow velocity in the right PCA strongly suggested a focal lesion involving the PCA. Intracranial MRA excluded an ICVA lesion and identified the intrinsic lesion within the right PCA. The preceding spells of left visual field loss favored an intrinsic right PCA occlusive lesion.[146] Even if more extensive infarction were to occur in the right PCA territory, the likelihood of serious disability was small. The risk to the patient of further, serious, neurologic disability did not, in my opinion, warrant invasive diagnostic procedures or hazardous therapy. I elected to prescribe aspirin.

DIFFERENTIAL DIAGNOSIS OF POSTERIOR CIRCULATION ISCHEMIA

Advances in technology, especially the introduction of MRI, echocardiography, ultrasound, TCD, and CTA and MRA, have now made it possible to investigate patients with posterior circulation ischemia safely and quickly and identify the causative vascular mechanism. Diffusion and perfusion-weighted MRI can also be helpful within the posterior circulation by showing regions that are hypoperfused and identifying infarcts earlier than T2-weighted standard MRI scans.

I have found it useful to divide the posterior circulation into smaller territories that reflect the vascular distribution of the main arteries.[1,2,25,58,175] The ICVAs join at the medullopontine junction to form the basilar arteries. The territory usually perfused by the ICVAs includes the medulla and the cerebellum supplied by the PICA branch of the ICVAs. This region is designated as proximal intracranial posterior circulation territory. The basilar artery bifurcates at the pontomesencephalic junction. The territory supplied by the basilar artery, including the pons and the portion of the cerebellum supplied by the AICA branch, is designated as middle-intracranial posterior circulation territory. The portion of the posterior circulation supplied by the distal basilar artery and its SCA, PCA, and penetrating artery branches

is referred to as distal intracranial posterior circulation territory. The distal territory includes the midbrain, thalamus, SCA-supplied cerebellum, and the occipital and temporal lobe regions supplied by the PCAs. Figure 7-26 shows these posterior circulation territories.

Designation of brain territory is made by using clinical and imaging data. For example, suppose a patient has clinical findings of a left lateral medullary syndrome and a right hemianopia. MRI shows only a left occipital-lobe infarct. This patient must have proximal and distal intracranial posterior circulation territory ischemia. Moreover, the left proximal-territory lesion means that the left ICVA must have been involved at some point. The combination of proximal and distal-territory infarction is most often explained by an embolus that first landed at the ICVA and then traveled to the basilar artery bifurcation region, or an occlusive lesion of the ICVA with distal embolism. Designation of the involved posterior circulation territory tells the clinician the rostro-caudal localization of the vascular lesion. Vascular diagnostic technology, including extracranial and transcranial ultrasound, CTA, MRA, standard angiography, and echocardiography can then be used to define the causative vascular lesions.

In the New England Medical Center Posterior Circulation Registry, distal territory lesions were the most common, either ischemia limited to the distal territory or ischemia that included the distal territory.[1,2,25,175] In other registries, the distal territory was also often involved. In the Lausanne Stroke Registry, 164/401 (41%) posterior circulation patients had infarcts that involved the thalamus or PCA territory.[175-178] Among 70 patients in the Lausanne Stroke registry in whom MRA was reported, 37% had distal territory infarcts while 27% had proximal territory infarcts and 23% had middle territory infarcts.[177] In the Besancon[179,180] and Athens[181] Stroke Registries, posterior circulation lesion localization was characterized as brainstem, cerebellum, and PCA territories. In the Besancon Stroke Registry, among 251 patients with posterior circulation ischemia, 34% were PCA, 39% brainstem, and 27% cerebellar.[179,180] In the Athens Registry, among 259 patients with posterior circulation ischemia, 27% included PCA territory, and 28% were brainstem and 24% cerebellar.[181]

In the New England Medical Center Posterior Circulation Registry, the PCA territories were the most commonly affected regions within the posterior circulation either when affected alone or when associated with other intracranial territory lesions; however, a significant number of patients with distal territory ischemia also had

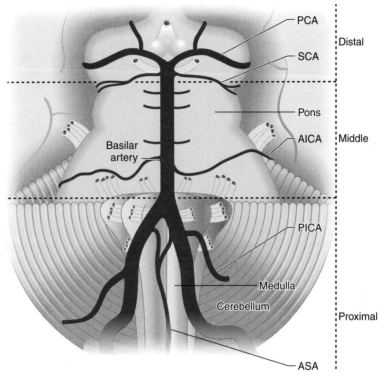

Figure 7-26. Sketch of base of the brain showing the intracranial vertebral and basilar arteries and respective branches. The brain regions are divided into proximal, middle, and distal intracranial territories. ASA, anterior spinal artery; PICA, posterior inferior cerebellar artery; AICA, anterior inferior cerebellar artery; SCA, superior cerebellar artery; PCA, posterior cerebral artery.

rostral brainstem and superior cerebellar artery territory infarcts.[175] If rostral brainstem and SCA cerebellar infarcts are added to the PCA infarcts tabulated in the Lausanne, Besancon, and Athens Registries, it is very highly probable that the frequency of distal territory infarction would parallel that found in the New England Medical Center Posterior Circulation Registry.

In the New England Medical Center Posterior Circulation Registry, the proximal intracranial territory that included lesions involving the medulla and/or the PICA-supplied cerebellum was the next most commonly affected intracranial territory. This territory was involved mostly in patients with ECVA and ICVA occlusive disease and cardiac embolism to PICA-cerebellar territory. The middle intracranial territory which comprised the pons and AICA-supplied cerebellum was least often involved. Middle territory lesions were caused mostly by basilar artery or basilar artery branch disease. Multiple territories were involved in a large number of patients in the Lausanne, Besancon, and Athens Stroke Registries,

just as they were in the New England Medical Center Posterior Circulation Registry.[175]

Treatment has lagged far behind advances in diagnostic technology. Antiplatelet drugs, anticoagulants, surgery, angioplasty and stenting, thrombolysis, and mechanical clot extraction have all been applied but, to date, no randomized therapeutic trials have clarified optimal treatment in patients with fully characterized vascular and brain lesions. These treatments have been described in Chapter 5 and in various parts of this chapter. I hope that in the near future trials of various therapies in patients with documented vascular lesions will shed more light on treatment.

References

1. Caplan LR: Posterior Circulation Disease: Clinical Findings, Diagnosis, and Management. Boston: Blackwell, 1996.
2. Caplan, LR: Posterior circulation ischemia: Then, now, and tomorrow [Thomas Willis Lecture—2000]. Stroke 2000;31:2011-2013.

3. Millikan C, Siekert R: Studies in cerebrovascular disease. The syndrome of intermittent insufficiency of the basilar arterial system. Mayo Clin Proc 1955; 30:61-68.

4. Denny-Brown D: Basilar artery syndromes. Bull N Engl Med Center 1953;15:53-60.

5. Fang H, Palmer J: Vascular phenomena involving brainstem structures. Neurology 1956;6:402-419.

6. Williams D, Wilson T: The diagnosis of the major and minor syndromes of basilar insufficiency. Brain 1962;85:741-774.

7. Millikan C, Siekert R, Shick R: Studies in cerebrovascular disease: The use of anticoagulant drugs in the treatment of insufficiency or thrombosis within the basilar arterial system. Mayo Clin Proc 1955;30:116-126.

8. Caplan LR: Vertebrobasilar disease: Time for a new strategy. Stroke 1981;12:111-114.

9. Caplan LR: Vertebrobasilar disease: Should we continue the double standard of managing patients with brain ischemia? Heart Stroke 1993;2:377-381.

10. Reivich M, Holling E, Roberts B, et al: Reversal of blood flow through the vertebral artery and its effects on cerebral circulation. N Engl J Med 1961;265:878-885.

11. Heyman A, Young W, Dillon M, et al: Cerebral ischemia caused by occlusive disease of the subclavian or innominate arteries. Arch Neurol 1964;10:581-589.

12. North R, Fisher W, DeBakey M, et al: Brachial-basilar insufficiency syndrome. Neurology 1962;12:810-820.

13. Patel A, Toole J: Subclavian steal syndrome: Reversal of cephalic blood flow. Medicine 1965; 44:289-303.

14. Hennerici M, Klemm C, Rautenberg W: The subclavian steal phenomenon: A common vascular disorder with rare neurologic deficits. Neurology 1988;38:669-673.

15. Pollock M, Blennerhassett J, Clark A: Giant cell arteritis and the subclavian steal syndrome. Neurology 1973;23:653-657.

16. Hall S, Barr W, Lie JT, et al: Takayasu arteritis. Medicine 1985;64:89-99.

17. Shinohara Y: Takayasu disease. In Caplan LR (ed): Uncommon Causes of Stroke, 2nd ed. Cambridge: Cambridge University Press, 2008, pp 27-31.

18. Brewster DC, Moncure AC, Darling C, et al: Innominate artery lesions: Problems encountered and lessons learned. J Vasc Surg 1985;2:99-112.

19. Hennerici M, Aulich A, Sandemann W, Freund H-J: Incidence of asymptomatic extracranial occlusive disease. Stroke 1981;12:750-758.

20. Symonds C: Two cases of thrombosis of subclavian artery with contralateral hemiplegia of sudden onset, probably embolic. Brain 1927;50:259-260.

21. Martin R, Bogousslavsky J, Miklossy J, et al: Floating thrombus in the innominate artery as a cause of cerebral infarction in young adults. Cerebrovasc Dis 1992;2:177-181.

22. Ferriere M, Negre G, Bellecoste JF, et al: Thrombus flottant sous-clavier responsible d'un syndrome encephalo-digital, deux observations. La Presse Med 1984;13:27-29.

23. Fields WS, LeMak NA, Ben-Menachem Y: Thoracic outlet syndrome: Review and reference to a stroke in a major league pitcher. AJNR Am J Neuroradiol 1986;7:73-78.

24. Baker R, Rosenbaum A, Caplan L: Subclavian steal syndrome. Contemp Surg 1974;4:96-104.

25. Caplan LR, Wityk RJ, Glass TA, et al: New England Medical Center posterior circulation registry. Ann Neurol 2004;56:389-398.

26. Caplan LR, Wityk RJ, Pazdera L, et al: New England Medical Center posterior circulation stroke registry: II. Vascular lesions. J Clin Neurol 2005;1:31-49.

27. Ekestrom S, Eklund B, Liljequist L, et al: Noninvasive methods in the evaluation of obliterative disease of the subclavian or innominate artery. Acta Med Scand 1979;206:467-471.

28. Berguer R, Higgins R, Nelson R: Noninvasive diagnosis of reversal of vertebral artery blood flow. N Engl J Med 1980;302:1349-1351.

29. von Reutern GM, Pourcelot L: Cardiac cycle-dependent alternating flow in vertebral arteries with subclavian artery stenosis. Stroke 1978;9: 229-236.

30. Liljequist L, Ekestrom S, Nordhus O: Monitoring direction of vertebral artery blood flow by Doppler shift ultrasound in patients with suspected subclavian steal. Acta Chir Scand 1981;147:421-424.

31. von Reutern G-M, von Budingen H-J: Ultrasound diagnosis of cerebrovascular disease. In Ultrasound Diagnosis of Cerebrovascular Disease: Doppler Sonography of the Extracranial and Intracranial Arteries: Duplex Scanning. Stuttgart: Georg Thieme, 1993, pp 129-175.

32. von Budingen H-J, Staudacher T: Evaluation of vertebrobasilar disease. In Newell DW, Aaslid R (eds): Transcranial Doppler. New York: Raven Press, 1992, pp 167-195.

33. Ackerstaff RGA: Duplex scanning of the aortic arch and vertebral arteries. In Bernstein EF (ed): Vascular Diagnosis, 4th ed. St Louis: Mosby, 1993, pp 315-321.

34. Hadjipetrou P, Cox S, Piemonte T, Eisenhauer A: Percutaneous revascularization of atherosclerotic obstruction of aortic arch vessels. J Am Coll Cardiol 1999;33:1238-1245.

35. Dorros G, Lewin RF, Jamnadas P, Mathiak LM: Peripheral transluminal angioplasty of the subclavian and innominate arteries utilizing the brachial approach: Acute outcome and follow-up. Catheter Cardiovasc Diagn 1990;19:71-76.

36. Hebrang A, Maskovic J, Tomac B: Percutaneous transluminal angioplasty of the subclavian arteries: Long-term results in 52 patients. AJR Am J Roentgenol 1991;156:1091-1094.

37. Henry M, Amor M, Henry I, et al: Percutaneous transluminal angioplasty of the subclavian arteries. J Endovasc Surg 1999;6:33-41.

38. Millaire A, Trinca M, Marache P, et al: Subclavian angioplasty: Immediate and late results in 50 patients. Catheter Cardiovasc Diagn 1993;29:8-17.

39. Motarjeme A: Percutaneous transluminal angioplasty of supra-aortic vessels. J Endovasc Surg 1996;3:171-181.

40. Motarjeme A, Keifer JW, Zuska AJ, Nabawi P: 1985. Percutaneous transluminal angioplasty for treatment of subclavian steal. Radiology 1985;155:611-613.

41. Vitek JJ: Subclavian artery angioplasty and the origin of the vertebral artery. Radiology 1989;170: 407-409.

42. Schillinger M, Haumer M, Schillinger S, et al: Risk stratification for subclavian artery angioplasty: Is there an increased rate of restenosis after stent implantation? J Endovasc Ther 2001;8:550-557.

43. Fisher CM, Gore I, Okabe N, et al: Atherosclerosis of the carotid and vertebral arteries: Extracranial and intracranial. J Neuropathol Exp Neurol 1965;24:455-476.

44. Hutchinson EC, Yates PO: The cervical portion of the vertebral artery, a clinicopathological study. Brain 1956;79:319-331.

45. Hutchinson E, Yates P: Carotico-vertebral stenosis. Lancet 1957;1:2-8.

46. Gorelick PB, Caplan LR, Hier DB, et al: Racial differences in the distribution of posterior circulation occlusive disease. Stroke 1985;16: 785-790.

47. Fisher CM: Vertigo in cerebrovascular disease. Arch Otolaryngol 1967;85:529-534.

48. Kerber KA, Brown D, Lisabeth LD, et al: Stroke among patients with dizziness, vertigo, and imbalance in the emergency department. A population-based study. Stroke 2006;37:2484-2487.

49. Lee H, Sohn S-I, Cho Y-W, et al: Cerebellar infarction presenting isolated vertigo. Frequency and vascular topographical patterns. Neurology 2006;67:1178-1183.

50. Moosy J: Morphology, sites, and epidemiology of cerebral atherosclerosis. Res Publ Assoc Res Nerv Ment Dis 1966;51:1-22.

51. Imparato A, Riles T, Kim G: Cervical vertebral angioplasty for brainstem ischemia. Surgery 1981;90:842-852.

52. Pelouze GA: Plaque ulcerie de l'ostium de l'artere vertebrale. Rev Neurol 1989;145:478-481.

53. Fisher CM: Occlusion of the vertebral arteries. Arch Neurol 1970;22:13-19.

54. Wityk RJ, Chang H-M, Rosengart A, et al: Proximal extracranial vertebral artery disease in the New England Medical Center posterior circulation registry. Arch Neurol 1998;55:470-478.

55. George B, Laurian C: Vertebrobasilar ischemia with thrombosis of the vertebral artery: Report of two cases with embolism. J Neurol Neurosurg Psychiatry 1982;45:91-93.

56. Caplan LR, Tettenborn B: Embolism in the posterior circulation. In Bergner R, Caplan LR (eds): Vertebrobasilar Arterial Disease. St Louis: Quality Medical Publishers, 1991, pp 50-63.

57. Caplan LR, Amarenco P, Rosengart A, et al: Embolism from vertebral artery origin occlusive disease. Neurology 1992;42:1505-1512.

58. Glass TA, Hennessey PM, Pazdera L, et al: Outcome at 30 days in the New England Medical Center posterior circulation registry. Arch Neurol 2002;59:369-376.

59. Moufarrij N, Little JR, Furlan AJ, et al: Vertebral artery stenosis: Long-term follow-up. Stroke 1984;15:260-263.

60. Callow A: Surgical management of varying patterns of vertebral artery and subclavian artery insufficiency. N Engl J Med 1964;270:546-552.

61. Roon A, Ehrenfeld W, Cooke P, et al: Vertebral artery reconstruction. Am J Surg 1979;138:29-36.

62. Berguer R: Surgical indications for reconstruction of the vertebral artery. In Berguer R, Caplan (eds): Vertebrobasilar Arterial Disease. St Louis: Quality Medical Publishers, 1991, pp 201-210.

63. Berguer R, Flynn LM, Kline RA, et al: Surgical reconstruction of the extracranial vertebral artery: Management and outcome. J Vasc Surg 2000;31: 9-18.

64. Kieffer E, Koskas F, Bahnini A, et al: Long-term results after reconstruction of the cervical vertebral artery. In Caplan LR, Shifrin EG, Nicolaides AN, Moore WS (eds): Cerebrovascular Ischaemia: Investigations and Management. London: Med-Orion, 1996, pp 617-625.

65. Myers PM, Schumacher HC, Higashida RT, et al: Use of stents to treat extracranial cerebrovascular disease. Ann Rev Med 2006;57:437-454.

66. Higashida R, Tsai F, Halbach V, et al: Transluminal angioplasty, thrombolysis, and stenting for extracranial and intracranial cerebral vascular disease. J Interv Cardiol 1996;9:245-255.

67. Chastain 2nd HD, Campbell MS, Iyer S, et al: Extracranial vertebral artery stent placement: In-hospital and follow-up results. J Neurosurg 1999;91:547-552.

68. Piotin M, Spelle L, Martin JB, et al: Percutaneous transluminal angioplasty and stenting of the proximal vertebral artery for symptomatic stenosis. AJNR Am J Neuroradiol 2000;21:727-731.

69. Stenting of Symptomatic Atherosclerotic Lesions in the Vertebral or Intracranial Arteries (SSYLVIA): Study results. Stroke 2004;35:1388-1392.

70. Caplan LR, Zarins C, Hemmatti M: Spontaneous dissection of the extracranial vertebral arteries. Stroke 1985;16:1030-1038.

71. Caplan LR, Tettenborn B: Vertebrobasilar occlusive disease, review of selected aspects:1. Spontaneous dissection of extracranial and intracranial posterior circulation arteries. Cerebrovasc Dis 1992;2:256-265.

72. Mokri B, Houser OW, Sandok BA, Piepgras DG: Spontaneous dissections of the vertebral arteries. Neurology 1988;38:880-885.

73. Silbert PL, Mokri B, Schievink WI: Headache and neck pain in spontaneous internal carotid and vertebral artery dissection. Neurology 1995;45:1517-1522.

74. Saeed AB, Shuaib A, Al-Sulaiti G, Emery D: Vertebral artery dissection: Warning symptoms, clinical features, and prognosis in 26 patients. Can J Neurol Sci 2000;27:292-296.

75. Arnold M, Bousser M-G: Clinical manifestations of vertebral artery dissection. In Baumgartner RW, Bogousslavsky J, Caso V, Paciaroni M (eds): Handbook on Cerebral Artery Dissection Basel: Karger, 2005, pp 77-86.

76. Arnold M, Bousser M-G, Fahrni G, et al: Vertebral artery dissection. Presenting findings and predictors of outcome. Stroke 2006;37:2499-2503.

77. Wilkinson I, Russel R: Arteries of the head and neck in giant cell arteritis. Arch Neurol 1972;27:378-391.

78. Bickerstaff E: Neurological Complications of Oral Contraceptives. Oxford: Clarendon Press, 1975.

79. Muller-Kuppers M, Graf KJ, Pessin MS, et al: Intracranial vertebral artery disease in the New England Medical Center posterior circulation registry. Eur Neurol 1997;37:146-156.

80. Shin H-K, Yoo K-M, Chang HM, Caplan LR: Bilateral intracranial vertebral artery disease in the New England Medical Center posterior circulation registry. Arch Neurol 1999;56:1353-1358.

81. Fisher CM, Karnes W, Kubik C: Lateral medullary infarction: The pattern of vascular occlusion. J Neuropathol Exp Neurol 1961;20:323-379.

82. Stephens RB, Stilwell DL: Arteries and Veins of the Human Brain. Springfield, Ill: Charles C Thomas, 1969.

83. Duvernoy HM: Human Brainstem Vessels. Berlin: Springer, 1978.

84. Kommerall G, Hoyt W: Lateropulsion of saccadic eye movements. Arch Neurol 1973;28:313-318.

85. Meyer K, Baloh R, Krohel G, et al: Ocular lateropulsion: A sign of lateral medullary disease. Arch Ophthalmol 1980;98:1614-1616.

86. Matsumoto S, Okuda B, Imai T, Kameyama M: A sensory level on the trunk in lower lateral brainstem lesions. Neurology 1988;38:1515-1519.

86a. Song I-U, Kim J-S, Lee D-G, et al: Pure sensory deficit at the T4 sensory level as an isolated manifestation of lateral medullary infarction. J Clin Neurol 2007;3:112-115.

86b. Kim JS, Lee JH, Lee MC: Patterns of sensory dysfunction in lateral medullary infarction: Clinical-MRI correlation. Neurology 1997;49:1557-1563.

87. Devereaux M, Keane J, Davis R: Automatic respiratory failure associated with infarction of the medulla: Report of two cases with pathologic study of one. Arch Neurol 1973;29:46-52.

88. Levin B, Margolis G: Acute failure of automatic respirations secondary to a unilateral brainstem infarct. Ann Neurol 1977;1:583-586.

89. Bogousslavsky J, Khurana R, Deruaz JP, et al: Respiratory failure and unilateral caudal brainstem infarction. Ann Neurol 1990;28:668-673.

90. Currier R, Giles C, Westerberg M: The prognosis of some brainstem vascular syndromes. Neurology 1958;8:664-668.

91. Caplan LR, Pessin M, Scott RM, et al: Poor outcome after lateral medullary infarcts. Neurology 1986;36:1510-1513.

92. Caplan LR: Bilateral distal vertebral artery occlusion. Neurology 1983;33:552-558.

93. Hauw J, Der Agopian P, Trelles L, et al: Les infarctes bulbaires. J Neurol Sci 1976;28:83-102.

94. Sawada H, Seriu N, Udaka F, Kameyama M: Magnetic resonance imaging of medial medullary infarction. Stroke 1990;21:963-966.

95. Tyler KL, Sandberg E, Baum KF: Medial medullary syndrome and meningovascular syphilis: A case report in an HIV-infected man and a review of the literature. Neurology 1994;44:2231-2235.

96. Kim JS, Kim HG, Chung CS: Medial medullary syndrome: Report of 18 new patients and a review of the literature. Stroke 1995;26:1548-1552.

96a. Hagiwara N, Toyoda K, Torisu R, et al: Progressive stroke involving bilateral medial medulla expanding to spinal cord due to vertebral artery dissection. Cerebrovasc Dis 2007;24:540-542.

96b. Kumral E, Afsar N, Kirbas D, et al: Spectrum of medial medullary infarction: Clinical and magnetic resonance imaging findings. J Neurol 2002;249:85-93.

97. Sypert G, Alvord E: Cerebellar infarction: A clinicopathological study. Arch Neurol 1975;32:351-363.

98. Amarenco P, Hauw JJ, Henin D, et al: Les infarctus du territoire de l'artere cerebelleuse posteroinferieure: Etude clinico-pathologique de 28 cas. Rev Neurol 1989;145:277-286.

99. Amarenco P, Hauw JJ, Gautier JC: Arterial pathology in cerebellar infarction. Stroke 1990;21:1299-1305.

100. Amarenco P, Caplan LR: Vertebrobasilar occlusive disease, review of selected aspects: 3. mechanisms of cerebellar infarctions. Cerebrovasc Dis 1993;3:66-73.

101. Caplan LR: Cerebellar infarcts: Key features. Rev Neurol Dis 2005;2:51-60.

102. Fisher CM, Picard E, Polak A, et al: Acute hypertensive cerebellar hemorrhage: Diagnosis and surgical treatment. J Nerv Ment Dis 1965;140:38-57.

103. Lehrich J, Winkler G, Ojemann R: Cerebellar infarction with brainstem compression: Diagnosis and surgical treatment. Arch Neurol 1970;22:490-498.

104. Fairburn B, Oliver L: Cerebellar softening: A surgical emergency. BMJ 1956;1:1335-1336.

105. Hornig CR, Rust DS, Busse O, et al: Space-occupying cerebellar infarction. Clinical course and prognosis. Stroke 1994;25:372-374.

106. Seelig J, Selhorst J, Young H, et al: Ventriculostomy for hydrocephalus in cerebellar hemorrhage. Neurology 1981;31:1537-1540.

107. Rieke K, Krieger D, Adams H-P, et al: Therapeutic strategies in space-occupying cerebellar infarction based on clinical, neuroradiological and neurophysiological data. Cerebrovasc Dis 1993;3:45-55.

108. Castaigne P, Lhermitte F, Gautier J, et al: Arterial occlusions in the vertebral-basilar system. Brain 1973;96:133-154.

109. Koroshetz WJ, Ropper AH: Artery-to-artery embolism causing stroke in the posterior circulation. Neurology 1987;37:292-296.

110. Sundt T, Whisnant J, Piepgras D, et al: Intracranial bypass grafts for vertebral-basilar ischemia. Mayo Clin Proc 1978;53:12-18.

111. Ausman J, Diaz F, de los Reyes R, et al: Anastomosis of occipital artery to AICA for vertebrobasilar junction stenosis. Surg Neurol 1981;16:99-102.

112. Roski R, Spetzler R, Hopkins L: Occipital artery to posterior-inferior cerebellar artery bypass for vertebrobasilar ischemia. Neurosurgery 1982;10:44-49.

113. Allen G, Cohen R, Preziosi T: Microsurgical endarterectomy of the intracranial vertebral artery for vertebrobasilar transient ischemic attacks. Neurosurgery 1981;81:56-59.

114. Takis C, Kwan ES, Pessin MS, et al: Intracranial angioplasty: Experience and complications. AJNR Am J Neuroradiol 1997;18:1661-1668.

115. Myers PM, Schumacher HC, Tanji K, et al: Use of stents to treat intracranial cerebrovascular disease. Ann Rev Med 2007;58:207-122.

116. Kubik C, Adams R: Occlusion of the basilar artery: A clinical and pathologic study. Brain 1946;69:73-121.

117. Caplan LR: Occlusion of the vertebral or basilar artery. Stroke 1979;10:272-282.

118. Voetsch B, DeWitt LD, Pessin MS, et al: Basilar artery occlusive disease in the New England Medical Center posterior circulation registry. Arch Neurol 2004;61:496-504.

119. Schonewille W, Wijman C, Michel P: BASICS investigators. Treatment and clinical outcome in patients with basilar artery occlusion. Stroke 2006;37:922-928.

120. Baird TA, Muir KW, Bone I: Basilar artery occlusion. Neurocritical care 2004;1:319-329.

121. Pessin MS, Gorelick PB, Kwan ES, et al: Basilar artery stenosis: middle and distal segments. Neurology 1987;37:1742-1746.

122. LaBauge R, Pages C, Marty-Double JM, et al: Occlusion du tronc basilaire. Rev Neurol 198 1;137:545-571.

123. Amarenco P, Hauw JJ: Cerebellar infarction in the territory of the anterior inferior cerebellar artery: A clinicopathological study of 20 cases. Brain 1990;118:139-155.

124. Amarenco P, Rosengart A, DeWitt LD, et al: Anterior inferior cerebellar artery territory infarcts. Mechanisms and clinical features. Arch Neurol 1993;50:154-161.

125. Fisher CM: Some neuro-ophthalmological observations. J Neurol Neurosurg Psychiatry 1967;30:383-392.

126. Chase T, Moretti L, Prensky A: Clinical and electroencephalographic manifestations of a vascular lesion of the pons. Neurology 1968; 18:357-368.

127. Biller J, Yuh W, Mitchell GW: Early diagnosis of basilar artery occlusion using magnetic resonance imaging. Stroke 1988;19:297-306.

128. Fisher CM: Bilateral occlusion of basilar artery branches. J Neurol Neurosurg Psychiatry 1977;40:1182-1189.

129. Klein IF, Lavallee PC, Schouman-Claeys E, Amarenco P: High-resolution MRI identifies basilar artery plaques in paramedian pontine infarct. Neurology 2005;64:551-552.

130. Caplan LR: Thrombolysis in vertebrobasilar occlusive disease. In Lyden PD (ed): Thrombolytic Therapy for Acute Stroke, 2nd ed. Totawa NJ: Humana Press, 2005, pp 203-209.

131. Lindsberg PJ, Mattle HP: Therapy of basilar artery occlusion: A systematic analysis comparing intra-arterial and intravenous thrombolysis. Stroke 2006;37:922-928.

131a. Smith WS: Intra-arterial thrombolytic therapy for acute basilar occlusion. Pro Stroke 2007;38:701-703.

132. Caplan LR, Sergay S: Positional cerebral ischemia. J Neurol Neurosurg Psychiatry 1976;39:385-391.

133. Bogousslavsky J, Regli F, Maeder P, et al: The etiology of posterior circulation infarcts: A prospective study using magnetic resonance imaging and magnetic resonance angiography. Neurology 1993;43:1528-1533.

134. Roether J, Wentz K-U, Rautenberg W, et al: Magnetic resonance angiography in vertebrobasilar ischemia. Stroke 1993;24:1310-1315.

135. Bash S, Villablanca JP, Duckwiler G, et al: Intracranial vascular stenosis and occlusive disease. Evaluation with CT angiography, MR angiography, and digital subtraction angiography. AJNR Am J Neuroradiol 2005;26:1012-1021.

136. Caplan LR: Top of the basilar syndrome: Selected clinical aspects. Neurology 1980;30: 72-79.

137. Mehler MF: The rostral basilar artery syndrome: Diagnosis, etiology, prognosis. Neurology 1989;39:9-16.

138. Mehler MF: The neuro-ophthalmologic spectrum of the rostral basilar artery syndrome. Arch Neurol 1988;45:966-971.

139. Fisher CM: Oval pupils. Arch Neurol 1980;37:502-503.

140. Hommel M, Bogousslavsky J: The spectrum of vertical gaze palsy following unilateral brainstem stroke. Neurology 1991;41:1229-1234.

141. Alemdar M, Kamaci S, Budak F: Unilateral midbrain infarction causing upward and downward gaze palsy. J Neuro-Ophthalmol 2006;26:173-176.

142. Hommel M, Besson G: Midbrain infarcts. In Bogousslavsky J, Caplan LR (eds): Stroke Syndromes, 2nd ed. Cambridge: Cambridge University Press, 2001, pp 512-519.

142a. Hermann DM, Siccoli M, Brugger P, et al: Evolution of neurological, neuropsychological and sleep-wake disturbances after paramedian thalamic stroke. Stroke 2008;39:62-68.

143. Pessin MS, Lathi E, Cohen M, et al: Clinical features and mechanism of occipital infarction. Ann Neurol 1987;21:290-299.

144. Chaves CJ, Caplan LR: Posterior cerebral artery. In Bogousslavsky J, Caplan LR (eds): Stroke Syndromes, 2nd ed. Cambridge: Cambridge University Press, 2001, pp 479-489.

145. Yamamoto Y, Georgiadis AL, Chang HM, Caplan LR: Posterior cerebral artery territory infarcts in the New England Medical Center (NEMC) posterior circulation registry. Arch Neurol 1999;56:824-832.

146. Pessin MS, Kwan E, DeWitt LD, et al: Posterior cerebral artery stenosis. Ann Neurol 1987;21:85-89.

147. Mohr JP, Pessin MS: Posterior cerebral artery disease. In Barnett HJM, Mohr JP, Stein BM, Yatsu F (eds): Stroke Pathophysiology, Diagnosis, and Management, 3rd ed. New York: Churchill Livingstone, 1998, pp 481-502.

148. Barton JS, Caplan LR: Cerebral visual dysfunction. In Bogousslavsky J, Caplan LR (eds): Stroke Syndromes, 2nd ed. Cambridge: Cambridge University Press, 2001, pp 87-110.

149. Georgiadis AL, Yamamoto Y, Kwan ES, et al: Anatomy of sensory findings in patients with posterior cerebral artery (PCA) territory infarction. Arch Neurol 1999;56:835-838.

150. Caplan LR, DeWitt LD, Pessin MS, et al: Lateral thalamic infarcts. Arch Neurol 1988;45:959-964.

151. Benson DF, Tomlinson EB: Hemiplegic syndrome of the posterior cerebral artery. Stroke 1971;2:559-564.

152. Hommel M, Besson G, Pollak P, et al: Hemiplegia in posterior cerebral artery occlusion. Neurology 1990;40:1496-1499.

153. Hommel M, Moreaud O, Besson G, Perret J: Site of arterial occlusions in the hemiplegic posterior cerebral artery syndrome. Neurology 1991;41:604-605.

154. Dejerine J: Contribution a l'etude anatomo-pathologique et clinique des differnetes varietes de cecite verbale. Memoires de la Societe Biologique 1892;4:61-90.

155. Geschwind N, Fusillo M: Color naming defect in association with alexia. Arch Neurol 1966;15:137-146.

156. Caplan LR, Hedley-White T: Cueing and memory dysfunction in alexia without agraphia. Brain 1974;97:25-262.

157. Kertesz A, Sleppard A, MacKenzie R: Localization in transcortical sensory aphasia. Arch Neurol 1982;39:475-479.

158. Victor M, Angevine J, Mancall E, et al: Memory loss with lesion of hippocampal formation. Arch Neurol 1961;5:244-263.

159. Ferro JM, Martins IP: Memory loss. In Bogousslavsky J, Caplan LR (eds): Stroke Syndromes, 2nd ed. Cambridge: Cambridge University Press, 2001, pp 242-251.

160. Benson F, Marsden C, Meadows J: The amnestic syndrome of posterior cerebral artery occlusion. Acta Neurol Scand 1974;50:133-145.

161. Mohr JP, Leicester J, Stoddard L, et al: Right hemianopia with memory and color deficits in circumscribed left posterior cerebral artery territory infarction. Neurology 1971;21:1104-1113.

162. Ott B, Saver JL: Unilateral amnestic stroke. Six new cases and a review of the literature. Stroke 1993;24:1033-1042.

163. Rubens A, Benson F: Associative visual agnosia. Arch Neurol 1971;24:305-316.

164. Grusser OJ, Landis T: Visual Agnosias and Other Disturbances of Visual Perception and Cognition. Boston: CRC Press, 1991.

165. Damasio A, Damasio H, Van Hoesen G: Prosopagnosia: Anatomic basis and behavioral mechanisms. Neurology 1982;32:331-341.

166. Tranel D, Damasio AR: Intact recognition of facial expression, gender, and age in patients with impaired recognition of face identity. Neurology 1988;38:690-696.

167. Fisher CM: Disorientation to place. Arch Neurol 1982;39:33-36.

168. Symonds C, McKenzie I: Bilateral loss of vision from cerebral infarction. Brain 1957;80:415-455.

169. Medina J, Rubino F, Ross E: Agitated delirium caused by infarctions of the hippocampal formation and fusiform and lingual gyri: A case report. Neurology 1974;24:1181-1183.

170. Horenstein S, Chamberlain W, Conomy J: Infarction of the fusiform and calcarine regions: Agitated delirium and hemianopsia. Trans Am Neurol Assoc 1962;92:357-367.

171. Meadows J: Disturbed perception of colors associated with localized cerebral lesions. Brain 1974;97:615-632.

172. Damasio A, Yamada T, Damasio H, et al: Central achromatopsia: behavioral, anatomic, and physiologic aspects. Neurology 1980;30:1064-1071.

173. Kinkle W, Newman R, Jacobs L: Posterior cerebral artery branch occlusions: CT and anatomical considerations. In Berguer R, Bauer R (eds): Vertebrobasilar Arterial Occlusive Disease. New York: Raven Press, 1984, pp 117-133.

174. Goto K, Tagawa K, Uemma K, et al: Posterior cerebral artery occlusion. Radiology 1979;132:357-368.

175. Caplan, LR, Chung, C-S, Wityk, RJ, et al: New England Medical Center posterior circulation stroke registry: I. Methods, data base, distribution of brain lesions, stroke mechanisms, and outcomes. J Clin Neurol 2005;1:14-30.

176. Bogousslavsky J, Cachin C, Regli F, et al: Cardiac sources of embolism and cerebral infarction-clinical consequences and vascular concomitants: The Lausanne Stroke Registry. Neurology 1991;41:855-859.

177. Bogousslavsky J, Regli F, Maeder P, Meuli R, Nader J. The etiology of posterior circulation infarcts: A prospective study using magnetic resonance angiography. Neurology 1993;43:1528-1533.

178. Bogousslavsky J, Van Melle G, Regli F. The Lausanne Stroke Registry: Analysis of 1000 consecutive patients with first stroke. Stroke 1988;19:1083-1092.

179. Moulin T, Tatu L, Crepin-Leblond T, et al: The Besancon Stroke Registry: An acute stroke registry of 2500 consecutive patients. Eur Neurol 1997;38:10-20.

180. Moulin T, Tatu L, Vuillier F, et al: Role of a stroke data bank in evaluating cerebral infarction subtypes: Patterns and outcome of 1776 consecutive patients from the Besancon Stroke Registry. Cerebrovasc Dis 2000;10:261-271.

181. Vemmos K, Takis C, Georgilis K, et al: The Athens Stroke Registry: Results of a five-year hospital-based study. Cerebrovasc Dis 2000;10:133-141.

Penetrating and Branch Artery Disease

8

Occlusions or stenoses of large extracranial and intracranial arteries are traditional lesions generally recognized by physicians and surgeons caring for stroke patients. Abnormalities in larger arteries are easily confirmed by angiography and noninvasive tests and are readily verified by inspection of arteries removed at surgery or necropsy. In contrast, lesions in microscopic intracranial arteries, although acknowledged as genuine pathologic findings, are a more controversial cause of stroke. Miller Fisher (see Figs. 1-6, 1-7, and 1-8) reviewed the history of lacunar infarctions,[1] defined the nature and etiology of the vascular pathology causing lacunes,[2] and described many clinical syndromes that can be readily and reliably diagnosed as lacunar. Fisher almost single-handedly brought this disorder to the attention of the neurologic community. Yet, some clinicians still fail or refuse to integrate the concept of lacunar infarction into their differential diagnosis of stroke, and others are skeptical that lacunes can be diagnosed clinically. Even in 2008, lacunes remain controversial.[3]

Durand-Fardel first introduced the term *lacunes* in 1843 to describe small holes, usually found in the striatum, which contain fine meshwork of tissues and vessels.[3-5] The clinical findings in patients with lacunar infarction were first described by Ferrand,[6] working in the laboratory of Pierre Marie, and by Marie himself.[7] These French authors noted that lacunes were most often located in the lentiform nuclei, thalamus, pons, internal capsule, and cerebral white matter. Hemiplegia was the major finding in acute lacunar infarction. The clinical condition of multiple lacunes was termed *état lacunaire* (lacunar state) by Marie and was characterized by pseudobulbar palsy and an abnormal small-stepped gait. Foix and colleagues added clinical details about the findings in capsular and pontine lacunar infarcts.[8-10] Little was added after Foix until Fisher's work on the pathology and clinical findings in lacunar infarction.[3,4]

PATHOLOGY

Lacunar infarcts are small, discrete, often irregular lesions, ranging from 1 to 20 mm in size. Only 17% of lacunes are smaller than 1 cm.[1] Inspection of the tiny cavities usually reveals fine strands of connective tissue resembling cobwebs. Marie recognized that true lacunar infarcts had to be differentiated from dilated perivascular spaces, so-called *état criblé*, and from postmortem holes produced by gas-forming bacilli (*état vermoulu*).[7] At necropsy, gas cavities are usually numerous, perfectly round, with no cobwebs, and often retain a characteristic bad smell. Magnetic resonance imaging (MRI) often reveals dilated perivascular état criblé lesions as discrete loci of increased signal.[11] The most common locations of lacunar infarcts are the putamen and the pallidum, followed by the pons, thalamus, caudate nucleus, internal capsule, and corona radiata. Rarer are lacunes in the cerebral peduncles, pyramids, and subcortical white matter. These lesions are not found in the cerebral or cerebellar cortices.

Serial sections of the penetrating arteries that supply the territory of lacunar infarcts shows a characteristic vascular pathology.[2] These tiny vessels often have focal enlargements and small hemorrhagic extravasation through the walls of the arteries. Subintimal foam cells sometimes obliterate the lumens, and pink-staining fibrinoid material lies within the vessel walls (Fig. 8-1). The arteries in spots are often replaced by whorls, tangles, and wisps of connective tissue that

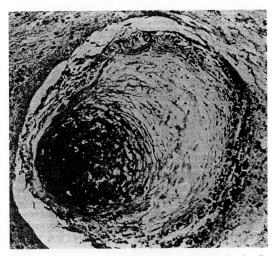

Figure 8-1. Small penetrating artery showing lipohyalinosis and fibrinoid necrosis; lumen is considerably compromised. (Courtesy of C. Miller Fisher, MD.)

8

obliterate the usual vascular layers. Fisher called these processes *segmental arterial disorganization, fibrinoid degeneration,* and *lipohyalinosis.* Fisher also recognized that sometimes larger deep infarcts, which he dubbed *giant lacunes,* could be caused by occlusion of parent vessels, such as the middle cerebral artery (MCA) stem, causing obstruction of the orifices of lateral lenticulostriate arteries.[12] Figure 8-2 shows a cartoon modeled after Fisher of a lipohyalinatic lesion that disrupts arterial flow causing a pontine infarct.[2]

Fisher,[13,14] Cole and Yates,[15] and Rosenblum[16] recognized that small aneurysmal dilatations of these lipohyalinotic penetrating arteries could potentially rupture, causing intracerebral hemorrhage. These lesions were probably similar to those recognized by Charcot and Bouchard[20] as the cause of parenchymatous bleeding. The distribution of deep hypertensive hemorrhages was the same as the locations of lacunes (putamen, capsule, thalamus, and pons). Lipohyalinotic arteries could occlude, leading to lacunar infarction, or rupture, causing intracerebral hemorrhage.[13] Fisher reviewed the charts of 114 patients who had lacunes at necropsy. All but three patients had hypertension defined by a prior history of this disease, elevated blood pressure recorded on examination, or heart weight exceeding 400 g without another explanation.[1] Fisher attributed segmental arterial disorganization and lipohyalinosis to hypertension.

A hereditary disorder, cerebral autosomal dominant arteriopathy with subcortical infarcts

and leukoencephalopathy (CADASIL), has now been convincingly shown to be a disorder of the small penetrating arteries within the brain.[18-20] The penetrating arteries in this condition contain a granular material in the media that extends into the adventitia. Periodic acid-Schiff (PAS) staining suggests the presence of glycoproteins, but staining for elastin and amyloid are invariably negative. Smooth muscle cells in the media are swollen and often degenerated.[20] The endothelium may be absent and replaced by collagen fibers. At times abnormalities seen in hypertensive patients are also found, including duplication and splitting of the internal elastic lamina, adventitial fibrosis and hyaline change, and fibrosis and hypertrophy of the arterial media. This hereditary condition causes lacunar infarcts in the basal ganglia and cerebral white matter similar to those found in hypertensive patients.

Another hereditary angiopathic condition, now known to be associated with mutations in a gene that encodes procollagen type IV alpha 1 (Col4A1), has been identified within the past decade. This genetic mutation affects small brain arteries as well as larger retinal and cerebral arteries.[20a-d] The clinical findings are heterogeneous and include: perinatal hemorrhages and porencephaly, tendency to brain hemorrhage after trauma, retinal artery tortuosity, cerebral aneurysms, penetrating artery related infarcts, white-matter gliosis, and kidney disease.[20a-d]

Detailed anatomic dissections during the late 19th century[21,22] and early 20th century[9,10,23-27] defined the locations, anatomy, and territories of arteries that branched from the parent cerebral and basilar arteries. Pullicino reviewed and illustrated in detail the anatomy of these arteries and their usual territories of supply.[28,29] Some of these penetrating arteries are shown in Figures 2-21 and 2-31.

Foix recognized that infarcts were often limited to the territories of one of these branches. The orifices of these branches were often obstructed by a pathology that differed from lipohyalinosis. Fisher and Caplan,[30] Fisher,[31] and Caplan[32] described the vascular pathology in these branches. Fisher and Caplan[30] reported vascular lesions causing ischemia limited to the territory of basilar artery branches, separating this vasculopathy from lipohyalinosis. This pathology is referred to as *intracerebral branch atheromatous disease* Figures 2-32, 8-3, and 8-4 contain cartoons that illustrate the location and mechanism of the pathology in the parent artery.[32] The orifices of the penetrating branches could be blocked by atheroma in the parent artery, atheroma could originate in the parent

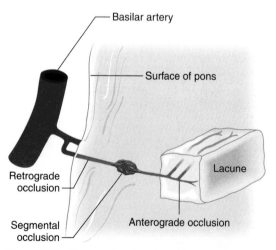

Figure 8-2. Diagram showing the relationship of a lacune in the pons to the causative penetrating artery vascular lesion. The artery beyond the region of arterial disorganization is thrombosed and thrombus has also formed in a retrograde manner extending toward the parent basilar artery. (Adapted from Fisher CM: The arterial lesion underlying lacunes. Acta Neuropathol 1969;12:1-15.)

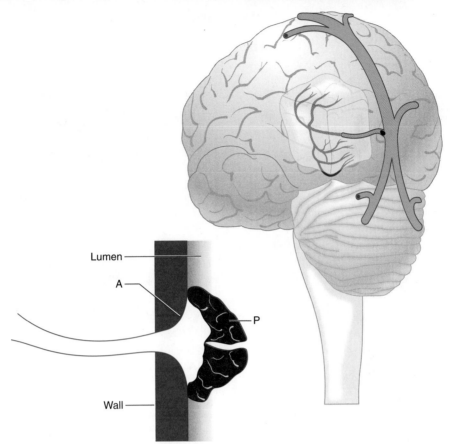

Lumen

A

P

Wall

Figure 8-3. Basilar-branch occlusion: The diagram at the bottom shows a close-up of the artery shown within the cube above; a plaque is seen extending into the branch. A, atheroma; P, plaque. (Adapted from Fisher CM and Caplan LR: Basilar artery branch occlusion: A cause of pontine infarction. Neurology 1971;21:900-905.)

artery and extend into the branch (so-called junctional atheromatous plaques), or microatheroma could arise at the origin of the branch itself. Thrombus was sometimes superimposed on the atheromas. This vasculopathy is sometimes referred to as microatheroma and is clearly distinct on pathologic grounds from the lipohyalinotic arteriopathy that also causes small deep infarcts.[33]

Recently it has become possible to image intracerebral branch atheromatous disease using high resolution MRI. Plaques in the middle cerebral artery[34,35] and basilar artery[36] (Fig. 8-5) can be shown to impinge upon or occlude penetrating branches by MRI techniques that show axial sections of the origins of branches from the parent arteries.

Pontine infarcts are the most frequent pathologic lesion found in necropsies of diabetics and are, in most cases, caused by atheromatous branch disease.[37] Infarcts limited to the territories of the anterior choroidal arteries (AChA) and the thalamogeniculate arteries are also most often

explained by atheromatous branch disease. Microatheromas, parent-artery plaques, and occlusion of parent arteries by in-situ thrombosis or embolism probably explain deep infarcts in normotensive patients.

The major important condition to separate from these "micropathologies" is occlusion of the parent artery blocking flow in penetrating artery branches. In patients of Asian origin, especially Japan, Korea, and China, small deep infarcts are often caused by occlusive disease of the large intracranial parent arteries, the occlusive lesions blocking the orifices of penetrating arteries.[38,39] In patients whose small deep infarcts are caused by severe occlusive disease of the intracranial large parent arteries, the infarcts are slightly larger, the neurologic signs are slightly worse, and recurrence is more common than in infarcts caused by intrinsic disease of the penetrating arteries.[40,41] Vascular imaging (CTA, MRA, TCD, and catheter contrast angiography) can readily show occlusion of the major intracranial large arteries.

Middle cerebral

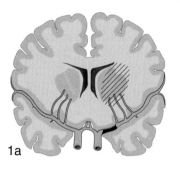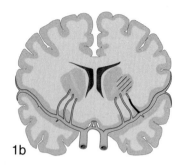

1a   1b

Posterior cerebral

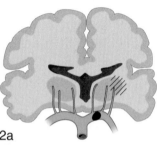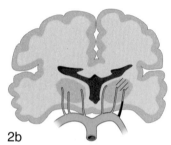

2a   2b

Figure 8-4. Mechanisms of deep infarction. **1A,** Basal ganglionic capsular infarct due to MCA occlusion. **1B,** Smaller deep capsular infarct due to lenticulostriate artery occlusion. **2A,** Lateral thalamic infarct due to PCA occlusion. **2B,** Lateral thalamic infarct due to thalamogeniculate artery occlusion. (Adapted from Caplan LR, DeWitt LD, Pessin MS, et al: Lateral thalamic infarcts. Arch Neurol 1988;45:959-964.)

Although lipohyalinosis and microatheroma are readily separated by meticulous pathologic examination, the distinction is difficult clinically. Boiten separated 100 patients with lacunes into two distinct groups.[42] One group had atherosclerotic risk factors and single symptomatic lacunes; the other group had hypertension, multiple lacunes (some of which were asymptomatic) and white-matter abnormalities on neuroimaging scans. He posited that the former group had atheromatous branch disease and the latter group had lipohyalinosis.[42] Because the prognosis for branch occlusions and lacunes is probably identical and treatment is similar, there is little practical reason to clinically separate lacunes from penetrating branch infarcts.

GENERAL CLINICAL FINDINGS

A 56-year-old, African-American man, RB, awakened with weakness of his right arm. As he stood to go to the bathroom, he became aware that his right leg was also weak. He called his wife, who noted that his voice was slightly thick. He did not have a headache, nor did he feel dizzy or otherwise unwell. As the day progressed, the weakness in his arm and leg seemed to fluctuate. By nightfall, however, he could not move

his right arm or right leg. He had no prior history of stroke, heart disease, or claudication, and did not recognize any warnings during the days before the episode. Two months earlier, a physician told him that his blood pressure was high and "bore watching," but did not prescribe medication.

Fisher repeatedly emphasized in his writings that hypertension was the major cause of fibrinoid degeneration and lipohyalinosis, the arteriopathy that leads to lacunar infarcts. Fisher noted that the same arteriopathy that caused lacunar infarcts also caused deep intracerebral hemorrhages and that these hemorrhages and lacunes involved the very same brain regions. Although Fisher attributed the arteriopathy to hypertension, others have noted a lower frequency of hypertension in patients, in whom computed tomography (CT) verified the diagnosis of lacunar infarcts (52.5%,[43] 57%,[44] 65%,[45] 72%[46]). Seventy-five percent of patients clinically diagnosed as having lacunar infarcts in the Harvard Stroke Registry had hypertension.[47] In a necropsy study, 64% of patients with lacunes at postmortem had a history of hypertension.[48] These frequencies, however, are not importantly different from the incidence of hypertension in

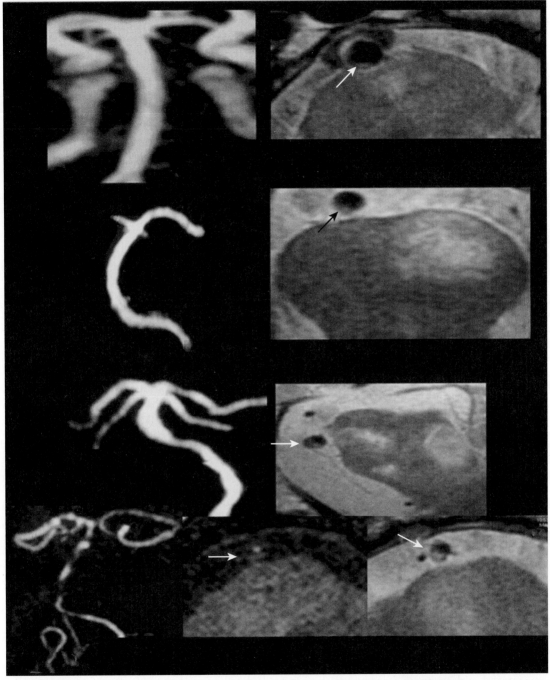

Figure 8-5. High-resolution MRI that shows a plaque in the parent basilar artery *(arrows)* obstructing a penetrating branch causing an infarct in the basis pontis. (Adapted from Klein IF, Lavallee PC, Schouman-Claeys E, Amaraenco P: High-resolution MRI identifies basilar artery plaques in paramedian pontine infarct. Neurology 2005; 64:551-552.)

large registries of patients with ischemic strokes. In the Northern Manhattan Study that included a multiethnic cohort of individuals, lacunar infarct patients tended to be older, and were more likely to have diabetes and elevated cholesterol levels than those with deep intracerebral hemorrhages.[48a]

For a more thorough evaluation, Fisher used pathologic criteria to diagnose lacunes and hypertension (heart weight 400 g with no other cause), and carefully searched hospital and doctors' notes for past blood-pressure recordings. Although clearly not all patients with deep infarcts are hypertensive, a diagnosing physician should be wary of attributing a lesion to intrinsic penetrating artery occlusive disease if there is no past or current evidence of hypertension or diabetes. Systolic hypertension, a finding very common in elderly individuals, may be particularly important in causing penetrating artery damage related to increased vascular pulsitivity. I have also seen normotensive patients with elevated hematocrits who have a clinical picture of lacunar infarction, possibly caused by clotting within small arteries. Kidney disease[48b] and dilatative arteriopathy[48c] (large intracranial dolichoectasia) (see Chapter 11) have also been found to be associated with small-vessel brain arterial disease.

Fisher found severe large-vessel atherosclerosis in 64% of the 114 patients with lacunes, a frequency far exceeding the usual 9% found in a population without lacunes.[1] Hypertension is known to predispose patients to premature atherosclerosis of larger extracranial and intracranial arteries. Large- and small-vessel diseases frequently coexist, so the mere presence of clinical, noninvasive, or angiographic evidence of atherosclerotic stenosis does not exclude a lacunar etiology of stroke.

Lacunes are small and deep. Because there is no accompanying overdistension of superficial arteries and deep arteries have no pain fibers, headache caused by vascular distension does not occur in patients with lacunes. These small lesions produce no mass effect that might cause headache or decreased alertness. Lacunes are far from the cortex and do not produce seizures[47] or affect the surface-recorded electroencephalogram (EEG).[49] The presence of decreased alertness, unaccustomed headache, or seizures argues against a lacunar etiology of a stroke.

The course of illness in patients with lacunar infarction is also different from patients with large-artery occlusive disease and brain embolism.[47,50] Prior transient ischemic attacks (TIAs) occur in approximately 20% of patients with lacunes,[50-52] a frequency far below that for large vessel disease but more often than in patients with brain embolism. When TIAs do occur in patients with lacunar infarcts, they span a shorter time interval and are more stereotyped than in other ischemic etiologies. Brief, stereotyped TIAs may occur many times during a day. The occurrence of repeated episodes of hemiplegia preceding a pure-motor stroke was labeled the "capsular warning syndrome" by Donnan and colleagues.[53] However, these repeated TIAs can occur in subcortical lesions in other areas and in the brainstem and are not limited to the internal capsule.

The neurologic deficit often evolves gradually in patients with lacunar infarcts, with frequent fluctuations and progression during the initial 72 hours of the stroke. Sudden deficits, maximal at onset, are less frequent than in patients with other causes of ischemic stroke. Gradual worsening of paralysis over a few days is a characteristic course in some patients with pure-motor hemiparesis caused by lacunar infarction. Lacunar infarction is the most common cause of worsening of clinical neurologic signs during the first week after stroke onset.[54,55]

> On examination of patient RB, the blood pressure was 165/95 mm Hg. He was alert and understood, repeated, and used language normally. The patient read, wrote, and spelled words correctly. His voice was slightly slurred. His right face, shoulder, arm, hand, thigh, and foot were moderately weak. Deep tendon reflexes were exaggerated on the right, and the right plantar response was extensor. He felt touch normally in his right limbs and could identify accurately the nature of objects in his right hand. He could also localize spots touched on his right limbs. Visual fields were normal.

Lacunes have a predilection for particular anatomic sites—those nourished by penetrating arteries. Some of these deep lesions produce characteristic clinical syndromes, whereas others are clinically silent or produce findings difficult to distinguish from superficial infarction. In a necropsy series of 167 patients with lacunes, 93 patients (56%) had no reported related symptoms.[48] Anatomic localization is probably most helpful in the diagnosis of lacunes. RB had paralysis of face, arm, and leg with exaggerated reflexes and an extensor toe sign. A lesion of the motor cortex causing these findings would have to extend from the face area near the sylvian fissure, a region fed by the MCA, to the paramedian frontal lobe foot area, which is fed by the anterior cerebral artery. Such a lesion would invariably affect language, sensation, or vision. A sizable superficial or deep frontal-lobe lesion would not only produce motor dysfunction, but would also likely cause conjugate eye deviation to the side of the lesion and abulia. Marie emphasized hemiplegia as the sign of lacunar infarction.[7] Fisher termed the syndrome of isolated weakness of the face, arm, and leg, *pure-motor hemiplegia*,[12] and taught that these findings are diagnostic of lacunar infarction in the pons or internal capsule.

Some authors, using radioisotope studies or CT, found lesions other than lacunes in patients with pure-motor hemiplegia.[45,56,57] MRI is more sensitive and shows cortical lesions in some patients clinically thought to have a lacunar syndrome. Remember that Fisher examined the patients thoroughly. When he called the patient's syndrome *pure motor*, he had compulsively tested sensation, visual fields, and cortical function and found them normal. Fisher also demanded that weakness include the face, arm, and leg, and that hypertension be present to make the diagnosis of a pure-motor stroke. Patient RB fulfills Fisher's criteria for pure-motor hemiplegia. Were patients with CT lesions, other than lacunes, examined in the same compulsive and thorough manner as an important requisite for the clinical diagnosis of lacunes in these other radiographic studies?

I advise a strategy similar to that taught in high school geometry: Try to prove your original diagnostic impression wrong. Seek out features (i.e., sensory, visual, or intellectual abnormalities) that would disprove your diagnosis. Mental status testing is key because most pure-motor hemiplegia patients with lesions other than lacunes have some alteration in alertness, behavior, or intellect that suggests frontal lobe disease.

Even when the lacunar syndromes are apparently pure, some patients have a small hematoma as the cause of the syndrome. Small putaminal, capsular, and pontine hematomas are known to cause pure-motor hemiparesis and other syndromes most often caused by lacunar infarction.[50,52,58-60] Before clinicians can be secure in their diagnosis of lacunar infarction, I believe neuroimaging tests (CT or MRI), which show a lacune or exclude parenchymatous hemorrhage and surface infarction, are mandatory. Diffusion-weighted MRI has the capacity for separating recent lacunar infarcts from old lesions. Vascular imaging is also important in excluding parent artery occlusive disease.

LOCATION OF LESIONS AND CLINICAL SYNDROMES

Hemispheral Lesions within the Anterior Circulation

Probably the most commonly recognized clinical syndrome in patients with lacunes in the cerebral hemispheres is pure-motor hemiparesis. Patient RB had this syndrome. The causative lesion is usually found in the internal capsule. Figure 8-6 is a necropsy specimen that shows a lacunar infarct that involves the basal ganglia and cuts through the internal capsule. The three types of capsular lesions causing pure-motor hemiparesis distinguished by Rascol and colleagues are (1) large lesions spanning the anterior and posterior limbs of the internal capsule, caused by occlusion of large lateral lenticulostriate arteries, (2) capsulopallidal infarcts located predominantly in the posterior limb of the capsule in the territory of medial lenticulostriate arteries, and (3) lesions in the anterior limb of the internal capsule and the caudate nucleus in the supply region of the lateral lenticulostriate arteries or the

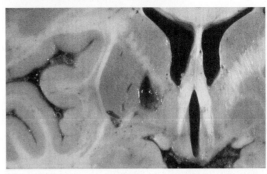

Figure 8-6. A necropsy specimen showing a cavity due to an old lacunar infarct located in and the medial basal ganglia (mostly the globus pallidus) and extends through the internal capsule in a patient with a pure motor hemiplegis during life.

recurrent arteries of Heubner.[50,52] MRI studies show that patients with pure-motor hemiparesis can also have lesions in the midbrain, pons, and medulla, affecting descending corticospinal fibers in the cerebral peduncle, basis pontis, and the medullary pyramid.[61,62]

Motor weakness does not always equally affect the face, arm, and leg. Often, the face is at least partially spared.[50] At times, almost a pure monoparesis of the arm or leg is present with only minimal weakness or hyperreflexia of the other limb. In the Stroke Data Bank, the clinical findings related to the degree of involvement of face, arm, and leg did not correlate with the location of the lesion in the internal capsule.[50,63] Mohr summarized as follows:

> There no longer seems much reason to adhere to the older dogma[64] that the motor fibers occupy the anterior half of the posterior limb of the internal capsule.... Further, the available case material does not document a series of cases with an homunculus whose face is anterior and whose leg is posterior in the plane of the internal capsule.[50]

In some patients with lacunar infarction, the clinical picture includes a combination of weakness, pyramidal signs, cerebellar-type ataxia, and incoordination of the limbs on one side of the body. This syndrome was first called *homolateral ataxia and crural paresis* in patients in whom the predominant involvement was in the lower limbs.[65] Later, Fisher dubbed the syndrome *ataxic hemiparesis*, indicating that the arm and leg could be variously involved, but the major signature of the syndrome was the combination of cerebellar and motor signs in the limbs on the same side of the body.[66] In some patients, there are also sensory symptoms ipsilateral to the motor abnormalities.[67] The relative severity of ataxia compared to weakness varies considerably, as does the relative involvement of the arm compared to the leg. Localization of lesions causing ataxic hemiparesis varies widely. Many lesions are in the posterior limb of the internal capsule. Lacunes in the midbrain and pons, however, can also cause this clinical syndrome.

At times, the clinical findings show abnormalities of motor function on one side of the body, but there is no true paralysis, reflexes are not exaggerated, and the plantar response is flexor. I refer to these findings as a *nonpyramidal hemimotor syndrome*. Some lesions that cause these clinical findings involve the striatum and the globus pallidus. Decreased spontaneous and associated movements, clumsiness, slight increased resistance to passive movement, and slowness of the affected limbs are often found. Some patients have a minor degree of hemiparkinsonism. Others have a movement disorder with choreic features. Some patients with hemichorea have had striatal infarcts.[68,69]

Sometimes, the predominant dysfunction in patients with hemispheral lacunes is bulbar. Dysarthria, dysphagia, and even mutism may occur, caused by interruption of corticobulbar fibers in the white matter underlying the motor cortex, capsule, striatum, or pons. Limb symptoms may be minor or absent. Tapping the corner of the mouth may show heightened contraction of the orbicularis oris and the orbicularis oculi on the side of the bulbar dysfunction, or on both sides of the face. Often, the tongue and face are weak on one side. In patients with predominantly bulbar signs, the lesions are often bilateral and the syndrome is pseudobulbar.[70] The initial lesion sometimes produces no symptoms or only minor hemimotor signs. When the contralateral side of the brain becomes involved, the bilateral disturbance in corticobulbar fibers causes predominantly bulbar abnormalities, especially dysarthria and dysphagia, sometimes with exaggerated laughing and crying.

In Chapter 6, I discuss caudate[71,72] and anterior choroidal artery (AChA)–territory infarcts.[70,73-76] Infarcts in these regions can be quite small, readily qualifying as lacunes, or they can be more extensive deep infarcts. Caudate lesions can be limited to the caudate nucleus or extend into the anterior limb of the internal capsule and anterior putamen.[71,72] AChA-territory infarcts can involve the globus pallidus or the posterior limb of the internal capsule.[70,73-76] Infarcts in these areas are probably caused by intracranial-branch atheromatous disease, affecting one or more of Heubner's arteries and the AChA.[32]

Involvement of small penetrating branches of these arteries is probably most often caused by microatheromas or lipohyalinosis. Neuropathologic studies of patients with lesions in the distribution of Heubner's artery and the AChA are too scanty to document or refute this hypothesis.[32] Some patients with caudate infarcts have prominent dysarthria and cognitive and behavioral abnormalities, especially abulia and restlessness.[71,72,77,78] Some patients with left caudate infarcts have aphasia, usually slight and transient. In a necropsy series of patients with lacunes found at postmortem, aphasia with right hemiparesis was one of the most frequent clinical syndromes correlating with lacunar infarction.[48] The responsible lesions were in the striatum and anterior limb of the internal capsule or thalamus.

Posterior Circulation, Brainstem, Thalamic Lacunes, and Branch Occlusions

Pons and Medulla

Lacunes and branch-territory infarcts are often found in the pons.[61,62,79,80] In a prospective study of MRI scans in 100 patients hospitalized with lacunar infarcts in Grenoble, France, 38 of the lesions (25%) were in the pons.[61] Among 12 patients in another series studied acutely with MRI, 6 of 11 lesions were located in the pons and had symptoms appropriate to that localization.[81] The most common site of the pontine lesions is in the basis pontis on one side, most often medially in the distribution of one of the paramedian branches of the basilar artery.[79,80] The penetrating branches of the basilar artery are shown in Figure 2-21. Occlusive changes in these vessels cause pontine infarcts in the supply zone of each of these branches. Few necropsy specimens of patients with infarcts in this location have been studied. The pathology in some has been lipohyalinosis and segmental arterial disorganization of penetrating arteries within the basis pontis.[2,12]

In three patients, arterial lesions involving basilar-artery branches were studied in more detail by serially sectioning the pons, with the basilar artery and its branches still attached to the pons.[30,31] In one patient, an atheromatous plaque within the basilar artery obstructed the intramural part of the 0.5-mm-diameter basilar-artery branch.[30] Distally, in the blocked branch, there was a mass of agglutinated platelets, which arose as a tiny intra-arterial embolus from the lesion in the parent artery or formed in situ because of reduced flow. In another patient, a plaque arising in the lumen of the basilar artery extended into the mouth of a 0.5-mm-diameter branch, forming a junctional plaque.[30] In a third patient, basilar-artery branches were blocked bilaterally.[31] At the orifice of a basilar branch in this patient, a microdissection made a crevice in a plaque, and a superimposed thrombus obstructed the branch. The mechanisms of blockage of branches are depicted in Figures 2-32, 8-3, and 8-4. Flat or elevated plaques in the parent basilar artery can block the orifices of branches or provide a nidus for small embolic fragments that extend into the branches. A dilatated dolichoectatic basilar artery can also distort branch orifices.

Infarction of the medullary pyramid can give rise to a pure-motor hemiparesis, often sparing the face.[12,79,82-84,84a] At times the medial lemniscus is also involved causing tingling of contralateral limbs. Nerve XII may be ischemic as it passes through the medullary base. Figure 8-7 is a necropsy specimen showing an infarct in the medullary pyramid on one side cause by an occlusion of a penetrating artery branch of the anterior spinal artery.

Lesions are basomedial in the territory of anterior spinal artery branches.

Infarcts in the pontine base caused by lipohyalinatic lesions within the course of a penetrating artery are often located within the pontine parenchyma sparing the basal pial border of the pons while occlusion of the mouth of a penetrating artery most often causes an infarct that begins at the basal pial surface. Figure 8-8 is a cartoon that illustrates the various locations of these two pathologies. Figure 8-9 is an MRI that shows an infarct in the paramedian basis pontis on one side caused by a basilar branch occlusion. Note that the infarct extends to the basal pial surface. Figure 8-10 is a necropsy specimen of a lacune in the dorsal portion of the basis pontis near the tegmental border.

The three major syndromes in the pons related to infarcts in the basis pontis are pure-motor

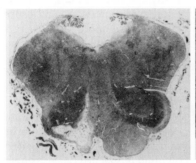
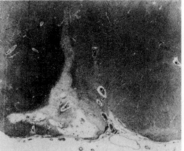

Figure 8-7. Infarct in the medial medulla. The left pyramid is destroyed and replaced by an empty cystic space. The old infarct extends dorsally in a linear fashion. The infarct involves also the ventromedial portion of the inferior olivary nucleus, the lateral part of the medial lemniscus, and the hypoglossal nerve. Cut section of a necropsy specimen showing an infarct in the medullary pyramid on the left of the figures. (From Ho KL, Meyer KR: The medial medullary syndrome. Arch Neurol 1981;38:385-387.)

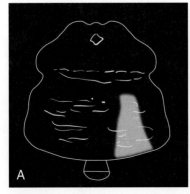
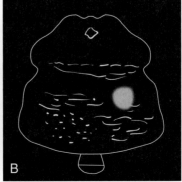

Figure 8-8. Cartoon showing pontine infarcts. **A,** Basilar artery branch infarct extending to the pial surface at the base of the pons. **B,** Infarct within the pontine parenchyma due to a lipohyalinatic lesion within the penetrating artery supplying this region. (From Caplan LR: Intracranial branch atheromatous disease: A neglected understudied, and underused concept. Neurology 1989;39:1246-1250.)

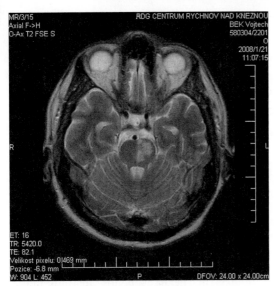

Figure 8-9. MRI T2-weighted image showing an infarct in the paramedian pons. The basilar artery flow void looks normal. (Courtesy of Ladislav Pazdera, MD.)

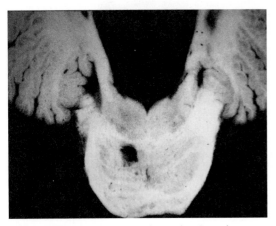

Figure 8-10. A necropsy specimen showing a lacunar infarct in the dorsal portion of the basis pontis on one side.

hemiparesis, ataxic hemiparesis, and dysarthria clumsy-hand syndromes.[79,80,85-88] Pure-motor hemiplegia is probably the most common of the syndromes and occurs most often when the pontine infarcts are in the paramedian basis pontis. In some patients, additional findings help identify the infarct as pontine. An ipsilateral VI– nerve palsy or intranuclear ophthalmoplegia are occasionally associated with the contralateral hemiparesis.[30,79,85] Involvement of the tegmentum and base can include the paramedian pontine reticular formation, causing a conjugate-gaze palsy toward the side of the lesion, accompanied by contralateral limb weakness and pyramidal signs. At times, although there is no gaze palsy, conjugate-gaze movements are asymmetric with

slight abnormalities of ipsilateral conjugate gaze. Involvement of the medial lemniscus, as well as pyramidal tract fibers, leads to some sensory symptoms and signs on the side of the hemiparesis.[85,86,88] Usually, patients report minor paresthesias and sensory examination shows only slight loss of vibration sense, with preserved pinprick and temperature sensation.

The basis pontis carries fibers crossing into the brachium pontis, traveling toward the cerebellum. Interruption of pontocerebellar fibers can cause cerebellar-type incoordination and ataxia. Ataxic hemiparesis is often caused by a pontine lesion.[65,66,79,80,85,86,88] The infarcts that cause ataxic hemiparesis are usually smaller and more rostral, dorsal, and lateral than the lesions associated with pure-motor hemiparesis.[79,80,86] Subtle, minor incoordination of the ipsilateral limbs can provide a clue to this localization because pontocerebellar-crossing fibers are involved bilaterally, to some extent. The dysarthria clumsy-hand syndrome is usually caused by a small lacune in the more dorsal portion of the basis pontis, affecting corticobulbar fibers near the medial lemniscus.[79,80,86-88] Often, associated facial and tongue weakness is severe, but examination of the hand and arm is nearly normal, despite the patient's report of awkwardness.

Occasionally, lacunes are located in the medial or lateral pontine tegmentum in the distribution of branches that penetrate horizontally from long, circumferential arteries or penetrate from the base of the pons.[79,80,88,89] These lacunes are the ischemic counterpart of lateral tegmental brainstem hematomas.[88,90] These lesions usually involve the sensory lemniscus that has formed from the joining of the medial lemniscus and lateral spinothalamic tracts in the rostral pons. Or these lesions may involve the medial lemniscus or the spinothalamic tract before formation of the sensory lemniscus. A pure, sensory, stroke-like syndrome occurs with subjective paresthesias or numbness (or both) in the contralateral face, arm, and leg. Dizziness, gait ataxia, dysarthria, and nystagmus are variable accompaniments.[88,89,91,92]

Midbrain

In the midbrain, penetrating-artery lesions involve primarily the cerebral peduncle and the paramedian zones. Figure 8-11 is an MRI that shows a cerebral peduncle infarct. Few examples have been reported in detail.[79,93-96] Some infarcts in this distribution are caused by occlusion of the parent posterior cerebral artery (PCA).[96,97] The distribution of the penetrating branches of the PCA is diagrammed in Figure 7-24. One clinical syndrome includes a third nerve palsy

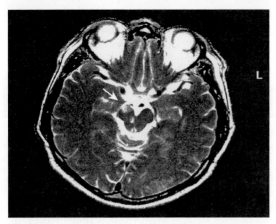

Figure 8-11. A T2-weighted MRI showing an infarct in the cerebral peduncle of the midbrain on one side.

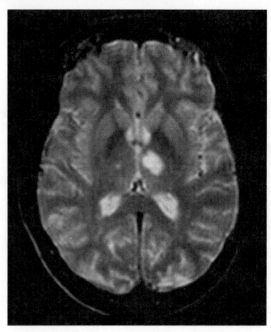

Figure 8-12. MRI T2-weighted image showing a left anterolateral polar artery territory infarct. (From Bogousslavsky J, Caplan LR: Vertebrobasilar occlusive disease: Review of selected aspects. III. Thalamic infarcts. Cerebrovasc Dis 1993;3:193-205.)

ipsilaterally, caused by involvement of the fascicles of the third nerve within the midbrain, accompanied by a contralateral hemiparesis (Weber's syndrome). In some patients, involvement of the red nucleus, as well as the cerebral peduncle on the same side, gives rise to a combination of motor weakness and tremor. The tremor usually develops as the hemiparesis improves and is present at rest and on intention. The affected arm is usually also quite incoordinated and ataxic. Some patients with focal lesions involving the decussation of the brachium conjunctivum in the midbrain present with bilateral limb ataxia and tremor. This syndrome is often referred to as the Wernekinck commissure syndrome and is quite rare.[97a,97b] Few cases of midbrain branch lesions with neuropathologic confirmation have been reported.[96-98]

Thalamus

Thalamic lacunes are quite common. In the MRI study by Hommel and colleagues, thalamic lesions accounted for 14% of the lacunes.[61] Penetrating-artery territory infarcts are located paramedially in the distribution of the various thalamoperforating arteries and laterally in the distribution of the thalamogeniculate artery or the lateral posterior choroidal artery. The two most important and consistent paramedian thalamoperforating arteries are the polar (tuberothalamic) artery and the thalamic-subthalamic arteries.[79,98-107]

The polar artery arises on each side from the middle third of the posterior communicating artery and supplies the anteromedial and anterolateral thalamic nuclei. Figure 8-12 is an MRI that shows a polar artery territory thalamic infarct. At times, this vessel is absent, in which case its territory is supplied by the thalamic-subthalamic arteries. The predominant findings in infarcts fed by the thalamoperforating arteries are cognitive and behavioral, but the syndromes do differ, depending on the artery involved.[62,79,100,102-104,106,107] Unilateral anterolateral thalamic infarction in the distribution of the polar artery on the left or right side usually causes abulia, facial asymmetry, transient minor contralateral motor abnormalities and, at times, aphasia (left lesions) or visual neglect (right lesions). Abulia—with slowness, decreased amount of activity and speech, and long delays in responding to queries or conversation—is the predominant abnormality. Some patients are disorganized and dress in a slovenly manner. Usually, in patients with unilateral lesions, abulia and cognitive and behavioral abnormalities improve after 3 to 6 months. Occasionally, bilateral infarcts are found in the territory of the polar artery of each side.[108] This means that bilateral arteries probably occasionally arise from a single or loop artery, or a common rete. When the polar artery is affected bilaterally, the behavioral abnormality is more severe and persistent. Memory may also be affected.[108] The behavioral effects are probably explained by the synaptic corticothalamic relationship with the frontal lobe and other cortical regions.

The thalamic-subthalamic arteries originate from the proximal PCAs and supply the most posteromedial portion of the thalamus near the posterior commissure. The right and left-sided arteries may arise separately, but can originate from a single unilateral artery or a common pedicle.[79,98,99,105] Unilateral lesions are usually characterized by paresis of vertical gaze (upward or both upward and downward) and by amnesia. Motor and sensory signs and symptoms are absent. The pathway for vertical gaze includes the rostral interstitial nucleus of the medial longitudinal fasciculi and connections between the two eyes for vertical eye movements that travel through the commissure at the diencephalic-mesencephalic junction. A unilateral lesion interrupts these commissural fibers, thus causing conjugate vertical-gaze palsy.[109] Memory loss may be severe, with profound difficulty in forming new memories and encoding recent events. The amnesia often improves within 6 months in unilateral-infarct patients. Bilateral butterfly-shaped paramedian posterior thalamic infarction can result from a branch occlusion of a single supplying artery or pedicle, although scant necropsy data are available from well-studied cases.[79,98,99,105,110] Hypersomnolence and bilateral third-nerve palsies can occur in patients with bilateral infarcts.[110] The same syndrome can result from occlusion of the rostral basilar artery most often caused by brain embolism, a topic discussed in Chapters 7 and 9.

Lacunes and branch-territory infarcts are especially common in the lateral thalamus. This region which includes the somatosensory nuclei (ventral posterior lateral and ventral posterior medial) and the ventral lateral and ventral anterior nuclei, is supplied by the thalamogeniculate group of arteries. These vessels arise from the PCA and are the posterior circulation counterpart of the lenticulostriate branches of the MCA. Occlusion of these arteries or their branches leads to a variety of different clinical syndromes.[79,111]

Larger lateral thalamic infarcts were first described by Dejerine and Roussy, and the clinical findings have long been referred to as *le syndrome thalamique*.[112] The essential features of this syndrome, almost always caused by atheromatous-branch disease in my experience, are contralateral hemisensory symptoms accompanied by contralateral limb ataxia. At times, there are jumpy adventitious hemichoreic movements of the contralateral arm, and the hand may tend to assume a fisted posture. Some patients have a transient hemiparesis at onset that improves quickly.[111]

Usually, the sensory phenomena are mostly paresthesias, which involve the face, neck, trunk, and limbs. Sensory loss is usually slight. The sensory signs relate to ischemia of the somatosensory nuclei. The ataxia is caused by interruption of cerebellofugal fibers going to the ventral anterior and ventral lateral nuclei. Also interrupted are fibers from the striatum (the ansa lenticularis) that project toward these motor nuclei. Dystonia, chorea, and hemiparkinsonian-like features are probably caused by interruption of these extrapyramidal-system projections. Pain in the affected limbs and trunk may develop months after the original stroke and was one of the cardinal features mentioned by Dejerine and Roussy.[112] Many patients never have pain. Pain is almost never noted at or shortly after onset. Figure 8-13 contains MRIs that show lateral thalamic infarcts.

Occlusion of branches of the thalamogeniculate arteries supplying the somatosensory nuclei is responsible for the vast majority of patients with so-called pure sensory stroke.[113-116] The infarcts are usually smaller than those found in patients with the broader lateral thalamic syndrome. Figure 8-14 is an MRI that shows a small lateral thalamic infarct in a patient with pure sensory stroke. In this condition, the patient has somatosensory complaints without other signs or symptoms. Most often, the patient describes numbness, tingling, or pins-and-needle sensations in the face, limbs, and trunk. All hemicorporeal sensations are represented in the thalamic somatosensory-relay nuclei. In the somatosensory cortex, the hand and face have large representations, whereas little space is accorded to the trunk, scalp, and other regions not capable of fine sensory distinctions. Thus, numbness of the inner mouth, eye, ear, scalp, chest, back, abdomen, and genitalia is much more common in thalamic lacunes than in superficial lesions of the parietal cortex.[114,115]

After a few days, the somatic sensations may take on an unpleasant quality and may be characterized as burning, tightness, or soreness.[113,114] Sensory symptoms may be persistent or transient, even when lacunar infarction is present on MRI. Usually, subjective sensory complaints are more prominent than objective loss of sensation. Many patients with pure sensory stroke have no detectable loss of threshold to any sensory modality, whereas others show only a minimal qualitative or quantitative difference between the two sides of the body. Motor, visual, and intellectual functions are normal. Occasionally, pure sensory stroke can be caused by lateral or medial tegmental pontine or midbrain infarcts.[79,89,91,94,95,117]

Occlusion of thalamogeniculate branches, on occasion, can cause a syndrome referred to as sensory motor stroke.[118] This condition is characterized by the sensory symptoms and signs described in relation to pure sensory stroke, accompanied by paresis and pyramidal signs in the same limbs as the sensory symptoms. Few such cases have been studied at necropsy. In one well-studied case, the responsible infarct involved the somatosensory nuclei. Pallor of the adjacent posterior limb of the internal capsule was evident.[118] Review of the

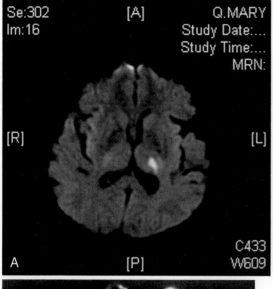

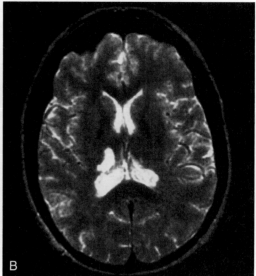

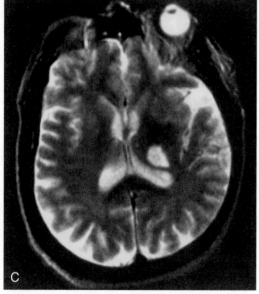

Figure 8-13. A montage of lateral thalamic infarcts. **A,** MRI-DWI image showing an acute left lateral thalamic infarct. **B, C,** T2-weighted MRIs that show lateral thalamic infarcts.

drawings from the original Dejerine-Roussy article clearly shows that lateral thalamic infarcts often affect the adjacent internal capsule.[79,111,112] The thalamogeniculate arteries must sometimes supply this zone, contrary to the teachings in some neuroanatomy texts. Ischemia of the internal capsule is probably responsible for the transient paresis found in some patients with lateral thalamic infarcts and for the motor abnormalities in patients with sensory motor stroke.

Infarcts in the territory of the medial and lateral posterior choroidal arteries are the least well known and most rarely reported of all thalamic infarcts. The lateral posterior choroidal arteries supply mostly the pulvinar, a portion of the lateral geniculate body, and then loop around the superior portion of the thalamus to supply the anterior nucleus. The medial arteries supply the habenula, anterior pulvinar part of the center median nucleus, and the paramedial nuclei.[79] There have been few clinical pathologic and neuroimaging reports of patients with posterior choroidal territory infarcts.[79,100,107,119-122]

Hemianopia, hemisensory symptoms, and behavioral abnormalities may occur in patients with posterior choroidal artery territory infarcts. The most specific and well-defined abnormality relates to the visual fields. The posterior choroidal arteries and their lateral choroidal artery branches supply a portion of the lateral geniculate body reciprocal to that supplied by the AChAs. The characteristic visual field defect in patients with posterior choroidal artery territory infarcts is a sectoranopia, involving a wedge-shaped defect on each side of the

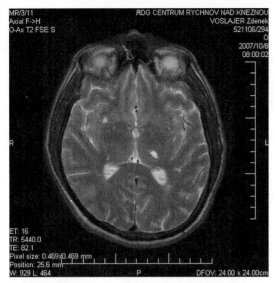

MR/3/11
Axial F->H
O-Ax T2 FSE S
RDG CENTRUM RYCHNOV NAD KNEZNOU
VOSLAJER Zdenek
521106/294
O
2007/10/8
08:00:02

R
L

ET: 16
TR: 5440.0
TE: 82.1
Pixel size: 0.469x0.469 mm
Position: 25.6 mm
W: 929 L: 464
P
DFOV: 24.00 x 24.00cm

Figure 8-14. T2-weighted MRI showing a small lateral thalamic infarct in a patient with pure sensory stroke.

horizontal meridien.[120-122] In contrast, the visual field defect in patients with AChA-territory infarcts can include loss of the upper and lower quadrants, with sparing of vision in a line along the median horizontal meridian. Patients with posterior choroidal territory infarcts can also have an upper or lower quadrantanopia.[107,122] Hemisensory symptoms, usually in the form of hemianesthesia and slight hemiparesis also occur due to lesions involving or adjacent to the ventral posterior nuclei. Amnesia and transient aphasia have also been described in patients with infarcts that involve the posterior choroidal artery territory.[107,122]

LABORATORY INVESTIGATIONS IN PATIENTS SUSPECTED OF HAVING LACUNAR STROKES

Having described the known lacunar syndromes and their usual responsible lesions, I return to patient RB, who had hypertension and the clinical findings of pure-motor hemiparesis.

> In RB, a complete blood cell count was normal. EEG showed minor symmetric slowing. CT showed a small infarct in the posterior limb of the internal capsule on the left and a tiny lesion in the right putamen. MRI also showed these lesions and another tiny lacune in the right thalamus. Magnetic resonance diffusion-weighted scans showed a bright lesion in the posterior limb of the internal capsule. Magnetic resonance angiography and ultrasound of the carotid and vertebral arteries were normal.

Because lacunes are small and deep in the hemisphere or are located in the brainstem, they usually

do not have a major influence on the EEG recorded from the convexity.[49] CT findings depend on the location and size of the lesion. Acute pontine lacunes are seldom imaged well by CT, but can nearly always be seen on MRI scans. Pure-motor hemiplegia probably has the highest frequency of CT positivity among the lacunar syndromes. Rascol et al found hypodense lesions on CT in 29 of 30 patients with pure-motor stroke.[52] They divided the lesions into large capsulo-putamino-caudate infarcts, and smaller capsulo-pallido or capsulo-caudate infarcts.[52] Some patients with larger infarcts had angiographic abnormalities in the lenticulostriate arteries. Others have reported MCA occlusive disease in patients with large basal ganglionic and capsular infarctions.[123-126] In contrast, patients with pure-sensory stroke seldom have lesions visible on CT.[115]

MRI is undoubtedly superior to CT in imaging small brainstem and thalamic infarcts.[61,62,79,81,127] Rothrock and colleagues evaluated 31 patients with the clinical diagnosis of lacunar infarction. Twenty-three patients (74%) had appropriate lesions on MRI.[81] When CT and MRI were performed, MRI was superior in imaging lesions appropriate to the symptoms. In another study among 110 patients, MRI was effective in imaging one or more possibly responsible lacunar infarcts in 89 patients.[61] When gadolinium-diethylene-triamine penta-acetic acid enhancement is given, acute lacunar infarcts are generally enhanced.[127] Use of enhancement may be helpful when the clinicians find more than one lesion and are uncertain of the age of the lesions. Generally, only acute lesions are enhanced. Although an upper limit of size of lacunes has traditionally been considered to be 15 mm, a study of 890 Korean stroke patients found that the size of the lesions alone on MRI was not indicative of a lacunar or nonlacunar etiology.[127a]

Diffusion-weighted MRI is especially useful in showing lacunar infarcts soon after symptoms begin, and in separating recent infarcts from old infarcts. Only recent lesions are shown well on diffusion-weighted MRI. CT or MRI is essential for excluding small hemorrhages from the differential diagnosis; such hemorrhages can cause findings identical to lacunar syndromes. Rajajee and colleagues compared acute CT scans and a modern multimodal MRI protocol in the diagnosis of lacunar infarction in patients presenting within 6 hours of symptom onset.[127b] Among 15 patients in this series diagnosed as acute lacunar infarct disease using clinical and CT criteria, MRI detected a different diagnosis in 5. However, large-artery occlusions were not found by MRA in any of the 15 patients implying that CT and clinical criteria are not specific for penetrating artery disease but may effectively in most instances exclude large-artery occlusion.[127a] By imaging hemosiderin, MRI is more effective than CT in determining whether old lesions were small hematomas or lacunar infarcts.

Angiographic abnormalities have been shown in some patients with lacunar infarcts, and include carotid artery and MCA disease.[126] Some large-artery lesions are probably incidental and unrelated to the cause of the stroke. Necropsy studies have shown that most patients with hypertension and lacunes have a high incidence of coexisting atherosclerosis. Angiography in apparently healthy prisoners also shows a high frequency of atherosclerosis.[128] Atherosclerotic plaques and stenosis in both extracranial and intracranial arteries are also found in patients with lacunar infarcts.[129] Thus, the finding of atherosclerotic occlusive disease in larger extracranial and intracranial arteries does not prove an etiologic relationship to the lacunar infarct. In some cases, blockage of parent arteries can produce infarction in territories of lenticulostriate, thalamogeniculate, and pontine penetrating arteries. Figure 8-4 diagrammatically depicts the vascular lesions in occlusion of penetrating and parent arteries. The lesion in the parent artery can be a plaque, in-situ thrombosis, or an embolus.[32] Parent-artery lesions are especially important to consider in patients with lacunes exceeding 20 mm that involve the basal ganglia and capsule. In my experience, the clinical syndrome usually includes more features than the usual lacunar syndrome.[32,125] Echocardiography and cardiac rhythm monitoring are also important to exclude cardiac-origin embolism to parent arteries in some patients. Larger deep infarcts are less often caused by lipohyalinosis.

Neuroimaging, preferably with MRI, is important in every patient. The need for thorough laboratory testing depends on the (1) presence of appropriate risk factors, such as hypertension, polycythemia, or diabetes; (2) typicality of the neurologic findings; (3) thoroughness of the neurologic examination and the experience of the examining physician[130]; and (4) the neuroimaging results. If the patient has no evidence of past or present hypertension, physicians should be skeptical of lipohyalinosis as the cause of infarction. Atypical neurologic findings or the presence of unaccustomed headache, reduced alertness, or seizures argue for more complete laboratory investigations. At times, unexpected superficial infarcts, small hemorrhages, and even nonvascular conditions, such as tumors, are discovered by CT or MRI.

When the clinical diagnosis is uncertain, extracranial and transcranial ultrasound, computed tomography angiography, magnetic resonance angiography, or standard angiography may be indicated. Usually, after preliminary evaluation, which should include a detailed history and examination, blood studies, EEG, and either CT or MRI, physicians are able to place the patient with brain ischemia into one of three categories: (1) high certainty of lacune; (2) lesion consistent with a lacune but not diagnostic (atypical lacune); or (3) findings not compatible with a lacunar etiology. Examples of possible findings in these three groups are listed in Table 8-1. Patients in categories two and three require more evaluation than those in category one.

RB was kept at bed rest. Weakness began to improve during the 2nd week, when he was transferred to a rehabilitation hospital. He was discharged on atorvastatin 40 mg/day and a combination of 25 mg of aspirin and 200 mg of modified-release dipyridamole, taken twice a day. While he was in rehabilitation hospitalization, he was referred to an internist who carefully followed him and instituted antihypertensive treatment.

Table 8-1.	**Findings in Patient with Suspected Lacunar Infarction (Right Limbs Involved)**		
	Diagnosis Highly Probable	**Diagnosis Likely but Uncertain**	**Lacune Unlikely or Excluded**
Ecology	Hypertension	Diabetic, slight hypertension	No hypertension
Neurologic signs	Paralysis of right face, arm, leg	Sparing or unequal involvement of face, arm, leg	Paralysis of right hand
Other symptoms	None	Slight unaccustomed headache	Severe headache, seizure at onset
Laboratory	Compatible small deep infarct CT or MRI	Normal CT or MRI	Hypodensity left frontal on CT or MRI; hemorrhage on CT or MRI

TREATMENT

No treatment has been shown to modify the acute course of lacunar infarction. The morphologic nature of lipohyalinosis and fibrinoid degeneration, both of which involve lesions of the vessel wall and not the arterial intima, make it theoretically unlikely that thrombolytic agents or anticoagulants, would be effective treatments. Unfortunately, there are insufficient data from trials concerning thrombolysis in patients with acute brain ischemia due to penetrating artery disease. Although the report of the NINDS thrombolytic trial claimed that all stroke subgroups including lacunar infarcts responded favorably to tPA,[131] their data in relation to lacunar infarction are clearly not credible. In that trial, history and examinations were hurried and not thorough, there was no vascular imaging, only CT was used and it did not show acute infarcts well, and no follow-up imaging was mandated or reported. Furthermore, the numbers of patients in the placebo and treatment groups were very dissimilar. A committee appointed to review the data and conclusions of the NINDS study affirmed that the conclusions about stroke subgroups were not supported by the data.[132] Anecdotal reports indicate that heparin anticoagulation is not effective during acute lacunar stroke.[133] My own personal experience confirms that patients continue to progress while receiving heparin. The disease is far beyond the reach of the surgeon's knife.

Infarction is most likely related to impaired blood flow beyond the region of penetrating artery obstruction. Logical treatment is maximization of blood pressure, blood volume, and blood flow. Because the lesion is caused by hypertension, the most logical therapy to prevent new lipohyalinotic disease is to carefully control the blood pressure. Overzealous reduction of blood pressure during the acute ischemia, however, can decrease flow in collateral arteries and expand the region of infarction.[30,31] I prefer to wait until after the first 2 to 3 weeks after the stroke to institute major reductions in blood pressure. Blood pressure management is extremely important in prevention of further lacunar strokes. Twenty-four-hour blood pressure monitoring shows that excessively high blood pressures at night with failure to show the normal nocturnal blood pressure dipping is predictive of further development of lacunes and white-matter abnormalities.[134] Excessive drops in nocturnal blood pressure are also problematic. Preliminary studies suggests that perindopril and other ACE inhibitors may have salutary effects on vasomotor function and be preferred over other classes of antihypertensives.[135] I try to maximize blood flow during the first days and keep the patient at rest with the head flat to augment cranial flow. If the vascular etiology of the lesion is parent-vessel disease and not lipohyalinosis, then treatment of that condition is appropriate.

Some findings support the use of antiplatelet agents, especially dipyridamole and cilostazole, and statins as prophylactic agents aimed at preventing further lacunar infarction and white-matter disease. In many trials, patients with lacunar infarction are overrepresented. Other causes of ischemic strokes such as cardiac embolism and carotid artery disease are usually excluded, and many patients with severe intracranial disease, such as basilar artery occlusion, are treated with anticoagulants. In the WARRS trial, lacunes made up about 40% of the patients and aspirin was effective.[136] In the ESPS-II trial, a combination of aspirin and modified-release dipyridamole was more effective than aspirin or dipyridamole alone.[137] Lacunes were considered the most prevalent stroke type in that trial. In a Japanese trial of patients with predominantly lacunar ischemic stroke, cilostazol, a putative antiplatelet aggregant, proved quite effective.[138] Cilosatazol and dipyridamole have potent vasodilator effects, and this capability might make them especially useful in patients with penetrating artery disease.

Statins also have vasodilator effects and can augment blood flow in patients with penetrating artery disease,[139,140] although there are no therapeutic trials to date of statins in patients with lacunar infarcts. A trial of intravenous magnesium in patients with acute ischemic strokes (Intravenous Magnesium Efficacy in Stroke [IMAGES]) suggested that magnesium seemed to be of benefit in patients with a lacunar stroke etiology.[140a,b] Magnesium is known to have vasoactive as well as neuroprotective properties and these may relate to the salutary effect in this population.[140b]

Some authors and physicians do not include lacunar infarction in their differential diagnosis of brain ischemia because they believe clinical recognition of the disorder is unreliable. I believe that its inclusion is important for two reasons. First, the disorder is common; to omit a lesion found in 10% of all brains is foolhardy. Second, recognition of this etiology has a direct behavioral result (i.e., no aggressive diagnostic testing, and no anticoagulant or surgical treatment is prescribed). Randomized trials of various treatments are needed in patients with well-defined lacunar infarction to test these hypotheses. The investigation and treatment of other causes of cerebral ischemia—large-artery occlusive disease, brain embolism, and systemic hypotension—are quite different. In addition, technological advances, especially MRI, have greatly improved the clinical diagnosis of lacunar infarction.

CHRONIC PENETRATING ARTERY DISEASE

Historical Background

The disorders that lead to single lacunar infarcts often involves multiple penetrating arteries. As a result, multiple lacunar infarcts are often found in the brain at necropsy or are visible on MRI scans. In the necropsy study of Tuszynski and colleagues, 169 patients had 327 lacunes, an average of 1.9 lacunes per patient.[48] Less than one half of the patients (46%) had only one lacune, 16% had two, and 38% had three or more lacunes. Early investigators found an even higher frequency of multiple lesions,[1-7] but more widespread control of hypertension has likely altered this tendency. Most often, lacunes involve the striatum, capsule, thalamus, cerebral white matter, and pons. When extensive, they give the deeper portions of the brain a Swiss cheese-like appearance. This condition was often referred to as *état lacunaire* after Pierre Marie.[7] Traditionally, the clinical findings have been described as including (1) pseudobulbar abnormalities of speech, swallowing, and emotional control; (2) small-stepped gait; (3) Parkinsonian-like rigidity; (4) hyperreflexia; (5) extensor plantar reflexes; (6) dementia with slow thinking and responses; and (7) variable weakness and sensory signs and symptoms. More recent experience, especially from CT and MRI, raises questions about this traditional view. First, many patients with multiple lacunes seem quite well preserved and function normally. Second, patients with the syndrome described almost always have associated, rather severe changes in the cerebral white matter and ventricular enlargement. Most clinicians and investigators are inclined to ascribe the dementia and clinical signs more to the white-matter disease (dubbed leukoaraiosis by Hachinski)[141] than to the lacunes. The combination of lacunes, white-matter gliosis, and atrophy almost invariably occur together and are associated with widespread abnormalities of penetrating small arteries.[142,143] The combination should be considered a chronic brain microvasculopathy.

Pathology

The chronic white-matter abnormalities were initially described by Binswanger.[143-145] Olszewski, in a review of the history and pathology of the condition, used the term *subcortical arteriosclerotic encephalopathy*.[143,146,147] Babikian and Ropper reviewed the pathologic features in more than 40 cases described in the literature,[148] and other reviews discuss the usual pathologic findings.[143,147,149,150] Grossly visible in the cerebral white matter are confluent areas of soft, puckered, and granular tissue. These areas are patchy and emphasize the occipital lobes and periventricular white matter, especially anteriorly and close to the surface of the ventricles.[143,146-150] The cerebellar white matter is also often involved. The ventricles are enlarged, and, at times, the corpus callosum is small. The volume of white matter is reduced, but the cortex is generally spared. The ventricles are enlarged as a result of atrophy of the white matter. The white-matter abnormalities surrounding the ventricles may reduce the strength of the supporting tissue and allow mechanically more ventricular distension.

The white-matter abnormalities are nearly always accompanied by some lacunes. These were present in one series in 39 of 42 necropsy cases of Binswanger's disease.[148] Microscopic study shows myelin pallor. Usually, the myelin pallor is not homogeneous, but islands of decreased myelination are surrounded by normal tissue. At times, the white-matter abnormalities are so severe that necrosis and cavitation occur. Gliosis is prominent in zones of myelin pallor.

The walls of penetrating arteries are thickened and hyalinized. Occlusion of the small arteries is rare.[149] Some patients have a pathologically different disorder characterized by dilated perivascular spaces, the condition called état criblé by Pierre Marie.[7] Multiple dilated perivascular spaces can be accompanied by white-matter changes and be accompanied by cognitive and behavioral abnormalities and basal ganglionic clinical dysfunction resembling Parkinson's disease.[150a,b]

Occasional patients with Binswanger white-matter changes have had amyloid angiopathy as the underlying vascular pathology.[151-154] In these patients, arteries within the cerebral cortex and leptomeninges are thickened and contain a congophilic substance that stains for amyloid. Arteries within the white matter and basal ganglia are also concentrically thickened but characteristically do not contain amyloid. In a few reported patients, a granulomatous arteritis complicates amyloid angiopathy.[155,156]

Similar microangiopathic abnormalities in the cerebral white matter and lacunar infarcts can also be found in CADASIL (cerebral autosomal dominant arteriopathy with subcortical infarcts).[18-20,157-160] The white-matter abnormalities are often evident early. Relatives of patients with clinical CADASIL can show white-matter abnormalities before symptoms develop. Usually localized, often nodular focal white-matter lesions are found early in the course of illness. Later the white-matter abnormalities become more diffuse, especially in the occipital and frontal periventricular white

8

matter. White-matter lesions in the external capsule and anterior temporal lobes are particularly characteristic of CADASIL.[20,161]

Clinical Findings

The clinical picture in patients with microangiopathies is quite variable. Most patients have some abnormalities of cognitive function and behavior.[143,147,148] Most often, patients become slow and abulic. Memory loss, aphasic abnormalities, and visuospatial dysfunction are also found. Executive functions such as planning and performing sequential tasks are affected. Pseudobulbar palsy, pyramidal signs, extensor plantar reflexes, and gait abnormalities are also common. The clinical findings often progress gradually or stepwise, with worsening during periods of days to weeks. Often, there are long plateau periods of stability of the findings.[143,147,148] Most patients also have acute lacunar strokes.

Patients with cerebral amyloid angiopathy most often present with recurrent brain hemorrhages, predominantly in the cerebral white matter. Some patients present with transient ischemic attacks and others show a progressive stepwise syndrome indistinguishable from the clinical picture in Binswanger disease related to hypertension.[162] Some patients with cerebral amyloid angiopathy have an accompanying granulomatous angiitis and present with progressive neurologic signs.[162a,b,c] The diagnosis is difficult to make without a brain biopsy. I wonder if breakdown of blood vessels containing amyloid results in amyloid being introduced into the cerebrospinal fluid and this induces an inflammatory response. Arteries containing amyloid often show cracks and disruptions in their walls. Occasional patients with cerebral amyloid associated angiitis have responded to corticosteroid treatment.[162d,e]

CADASIL has a rather early age of onset—the average is approximately 40 years of age.[158] Acute strokes and progressive cognitive, behavioral, and motor signs predominate. Depression and headache, often meeting criteria for migraine, are also frequently present in patients with CADASIL and their relatives.[158,159] Tournier-Lasserve and colleagues have shown linkage of the CADASIL disease gene to the D19S226 locus on chromosome 19q12.[160] The clinical findings vary considerably in severity. Some patients are devastated rather early in their middle years, while others have relatively slight neurologic findings.

Imaging

CT often shows periventricular hypodensity. On MRI, the findings are more obvious and dramatic, with zones of periventricular increased density on T2-weighted images and patchy white-matter abnormalities.[143,148,161] Figure 8-15 is an MRI of a patient with Binswanger white-matter abnormalities. I prefer not to use the term leuko-araiosis for these white-matter changes. Leuko-araiosis is a

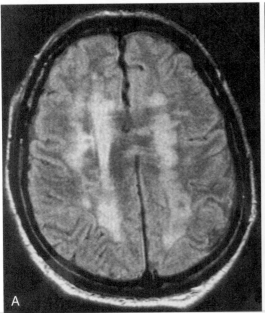 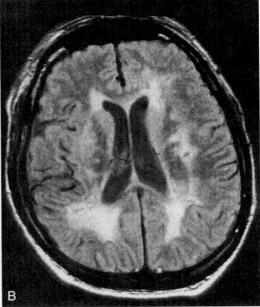

Figure 8-15. MRI T2-weighted images. Axial sections (**A**) and (**B**) show increased signal around the ventricles and large areas of abnormal signal in the white matter of the centrum semiovale in a patient with Binswanger disease.

general term and many patients with white-matter abnormalities do not have vascular disease. Several different patterns of white-matter abnormalities include (1) caps that occur around the ventricular system, especially in the region of the anterior horns and the occipital region; (2) a rim of abnormal white matter signal often surrounds the ventricle diffusely or more focally; and (3) discrete, small foci or patchy or confluent regions of abnormal signal are also noted and vary from single to many lesions. Awad and colleagues attempted to correlate these various lesions with the neuropathology.[11] In general, diffuse periventricular rims represent gliosis that is probably caused by transependymal flow of cerebrospinal fluid.[11] Tiny foci often are caused by état criblé. Lesions in the centrum semiovale and corona radiata are generally regions of chronic partial ischemia.[11]

Pathogenesis of Lacunar Infarcts and Chronic White-Matter Abnormalities

The mechanism of discrete infarcts in the territory of a single penetrating artery is quite straightforward. The compromised penetrator has a reduced luminal size and further obstruction of the lumen by plaque, microdissection, or thrombus diminishes blood flow in the brain region supplied by that penetrator. Hemorheologic factors could also reduce flow in that penetrator sufficiently to cause an infarct.

The mechanism of white-matter abnormalities larger than the territory of a single penetrator is more difficult to explain, and may have a number of different mechanisms. The two major types of posited mechanisms involve either ischemia or vascular permeability.

1. Ischemia related to tandem penetrating arterial lesions. This explanation posits severe flow limiting luminal compromise involving a number of parallel penetrating arteries. Then, hemorheologic changes that reduce cerebral blood flow could produce ischemia and white-matter damage in an area supplied by the group of compromised arteries. Cerebral blood-flow reduction could be caused by: decreased blood pressure, diminished cardiac output, decreased blood volume, or increased whole-blood viscosity. Similarly, consider the circumstance of several penetrators that were previously occluded or nearly occluded, and a single penetrator had provided collateral circulation to the region supplied by the previously compromised penetrators. Then the penetrator that supplied collateral flow

becomes occluded. The resulting infarct would be larger than the supply of any of the individual penetrators.
2. Increased vascular permeability. Leakage of fluid, transudation, could occur when the blood pressure within the penetrating arteries is very high. This condition when acute is called *hypertensive encephalopathy*. This condition is characterized by transudation of fluid from small arteries and arterioles causing brain edema as well as petechial and sometimes larger intracerebral hemorrhages. When chronic, the transudated fluid could cause gliosis and damage to the cerebral white matter and basal ganglia. Some have posited that white-matter damage is due to a chronic or recurrent hypertensive encephalopathy.

Some patients with chronic white-matter abnormalities do not have important hypertension. The media and adventitia may, in these patients, become so abnormal that fluid leaks from the damaged arteries even when the blood pressure in the arteries is normal.

Some studies support each of these two posited mechanisms. Yamamoto and colleagues analyzed the results of 24-hour blood-pressure monitoring among Japanese patients with lacunar infarcts and subcortical white-matter abnormalities.[163-165] Poor control of blood pressure with high-average ambulatory blood pressures and reduced nighttime dips in blood pressure indicating excessive night time blood pressure predicted progression of both lacunar infarcts and white-matter lesions. Others have also shown the importance of too-high and too-low blood pressures on progression of white-matter lesions and lacunar infarcts.[166,167] Suboptimal treatment of hypertension can clearly contribute to worsening of white-matter abnormalities.

Increased whole-blood viscosity and fibrinogen levels are present in many patients with chronic severe white-matter abnormalities and Binswanger disease.[143,168,169] Increased blood viscosity and slow flow through the microvasculature could compound the vascular lesions, leading to hypoperfusion in the territories of deep penetrating arteries.

Rosenberg and colleagues have shown the importance of matrix metalloproteins in understanding vascular permeability.[170-172] Matrix metalloproteinase-9 levels are significantly elevated in the white matter and cerebrospinal fluid of patients with Binswanger-type pathology.[170,171] Matrix metalloproteinases disrupt the blood-brain barrier by degrading tight junction proteins found within blood vessels.[172] These increased levels of metalloproteinases in thickened penetrating arteries could promote leakage of fluid from these blood vessels. Chronic edema in perivascular areas could stimulate gliosis.

Treatment

Treatment of the chronic microangiopathies is unknown. Clearly blood pressure control is very important. Twenty-four-hour ambulatory blood pressure monitoring is a very useful way to study blood pressure levels and variations. Nocturnal blood pressure may be very important. Impressed by the preliminary data about hyperviscosity, I have begun to treat patients with lacunar infarcts and chronic microvascular white-matter disease by attempting to reduce their hematocrits (by blood donation and stopping smoking) and by reducing their fibrinogen levels by prescribing eicosapentaenoic-rich fish oil preparations and other strategies. I also encourage liberal fluid intake.

This microvasculopathy must be differentiated from multiple infarcts caused by large-artery occlusive disease and from multiple cerebral emboli as causes of vascular dementia. In these two other conditions, most of the infarcts are cortical or cortical and subcortical, and the history usually includes acute strokes. In these latter causes of vascular dementia, extracranial and transcranial ultrasound, echocardiography, cardiac rhythm monitoring, hematologic screening for coagulopathies, and vascular imaging studies usually show a cardiac-origin embolic source or multiple large-artery occlusive disease.

References

1. Fisher CM: Lacunes, small deep cerebral infarcts. Neurology 1965;15:774-784.
2. Fisher CM: The arterial lesions underlying lacunes. Acta Neuropathol 1969;12:1-15.
3. Besson G, Hommel M: Historical aspects of lacunes and the "lacunar controversy". In Pullicino PM, Caplan LR, Hommel M (eds): Cerebral Small Artery Disease. New York: Raven Press, 1993, pp 1-10.
4. Hauw J-J: The History of Lacunes. In Donnan G, Norrving B, Bamford J, Bogousslavsky J (eds): Lacunar and Other Subcortical Infarcts. Oxford: Oxford University Press, 1995, pp 3-15.
5. Durand-Fardel M: Traite des ramollissements du cerveau. Paris: Bailliere, 1843.
6. Ferrand J: Essai Sur l'Hemiplegie des Vieillards: Les Lacunes de Desintegration Cerebrale [thesis]. University of Paris, Paris, 1902.
7. Marie P: Des foyers lacunaires de desintegration et des differents autres etats cavitaires du cerveau. Rev Med (Paris) 1901;21:281.
8. Foix C, Levy M: Les ramollissements sylviens. Rev Neurol 1927;43:1-51.
9. Foix C, Hillemand P: Contribution a l'etude des ramollisements protuberantiels. Rev Med 1926;43:287-305.
10. Caplan LR: Charles Foix-the first modern stroke neurologist. Stroke 1990;21:348-356.
11. Awad I, Johnson PC, Spetzler RF, Hodak JA: Incidental subcortical lesions identified on magnetic resonance imaging in the elderly: II. Postmortem pathological correlations. Stroke 1986;17:1090-1097.
12. Fisher CM: Pure motor hemiplegia of vascular origin. Arch Neurol 1965;13:30-44.
13. Fisher CM: Pathological observations in hypertensive cerebral hemorrhage. J Neuropathol Exp Neurol 1971;30:536-550.
14. Fisher CM: Cerebral miliary aneurysms in hypertension. Am J Pathol 1972;66:313-324.
15. Cole F, Yates P: Intracerebral microaneurysms and small cerebrovascular lesions. Brain 1966;90:759-767.
16. Rosenblum WJ: Miliary aneurysms and "fibrinoid" degeneration of cerebral blood vessels. Hum Pathol 1977;8:133-139.
17. Baudrimont M, Dubas F, Joutel A: Autosomal dominant leukoencephalopathy and subcortical ischemic strokes: A clinicopathological study. Stroke 1993;24:122-125.
18. Lammie GA, Rakshi J, Rossor MN, et al: Cerebral autosomal dominant arteriopathy with subcortical infarcts and leukoencephalopathy—Confirmation by cerebral biopsy in e cases. Clin Neuropathol 1995;14:201-206.
19. Chabriat H, Bousser M-G: Cerebral autosomal dominant arteriopathy with subcortical infarcts and leukoencephalopathy. In Donnan G, Norrving B, Bamford J, Bogousslavsky J (eds): Subcortical Stroke, 2nd ed. Oxford: Oxford University Press, 2002, pp 111-120.
20. Charcot J, Bouchard C: Nouvelles recherches sur la pathogenie de l'hemorrhagie erebrale. Arch Phys Norm Pathol 1868;1:110-127, 643-665.
20a. Gould DB, Phalan FC, Breedveld GI, et al: Mutations in Col4a1 cause perinatal cerebral hemorrhage and porencephaly. Science 2005;308:1167-1171.
20b. van der Knaap MS, Smit LM, Barkhof F, et al: Neonatal porencephaly and adult stroke related to mutations in collagen IVA1. Ann Neurol 2006;59:504-511.
20c. Gould DB, Phalan FC, van Mil SE, et al: Role of Col4A1 in small-vessel disease and hemorrhagic stroke. N Engl J Med 2006;354:1489-1496.
20d. Plaisir E, Gribouval O, Alamowitch S, et al: Col4A1 mutations and hereditary angiopathy, nephropathy, aneurysms, and muscle cramps. N Engl J Med 2007;357:2687-2695.
21. Düret H: Conclusion d'un memorie sur la circulation bulbaire. Arch Phys Norm Pathol 1873;50:88-89.
22. Düret H: Recherches anatomiques sur la circulation de l'encephale. Arch Phys Norm Pathol 1874;1:60-91, 316-353.

23. Foix C, Hillemand P: Irrigation de la protuberance. Compt Rendu Soc Biol (Paris) 1925; 42:35-37.

24. Foix C, Hillemand P: Les arteres de l'axe encephalique jusqu'a diencephale inclusivement. Rev Neurol 1925;41:705-739.

25. Foix C, Hillemand P: Irrigation du bulbe. Compt Rendu Soc Biol (Paris) 1924;42:33-35.

26. Stopford J: The arteries of the pons and medulla oblongata: I. J Anat Physiol 1915;50:131-164.

27. Stopford J: The arteries of the pons and medulla oblongata: II. J Anat Physiol 1916;50:255-280.

28. Pullicino PM: The course and territories of cerebral small arteries. In Pullicino PM, Caplan LR, Hommel M (eds): Cerebral Small Artery Disease. New York: Raven Press, 1993, pp 11-39.

29. Pullicino PM: Diagrams of perforating artery territories in axial, coronal, and sagittal planes. In Pullicino PM, Caplan LR, Hommel M (eds): Cerebral Small Artery Disease. New York: Raven Press, 1993, pp 41-72.

30. Fisher CM, Caplan LR: Basilar artery branch occlusion: A cause of pontine infarction. Neurology 1971;21:900-905.

31. Fisher CM: Bilateral occlusion of basilar artery branches. J Neurol Neurosurg Psychiatry 1977;40:1182-1189.

32. Caplan LR: Intracranial branch atheromatous disease: A neglected, understudied and underused concept. Neurology 1989;39:1246-1250.

33. Ostrow PT, Miller LL: Pathology of Small Artery Disease. In Pullicino PM, Caplan LR, Hommel M (eds): PM Pullicino, LR Caplan, M Hommel (eds): Cerebral Small Artery Disease. New York: Raven Press, 1993, pp 93-123.

34. Klein IF, Lavallee PC, Touboul P-J, et al: In vivo middle cerebral artery plaque imaging by high-resolution MRI. Neurology 2006;67:327-329.

35. Lam WW, Wong KS, So NM, et al: Plaque volume measurement by magnetic resonance imaging as an index of remodeling of middle cerebral artery: Correlation with transcranial color Doppler and magnetic resonance angiography. Cerebrovasc Dis 2004;17:166-169.

36. Klein IF, Lavallee PC, Schouman-Claeys E, Amaraenco P: High-resolution MRI identifies basilar artery plaques in paramedian pontine infarct. Neurology 2005;64:551-552.

37. Peress N, Kane W, Aronson S: Central nervous system findings in a tenth-decade autopsy population. Prog Brain Res 1973;40:473-484.

38. Bang OY, Heo JH, Kim JY, et al: Middle cerebral artery stenosis is a major clinical determinant in striatocapsular deep infarction. Arch Neurol 2002;59:259-263.

39. Wong KS, Gao S, Chan YL, et al: Mechanisms of acute cerebral infarctions in patients with middle cerebral artery stenosis: A diffusion-weighted imaging and microemboli monitoring study. Ann Neurol 2002;52:74-81.

40. Bang OY, Joo SY, Lee PH, et al: The course of patients with lacunar infarcts and a parent arterial lesion: Similarities to large artery vs small artery disease. Arch Neurol 2004;61:514-519.

41. Baumgartner RW, Sidler C, Mosso M, Georgiadis D: Ischemic lacunar stroke in patients with and without potential mechanism other than small-artery disease. Stroke 2003;34:653-659.

42. Boiten J: Lacunar Stroke: A Prospective Clinical and Radiologic Study [thesis]. Maastricht, 1991.

43. Norrving B, Cronqvist S: Clinical and radiologic features of lacunar versus nonlacunar minor stroke. Stroke 1989;20:59-64.

44. Pullicino P, Nelson R, Kendall B, et al: Small deep infarcts diagnosed on computed tomography. Neurology 1980;30:1090-1096.

45. Weisberg L: Computed tomography and pure motor hemiparesis. Neurology 1979;29:490-495.

46. Donnan G, Tress B, Bladin P: A prospective study of lacunar infarction using computed tomography. Neurology 1982;32:47-56.

47. Mohr JP, Caplan LR, Melski J: The Harvard Cooperative Stroke Registry: A prospective registry. Neurology 1978;28:754-762.

48. Tuszynski MH, Petito CK, Levy DB: Risk factors and clinical manifestations of pathologically verified lacunar infarctions. Stroke 1989;20: 990-999.

48a. Labovitz DL, Boden-Albala B, Hauser WA, Sacco RL: Lacunar infarct or deep intracerebral hemorrhage. Who gets which? The Northern Manhattan Study. Neurology 2007;68:606-608.

48b. Ikram MA, Vernooji MW, Hofman A, et al: Kidney function is related to cerebral small vessel disease. Stroke 2008;39:55-61.

48c. Pico F, Labreuche J, Seilhean D, et al: Association of small-vessel disease with dilatative arteriopathy of the brain. Neuropathologic evidence. Stroke 2007;38:1197-1202.

49. Caplan LR, Young R: EEG findings in certain lacunar stroke syndromes. Neurology 1972;22:403.

50. Mohr JP: Lacunes. Stroke 1982;13:3-11.

51. Miller V: Lacunar stroke, a reassessment. Arch Neurol 1983;40:129-134.

52. Rascol A, Clanet M, Manelfe C, et al: Pure motor hemiplegia: CT study of 30 cases. Stroke 1982;13:11-17.

53. Donnan GA, O'Malley HM, Quang L, et al: The capsular warning syndrome and lacunar TIAs. In Donnan G, Norrving B, Bamford J, Bogousslavsky J (eds): Subcortical Stroke, 2nd ed. Oxford: Oxford University Press, 2002, pp 175-184.

54. Steinke W, Ley S: Lacunar stroke is the major cause of progressive motor deficits. Stroke 2002;33:1510-1516.

55. Caplan LR: Worsening in ischemic stroke patients: Is it time for a new strategy? Stroke 2002;33:1443-1445.

56. Nelson R, Pullicino P, Kendall B, et al: Computed tomography in patients presenting with lacunar syndromes. Stroke 1980;11: 256-261.

57. Richter R, Bruse J, Bruun B, et al: Frequency and course of pure motor hemiparesis: A clinical study. Stroke 1977;8:58-60.

58. Gobernado JM, de Molina AR, Gimeno A: Pure motor hemiplegia due to hemorrhage in the lower pons. Arch Neurol 1980;37:393.

59. Mori E, Tabuchi M, Yamadori A: Lacunar syndrome due to intracerebral hemorrhage. Stroke 1985;16:454-459.

60. Kase CS: Subcortical haemorrhages. In Donnan G, Norrving B, Bamford J, Bogousslavsky J (eds): Subcortical Stroke, 2nd ed. Oxford: Oxford University Press, 2002, pp 347-377.

61. Hommel M, Besson G, LeBas JF, et al: Prospective study of lacunar infarction using magnetic resonance imaging. Stroke 1990;21:546-554.

62. Besson G: Les Infarctus Lacunaires: Evaluation Clinique et par l'Imagerie par Resonance Magnetique [thesis]. University of Grenoble, France, 1989.

63. Kase CS, Wolf PA, Hier DB, et al: Lacunar infarcts: Clinical and CT aspects. The Stroke Data Bank experience. Neurology 1986;36:178-179.

64. Dejerine J, Dejerine-Klumpke H: Anatomie des Centres Nerveux, vol 2. Paris: Rueff, 1901.

65. Fisher CM, Cole M: Homolateral ataxia and crural paresis, a vascular syndrome. J Neurol Neurosurg Psychiatry 1965;28:48-55.

66. Fisher CM: Ataxic hemiparesis. Arch Neurol 1978;35:126-128.

67. Helgason CM, Wilbur AC: Capsular hypesthetic ataxic hemiparesis. Stroke 1990;21:24-33.

68. Goldblatt D, Markesbury W, Reeves AG: Recurrent hemichorea following striatal lesions. Arch Neurol 1974;32:51-54.

69. Kase C, Maulsby G, DeJaun E: Hemichorea-hemiballism and lacunar infarction in the basal ganglia. Neurology 1981;31:452-455.

70. Helgason C, Wilbur A, Weiss A, et al: Acute pseudobulbar mutism due to discrete bilateral capsular infarction in the territory of the anterior choroidal artery. Brain 1988;111:507-524.

71. Caplan LR, Schmahmann JD, Kase CS, et al: Caudate infarcts. Arch Neurol 1990;47:133-143.

72. Caplan LR: Caudate infarcts. In Donnan G, Norrving B, Bamford J, Bogousslavsky J (eds): Subcortical Stroke, 2nd ed. Oxford: Oxford University Press, 2002, pp 209-223.

73. Fisher FM: Capsular infarcts. Arch Neurol 1979;36:65-73.

74. Helgason C, Caplan LR, Goodwin J, Hedges T: Anterior choroidal artery territory infarction: Case reports and review. Arch Neurol 1986;43:681-686.

75. Mohr JP, Steinke W, Timsit SG, et al: The anterior choroidal artery does not supply the corona radiata and lateral ventricular wall. Stroke 1991;22:1502-1507.

76. Caplan LR: Anterior choroidal artery territory infarcts. In Donnan G, Norrving B, Bamford J, Bogousslavsky J (eds): Subcortical Stroke, 2nd ed. Oxford: Oxford University Press, 2002, pp 225-240.

77. Kumral E, Evyapan D, Balkir K: Acute caudate vascular lesions. Stroke 1999;30:100-108.

78. Mendez M, Adams N, Lewandowski K: Neurobehavioral changes associated with caudate lesions. Neurology 1989;39:349-354.

79. Caplan LR: Posterior Circulation Disease: Clinical Findings, Diagnosis, and Management. Boston: Blackwell Science, 1996.

80. Bassetti C, Bogousslavsky J, Barth A, Regli F: Isolated infarcts of the pons. Neurology 1996;46:165-175.

81. Rothrock JF, Lyden PD, Hesselink JF, et al: Brain magnetic resonance imaging in the evaluation of lacunar stroke. Stroke 1987;18:781-786.

82. Leestra JE, Noronha A: Pure motor hemiplegia, medullary pyramid lesion, and olivary hypertrophy 1976;39:877-884.

83. Ropper AH, Fisher CM, Kleinman GM: Pyramidal infarction in the medulla: A cause of pure motor hemiplegia sparing the face. Neurology 1979;29:91-95.

84. Milandre L, Arnaud O, Khalil R: Infarction of the medullary pyramid identified on MRI. Cerebrovasc Dis 1992;2:183-184.

84a. Ho KL, Meyer KR: The medial medullary syndrome. Arch Neurol 1981;38:385-387.

85. Kataoka S, Hori A, Shirakawa T, Hirose G: Paramedian pontine infarction, neurological/topographical correlation. Stroke 1997;28:809-815.

86. Kim JS, Lee JH, Im JH, Lee MC: Syndromes of pontine base infarction, a clinical-radiological correlation study. Stroke 1995;26:950-955.

87. Fisher CM: A lacunar stroke, the dysarthria-clumsy hand syndrome. Neurology 1967;17:614-617.

88. Chung C-S, Caplan LR: Pontine infarcts and hemorrhages. In Bogousslavsky J, Caplan LR (eds): Stroke Syndromes, 2nd ed. Cambridge: Cambridge University Press, 2001, pp 520-533.

89. Helgason CM, Wilbur AC: Basilar branch pontine infarctions with prominent sensory signs. Stroke 1991;22:1129-1136.

90. Caplan LR, Goodwin J: Lateral segmental brainstem hemorrhages. Neurology 1982;32:252-260.

91. Shintani S, Tsuroka S, Shiigai T: Pure sensory stroke caused by a pontine infarct. Clinical, radiological, and physiological features in four patients. Stroke 1994;25:1512-1515.

92. Kim JS, Bae YH: Pure or predominant sensory stroke due to brainstem lesion. Stroke 1997;28:1761-1764.

93. Ho K-L: Pure motor hemiplegia due to infarction of the cerebral peduncle. Arch Neurol 1982;39:524-526.

94. Bogousslavsky J, Maeder P, Regli F, et al: Pure midbrain infarction: Clinical syndromes, MRI, and etiologic patterns. Neurology 1994;44:2032-2040.

95. Martin PJ, Chang H-M, Wityk R, Caplan LR: Midbrain infarction: Associations and aetiologies in the New England Medical Center posterior circulation registry. J Neurol Neurosurg Psychiatry 1998;64:392-395.

96. Hommel M, Besson G: Midbrain infarcts. In Bogousslavsky J, Caplan LR (eds): Stroke Syndromes, 2nd ed. Cambridge: Cambridge University Press, 2001, pp 512-519.

97. Hommel B, Besson G, Pollak P, et al: Hemiplegia in posterior cerebral artery occlusion. Neurology 1990;40:1496-1499.

97a. Mossuto-Agatiello L: Caudal paramedian midbrain syndrome. Neurology 2006;66:1668-1671.

97b. Sato S, Toyoda K, Kawase K, et al: A caudal mesencephalic infarct presenting only tetra-ataxia and tremor. Cerebrovasc Dis 2008;25:187-189.

98. Castaigne P, Lhermitte F, Buge A, et al: Paramedian thalamic and midbrain infarcts: Clinical and neuropathological study. Ann Neurol 1981;10:127-148.

99. Percheron G: Les arteres du thalamus humain: II. Arteres et territoires thalamique paramedians de l'arterie basilarie communicante. Rev Neurol (Paris) 1976;132:309-324.

100. Barth A, Bogousslavsky J, Caplan LR: Thalamic infarcts and hemorrhages. In Bogousslavsky J, Caplan LR (eds): Stroke Syndromes, 2nd ed. Cambridge: Cambridge University Press, 2001, pp 461-468.

101. Bogousslavsky J, Miklossy J, Deruaz J, et al: Unilateral left paramedian infarction of thalamus and midbrain: A clinicopathological study. J Neurol Neurosurg Psychiatry 1986;49:686-694.

102. Graff-Radford NR, Damasio H, Yamada T, et al: Nonhaemorrhagic thalamic infarction. Brain 1985;108:495-516.

103. Bogousslavsky J, Regli F, Assal G: The syndrome of tuberothalamic artery territory infarction. Stroke 1986;17:434-441.

104. Bogousslavsky J, Regli F, Uske A: Thalamic infarcts: Clinical syndromes, etiology, and prognosis. Neurology 1988;38:837-848.

105. Tatemichi T, Steinke W, Duncan C, et al: Paramedian thalamo-peduncular infarction: Clinical syndromes and magnetic resonance imaging. Ann Neurol 1992;32:162-171.

106. Bogousslavsky J, Caplan LR: Vertebrobasilar occlusive disease, review of selected aspects. III: Thalamic infarcts. Cerebrovasc Dis 1993;3:193-205.

107. de Freitas GR, Bogousslavsky J: Thalamic infarcts. In Donnan G, Norrving B, Bamford J, Bogousslavsky J (eds): Subcortical Stroke, 2nd ed. Oxford: Oxford University Press, 2002, pp 255-285.

108. Kaplan RF, Estol CJ, Damasio H, et al: Bilateral polar artery thalamic infarcts. Neurology 1991;41(suppl 1):329.

109. Wall M, Slamovits TL, Weisberg LA, Trufant SA: Vertical gaze ophthalmoplegia from infarction in the area of the posterior thalamo-subthalamic paramedian artery. Stroke 1986;17:546-555.

110. Meissner I, Sapir S, Kokmen E, Stein SD: The paramedian diencephalic syndrome: A dynamic phenomenon. Stroke 1987;18:380-385.

111. Caplan LR, DeWitt LD, Pessin MS, et al: Lateral thalamic infarcts. Arch Neurol 1988;45:959-964.

112. Dejerine J, Roussy G: Le syndrome thalamique. Rev Neurol 1906;14:521-532.

113. Fisher CM: Pure sensory stroke involving face, arm, and leg. Neurology 1965;15:76-80.

114. Fisher CM: Thalamic pure sensory stroke: A pathologic study. Neurology 1978;28:1141-1144.

115. Fisher CM: Pure sensory stroke and allied conditions. Stroke 1982;13:434-447.

116. Fisher CM: Lacunar strokes and infarcts: A review. Neurology 1982;32:871-876.

117. Hommel M, Besson G, Pollak P, et al: Pure sensory stroke due to a pontine lacune. Stroke 1989;20:406-408.

118. Mohr JP, Kase C, Meckler R, et al: Sensorimotor stroke. Arch Neurol 1977;34:734-741.

119. Mohr JP, Timsit S: Choroidal artery disease. In Barnett HJM, Mohr JP, Stein BM, Yatsu F (eds): Stroke, Pathophysiology, Diagnosis, and Management, 3rd ed. New York: Churchill Livingstone, 1998, pp 503-512.

120. Besson G, Bogousslavsky J, Regli F: Posterior choroidal-artery infarct with homonymous horizontal sectoranopia. Cerebrovasc Dis 1991;1:117-120.

121. Frisen I, Holmegaard L, Rosencrantz M: Sectorial optic atrophy and homonymous, horizontal sectoranopia: A lateral posterior choroidal artery syndrome. J Neurol Neurosurg Psychiatry 1978;41:374-380.

122. Neau JP, Bogousslavsky J: The syndrome of posterior choroidal artery territory infarction. Ann Neurol 1996;39:779-788.

123. Adams H, Damasio H, Putnam S, et al: Middle cerebral artery occlusion as a cause of isolated subcortical infarction. Stroke 1983;14:948-952.

124. Maki G, Mihara H, Shizuka M, et al: CT and arteriographic comparison of patients with transient ischemic attacks: Correlation with small infarcts of basal ganglia. Stroke 1983;14:276-280.

125. Caplan LR, Babikian V, Helgason C, et al: Occlusive disease of the middle cerebral artery. Neurology 1985;35:975-982.

126. Bogousavsky J, Regli F, Maeder P: Intracranial large-artery disease and "lacunar" infarction. Cerebrovasc Dis 1991;1:154-159.

127. Miyashita K, Naritomi H, Sawada T, et al: Identification of recent lacunar lesions in cases of multiple small infarction by magnetic resonance imaging. Stroke 1988;29:834-839.

127a. Bang OY, Yeo SH, Yoon JH, et al: Clinical MRI cutoff points for predicting lacunar stroke may not exist: Need for a grading rather than a dichotomized system. Cerebrovasc Dis 2007;24:520-529.

127b. Rajajee V, Kidwell C, Starkman S, et al: Diagnosis of lacunar infarcts within 6 hours of onset by clinical and CT criteria versus MRI. UCLA MRI Acute Stroke Investigators. J Neuroimag 2008;18:66-72.

128. Faris A, Poser C, Wilmore D, et al: Radiologic visualization of neck vessels in healthy men. Neurology 1963;13:386-396.

129. Takahashi W, Fujii H, Ide M, et al: Atherosclerotic changes in intracranial and extracranial large arteries in apparently healthy persons with asymptomatic lacunar infarction. J Stroke Cerebrovasc Dis 2005;14:17-22.

130. Lodder J, Bamford J, Kappelle J, Boiten J: What causes false clinical prediction of small deep infarcts. Stroke 1994;25:86-91.

131. National Institute of Neurological Disorders and Stroke rt-PA Study Group: Tissue plasminogen activator for acute ischemic stroke. N Engl J Med 1995;333:1581-1587.

132. Ingall TJ, O'Fallon WM, Asplund K, et al: Findings from the reanalysis of the NINDS tissue plasminogen activator for acute ischemic stroke treatment trial. Stroke 2004;35:2418-2424.

133. Dobkin B: Heparin for lacunar stroke in progression. Stroke 1983;14:421-423.

134. Yamamoto Y, Akiguchi I, Oiwa K, et al: Twenty-four-hour blood pressure and MRI as predictive factors for different outcomes in patients with lacunar infarct. Stroke 2002;33:297-305.

135. Walters M, Muir S, Shah I, Lees K: Effect of perindopril on cerebral vasomotor reactivity in patients with lacunar infarction. Stroke 2004;35:1899-1902.

136. Mohr JP, Thompson JLP, Lazar RM, et al: A comparison of warfarin and aspirin for the prevention of recurrent ischemic stroke. Warfarin-Aspirin Recurrent Stroke Study Group. N Engl J Med 2001;345:1444-1451.

137. Diener HC, Cunha L, Forbes C, et al: European Stroke Prevention Study 2. Dipyridamole and acetylsalicylic acid in the secondary prevention of stroke. J Neurol Sci 1996;143:1-13.

138. Gotoh F, Tohgi H, Hirai S, et al: Cilostazole Stroke Prevention Study: A placebo-controlled double-blind trial for secondary prevention of cerebral infarction. J Stroke Cerebrovasc Dis 2000;9:147-157.

139. Carod-Artal FJ: Statins and cerebral vasomotor reactivity. Implications for a new therapy. Stroke 2006;37:2446-2448.

140. Pretnar-Oblak J, Sabovic M, Sebestjen M, et al: The influence of atorvastatin treatment on L-arginine cerbrovascualr reactivity and flow-mediated dilatation in patients with lacunar infarction. Stroke 2006;37:2540-2545.

140a. Intravenous Magnesium Efficacy in Stroke (IMAGES) Study Investigators: Magnesium for acute stroke (Intravenous Magnesium Efficacy in Stroke trial): Randomized controlled trial. Lancet 2004;363;439-445.

140b. Aslanyan S, Weir CJ, Muir KW, Lees KR: Magnesium for treatment of acute lacunar stroke syndromes. Further analysis of the IMAGES trial. Stroke 2007;38:1269-1273.

141. Hachinski V, Potter P, Merskey H: Leuko-araiosis. Arch Neurol 1987;44:21-23.

142. Okeda R: Morphometrische Vergleichsuntersuchungen an Hirnarterien bei Binswangerscher Encephalopathie und Hochdruckencephalopathie. Acta Neuropathol (Berlin) 1973;26:23-43.

143. Caplan LR: Binswanger's disease-revisited. Neurology 1995;45:626-633.

144. Binswanger O: Die abgrenzung der allgemeinen progressiven paralyse. Klin Wochenschr 1894;49:1103-1105, 1895;50:1137-1139, and 1895;52:1180-1186.

145. Blass JP, Hoyer S, Nitsch R: A translation of Otto Binswanger's article: The delineation of the generalized progressive paralysis. Arch Neurol 1991;48:961-972.

146. Olszewski J: Subcortical arteriosclerotic encephalopathy. World Neurol 1965;3:359-374.

147. Caplan LR, Schoene WC: Clinical features of subcortical arteriosclerotic encephalopathy (Binswanger's disease). Neurology 1978;28:1206-1215.

148. Babikian V, Ropper AH: Binswanger disease: A review. Stroke 1987;18:1-12.

149. Fisher CM: Binswanger's encephalopathy: A review. J Neurol 1989;236:65-79.

150. Ward NS, Brown MM: Leukoaraiosis. In Donnan G, Norrving B, Bamford J, Bogousslavsky J (eds): Subcortical Stroke, 2nd ed. Oxford: Oxford University Press, 2002, pp 47-66.

150a. Maclullich AM, Wardlaw JM, Ferguson KJ, et al: Enlarged perivascular spaces are associated with cognitive function in healthy elderly men. J Neurol Neurosurg Psychiatry 2004;75:1519-1523.

150b. Kim D-G, Oh S-H, Kim J: A case of disseminated polycystic dilated perivascular spaces presenting with dementia and parkinsonism. J Clin Neurol 2007;32:96-100.

151. Gray F, Dubas F, Roullet E, Escourolle R: Leukoencephalopathy in diffuse hemorrhagic cerebral amyloid angiopathy. Ann Neurol 1985;18:54-59.

152. Dubas F, Gray F, Roullet E, Escourolle R: Leukoencephalopathies arteriopathiques. Rev Neurol 1985;141:93-108.

153. Loes D, Biller J, Yuh WT, et al: Leukoencephalopathy in cerebral amyloid angiopathy: MR imaging in four cases. AJNR Am J Neuroradiol 1990;11:485-488.

154. DeWitt LD, Louis DN: Case records of the Massachusetts General Hospital: Case 27-1991. N Engl J Med 1991;325:42-54.

155. Fountain NB, Eberhard DA: Primary angiitis of the central nervous system associated with cerebral amyloid angiopathy: Report of two cases and review of the literature. Neurology 1996;46:190-197.

156. Caplan LR: Case records of the Massachusetts General Hospital. Case 10-2000. N Engl J Med 2000;342:957-964.

157. Baudrimont M, Dubas F, Joutel A, et al: Autosomal dominat leukoencephalopathy and subcortical ischemic stroke: A clinicopathological study. Stroke 1993;24:122-125.

158. Davous P: CADASIL: A review with proposed diagnostic criteria. Eur J Neurology 1998;5:219-233.

159. Dichgans M, Mayer M, Uttner I, et al: The phenotypic spectrum of CADASIL: Clinical findings in 102 cases. Ann Neurol 1998;44:731-739.

160. Tournier-Lasserve E, Joutel A, Melki J, et al: Cerebral autosomal dominant arteriopathy with subcortical infarcts and leukoencephalopathy maps on chromosome 19q12. Nat Gen 1993;3:256-259.

161. Chabriat H, Levy C, Taillia H, et al: Patterns of MRI lesions in CADACIL. Neurology 1998;51:452-457.

162. Greenberg SM, Vonsattel JPG, Stakes JW, et al: The clinical spectrum of cerebral amyloid angiopathy: Presentations without lobar hemorrhage. Neurology 1993;43:2073-2079.

162a. Scolding NJ, Joseph J, Kirby PA, et al: Alpha-Beta related angiitis: Primary angiitis of the central nervous system associated with cerebral amyloid angiopathy. Brain 2005;128:500-515.

162b. Eng JA, Frosch MP, Choi K, et al: Clinical manifestations of cerebral amyloid-related inflammation. Ann Neurol 2004;55:250-256.

162c. Caplan LR: (Case Record of the Massachusetts General Hospital) Case 10-2000. N Engl J Med 2000;342:957-964.

162d. Ginsberg L, Geddes J, Valentine A: Amyloid angiopathy and granulomatous angiitis of the central nervous system: A case responding to corticosteroid treatment. J Neurol 1998;235:438-440.

162e. McHugh JC, Ryan AM, Lynch T, et al: Steroid-responsive recurrent emcephalopathy in a patient with cerebral amyloid angiopathy. Cerebrovasc Dis 2007;23:66-69.

163. Yamamoto Y, Akiguchi I, Oiwa K, et al: Adverse effect of nightime blood pressure on the outcome of lacunar infarct patients. Stroke 1998;29:570-576.

164. Yamamoto Y, Akiguchi I, Oiwa K, et al: Twenty-four-hour blood pressure and MRI as predictive factors for different outcomes in patients with lacunar infarct. Stroke 2002;33:297-305.

165. Yamamoto Y, Akiguchi I, Oiwa K, et al: The relationship between 24-hour blood pressure readings, subcortical ischemic lesions and vascular dementia. Cerebrovasc Dis 2005;19:302-308.

166. Hoshide Y, Kario K, Schwartz JE, et al: Incomplete benefit of antihypertensive therapy on stroke reduction in older hypertensives with abnormal nocturnal blood pressure dipping (extreme-dippers and reverse-dippers). Am J Hypertens 2002;15:844-850.

167. Chamorro A, Pujol J, Saiz A, et al: Periventricular white matter lucencies in patients with lacunar stroke. A marker of too high or too low blood pressure. Arch Neurol 1997;54:1284-1288.

168. Schneider R, Ringelstein EB, Zeumer H, et al: The role of plasma hyperviscosity in subcortical arteriosclerotic encephalopathy (Binswanger's disease). J Neurol 1987;234:67-73.

169. Chung C-S, Caplan LR, van Swieten J, et al: White matter changes in stroke and fibrinogen levels. Ann Neurol 1993;34:260.

170. Rosenberg GA, Sullivan N, Esiri MM: White matter damage is associated with matrix metalloproteinases in vascular dementia. Stroke 2001;32:1162-1168.

171. Adair JC, Charlie J, Dencoff JE, et al: Measurement of gelatinase B (MMP-9) in the cerebrospinal fluid of patients with vascular dementia and Alzheimer disease. Stroke 2004;35: e159-162.

172. Yang Y, Estrada EY, Thompson JF, et al: Matrix metalloproteinase-mediated disruption of tight junction proteins in cerebral vessels is reversed by synthetic matrix metalloproteinase inhibitor in focal ischemia in rat. J Cereb Blood Flow Metab 2007;27:697-709.

Embolism is the most common cause of brain ischemia. A variety of embolic particles arise from the heart, aorta, and cervicocranial arteries to reach the intracranial arteries, and other substances such as air, fat, tumor cells, and foreign objects are also occasionally introduced into the vascular system and reach the brain and other organs.[1] Doctors in the past thought that release of embolic materials into the circulation was unusual and had a high hit rate (i.e., that emboli reaching intracranial arteries had a strong likelihood of causing stroke and brain infarction). Newer diagnostic testing, including emboli monitoring using transcranial Doppler ultrasound (TCD), has shown high rates of brain embolism.[2-9] Embolic particles are often found in the circulation, but the hit rate is low.[9]

CLINICAL FINDINGS

Embolism requires a donor source and a recipient artery (see Fig. 2-5). The clinical presentation of a patient with brain embolism relates to the recipient site; symptoms and signs depend on the nature and size of the embolus, location of the recipient artery, and how long the embolus continues to block blood flow at the recipient site.[10] The recipient artery, of course, cannot distinguish the source and composition of the embolic material, nor do the clinical neurologic findings differ among emboli of cardiac, intra-arterial, or venous origin.

> A 31-year-old carpenter, TL, was evaluated after the sudden onset of confusion and right-hand weakness. The symptoms began suddenly at work. Three years earlier, he had what he called a minor stroke, characterized by numbness and weakness of the left arm and leg. Cerebral angiography was normal, but he was given warfarin during the 2 years after this event. Approximately 3 months after stopping coumadin, he had a brief attack of dizziness and veered to the left when he walked for approximately 1 week. He gave no history of cardiac or vascular disease, and examination of the heart and neck arteries was normal, except for a slight tachycardia. Blood pressure was 130/60 mm Hg. On neurologic examination, his speech was fluent but contained many paraphasic errors. He had difficulty repeating spoken language and he read,

wrote, and spelled poorly. His right arm was weak, and he could not recognize objects placed in his right hand. His left plantar response was extensor.

TL's recent event involved the left cerebral hemisphere and most likely included the precentral and postcentral gyri and the inferior parietal lobe. The event that occurred 3 years earlier was also of sudden onset and involved the right cerebral hemisphere. The dizziness and veering to one side probably represented ischemia in the left cerebellum. The three events in three different locations and vascular territories makes embolism by far the most likely diagnosis, but the source is not obvious from the clinical data.

Embolic strokes most often begin suddenly. The clinical signs evolve during seconds or a few minutes. The deficit may begin during physical activity but more often occurs during rest or activities of daily life.[10-12] Traditionally, the neurologic deficit in patients with embolic stroke is described as maximal at onset. As soon as an embolus blocks a recipient brain artery, collateral circulation begins to develop and some improvement may occur. Unlike thrombi formed locally at sites of prior atherosclerotic narrowing, emboli only loosely adhere to blood vessel walls. They readily fragment, dislodge, and move to more distal arteries. The breakup and distal movement of emboli strongly affects the subsequent clinical course. Movement of emboli most often occurs during the first 48 hours after symptom onset.

Fragmentation and distal movement of emboli before the development of irreversible brain damage allows reperfusion ("recanalization") of ischemic brain tissue and is usually accompanied by clinical improvement. In some patients, however, the embolus or its fragments block an important distal branch, leading to further ischemia and worsening of symptoms. For example, a patient with an embolus to the left mainstem middle cerebral artery (MCA) might have the sudden onset of aphasia and right hemiplegia and hemisensory loss. When the embolus passes and the lenticulostriate arteries supplying the internal capsule and basal ganglia regions are reperfused, the hemiparesis might improve. Increased cortical blood flow could lead to better language function. If the embolus passed into the inferior division of the MCA supplying the temporal lobe and occluded a temporal artery branch, the patient might then develop a fluent Wernicke-type aphasia. When there is further worsening after initial improvement in patients with embolism, the worsening usually occurs in a single step and nearly always occurs during the first 48 hours. Multiple, stepwise worsening; gradual, smooth worsening; and delayed worsening are unusual. Late worsening after 48 hours is explained by the development of brain edema or hemorrhage into the area of infarction because hemorrhagic transformation often occurs between days 2 and 7 after stroke onset.

Another pattern quite characteristic of brain embolism has been called *spectacular shrinking deficit* by Mohr.[13,14] This term describes sudden, complete or nearly complete clearing of sudden-onset severe neurologic signs. Most often, the patient has had rapid recanalization of a mainstem MCA or basilar artery embolus.[14]

Approximately four out of every five emboli that arise from the heart go into the anterior circulation equally divided between the two sides. The remaining one fifth of emboli go into the posterior circulation,[10-12,15-17] a rate about equal to the proportion of the blood supply that goes into the vertebrobasilar arteries. The recipient artery destination depends on the size and nature of the particles. Calcific particles from heart valves and mitral annular calcifications are less mobile and adapt less well to the shape of their recipient artery than red (erythrocyte-fibrin) and white (platelet-fibrin) thrombi. Figure 9-1 shows a red thrombus that was removed from the middle cerebral artery at necropsy. The circulating bloodstream seems able to somehow bypass,

obstructing cholesterol crystal emboli, especially in the retinal arteries.

Within the anterior and posterior circulations, there are predilection sites for the destination of embolic particles.[10,16-18] Large emboli entering a common carotid artery (CCA) could become lodged in the CCA or internal carotid artery (ICA), especially if atheromatous plaques had already narrowed the lumens of these arteries. If the emboli successfully traversed the ICAs in the neck, the next common lodging place is the intracranial bifurcation of the ICAs into the anterior cerebral arteries (ACAs) and MCAs. Arterial bifurcations are common resting places for emboli. Emboli that pass through the carotid intracranial bifurcations most often go into the MCAs and their branches. Gacs et al showed that balloon emboli placed in the circulation nearly always followed the same pathway and ended up in the MCAs and their branches.[16] Embolism in experimental animals caused by the introduction of silicone cylinders or spheres, elastic cylinders, and autologous blood clots also showed a high incidence of MCA-territory localization.[17] Emboli often pass into the superior and inferior divisions of the MCA and their cortical branches. The superior division supplies the cortex and white matter above the sylvian fissure, including the frontal and superior parietal lobes. The inferior division supplies the area below the sylvian fissure, including the temporal and inferior parietal lobes. TL's recent event most likely involved the inferior division of the left MCA. His first attack probably involved the right MCA. Emboli seldom go into the MCA penetrating artery (lenticulostriate arteries) branches because these arteries originate at a nearly 90-degree angle from the parent arteries.

Embolism into the MCAs can cause a variety of patterns of infarction[4,10] (see Fig. 2-36). Cortical and cortical-subcortical infarcts are most common. In young patients whose mainstem MCA is acutely occluded, the rapid development of collateral circulation over the convexity of the brain often leads to sparing of the superficial territory of the MCA. The lenticulostriate branches are blocked by the embolus in the mainstem MCA, and collateral circulation to the deep MCA territory is poor. The resultant infarct is limited to the basal ganglia and surrounding white matter and is usually called a striatocapsular infarct. Occasionally, emboli block an ACA or its distal branches, causing an infarct in the paramedian area of one frontal lobe.

Emboli that enter the posterior circulation can block the vertebral arteries in the neck or intracranially. Emboli that are able to pass through the intracranial vertebral arteries (ICVAs) usually pass through the proximal and middle portions of the

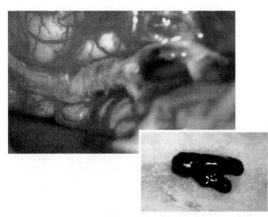

Figure 9-1. An embolus within the middle cerebral artery at necropsy. The inset shows the red thrombus removed from the artery. (From Caplan LR, Manning WJ: Brain Embolism. New York: Informa Healthcare, 2006, with permission.)

basilar artery, which are wider than the ICVAs. The basilar artery becomes narrower as it courses craniad. Emboli often block the distal basilar artery bifurcation (top of the basilar) or one of its branches—the penetrating arteries to the medial portions of the thalami and midbrain, the superior cerebellar artery (SCA), which supplies the upper surface of the cerebellum, and the posterior cerebral arteries (PCAs), which supply the lateral portions of the thalami and the temporal and occipital lobe territories of the PCAs.[18-20] The cartoon in Figure 9-2 shows the major sites of embolic occlusion within the vertebrobasilar arterial system. Figure 9-3 shows a basilar artery embolus found at necropsy. The most frequent brain areas infarcted are the (1) posterior inferior portion of the cerebellum in the territory of the posterior inferior cerebellar artery branch of the ICVA, (2) the superior surface of the cerebellum in the territory of the SCA, and (3) the thalamic and hemispheral territories of the PCAs.[18] TL's second attack probably represented cerebellar ischemia.[18,21]

The clinical neurologic signs depend on the location of the occluded artery and are similar to the signs described in Chapters 6 and 7. An occluded ACA causes leg weakness, abulia, and

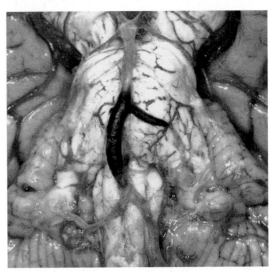

Figure 9-3. The base of the brain at necropsy showing a red embolus distending the basilar artery.

left-arm apraxia. When the occluded vessel is the upper trunk of the left MCA, Broca's aphasia and weakness of the right side of the face, and the right hand and arm result. An occluded left MCA inferior trunk causes Wernicke's aphasia and a right homonymous hemianopia. An occluded PCA causes a homonymous hemianopia, whereas an embolus at the top of the basilar artery can cause cortical blindness, lethargy or agitation, and abnormal eye movements. At times, emboli may be large enough to occlude a normal or an already stenotic ICA, MCA stem, ICVA, or basilar artery, causing more severe neurologic deficits.

Emboli of cardiac origin are often larger than those arising in the cervicocranial arteries, so the infarcts are, on average, larger than artery-to-artery infarcts.[10,22-25] In the Stroke Data Bank, the average volume of infarction on computed tomography (CT) in patients with cardiac origin embolism was 2.4 times greater than in patients with intra-arterial embolism, a highly significant difference ($P < .01$).[24,26] In a study of more than 2000 stroke patients, the average size of brain infarcts caused by cardiac-source embolism was 73.7 cm^3 versus 48.9 cm^3 for nonembolic infarcts.[25] Decreased level of consciousness early during the course of the stroke, a finding probably related to the size of infarction among other factors, was also significantly more common in Stroke Data Bank patients with cardiogenic embolism, as compared with those with intra-arterial embolism (29.8% vs 6.1%, $P < .01$).[26]

TL had no history of systemic embolism. Embolism to systemic arteries has traditionally been considered an important criterion for the clinical diagnosis of brain embolism. Necropsy studies of

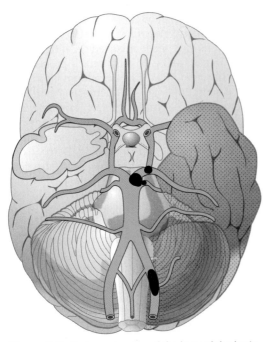

Figure 9-2. Cartoon drawing of the base of the brain showing the most frequent sites of embolism within the posterior circulation. The *black clots* are located within the left intracranial vertebral artery and in the distal basilar artery and its left superior cerebellar and posterior cerebral artery branches. The left temporal lobe and left cerebellum are shaded *gray* to show infarction.

patients with brain embolism of cardiac origin and those with fatal strokes nearly always show embolic infarcts in other organs, especially the spleen and kidneys.[27,27a] In contrast, the frequency of clinical recognition of systemic embolism is quite low. The frequency of diagnosis of systemic embolism in various stroke registries was 2% in the Harvard Stroke Registry, 2.3% in the Michael Reese Stroke Registry, 3.6% in the Stroke Data Bank, and 3% in the Lausanne Stroke Registry.[4,10-12,15,26] Eight percent, the highest frequency of systemic embolism, was found in a study of 60 patients with cardiogenic brain embolism in whom two patients had kidney embolism and three patients had peripheral limb embolism.[28]

Embolism to the brain that causes ischemia usually produces transient or persistent neurologic symptoms. The brain is like litmus paper and is sensitive to perturbations. Systemic embolism also causes ischemia, but the symptoms are much less specific. Embolism to a limb might cause arm pain, leg cramps, or other transient discomfort. These symptoms are common and usually result from activity, positioning of the limb, or some other banal, everyday occurrence. Similarly, embolism to the intestinal tract might cause stomach cramps, bowel irregularity, or a stomachache. These are rather common and nonspecific symptoms. Embolism to the kidneys or spleen causes flank or abdominal discomfort and is rarely diagnosed as related to systemic embolism. Hematuria and sudden-onset severe limb ischemia are probably the only two situations that usually lead to recognition of systemic embolism, especially in patients with known heart disease. An analysis of the findings on urinalysis and renal function among 324 acute ischemic stroke patients found that patients with high urine white and red blood-cell counts and serum creatinine determinations had a high frequency of cardiac origin embolism.[28a] Imaging using CT or MRI of the abdomen may help in differentiating embolism from a central source (heart or aorta) from intravascular lesions by showing embolic infarcts in the spleen and kidneys and other abdominal viscera.

IMAGING AND LABORATORY FINDINGS RELATED TO THE RECIPIENT ARTERY AND ITS SUPPLY

Brain imaging using CT, magnetic resonance imaging (MRI), or both, and vascular imaging using CT angiography (CTA), magnetic resonance angiography (MRA), standard catheter angiography, and TCD can yield information in relation to the recipient artery and the presence, location, and size of embolic brain infarcts.

> A CT scan in TL showed a region of lucency involving the left angular and postcentral gyri. Within the lucent areas were small regions of stippling caused by hemorrhagic transformation. There were also small, old infarcts in the right frontal lobe and left cerebellum. Hematologic, serologic, and coagulation studies were normal. MRI confirmed the same regions of infarction. The hemorrhagic changes in the recent inferior parietal lobe infarct were more evident on MRI than CT. Angiography on the third hospital day revealed a sharp cutoff of the left angular artery. The proximal arteries were normal.

Brain imaging with CT and MRI can suggest brain embolism. Because emboli most often lodge in distal arteries that supply cortical zones, embolic infarcts are often V-shaped and abut on the superficial cortical surface. Multiple cortical infarcts in various vascular supply regions suggest cardiac-origin embolism. Ringelstein and colleagues analyzed the CT pattern of infarction among 60 patients with cardiogenic embolism[29] (see Fig. 2-36). Most infarcts were large and cortically based (41 lesions). Some patients had small cortical, subcortical, and insular infarcts. A few patients had deep infarcts in the striatocapsular region.[29] Multiple cortical and cortical-subcortical infarcts in different vascular territories are especially suggestive of brain embolism from a cardiac or aortic source. At times, acute emboli are imaged as hyperdense arteries on noncontrast CT[30,31] (see Fig. 4-19). Most often, the hyperdensity takes the course and shape of the MCA. Occasionally, calcific fragments can also be seen within arteries on noncontrast CT scans (see Fig. 4-20). Emboli monitoring using TCD (see Figs. 4-17 and 4-18) has shown high rates of brain embolism.[2,5-10]

Embolic infarcts may be pale, spotted with small petechial hemorrhages, or frankly hemorrhagic. The necropsy specimen in Figure 9-4 shows a typical hemorrhagic infarct. Fisher and Adams extensively studied their necropsy material to define the mechanism of hemorrhagic infarction in the brain.[32,33] Obstruction of a nutrient artery causes brain ischemia to neurons and ischemic damage to the blood vessels within the area of ischemia. When the obstructing embolus moves distally, the previously ischemic region is reperfused with blood. The damaged capillaries and arterioles within that region are no longer competent, and blood leaks into the surrounding infarcted tissue. An example of this from the Fisher and Adams study is shown in Figure 9-5. This patient had an embolus that initially blocked the mainstem MCA before its lenticulostriate branches, causing ischemia to the basal ganglia,

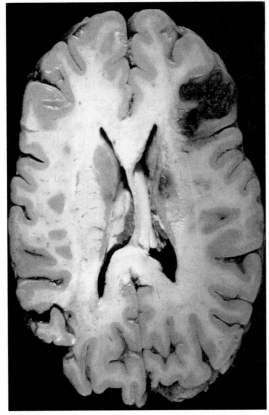

Figure 9-4. A hemorrhagic infarct involves the territory of an anterior branch of the superior division of the middle cerebral artery at necropsy. There is also a small region of hemorrhagic infarction in the basal ganglia. (From Caplan LR, Manning WJ: Brain Embolism. New York: Informa Healthcare, 2006, with permission.)

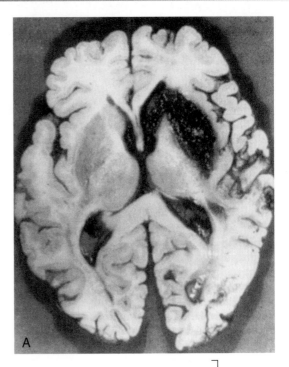

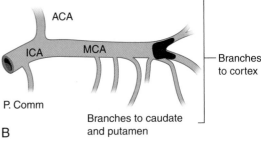

Figure 9-5. A, Coronal section of the brain at necropsy showing a hemorrhagic infarction on the right involving the caudate nucleus and putamen, regions supplied by the lenticulostriate branches of the right MCA. **B,** Cartoon of the intracranial ICA and its branches at necropsy. An embolus *(hatched region)* was found in the distal portion of the mainstem MCA beyond the lenticulostriate branches that supply the caudate nucleus and putamen. This embolus must have previously blocked these penetrating branches and then moved more distally in the artery. (From Fisher CM, Adams RD: Observations on Brain Embolism with Special Reference to Hemorrhagic Infarction. In AJ Furlan (ed): The Heart and Stroke. London: Springer, 1987, pp 17-36, with kind permission of Springer Science+Business Media.)

internal capsule, and the superficial cortical territories supplied by the MCA. The embolus then moved and had passed beyond the lenticulostriate branches at necropsy but continued to obstruct the MCA more distally. The reperfused deep basal ganglionic region was hemorrhagic at necropsy, whereas the superficial territory of the MCA that was never reperfused showed a bland infarct. Figure 9-6 shows a similar instance of hemorrhagic infarction in a reperfused region.

The essential cause of hemorrhagic infarction is reperfusion of previously ischemic tissue. The other stroke mechanism that causes hemorrhagic infarction is systemic hypoperfusion. After cardiac arrest or shock, the reinstitution of effective circulation after a prolonged period of brain hypoperfusion can cause hemorrhage within border-zone infarcts. Hemorrhagic changes are very common in patients with brain embolism. In two series, investigators prospectively studied the frequency of hemorrhagic infarction on sequential brain-imaging scans.[34,35] Yamaguchi et al compared the findings on CT scans performed 3-10 days after stroke in 120 patients who had embolic brain infarcts with 109 patients whose infarcts were believed to be caused by local thrombotic occlusive disease.[34] Hemorrhagic infarcts were found in 45 patients (40%) with embolic infarcts, as compared with two patients (1.8%) with local-related infarcts. Okada and colleagues performed CT scans every 10 days in 160 patients who had presumed embolic brain infarcts.[35] Hemorrhagic infarction

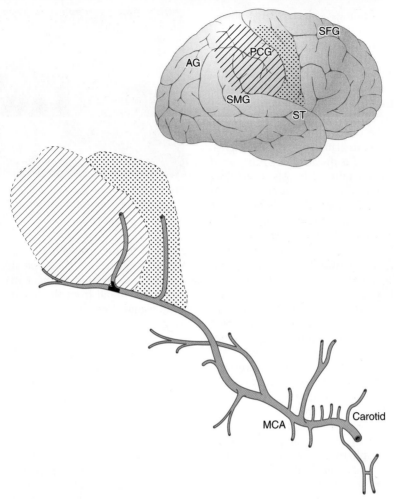

Figure 9-6. On the right is a lateral view of the right side of the brain. The stippled dotted area represents hemorrhagic transformation while the more solid grey area represents bland nonhemorrhagic infarction at necropsy. The figure on the left shows an embolus found within a branch of the middle cerebral artery. The region beyond the embolus shows a bland infarct, while the area reperfused is hemorrhagic. AG, angular gyrus; SMG, supramarginal gyrus; ST, superior temporal gyrus; SFG, superior frontal gyrus; PCG, postcentral gyrus. (Adapted from Fisher CM, Adams RD: Observations on Brain Embolism with Special Reference to Hemorrhagic Infarction. In AJ Furlan (ed): The Heart and Stroke. London: Springer, 1987, pp 17-36, with kind permission of Springer Science+Business Media.)

was found on CT at some time during the course in 65 patients (40.6%). Hemorrhagic changes were found on the initial CT scan performed during the first 4 days in only 10 patients (6%), whereas the remainder of the hemorrhagic infarcts were found on follow-up CT scans.[35] Studies at the New England Medical Center in Boston showed that all patients with cerebral and cerebellar hemorrhagic infarcts reported had embolic causes.[36,37] MRI is more sensitive than CT in showing hemorrhagic changes, therefore sequential MRI probably would show a frequency greater than 50% for hemorrhagic changes in patients with embolic brain infarcts.

In most patients, hemorrhagic infarction consists of diapedesis of red blood cells into infarcted tissue. The appearance is that of scattered petechial hemorrhages or a confluent purpuric pattern scattered throughout the infarct. In some brain infarcts, especially large ones involving more than one lobe, localized homogeneous collections of blood (hematomas) can develop within the region of hemorrhagic infarction.[38] In most patients with hemorrhagic infarcts, the hemorrhagic transformation does not cause worsening of the clinical symptoms and signs. The hemorrhagic changes are usually found on routine follow-up scans. Bleeding into dead tissue does

9

not alter clinical findings unless a large space-occupying hematoma develops.

Experience with acute angiography since the late 1980s has shown a high rate of demonstration of intracranial emboli in patients with cardiac-origin sources and extracranial occlusive disease.[39-41] CTA, MRA, and standard catheter angiography, especially if performed within 48 hours of stroke onset, often shows findings characteristic of embolism. A sudden sharp, abrupt termination of a distal or medium-sized vessel without visible atherosclerosis or a filling defect in the lumen of a symptomatic recipient artery is diagnostic of embolization. Figures 4-31 and 4-32 show acute multimodal MRI and CT studies. In each patient, the vascular occlusive embolus was shown on vascular imaging (MRA and CTA), and the perfusion abnormality exceeded the diffusion abnormality, indicating the presence of brain tissue that was ischemic but not yet infarcted. Disappearance of the obstruction in subsequent films or on later angiograms substantiates the diagnosis. Dalal et al reported nine patients who had emboli seen on initial angiography that later disappeared.[42] Others have also shown disappearance or movement of emboli.[43,44] The finding of a normal artery that supplies a region of cortical and subcortical infarction is also highly suggestive of embolism.

TCD ultrasound insonation of patients with sudden-onset hemispheric strokes has shown frequent MCA occlusion. Sequential TCD examinations that show clearing of an obstruction suggest embolism.[2,35-37,45] A very important but underutilized capability has entered the diagnostic arsenal of clinicians during the last decade—emboli monitoring using TCD.[2,45] Ultrasound probes are positioned over brain arteries, most often the MCA and PCA on each side. When particles pass through the arteries being monitored, they produce an audible chirping noise and high-intensity transient signals (HITS) are visible on an oscilloscope. The signal character depends on the nature of the particles (gas, thrombus, calcium, cholesterol crystal, and so forth), particle size, and particle transit time. Figures 4-17 and 4-18 show microembolic signals captured by TCD monitoring. Figure 9-7 shows a flurry of microembolic signals in an MCA in a patient during carotid artery angioplasty. Monitoring probes can be placed on the neck and brain arteries. Emboli that arise from the heart or aorta should go equally to each side, proportionately to the anterior and posterior circulation arteries. About 40% should go to each MCA and 20% to the posterior circulation. The signals should appear in the neck before appearing intracranially. In contrast, emboli that originate from a carotid artery should

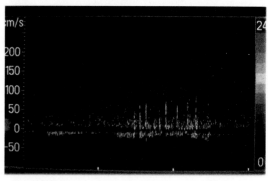

Figure 9-7. TCD monitoring during carotid angioplasty shows a flurry of microembolic signals in the MCA.

go only to the intracranial anterior circulation arterial branches on the same side. Embolic signals do not appear in the neck over that ICA. For example, emboli from the left ICA generate embolic signals detectable in the left MCA and not in the neck, PCAs, or right-sided arteries. Emboli that originate in a vertebral artery could go to either PCA. This ultrasound monitoring technique allows better identification of the nature of embolic materials and their sources. This technique also allows some quantification of the emboli load and a means of monitoring the effect of various therapies on lessening that load.

In one study, Daffertshofer and colleagues monitored 280 patients who had acute MCA-territory ischemic events, as well as 118 asymptomatic controls, for periods of 30 to 60 minutes.[7] Only two control patients (1.7%) had microembolic signals. No microembolic signals were detected among 78 patients who had no identified sources of embolism, whereas 12.9% of patients with sources of emboli had microembolic signals.[7] Microemboli were found more often in patients with vascular sources of embolism, such as ICA stenosis (17.1%), as compared with 6.2% in patients with cardiac sources of embolism. One fifth of patients with ICA stenosis greater than 70% had microembolic signals, as compared with 13% in patients with less than 70% ICA stenosis.[7]

Sliwka et al, during a 6-month period, monitored 109 consecutive patients with atrial fibrillation or other potential cardiac sources of embolism.[8] Nine of the patients had insufficient temporal windows and could not be monitored with TCD. Microembolic signals were detected in 36 of the 100 patients successfully monitored. The average number of microembolic signals was 2.69 (± 2.7) per 30 minutes (range, 1 to 12). Patients with atrial fibrillation who had coronary atherosclerotic heart disease with ejection fractions of less than 30%, dilatated cardiomyopathy, or mitral stenosis had the highest percentage of microemboli detection.[8]

Georgiadis and colleagues monitored 300 patients with potential cardiac sources of emboli and 100 patients with severe ICA disease using TCD.[48] They found the following frequencies of microembolic signals among their monitored patients: 43%, infective endocarditis; 34%, left ventricular aneurysm; 26%, intracardiac thrombus; 26%, dilatated cardiomyopathy; 21%, non-valvular atrial fibrillation; 15%, native valvular disease; 55% prosthetic valves; 28%, ICA disease (52% symptomatic ICA disease, 7% asymptomatic disease); and 5% among controls.[48]

> In TL, echocardiography showed an enlarged heart with a reduced ejection fraction suggestive of a cardiomyopathy. Myocardial biopsy later revealed cardiac sarcoidosis. Over the next year, TL had no further brain emboli while taking warfarin.

In this patient, the multiple acute onset brain infarcts in different vascular territories, the negative hematologic studies, absence of risk factors for atherosclerosis, and normal proximal extracranial and intracranial arteries suggested the likelihood of cardiac origin brain embolism despite the absence of known cardiac disease. Cardiac evaluation finally clarified the diagnosis.

SOURCES OF EMBOLI

The great majority of emboli to the brain arise from the heart, aorta, and cervicocranial arteries. Figure 2-5 illustrates these major sources. A variety of particles with different physical properties can arise from the heart, arteries, or circulation.[1,4,50] Table 9-1 lists the various particles

that arise from cardiac and intra-arterial sources. Occasionally, foreign materials, such as air, fat, and cancer cells, enter the circulation and embolize to various systemic organs. Importantly, pharmacologic prophylaxis to prevent recurrent embolization depends mostly on the nature of the substance that makes up the embolus rather than its source. It's not the nest alone, but the bird that flew from the nest that deserves attention.

Cardiac Sources

During the 1950s, the only two cardiac conditions accepted as having an important risk of causing embolism were rheumatic mitral stenosis with atrial fibrillation and recent myocardial infarction. Many cardiac lesions and disorders carry a risk of cardiac thrombosis and embolism. More modern cardiac diagnostic testing has made it possible to diagnose cardiac disorders more definitively and to attempt to quantify the risk of embolism. Cardiac disorders that carry a risk of brain embolism can be divided into six groups:[4,51,52]

1. Arrhythmias, especially atrial fibrillation and sick sinus syndrome
2. Valvular heart diseases, especially mitral stenosis, prosthetic heart valves, infective endocarditis, and marantic endocarditis
3. Ventricular myocardial abnormalities, especially related to coronary artery disease, myocarditis, and other dilatated cardiomyopathies
4. Lesions within the cavity of the ventricles, especially tumors, such as myxomas and thrombi
5. Shunts, especially intra-atrial septal defects and patent foramen ovale (PFO) that allow

Table 9-1.   Types of Embolic Materials from Various Sources

Cardiac Origin	Arterial Origin	Systemic
Red fibrin-dependent thrombi	Red fibrin-dependent thrombi	Air
White platelet-fibrin thrombi	White platelet-fibrin thrombi	Fat
Fibrin strands and bland valve vegetations (NBTE)	Combined white and red thrombi	Mucin from tumors
Bacteria from infective endocarditis	Cholesterol crystals	Talc and microcrystalline cellulose (drug injections)
Calcium from valve calcifications	Atheromatous plaque debris	Foreign bodies
Tumor (myxoma and other cardiac neoplasms)	Calcium from areas of arterial calcification	

passage of emboli forming in the peripheral veins to enter the systemic circulation, causing so-called paradoxical embolism

6. Atrial lesions, such as dilatated atria, atrial infarcts and thrombi, and atrial septal aneurysms

Table 9-2 lists the major cardiac donor sources of embolism.

Virchow, in 1856, described three antecedent conditions for the development of thrombi within blood vessels and the chambers of the heart.[53] These three conditions are (1) a region of circulatory stasis, (2) injury to an endothelial surface, and (3) increased blood coagulability. In areas of stasis, a low shear rate and other factors activate the classical coagulation cascade, leading to the formation of erythrocyte-fibrin thrombi. Stasis

occurs most often in the atria and atrial appendages in patients with atrial fibrillation. Stasis also occurs in the ventricular chambers in patients with global and focal regions of decreased myocardial contractility. Altered myocardial endothelium occurs in patients with myocardial infarcts, ventricular aneurysms, inflammatory and other myocardiopathies, and endocardial disorders. Valvular endothelium can be damaged by many different conditions. Loss of a protective endothelial surface exposes circulating blood to the underlying tissues and causes platelet activation, adhesion, and secretion, as well as activating the coagulation cascade. Studies show increased platelet activation and blood coagulability in patients with cardiac-source embolism.[54-58]

Arrhythmias

ATRIAL FIBRILLATION

Atrial fibrillation is characterized by loss of organized atrial electrical and mechanical activity resulting in stasis of blood within the body of the atria and especially within the left atrial appendage.[52] The ejection velocity in the left atrial appendage is markedly depressed (<20 cm/second) in patients with atrial fibrillation, and the risk of thrombus formation is inversely related to the left atrial appendage ejection velocity.[52,59] In addition to stasis, hematologic studies suggest that atrial fibrillation is associated with an increased blood coagulability state.[56]

Atrial fibrillation is one of the most common heart conditions. Over 2.5 million people in the United States have atrial fibrillation, a population that greatly exceeds those with rheumatic mitral stenosis. Approximately 0.4% of the population has atrial fibrillation and the disorder becomes much more common as patients age. Perhaps as many as 5% of individuals older than 60 years have atrial fibrillation. Epidemiologic studies performed since the 1970s have firmly established that atrial fibrillation is an important risk factor for stroke, that stroke in patients with atrial fibrillation is most often caused by cardiogenic embolism, and that standard antithrombotic treatment substantially reduces the frequency of brain embolism in patients with atrial fibrillation. The etiology of atrial fibrillation and associated cardiac and other medical factors affect the risk of stroke in patients with atrial fibrillation. In the Framingham Study, the presence of rheumatic heart disease and atrial fibrillation conveyed 17.6 times the risk of stroke compared with the lone atrial fibrillation rate of 5.6 times.[60,61] Advanced age, congestive heart failure, history of hypertension, previous myocardial infarction, and prior thromboembolism increase the risk of

Table 9-2.	Some Cardiac Sources of Emboli

Coronary Artery Disease

Mural thrombi
Ventricular aneurysms
Hypokinetic zones

Arrhythmias

Atrial fibrillation
Sick-sinus syndrome

Valvular Disease

Mitral stenosis, rheumatic
Aortic stenosis, rheumatic
Bicuspid aortic valve
Mitral annulus calcification
Calcific aortic stenosis
Mitral valve prolapse
Bacterial endocarditis
Nonbacterial thrombotic endocarditis

Cardiomyopathies or Endocardiopathies

Endocardial fibroelastosis
Alcoholic cardiomyopathy
Cocaine cardiomyopathy
Myocarditis
Sarcoidosis
Fabry's disease
Amyloidosis

Intracardiac Lesions

Myxomas
Fibroelastomas
Malignant cardiac tumors
Metastatic tumors
Ball-valve thrombi

Septal Abnormalities (Paradoxic Embolism)

Atrial septal defects
Patent foramen ovale
Atrial septal aneurysms

stroke in patients with atrial fibrillation.[62-64] These features should be known from the medical history. A collaborative analysis of five atrial fibrillation stroke prevention studies analyzed the contribution of various historical risk factors on the development of stroke during follow-up.[65] The relative risks (RRs) determined by multivariate analysis of all the data were history of previous stroke or transient ischemic attack (TIA) (RR, 2.5), diabetes mellitus (RR, 1.7), history of hypertension (RR, 1.6), and increasing age (RR, 1.4 for each decade).[65] These calculated RRs were for the occurrence of any stroke and were not limited to those attributable to cardiogenic embolism.

Echocardiography findings are also helpful in assessing the risk of brain embolism in individual patients with atrial fibrillation.[52,66-74] Transesophageal echocardiography (TEE) can detect left atrial and left atrial appendage thrombi. Figure 4-35 is a TEE that shows a left atrial thrombus in an atrial fibrillation patient. In patients with atrial fibrillation who do not have valvular disease, thrombi often form in, and dislodge from, the left atrial appendage, whereas patients with atrial fibrillation and valvular disease have more left atrial thrombi. In patients with valvular disease and atrial fibrillation, thrombi have been detected in 9% to 29% of patients, compared with 10% prevalence in patients without valvular disease.[51] Small thrombi (<2 mm) and those that have already dislodged are not readily detected. Left atrial enlargement and abnormal left atrial appendage function, as determined by Doppler TEE, also convey an increased risk for cardioembolic stroke.[59,69,70] The presence of mitral annulus calcification (MAC) and left ventricular dysfunction also increase the risk of stroke in patients with atrial fibrillation.

Spontaneous echo contrast (also called *smoke*) is probably one of the most important factors that predict the likelihood of cardiogenic embolism in patients with atrial fibrillation.[71-76] Figure 9-8 is a TEE that shows this abnormality. First described in patients with mitral valve disease, spontaneous echo contrast refers to swirling hazes of echogenicity within the cardiac chambers. The echogenic swirls can move repeatedly within the cavity and may disappear when blood flow increases or when local stasis resolves. The intensity can vary from a faint cloud-like appearance to bright echo contrast. Spontaneous echo contrast is probably caused by the interaction between plasma proteins and erythrocytes at low shear rates. It is a marker of stasis within the left atrium. The major determinants of spontaneous echogenicity are the hematocrit, fibrinogen levels, and slow intracardiac flow. Chimowitz and colleagues showed that

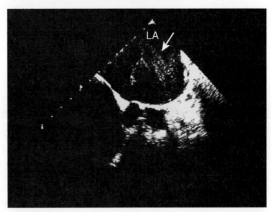

Figure 9-8. TEE in a patient with a swirling pattern of spontaneous echo contrast *(white arrow)* in the body of the left atrium (LA) indicating slow/stagnant flow. (From Caplan LR, Manning WJ: Brain Embolism. New York: Informa Healthcare, 2006, with permission.)

the presence of spontaneous echo contrast was highly associated with prior strokes in patients who had either atrial fibrillation or mitral valve stenosis.[74] Spontaneous echo contrast may be seen in 60% of patients with atrial fibrillation and more than 85% of those with atrial fibrillation and left atrial thrombi.[75,76] Prospective TEE studies show left atrium (LA) thrombi in 14% of patients with new-onset atrial fibrillation,[77,78] increasing to 27% of those with chronic atrial fibrillation,[79] and 45% in those presenting with atrial fibrillation and recent clinical thromboembolism.[80]

Table 9-3 tabulates the results of the major trials of anticoagulation and antiplatelet aggregants in patients with atrial fibrillation who do not have valvular disease.[81-88] Warfarin is approximately 50% more effective than aspirin in reducing the rate of stroke in patients with atrial fibrillation without valvular disease.[89] There is an overwhelming consensus among neurologists that warfarin is the drug of choice in the great majority of patients with atrial fibrillation unless there are compelling contraindications to anticoagulation. General physicians and internists are often reluctant to anticoagulate elderly patients but studies show that warfarin is effective and relatively safe in older individuals.[89a,b] In one randomized trial that included 973 patients with a mean age of 81.5, warfarin (INR range, 2 to 3) was associated with half the brain infarcts and hemorrhages compared to aspirin (75 mg/day), and less extracranial bleeding (annual risk 1.4% for warfarin vs 1.6% for aspirin).[89b] Ximelagatran, a direct thrombin inhibitor, has also been evaluated in randomized therapeutic trials that compared its effectiveness and hemorrhage rate with warfarin in patients with atrial fibrillation.[90,91] Ximelagatran proved as effective in reducing the development of new

Table 9-3.   Trials of Prophylactic Therapy in Patients with Atrial Fibrillation without Valvular Disease

Trial	Design	Results
Copenhagen AFASKA[84]	1007 patients; mean age 73; Coumadin (INR 2.8-4.2) vs aspirin (75mg/day) vs placebo	Thromboemboli (stroke, TIA, systemic embolism) Coumadin 2%/year; Aspirin 5.5%/year; placebo 5.5%/year
BAATAF[84]	628 patients; mean age 68; Coumadin (INR 1.5-2.7) vs other medical Rx (could include aspirin)	Coumadin 2 strokes (0.4%/year); control 13(3%/year). No benefit of aspirin (8 of 13 strokes in controls on aspirin); 2 hemorrhages-1 each group
SPAF[85]	1330 patients; mean age 67; warfarin-eligible patients randomized to warfarin (INR 2-3.5), aspirin (325 mg/day), or placebo. Warfarin-ineligible patients randomized to aspirin or placebo	Warfarin 2.3%/year vs 7.4%/year placebo; stroke in warfarin-ineligible aspirin group 3.6%/year vs 6.3% in placebo group. Major bleeding 1.5%, 1.4%, 1.6% in warfarin, aspirin, placebo groups
EAFT[83]	1007 patients, mean age 73; warfarin-eligible patients randomized to warfarin (INR 2.5-4), aspirin (300 mg), or placebo. Warfarin-ineligible to aspirin or placebo	Strokes in 8% of 225 in warfarin group, 15% of 404 in aspirin group, 19% of 378 in placebo group. Major bleeding 2.8%/year warfarin group and 0.9%/year aspirin group
SPAF II[86]	1100 patients; mean age 69.6; warfarin (INR 2-4.5) vs aspirin (325 mg/day) compared in patients <75 and patients >75	715 patients <75; ischemic stroke and systemic embolism 1.3%/year warfarin vs 1.9%/year aspirin; major hemorrhage 0.9%/year aspirin, 1.7%/year warfarin; 385 >75; ischemic stroke and systemic embolism 3.6%/year warfarin, 4.8%/year aspirin; major bleeds 4.2% warfarin,[a] 1.6% aspirin
SPAF III[87] SPAF III[88]	1044 patients with 1 or more risk factors; mean age 72; low-intensity fixed dose warfarin (INR 1.2-1.5) plus aspirin (325 mg/day) vs adjusted dose warfarin (INR 2-3) 892 patients with posited low risk were given 325 mg aspirin	INR 1.3 fixed dose warfarin vs INR target 2.4 adjusted group. Ischemic stroke and systemic embolism in 7.9% of fixed dose and aspirin vs 1.9% in adjusted dose group The rate of ischemic stroke was low (2%/year) and disabling ischemic stroke only 0.8%/year. The rate of major bleeding was 0.5%/year
BAFTA[89b]	973 elderly (mean age 81.5) warfarin (INR 2-3) vs aspirin 75mg/day	50% less of combined ischemic stroke, intracranial hemorrhage, systemic emboli in warfarin group; annual risk of extracranial hemorrhage 1.4% warfarin vs 1.6% aspirin

[a] Seventy-one percent of intracranial hemorrhages fatal; 29% had residual deficit.

AFASAK, Copenhagen Atrial Fibrillation Aspirin Anticoagulation Study; BAATAF, Boston Area Anticoagulation Trial for Atrial Fibrillation; EAFT, European Atrial Fibrillation Trial; SPAF, Stroke Prevention in Atrial Fibrillation study.

strokes and caused less hemorrhages. Even in high-risk patients 75 years of age or older, ximelagatran was as effective as warfarin in preventing strokes and systemic emboli and was accompanied by less bleeding.[91a] Unfortunately, the occurrence of liver function abnormalities led to the Food and Drug Administration (FDA) refusing to approve the drug in the United States. Aspirin is also an effective treatment; aspirin probably conveys a stroke risk reduction of 20% to 25% with no clear relationship to aspirin dose. Treatment should be decided on an individual basis. Clinicians should weigh the risk of stroke without warfarin versus the risk of important hemorrhage during warfarin treatment.

Other treatment strategies have also been explored in patients with atrial fibrillation. Five randomized clinical trials compared the effectiveness of rate control versus rhythm control.[92] Surprisingly the risk of thromboemboli was greater in the rhythm control group than in those whose rate was controlled (2.9% to 7.9% vs 0% to 0.5%).[92] Rate was controlled pharmacologically, and rhythm control was by electrical conversion and/or medications. The results show that recurrent episodes of atrial fibrillation are probably common even in patients who are treated with rhythm control measures.

Surgeons and cardiology interventionalists have also attempted to decrease stroke risk in patients with atrial fibrillation by producing various ablations and lesions in the pulmonary vein and left atrial region to maintain the heart in normal sinus rhythm.[93] The left atrial appendage has also been removed to prevent thrombi from developing there and later embolizing.[93,94,94a] These ablation procedures were first performed in patients who were having open heart surgeries for valvular heart disease at the time of the heart surgery. More recently a variety of different percutaneous interventional techniques have been explored to control the atrial arrhythmia and to exclude the left atrial appendage.[94,94a]

SICK SINUS SYNDROME

Although sinus node dysfunction has been recognized clinically since the beginning of the twentieth century, identification of the malfunctioning atrium as a source of embolism was first recognized during the 1970s.[95,96] A variety of names are used for this condition, including sick sinus syndrome, sinoatrial disorder, and bradycardia-tachycardia syndrome. Essential for the diagnosis is demonstration of sinus node dysfunction. Patients often present with slow or fast cardiac rhythms, or both. Lown characterized the disorder as consisting of chaotic atrial activity, changing p-wave contour, and bradycardia,

admixed with multiple and recurrent ectopic beats and runs of atrial and nodal tachycardia.[97] Many patients also have atrial fibrillation or flutter with a relatively slow ventricular response (<70 beats/minute).[98] An analysis of cardiovascular disease in Rochester, Minnesota showed that 2.9% of men and 1.5% of women aged 75 years or older had the sick sinus syndrome.[99]

Systemic emboli mostly to the brain occurred in approximately 14% to 18% of patients with the sick sinus syndrome.[100,101] Patients with tachyarrhythmias are more likely to embolize than those with just bradyarrhythmias. As in patients with atrial fibrillation, increasing age is associated with an increased frequency of embolism. The use of pacemakers (atrial single-chamber pacing or ventricular single-chamber pacing) does not seem to reduce the frequency of stroke or stroke death.[102]

As in patients with atrial fibrillation, dysfunction of the LA probably promotes thrombus formation. Tachycardia may precipitate dislodging of thrombi from the heart into the systemic circulation. Activation of platelets and increased blood coagulability probably contribute to the likelihood of thromboembolism. Although no formal, prospective, randomized trials of anticoagulation or aspirin therapy have been performed in patients with sinus node dysfunction, the therapeutic responses and treatment considerations are probably the same as those for patients with atrial fibrillation, although the frequency of brain embolism is lower.

CARDIAC VALVE DISEASE

One fifth to one tenth of all patients with cardiac valve disease have cardioembolic strokes.[103] Abnormalities of valve surfaces and changes in valve function and cardiac physiology that result from valve disease, promote the formation of white platelet-fibrin thrombi and red clots on valve surfaces and in the adjacent heart chambers. Stenotic valves have decreased pliability and irregular surfaces; progressive commisural adhesions and valve leaflet dystrophic calcification develops, leading to progressive narrowing of the cross-sectional area of valve orifices. Valvular outlet obstruction causes increased turbulence of blood flow. The intensity of turbulence is markedly increased in the jet stream of blood distal to a stenotic valve.[104] Platelets are activated in regions of increased turbulence; the amount of thrombus formed is directly related to valve orifice turbulence.

Distal to stenotic valves, blood flow consists of a central jet stream surrounded by annular eddies that course between the outflow tract walls and the mainstream. These eddies permit blood to remain closer to the irregular valve surfaces than occurs in regions of normal laminar flow.

Platelets activated by the turbulent jet stream have prolonged contact with dystrophic irregular valve surfaces, causing adhesion of platelet-fibrin thrombi to valve surfaces, further platelet activation, and formation of thrombi. Valve incompetence also prolongs the time that blood is in contact with abnormal valve surfaces and also promotes thrombus formation. Valve disease often leads to atrial and ventricular enlargement. Left atrial enlargement is especially common in patients with mitral stenosis and mitral insufficiency and can be severe. Enlargement of the LA is accompanied by stasis and thrombus formation, especially in the left atrial appendage and in patients who develop atrial fibrillation.

RHEUMATIC MITRAL VALVE DISEASE

Although the incidence of rheumatic fever and rheumatic heart disease has dramatically declined, rheumatic heart disease is still an important cause of brain embolism. The mitral valve is most often involved. Second in frequency is involvement of the mitral and aortic valves. Isolated rheumatic aortic valve disease is unusual, and the pulmonic and tricuspid valves are seldom the site of important clinical rheumatic valvulitis. The strong association of rheumatic mitral stenosis and stroke has long been recognized.

The normal adult mitral valve cross-sectional area is 4 to 6 cm^2.[52] Clinical symptoms most often develop when the mitral valve area declines to less than 2 cm^2.[52] The predominant cause of mitral stenosis is rheumatic fever leading to predominant mitral stenosis (especially common among women), mixed mitral stenosis and mitral regurgitation, or predominant mitral regurgitation (more common among men). With rheumatic valvular disease, the mitral leaflets fuse at their edges with thickening of the chordae tendinae. The stenotic mitral valve is typically funnel shaped. Progressive mitral valve obstruction leads to increased intra-atrial pressure and progressive dilation of the LA. Fibrosis may also develop in the endothelium of the LA. Progressive left atrial dilation, blood stasis, and endocardial surface abnormalities promote thrombus formation, yet the incidence of thromboembolism does not appear to be related to the severity of mitral stenosis.[52,105] Large thrombi within the body of the LA, especially "ball" thrombi, are almost exclusively seen among patients with rheumatic mitral stenosis (and those with prosthetic mitral valve thrombosis). Although unusual, these ball thrombi are often readily appreciated by transthoracic echocardiography.

Before the availability of anticoagulation, autopsy and surgical series showed an increased risk of clinical thromboembolism in the mitral stenosis population.[106-108] Embolization, especially to the brain, may be the earliest clinical indication of rheumatic mitral stenosis. The frequency of embolism in patients with mitral stenosis ranges in series from 10% to 20%.[109-111] Approximately 50% to 75% of emboli detected clinically involve the brain. Embolism is more common in patients with mitral stenosis than in those with mitral insufficiency. Although embolism does occur in patients with mitral stenosis who have normal sinus rhythm, the development of atrial fibrillation greatly increases the risk of embolism. In 194 patients with rheumatic heart disease and systemic embolism, Daley et al found a mitral valve lesion in 97%, atrial fibrillation in 90%, and either a mitral valve lesion or atrial fibrillation in 100%.[112] In a study of 754 patients with chronic rheumatic heart disease followed for more than 5000 patient-years, the incidence of embolism was 1.5% per patient-year.[109] Embolism was seven times more frequent in patients with atrial fibrillation than in those with sinus rhythm. A third of recurrences of embolism occurred during the first month, and two thirds of recurrences were during the first year after the onset of atrial fibrillation.[109]

Anticoagulants clearly reduce the frequency of recurrent embolism.[113] Mitral valvuloplasty, the predominant treatment of mitral stenosis during the 1960s and 1970s, did not greatly influence the frequency of embolism. The atrial appendage was sometimes removed to prevent lodging of thrombi in this region. Modern diagnostic technology, especially echocardiography, has revolutionized the diagnosis of patients with mitral stenosis and other rheumatic valve lesions. Echocardiography allows quantification of the valve orifice, as well as the effects of the mitral valve disease on the LA and left ventricle. These measurements can be performed sequentially to study disease progression and response to treatment. Left atrial and left atrial appendage thrombi are also reliably detected. Superimposed bacterial endocarditis can precipitate brain embolism, although the occurrence of endocarditis in patients with isolated mitral stenosis is unusual.

Rheumatic mitral regurgitation is a less frequent cause of brain embolism than mitral stenosis. Among individuals with embolism, mitral insufficiency is often accompanied by progressive left ventricular hypertrophy. Mitral valve repair and mitral valve replacement are probably important considerations in the prevention of embolism in patients with rheumatic mitral insufficiency.

AORTIC VALVE DISEASE

Most often, the cause of acquired aortic valve disease is not determined. Progressive calcific aortic stenosis commonly develops in patients with congenital bicuspid aortic valves and can also follow rheumatic valvulitis. Calcific degenerative changes are usually well developed during the 4th and 5th decades of life in patients with bicuspid valves, whereas idiopathic calcific aortic stenosis is more prevalent during the sixth to eighth decades.[114] Idiopathic calcific aortic valve disease of the elderly may be caused by an atherosclerotic degenerative process, although definite proof of this hypothesis is not yet available. Microthrombi with evidence of organization have been found at necropsy in about half of stenotic aortic valves. Changes in the aortic valve are progressive. Thickening of previously diseased valves is thought to result from the deposition of fibrin. Fibrin deposits become organized and calcified with resultant distortion of the normal valve architecture. Bicuspid and calcific aortic valves are not able to open freely. Narrowing and irregularity of the valve orifice contributes to turbulent blood flow. Abnormal flow and valve surfaces activate platelets and induce fibrin deposition, accounting for the prevalence of microthrombi along valve surfaces.

Embolism is a much less common occurrence in patients with aortic valve disease when compared with mitral valve disease. Some clinical and necropsy studies show that embolism from calcific aortic valves is probably not rare. Soulie et al found emboli in 33% of 81 patients with calcific aortic stenosis.[115] In another autopsy study, calcific emboli were found in 37 of 165 patients (22%) with calcific aortic stenosis.[116] Thirty-two emboli were found in the coronary arteries, 11 in the renal vessels, 1 in the central retinal artery, and 1 in the MCA. Although the MCA was occluded by a calcific embolus in one patient, no neurologic signs were recorded and no infarct was found.[116] During life, calcific emboli have often been identified in the eye because of their typical morphology on funduscopic examination of the retina. Calcific retinal emboli appear as white, irregular, immovable densities, and are usually distinguishable from bright cholesterol crystals and fibrin-platelet plugs.

In all clinical studies, symptoms that reflect embolization occur more often after cardiac procedures (catheterization and surgery) than occur spontaneously. Aortic valve surgery is especially associated with a high frequency of embolism. Embolism is also more common in patients with bacterial endocarditis superimposed on bicuspid or calcific aortic valves than it is in noninfected valves. The discrepancy between the relatively high frequency of calcific emboli found at necropsy and in the eye and the low frequency of

clinically symptomatic brain and visceral organ ischemic events is probably explained by the small size of the embolic particles and the fact that visceral emboli are much harder to diagnose than brain emboli.

Hypertrophic cardiomyopathy, also called idiopathic hypertrophic subaortic stenosis, has become more frequently recognized since the advent of echocardiography. This disorder is characterized by disproportionate and asymmetric hypertrophy of the left ventricular myocardium in the region of the ventricular septum, as compared with the left ventricular free wall. Septal hypertrophy is associated with systolic anterior motion of the mitral valve and variable left ventricular outflow obstruction, depending on myocardial contractility. Structural abnormalities of the mitral valve often accompany the hypertrophic cardiomyopathy.[117] The rate of stroke in patients with hypertrophic cardiomyopathy is low. Stroke rarely occurs early in the course of the disease. When stroke occurs, it is usually a result of embolism in relation to atrial fibrillation, bacterial endocarditis, mitral valve dysfunction, or mitral annular calcification. Atrial fibrillation tends to develop late in patients with hypertrophic cardiomyopathy, and is often accompanied by left atrial enlargement.[117-119] Mitral annulus calcification is also associated with idiopathic hypertrophic subaortic stenosis.[120]

Little has been written about embolism in patients with aortic insufficiency. Aortic regurgitation is caused by dysfunction of the aortic valve leaflets or aortic root. Rheumatic valvulitis and infective endocarditis are probably the most common causes of aortic leaflet disease causing aortic insufficiency, whereas Marfan syndrome, aortic dissection, and annulo-aortic ectasia caused by aging and hypertension are the usual causes of aortic root disease. Syphilis was formerly a common cause of aortic valve insufficiency but is rare. Rheumatic aortic valvulitis and vegetations on the aortic valve are potential sources of brain and systemic embolism in patients with aortic regurgitation.

MITRAL VALVE PROLAPSE

Barlow and Bosman, in an early report of the midsystolic click (mitral valve prolapse [MVP]) syndrome, reported a 23-year-old woman who had transient left arm weakness. Evaluation showed MVP.[121,122] No details of the neurologic symptoms or signs were included and the relationship of the neurologic event to her heart condition was not considered.[121,122] Since then, a number of case control and necropsy studies have shown that patients with MVP may have cardiogenic embolism, but rarely. Cerebrovascular events in patients with MVP have a relatively low recurrence rate, even without treatment.

MVP is the single most frequently diagnosed cardiac valvular abnormality. Estimates of prevalence range from 5% to 21%, with the rate being slightly higher in girls and women.[123] The basic pathologic process is disruption of collagen and infiltration of the valve by a myxomatous substance rich in mucopolysaccharide. The mitral valve is often thickened and the chordae tendineae and mitral annulus may also contain myxomatous deposits that can cause elongation of the chordae, sometimes with rupture and dilatation of the mitral valve annulus. Abnormal mitral valve leaflet motion can cause fibrosis and thickening of the endocardial surface of the valve leaflets.[124] The tricuspid and aortic valves sometimes also show myxomatous degeneration. When there is enough slippage, so that a portion of the mitral valve fails to coapt against the rest of the leaflet, then mitral regurgitation develops.

Patients with MVP sometimes have abnormal left ventricular contractions. At necropsy, thrombi have been found, especially in the angle between the posterior leaflet of the mitral valve and the left atrial wall.[122,125,126] Transformation of the normally rigid valve into loose myxomatous tissue results in stretching of the valve leaflets, loss of endothelial continuity, and rupture of subendothelial connective tissue fibers. These changes could promote the formation of platelet-fibrin thrombi on the valve surface.

MVP is diagnosed by echocardiography when there is abnormal posterior movement of the coapted anterior or posterior leaflets (or both) of 2 mm or more, and one or both of the mitral valve leaflets are displaced during systole into the LA above the plane of the mitral annulus.[122] Midsystolic "buckling" or pansystolic "hammocking" of the valve leaflets is also sometimes found.[123] Mitral valve thickening and redundancy and the presence of mitral regurgitation are important additional criteria for the presence of important myxomatous mitral valve changes.[127,128] Approximately 8% of patients with MVP develop severe mitral regurgitation, which leads to congestive heart failure and necessitates mitral valve replacement. Atrial fibrillation can occur at any time but is more common in older patients, especially those with mitral regurgitation and large left atria. Myxomatous valves can become infected during bacteremia but the frequency of infective endocarditis is low. MVP occurs in patients with inherited connective tissue disorders, such as Marfan syndrome, Ehlers-Danlos syndrome, and osteogenesis imperfecta.[122]

The first report of a possible relation between MVP and brain ischemia was by Barnett in 1974.[129] The initial report outlined four patients, but Barnett and his colleagues later expanded the number of cases to 14 patients.[126,130] All patients were relatively young (age 10 to 48 years), and none had cardiovascular risk factors or occlusive vascular lesions. Barnett and colleagues later published a case-control series that provided further evidence of a relationship between MVP and brain ischemia in young patients.[121]

Among six series of patients with MVP and brain ischemic events reviewed by Lauzier and Barnett,[122] there were 114 patients, including 46 men and 68 women. Two-thirds of the events were strokes. The remainder were TIAs. Single attacks were more common than multiple ischemic events. Sixteen of the patients had an arrhythmia detected by rhythm monitoring, including eight with atrial fibrillation.[122]

Abnormalities of platelet function have been shown in patients with MVP and thromboembolism. Shortened platelet survival time, an increase in circulating platelet aggregates, and increased levels of beta-thromboglobulin and platelet factor IV were found in patients with MVP.[122] Interaction of circulating platelets with abnormal endocardial and valve structures in patients with myxomatous valve degeneration causes increased platelet aggregation, adhesion, and secretion. Platelet fibrin aggregates adhere to abnormal valve surfaces and later embolize or promote formation of erythrocyte-fibrin clots.

The recurrence rate of stroke in patients with MVP is low. In patients with mitral regurgitation and large left atria, and in those with atrial fibrillation and atrial or valvular thrombi shown by echocardiography, warfarin anticoagulation is probably indicated. In patients who do not have atrial fibrillation, endocarditis, or severe mitral insufficiency, the treatment of choice is probably an antiplatelet aggregant, such as aspirin, aspirin combined with modified-release dipyridamole, or clopidogrel.

MITRAL ANNULUS CALCIFICATION (MAC)

MAC is a degenerative disorder of the fibrous support structure of the mitral valve that occurs rather commonly in the elderly, especially in women. The most common TTE finding among elderly patients referred for a cardiac source of embolism is a high reflective area in the posterior portion of the mitral annulus representing mitral annular calcification.[52,132,133] MAC is very common in the elderly. A study of over 2000 patients (mean age 81 years) found that 48% had MAC with an increased prevalence of atrial fibrillation (22% vs 8% without MAC).[132] In addition to age,

MAC is associated with hypertension and aortic atherosclerosis.

In the original description of MAC, four of the 14 patients described by Korn and colleagues had brain infarcts, and three of those four had multiple infarcts.[134] The first important description of MAC as a potential cause of stroke was by DeBono and Warlow who studied 151 patients with retinal or brain ischemia and found MAC in eight patients, as compared with no instances of MAC in age and sex-matched controls who did not have brain or eye ischemia.[135] In 1979 to 1981, a total of 426 men and 733 women in the Framingham Study Cohort (average age, 70 years) who did not have strokes had M-mode echocardiograms.[136] Among these 1159 patients, 44 men (10.3%) and 116 women (15.8%) had MAC. During 8 years of follow-up, 51 patients without MAC (5.1%) had strokes, as compared with 22 patients with MAC (13.8%); MAC was associated with a 2.1 RR of stroke (95% confidence interval [CI], 1.24 to 3.57; $P = .006$).[136] A continuous relation was found in this study between frequency of stroke and severity of MAC; each millimeter of thickening on the echocardiogram represented a RR for stroke of 1.24. Even when patients with atherosclerotic heart disease and congestive heart failure were excluded, patients with MAC still had a stroke risk that was two times as high as those without MAC.[136] A recent study explored the role of MAC among 2723 Native Americans who did not have known cardiovascular disease.[137] The presence of MAC but not aortic valve sclerosis proved to be a strong risk factor for incident stroke even after adjusting for multiple other risk factors.[137]

Calcification has a predilection for the posterior portion of the mitral annulus ring. Calcific masses often extend as far as 3.5 cm into the adjacent myocardium and often project superiorly toward the atrium and centrally into the cavity of the left ventricle.[134] Ulceration and extrusion of the calcium through the overlying cusp into the ventricular cavity is found in some patients with MAC studied at necropsy, and thrombi are sometimes attached to the ulcerated regions.[138] Thrombi attached to calcified mitral annuli have also been shown by echocardiography.[137,139,140] Embolic material in patients with MAC can be calcium (as shown in calcific aortic stenosis) or thrombus.

MAC is common and is often accompanied by mitral regurgitation, atrial fibrillation, and aortic atheromas. Bacterial endocarditis can be superimposed. Hypertension, coronary atherosclerotic heart disease, and occlusive cerebrovascular disease are also often present in the population of patients with MAC. There are no data on the use of any prophylactic treatment on the prevention of brain or arterial embolism in patients with MAC. The association of MAC and aortic atheroma (84% vs 33% without MAC) may partially explain the association of MAC with stroke.[141]

PROSTHETIC CARDIAC VALVES

Advances in cardiac diagnosis and surgery have led to increasingly frequent replacement of heart valves. There are more than 80 different models of prosthetic valves, and more than 60,000 valve replacements are performed annually in the United States alone.[142] Mechanical valves are made primarily with metal and carbon alloys and are quite thrombogenic. Bioprosthetic valves are most often heterografts derived from pig or cow pericardial or valve tissues mounted on metal supports. Homografts, in the form of preserved human valves, are occasionally used for valve replacements. Bioprosthetic valves have low thrombogenic tendencies (but still higher than native valves), so long-term anticoagulation is ordinarily not prescribed. Bioprosthetic valves are less durable than mechanical valves.[142]

Valve thrombosis is an important complication in patients with both mechanical and bioprosthetic valves. Important valve thrombosis causes pulmonary congestion, reduced cardiac output, and brain and systemic embolism. The frequency of prosthetic-valve thrombosis is estimated to be between 0.1% and 5.7% per year.[143,144] Alteration of blood flow related to mechanical valves, as well as the inherent thrombogenicity of the materials used, promotes thrombosis and thromboembolism. Hematologic studies in patients with mechanical valves show elevation of platelet-specific proteins, which indicate platelet activation and decreased platelet survival in patients with artificial heart valves.[145]

Thrombus formation and subsequent embolization are found most often in mechanical valve prostheses in the mitral or tricuspid position in the setting of suboptimal anticoagulation.[146,147] Evaluation of prosthetic valves, especially prostheses in the mitral position, is best performed by TEE. It is often assumed clinically that patients with mechanical prostheses who present with systemic embolization have prosthetic valve thrombi, especially if there is no other obvious cause and/or the INR is suboptimal. In patients who have thromboembolism and a therapeutic INR, TEE is often helpful in distinguishing valve dysfunction related to pannus ingrowth from thrombus.[52]

The pathophysiologic events that promote thromboembolism begin during heart surgery. Prosthetic materials and injured perivalvular

9

tissues cause platelet activation as soon as circulation is restored. Dacron sewing rings, common to all prosthetic valves, form a fertile nidus for platelet activation and adhesion. Prosthetic material also activates the intrinsic pathway of the coagulation cascade. These events promote the formation of red erythrocyte-fibrin thrombi. Degenerative changes in bioprosthetic valves can also stimulate deposition of white platelet-fibrin thrombi. Late thrombosis is also found in the cusp sinuses of bioprosthetic mitral valves that have undergone fibrosis and calcification.

Embolism is an important complication in patients with mechanical and bioprosthetic valves. The frequency of major embolism in patients with mechanical valves is estimated to be 4% per year if no antithrombotic therapy is used.[148] This frequency is reduced to approximately 2% per year by medications that decrease platelet aggregation, and to 1% per year with warfarin anticoagulation.[148] Most symptomatic emboli go to the brain. Patients with mitral mechanical valves have a slightly higher frequency of embolization than those with aortic valves, probably related to the higher frequency of associated atrial fibrillation and large left atria in patients with mitral valve prostheses. Patients with bioprosthetic valves also have a risk of embolism. In one series of 128 patients with porcine bioprosthetic valves inserted during 5 to 8 years of follow-up, two of 43 patients with aortic valve replacement, nine of 62 with porcine mitral valves, and four of 18 with both mitral and aortic prosthetic valves had clinical thromboemboli.[149] Most patients with thromboemboli in this series had atrial fibrillation or heart block.[149] Large left atria, atrial fibrillation, left ventricular dysfunction, and infective endocarditis are important associated conditions in patients with prosthetic valves that cause thromboembolism.

Anticoagulation is recommended for all patients with prosthetic heart valves. Patients with bioprosthetic valves are often treated for the first 3 months after surgery using a target international normalized ratio (INR) of 2.0 to 3.0. Oral anticoagulant therapy reduces the frequency of embolism in patients with mechanical valve prostheses and the intensity of anticoagulation has been recommended to be higher than that used with bioprosthetic valves. Patients with caged-ball prostheses may require a higher intensity of anticoagulation than those with bileaflet disk valves and those with single-tilting disk valves. Adding antiplatelet medications, such as dipyridamole, aspirin, or clopidogrel, can further reduce the frequency of embolism. Aspirin and lower-intensity anticoagulation (INR of 2.0 to 3.0) are probably as effective

as high-intensity anticoagulation and have less risk of serious bleeding. Because prosthetic valves induce formation of white platelet-fibrin and red erythrocyte-fibrin clots, the use of combined antiplatelet aggregant and anticoagulant therapy makes sense. Pregnant women with prosthetic valves should be treated with heparin or low-molecular-weight heparin because the incidence of thromboemboli is increased while pregnant and also in the puerperium.

INFECTIVE ENDOCARDITIS

Although neurologic complications of infective endocarditis have been well recognized since the time of Osler,[150] the clinical spectrum of endocarditis has changed dramatically in recent decades. Compared with series of endocarditis patients performed in the 1960s, series of patients with infective endocarditis performed more recently contain older patients, more drug addicts, more examples of tricuspid valve involvement (usually in intravenous drug addicts), and more patients with infection of prosthetic valves. Diagnostic capabilities have also changed. Echocardiography and newer brain and cerebrovascular imaging techniques allow better clarification of the cardiac and brain pathology and pathophysiology. Brain ischemia, intracerebral hemorrhage, subarachnoid hemorrhage, encephalopathy, and meningitis are the major neurologic complications found in series of patients with native valve and prosthetic valve endocarditis.[151-157]

Brain ischemia is invariably caused by embolism. Approximately one fifth of patients with endocarditis develop brain infarcts. At necropsy, small, usually multiple, cortical or subcortical bland infarcts are found. The larger infarcts are usually found in patients with *Staphylococcus aureus* endocarditis. Ischemia can take the form of TIAs that involve the brain or retina. Brain ischemia may be the presenting sign of endocarditis and is most common early in the course of the disease. Ischemic strokes can also occur days after antibiotic treatment has begun. Monitoring of patients with endocarditis using TCD shows that microemboli continue to occur even after antibiotic treatment, although more emboli are detected before and shortly after antibiotics are given. Brain ischemia was described in 17%,[152] 19%,[153] and 15%[156] of patients in various infective endocarditis series.

After congestive heart failure, arterial embolism is the most common life-threatening complication in patients with infective endocarditis. Embolization during the first week of antibiotic treatment is most common,[157] and becomes less frequent thereafter.[158] Late thromboembolism after completion of antibiotic treatment is rare unless recurrent infection develops. Staphylococci and streptococcus species account for more than 80% of native valve endocarditis.[159] Staphylococcal endocarditis poses a higher risk of clinical thromboembolism compared with other bacterial causes.[152,157,158,160] Fungal endocarditis is also associated with frequent embolism. Mitral valve vegetations have a higher frequency of clinical thromboemboli than aortic valve lesions.[157,161,162]

Infective vegetations appear at echocardiography as bright, usually mobile echo-dense lesions attached to valve leaflets. Figure 4-36 shows a large vegetation on the mitral valve in a patient with infective endocarditis. Figure 9-9 shows bacterial vegetations in a number of valve regions. The frequency of detection of vegetations on echocardiography depends on the technique used and the frequency of examinations. Lesions smaller than 2 mm are not reliably identified by echocardiography. In the series of Hart et al (using M-mode and two-dimensional transthoracic echocardiography [TTE]), vegetations were found on 41% of initial echocardiograms in patients with *S. aureus* endocarditis, compared with 57% of initial studies in patients with streptococcal species endocarditis.[153] An echocardiogram that fails to show a vegetation does not exclude the diagnosis of endocarditis. A negative TTE should be followed by TEE (with superior spatial resolution) if the clinical suspicion is high or moderate.[163,164] TEE evidence for large (>10 mm) vegetations and increased mobility identify patients at high risk for clinical thromboembolism.[164]

Brain hemorrhage is much less frequent than ischemia, but the effects of hemorrhage can be devastating and fatal. Intracerebral hemorrhage was found in 6%,[152] 7%,[153] 2.8%,[155] and 5.6%[156] of patients in various endocarditis series. Series that included modern brain imaging and necropsy studies clarified the mechanisms of intracerebral hemorrhage in endocarditis.[154,165,166] Some patients bleed into bland infarcts. This usually takes the form of hemorrhagic infarction characterized by petechial and larger regions of hemorrhagic mottling within infarcts, without formation of frank, discrete hematomas. In some patients, large hematomas develop. Hematomas are often found in patients treated with anticoagulants. In other patients, intracerebral hemorrhage results from rupture of a septic arteritis caused by embolization of infected material to the artery with necrosis of the arterial wall.[165,166] In a minority of patients, intracerebral hemorrhage is caused by rupture of a mycotic aneurysm into the

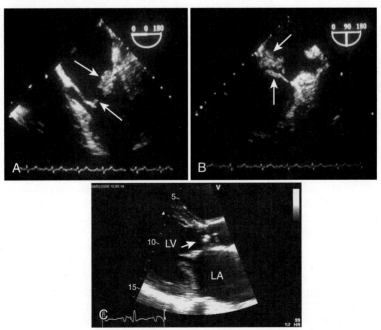

Figure 9-9. Echocardiography showing bacterial vegetations in a patient with infective endocarditis. **A,** TEE showing a large vegetation protruding from the posterior mitral leaflet *(white arrow)* and **B,** a much smaller vegetation at the tip of the anterior mitral leaflet *(white arrow)*. **C,** Transthoracic echocardiogram in the parasternal long axis view. Note the vegetation *(white arrow)* on the left ventricular outflow tract side of the aortic valve. The left ventricle (LV) and left atrium (LA) are identified. (From Caplan LR, Manning WJ: Brain Embolism. New York: Informa Healthcare, 2006, with permission.)

brain substance. Brain hemorrhage, similar to the situation in patients with brain ischemia, is most common at or near presentation and is less common after effective antibiotic treatment. Many patients who develop brain hemorrhages have had an attack of transient or persistent brain ischemia in the hours or days before the hemorrhage. This prodromal ischemia is explained by an arterial embolus causing brain infarction. Hemorrhage into an infarct or rupture of the artery that received the infected embolus causes the hemorrhage, which often proves fatal.[165,166]

The need for angiography to detect mycotic aneurysms and the indications for surgical treatment of aneurysms found by angiography remain controversial. In a review by Hart et al, among 2119 patients with endocarditis, only 5% of patients with brain hemorrhages had identified mycotic aneurysms.[165] Mycotic aneurysms are caused by embolization of infected material into the wall and adventitia of brain arteries. The aneurysms usually occur distally along arteries and tend to be multiple. The location of aneurysms in patients with infective endocarditis is similar to those found in patients with atrial myxomas, probably because of similar embolic etiologies. In contrast, ordinary saccular "berry" aneurysms occur proximally along the basal arteries of the circle of Willis. More recently, the advent of gradient echo recall images (T2*-weighted images) shows that some patients with infective endocarditis have tiny round dark regions of susceptibility usually referred to as "microbleeds."[166a,b] These are often located within sulci and probably represent small mycotic aneurysms. Angiography of patients without clinical or imaging evidence of intracranial hemorrhage seldom shows mycotic aneurysms. Mycotic aneurysms have been shown to disappear in some patients on sequential angiography performed after bacteriologic cure.[167-169] Mycotic aneurysms can rupture, however, sometimes after bacteriologic cure, and re-rupture can prove fatal. The decision as to whether to perform angiography and surgical treatment if an aneurysm is found must rest on the clinical findings in individual patients.

Diffuse brain-related symptoms, usually referred to as encephalopathy, are common in patients with endocarditis. Symptoms include lethargy and decreased level of consciousness, confusion, agitation, poor concentration, and reduced memory. Encephalopathy has different explanations. Often, the cause is toxi-metabolic and explained by systemic factors, such as azotemia, pulmonary dysfunction, hyponatremia, and so forth. In many patients, encephalopathy is a toxic effect related to fever and the acute infection. Patients with *S. aureus* acute endocarditis are more often encephalopathic than in endocarditis caused by other organisms. Necropsy, CT, and MRI studies of patients with encephalopathy often show multiple, small, scattered brain infarcts, microabscesses, or both.[154,170] Encephalopathy usually develops during uncontrolled infection with virulent organisms, supporting the role of microscopic septic emboli as the cause.[154]

Meningitis also occurs in patients with endocarditis. Meningeal infection is caused by embolization of infected vegetations to meningeal arteries. The presentation is often headache with fever. Because the usual infecting organism is not virulent, the patient is not as ill as in other acute forms of bacterial meningitis. Meningitis occurred in 6.4%[151] and 1.1%[152] in two series of patients with endocarditis.

Valvular vegetations in patients with infective endocarditis are composed of platelets, fibrin, erythrocytes, and inflammatory cells attached to damaged endothelium of native and prosthetic valves. Organisms are enmeshed within the fibrinous material, often deep within the vegetations, explaining why antibiotics have difficulty sterilizing the lesions. Vegetations range in size from several millimeters to several centimeters, and their potential for embolization relate to their size and friability. The mitral valve is most often involved. Mitral valve disease, however, is also more frequent than other valve disease. In the past, the predominant underlying valve disease was rheumatic; calcified valves, MVP, and prosthetic valves now make up a higher proportion of cases than in the past. The neurologic complications of native valve and prosthetic valve endocarditis are the same.[152,154,155]

Laboratory studies are helpful in diagnosis, but the clinical findings remain protean, and most important for recognition of infective endocarditis is a strong clinical suspicion. The disease should be suspected in any patient with unexplained fever and a heart murmur. Multiple blood cultures are important in all patients suspected of having infective endocarditis. The spinal fluid may be normal or contain slightly increased protein levels and increased numbers of erythrocytes and leukocytes. Usually, the pleocytosis is moderate (<300 cells/mL) and may be predominantly lymphocytic or polymorphonuclear. When a clinical picture of meningitis is present, there may be more white blood cells. Echocardiography is an important diagnostic test, but, as indicated above, a negative echocardiographic examination does not exclude the diagnosis of infective endocarditis.

The most important treatment is the rapid introduction of specific antimicrobial drugs. Most neurologic complications occur before or near the time of diagnosis and initial antibiotic treatment. Recurrent strokes do occur after bacteriologic cure, but rarely. In one series among 147 patients discharged from the hospital after treatment of infective endocarditis, 15 developed strokes after discharge; all except one of the stroke patients had prosthetic valve endocarditis.[152] Strokes in this series occurred long after discharge (median, 22 months) and were better explained by recurrence of endocarditis, complications of anticoagulants, and noninfective disease of the prosthetic valves than by cerebrovascular complications of the original endocarditic episode.[152]

Native valve endocarditis is not an indication for anticoagulation, even when brain or systemic embolism has occurred. Controversy surrounds the issue of maintenance of anticoagulation in patients who have mechanical valve endocarditis, but most clinicians favor cautious continuation of anticoagulants unless a brain hemorrhage develops. When a hemorrhagic infarct or brain hemorrhage develops, anticoagulation with warfarin is usually stopped for 1 to 2 weeks. In patients with a major risk of recurrent embolization, it may be safe to use heparin beginning soon after the hemorrhage is discovered and later switch back to warfarin. Cardiac surgery to debride or replace infected valves is performed for cardiac indications. These include mostly heart failure related to valve dysfunction, lack of control of infection, valve infection with fungal or other virulent organism not controllable by antimicrobial drugs, and valve or chordae tendineae rupture.

Noninfective Fibrous and Fibrinous Endocardial Lesions (Including Valve Strands)

In a variety of other circumstances, fibrous valve thickening, often with grossly visible vegetations that contain mixtures of platelets and fibrin, are found on the heart valves and adjacent endocardium in patients who have no evidence of rheumatic fever or bacterial endocarditis. The first detailed description of such lesions was by Libman and Sacks, who reported four patients studied clinically and pathologically with an "atypical verrucous endocarditis."[171] Necropsy showed fibrous thickening of valves with vegetations, especially along the closure lines of the valves and on the valve leaflets. The vegetations spread to the papillary muscles and ventricular endocardium. Only one patient had prominent clinical neurologic abnormalities, a unilateral paralysis and seizures that developed just before death. The authors speculated that these findings might be caused by emboli from the valvular vegetations. Libman and Sacks were uncertain of the diagnosis but noted that the clinical findings resembled some of the erythematous diseases. The next year, Klemperer, Pollack, and Baehr published the pathologic findings in disseminated lupus erythematosus.[172] In 1935, Baehr and colleagues reported a series of 23 patients who had acute disseminated lupus erythematosus, among whom 13 patients had a nonrheumatic verrucous endocarditis similar to that described by Libman and Sacks.[173] These clinical and pathologic reports brought the disease systemic lupus erythematosus (SLE), known previously as predominantly a skin disorder, to the attention of the medical community as an acute disseminated systemic disease.

Gross, a younger colleague of Libman and Sacks at Mount Sinai Hospital in New York in 1940, reported a detailed study of 27 hearts, 23 of which were fatal cases of SLE.[174] Gross pointed out that the patients in the original report from the Mount Sinai Hospital had the typical clinical findings of lupus erythematosus and suggested that the verrucous endocardial lesions were diagnostic of that disease.[174] Libman and Sacks[171] and Gross[174] were aware that similar endocarditic lesions also occurred in terminal or cachectic diseases, such as carcinoma, tuberculosis, and leukemia, and were called nonbacterial thrombotic endocarditis. Since these early reports, similar lesions of the cardiac valves and endocardium are known to occur in patients with SLE, the antiphospholipid antibody (APLA) syndrome, and marantic nonbacterial thrombotic endocarditis (NBTE). All likely have a similar pathogenesis.

Valvular lesions are common in patients with SLE. Roldan et al performed TEE on 69 SLE patients on two occasions, averaging 29 months between echocardiograms.[175] Valvular abnormalities were found in 61% of patients on the initial TEE, and in 53% on the second echocardiographic study. Valve thickening (61%), vegetations (43%), valve regurgitation (25%), and stenosis (4%) were found on the initial echocardiograms. The mitral valve was most often involved, followed closely by involvement of the aortic valve; tricuspid valve disease occurred occasionally, but pulmonic valve involvement was rare. The combined incidence of stroke, peripheral embolism, heart failure, and superimposed infective endocarditis was 22% in those with valvular disease found on TEE.[175] In a recent review of 38 SLE patients who had Libman-Sacks endocarditis, valvular involvement correlated with the duration of SLE and the presence of APLA and clinical thromboses.[175a]

The APLA syndrome was first recognized during the 1970s as a prothrombotic syndrome separate from SLE. The APLA syndrome is characterized by frequent fetal loss, strokes, myocardial infarcts, phlebothrombosis, pulmonary emboli, and thrombocytopenia. Serologic testing reveals positive assays for the lupus anticoagulant, anticardiolipin antibodies, or both. Echocardiographic studies have shown that there is a relatively high frequency of cardiac valvular lesions in patients with the APLA syndrome, and that the valve lesions are indistinguishable from those found in patients with SLE. Figure 9-10 is a TEE and surgical specimen of a valve with a fibrinous vegetation in a young man with the APLA syndrome. Barbut et al studied the prevalence of antiphospholipid antibodies among 87 patients in whom echocardiography showed mitral or aortic regurgitation, or both[176]; 26 patients (30%) had immunoglobulin G or M anticardiolipin antibodies. Focal brain ischemic events occurred in eight of these patients (seven judged embolic), including seven of the immunoglobulin G anticardiolipin-positive patients.[176] In another report, Barbut and colleagues studied 21 patients with APLA antibodies who had focal brain ischemic events.[177] Twelve of 14 stroke patients (86%), and 3 of 7 non-stroke patients (42%) had echocardiographic evidence of mitral or aortic valve abnormalities. Eight of the 21 patients with APLA had SLE in this study.[177] In a large cooperative study performed by the Antiphospholid Antibodies in Stroke Study Group among 128 patients who had brain or ocular ischemia and were APLA positive, 16 patients (22.2%) had mitral valve abnormalities on echocardiograms, and 2 patients had aortic valve lesions.[178] Phospholipids are important constituents of cardiac valve endothelium, blood platelets, vascular endothelium, and coagulation proteins. At present, most assays for antiphospholipid antibodies only include testing for lupus anticoagulant and anticardiolipin antibodies. Some patients with the clinical features of the APLA syndrome

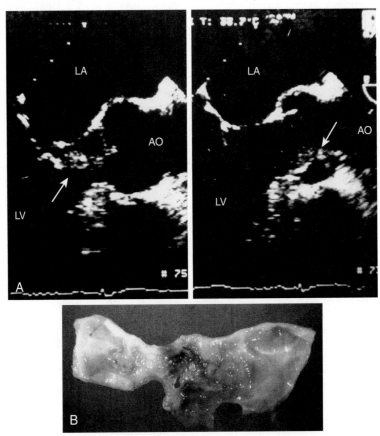

Figure 9-10. Mitral valve vegetations in a patient with APLA antibody syndrome and multiple brain emboli. **A,** Echocardiography showing a pedunculated, mobile lesion on the mitral valve *(white arrows).* **B,** The valve lesion removed at surgery showing vegetation. LA, left atrium, LV, left ventricle, AO, aorta. (**A,** From Caplan LR, Manning WJ: Brain Embolism. New York: Informa Healthcare, 2006, with permission.)

have valve vegetations and cardiogenic brain embolism, but antibody assays are negative.

Hypercoagulability and NBTE have long been known to occur in patients with cancer and other debilitating chronic diseases. Most often, the cancers are mucinous adenocarcinomas.[179] In one study of 20 cancer patients who had thromboembolic disease of the brain and other organs, 16 patients (80%) had NBTE at necropsy.[180] Edoute et al performed prospective echocardiograms on 200 cancer patients and found a 19% frequency of NBTE.[181] The valve lesions equally involved the mitral and aortic valves. Elevated plasma D-dimer levels, a marker for hypercoagulability, was also often found in cancer patients with clinical thromboembolism.[181] NBTE is characterized by friable white or tan vegetations, usually along lines of valve closure. The vegetations can be large. Microscopy usually shows degenerating platelets interwoven with strands of fibrin and some leukocytes, forming eosinophilic masses of tissue. All three conditions—SLE, APLA syndrome, and NBTE—are associated with hypercoagulability, strokes, and thrombocytopenia. The cardiac valve and endothelial lesions in these three conditions are similar and probably indistinguishable grossly and microscopically. Platelet deposition, incorporation of fibrin, and the formation of platelet thrombi on valve and endocardial surfaces are common to all three conditions. Treatment of these conditions has not been formally studied. In theory, drugs that alter platelet aggregation, secretion, and adhesion might be effective. In patients with SLE and APLA syndrome who have hypercoagulability, heparin and warfarin compounds are usually prescribed to treat the hypercoagulability and prevent venous and arterial occlusions.

Noninfective valve lesions are also found in patients with carcinoid tumors (probably causally related to elevated serotonin levels in the blood) and after the use of some drugs (ergotamine, methysergide, dexfenfluramine, and fenfluramine and phentermine, cabergoline, and pergolide).[182,183] The valve and endocardial lesions that result are similar to each other morphologically and consist of fibrotic thickening of the valves with reduced pliability.

Echocardiographic examinations often show strands of mobile tissue attached to valve surfaces. The cause and significance of these strands remains uncertain. In 1856, Lambl had originally described such filamentous outgrowths from the ventricular surfaces of the aortic valves sometimes found at necropsy,[184] so these fibrous strand-like lesions have often been called Lambl excrescences. Later, Magarey found similar filiform strands on the atrial surface of mitral valves.[185] The strands, which were composed of a cellular connective tissue core covered by endothelium, were usually less than 1 mm thick and ranged in length from 1 to 10 mm.[185] Magarey related the strands to mitral valve thickening and posited that they originated from fibrinous deposits on valve surfaces.[185] Echocardiographic examinations show these valve excrescences as thin, elongated, mobile echoreflective structures with independent undulating hypermobility seen near the leaflet's line of closure. They are found on the atrial side of the mitral valve, and the ventricular side of the aortic valve and are increasingly recognized in elderly patients undergoing echocardiography.[186]

Freedberg et al performed a retrospective review of 1559 patients with TEEs during a 2-year period and found mitral valve strands in 63 patients (4%) and aortic valve strands in 26 patients (1.7%).[187] Strands were found in 10.6% of patients referred because of suspected recent embolic events, compared with 2.3% of those referred for other indications.[187]

Roberts and colleagues compared the frequency of strands among patients referred for TEE because of brain ischemia and those referred for other indications and also found an association between brain ischemia and strands.[188] The association was strongest for younger patients and those with mitral and aortic valve strands.[188] Cohen et al found strands in 22.5% of 338 brain ischemia patients versus 12.1% of 276 patients who had no history of brain ischemia (odds ratio, 2; 95% CI, 1.3 to 3.4; $P < .005$).[189] The risk of recurrent stroke in patients with strands was low.[189] Strands are often found in patients with mitral valve thickening.[189,190] Strands probably form because of a degenerative process that causes fibrinous deposits on valve surfaces. Emboli can arise from the abnormal valves, strands, or thrombi formed on the surface of the valve or on the strands. In some patients, strands may share a pathogenesis with valve lesions found in patients with SLE, APLAs, and cancer.

Nighoghossian et al reported three patients who had brain ischemic events presumably related to mitral valve strands who had cardiac surgery.[191] Extensive evaluation including cerebral angiography and serological testing showed no cause for stroke other than the valve lesions. The valve lesions were described as a floating mass 6 mm thick on the ventricular surface of the mitral valve; a 6-mm lesion on the anterior mitral valve leaflet; and a sessile 5-mm lesion on the anterior mitral valve leaflet.[191] One patient had urgent cardiac surgery when the valve lesion was found; the other two patients had surgery when

9

they had recurrent strokes despite anticoagulant therapy. Histopathologic examinations showed that the lesions were composed of an acellular fibrous core with rings of granular material and endothelial cells. In two patients, thrombi were attached to the lesions.[191]

Treatment of patients with strands has not been formally studied, but anticoagulants were unsuccessful in preventing brain emboli in two of the patients of Nighoghossian et al[191] and may not be effective in patients with NBTE. Antiplatelet aggregants, or a combination of antiplatelet aggregants and anticoagulants, might be more effective in preventing thrombus formation and embolism than either agent alone.

Myocardial and Cardiac Chamber Lesions

MYOCARDIAL INFARCTION AND CORONARY ARTERY DISEASE

Systemic embolism is apparent clinically in approximately 3% (range, 0.6% to 6.4%) of patients with acute myocardial infarction.[2,51,192,193] Most clinically detected emboli involve the brain. Most strokes that occur in patients with acute myocardial infarcts are caused by embolization of thrombi formed in the left ventricle, but some strokes are caused by left atrial thrombi, hypotension, and extracranial occlusive vascular disease. Coronary artery thrombosis can cause an increase in acute phase reactants, including serine protease coagulation proteins. Venous thromboses and occlusion of atherostenotic craniocervical arteries develop in the days and weeks after myocardial infarction because of this hypercoagulability.

The risk of stroke and thrombus formation is related to infarct location (anterior at higher risk) and infarct size. In the GISSI-3 trial, the incidence of LV thrombus among those with an anterior infarction increased to almost 18% for patients with a LV ejection fraction of less than 40% as compared with less than 10% of those with a higher ejection fraction.[194] The corresponding frequency for infarctions at nonanterior sites ranges between 1.8% to 5.4%.[51,194-197] Most thrombi form on the apical wall of the left ventricle in regions of reduced ventricular contractility. Mural thrombi are more likely to form in patients with transmural and large anterior myocardial infarcts than in those with small infarcts. Areas of decreased ventricular contractility, low ejection fraction, and development of a left ventricular aneurysm predispose to thrombus formation. Figure 9-11 shows a large thrombus in the left ventricle of a patient with a fatal recent myocardial infarct.

Cardiac thrombi often develop within the first 3 days after myocardial infarction, especially in

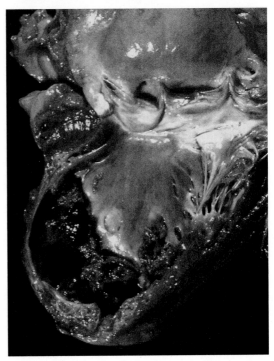

Figure 9-11. Heart at necropsy in a patient with a massive brain embolus. There is a large clot overlying a recent myocardial infarct.

patients with large infarcts, but can develop later. Using serial TTE, most thrombi are found to develop within the first two weeks after infarction (median 5 to 6 days).[198-200] While some patients develop a new LV thrombus, most often it is in association with worsening LV systolic function.[200,201] Thrombus mobility and protrusion are associated with increased risk of stroke.[202]

Systemic embolization occurs, on average, 14 days after myocardial infarction and is unusual after 4 to 6 weeks.[203] Anticoagulants reduce the frequency of stroke in patients with acute myocardial infarcts. Among 999 patients with acute myocardial infarction, short-term warfarin treatment for 28 days reduced the rate of stroke (0.8% vs 3.8% in nonanticoagulated controls, $P < .001$).[204]

Regions of decreased ventricular contraction and frank ventricular aneurysms often persist after acute myocardial infarction. In the Coronary Artery Surgery Study (CASS), 7.6% of patients had angiographically defined left ventricular aneurysms.[205] Although aneurysms are relatively common and mural thrombi often form within aneurysms, the risk of stroke is relatively low, at approximately 5%.[206] The risk of stroke in patients with impaired left ventricular function after myocardial infarction is substantial. In one study of 2231 patients with left ventricular dysfunction after acute myocardial infarction who were followed for an average of 42 months, 103 patients (4.6%) developed strokes.[207] Patients with ejection fractions of less than 28% were at highest risk, and for every absolute decrease of 5% in the left ventricular ejection fraction, the risk of stroke increased by 18%.[207]

Some patients with brain embolism are unexpectedly found to have thrombi within their left ventricles. These thrombi are most often detected with TTE, which has a reported sensitivity and specificity greater than 90%.[51,208-210] The use of intravenous echo contrast agents may assist with the discrimination between apical trabeculations and thrombus.[51] While detection of apical LV thrombi have been reported,[195] the frequent inability of TEE to visualize the true LV apex makes TEE a less appropriate imaging test for suspected LV apical thrombi. Delayed enhancement cardiac magnetic resonance may be superior to both TTE and TEE for identifying left ventricular thrombi.

Some patients with left ventricular thrombi do not have a history of acute myocardial infarction, and the cardiac cavity lesions may be mistaken for myxomas or other cardiac tumors. Sequential echocardiography shows that these thrombi can gradually regress or suddenly disappear,[4] often without development of neurologic or other symptoms of embolism. Thrombus formation, spontaneous endogenous fibrinolysis, and fragmentation of thrombi are dynamic processes. Thrombolytic treatment of patients with cardiac thrombi poses the theoretical risk of fragmentation of large thrombi into portions that could embolize and cause stroke, myocardial infarction, and systemic embolism. Thrombi may disappear during anticoagulation without symptoms or signs of embolism.

MYOCARDIOPATHIES

Conditions that affect the endocardium and myocardium promote the formation of cardiac mural thrombi and systemic and brain embolism. The three most important factors that determine thrombus formation are (1) involvement of the endocardial surface, (2) ventricular contractility and blood flow and ejection patterns within the ventricles, and (3) activation of platelets and the coagulation system. Among the three categories of cardiomyopathies—dilatated, restrictive, and hypertrophic—mural thrombus formation and embolism are most common among the dilatated cardiomyopathies. Intraventricular thrombus formation is enhanced by stasis of blood and the loss of normal subendocardial trabeculation. The network of subendocardial trabeculae functions as many small compartments that produce high levels of force within the ventricle, propelling blood away from the endocardial surface.[211]

Conditions as diverse as muscular dystrophies, cardiac amyloidosis, peripartum cardiomyopathy, Fabry's disease, cocaine-related cardiomyopathy, noncompaction of the myocardium, and cardiac sarcoidosis are sources of cardiac-origin embolism. Morbid obesity is also associated with a myocardiopathy.[211a] Recently, Japanese researchers and others have described a myocardiopathy associated with emotional distress referred to as Takotsubo cardiomyopathy.[211b,211c] Takotsubo is the Japanese name of an octopus trap shaped like an ampulla. This name has been applied to the cardiomyopathy because acute emotional stress and trauma cause a characteristic apical ballooning of the heart recognizable on echocardiography that resembles the Japanese octopus trap. Like other disorders of the heart muscle, takotsubo cardiomyopathy is occasionally a source of brain embolism.

In patients with cardiomyopathies, mural thrombi form mostly within the trabeculae carneae near the cardiac apex. Atrial fibrillation develops in some patients with cardiomyopathies and further increases the frequency of embolism. Embolism is unusual in patients with hypertrophic cardiomyopathies unless they develop atrial fibrillation.

CARDIAC MYXOMAS AND OTHER TUMORS

Primary cardiac tumors are rare, occurring in fewer than 0.03% of autopsy studies, with myxomas constituting almost 60% of these lesions.[212] Although cardiac tumors are rare, they are an important cause of brain embolism. Myxomas are the most common heart tumor. Myxomas are histologically benign tumors that most often are found within the body of the LA and attached to the midportion of the interatrial septum at the edge of the fossa ovalis, but some originate from the posterior or anterior atrial walls or the auricular appendage.[213] Figure 9-12 is a TEE that shows a typical left atrial myxoma attached to the interatrial septum. Approximately 75% are located in the LA and 15% to 20% in the right atrium.[213] Approximately 6% to 8% of myxomas are found in the ventricles equally divided between the left and right ventricles.[213] Myxomas rarely arise from the heart valves. Biatrial myxomas have been described, in which case the tumor usually projects into the contralateral atrium through a PFO. Myxomas project from their endocardial attachments into cardiac chambers. Myxomas are most often found in patients between the ages of 30 and 60 years; women are affected slightly more than men, and there are instances of familial occurrence of myxomas.

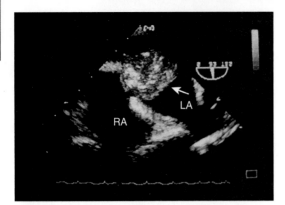

Figure 9-12. TEE in a patient with a large left atrial myxoma (*white arrow*) within the LA attached to the interatrial septum in the area of the foramen ovale. LA, left atrium; RA, right atrium. (From Caplan LR, Manning WJ: Brain Embolism. New York: Informa Healthcare, 2006, with permission.)

Embolism occurs in 30% to 50% of patients with cardiac myxomas.[213,214] Most emboli arise from the LA and travel to the brain or systemic organs. The mobility of the myxomas is related more to the likelihood of embolism than the size of the tumors.[214a] Occasionally, right atrial myxomas cause systemic embolism in the presence of a PFO. Both white and red thrombi tend to form on the surface of the myxomas. Emboli consist of tumor fragments, particles of thrombi, or both.

Occasionally, patients with brain emboli from myxomas have subarachnoid or intracerebral hemorrhage. Bleeding is related to the development of hemorrhagic infarction or rupture of aneurysms. Embolism from myxoma tissue to the wall of brain arteries causes aneurysms that are identical to mycotic aneurysms found in patients with bacterial endocarditis. Usually, the aneurysms are relatively small, multiple, and located on peripheral branches of brain arteries. Some aneurysms are quite large. The peripheral location of aneurysms in patients with myxomas and endocarditis differs from that usually found in patients with saccular ("berry") aneurysms. Delayed progressive brain ischemia and enlargement of aneurysms can develop after the initial embolic event. Although delayed growth and rupture of aneurysms and metastatic tumor growth do occur, their frequency is low. In a review of 35 patients followed at the Mayo Clinic after surgical removal of atrial myxomas, none had subsequent delayed neurologic events attributable to their myxomas.[215] Recurrent cardiac tumors after surgery can, however, give rise to recurrent embolization.

Papillary fibroelastomas are another type of cardiac tumor that often give rise to brain embolism.[214,216-219,219a] The lesions consist of multiple papillary fronds that radiate from an avascular fibrocollagenous core attached by a short pedicle to the endothelium. These tumors are usually highly spherical, highly mobile pedunculated tumors most commonly located on the aortic or mitral valves. Less often, they are found on endocardial surfaces. Echocardiographically, papillary fibroelastomas appear speckled with echolucencies near the edges.[219] These tumors classically are not associated with valvular dysfunction, but they may be a source of systemic embolization due to migration of thrombus from the tumor surface[219] or tumor embolization.[216] Angina and coronary ischemia are caused by embolism to the coronary arteries. Multiple brain infarcts usually occur before the diagnosis is made by echocardiography.

Both TTE and TEE are highly sensitive in detecting myxomas and papillary fibroelastomas, though TEE may provide more accurate anatomical details, such as the site of attachment, and, in selected patients, may help to differentiate these tumors from thrombi.[51] Rhabdomyomas are often multiple, arise from the ventricular myocardium, and project into the ventricular cavity. Tuberous sclerosis and neurofibromatosis predispose to the development of cardiac rhabdomyomas.

Emboli are often composed of tumor fragments. Theoretically, white platelet-fibrin nidi might develop on the surface and crevices of cardiac tumors, as might red erythrocyte-fibrin thrombi. For this reason, agents that affect platelet aggregation and function and standard anticoagulants might have some therapeutic effect, but no studies of their use in patients with myxomas or other cardiac neoplasms have been performed. The only definitive treatment is surgery.

Paradoxical Embolism and Cardiac Septal Lesions

Recently the topics of paradoxical embolism and patent foramen ovale (PFO) have received much greater attention than in the past, largely because of the improved cardiac technology that can recognize the presence of a PFO. Paradoxical emboli are those that enter the systemic circulation through right-to-left shunting of blood. By far, the most common potential intracardiac shunt is a residual PFO. The high frequency of PFOs in the normal population makes it difficult to be certain in an individual stroke patient with a PFO whether paradoxic embolism through the PFO was the cause of their stroke or whether the PFO was merely an incidental finding.

Because the nomenclature is confusing it is worthwhile to review the embryology of the division of the common atrium into left and right atria. The interatrial septum begins to form during the 5th week of uterine life.[220] The septum primum grows caudally from the superior portion of the single atrium and fuses with the endocardial cushion closing the defect called the ostium primum. Another potential defect forms from partial resorption of the septum primum and is called the ostium secundum. A second septum, the septum secundum, arises from the superior portion of the atrium and descends on the right side of the septum primum to cover the ostium secundum. The ostium secundum is not covered completely because of the presence of the foramen ovale. The foramen ovale consists of the septum primum and septum secundum which are joined parallel to a slit-like valve. This valve allows oxygenated blood to bypass the pulmonary circulation of the fetus during intrauterine life.[220] A PFO is necessary during fetal life to facilitate shunting of blood from the right atrium to the LA, thereby bypassing the high resistance pulmonary circuit. The lungs are not aerated during intrauterine existence. At birth or shortly thereafter, the septum primum and the septum secundum usually fuse, closing the interatrial septum to the flow of blood. Ostium secundum atrial septal defects occur when there is excess resorption of the septum primum or inadequate formation of the septum secundum. A PFO occurs when fusion of the septum primum with the septum secundum is inadequate.

In a significant number of individuals the foramen ovale remains somewhat patent during adult life. The prevalence of a PFO varies depending on its definition. Autopsy series have shown that approximately 30% of adults have a probe PFO at necropsy.[221] Hagen et al studied 956 patients with clinically and pathologically normal hearts and found a PFO in 27.3%.[221] The frequency of PFOs declined with age—34.3% during the first 3 decades of life, 25.4% during the 4th through 8th decades, and 20.2% during the 9th and 10th decades. The average diameter of PFOs was 4.9 mm, and the size tended to increase with age.[221] Echocardiographic studies have shown that PFOs are found more often in patients with stroke than in controls, and PFOs are more common in patients with an undetermined cause of stroke ("cryptogenic stroke") than in those in whom another etiology has been defined.[222-224]

I use the following five criteria for paradoxic embolism: (1) situations that promote thrombosis of leg or pelvic veins (e.g., sitting in one position for a long period, recent surgery, and so forth) (Table 9-4 lists the major risk factors for venous thrombosis); (2) increased coagulability (e.g., the use of oral contraceptives, presence of Leiden factor with resistance to activated protein C, dehydration); (3) sudden onset of stroke

Table 9-4. Conditions Predisposing to Venous Thrombosis and Pulmonary and Paradoxical Embolism

Blood coagulation disorders
- Deficiencies of antithrombin III, protein C, protein S, plasminogen
- Activated protein C resistance with or without factor V Leiden
- Prothrombin gene mutation
- Dysfibrinogenemia
- Elevated levels of factors VIII, IX, XI
- Very high blood fibrinogen levels
- Very high homocysteine levels

Lower limb paralysis
Prolonged sitting, such as airplane or car trip
Cancer
Acute inflammatory conditions (e.g., Crohn's disease, ulcerative colitis)
Surgery
Limb trauma
Pregnancy
Antiphospholipid antibody syndrome
Female hormone use
Immobilization often with a cast
Obesity
Central venous catheters

during sexual intercourse, straining at stool, or other activity that includes a Valsalva maneuver or promotes right-to-left shunting of blood; (4) pulmonary embolism within a short time before or after the neurologic ischemic event; and (5) the absence of other putative causes of stroke after thorough evaluation. When at least four of these criteria are met, the diagnosis of paradoxical embolism is highly probable.

One typical patient was a 29-year-old woman who, with her husband and four children, returned home from a trip. The day was hot and she had had nothing to drink during the 8-hour car ride. Much of the ride was spent disciplining the children while she kneeled on her seat facing the children, who cavorted in the back of the station wagon. When she and her husband got home, they fed the children and put them to bed. She showered and, immediately thereafter, had sex with her husband. At the point of climax, she became unable to speak and her right arm was weak and numb. Examination showed a right hemiparesis and aphasia. CT showed a left upper-division, MCA-territory infarct. Echocardiography showed a large PFO with increased flow during a Valsalva's maneuver. The heart and aorta were otherwise normal, and an MRA examination of the cervicocranial arteries was normal. She made a good recovery

9

but had residual right hand numbness and dysnomia.

Gautier and colleagues reported on 29 patients who had paradoxical embolism and reviewed 31 patients reported by others.[225] Situations that promoted venous occlusions among these 60 patients included surgery, postpartum, lower extremity injury, and jugular vein catheterization. Strokes occurred after sex, straining at stool, weight lifting, vigorous nose blowing, asthmatic attacks, gymnastics, decompressing the ears, and martial arts. Venous thrombosis was detected in few patients, and few had clinical pulmonary emboli. Pulmonary radionuclide scans, angiography, and necropsy showed pulmonary emboli in many patients.[225] The most common territory of stroke was the MCA, which was involved in 25 patients. Fifteen patients (37.5%) had vertebrobasilar-territory embolic infarcts, a proportion more than expected by chance, because only 20% of blood flow to the brain goes through the posterior circulation. A study of the distribution of microemboli in patients with PFOs also showed that there is an unexplained predilection for embolic material to go to posterior circulation arteries.[226]

Paradoxic embolism also occurs through ventricular septal defects, atrial septal defects, and pulmonary arteriovenous fistulas. Venous thrombosis can be detected if studies are performed early in the course. Some venous thrombi involve the pelvic veins and might be detected by abdominal and pelvic imaging techniques.

A PFO can be identified noninvasively using TTE and/or TEE with intravenous agitated saline contrast. Microbubbles appear in the LA within three to five beats of full opacification of the right atrium. Imaging is usually performed at rest and with maneuvers that transiently increase right atrial pressure so as to promote right-to-left shunting, including Valsalva maneuver release and cough. Imaging with cough provides the highest sensitivity. The size of the shunt is graded semiqualitatively with less than 10 bubbles considered "trivial," 10 to 30 bubbles considered a "small shunt" and more than 30 bubbles suggesting a large shunt.[222] TEE is more sensitive than TTE.[51,227] Administration of saline contrast from the groin is probably superior to introduction from the antecubital fossa.[228] The relative quantity of contrast (or severity of right-to-left shunting) appearing in the LA after venous injection appears to be associated with increased risk.[229,230] Occasionally an echocardiogram can capture the presence of a thrombus traversing a PFO as is shown in Figure 9-13.

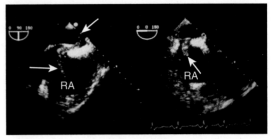

Figure 9-13. TEE in a patient who presented with an ischemic stroke. A thrombus *(white arrows)* is imaged in transit through the intraatrial septum. (From Caplan LR, Manning WJ: Brain Embolism. New York: Informa Healthcare, 2006, with permission.)

TCD has also been used effectively to diagnose the presence of right-to-left cardiac or pulmonary shunting.[231-233] The technique involves injection of a small amount of saline that has been agitated vigorously with a small amount of air, or mixed with a polygeline contrast agent, and injected into a cubital vein.[232] During and after the injection, the MCA is insonated using TCD. Appearance of microbubbles in the MCA within the first three to five cardiac cycles (<10 seconds) indicates the presence of right-to-left shunting of blood. Figure 4-18 shows the appearance of microembolic signals produced by air bubbles during a test for the presence of right to left blood shunting. The test is usually done with and without a Valsalva's maneuver. The technique has the advantage of being able to be used at the bedside because TCD is portable. Real-time MRI during injection of a gadolinium-based contrast agent is another method of showing a right-to-left shunt.[234]

Atrial septal aneurysms (ASAs) have recently received increased attention in relation to their possible role in contributing to brain embolism. Fusion of the septum primum closes the foramen ovale and leads to a depression on the right side of the interatrial septal wall. Bulging of the septum primum tissue of the atrial septum through the fossa ovalis into either the right or left atria is called an atrial septal aneurysm. A strong association exists between atrial septal aneurysms and interatrial shunts. Atrial septal aneurysms are less common than PFOs and are usually defined by echocardiography as a bulging/septal mobility in the region of the fossa ovalis due to redundant atrial septal tissue.[235] The amount of septal excursion for an ASA is usually defined as the sum of the greatest leftward and rightward deflections of at least 10 or 15 mm. Prevalence in the normal population is estimated to be 0.5% by TTE[236] and up to 5% by TEE.[237,238] An ASA is often associated with a PFO, and more than 50% of patients with an ASA have a coexistent PFO.[239,240] The mechanism for stroke in ASA has been ascribed to coexistent PFO, tendency for atrial arrhythmias,[241] and formation of a thrombus in the neck of the aneurysm due to an irregular surface.[242] The risk of ASA in the absence of PFO is uncertain.

Cabanes et al studied the frequency of atrial septal aneurysms, PFO, and MVP among 100 fully evaluated stroke patients younger than 55 years and 50 controls.[243] Atrial septal aneurysms were found in 28% of stroke patients and 8% of controls. A PFO was found in 72% of patients with atrial septal aneurysms and 25% of patients without atrial septal aneurysms. The presence of an atrial septal aneurysm (odds ratio, 4.3; 95% CI, 1.3 to 14.6; P = .01) or a PFO (odds ratio, 3.9; 95% CI, 1.5 to 10.0; P = .003) was strongly associated with cryptogenic stroke. The stroke odds ratio of a patient with both an atrial septal aneurysm and a PFO were 33.3 times (95% CI, 4.1 to 270.0) the stroke odds of a patient who had neither. Atrial septal aneurysms with more than 10 mm excursion were eight times more likely to be associated with stroke than those with smaller excursions.[243] The presence of MVP in this study did not increase the odds of cryptogenic stroke. One prospective intraoperative study found that the incidence of embolic strokes associated with an atrial septal defect was quite low.[238]

Predictors for the likelihood of paradoxic embolism through PFOs have been sought using TEE.[230,244] In one study, the presence of an atrial septal aneurysm accompanying the PFO was an important finding, favoring the presence of paradoxic embolism.[244] In another study, PFOs were significantly larger, and more microbubbles were present in patients with cryptogenic stroke than in those with identified causes of stroke.[230] Electrocardiographic findings can also suggest the presence of PFOs and ostium secundum atrial septal defects. An M-shaped notch on the ascending branch or on the peak of the R-wave in inferior electrocardiographic leads (II, III, aVF) is often found in patients with PFOs or atrial septal defects.[245] This notched pattern has been called *crochetage* because of its resemblance morphologically to a crochet needle.

Some studies have analyzed the recurrence rate of stroke in patients with PFOs and the effect of various treatments on recurrence.[4,246,247] Bogousslavsky and his Swiss colleagues studied stroke recurrence among 140 consecutive patients who had PFOs and brain ischemic events.[246] One fourth of the patients also had atrial septal aneurysms. During a mean follow-up period of 3 years, the stroke or death rate was 2.4% per year. Only eight patients had a recurrent brain infarct (1.9% per year).[246] Ninety-two patients (66%) took aspirin (250 mg/day), whereas 37 patients (26%) were given anticoagulants, and 11 patients (8%) had surgical closure of the PFO within 12 weeks of the stroke after being treated with anticoagulants. No significant difference was found in the effect of any of the treatments on recurrence. The relatively low rate of recurrence contrasted with the severity of the initial stroke, which left disabling effects in one half of the patients.[246]

In a French multicenter study, among 132 patients with PFOs, atrial septal aneurysms, or both, and cryptogenic stroke were followed for an average of 22.6 months.[247] The recurrence rate was approximately 2% to 3% at 2 years, and was higher in patients with both PFOs and atrial septal aneurysms. Recurrences occurred in four patients who were taking antiplatelet agents, and in one patient treated with anticoagulants.[247] Lausanne investigators found no recurrence of stroke during an average follow-up of 2 years among 30 patients who had suture closure of PFOs during cardiopulmonary bypass surgery.[248] None of the patients were given antiaggregants or anticoagulants after surgery. No serious surgical complications occurred. After surgery, two patients had interatrial shunting determined by TCD and TEE, but the shunts were much smaller than before surgery.[248] Now some cardiothoracic surgeons are closing PFOs through small incisions—so-called minimally invasive surgery but the success and complication rates are unknown as yet.

PFOs have also been increasingly closed percutaneously using a variety of different devices.[249,250] The available data regarding treatment are inconclusive, but all studies have shown a low recurrence rate (approximately 2% per year) among stroke patients with PFOs. The presence of both a PFO and an atrial septal aneurysm substantially increases the risk of stroke recurrence. Warfarin and surgical or transcatheter closure are posited to be more effective than drugs that affect platelet functions, but retrospective studies have not shown their superiority. Debate and controversy surround decisions on whether or not to close PFOs and by what method.[250a]

Most Common Cardiac Sources

Atrial arrhythmias, congestive heart failure, and akinetic regions were the most common cardiac sources of brain embolism in the Stroke Data Bank.[24] Atrial arrhythmias and left ventricular akinetic regions were the most frequent potential cardiac sources of brain emboli in the Lausanne Stroke Registry.[15,251] Atrial arrhythmias, myocardial abnormalities related to coronary artery disease, and congestive heart failure with low cardiac ejection fractions are probably the most important cardiac abnormalities that predispose to embolism.

AORTA

Studies of patients with stroke and TIAs have firmly established that the thoracic aorta is an important source of brain embolism. Although it was well known that the aorta was an important site of atheromatous disease, almost no mention was made of aortic atherosclerotic disease as an important cause of stroke until the 1990s. Tunick and colleagues reported four patients with unexplained brain ischemic events in whom TEE showed large, protruding, often mobile atheromas.[252,253] Tunick and colleagues then reported the TEE results among 122 patients who had stroke, TIAs, or peripheral emboli, and 122 age- and gender-matched controls.[254] Protruding atheromas were strongly related to the occurrence of embolic events (odds ratio, 3.2; 95% CI, 1.6 to 6.5; $P < .001$), and atheromas with mobile components were only found in patients with embolic events.[254]

Observational studies and case reports alerted the medical community to the possible importance of aortic atheromas as a cause of stroke and peripheral embolism. In 1992, Pierre Amarenco and his Paris colleagues published two reports that showed definitively that aortic atheromatous disease was an important cause of stroke and could be identified clinically.[255,256] Amarenco et al first published a necropsy study of 500 patients who had stroke or other neurologic diseases. Ulcerated aortic plaques were found in 26% of 239 patients with cerebrovascular disease, compared with only 5% of 261 patients with other neurologic diseases ($P < .001$).[255] The prevalence of aortic atheromas was 61% among patients with brain infarcts and no demonstrated cause and 22% among those with other defined causes ($P < .001$).[255] The presence of ulcerated plaques in the aortic arch did not correlate with the presence of carotid artery stenosis, suggesting that aortic and carotid artery disease were independent stroke risk factors. Amarenco and colleagues also reported a study of 12 consecutive patients with cryptogenic stroke studied by TEE.[256] Six patients (50%) had intraluminal echogenic masses in the aortic arch, most often at the junction of the ascending aorta and the arch. In one patient, the mass was pedunculated, but in the other five patients, the attachment was broad-based with an irregular surface. The masses extended from 3 to 15 mm into the aortic lumens. Cholesterol emboli were found in quadriceps muscle biopsies in two patients with aortic masses.[256]

Tobler et al studied at necropsy the presence and distribution of atherosclerotic plaques in the ascending aorta.[257] Among 97 ascending aortas, 38% had atherosclerotic plaques larger than 8 mm in diameter; the average diameter of plaques was 19 mm. Most of the 66 plaques were distributed anteriorly or posteriorly on the right side of the ascending aorta, and the upper and lower halves of the ascending aorta were equally involved.[257] Plaques were also often found in the aortic arch, especially at the orifice of the innominate artery (21% of 48 arch specimens).[257]

Two studies investigated the frequency of occurrence of vascular events in patients who had TEE-documented aortic arch atherosclerosis.[258,259] The French Study of Aortic Plaques in Stroke Group followed 331 patients who presented with brain infarcts for 2 to 4 years.[259] The frequency of subsequent brain infarction and other vascular events was closely correlated with the thickness of the aortic wall. After controlling for other confounding factors, the RR of brain infarction was 3.8 (95% CI, 1.8 to 7.8; $P = .0012$), and of all vascular events, 3.5 (95% CI, 2.1 to 5.9; $P < .001$) in patients with aortic wall plaques larger than 4 mm.[258] In a prospective study conducted in two German university hospitals, physicians followed 136 patients with flat plaques less than 5 mm in thickness and 47 patients with thick plaques more than 5 mm thick or complex plaques with mobile components, for an average of 16 months.[260] Embolic events occurred in 15 patients; the incidence was 4.1 out of 100 patient-years in patients with flat plaques versus 13.7 out of 100 patient-years in those with complex, thick, or mobile plaques.[260]

TEE has become the standard way to image the aorta. Figure 4-37 illustrates a number of different aortic plaques imaged by TEE. There is very good concordance between TEE images and pathology of the aorta.[261] The limitations of TEE are that it is invasive, and there is an area of the aorta that is obscured because of the bronchus and is not readily imaged. TEE can show large plaques and floating mobile thrombi within the lumen of the aorta. Figures 9-13 and 9-14 show various aortic plaques shown by TEE. Vaduganathan et al showed a 73% agreement between intraoperative TEE imaging of the thoracic aorta and histology.[262] TEE does not always detect ulceration but is able to show complex atheroma and mobile debris. Epiaortic ultrasound applied at the beginning of surgery is also a useful method for detecting severe atheromas and intima-medial thickness of the aorta at various locations.[261]

The ascending aorta can also be insonated using a duplex ultrasound probe placed in the right

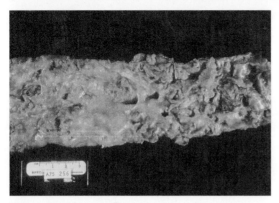

Figure 9-14. Descending aorta at necropsy from a patient whose TEE before surgery showed severe disease of the ascending aorta and aortic arch with mobile protruding plaques. This patient died after CABG surgery, having never awakened after the procedure. (Courtesy of Denise Barbut, MD.)

supraclavicular fossa; the arch and proximal descending thoracic aorta can be imaged using a left supraclavicular ultrasound probe.[263] The results are preliminary but promising. The technique requires training to master and is not used in most centers. Most plaques are located in the curvature of the arch from the distal ascending aorta to the proximal descending aorta, regions well shown using B-mode ultrasound.[263] The aorta has also been imaged by a suprasternal approach during transthoracic echocardiography using harmonic imaging. In one study large protruding plaques were found with a 91% positive predictive value and negative findings had a 98% predictive value, but unfortunately adequate image quality for interpretation could only be obtained in 89% of patients studied.[264]

Magnetic resonance angiography (MRA) and MRI have also been used to image the proximal aorta. Kutz et al compared the sensitivity of detection of large plaques (>5 mm) using gadolinium-enhanced MRA during breath-holding versus TEE.[265] The sensitivity was 54% with MRA versus 92% with TEE. Techniques that show the lumen of the aorta such as MRA and standard angiography usually do not show the wall of the aorta and so underestimate atherosclerotic plaques. Some researchers have experimented with techniques that enhance atherosclerotic plaques and the vascular endothelium. In a rabbit model gadofluorine enhances plaques and allows for detection of early atherosclerotic lesions.[266] In a recent study, 3-tesla MRI was superior to TEE in recognizing important aortic abnormalities.[266a] MRI showed high-risk aortic lesions larger than 4 μm in 37 of 74 patients compared with 23 by TEE ($P = .029$).[266a] High-resolution MRI using plaque and endothelial enhancing agents has great promise for becoming the preferred imaging technique for detecting and quantifying aortic atherosclerosis in the near future.

Treatment of aortic atheromatous disease is unsettled. Although anticoagulants have been posited to aggravate cholesterol crystal embolism in several patients, aortic thrombotic masses have disappeared after anticoagulant therapy.[267,268] By preventing the formation of thrombi over ulcerated areas of aortic atheromas, heparin, coumadin, or direct thrombin inhibitors could theoretically facilitate contact of the atheromatous material with the lumen and promote cholesterol embolism. Cholesterol embolism has also been described after thrombolytic treatment of patients with acute myocardial infarction.[269] Similar to anticoagulants, thrombolytic agents could expose ulcerated areas to the circulation if thrombi were lysed. Intravenous thrombolytic treatment[270] and surgical removal of protruding atheromas[271] have also been reported to be successful in treating patients with aortic atheromas. Agents that affect platelet aggregation and function and combinations of antiplatelet drugs and anticoagulants might be effective in preventing embolism from aortic plaques, but they have not been systematically studied. Antiplatelet agents might be successful in preventing white platelet-fibrion thrombi which, in turn, stimulate the development of superimposed red thrombi. A trial of antiplatelet agents versus anticoagulants is now underway. Until the results are known, I suggest treating patients with large protruding (>4 mm), and mobile atheromata with anticoagulants and patients with flat and smaller plaques with antiplatelet agents.

COMPLICATIONS OF CARDIAC SURGERY

The section on complications of cardiac surgery is located here because most complications are due, at least in part, to brain embolism, and because the aorta and the heart are the major donor sources of that embolism. The reported incidence of neurologic abnormalities during the postoperative period varies from 7% to 61% for transient, and from 1.6% to 23% for permanent complications.[272-274] The complication rate is much higher in prospective series, in which patients are routinely examined postoperatively, rather than in retrospective reviews of charts. In one study of 312 patients, transient complications were noted in fully 61% of patients.[274] At the Cleveland Clinic among a series of 421 CABG patients, 16.8% had prolonged encephalopathy or stroke.[275] Complications can be readily divided into four groups: (1) encephalopathy, (2) stroke,

(3) cognitive dysfunction, and (4) peripheral nervous system complications.

Encephalopathy and Stroke

A wide spectrum of neuropsychiatric findings, including delirium, confusion, disorientation, drowsiness, and altered behavior without focal neurologic abnormalities, are often bundled together under the broad term *encephalopathy*. Imaging tests in these patients usually do not show new large focal brain infarcts. In the Cleveland Clinic series of CABG operations, 11.6% of patients were considered encephalopathic on the fourth postoperative day.[275] In another large series, 57 of 1669 CABG patients (3.4%) had severe postoperative mental changes, including delirium and encephalopathy.[276] Undoubtedly, the causes are multiple. Microembolism is a major cause. Encephalopathy is especially common among older patients and those with a history of alcohol abuse and renal disease. Some patients have a hypoxic-ischemic encephalopathy caused by prolonged time on the pump, during which their brain was poorly perfused. An important number of cases are explained by medications. Sedatives; analgesics, especially narcotics; and, most important, haloperidol and other antipsychotics are common offenders. Haloperidol often produces depressed alertness, stiffness, inertia, and drowsiness, and the drug stays in the body a long time. Haloperidol has been shown to retard recovery in animals with brain lesions.[277,278] In my opinion, this drug should not be used in older surgical and medical patients, especially those with abnormal brains.

The initial recognition that the neurobehavioral changes were not psychiatric in origin was made by Gilman in 1965, when he prospectively followed a series of open heart surgery patients.[273] Early research drew the conclusion that embolization of particulate matter related to the pump and its filters leads to encephalopathy.[279] The introduction of membrane, rather than bubble, oxygenators and in-line filtration led to a decrease in the risk of large macroembolic particles reaching the systemic circulation.[279]

A 1990 report of the necropsy findings in five patients and six dogs who had cardiac surgery aroused new interest in this subject.[280] Focal small capillary and arteriolar dilatations were widely scattered in 10 of these 11 brains. Approximately one half of the focal small capillary and arteriolar dilatations contained birefringent crystalline material within the dilatated capillary regions.[280] The vascular lesions affected medium-sized arterioles, terminal arterioles, and capillaries; they were often distributed in multiples in the same vessels or in clusters near each other. Two other patients had a small number of focal small capillary and arteriolar dilatations. The authors thought that the findings were most consistent with iatrogenically induced release into the system of small particles of air or fat.[280] Microemboli are likely to be an important cause of encephalopathy and persistent cognitive abnormalities after cardiopulmonary bypass surgery.

During and shortly after cardiac surgery, many microemboli are detectable and correlate with the occurrence of strokes, encephalopathy, and cognitive abnormalities.[281-284] When patients are monitored using echocardiography and transcranial Doppler ultrasound, a myriad of microemboli are detected in the MCAs and in the aortic lumen. Most of the microembolic particles are recorded during clamping and unclamping of the aorta, but flurries of emboli are also detected during cannulation of the aorta and at the beginning and end of cardiac bypass.[282,283] The particles are of diverse composition and probably consist of air, atheromatous debris, lipid, and platelet-fibrin thrombi. Cardiac and aortic-origin embolisms undoubtedly contribute to the brain damage often noted after cardiac surgery. Brain perfusion during cardiac surgery is also an important factor in predicting the presence and severity of ischemic brain damage after surgery.[282]

Hypoperfusion likely augments brain ischemia by lessening the throughput and washout of these microemboli. Among 100 cardiopulmonary bypass surgery patients, Tufo et al found neurologic signs in 78% of patients maintained at a mean arterial pressure of 40 mm Hg, but in only 27% of those whose mean pressure was 60 mm Hg.[284] The duration of hypotension below 60 mm Hg averaged 46 minutes in patients with neurologic signs compared to 21 minutes in those without signs.[285] In another study, the importance of both the severity and duration of hypotension below a mean arterial pressure of 50 mm Hg were important factors in the development of neurologic abnormalities after cardiac surgery.[286] In a randomized study, patients whose mean arterial pressure was maintained in the 50 to 60 mm Hg range had a stroke frequency of 7.2% compared to 2.4% in patients whose mean arterial pressures were maintained in the 80 to 100 mm Hg range.[287] In a review of 15 patients who were considered at high risk for postoperative stroke who had on-pump coronary artery bypass surgery, a drop in mean arterial pressure from a preoperative baseline predicted cognitive dysfunction found early after surgery.[287a]

Monitoring of basal cerebral artery blood flow velocities by TCD provides a better measure of brain perfusion than mean arterial blood pressure. Among 100 patients continuously monitored using TCD during heart surgery, the reduction in baseline blood flow velocities was 17% for patients who had no neurologic deficits, 34% for those who had diffuse encephalopathy, and 43% for patients who had strokes.[282] The duration in minutes of perfusion at less than 50% of baseline was 36 minutes for those without neurologic signs compared with 71 minutes for those with encephalopathy, and 105 minutes for those with strokes.[282]

Pugsley and colleagues studied 100 patients who had cardiopulmonary bypass, 50 with an arterial line filter and 50 without a filter.[281] TCD was used to monitor microemboli. All patients were given neuropsychological tests before and after surgery. Neuropsychological deficits at 8 days and 8 weeks postoperatively were more common in patients who had cardiopulmonary bypass without the arterial filter, and neuropsychological abnormalities correlated with the number of microemboli.[281]

The frequency of clinical focal deficits that qualify as strokes ranges from 4.7% to 5.2% in various series.[273-275,282] Intracardiac operations, such as valve replacements, carry a higher risk of postoperative strokes, ranging from 4.2% to 13%.[282] Among 2264 patients having CABG with and without intracardiac procedures, the frequency of neurologic deficits was approximately doubled in those who had intracardiac procedures in addition to CABG.[282] Among the Cleveland Clinic series were 22 of 421 patients (5.2%) who had postoperative strokes, but the deficits were severe in only 2% of the total series.[275] Twelve infarcts involved a cerebral hemisphere (seven right, five left), five involved the brainstem, five involved the retina, and two involved an optic nerve.[275] Using neuroimaging data, infarcts are multiple in 65% of patients. Infarcts are typically small and numerous and involve preferentially the cerebellum, occipital lobes, borderzone territories between the MCAs and posterior cerebral arteries, and territories supplied by MCA branches.[282] Many strokes are first noted after the patient awakens from anesthesia, but strokes also often develop during the first few postoperative days.

The vast majority of brain infarcts after cardiac surgery are caused by embolism from the heart and aorta. A major worry of cardiac surgeons, cardiologists, and neurologists has been that hemodynamic circulatory stress during heart surgery might lead to underperfusion of tenuous zones of pre-existing extracranial vascular stenosis. This concern was the driving force behind early use of preoperative auscultation for bruits and later use of noninvasive and angiographic demonstration of the extracranial vascular system before cardiac surgery. If carotid artery disease was found, carotid artery surgery was performed before or during the same anesthetic as cardiac surgery. The morbidity and mortality of this approach proved high.[289]

Studies show that patients with carotid stenosis documented by ultrasound had a low rate of ipsilateral ischemic infarcts in the perioperative periods.[290-292] In a retrospective study of CABG patients with known carotid artery disease, 144 patients had severe atherostenosis (>50% luminal narrowing) affecting 155 arteries, as shown by preoperative angiography.[293] Strokes ipsilateral to the stenosis occurred in only 1.1% of arteries with 50% to 90% stenosis, in 6.2% of arteries with greater than 90% stenosis, and in only 2% of arteries with carotid occlusion.[293] Von Reutern and colleagues monitored the MCA of patients using TCD during cardiac surgery. Even patients with severe carotid stenosis usually showed no important changes during surgery.[294]

Brain infarcts often develop in the period after cardiac surgery. Because hemodynamic stress is maximal intraoperatively, underperfusion should cause damage noted on awakening after surgery. In one study, 5 of 30 postoperative strokes (17%) were noted immediately after cardiac surgery,[295] 14 others developed deficits within 24 hours, and seven did so during the subsequent 24- to 48-hour period. In two patients, strokes occurred 5 and 11 days, respectively, after surgery. The distribution and multiplicity of the postoperative infarcts on CT scans were most consistent with embolism.[295] Some emboli originate from cardiac lesions known to exist before heart surgery, such as valve lesions, ventricular aneurysms, and myocardial akinetic zones. Atrial fibrillation and other arrhythmias may have been present before surgery or may first appear during the postoperative period. Atrial fibrillation often develops after surgery and may be transient. Some patients had taken warfarin or aspirin before surgery, but this was discontinued before and during the operation and was not restarted until after the embolic stroke had occurred.

Mounting evidence links postoperative embolism to ulcerative atherosclerotic lesions of the ascending aorta.[282,296-302] Aortotomy or cross-clamping of the aorta to anastomose the vein graft may liberate cholesterol crystals and calcific plaque debris. Yellow aortic plaques are often visible and can be palpated by the surgeon. When the aorta is clamped, an audible crunch is often heard. Figure 9-14 is a photograph of the descending aorta at necropsy that contains many

9

ulcerative lesions in a patient who did not awaken after CABG surgery. The transesophageal echocardiography of this patient showed severe aortic disease with multiple mobile plaques. Atheromatous material from the proximal portion of the descending aorta can be carried retrograde into the aortic arch and embolize to the brain.

The most important risk factor for stroke after cardiopulmonary bypass surgery is aortic atheromatosis. The frequency of aortic atheromas increases dramatically with age, from 20% in the 5th decade at necropsy, to 80% in patients older than 75 years.[282,303] The stroke rate after CABG also increases sharply with age, from 1% in patients age 51 to 60 years, to 9% in patients older than 80 years.[283] The correlation between aortic atheromas and stroke after CABG was first shown at necropsy in a study that involved 221 patients.[303] Atheroemboli were found in 37% of patients who had severe atherosclerosis of the ascending aorta, but in only 2% of patients who did not have significant ascending aortic atheromas.[303] In another study, cardiac surgeons retrospectively reviewed the records of 3279 consecutive patients with CABG at Johns Hopkins, seeking risk factors for postoperative stroke.[302] Severe atherosclerosis of the ascending aorta was one of the most definitive risk factors found.[302]

Embolization can be detected and quantified before, during, and after surgery using ultrasound. TCD recording over the MCAs can detect the arrival of microemboli in the cranial arteries. Figures 9-15 and 9-16 represent TCD recordings taken during cardiac surgery at various times during the procedure. Intraoperative transesophageal echocardiography can be used to detect the passage of emboli into and through the aorta. Figure 9-17 is a transesophageal echocardiography recorded during cardiac surgery that shows a shower of emboli entering the aortic lumen.

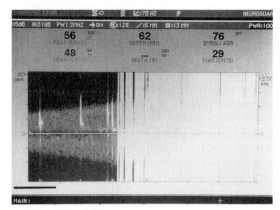

Figure 9-16. TCD recording from the MCA during cardiac bypass surgery. A few distinct emboli (white streaks at left of figure) are followed by a massive shower of emboli ("white-out") at the time of the release of aortic clamps. (Courtesy of Denise Barbut, MD.)

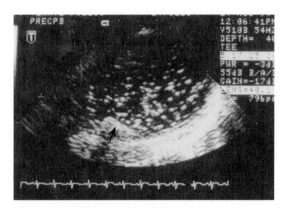

Figure 9-17. TEE recording during cardiac surgery from the aorta at the level of origin of the left subclavian artery. A mobile plaque is seen protruding into the aortic lumen (*small black arrow*). This recording was taken after the release of aortic clamps and shows a "shower" of emboli within the aortic lumen beyond where the aorta was previously clamped. (Courtesy of Denise Barbut, MD.)

More emboli are detected during intracardiac surgery because these patients often have valve calcifications, valve vegetations, and intracardiac thrombi. By using TCD monitoring during closed cardiac operations, the number of microemboli vary from 0 to 1200 within one MCA (average, 130).[282] The numbers of emboli detected in the aorta by transesophageal echocardiography is in the thousands, reflecting the fact that only a fraction of the microembolic particles reach the brain.[282,304]

Embolization is not evenly distributed during the various stages of surgery. Maneuvers that involve manipulation of the aorta, such as clamping and unclamping, account for more than 60% of the total number of emboli.[282,304] Flurries of emboli are detected during aortic cannulation

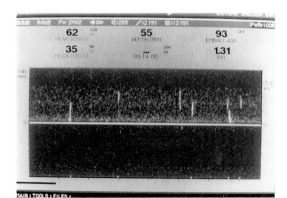

Figure 9-15. TCD recording from the MCA during steady state cardiac bypass surgery at a time when the aorta was being manipulated. The white streaks represent microemboli. (Courtesy of Denise Barbut, MD.)

and at the start and termination of cardiopulmonary bypass. During open cardiac procedures, the number of emboli detected by TCD is especially high during cardiac ejection, after the release of aortic cross-clamps, and immediately after bypass.[282] Figure 9-16 is a TCD recording during cardiac surgery that shows a "white-out" created by a massive shower of emboli that occurred immediately after release of aortic clamps. Many of the microemboli are gaseous particles. Aortic clamping and clamp release are followed by a snowstorm-like appearance of intensely echogenic, well-defined particles within the aorta and a corresponding flurry of particles within the brain arteries.[282] The mean diameter of these particles is 0.85 mm. These microembolic particles are most likely atheromatous debris from the aorta. They are small enough to enter the brain circulation, although only a small fraction do so. Off-pump coronary artery bypass surgery in which the aorta is not clamped is associated with a much smaller quantity of microembolic signals.[304a]

Transesophageal echocardiography can detect and quantitate ulcerative aortic plaques before surgery (see Fig. 4-37) Some cardiac surgeons use transesophageal echocardiography during surgery (before clamping) to detect aortic atheromas and so indicate the regions of the aorta to avoid during clamping. Marshall and colleagues used an intraoperative B-mode ultrasound probe placed on the aorta to search for protruding plaques.[305] Ultrasonic imaging was more effective in showing plaques than visual inspection and palpation. Furthermore, the amount and location of plaque often altered the procedure performed.[305] Cardiac surgeons have begun to introduce filter devices into the aorta when the aortic clamps are removed to catch debris and cholesterol crystals. Figure 9-18 shows cholesterol crystals and other particulate debris caught in one of these filters.

Cognitive dysfunction without accompanying focal motor, sensory, or visual dysfunction is the most common complication of CABG surgery. Some patients have obvious loss of intellect, whereas others have subtle problems detectable only by formal neuropsychological evaluation.

Advanced age and length of bypass are important risk factors for cognitive dysfunction after cardiopulmonary bypass.[306] Prospective studies provide evidence that microembolism is the most important cause of cognitive deficits after cardiac surgery using cardiopulmonary bypass.[281,282,307,308] Patients with cognitive deficits have more microemboli during surgery, compared with patients who have no cognitive decline. Pugsley and colleagues found that 43% of patients with

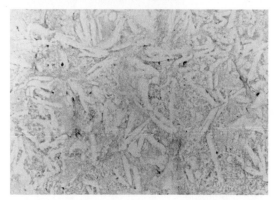

Figure 9-18. Cholesterol crystals and other particulate debris are caught in a filter placed in the aorta at the time that aortic clamps are removed. (Courtesy of Denise Barbut, MD.)

intraoperative embolic counts greater than 1000 had cognitive abnormalities at 8 weeks after cardiac surgery, compared with only 8% of patients with less than 200 emboli.[281] Barbut et al found that the average number of microemboli at the time of removal of aortic clamps was 166 in six patients with cognitive abnormalities, compared with 73 microemboli in 11 patients who showed no loss of cognitive function.[307]

Another syndrome that has been found occasionally after cardiac surgery is a selective paralysis of saccadic eye movements.[308a-d] Shortly after awakening from surgery the patients cannot voluntarily initiate conjugate horizontal eye movements. Vertical eye movements are also sometimes involved. Smooth pursuit and reflex eye movements are preserved. The patients often initiate eye movements by moving their heads inducing a passive reflex eye movement. At times other deficits coexist. Some patients have had small localized infarcts in the paramedian pontine tegmentum.[308a-d]

In my opinion, all patients who are going to have cardiac surgery should have preoperative transesophageal echocardiography. This should allow detection of potential cardiac and aortic sources of embolization. At the same time left ventricular function, atrial size, and ejection fraction can be measured. When the chest is opened, epiaortic ultrasound is also helpful. The presence of potential cardiac sources helps guide the use of heparin during and after surgery. Knowledge of aortic disease guides clamping sites and technique. Some patients can be operated on without aortic clamping—so-called off-pump surgery.[292] A recent study that compared on and off pump surgery showed no difference in late cognitive effects but no data about the aorta and left ventricular function were included.[309] Off-pump surgery takes a bit longer than on-pump operations but does not involve aortic clamping. On pump surgery is quicker but does involve clamping of the aorta. It seems likely that patients with severe aortic disease and good ventricular function would do best with off-pump surgery. Those with normal aortas and impaired ventricular function might do better with on-pump bypass surgery. Knowledge of left ventricular function and ejection fraction and of the aorta should be very useful information in addition to the location of the occlusive coronary artery disease in planning and carrying out surgery. Placement of a filtering device in the aorta during and after release of aortic clamps is another useful maneuver to prevent microemboli from reaching the brain and other organs.

ARTERIAL SOURCES OF EMBOLISM

Extracranial and intracranial large arteries often serve as the donor source for embolism to the brain. Arterial-source embolism is referred to as artery-to-artery, intra-arterial, or local embolism. The location and frequency of atherosclerotic lesions within the large arteries of the anterior and posterior circulations are discussed in Chapters 6 and 7. Ulcerated and stenotic lesions and recent occlusions within the proximal extracranial and intracranial arteries are most often incriminated as embolic sources.

Although atherosclerosis is by far the most common condition that leads to intra-arterial embolism, other vascular diseases can also serve as donor sources. Trauma and dissections of arteries leads to local thrombus formation and embolism. Dissections are probably the second most frequent source of intra-arterial embolism. Occasionally, inflammatory diseases of the brachiocephalic branches of the aortic arch, such as temporal arteritis and Takayasu disease, can lead to intra-arterial embolism. Thrombi sometimes form within arterial aneurysms, saccular,[310,311] dissecting, and fusiform dolichocephalic aneurysms,[312] and can then break off and embolize to distal-branch arteries.

Fibromuscular dysplasia is an important but relatively uncommon vascular disease that affects the pharyngeal and occasionally the intracranial portions of the carotid and vertebral arteries, which also can serve as a source of distal intra-arterial embolism. Thrombi can, on occasion, form within large arteries in the absence of important arterial disease in patients with cancer and other causes of hypercoagulability.[313] These luminal thrombi then embolize to intracranial arteries, causing strokes. Figure 9-19 shows a large thrombus within the ICA.

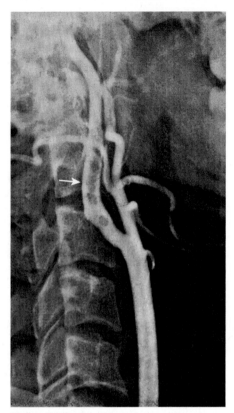

Figure 9-19. Carotid arteriogram, lateral view. Dark filling defects within the artery *(white arrow)* represent luminal clots.

IMAGING AND LABORATORY EVALUATION OF POTENTIAL DONOR SOURCES

When the clinical findings, brain imaging, and vascular tests suggest brain embolism, a thorough evaluation of all potential sources—cardiac, aortic, and cerebrovascular—is usually indicated. Clinical distinction between brain embolism and in situ thrombosis are discussed in Chapter 3. Table 9-5 lists the common differential diagnostic features of these two stroke mechanisms. Some patients have more than one potential embolic donor source. Atherosclerotic plaques and occlusive lesions often coexist in the heart, aorta, and brachiocephalic arteries. Patients with cerebrovascular occlusive lesions have a high frequency of coronary atherosclerotic heart disease, and their coronary disease is often a more serious threat for mortality and disability than cerebrovascular disease. Also, patients with coronary atherosclerotic heart disease have a high frequency of occlusive lesions within their extracranial and intracranial vascular beds. Prophylactic treatment to prevent subsequent thromboembolism should include measures to prevent embolism from all potential

Table 9-5.	Differentiating Signs of Thrombosis and Embolism	
Thrombosis	**Embolism**	
1. Preceding brief, frequent, shotgun-like TIAs	1. Single or infrequent but longer-lasting TIAs or strokes	
2. TIAs all in same vascular territory	2. Deficits maximal at onset	
3. Onset of stroke after sleep	3. Onset during activity or sudden strain, cough, or sneeze	
4. Postural sensitivity of symptoms	4. Infarcts in multiple vascular territories	
5. Occlusion or severe stenosis of large artery	5. Presence of distal intra-arterial emboli	
6. Absence of distal embolus by angiography	6. Hemorrhagic brain infarct	
7. Infarct near border zone of affected artery	7. Infarct in heart of vascular territory, wedge-shaped, and abutting on cortical surface	
8. Presence of risk factors for atherosclerosis: hypertension, hypercholesterolemia, angina, etc.	8. Presence of known cardiac, arterial, or venous source of embolus	

donor sources, not only the one that caused the present embolism.

Many patients with severe heart disease have abnormalities uncovered by history, physical examination, electrocardiograms, and chest x-ray. A TTE, including Doppler insonation and the injection of microbubbles searching for intracardiac shunts, is ordinarily indicated. Some patients, especially young adults who have a well-defined vascular donor source of embolism, such as a cervical dissection, do not need echocardiography.

In order to decide on the utility of echocardiography and to choose between a transthoracic and transesophageal approach, it is useful to review cardiac anatomy.[52] The LA is a thin-walled, ovoid chamber that lies immediately behind the ascending aorta. The endocardial surface of the LA is usually smooth and continuous as it developed from the fetal common pulmonary vein.[52,314] Body-size normograms for transthoracic left atrial measurements in men and women have been published, but absolute dimension and length value are reported by most clinical echocardiographic laboratories.

With normal aging, the left atrial cavity dimensions increase. The body of the LA is well visualized from multiple perspectives on TTE.[52] The left atrial appendage is a highly trabeculated and often multilobulated cul-de-sac that arises from the midportion of the lateral wall of the left atrium near the entrance of the left upper pulmonary vein. The left atrial appendage is often not visualized on TTE, but the close proximity of the esophagus to the posterior portion of the LA and the absence of intervening bone or lung makes TEE the ideal imaging tool for visualization of both the LA and the left atrial appendage. Several studies have documented the very high accuracy of TEE in showing left atrial and left atrial appendage thrombi when echocardiography has been compared with intraoperative visualization of these structures.[52,315,316]

TTE performed with saline contrast is a minimally invasive procedure, while TEE is a moderately invasive procedure during which a modified gastroscope (containing an ultrasound crystal at its tip) is positioned within the esophagus. Imaging is performed within the esophagus and the gastric fundus. The close proximity of the esophagus to the posterior portion of the heart, the lack of intervening lung and bone, and the use of higher-frequency imaging transducers results in enhanced spatial resolution.[52] TEE is preferred for identification or exclusion of pathology that is particularly relevant for detecting cardiac and aortic sources of thromboembolism, including identification of intra-atrial thrombi and tumors, PFOs, valvular vegetations, atheromatous plaques within the aorta, and spontaneous echo contrast.[52] TTE remains preferred for identification of left ventricular regional systolic function and apical left ventricular thrombi. Thus, for many patients, direct TEE (with omission of the TTE) may be the most expeditious route to identify a cardiac source of embolism.[52,317-320]

TEE sometimes fails to identify cardiac sources of emboli. Some thromboemboli are too small to be detected. An embolus that is 1 to 2 mm can cause a devastating neurologic deficit. A particle this size is often beyond the resolution of echocardiography. The other major reason for failure is that thrombosis and embolism are dynamic processes. When a thrombus leaves the heart to go to the brain, echocardiography may not show a thrombus within the heart if performed soon after the clinical event. Later, the thrombus may re-form.

TEE also yields important information about the proximal aorta, a region not imaged by TTE. TEE is important in all patients in whom TTE suggests, but does not adequately define, the cardiac pathology and in all patients in whom other studies (cerebrovascular, hematologic, and other cardiac investigations) do not show the cause of brain embolism and brain ischemia. Radionuclide testing, including gated blood pool imaging (multigated acquisition scans), may also be helpful in selected patients, as might other cardiac imaging techniques.[321] Platelet scintigraphy is sometimes helpful in defining the presence of cardiac thrombi.[322]

TEE is the only effective, established way to image the aorta for plaques and thrombi. The ascending aorta can also be insonated using a duplex ultrasound probe placed in the right supraclavicular fossa, and the arch and proximal descending thoracic aorta can be imaged using a left supraclavicular probe.[263] Newer magnetic resonance techniques can also show the aorta well.[265]

The extracranial and intracranial arteries should be studied to define potential arterial donor sources of embolism, provide information about blockage of recipient arteries by emboli, or both. The four most common and effective means of studying the brachiocephalic arteries are by MRA, CTA, ultrasound, and cerebral catheter-dye angiography. Brain imaging always should accompany the vascular studies to show the location, severity, and distribution of related brain ischemia. These diagnostic tests and their use in diagnosing large artery lesions in the anterior and posterior circulations have been extensively reviewed in Chapters 4, 6, and 7.

Hematologic studies are also important in the evaluation of patients suspected of having brain embolism. Why does a patient with a chronic lesion, such as an aortic protruding atheroma, atrial fibrillation, or ICA stenosis develop a superimposed thrombus at a given time? In many patients, the explanation lies in activation of platelets, the coagulation system, or both.[323] The two processes, an intimal-endothelial lesion and heightened coagulation, interact to explain the thromboembolic event. Various conditions affect the coagulation system. Coexisting infection, cancer, dehydration, and congenital or acquired hypercoagulability (i.e., in patients with resistance to activated protein C or decreased antithrombin III activity) can activate the coagulation cascade that, in the presence of a suitable lesion, can lead to thrombus formation and embolism. Coagulation studies should be an integral part of the evaluation of patients with suspected brain embolism and those with potential sources of embolism who have not, as yet, had clinical events.

TREATMENT OF PATIENTS WITH BRAIN EMBOLISM

The goals of treatment are minimization of brain ischemic injury caused by brain embolism and prevention of acute recurrent embolism. Strategies for accomplishing this fall into four broad categories: (1) reperfusion of the brain region rendered ischemic by the embolus; (2) acute anticoagulation to prevent propagation and further embolization of thromboemboli; (3) making the brain more resistant to ischemia, allowing survival of nerve cells despite ischemia; and (4) managing complications of embolic infarction such as brain edema and brain hemorrhage.[324]

Reperfusion

The most important predictor of recovery from brain embolism is whether brain tissue rendered ischemic by an embolus blocking a recipient artery is reperfused with blood before irreversible damage occurs, and how quickly reperfusion develops. Reperfusion occurs in two different complementary ways: recanalization of the occluded artery when an embolus moves distally, either spontaneously or after treatment, and augmentation of blood flow through collateral circulation sufficient to restore adequate nutrition to ischemic tissue.

Opening of Blocked Recipient Arteries

Angiographic opacification of cervicocranial arteries soon after onset of brain ischemic symptoms shows that the intracranial arteries in a very high percentage of patients are occluded when angiography is performed within 6 to 8 hours of symptom onset.[39,40,325] Clinical and angiographic studies proved that emboli often passed distally from their initial resting place within recipient arteries.[13,14,42,43,326] In some patients passage of emboli was accompanied by dramatic clinical recovery.[13,14] When angiograms were performed 48 hours or more after neurologic symptom onset in patients in the Harvard Stroke Registry, emboli had mostly passed and were not visible angiographically.[11,327] TCD can effectively show opening and reocclusion of embolic brain artery occlusions.[2]

Acute studies using MRI protocols that include MRA and diffusion-weighted images have clearly shown that patients rarely develop progressive brain infarction when arteries have already recanalized.[328-331] Angiographic and transcranial Doppler studies of untreated patients and those treated with intravenous or intra-arterial thrombolytic agents also show clearly that patients whose arteries recanalize do much better than patients whose arteries remain occluded.[332-336] The extent of brain infarction and clinical recovery also correlate with the length of time that the recipient artery remained occluded.[332-336] The location, extent, and duration of arterial occlusion is the most important determinant of outcome.

Chemical or Mechanical Thrombolysis and Clot Removal

Opening of occluded arteries can be accomplished chemically by administering drugs that lyse clots, or mechanically using devices that extract thromboemboli. Thrombolytic drugs can be given either intravenously or intra-arterially. Each has advantages and disadvantages. Intravenous therapy can be given quickly and needs no special training. The amount of thrombolytic agent that reaches large obstructed arteries is, however, more limited than intra-arterial infusion of drug, which delivers the drug locally within the obstructing clot. Intra-arterial therapy requires a trained interventionalist. Angiography is ordinarily required before, during, and after thrombolysis. This delays treatment. The major advantage of intra-arterial therapy is that the interventionalist can physically manipulate the clot, a process that facilitates thrombolysis, and can perform angioplasty/stenting during the same procedure if necessary. Usually less drug is used during intra-arterial therapy and the rate of hemorrhagic complications is lower than with intravenous therapy. Another strategy employed is to begin with intravenous treatment. MRI studies including MRA are then performed. If the artery does not recanalize and the patient does not improve then angiography with intra-arterial therapy is given.[337,338] I have discussed thrombolysis in detail in Chapter 5.

Mechanical removal of thromboemboli can be used as an adjunct to chemical thrombolysis or pursued when there are absolute or relative contraindications for thrombolysis and thromboemboli are present.[339-344] A variety of different types of instruments can be used to mechanically remove thrombi: suction techniques, snares, nets, corkscrew retrievers, or direct angioplasty or stenting.[343,344] Laser energy (endovascular photoacoustic recanalization [EPAR]) can be used to emulsify and suction thrombi. Mechanical removal of thrombi has some theoretical advantages over chemical thrombolysis. Chemical thrombolysis, whether intravenous or intra-arterial, takes time. Recanalization can take 1 to 2 hours to accomplish after drug infusion.[16,71] Thrombi can be extracted solely mechanically or mechanical disruption could facilitate pharmacologic thrombolysis by fragmenting the nonthrombotic components of the thrombus and increasing the surface area contact with the thrombolytic drugs. Mechanical thrombolysis should pose less of a threat for bleeding since systemic or local fibrinolysis would not be used, and thus decreased coagulability would not occur. Mechanical clot removal could be pursued in patients who are presently excluded from chemical thrombolysis, such as those who have had a recent procedure and those already treated with anticoagulants. A variety of mechanical devices have been used and are now being studied.[32-38] Stent placement with suctioning of the clot can be performed in some patients without chemical thrombolysis.[29] Some devices simply snare the thrombus and then drag it back through the arterial catheter.[32,34,38] The major limitation of mechanical clot removal is the need for a trained and experienced interventionalist who has familiarity and experience with the device used.

Selection of patients for thrombolysis or mechanical clot removal depends on assessing the benefit/risk ratio of treatment. The three key elements in the decision are (1) whether an artery is occluded and where and how, (2) the extent of brain already infarcted, and (3) whether the brain is still at risk for further infarction. If there is a vascular occlusion, little or no infarction, and a sizable important area of brain is at risk for further ischemic damage, then every attempt should be made to open the arterial occlusion. The presence of good collateral circulation also is important because this makes successful reperfusion more likely. The longer the occlusion has been present, the more likely that ischemic damage has included blood vessels within the ischemic zone, and so the more likely that reperfusion could be associated with bleeding and/or edema. The imaging techniques—MRI, diffusion-weighted imaging (DWI), MRA and MR perfusion, CT, CTA, and CT perfusion—and extracranial and transcranial ultrasound that can define the brain region infarcted, the vascular occlusion, and the region still at risk of further damage are discussed at length in Chapter 4. Recommendations for thrombolysis in acute stroke are noted in Table 5-10.

Augmenting Brain Blood Flow and "Neuroprotection"

Various medical strategies are available to try to improve circulation to brain regions rendered ischemic by a brain embolus. Optimal management of blood pressure, blood volume, and cardiac output can improve blood flow to the ischemic region. Cerebral blood flow increases with rising blood pressure until the pressure becomes very high, approaching the malignant range. During the acute period of brain ischemia, it is unwise to lower the systemic pressure unless it is extremely high—for example, above 200/120 torr.

In some patients with low blood pressure, elevation of blood pressure with phenylephrine, ephedrine or other catecholaminergic drugs might augment brain circulation. Blood volume also affects perfusion pressure and blood flow. Some patients who cannot eat normally will become dehydrated and relatively hemoconcentrated. Other factors—such as vomiting, restrictions on eating because of concern for aspiration, or simply the rush of diagnostic testing occupying patients at mealtimes—all contribute to reduced fluid intake during the early hours and days after the onset of brain embolism. It is best to keep blood volume, especially plasma volume, high. Fluids must often be given intravenously or by nasogastric or stomach tubes. Care, however, must be taken to avoid fluid overload and the complications of cardiac failure and brain edema. Careful monitoring of cardiac and cerebral function should accompany attempts to increase fluid volume.[52]

Many patients with brain embolism also have cardiac dysfunction. A strong pump helps maximize cerebral blood flow. Attention to cardiac rhythm and pump function is important, especially during the acute, fragile period of brain ischemia after embolism. Cardiac output can sometimes be improved by the use of digitalis or vasodilators, use of pacemakers or medications to treat slow rhythms and heart block, adjustment of already prescribed drugs such as digitalis and diuretics, correction of abnormal serum K^+ and Ca^{++} levels, and control of tachyarrhythmias. Cardiac-ejection fractions and output can be monitored by echocardiography.

Clinicians and researchers have explored the use of drugs that have the potential to make the brain more resistant to ischemia. This type of therapy is usually called neuroprotective treatment. Neuroprotective therapy attempts to ameliorate the cellular metabolic consequences of ischemic injury. Unfortunately, all agents studied in randomized trials in humans have failed to show efficacy. However trials and studies have not been optimal. Neuroprotection is discussed at length in Chapter 5. Perhaps in the future, agents will be found that ameliorate the effects of brain ischemia.

Anticoagulation

Heparin and heparin-like compounds are often prescribed as a treatment for patients with acute thromboembolism. The posited purpose of heparinization is to prevent propagation of thrombi and break-off of the tail of existing thrombi and so prevent further embolization. As far as is known, heparin does not lyse existing thrombi, although cardiac clots often disappear during heparin treatment. The arguments used to recommend acute heparinization are twofold: preventing further activity in the embolus already present intracranially and preventing further clot

formation in the original donor source region where the thrombus developed. Heparin is also often used after thrombolysis to maintain arterial patency.

Once an embolus has reached an intracranial artery recipient site, it most often fragments at some point in time and does not usually accrue further clot material. The embolus that has already occurred is not the main focus of heparin treatment. The decision on whether to prescribe heparin acutely to prevent the next thromboembolic stroke should depend on weighing the risk of acute reembolization versus the risk of hemorrhage related to heparin therapy. The risk of further acute thrombus formation and embolization depends primarily on the nature of the cardiac and arterial source of the original thromboembolus.

In patients with cardiac lesions that carry high rates of reembolization, such as mitral stenosis with atrial fibrillation, atrial fibrillation with atrial thrombi or large left atria, and, acute myocardial infarction with mural thrombi, then acute heparinization is probably warranted. In patients with cardiac sources that have a low risk of acute reembolization, such as chronic atrial fibrillation or mitral annulus calcification, heparin can be withheld during the acute period.

Acute carotid and vertebral artery occlusions in the neck are important sources of intra-arterial embolism. When a thrombus first forms in a region of atherostenosis, the clot is not well organized and does not adhere to the arterial wall. The thrombus often extends and new thrombus forms especially since flow is reduced above the thrombus. With time, probably 3 to 4 weeks, the thrombus becomes well organized and adherent and further thrombus formation seems not to develop. Also during these weeks collateral circulation develops and stabilizes. An argument can be made to use heparin and subsequently warfarin during the 3- to 6-week period during which further thrombus development and embolization is a concern.

The other aspect of the decision regarding acute anticoagulation relates to the risk of bleeding into the brain or other organs. The major risks factors are: hypertension, the presence of potential bleeding lesions, such as peptic ulcer disease or hemorrhagic colitis, and the extent of brain infarction. If the patient has a large brain infarct then the risk of brain hemorrhage after acute anticoagulation is higher than when there is no brain infarct or a small brain infarct.

Reintroduction of anticoagulation in patients who have had an intracerebral hemorrhage while taking anticoagulants is a special problem.[346,347] The decision on if and when to restart anticoagulants depends on the risk of embolization from the donor source (atrial fibrillation, prosthetic heart valves, etc.) and the risk of further intracranial bleeding. Studies seem to show that the risk of embolization while anticoagulants are stopped is less than predicted and the risk of hemorrhage if anticoagulants are reintroduced is also less than expected.[346,347] I suggest that waiting a week or 10 days seems practical, and begin with heparin rather than coumadin.

The introduction of direct inhibitors of thrombin such as ximelagatran, dabigatran, and argatroban into clinical care might change the method and risks of anticoagulation. Ximelagatran and other orally administered direct thrombin inhibitors produce rapid anticoagulant effects. These agents are usually given in a fixed dose and need not be monitored by either APTT or INR determinations, making them easier to use and control. Direct thrombin inhibitors could replace both heparin and warfarin in treating stroke patients.

Managing Brain Edema and Mass Effect

Brain edema also is an early occurrence in patients with embolic strokes. Ischemic edema can be intracellular (so-called cytotoxic edema or dry edema) or exist mostly in the extracellular spaces and connective tissue (vasogenic edema or wet edema).[348] Brain edema that lies in the interstices outside of cells might be posited to respond to osmotic diuretics such as hypertonic saline, mannitol and glycerol, or to corticosteroids. However, studies have shown that these agents are not very effective in series of stroke patients with large brain infarcts or hemorrhages. Most edema is probably within cells and indicates that the cells are sick. Restitution of the normal metabolic functions of these cells is likely to be more therapeutic than so-called antiedema agents. There are some individuals, mostly young patients, who quickly develop extensive vasogenic, extracellular brain edema with the consequences of increased intracranial pressure and displacement and herniations of brain compartments. In these patients, a therapeutic trial of osmotic agents and/or corticosteroids is warranted since the situation is often desperate.

In some patients with massive brain swelling and increased intracranial pressure, removal of the skull overlying the side of the infarct (hemicraniectomy) can be life-saving but patients are sometimes left with severe neurologic residual deficits.[349-352] Surprisingly, some patients make extraordinary recoveries after hemicraniectomies and survive with very little neurologic deficit.

> ML is a 46-year-old woman who suddenly developed aphasia and weakness of the right hand. She had a chronic myocardiopathy and during the preceding months reported increasing dyspnea and pedal edema. Examination 3.5 hours after onset of the neurologic symptoms showed slight right-hand clumsiness and occasional word errors. She made reading, writing, and spelling errors. MR studies performed 4 hours after onset showed an occluded left MCA on MRA, a small elliptical zone of abnormal diffusion on DWI, and a normal T2-weighted MRI scan. TCD after intravenous recombinant tissue plasminogen activator showed reperfusion in the MCA territory. MRI and MRA studies were repeated 18 hours after thrombolysis. The MCA obstruction had improved, but there was still a residual filling defect. The infarct was seen on T2-weighted MRI and DWI, but had not expanded. Perfusion imaging showed a defect larger than the infarct. On a later study, the MCA completely recanalized and the perfusion deficit cleared. The infarct remained the same but her examination returned to normal, except for minor loss of dexterity with her right hand when she played the piano.

The timing of thrombolysis is important if brain tissue is to be saved. Experimental studies in animals show that after 3 hours, irreversible brain ischemia (infarction) has already developed. However, salvageability of ischemic brain tissue varies considerably from patient to patient. Sometimes ischemic but salvageable brain tissue persists for many hours. This hypoperfused tissue has inadequate blood supply to function but is not irreversibly damaged. Stunned brain and ischemic penumbra are terms used for ischemic nonfunctioning brain that is not yet infarcted. The major danger of thrombolysis and of spontaneous reperfusion is that reperfusion of damaged vessels in the ischemic zone could cause major bleeding. Ideally, the decision on whether to pursue thrombolysis or other means of reperfusion, such as angioplasty, should rest on the presence of viable salvageable penumbral tissue and the extent of brain that is already infarcted, not on the time that has expired since symptom onset. The extent of infarction determines the risk of treatment; the presence and size of penumbral, stunned tissue determines the potential benefit of thrombolysis that accomplishes reperfusion. The newer magnetic resonance techniques of diffusion-weighted and perfusion MR scans performed with echoplaner equipment, when coupled with MRA, give clinicians a quantitative estimate of these factors.

The case of ML illustrates the power of this imaging tool. Despite the more than 4 hours that transpired after symptom onset, the imaging showed that there was considerable potential benefit of trying to recanalize the recipient artery and much risk of leaving the clot where it was. Had the artery not recanalized after intravenous treatment, we would have performed an arteriogram and attempted to remove the clot by intra-arterial thrombolysis and/or mechanical means.

Clinicians should estimate the extent of normal, infarcted and stunned brain supplied by the occluded artery by using brain imaging (CT and T2-weighted MRI scans), vascular studies (CTA, MRA, TCD, angiography), and neurologic examination. If the patient has a severe neurologic deficit and a large infarct is present on brain scans, then much of the brain is infarcted and there is little to gain by thrombolysis, which carries a substantial risk of hemorrhage in this circumstance. If the patient has a severe neurologic deficit and brain scans are normal, however, then there could be considerable stunned, salvageable brain, which could be restored to function if thrombolysis were successful.

Chronic Prophylactic Treatment to Prevent Re-embolization

Almost immediately, physicians caring for patients with brain embolism must think of preventing the next embolus. The three strategies used for prophylaxis are (1) removal of the donor source of embolism whenever possible, (2) modification of risk factors that relate to disease at the donor site, and (3) modification of coagulation functions to prevent the formation of new thromboemboli. Some donor site lesions can be corrected, or at least ameliorated surgically, or by using interventional radiologic techniques. Cardiac valve lesions, cardiac tumors, atrial septal defects, PFOs, and protruding, mobile, large aortic atheromas can be treated surgically. Newer interventional techniques may permit effective interventional percutaneous treatment of PFOs and aortic atheromas. Carotid and vertebral artery lesions can be corrected surgically (endarterectomy) or by stenting and angioplasty. Many patients with cardiac, aortic, and cerebrovascular donor site lesions have modifiable risk factors, such as smoking, hyperlipidemia, hypertension, inactive sedentary lifestyle, and obesity. Counseling and medical treatment of these risk factors are an important part of the care of patients with brain embolism.

Manipulation of coagulation to prevent future thromboemboli is a strategy applicable to the majority of patients with brain embolism. Embolic particles are diverse. White platelet thrombi, red erythrocyte-fibrin thrombi, cholesterol crystals, calcified particles from arteries and valves, myxomatous tissue, bacteria in patients with infective endocarditis, and bland fibrous vegetations in patients with noninfective endocarditis are the most important substances. Medical prophylactic treatment against reentry of these particles into the circulation depends much on the "stuff" in the emboli rather than the source of the materials.[1,4,50] It's the bird rather than the location of the nest that is important.[50] For example, the most effective prophylaxis for prevention of embolization in patients with bacterial endocarditis is effective antibiotic sterilization of the bacterial vegetations. Cholesterol crystals, calcific particles, bacterial vegetation, and myxomatous emboli do not, as far as is known, respond to treatment with anticoagulants or drugs that modify platelet function.

The two types of medicinal agents most often used to prevent thromboemboli are standard anticoagulants (heparin, low-molecular-weight heparins, heparinoids, and warfarin compounds) and agents that alter platelet adhesion, aggregation, and secretion, such as aspirin, ticlopidine, clopidogrel, dipyridamole, cilostazole, and omega-3 fish oils. Chapter 5 contains a detailed discussion of the use of these compounds. White platelet-fibrin thrombi are posited to form on irregular surfaces in fast-moving bloodstreams in widely patent arteries and cavities. Red erythrocyte-fibrin thrombi, on the other hand, tend to form in regions of stasis, such as leg veins, dilated cardiac atria, severely stenotic arteries, and so forth. At times, both white and red thrombi coexist because activated platelets are a stimulus for activation of the coagulation cascade and subsequent red-clot formation. I choose anticoagulant treatment for prophylaxis, first with heparin or low-molecular-weight heparin, and then coumadin, in patients who have lesions that promote red-clot formation and in patients whose imaging studies show thrombi. I continue coumadin as long as the situation that promotes red clots persists. These situations include persistent atrial fibrillation, myocardial aneurysm, prosthetic valves, and stenotic extracranial arteries. In patients with acute occlusive thrombi superimposed on preocclusive atherostenosis, I continue coumadin only for a short time (6 to 12 weeks), during which thrombi organize and no longer propagate or form fresh tails that embolize. During this time, collateral circulation has usually become maximal. Sometimes, lesions that caused the original thrombosis later improve (e.g., arterial dissections, regressing atheromas, or corrected cardiac right-to-left shunts), so anticoagulation can be stopped and replaced with antiplatelet drugs.

I use agents that alter platelet functions for patients with lesions posited to predispose to formation of white platelet-fibrin thrombi. Irregular nonstenosing atherosclerotic plaques and irregular, but nonstenotic valve surfaces are the most common situations. In patients who can tolerate aspirin, I usually prescribe 325 mg of coated aspirin daily or aspirin with modified-release dipyridamole, cilostazole, and clopidogrel are other antiplatelet agents that are often prescribed. High fibrinogen levels increase whole-blood viscosity and platelet aggregability and predispose to red clot formation. Drugs that lower fibrinogen levels are prescribed. In some situations, in which both red and white clots are likely to form, a combination of platelet antiaggregants and coumadin might be more effective than either agent alone.

EMBOLIC MATERIALS THAT ORIGINATE OUTSIDE THE VASCULAR SYSTEM

Some embolic materials that enter the systemic and brain circulations do not originate in the heart, aorta, or cervicocranial arteries and are not composed of blood elements or thrombi. Because the situations and nature of the emboli is so different from the much more common intravascular emboli, I discuss the major features of these emboli at the end of this chapter. The types of particles are diverse as are the clinical syndromes and circumstances of brain embolization.[353] Fat and gas bubbles cause microembolism to many small brain capillaries and arterioles causing an encephalopathy type syndrome while tumor and foreign body emboli usually block single discrete arteries causing strokes.

Fat Embolism

Fat embolism occurs most often after serious physical trauma that causes bone fractures. The frequency, clinical and laboratory features, and circumstances of the fat embolism syndrome have been extensively described.[3,353-357] The syndrome consists of a triad of respiratory distress, decreased alertness, and a petechial rash developing 24 to 48 hours after an injury. Table 9-6 lists the major findings in patients with the fat embolism syndrome. Fat embolism is most often found after blunt physical trauma with fractured bones but can occur after cardiac surgery and in patients who have bone infarctions. In patients with injuries, the long

Table 9-6. Fat Embolism
Major Clinical Features
Dyspnea and respiratory distress
Decreased alertness and cognitive function
Petechiae
Other Findings
Fever
Tachycardia
Retinal infarcts
Jaundice
Laboratory and Imaging
Anemia
Thrombocytopenia
Hypoxia
Abnormal chest x-ray
Fat globules and lipid in the urine
Microembolism during transcranial Doppler monitoring
Fat emboli visible during transesophageal echocardiography
MRI showing multiple infarcts and small hemorrhages

bones and pelvis are most often involved especially the femurs. The fat embolism syndrome is unusual in children and in patients with fractures limited to the upper extremities.[353] Often the cause is multiple fractures resulting from vehicular accidents. Investigators retrospectively reviewed 10 years of experience of the fat embolism syndrome found at one trauma center and found 27 instances among 3026 patients (0.9%) with long-bone fractures.[354]

Occasionally the fat embolism syndrome develops after cardiac surgery when the atria or ventricles are entered.[358,359] The mechanism of fat embolism after open heart surgery is unclear, but fat from the sternotomy or epicardial fat may directly enter the systemic circulation. Cardiotomy suction tubes draining the pericardium during cardiopulmonary bypass contain variable quantities of fat globules.

Fat embolism has also been reported in patients with sickle cell anemia (homozygous S-S and those who have S-C disease).[360-363] In sickle-cell-disease patients, the fat originates from bone and bone marrow infarcts. Bone and joint pain and crisis may precede fat embolism in some patients.

Fat embolism has also been described after therapeutic procedures that use lipid substances to form stable drugs for injection. Lipidol has been used to mix with anticancer drugs that are fat soluble to form stable covalent conjugates. This mixture is then injected into an artery feeding a tumor, such as in the liver. Fat embolism has been described after such therapeutic procedures.[364] The clinical findings included dyspnea and decreased alertness. Hypoxemia preceded or accompanied stupor. MRI showed multiple focal abnormalities mostly in border-zone regions. The neurologic signs were severe but transient and cleared completely within weeks. None of the three reported patients had cardiac shunts demonstrable by echocardiography.[364] Fat emboli can occasionally be introduced during placement of pumps designed to release pharmaceutical agents into the cerebrospinal fluid.[365] Parenteral nutrition containing high lipid content occasionally is infused into a cervicocranial artery when a catheter is misplaced into an artery rather than a vein.

The fat embolism syndrome usually develops after a delay of a few hours up to a few days after trauma. In one series of 14 patients, all of whom had traumatic injuries with long bone fractures, the latency of onset of signs of fat embolism after trauma ranged from 12 to 72 hours (mean 41 hours).[356] At times the clinical manifestations of fat embolism can be delayed for as long as 5 days.[357] Most patients have symptom onset between 24 and 72 hours after injury.

The major clinical manifestations of the fat embolism syndrome are dyspnea, tachypnea, fever, tachycardia, petechiae, and neurologic dysfunction.[1] Jaundice can also occur. Neurologic symptoms and signs may precede or follow respiratory distress and are characterized as confusion with delirium often followed by a decrease in the level of consciousness. Neurologic symptoms and signs are present in more than 80% of patients. Most often patients develop an encephalopathy characterized by restlessness, agitation, confusion, poor memory, and decreased alertness. This state often passes into stupor or coma. Seizures are common at onset or early during the course of illness. Seizures can be focal or generalized. Focal neurologic signs are also common and include hemiparesis, conjugate eye deviation, aphasia and visual field abnormalities. Motor abnormalities including increased tone in the lower extremities, Babinski signs, and decerebrate rigidity are often found. Focal neurologic signs were noted in 33% of patients in one series.[357] Some patients have scotomas and other visual abnormalities related to retinal dysfunction caused by fat embolism.

Pulmonary symptoms develop shortly after or concurrent with the neurologic symptoms. Dyspnea and tachypnea are prominent and patients may become cyanotic. Tachycardia, high fever, and circulatory collapse also occur; hypotension is often related to blood loss, hypoxemia, and hypovolemia. Renal failure can develop. The pulmonary emboli can result in increased resistance in the pulmonary artery bed and increased

pressures in the right side of the heart. In patients with a PFO, pulmonary hypertension may promote extensive right-to-left passage of fat emboli through the PFO.

An important clue to the presence of fat microemboli is the presence on physical examination of petechiae. Petechiae are found in 50% to 75% of patients with the fat embolism syndrome. They are most often found in the lower palpebral conjunctivae and the skin of the neck, shoulder, and the axillary folds.[1,353,354] Another important clinical clue is the appearance of fat emboli within the arteries of the eye. Microinfarcts are sometimes visible in the optic fundus especially in the perimacular regions. Small hemorrhages sometimes with white pale centers are also found. Fat globules can sometimes be seen within retinal arteries. Papilledema is occasionally found.

Laboratory tests are often helpful in diagnosis. Many patients develop abnormal chest x-rays. Fine stippling and fluffy lung infiltrates are common and are seen diffusely through the lung fields. Most patients have a drop in hemoglobin and hematocrit due to traumatic loss of blood and hemolysis. Thrombocytopenia and prolonged prothrombin and activated partial thromboplastin times are common, and are attributed to a consumptive coagulopathy. Frank disseminated intravascular coagulation may also occur. TCD monitoring of patients with long-bone fractures can document fat emboli.[364,365] Brain imaging may show small hemorrhages, brain edema, and focal infarcts usually manifested by regions of gyral enhancement on CT or MRI scans. CT scans are most often normal but may show areas of hypodensity and small hemorrhages. MRI is much more sensitive and often shows abnormalities within the white matter and in border-zone regions.[366] FLAIR and contrast-enhanced images are particularly helpful in showing microinfarcts.[366] Figure 9-20 is an MRI FLAIR image that shows many small brain infarcts due to fat embolism in a patient who became stuporous after a leg fracture. Magnetic resonance spectroscopy can also be used to identify the presence of fat.[367] In one reported patient who had fat embolism develop after a femoral fracture, magnetic resonance spectroscopy performed 35 hours after the onset of coma showed the presence of long-chain lipid resonance in high quantities in the periventricular white matter and occipital cerebral cortices of the patient with no associated lactate resonance. The lipid gradually disappeared on subsequent examinations.[367]

Lipid globules are sometimes found in the urine when fat stains are used. Skin, renal, and muscle biopsies may show fat globules within small skin, muscle, and renal vessels and in renal glomeruli. Cryostat frozen sections of blood also can show the

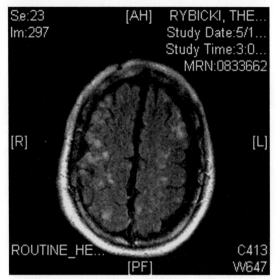

Figure 9-20. MRI FLAIR image showing multiple small infarcts in a patient with fat embolism after a leg fracture.

presence of neutral fat. Neutral fat is most often found in patients with hypoxemia and $PaCO_2$ of less than 60 mm Hg. Hypoxemia is very common in patients with the fat embolism syndrome. One of the most effective and specific tests for fat embolism is bronchopulmonary lavage.[368,369] The technique involves microscopic examination of cells recovered by lavage and stained with a specific stain for neutral fat, such as using oil red O dye.

The mortality rate in patients with the fat embolism syndrome is quite high (as much as 50%), although the mortality rate has declined over time.[1,353,356] When coma, severe blood loss, hypotension, high fever, and disseminated intravascular coagulation (DIC) are present, the mortality rate remains substantial. Necropsy of the brain of patients dying with the fat embolism syndrome shows many small-ball or ring-shaped, and perivascular hemorrhages, brain edema, and regions of microinfarction.[370] Stains for fat reveal fat globules within hemorrhagic lesions and in small vessels throughout the brain. Small hemorrhages, edema, and hyaline membranes are often found in the lungs. Fat globules are also often visible in renal glomeruli, myocardium, liver, pancreas, spleen, and gastrointestinal mucosa.

Treatment of patients with the fat embolism syndrome has not been formally studied in therapeutic trials. Supportive care including oxygen administration often with assisted respiration and fluid and blood replacement is very important. Corticosteroids, heparin, and intravenous administration of 5% alcohol solutions have all been tried, but their effectiveness has not been well studied. Heparin has been used in patients with consumptive coagulopathies and also because of

its posited lipolytic effect. Alcohol is also believed to have a lipolytic capability. Among these treatments, corticosteroids administration has been most frequently used.

Air Embolism

Gas bubbles occasionally enter the systemic circulation and cause air embolism to the brain and other organs. The sources of air are quite diverse. Most often air is introduced iatrogenically during procedures and surgery. Air embolism can follow endoscopy laparoscopy and surgery on the gastrointestinal tract,[1,371-374] spontaneous pneumothorax and procedures and surgery in the thorax involving the lungs,[371,375] pneumo-orbitography, perineal and peritoneal air insufflation, pneumo-arthrography, and surgery on the heart, neck, brain, and axilla.[371] Air also can enter the cranium after fractures involving the cribriform plate and the paranasal sinuses[376] and after surgery on the sinuses. Venous and arterial catheterization and cardiopulmonary bypass are common causes of air embolism. Air can also be introduced during home infusion therapy.[377] Less often air embolism follows penetrating traumatic injuries to the thorax, lungs, or major blood vessels. Air introduction into the vascular system is quite common during cesarean deliveries.[378] Precordial Doppler can demonstrate some air embolism in about half of all cesarean deliveries.[378,379]

Another important and quite different circumstance that leads to air embolism is in relation to scuba diving and rapid ascents after descents into deep water.[380,381] During diving accidents, air becomes trapped in the alveoli of the lungs due to partial bronchial occlusion from mucous plugs and failure to exhale. Because the volume of a gas varies inversely with pressure (Boyle's law), pressurized air bubbles in the lungs increase dramatically in volume as the diver ascends and the ambient surrounding pressure falls.[371] The rapid expansion of air in the lungs causes entry of air into the pulmonary arterial and venous outflow systems.[381] Gas bubbles pass through the lung vasculature or through a patent foramen ovale into the systemic circulation. Similar to the situation in fat embolism, many small particles enter the circulation and block the microvasculature. The frequency of patent foramen ovale in divers with clinical decompression syndromes is higher than expected by chance.

Introduction of a large quantity of air into the venous system can result in sudden blockage of the pulmonary artery and right ventricular outflow tract with resultant cardiac arrhythmia and sudden death or circulatory collapse.[378] Dyspnea, cyanosis, chest pain, restlessness and a feeling of impending death can develop. When small amounts of air are released into the venous system filtering by the pulmonary vessels protects the coronary and brain circulations. Lung edema can result from air in the lungs especially when there is an increase in pulmonary artery pressure. Air can also stimulate the release of various thromboplastins, surfactants, and cytokines that cause lung injury and coagulopathy.

Air bubbles in arteries supplying the brain cause an immediate but transient block in blood flow. Air quickly moves through the capillary bed into the venules and dissipates.[1,371] The gas bubbles cause arterial vasoconstriction followed by dilatation and stasis of blood flow.[371]

Symptoms and signs of brain gas embolism have been studied most thoroughly in individuals who have had diving-related incidents.[371,381,382] These occur during scuba diving and have been well studied in naval personnel who escape too quickly from submerged submarines.[382] Loss of consciousness often develops suddenly after the diver emerges onto the surface of the water. Dizziness, chest discomfort, paresthesias, weakness, blurred vision, nausea, and headache are the most common symptoms and may precede the loss of consciousness. Seizures and focal neurologic signs, especially related to dysfunction of the brainstem and cerebellum are also quite common.[371-375,381]

Discrete focal collections of gas and multiple focal air collections are sometimes found in the brain on cranial CT examination.[372-375,383] Brain edema with compression of the ventricular system is another common and important finding on brain imaging examinations. DWI imaging using MRI can also show scattered areas of brain infarction.[383] TCD is quite sensitive for detection of air microemboli.[382,384] Treatment has usually consisted of inhalation of 100% oxygen as well as the use of hyperbaric decompression chambers.[378]

Tumor Embolism

Occasionally major arteries supplying the brain are occluded by tumor emboli. This occurs when a neoplasm directly erodes into a cervical artery, or a pulmonary vein, or when a tumor erodes into a systemic vein, embolizes to the heart, and then passes through a cardiac septal abnormality to enter the systemic circulation. The most frequent tumors that embolize are primary pulmonary neoplasms or tumors that have metastasized to the lungs.[385] Brain embolism has sometimes occurred after lung surgery for cancer. Necropsy has usually shown tumor invasion of pulmonary veins or invasion of the LA.[385] Surgical manipulation of the lungs in patients with lung tumors can promote systemic embolization of the tumor.

Although most often the clinical syndrome is that of a stroke, embolism to other systemic organs also occurs. Tumor emboli can also pass through a patent foramen ovale or another cardiac septal defect. Tumor emboli have also been reported in patients with thyroid and other neck cancers that eroded into neck arteries.[386]

Foreign Body Embolism

Occasionally foreign bodies enter the systemic vascular system and embolize to the brain. Foreign bodies that embolize to the brain must either enter the lungs and pulmonary veins, enter directly into the left side of the heart itself, enter the right side of the heart and traverse a defect in the cardiac septum, or penetrate the cervicocranial arteries that supply the brain. Bullets and pellets may penetrate the skin and land in the heart.[387] Shotgun pellets have been reported to puncture a carotid artery in the neck and become visible on cranial CT scans causing brain embolic infarction.[388,389] Langenbach et al described the case of a 52-year-old man whose right neck was penetrated by a small metal particle while hammering.[390] He soon developed a severe left hemiplegia. Plain skull films showed a 2×7-mm, metal-dense particle to the right of the pituitary fossa. CT showed a large right middle cerebral artery territory infarct, and angiography showed that the metal fragment was blocking the MCA.[390] Figure 9-21 is a CT scan showing a shotgun pellet proximal to a large MCA territory infarct, and Figure 9-22 contains arteriograms in the same patient that show 2-mm-sized pellets blocking the intracranial carotid artery and MCAs. These pellets originated from the heart in a patient who was shot in the chest during an argument.[393a] One reason that echocardiograms often fail to show an embolic source is the very small size of potentially devastating thromboemboli. Foreign bodies for a variety of reasons can gain entry into the heart and embolize to systemic arteries and the brain.[391-393]

Retinal and brain arteries can become blocked by foreign particles in patients who mash drugs manufactured for oral use and inject the drugs intravenously.[394-397] The most frequently reported particles are talc and methylcellulose that are used to bind drugs to maintain them in pill form. The particles first block lung vessels. Pulmonary vascular obliteration causes pulmonary hypertension and arteriovenous shunting develops in the lungs, allowing the particles to enter the pulmonary veins and then the systemic circulation.[394,395] Talc and cornstarch emboli can be seen in the retinal arteries of some of these drug abusers.[396] Strokes have also been described in patients who have injected drugs directly into neck arteries.[397,398]

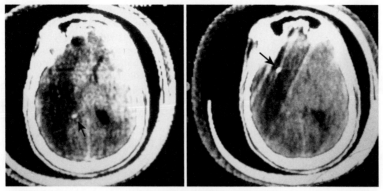

Figure 9-21. CT scans showing a large middle cerebral artery territory infarct on the right of the scans. *Black arrows* point to the pieces of shotgun pellet seen within the brain images. (From Kase CS, White R, Vinson TL, Eichelberger RP: Shotgun pellet embolism to the middle cerebral artery. Neurology 1981;31: 458-461, with permission.)

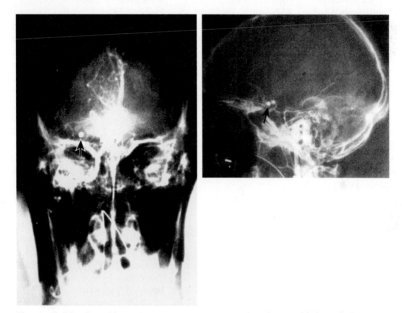

Figure 9-22. Carotid arteriograms, a anteroposterior view and b lateral view showing two pieces of buckshot *(black arrows)* blocking the middle cerebral artery. (From Kase CS, White R, Vinson TL, Eichelberger RP: Shotgun pellet embolism to the middle cerebral artery. Neurology 1981;31:458-461, with permission.)

References

1. Caplan LR: Embolic particles. In Caplan LR, Manning W (eds): Brain Embolism. New York:Informa Healthcare, 2006, pp 259-275.
2. Molina C, Alexandrov A: Transcranial Doppler ultrasound. In Caplan LR, Manning W (eds): Brain Embolism. New York: Informa Healthcare, 2006, pp 113-128.
3. Caplan LR: Brain embolism, revisited. Neurology 1993;43:1281-1287.
4. Caplan LR: Brain embolism. In Caplan LR, Hurtst JW, Chimowitz M (eds): Clinical Neurocardiology. New York: Marcel Dekker, 1999, pp 35-185.
5. Markus HS: Transcranial Doppler detection of circulating cerebral emboli: A review. Stroke 1993;24:1246-1250.
6. Sliwka U, Job F-P, Wissuwa D, et al: Occurrence of transcranial Doppler high-intensity transient signals in patients with potential cardiac sources of embolism: A prospective study. Stroke 1995;26: 2067-2070.
7. Daffertshofer M, Ries S, Schminke U, Hennerici M: High-intensity transient signals in patients with cerebral ischemia. Stroke 1996;27:1844-1849.
8. Sliwka U, Lingnau A, Stohlmann W-D, et al: Prevalence and time course of microembolic signals in patients with acute strokes, a prospective study. Stroke 1997;28:358-363.

9. Babikian VL, Caplan LR: Brain embolism is a dynamic process with variable characteristics. Neurology 2000;54:797-801.

10. Caplan LR: Recipient artery. In Caplan LR, Manning W (eds): Brain Embolism. New York: Informa Healthcare, 2006, pp 31-59.

11. Mohr JP, Caplan LR, Melski JW, et al: The Harvard Cooperative Stroke Registry: A prospective registry. Neurology 1978;29:754-762.

12. Caplan LR, Hier DB, D'Cruz I: Cerebral embolism in the Michael Reese Stroke Registry. Stroke 1983;14:530-536.

13. Mohr JP, Gautier JC, Hier DB, Stein RW: Middle cerebral artery. In Barnett HJM, Mohr JP, Stein BM, Yatsu FM (eds): Stroke, Pathophysiology, Diagnosis, and Management, vol 1. New York: Churchill Livingstone, 1986, pp 377-450.

14. Minematsu K, Yamaguchi T, Omae T: "Spectacular shrinking deficit": Rapid recovery from a major hemispheric syndrome by migration of an embolus. Neurology 1992;42:157-162.

15. Bogousslavsky J, van Melle G, Regli F: The Lausanne Stroke Registry: Analysis of 1000 consecutive patients with first stroke. Stroke 1988;19:1083-1092.

16. Gacs G, Merer FT, Bodosi M: Balloon catheter as a model of cerebral emboli in humans. Stroke 1982;13:39-42.

17. Helgason C: Cardioembolic stroke topography and pathogenesis. Cerebrovasc Brain Metab Rev 1992;4:28-58.

18. Caplan LR: Posterior Circulation Disease, Clinical Findings, Diagnosis, and Management. Boston: Blackwell, 1996.

19. Caplan LR: Top of the basilar syndrome: Selected clinical aspects. Neurology 1980;30:72-79.

20. Mehler MF: The rostral basilar artery syndrome: Diagnosis, etiology, prognosis. Neurology 1989;39:9-16.

21. Caplan LR: Cerebellar infarcts: Key features in Rev Neurol Dis 2005;2:51-60.

22. Lodder J, Krijne-Kubat B, Broekman J: Cerebral hemorrhagic infarction at autopsy: Cardiac embolic cause and the relationship to the cause of death. Stroke 1986;17:626-629.

23. Hart RG, Easton JD: Hemorrhagic infarcts. Stroke 1986;17:586-589.

24. Timsit SG, Sacco RL, Mohr JP, et al: Brain infarction severity differs according to cardiac or arterial embolic source. Neurology 1993;43:728-733.

25. Bladin CF: Seizures after Stroke [thesis]. Melbourne, Australia: University of Melbourne, 1997.

26. Kittner SJ, Sharkness CM, Price TR, et al: Infarcts with a cardiac source of embolism in the NINCDS Stroke Data Bank: Historical features. Neurology 1990;40:281-284.

27. Hinton RC, Kistler JP, Fallon JR, et al: Influence of etiology of atrial fibrillation on incidence of systemic embolism. Am J Card 1977;40:509-513.

27a. Abboud H, Labreuche J, Gongora-Riverra F, et al: Prevalence and determinants of subdiaphragmatic

visceral infarction in patients with fatal stroke. Stroke 2007;38:1442-1446.

28. Ringelstein EB, Koschorke S, Holling A, et al: Computed tomographic patterns of proven embolic brain infarctions. Ann Neurol 1989;26:759-765.

28a. Viehman JA, Saver JL, Liebeskind DS, et al: Utility of urinalysis in discriminating cardioembolic stroke mechanism. Arch Neurol 2007;64:667-670.

29. Ringelstein EB, Koschorke S, Holling A, et al: Computed tomographic patterns of proven embolic brain infarctions. Ann Neurol 1989;26:759-765.

30. Gacs G, Fox AJ, Barnett HJ, Vinuela F: CT visualization of intracranial arterial thromboembolism. Stroke 1983;14:756-763.

31. Tomsick T, Brott T, Barsan W, et al: Thrombus localization with emergency cerebral computed tomography. Stroke 1990;21:180.

32. Fisher CM, Adams R: Observations on brain embolism with special reference to the mechanism of hemorrhagic infarction. J Neuropathol Exp Neurol 1951;10:92-93.

33. Fisher CM, Adams RD: Observations on brain embolism with special reference to hemorrhagic infarction. In Furlan AJ (ed): The Heart and Stroke. London: Springer, 1987, pp 17-36.

34. Yamaguchi T, Minematsu K, Choki JI, Ikeda M: Clinical and neuroradiological analysis of thrombotic and embolic cerebral infarction. Jpn Circ J 1984;48:50-58.

35. Okada Y, Yamaguchi T, Minematsu K, et al: Hemorrhagic transformation in cerebral embolism. Stroke 1989;20:598-603.

36. Pessin MS, Estol C, Lafranchise F, Caplan LR: Safety of anticoagulation after hemorrhagic infarction. Neurology 1993;43:1298-1303.

37. Chaves CJ, Pessin MS, Caplan LR, et al: Cerebellar hemorrhagic infarction. Neurology 1996;46:346-349.

38. Garcia J, Ho K-L, Caccamo DV: Intracerebral hemorrhage: Pathology of selected topics. In Kase CS, Caplan LR (eds): Intracerebral Hemorrhage. Boston: Butterworth-Heinemann, 1994;45-72.

39. Fieschi C, Argentino C, Lenzi G, et al: Clinical and instrumental evaluation of patients with ischemic stroke within the first six hours. J Neurol Sci 1989;91:311-322.

40. del Zoppo GJ, Poeck K, Pessin MS, et al: Recombinant tissue plasminogen activator in acute thrombotic and embolic stroke. Ann Neurol 1992;32:78-86.

41. Wolpert SM, Bruckmann H, Greenlee R, et al: Neuroradiologic evaluation of patients with acute stroke treated with recombinant tissue plasminogen activator. The rt-PA Acute Stroke Study Group. AJNR Am J Neuroradiol 1993;14:3-13.

42. Dalal P, Shah P, Sheth S, et al: Cerebral embolism: Angiographic observations on spontaneous clot lysis. Lancet 1965;1:61-64.

43. Liebeskind A, Chinichian A, Schechter M: The moving embolus seen during cerebral angiography. Stroke 1971;2:440-443.

44. Caplan LR, Allam GJ, Teal PA: The moving embolus. J Neuroimaging 1993;3:195-197.

45. Sharma VK, Tsivgoulis G, Lao AY, Alexandrov AV: Role of transcranial Doppler ultrasonography in evaluation of patients with cerebrovascular disease. Curr Neurol Neurosci Rep 2007;7:8-20.

46. Thomassen L, Waje-Andreassen U, Naess H, et al: Doppler ultrasound and clinical findings in patients with acute ischemic stroke treated with thrombolysis. Eur J Neurol 2005;12:462-465.

47. Molina CA, Alexandrov AV, Demchuk AM, et al: Improving the predictive accuracy of recanalization on stroke outcome in patients treated with tissue plasminogen activator. Stroke 2004;35:151-156.

48. Askevold ET, Naess H, Thomassen L: Predictors of recanalization after intravenous thrombolysis in acute ischemic stroke. J Stroke Cerebrovasc Dis 2007;16:21-24.

49. Georgiadis D, Lindner A, Manz M, et al: Intracranial microembolic signals in 500 patients with potential cardiac or carotid embolic source and in normal controls. Stroke 1997;28:1203-1207.

50. Caplan LR: Of birds and nests and brain emboli. Rev Neurol 1991;147:265-273.

51. Caplan LR, Manning W: Cardiac sources of embolism: The usual suspects. In Caplan LR, Manning W (eds): Brain Embolism. New York: Informa Healthcare, 2006, pp 129-159.

52. Manning W: Cardiac sources of embolism: Pathophysiology and identification. In Caplan LR, Manning W (eds): Brain Embolism. New York: Informa Healthcare, 2006, pp 161-186.

53. Virchow R: Gesammelte Abhandlungen zur Wissenschaftlichenmedtezin. Frankfurt: Meidinger Sohn, 1856.

54. Harker LA, Slichter SL: Studies of platelet and fibrinogen kinetics in patients with prosthetic heart valves. N Engl J Med 1970;283:1302-1305.

55. Baumgartner HR, Haudenschild C: Adhesion of platelets to subendothelium. Ann N Y Acad Sci 1972;201:22-36.

56. Gustafsson C, Blomback M, Britton M, et al: Coagulation factors and the increased risk of stroke in nonvalvular atrial fibrillation. Stroke 1990;21:47-51.

57. Kumagai K, Fukunami M, Ohmori M, et al: Increased intracardiovascular clotting in patients with chronic atrial fibrillation. J Am Coll Cardiol 1990;16:377-380.

58. Hanna JP, Furlan AJ: Cardiac disease and embolic sources. In Caplan LR (ed): Brain Ischemia. London: Springer, 1995, pp 299-315.

59. Goldman ME, Pearce LA, Hart RG: Pathophysiologic correlates of thromboembolism in nonvalvular atrial fibrillation: I. Reduced flow velocity in the left atrial appendage (the Stroke Prevention in Atrial Fibrillation [SPAF-III] study). J Am Soc Echocardiogr 1999;12:1080-1087.

60. Wolf PA, Dawber TR, Thomas HE, Kannel WB: Epidemiologic assessment of chronic atrial fibrillation and risk of stroke: The Framingham Study. Neurology 1978;28:973-977.

61. Wolf PA, Abbott RD, Kannel WB: Atrial fibrillation: A major contribution to stroke in the elderly. The Framingham Study. Arch Intern Med 1987;147:1561-1564.

62. Cairns JA, Connolly SJ: Nonrheumatic atrial fibrillation. Risk of stroke and role of antithrombotic therapy. Circulation 1991;84:469-481.

63. Dunn M, Alexander J, DeSilva R, Hildner F: Antithrombotic therapy in atrial fibrillation. Chest 1989;95:S118-S127.

64. The Stroke Prevention in Atrial Fibrillation Investigators: Predictors of thromboembolism in atrial fibrillation: 1. Clinical features of patients at risk. Ann Intern Med 1992;116:1-5.

65. Atrial Fibrillation Investigators: Risk factors for stroke and efficacy of antithrombotic therapy in atrial fibrillation: Analysis of pooled data from five randomized controlled trials. Arch Intern Med 1994;154:1449-1457.

66. Caplan LR, D'Cruz I, Hier DB, et al: Atrial size, atrial fibrillation, and stroke. Ann Neurol 1986;19:158-161.

67. Stroke Prevention in Atrial Fibrillation Investigators: Predictors of thromboembolism in atrial fibrillation: II. Echocardiographic features of patients at risk. Ann Intern Med 1992;116:6-12.

68. DiPasquale G, Urbinati S, Pinelli G: New echocardiographic markers of embolic risk in atrial fibrillation. Cerebrovasc Dis 1995;5:315-322.

69. Vernhorst P, Kamp O, Visser CA, Verheught FWA: Left atrial appendage flow velocity assessment using transesophageal echocardiography in nonrheumatic atrial fibrillation and systemic embolism. Am J Cardiol 1993;71:192-196.

70. Garcia-Fernandez MA, Torrecilla EG, San Roman D, et al: Left atrial appendage Doppler flow patterns: Implications of thrombus formation. Am Heart J 1992;124:955-965.

71. Beppu S, Nimura Y, Sakakibara H: Smoke-like echo in the left atrial cavity in mitral valve disease: Its features and significance. J Am Coll Cardiol 1985;6:744-749.

72. Merino A, Hauptman P, Badiman L, et al: Echocardiographic 'smoke' is produced by an interaction of erythrocytes and plasma proteins modulated by shear forces. J Am Coll Cardiol 1992;20:1661-1668.

73. Black IW, Stewart WJ: The role of echocardiography in the evaluation of cardiac sources of embolism. Echocardiography 1993;10:429-439.

74. Chimowitz MI, DeGeorgia MA, Poole RM, et al: Left atrial spontaneous echo contrast is highly associated with previous stroke in patients with atrial fibrillation or mitral stenosis. Stroke 1993;24:1015-1019.

75. Manning WJ, Silverman DI, Gordon SPF, et al: Cardioversion from atrial fibrillation without prolonged anticoagulation with use of transesophageal echocardiography to exclude the presence of atrial thrombi. N Engl J Med 1993;328:750-756.

76. The Stroke Prevention in Atrial Fibrillation Investigators Committee on Echocardiography: Transesophageal echocardiographic correlates of thromboembolism in high-risk patients with nonvalvular atrial fibrillation. Ann Intern Med 1998;128:639-647.

77. Weigner MJ, Thomas LR, Patel U, et al: Transesophageal-echocardiography-facilitated early cardioversion from atrial fibrillation: Short-term safety and impact on maintenance of sinus rhythm at 1 year. Am J Med 2001;110:694-702.

78. Klein AL, Grimm RA, Murray RD, et al: Use of transesophageal echocardiography to guide cardioversion in patients with atrial fibrillation. N Engl J Med 2001;344:1411-1420.

79. Stoddard MF, Dawkins PR, Prince CR, Ammash NM: Left atrial appendage thrombus is not uncommon in patients with acute atrial fibrillation and a recent embolic event: A transesophageal echocardiographic study. J Am Coll Cardiol 1995;25:452-459.

80. Manning WJ, Silverman DI, Waksmonski CA, et al: Prevalence of residual left atrial thrombi in patients presenting with acute thromboembolism and newly recognized atrial fibrillation. Arch Intern Med 1995;155:2193-2197.

81. The Boston Area Anticoagulation Trial for Atrial Fibrillation Investigators: The effect of low-dose warfarin on the risk of stroke in patients with nonrheumatic atrial fibrillation. N Engl J Med 1990;323:1505-1511.

82. EAFT Study Group: Silent brain infarction in nonrheumatic atrial fibrillation. Neurology 1996;46:159-165.

83. EAFT (European Atrial Fibrillation Trial) Study Group: Secondary prevention in non-rheumatic atrial fibrillation after transient ischaemic attack or minor stroke. Lancet 1993;342:1255-1262.

84. Petersen P, Godtfredsen J, Boysen G, et al: Placebo-controlled, randomized trial of warfarin and aspirin for prevention of thromboembolic complications in chronic atrial fibrillation: The Copenhagen AFASAK study. Lancet 1989;1:175-179.

85. Stroke Prevention in Atrial Fibrillation Investigators: The stroke prevention in atrial fibrillation study: Final results. Circulation 1991;84:527-539.

86. Stroke Prevention in Atrial Fibrillation Investigators: Warfarin versus aspirin for prevention of thromboembolism in atrial fibrillation: Stroke Prevention in Atrial Fibrillation II study. Lancet 1994;343:687-691.

87. Stroke Prevention in Atrial Fibrillation Investigators: Adjusted-dose warfarin versus low-intensity, fixed-dose warfarin plus aspirin for high-risk patients with atrial fibrillation: Stroke Prevention in Atrial Fibrillation III randomised clinical trial. Lancet 1996;348:633-638.

88. Stroke Prevention in Atrial Fibrillation Investigators: Prospective identification of patients with nonvalvular atrial fibrillation at low risk of stroke during treatment with aspirin: Stroke Prevention in Atrial Fibrillation III Study. Circulation 1997;96(suppl):1-281(abst).

89. Albers G: Atrial fibrillation and stroke. Three new studies, three remaining questions. Arch Intern Med 1994;154:1443-1448.

89a. Rash A, Downes T, Portner R, et al: A randomized controlled trial of warfarin vs aspirin for stroke prevention in octogenarians with atrial fibrillation (WASPO). Age Ageing 2007;36:151-156.

89b. Mant J, Hobbs FD, Fletcher K, et al: Warfarin versus aspirin for stroke prevention in an elderly community population with atrial fibrillation (the Birmingham Atrial Fibrillation Treatment of the Aged study, BAFTA): A randomized controlled trial. Lancet 2007;370:493-503.

90. Olsson SB: Executive Steering Committee on Behalf of SPORTIF III Investigators. Stroke prevention with the oral direct thrombin inhibitor ximelagatran compared with warfarin in patients with non-valvular atrial fibrillation (SPORTIF III): Randomized controlled trial. Lancet 2003;362:1691-1698.

91. Albers GW, Diener HC, Frison L, et al: SPORTIF Executive Steering Committee for the SPORTIF V Investigators. Ximelagatran vs warfarin for stroke prevention in patients with nonvalvular atrial fibrillation: A randomized trial. JAMA 2005;293:690-698.

91a. Ford GA, Choy AM, Deedwania P, et al: Direct thrombin inhibition and stroke prevention in elderly patients with atrial fibrillation. Experience from the SPORTIF III and V trials. Stroke 2007;38:2965-2971.

92. Sherman DG: Stroke prevention in atrial fibrillation. Pharmacological rate vs rhythm control. Stroke 2007;38(part 2):615-617.

93. Gillinov AM: Advances in surgical treatment of atrial fibrillation. Stroke 2007;38(part 2):618-623.

94. Onalan O, Crystal E: Left atrial appendage exclusion for stroke prevention in patients with nonrheumatic atrial fibrillation. Stroke 2007;38 (part 2):624-630.

94a. Syed TM, Halperin JL: Left atrial appendage closure for stroke prevention in atrial fibrillation: State of the art and current challenges. Nat Clin Pract Neurol 2007;4:428-435.

95. Rubenstein JJ, Schulman CL, Yurchak PM, et al: Clinical spectrum of the sick sinus syndrome. Circulation 1972;46:5-13.

96. Fairfax AJ, Lambert CD, Leatham A: Systemic embolism in chronic sinoatrial disorder. N Engl J Med 1976;295:190-192.

97. Lown B: Electrical reversion of cardiac arrythmias. Br Heart J 1967;29:469-489.

98. Orencia AJ, Hammill SC, Whisnant JP: Sinus node dysfunction and ischemic stroke. Heart Dis Stroke 1994;3:91-94.

99. Phillips SJ, Whisnant JP, O'Fallon WM, Frye RL: Prevalence of cardiovascular disease and diabetes mellitus in residents of Rochester, Minnesota. Mayo Clin Proc 1990;65:344-359.

100. Radford DJ, Julian DG: Sick sinus syndrome. Experience of a cardiac pacemaker clinic. BMJ 1974;3:504-507.

101. Rosenqvist M, Vallin H, Edhag O: Clinical and electrophysiologic course of sinus node disease: Five-year follow-up study. Am Heart J 1985;109: 513-522.

102. Bathen J, Sparr S, Rokseth R: Embolism in sinoatrial disease. Acta Med Scand 1978;203:7-11.

103. Cerebral embolism task force: Cardiogenic brain embolism. Arch Neurol 1986;43:71-84.

104. Stein PD, Sabbah HN, Pitha JV: Continuing disease process of calcific aortic stenosis. Am J Cardiol 1977;39:159-163.

105. Casella L, Abelmann WH, Ellis LB: Patients with mitral stenosis and systemic emboli. Arch Intern Med 1964;114:773-781.

106. Weiss S, Davis D: Rheumatic heart disease: III. Embolic manifestations. Am Heart J 1933;9:45-52.

107. Wallach JB, Lukash L, Angrist AA: An interpretation of the incidence of mitral thrombi in the left auricle and appendage with particular reference to mitral commissurotomy. Am Heart J 1953;45:252-254.

108. Bannister RB: Risk of deferring valvotomy in patients with moderate mitral stenosis. Lancet 1960;2:329-332.

109. Szekely P: Systemic embolism and anticoagulant prophylaxis in rheumatic heart disease. BMJ 1964;1:1209-1212.

110. Keen G, Leveaux VM: Prognosis of cerebral embolism in rheumatic heart disease. BMJ 1958;2:91-92.

111. Coulshed N, Epstein EJ, McKendrick CS, et al: Systemic embolism in mitral valve disease. BMJ 1970;32:26-34.

112. Daley R, Mattingly TW, Holt CL, et al: Systemic arterial embolism in rheumatic heart disease. Am Heart J 1951;42:566-581.

113. Fleming HA, Bailey SM: Mitral valve disease, systemic embolism and anticoagulants. Postgrad Med J 1971;47:599-604.

114. Carabello BA, Crawford FA: Valvular heart disease. N Engl J Med 1997;337:32-41.

115. Soulie P, Caramanian M, Soulie J, et al: Les embolies calcaires des atteintes orificielles calcifees du coeur gauche. Arch Mal Coeur Vaiss 1969;12:1657-1684.

116. Holley KE, Bahn RC, McGoon DC, Mankin HT: Spontaneous calcific embolization associated with calcific aortic stenosis. Circulation 1963;27:197-202.

117. Klues HG, Maron BJ, Dollar AL, Roberts WC: Diversity of structural mitral valve alterations in hypertrophic cardiomyopathy. Circulation 1992;85:1651-1660.

118. Hardarson T, De la Calzada CS, Curiel R, Goodwin JF: Prognosis and mortality of hypertrophic obstructive cardiomyopathy. Lancet 1973;1462-1467.

119. Glancy DL, O'Brien KP, Gold HK, Epstein SE: Atrial fibrillation in patients with idiopathic hypertrophic subaortic stenosis. Br Heart J 1970;32:652-659.

120. Tajik AJ, Giuliani ER, Frye RL, et al: Mitral valve and/or annulus calcification associated with hypertrophic subaortic stenosis (IHSS). Circulation 1972;16(suppl II):228.

121. Barlow JB, Bosman CK: Aneurysmal protrusion of posterior leaflets of the mitral valve. An auscultatory-electrocardiographic syndrome. Am Heart J 1966;71:166-178.

122. Lauzier S, Barnett HJM: Cerebral ischemia with mitral valve prolapse and mitral annular calcification. In Furlan AJ (ed): The Heart and Stroke: Exploring Mutual Cerebrovascular and Cardiovascular Issues. London: Springer, 1987, pp 63-100.

123. Markiewicz W, Stoner J, London E, et al: Mitral valve prolapse in one hundred presumably healthy young females. Circulation 1976;53:464-473.

124. Cheitlin MD, Byrd RC: Prolapsed mitral valve: The commonest valve disease? Curr Probl Cardiol 1984;8:3-53.

125. Ranganatham N, Silver MD, Robinson T, et al: Angiographic-morphological correlation in patients with severe mitral regurgitation due to prolapse of the posterior mitral valve leaflet. Circulation 1973;48:514-518.

126. Kostuk WJ, Boughner DR, Barnett HJM, Silver MD: Strokes: A complication of mitral-leaflet prolapse? Lancet 1977;2:313-316.

127. Marks AR, Choong CY, Sanfilippo AJ, et al: Identification of high-risk and low-risk subgroups of patients with mitral-valve prolapse. N Engl J Med 1989;320:1031-1036.

128. Nishimura RA, McGoon MD, Shub C, et al: Echocardiographically documented mitral-valve prolapse: Long-term follow-up of 237 patients. N Engl J Med 1985;313:1305-1309.

129. Barnett HJM: Transient cerebral ischemia: Pathogenesis, prognosis, and management. Ann R Coll Phys Surg Can 1974;7:153-173.

130. Barnett HJM, Jones MW, Boughner DR, Kostuk WJ: Cerebral ischemic events associated with prolapsing mitral valve. Arch Neurol 1976;33:777-782.

131. Barnett HJM, Boughner DR, Taylor DW, et al: Further evidence relating mitral-valve prolapse to cerebral ischemic events. N Engl J Med 1980;302:139-144.

132. Aronow WS, Koenigsberg M, Kronzon I, Gutstein H: Association of mitral annular calcium with new thromboembolic stroke and cardiac events at 39-month follow-up in elderly patients. Am J Cardiol 1990;65:1511-1512.

133. Benjamin EJ, Plehn JF, D'Agostino RB, et al: Mitral annular calcification and the risk of stroke in an elderly cohort. N Engl J Med 1992;327:374-379.

134. Korn D, DeSanctis R, Sell S: Massive calcification of the mitral valve, a clinicopathological study of fourteen cases. N Engl J Med 1962;267:900-909.

135. DeBono D, Warlow C: Mitral annulus calcification and cerebral or retinal ischemia. Lancet 1979;2: 383-385.

136. Benjamin EJ, Plehn JF, D'Agostino RB, et al: Mitral annular calcification and the risk of stroke in an elderly cohort. N Engl J Med 1992;327:374-379.

137. Kizer J, Wiebers DO, Whisnant JP, et al: Mitral annular calcification, aortic valve sclerosis, and

incident stroke in adults free of clinical cardio-vascular disease. The Strong Heart Study. Stroke 2005;36:2533-2537.

138. Pomerance A: Pathological and clinical study of calcification of the mitral valve ring. J Clin Pathol 1970;23:354-361.

139. Stein JH, Soble JS: Thrombus associated with mitral valve calcification. A possible mechanism for embolic stroke. Stroke 1995;26:1697-1699.

140. Barnett HJM: Stroke by cause. Some common, some exotic, some controversial. Stroke 2005;36:2523-2525.

141. Adler Y, Shohat-Zabarski R, Vaturi M, et al: Association between mitral annular calcium and aortic atheroma as detected by transesophageal echocardiographic study. Am J Cardiol 1998;81:784-786.

142. Vongpatanasin W, Hillis D, Lange RA: Prosthetic heart valves. N Engl J Med 1996;335:407-416.

143. Edmunds Jr LH. Thromboembolic complications of current cardiac valvular prostheses. Ann Thorac Surg 1982;34:96-106.

144. Metzdorff MT, Grunkemeier GL, Pinson CW, Starr A: Thrombosis of mechanical cardiac valves: A qualitative comparison of the silastic ball valve and the tilting disc valve. J Am Coll Cardiol 1984;4:50-53.

145. Harker LA, Slichter SL: Studies of platelet and fibrinogen kinetics in patients with prosthetic heart valves. N Engl J Med 1970;283:1302-1305.

146. Silber H, Khan SS, Matloff JM, et al: The St Jude valve: Thrombolysis as the first line of therapy for cardiac valve thrombosis. Circulation 1993;87:30-37.

147. Vitale N, Renzulli A, Cerasuolo F, et al: Prosthetic valve obstruction: Thrombolysis versus operation. Ann Thorac Surg 1994;57:365-370.

148. Cannegieter SC, Rosendaal FR, Briet E: Thromboembolic and bleeding complications in patients with mechanical heart valve prostheses. Circulation 1994;89:635-641.

149. Cohn LH, Mudge GH, Pratter F, Collins Jr JJ: Five- to eight-year follow-up of patients undergoing porcine heart-valve replacement. N Engl J Med 1981;304:258-262.

150. Osler W: Gulstonian lectures on malignant endocarditis. Lancet 1885;1:459-465.

151. Jones HR, Siekert RG, Geraci J: Neurologic manifestations of bacterial endocarditis. Ann Intern Med 1969;71:21-28.

152. Salgado AV, Furlan AJ, Keys TF, et al: Neurologic complications of endocarditis: A 12-year experience. Neurology 1989;39:173-178.

153. Hart RG, Foster JW, Luther MF, Kanter MC: Stroke in infective endocarditis. Stroke 1990;21:695-700.

154. Kanter MC, Hart RG: Neurologic complications of infective endocarditis. Neurology 1991;41:1015-1020.

155. Keyser DL, Biller J, Coffman TT, Adams HP: Neurologic complications of late prosthetic valve endocarditis. Stroke 1990;21:472-475.

156. Matsushita K, Kuriyama Y, Sawada T, et al: Hemorrhagic and ischemic cerebrovascular complications of active infective endocarditis of native valve. Eur Neurol 1993;33:267-274.

157. Pruitt AA, Rubin RH, Karchmer AW, Duncan GW: Neurological complications of bacterial endocarditis. Medicine 1978;57:329-343.

158. Steckelberg JM, Murphy JG, Ballard D, et al: Emboli in infective endocarditis: The prognostic value of echocardiography. Ann Intern Med 1991;114:635-640.

159. Tunkel AR, Mandell GL: Infecting microorganisms. In Kay D (ed): Infective Endocarditis, 2nd ed. New York; Raven Press, 1992:85-97.

160. Garvey GJ, Neu HC: Infective endocarditis—an evolving disease. A review of endocarditis at the Columbia-Presbyterian Medical Center, 1968-1973. Medicine 1978;57:105-127.

161. Jaffe WM, Morgan DE, Pearlman AS, Otto CM: Infective endocarditis, 1983-1988: Echocardiographic findings and factors influencing morbidity and mortality. J Am Coll Cardol 1990:15:1227-1233.

162. Rohmann S, Erbel R, Gorge G, et al: Clinical relevance of vegetation localization by transesophageal echocardiography in infective endocarditis. Eur Heart J 1992;12:446-452.

163. Shively BK, Gurule FT, Roldan CA, et al: Diagnostic value of transesophageal compared with transthoracic echocardiography in infective endocarditis. J Am Coll Cardiol 1991;18:391-397.

164. Sanfilippo AJ, Picard MH, Newell JB, et al: Echocardiographic assessment of patients with infectious endocarditis: Prediction of risk for complications. J Am Coll Cardiol 1991;18:1191-1199.

165. Hart RG, Kagan-Hallet K, Joerns S: Mechanisms of intracranial hemorrhage in infective endocarditis. Stroke 1987;18:1048-1056.

166. Masuda J, Yutani C, Waki R, et al: Histopathological analysis of the mechanisms of intracranial hemorrhage complicating infective endocarditis. Stroke 1992;23:843-850.

166a. Klein I, Iung B, Wolff M, et al: Silent T2* cerebral microbleeds. A potential new imaging clue in infective endocarditis. Neurology 2007;68:2043.

166b. Nandigam K: Silent T2* cerebral microbleeds: A potential new imaging clue in infective endocarditis. Neurology 2008;70:323-324.

167. Morawetz RB, Karp RB: Evolution and resolution of intracranial bacterial (mycotic) aneurysms. Neurosurgery 1984;15:43-49.

168. Moskowitz MA, Rosenbaum AE, Tyler HR: Angiographically monitored resolution of cerebral mycotic aneurysms. Neurology 1974;24:1103-1108.

169. Bingham WF: Treatment of mycotic intracranial aneurysms. J Neurosurg 1977;46:428-437.

170. Bertorini TE, Laster RE, Thompson BF, Gelfand M: Magnetic resonance imaging of the brain in bacterial endocarditis. Arch Intern Med 1989;149:815-817.

171. Libman E, Sacks B: A hitherto undescribed form of valvular and mural endocarditis. Arch Intern Med 1924;33:701-737.

172. Klemperer P, Pollack AD, Baehr G: Pathology of disseminated lupus erythematosis. Arch Pathol 1941;32:569-631.

173. Baehr G, Klemperer P, Schifrin A: A diffuse disease of the peripheral circulation usually associated with lupus erythematosis and endocarditis. Trans Assoc Am Physicians 1935;50:139-155.

174. Gross L: The cardiac lesions in Libman-Sacks disease, with a consideration of its relationship to acute diffuse lupus erythematosis. Am J Pathol 1940;16:375-407.

175. Roldan CA, Shively B, Crawford MH: An echo-cardiographic study of valvular heart disease associated with systemic lupus erythematosus. N Engl J Med 1996;335:1424-1430.

175a. Moyssakis I, Tektonidou MG, Vassilios V, et al: Libman-Sacks endocarditis in systemic lupus erythematosis: Prevalence, associations, and evolution. Am J Med 2007;120:636-642.

176. Barbut D, Borer J, Gharavi A, et al: Prevalence of anticardiolipin antibody in isolated mitral or aortic regurgitation, or both, and possible relation to cerebral ischemic events. Am J Cardiol 1992;70:901-905.

177. Barbut D, Borer J, Wallerson D, et al: Anticardiolipin antibody and stroke: Possible relation of valvular heart disease and embolic events. Cardiology 1991;79:99-109.

178. The Antiphospholipid Antibodies in Stroke Study Group: Clinical and laboratory findings in patients with antiphospholipid antibodies and cerebral ischemia. Stroke 1990;21:1268-1273.

179. Amico L, Caplan LR, Thomas C: Cerebrovascular complications of mucinous cancer. Neurology 1989;39:522-526.

180. Reagan TJ, Okazaki H: The thrombotic syndrome associated with carcinoma. Arch Neurol 1974;31:390-395.

181. Edoute Y, Haim N, Rinkevich D, et al: Cardiac valvular vegetations in cancer patients: A prospective echocardiographic study of 200 patients. Am J Med 1997;102:252-258.

182. Connolly HM, Crary JL, McGoon MD, et al: Valvular heart disease associated with Fenflurmine-phentermine. N Engl J Med 1997;337:581-588.

183. Yamamoto M, Uesugi T, Nakayama T: Dopamine agonists and cardiac valvulopathy in Parkinson's disease: A case control study. Neurology 2006;67:1225-1229.

184. Lambl VA: Papillare exkreszenzen an der semilunar-klappe der aorta. Wien Med Wochenscshr 1856;6:244-247.

185. Magarey FR: On the mode of formation of Lambl's excrescences and their relation to chronic thickening of the mitral valve. J Pathol Bacteriol 1949;61:203-208.

186. Roldan CA, Shively BK, Crawford MH: Valve excrescences: Prevalence, evolution and risk for embolism. J Am Coll Cardiol 1997;30:1308-1314.

187. Freedberg RS, Goodkin GM, Perez JL, et al: Valve strands are strongly associated with systemic embolization: A transesophageal echocardiographic study. J Am Coll Cardiol 1995;26:1709-1712.

188. Roberts JK, Omarali I, Di Tullio MR, et al: Valvular strands and cerebral ischemia. Effect of demographics and strand characteristics. Stroke 1997;28:2185-2188.

189. Cohen A, Tzourio C, Chauvel C, et al: Mitral valve strands and the risk of ischemic stroke in elderly patients. Stroke 1997;28:1574-1578.

190. Lee RJ, Bartzokis T, Yeoh TK, et al: Enhanced detection of intracardiac sources of cerebral emboli by transesophageal echocardiography. Stroke 1991;22:734-739.

191. Nighoghossian N, Derex L, Loire R, et al: Giant Lambl excrescences. An ususual source of cerebral embolism. Arch Neurol 1997;54:41-44.

192. Vaitkus PT, Berlin JA, Schwartz JS, Barnathan ES: Stroke complicating acute myocardial infarction: A meta-analysis of risk modification by anticoagulation and thrombolytic therapy. Arch Intern Med 1992;152:2020-2024.

193. Konrad MS, Coffey CE, Coffey KS, et al: Myocardial infarction and stroke. Neurology 1984;34:1403-1409.

194. Chiarella F, Santoro E, Domenicucci S, et al: Predischarge two-dimensional echocardiographic evaluation of left ventricular thrombosis after acute myocardial infarction in the GISSI-3 study. Am J Cardiol 1998;81:822-827.

195. Meltzer RS, Visser CA, Fuster V: Intracardiac thrombi and systemic embolization. Ann Intern Med 1986;104:689-698.

196. Visser CA, Kan G, Meltzer RS, et al: Embolic potential of left ventricular thrombi after myocardial infarction: A two-dimensional echocardiographic study of 119 patients. J Am Coll Cardiol 1985;5:1276-1280.

197. Kouvaras G, Chronopoulas G, Soufras G, et al: The effects of long-term antithrombotic treatment on left ventricular thrombi in patients after an acute myocardial infarction. Am Heart J 1990;119:73-78.

198. Asinger RW, Mikell FL, Elsperger J, Hodges M: Incidence of left-ventricular thrombosis after acute transmural myocardial infarction. Serial evaluation by two-dimensional echocardiography. N Engl J Med 1981;305:297-302.

199. Nihoyannopoulos P, Smith GC, Maseri A, Foale RA: The natural history of left ventricular thrombus in myocardial infarction: A rationale in support of masterly inactivity. J Am Coll Cardiol 1989;14:903-911.

200. Greaves SC, Zhi G, Lee RT, et al: Incidence and natural history of left ventricular thrombus following anterior wall acute myocardial infarction. Am J Cardiol 1997;80:442-448.

201. Keren A, Goldberg S, Gottlieb S, et al: Natural history of left ventricular thrombi: Their appearance and resolution in the posthospitalization period of acute myocardial infarction. J Am Coll Cardiol 1990;15:790-800.

202. Domenicucci S, Chiarella F, Bellotti P, et al: Long-term prospective assessment of left ventricular thrombus in anterior wall acute myocardial infarction and implications for a rational approach to embolic risk. Am J Cardiol 1999;83:519-524.

203. Lapeyre AC III, Steele PM, Kazmier FJ, et al: Systemic embolism in chronic left ventricular aneurysm: Incidence and the role of anticoagulation. J Am Coll Cardiol 1985;6:534-538.

204. Anticoagulants in acute myocardial infarction: Results of a cooperative clinical trial. JAMA 1973;225:724-729.

205. Faxon DP, Ryan TJ, Davis KB, et al: Prognostic significance of angiographically documented left ventricular aneurysm from the coronary artery surgery study (CASS). Am J Cardiol 1982;50:157-164.

206. Reeder GS, Lengyei M, Tajik AJ, et al: Mural thrombus in left ventricular aneurysm. Incidence, role of angiography, and relation between anticoagulation and embolism. Mayo Clin Proc 1981;56:77-81.

207. Loh E, Sutton M, Wun C-C, et al: Ventricular dysfunction and the risk of stroke after myocardial infarction. N Engl J Med 1997;336: 251-257.

208. Stratton JR, Lighty GW, Pearlman AS, Ritchie JL: Detection of left ventricular thrombus by two-dimensional echocardiography: Sensitivity, specificity, and causes of uncertainty. Circulation 1982;66:156-166.

209. Ports TA, Cogan J, Schiller NB, Rapaport E: Echocardiography of left ventricular masses. Circulation 1978;58:528-536.

210. Chen C, Koschyk D, Hamm C, et al: Usefulness of transesophageal echocardiography in identifying small left ventricular apical thrombus. J Am Coll Cardiol 1993;21:208-215.

211. Oppenheimer SM, Lima J: Neurology and the heart. J Neurol Neurosurg Psychiatry 1998;64: 289-297.

211a. Wong C, Marwick TH: Obesity cardiomyopathy: Diagnosis and therapeutic implications. Nat Clin Pract Cardiovasc Med 2007;4:480-489.

211b. Grabowski A, Kilian J, Strank C, et al: Takotsubo cardiomyopathy—A rare cause of cardioembolic stroke. Cerebrovasc Dis 2007;24:146-148.

211c. Ziegelstein RC: Acute emotional stress and cardiac arrythmias. JAMA 2007;298:324-329.

212. Wold LE, Lie JT: Cardiac myxomas: A clinico-pathologic profile. Am J Pathol 1980;101: 219-240.

213. Reynen K: Cardiac myxomas. N Engl J Med 1995;333:1610-1617.

214. Blondeau P: Primary cardiac tumors: French study of 533 cases. Thorac Cardiovasc Surg 1990;38(suppl 2):192-195.

214a. Lee VH, Connolly HM, Brown Jr RD: Central nervous system manifestations of cardiac myxoma. Arch Neurol 2007;64:1115-1120.

215. Sandok BA, von Estorff I, Giuliani ER: Subsequent neurological events in patients with atrial myxoma. Ann Neurol 1980;8:305-307.

216. Edwards FH, Hale D, Cohen A, et al: Primary cardiac valve tumors. Ann Thorac Surg 1991;52:1127-1131.

217. Giannesini C, Kubis N, N'Guyen A, et al: Cardiac papillary fibroelastoma: A rare cause of ischemic stroke in the young. Cerebrovasc Dis 1999;9:45-49.

218. Brown RD, Khandheria BK, Edwards WD: Cardiac papillary fibroelastoma: A treatable cause of transient ischemic attack and ischemic stroke detected by transesophageal echocardiography. Mayo Clin Proc 1995;70:863-868.

219. Klarich KW, Enriquez-Sarano M, Gura GM, et al: Papillary fibroelastoma: Echocardiographic characteristics for diagnosis and pathologic correlation. J Am Coll Cardiol 1997;30:784-790.

219a. Gagliardi R, Franken R, Protti G: Cardiac papillary fibroelastoma and stroke in a young man—etiology and treatment. Cerebrovasc Dis 2008;185-187.

220. Azarbal B, Tobis J: Interatrial communications, stroke, and migraine headache. Appl Neurol 2005;1:22-36.

221. Hagen PT, Scholz DG, Edwards WD: Incidence and size of patent foramen ovale during the first 10 decades of life: An autopsy study of 965 normal hearts. Mayo Clin Proc 1984;59:17-20.

222. Lechat PH, Mas JL, Lascault G, et al: Prevalence of patent foramen ovale in patients with stroke. N Engl J Med 1988;318:1148-1152.

223. Di Tullio M, Sacco RL, Gopal A, et al: Patent foramen ovale as a risk factor for cryptogenic stroke. Ann Intern Med 1992;117:461-465.

224. Petty GW, Khanderia BK, Chu C-P, et al: Patent foramen ovale in patients with cerebral infarction. A transesophageal echocardiographic study. Arch Neurol 1997;54:819-822.

225. Gautier JC, Durr A, Koussa S, et al: Paradoxical cerebral embolism with a patent foramen ovale. A report of 29 patients. Cerebrovasc Dis 1991; 1:193-202.

226. Venketasubramanian N, Sacco RL, Di Tullio M, et al: Vascular distribution of paradoxical emboli by transcranial Doppler. Neurology 1993;43:1533-1535.

227. Konstantinides S, Kasper W, Geibel A, et al: Detection of left-to-right shunt in atrial septal defect by negative contrast echocardiography: A comparison of transthoracic and transesophageal approach. Am Heart J 1993;126:909-917.

228. Hamann GF, Schatzer-Klotz D, Frohlig G, et al: Femoral injection of echo contrast medium may increase the sensitivity of testing for a patent foramen ovale. Neurology 1998;50:1423-1428.

229. Hausmann D, Mügge A, Daniel WG: Identification of patent foramen ovale permitting paradoxic embolism. J Am Coll Cardiol 1995;26:1030-1038.

230. Homma S, Tullio MR, Sacco RL, et al: Characteristics of patent foramen ovale associated with cryptogenic stroke: A biplane transesophageal echocardiographic study. Stroke 1994;25: 582-586.

231. Chimowitz MI, Nemec JJ, Marwick TH, et al: Transcranial Doppler ultrasound identifies patients with right-to-left cardiac or pulmonary shunts. Neurology 1991;41:1902-1904.

232. Albert A, Muller HR, Hetzel A: Optimized transcranial Doppler technique for the diagnosis of cardiac right-to-left shunts. J Neuroimaging 1997;7:159-163.

233. Di Tullio M, Sacco RL, Venketasubramanian N, et al: Comparison of diagnostic techniques for the detection of a patent foramen ovale in stroke patients. Stroke 1993;24:1020-1024.

234. Mohrs OK, Petersen SE, Erkapic D, et al: Diagnosis of patent foramen ovale using contrast-enhanced dynamic MRI: A pilot study. AJR Am J Roetgenol 2005;184:234-240.

235. Ilercil A, Meisner JS, Vijayaraman P, et al: Clinical significance of fossa ovalis membrane aneurysm in adults with cardioembolic cerebral ischemia. Am J Cardiol 1997;80:96-99.

236. Belkin RN, Hurwitz BJ, Kislo J: Atrial septal aneurysm: Association with cerebrovascular and peripheral embolic events. Stroke 1987;18:856-862.

237. Schneider B, Hanrath P, Vogel P, Meinertz T: Improved morphologic characterization of atrial septal aneurysm by transesophageal echocardiography: Relation to cerebrovascular events. J Am Coll Cardiol 1990;16:1000-1009.

238. Burger AJ, Sherman HB, Charlamb MJ: Low incidence of embolic strokes with atrial septal aneurysms: A prospective, long-term study. Am Heart J 2000;139:149-152.

239. Agmon Y, Khandheria BK, Meissner I, et al: Frequency of atrial septal aneurysms in patients with cerebral ischemic events. Circulation 1999;99:1942-1944.

240. Zabalgoitia-Reyes M, Herrera C, Gandhi DK, et al: A possible mechanism for neurologic ischemic events in patients with atrial septal aneurysm. Am J Cardiol 1990;66:761-764.

241. Berthet K, Lavergne T, Cohen A, et al: Significant association of atrial vulnerability with atrial septal abnormalities in young patients with ischemic stroke of unknown cause. Stroke 2000;31:398-403.

242. Silver MD, Dorsey JS: Aneurysms of the septum primum in adults. Arch Pathol Lab Med 1978;102:62-65.

243. Cabanes L, Mas JL, Cohen A, et al: Atrial septal aneurysm and patent foramen ovale as risk factors for cryptogenic stroke in patients less than 55 years of age. A study using transesophageal echocardiography. Stroke 1993;24:1865-1873.

244. Hanna JP, Sun JP, Furlan AJ, et al: Patent foramen ovale and brain infarct. Echocardiographic predictors, recurrence, and prevention. Stroke 1994;25:782-786.

245. Ay H, Buonanno FS, Abraham S, et al: An electrocardiographic criterion for diagnosis of patent foramen ovale associated with ischemic stroke. Stroke 1998;29:1393-1397.

246. Bogousslavsky J, Garazi S, Jeanrenaud X, et al: Stroke recurrence in patients with patent foramen ovale: The Lausanne study. Neurology 1996;46:1301-1305.

247. French Study Group on Patent Foramen Ovale and Atrial Septal Aneurysm: Recurrent cerebrovascular events in patients with patent foramen ovale or atrial septal aneurysms and cryptogenic stroke or TIA. Am Heart J 1995;130:1083-1088.

248. Devuyst G, Bogousslavsky J, Ruchat P, et al: Prognosis after stroke followed by surgical closure of patent foramen ovale: A prospective follow-up study with brain MRI and simultaneous transesophageal and transcranial Doppler ultrasound. Neurology 1996;47:1162-1166.

249. Kim D, Saver JL: Patent foramen ovale and stroke: What we do and don't know. Rev Neurol Dis 2005;2:1-7.

250. Bridges ND, Hellensbrand W, Catson L, et al: Transcatheter closure of patent foramen ovale after presumed paradoxical embolism. Circulation 1992;86:1902-1908.

250a. Furlan AJ: Patent foramen ovale and stroke: To close or not to close? Cleveland Clin J Med 2007;74(suppl 1) S118-S120.

251. Bogousslavsky J, Cachin C, Regli F, et al: Cardiac sources of embolism and cerebral infarction. Clinical consequences and vascular concomitants. Neurology 1991;41:855-859.

252. Tunick PA, Kronzon I: Protruding atherosclerotic plaque in the aortic arch of patients with systemic embolization: A new finding seen by transesophageal echocardiography. Am Heart J 1990;120:658-660.

253. Tunick PA, Culliford AT, Lamparello PJ, Kronzon I: Atheromatosis of the aortic arch as an occult source of multiple systemic emboli. Ann Intern Med 1991;114:391-392.

254. Tunick PA, Perez JL, Kronzon I: Protruding atheromas in the thoracic aorta and systemic embolization. Ann Intern Med 1991;115:423-427.

255. Amarenco P, Duyckaerts C, Tzourio C, et al: The prevalence of ulcerated plaques in the aortic arch in patients with stroke. N Engl J Med 1992;326:221-225.

256. Amarenco P, Cohen A, Baudrimont M, Bousser M-G: Transesophageal echocardiographic detection of aortic arch disease in patients with cerebral infarction. Stroke 1992;23:1005-1009.

257. Tobler HG, Edwards JE: Frequency and location of atherosclerotic plaques in the ascending aorta. J Thorac Cardiovasc Surg 1988;96:304-306.

258. Bruns JL, Segel DP, Adler S: Control of cholesterol embolization by discontinuation of anticoagulant therapy. Am J Med Sci 1978;275:
105-108.

259. French Study of Aortic Plaques in Stroke
Group: Atherosclerotic disease of the aortic
arch as a risk factor for recurrent ischemic
stroke. N Engl J Med 1996;334:1216-1221.

260. Mitusch R, Doherty C, Wucherpfennig H, et al:
Vascular events during follow-up in patients
with aortic arch atherosclerosis. Stroke
1997;28:36-39.

261. Amarenco P, Cohen A: Update on imaging
aortic atherosclerosis. In Barnett HJM,
Bogousslavsky J, Meldrum H (eds): Advances
in Neurology, vol 82, Ischemic Stroke.
Philadelphia: Lippincott Williams & Wilkins,
2003, pp 75-89.

262. Vaduganathan V, Ewton A, Nagueh SF, et al:
Pathologic correlates of aortic plaques, thrombi
and mobile "aortic debris" imaged in vivo with
transesophageal echocardiography. J Am Coll
Cardiol 1997;30:357-363.

263. Weinberger J, Azhar S, Danisi F, et al: A new
noninvasive technique for imaging atherosclerotic plaque in the aortic arch of stroke
patients by transcutaneous real-time B-mode
ultrasonography. Stroke 1998;29:673-676.

264. Schwammenthal A, Schwammenthal Y, Tanne
D, et al: Transcutaneous detection of aortic
arch atheromas by suprasternal harmonic
imaging. J Am Coll Cardiol 2002;39:1127-1132.

265. Kutz SM, Lee VS, Tunick PA, et al: Atheromas
of the thoracic aorta: A comparison of transesophageal echocardiography and breath-hold
gadolinium enhanced 3-dimensional magnetic
resonance angiography. J Am Soc Echocardiogr
1999;12:853-858.

266. Barkhausen J, Ebert W, Heyer C, et al: Detection
of atherosclerotic plaque with gadofluorine-
enhanced magnetic resonance imaging.
Circulation 2003;108:605-609.

266a. Harloff A, Dudler P, Frydrychowicz A: Reliability of aortic MRI at 3 Tesla in patients with
acute cryptogenic stroke. J Neurol Neurosurg
Psychiatry 2007;79:540-549.

267. Blackshear JL, Jahangir A, Oldenberg WA,
Safford RE: Digital embolization from plaque-
related thrombus in the thoracic aorta: Identification with transesophageal echocardiography
and resolution with warfarin therapy. Mayo
Clin Proc 1993;68:268-272.

268. Freedberg RS, Tunick PA, Culliform AT, et al:
Disappearance of a large intraaortic mass in a
patient with prior systemic embolization. Am
Heart J 1993;125:1445-1447.

269. Fine MJ, Kapoor W, Falanga V: Cholesterol crystal embolization: A review of 221 cases in the
English literature. Angiology 1987;38:769-784.

270. Hausmann D, Gulba D, Bargheer K, et al: Successful thrombolysis of an aortic-arch thrombus in a patient after mesenteric embolism. N
Engl J Med 1992;327:500-501.

271. Belden JR, Caplan LR, Bojar RM, et al:
Treatment of multiple cerebral emboli from an
ulcerated, thrombogenic ascending aorta with
aortectomy and graft replacement. Neurology
1997;49:621-622.

272. Slogoff S, Girgis KZ, Keats AS: Etiologic factors
in neuropsychiatric complications associated
with cardiopulmonary bypass. Anesth Analg
1982;61:903-911.

273. Gilman S: Neurological complications of
open heart surgery. Ann Neurol 1990;28:
475-476.

274. Shaw PJ, Bates D, Cartledge NEF: Early neurological complications of coronary artery bypass
surgery. BMJ 1985;391:1384-1387.

275. Breuer AC, Furlan AJ, Hanson MR, et al: Central
nervous system complications of coronary artery
bypass graft surgery: Prospective analysis of
421 patients. Stroke 1983;14:682-687.

276. Coffey CE, Massey EW, Roberts KB, et al: Natural history of cerebral complication of coronary
artery bypass graft surgery. Neurology
1983;33:1416-1421.

277. Feeney DM, Gonzalez A, Law WA: Amphetamine,
haloperidol and experience interact to affect the
rate of recovery after motor cortex injury. Science
1982;217:855-857.

278. Houda DA, Feeney DM: Haloperidol blocks
amphetamine induced recovery of binocular
depth perception of the bilateral visual cortex
abilities in the cat. Proc West Pharmacol Soc
1985;28:209-211.

279. Sila C: Neuroimaging of cerebral infarction
associated with coronary revascularization.
AJNR Am J Neuroradiol 1991;12:817-818.

280. Moody DM, Bell MA, Challa VR, et al: Brain microemboli during cardiac surgery or aortography.
Ann Neurol 1990;28:477-486.

281. Pugsley W, Klinger L, Paschalis C, et al: The
impact of microemboli during cardiopulmonary
bypass on neuropsychological functioning.
Stroke 1994;25:1393-1399.

282. Barbut D, Caplan LR: Brain complications of cardiac surgery. Curr Probl Cardiol 1997;22:445-476.

283. Barbut D, Lo Y, Gold JP, et al: Impact of embolization during coronary artery bypass grafting on
outcome and length of stay. Ann Thorac Surg
1997;63:998-1002.

284. Clark RE, Brillman J, Davis DA, et al: Microemboli
during coronary artery bypass grafting: genesis
and effect on outcome. J Thorac Cardiovasc Surg
1995;25:1393-1399.

285. Tufo HM, Ostfeld AM, Shekelle R: Central
nervous system dysfunction following open-
heart surgery. JAMA 1970;212:1333-1340.

286. Stockard JJ, Bickford RG, Schauble JF: Pressure-
dependent cerebral ischemia during cardiopulmonary bypass. Neurology 1973;23:521-529.

287. Gold JP, Charlson ME, Williams-Russo P, et al:
Improvement of outcomes after coronary artery
bypass: A randomized trial comparing intraoperative high vs low mean arterial pressure. J
Thorac Cardiovasc Surg 1995;110:1302-1314.

287a. Gottesmann RF, Hillis AE, Grega MA, et al: Early postoperative cognitive dysfunction and blood pressure during coronary artery bypass graft operation. Arch Neurol 2007;64:1111-1114.

288. Wolman RL, Kanchuger MS, Newman MF, et al: Adverse neurological outcome following cardiac surgery. Anesth Analg 1994;78 (suppl):S484.

289. Dubinsky RM, Lai SM: Mortality from combined carotid endarterectomy and coronary artery bypass surgery in the US. Neurology 2007;68:195-197.

290. Breslau PJ, Fell G, Ivey TD, et al: Carotid arterial disease in patients undergoing coronary artery bypass operations. J Thorac Cardiovasc Surg 1981;82:765-767.

291. Turnipseed WD, Berkhoff HA, Belzer FO: Postoperative stroke in cardiac and peripheral vascular disease. Ann Surg 1980;192:365-368.

292. Chimowitz M: Neurological complications of cardiac surgery. In Caplan LR, Hurtst JW, Chimowitz M (eds): Clinical Neurocardiology. New York: Marcel Dekker, 1999, pp 226-257.

293. Furlan A, Craciun A: Risk of stroke during coronary artery bypass graft surgery in patients with internal carotid artery disease documented by angiography. Stroke 1985;16:797-799.

294. Von Reutern G, Hetzel A, Birnbaum D, et al: Transcranial Doppler ultrasound during cardiopulmonary bypass in patients with internal carotid artery disease documented by angiography. Stroke 1988;19:674-680.

295. Hise JH, Nipper MN, Schnitker JC: Stroke associated with coronary artery bypass surgery. AJNR Am J Neuroradiol 1991;12:811-814.

296. Barbut D, Gold JP: Aortic atheromatosis and risks of cerebral embolization. J Cardiothorac Vasc Anesth 1996;10:24-30.

297. Blauth CI, Cosgrove DM, Webb BW, et al: Atheroembolism from the ascending aorta. An emerging problem in cardiac surgery. J Thorac Cardiovasc Surg 1992;103:1104-1112.

298. Masuda J, Yutani C, Ogata J, et al: Atheromatous embolism to the brain: A clinicopathologic analysis of 15 autopsy cases. Neurology 1994;44:1231-1237.

299. Katz ES, Tunick PA, Rusinek H, et al: Protruding aortic atheromas predict stroke in elderly patients undergoing cardiopulmonary bypass: Experience with intraoperative transesophageal echocardiography. J Am Coll Cardiol 1992;20:70-77.

300. Mills NL, Everson CT: Atherosclerosis of the ascending aorta and coronary artery bypass. Pathology, clinical correlates and operative management. J Thorac Cardiovasc Surg 1991;102:546-553.

301. Yao FSF, Barbut D, Hager DN, et al: Detection of aortic emboli by transesophageal echocardiography during coronary artery bypass surgery. J Cardiothorac Vasc Anesth 1996;10:314-317.

302. Gardner TJ, Horneffer PJ, Manolio TA, et al: Stroke following coronary artery bypass grafting: A ten-year study. Ann Thorac Surg 1985;40:574-581.

303. Warehag TH, Davila-Roman VG, Barzilai B, et al: Management of the severely atherosclerotic aorta during cardiac operations. J Thorac Cardiovasc Surg 1992;103:453-462.

304. Barbut D, Yao FS, Hager DN, et al: Comparison of transcranial Doppler ultrasonography and transesophageal echocardiography during coronary artery bypass surgery. Stroke 1996;27:87-90.

304a. Dittrich R, Ringelstein EB: Occurrence and clinical impact of microembolic signals during or after cardiosurgical procedures. Stroke 2008;39:503-511.

305. Marshall WG, Barzilai B, Kouchoukos NT, et al: Intraoperative ultrasonic imaging of the ascending aorta. Ann Thorac Surg 1989;48:339-344.

306. Borowicz I, Goldsborough M, Selnes O, McKann G: Neuropsychologic change after cardiac surgery. A critical review. J Cardiothorac Vasc Anesth 1996;10:105-111.

307. Barbut D, Hinton R, Szatrowski, et al: Cerebral emboli detected during bypass surgery are associated with clamp removal. Stroke 1994;25:2398-2402.

308. Hammon J, Stump D, Kon N, et al: Risk factors and solutions for the development of neurobehavioral changes after coronary artery bypass grafting. Ann Thorac Surg 1997;63:1613-1618.

308a. Hanson MR, Hamid MA, Tomsak RL, et al: Selective saccadic palsy caused by pontine lesions: Clinical, physiological, and pathological correlations. Ann Neurol 1986;20:209-217.

308b. Tomsak RL, Volpe BT, Stahl JS, Leigh RJ: Saccadic palsy after cardiac surgery: visual disability and rehabilitation. Ann NY Acad Sci 2002;956:430-433.

308c. Eggers SDZ, Moster ML, Cranmer K: Selective saccadic palsy after cardiac surgery. Neurology 2008;70:318-320.

308d. Solomon D, Ramat S, Tomsak RL, et al: Saccadic palsy after cardiac surgery: Characteristics and pathogenesis. Ann Neurol 2008;63:355-365.

309. van Dijk D, Spoor M, Hijman R, et al: Cognitive and cardiac outcomes 5 years after off-pump vs on-pump coronary artery bypass graft surgery. Octopus Study Group. JAMA 2007;297:701-708.

310. Duncan A, Rumbaugh C, Caplan LR: Cerebral embolic disease, a complication of carotid aneurysms. Radiology 1979;133:379-384.

311. Fisher M, Davidson R, Marcus E: Transient focal cortical ischemia as a presenting manifestation of unruptured cerebral aneurysms. Ann Neurol 1980;8:367-372.

312. Pessin MS, Chimowitz MI, Levine SR, et al: Stroke in patients with fusiform vertebrobasilar aneurysms. Neurology 1989;39:16-21.

313. Caplan LR, Stein R, Patel D, et al: Intraluminal clot of the carotid artery detected radiographically. Neurology 1984;34:1175-1181.

314. Perloff JK: The Clinical Recognition of Congenital Heart Disease. Philadelphia: WB Saunders, 1987.

315. Manning WJ, Weintraub, RM, Waksmonski, CA, et al: Accuracy of transesophageal echocardiography for identifying left atrial thrombi. A prospective, intraoperative study. Ann Intern Med 1995;123:817-822.

316. Fatkin D, Scalia G, Jacobs N, et al: Accuracy of biplane transesophageal echocardiography in detecting left atrial thrombus. Am J Cardiol 1996;77:321-323.

317. Pearson AC, Labovitz AJ, Tatineni S, Gomez CR: Superiority of transesophageal echocardiography in detecting cardiac source of embolism in patients with cerebral ischemia of uncertain etiology. J Am Coll Cardiol 1991;17:66-72.

318. DeRook FA, Comess KA, Albers GW, Popp RL: Transesophageal echocardiography in the evaluation of stroke. Ann Intern Med 1992;117:922-932.

319. Daniel WG, Mugge A: Transesophageal echocardiography. N Engl J Med 1995;332:1268-1279.

320. Horowitz DR, Tuhrim S, Weinberger J, et al: Transesophageal echocardiography: Diagnostic and clinical applications in the evaluation of the stroke patient. J Stroke Cerebrovasc Dis 1997;6:332-336.

321. Johnson LL, Pohost GM: Nuclear cardiology. In RC Schlant, RW Alexander (eds): Hurst's The Heart, 8th ed. New York: McGraw-Hill, 1994, pp 2281-2323.

322. Ezekowiz MD, Wilson DA, Smith EO, et al: Comparison of indium-111 platelet scintigraphy and two-dimensional echocardiography in the diagnosis of left ventricular thrombi. N Engl J Med 1982;306:1509-1513.

323. Caplan LR, Feinberg WM, Fisher MJ, del Zoppo GJ: The blood. In Caplan LR (ed): Brain Ischemia. Basic Concepts and Clinical Relevance. London: Springer, 1995, pp 83-126.

324. Caplan LR: Treatment of the acute embolic event. In Caplan LR, Manning W (eds): Brain Embolism. New York: Informa Healthcare, 2006, pp 277-288.

325. Furlan A, Higashida R, Wechsler L, et al: Intraarterial prourokinase for acute ischemic stroke. The PROACT II Study: A randomized controlled trial. Prolyse in acute cerebral thromboembolism. JAMA 1999;282: 2003-2011.

326. Fisher CM, Perlman A: The nonsudden onset of cerebral embolism. Neurology 1967;17: 1025-1032.

327. Melski J, Caplan LR, Mohr JP, et al: Modeling the diagnosis of stroke at two hospitals. MD Computing 1989;6:157-163.

328. Staroselskaya I, Chaves C, Silver B, et al: Relationship between magnetic resonance arterial patency and perfusion-diffusion mismatch in acute ischemic stroke and its potential clinical use. Arch Neurol 2001;58:1069-1074.

329. Derex L, Nighoghossian N, Hermier M, et al: Early detection of cerebral arterial occlusion on magnetic resonance angiography: Predictive value of the baseline NIHSS score and impact on neurological outcome. Cerebrovasc Dis 2002;13:225-229.

330. Parsons MW, Barber PA, Chalk J, et al: Diffusion- and perfusion-weighted response to thrombolysis in stroke. Ann Neurol 2002;51:28-37.

331. Albers DEFUSE Ann Neurol.

332. Pessin MS, del Zoppo GJ, Furlan AJ: Thrombolytic Treatment in Acute Stroke: Review and Update of Selected Topics. In Caplan L(ed): Cerebrovascular Disease: 19th Princeton Conference, 1994. Boston: Butterworth-Heinemann, 1995, pp 409-418.

333. Caplan LR: Caplan's Stroke: A Clinical Approach. Boston: Butterworth-Heinemann, 2000.

334. Caplan LR: Thrombolysis 2004. The good, the bad, and the ugly. Rev Neurol Dis 2004;1:16-26.

335. Christoforidis G, Mohammad Y, Bourekas E, Slivka A: Initial severity of angiographic occlusion predicts subsequent volume of cerebral infarction following intra-arterial thrombolysis in acute ischemic stroke. Neurology 2004;62(suppl 5):A449.

336. Toni D, Fiorelli M, Zanette EM, et al: Early spontaneous improvement and deterioration of ischemic stroke patients: A serial study with transcranial Doppler ultrasonography. Stroke 1998;29:1144-1148.

337. Lewandowski C, Frankel M, Tomsick T, et al: Combined intravenous and intra-arterial r-tPA versus intra-arterial therapy of acute ischemic stroke: Emergency management of Stroke (EMS) Bridging Trial. Stroke 1999;30:2598-2605.

338. IMS Study Investigators: Combined intravenous and intra-arterial recanalization for acute ischemic stroke: The Interventional Management of Stroke Study. Stroke 2004;35:904-912.

339. Fourie P, Duncan IC: Microsnare-assisted mechanical removal of intraprocedural distal middle cerebral arterial thromboembolism. AJNR Am J Neuroradiol 2003;24:630-632.

340. Berlis A, Lutsep H, Barnwell S, et al: Mechanical thrombolysis in acute ischemic stroke with endovascular photoacoustic recanalization. Stroke 2004;35:1112-1116.

341. Starkman S: Results of the combined MERCI I-II (Mechanical Embolus Removal in Cerebral Ischemia) trials. Stroke 2004;35:240.

342. Gobin YP, Starkman S, Duckwiler GR, et al: MERCI I: A phase I study of mechanical embolus removal in cerebral ischemia. Stroke 2004;35:2848-2854.

343. Nesbit GM, Luh G, Tien R, Barnwell SL: New and future endovascular treatment strategies for acute ischemic stroke. J Vasc Interv Radiol 2004;15: S103-S110.

344. Fussell D, Schumacher C, Meyers PM, Higashida RT: Mechanical interventions to treat acute stroke. Curr Neurol Neurosci Rep 2007;7:21-27.

345. Alexandrov AV, Demchuk Am, Felberg RA, et al: High rate of recanalization and dramatic clinical

recovery during tPA infusion when continuously monitored with 2-Mhz transcranial Doppler monitoring. Stroke 2000;31:610-614.

346. Hacke W: The dilemma of reinstituting anticoagulation for patients with cardioembolic sources and intracranial hemorrhage: How wide is the strait between Skylla and Karybdis? Arch Neurol 2000;57:1682-1684.

347. Phan TG, Koh M, Wijdicks EF: Safety of discontinuation of anticoagulation in patients with intracranial hemorrhage at high thromboembolic risk. Arch Neurol 2000;57:1710-1713.

348. O'Brien MD: Ischemic cerebral edema in brain ischemia. In Caplan LR (ed): Basic Concepts and Clinical Relevance. London: Springer-Verlag, 1995, pp 43-50.

349. Delashaw JB, Broaddus WC, Kassell NF, et al: Treatment of right hemisphere cerebral infarction by hemicraniectomy. Stroke 1990;21:874-881.

350. Georgiadis D, Schwaqb S, Aschoff A, Schwab S: Hemicraniectomy and moderate hypothermia in patients with severe hemispheric stroke. Stroke 2002;33:1884-1888.

351. Schwab S, Rieke K, Aschoff A, et al: Hemicraniotomy in space-occupying hemispheric infarction:useful early intervention or desperate activism. Cerebrovasc Dis 1996;6:325-329.

352. Schwab S, Steiner T, Aschoff A, et al: Early hemicraniectomy in patients with complete middle cerebral artery infarction. Stroke 1998;29:1888-1893.

353. Parisi DM, Koval K, Egol K: Fat embolism syndrome. Am J Orthop 2002:507-512.

354. Bulger E, Smith DG, Maier RV, Jurkovich G: Fat embolism syndrome. A 10-year review. Arch Surg 1997;132:435-439.

355. Sevitt S: Fat embolism. London: Butterworth & Co, 1962.

356. Dines DE, Burgher LW, Okazaki H: The clinical and pathological correlation of fat embolism syndrome. Mayo Clin Proc 1975;50:407-411.

357. Jacobson DM, Terrence CF, Reinmuth OM: The neurologic manifestations of fat embolism. Neurology 1986;36:847-851.

358. Hill JD, Aguilar MJ, Baranco AP, Gerbode F: Neuropathological manifestations of cardiac surgery. Ann Thorac Surg 1969;7:409-517.

359. Ghatal NR, Sinnenberg RJ, DeBlois GG: Cerebral fat embolism following cardiac surgery. Stroke 1983;14:619-621.

360. Charache S, Page DL: Infarction of bone marrow in sickle cell disorders. Ann Intern Med 1967;67:1195-1200.

361. Vichinsky E, Williams K, Das M, et al: Pulmonary fat embolism: A distinct cause of severe acute chest syndrome in sickle cell anemia. Blood 1994;83:3107-3112.

362. Shelley WM, Curtis EM: Bone marrow and fat embolism in sickle cell anemia and sickle cell-hemoglobin C disease. Bull Johns Hopkins Hosp 1958;103:8-25.

363. Chmel H, Bertles J: Hemoglobin S/C disease in a pregnant woman with crisis and fat embolization syndrome. Am J Med 1975;58:563-566.

364. Forteza AM, Rabinstein A, Koch S, et al: Endovascular closure of a patent foramen ovale in the fat embolism syndrome. Changes in the embolic pattern as detected by transcranial Doppler. Arch Neurol 2002;59:455-459.

365. Forteza AM, Koch S, Romano JG, et al: Transcranial Doppler detection of fat emboli. Stroke 1999;30:2687-2691.

366. Simon A, Ulmer JL, Strottman JM: Contrast-enhanced MR imaging of cerebral fat embolism: Case report and review of the literature. AJNR Am J Neuroradiol 2003;24:97-101.

367. Guillevin R, Vallee JN, Demeret S, et al: Cerebral fat embolism: Usefulness of magnetic resonance spectroscopy. Ann Neurol 2005;57:434-439.

368. Chastre J, Fagon J-Y, Soler P, et al: Bronchoalveolar lavage for rapid diagnosis of the fat embolism syndrome in trauma patients. Ann Intern Med 1990;113:583-588.

369. Godeau B, Schaeffer A, Bachir D, et al: Bronchoalveolar lavage in adult sickle cell patients with acute chest syndrome: value for diagnostic assessment of fat embolism. Am J Resp Care Med 1996;153:1691-1696.

370. Kamenar E, Burger PC: Cerebral fat embolism: A neuropathological study of a microembolic state. Stroke 1980;11:477-484.

371. Menkin M, Schwartzman RJ: Cerebral air embolism. Report of five cases and review of the literature. Arch Neurol 1977;34:169-170.

372. Valentino R, Hilbert G, Vargas F, Gruson D: Computed tomographic scan of massive cerebral air embolism. Lancet 2003;361:1848.

373. Demaerel P, Gevers A-M, De Brueker Y, et al: Stroke caused by cerebral air embolism during endoscopy. Gastrointest Endosc 2003;1:134-135.

374. Weber M-A, Fiebach JB, Lichy MP, et al: Bilateral cerebral air embolism. J Neurol 2003;250:1115-1117.

375. Hodics T, Linfante I: Cerebral air embolism. Neurology 2003;60:112.

376. Hertz JA, Schinco MA, Frykberg ER: Extensive pneumocranium. J Trauma Inj Infect Crit Care 2002;52:188.

377. Laskey AL, Dyer C, Tobias JD: Venous air embolism during home infusion therapy. Pediatrics 2002;109:e15.

378. Gei AF, Vadhera, Hankins GDV: Embolism during pregnancy: Thrombus, air, and amniotic fluid. Anesthesiol Clin North Am 2003;21:165-182.

379. Malinow AM, Naulty JS, Hunt CO, et al: Precordial ultrasonic monitoring during cesarean delivery. Anesthesiology 1987;66:816-819.

380. Spencer MP, Campbell SD: Development of bubbles in venous and arterial blood during hyperbaric decompression. Bull Mason Clin 1968;22:26-32.

381. Gillen HW: Symptomatology of cerebral gas embolism. Neurology 1968;18:507-512.

382. Cantais E, Louge P, Suppini A, et al: Right-to-left shunt and risk of decompression illness with cochleovestibular and cerebral symptoms in divers: Case control study in 101 consecutive dive accidents. Crit Care Med 2003;31:84-88.

383. Jeon S-B, Kim JS, Lee DK, et al: Clinicoradiological characteristics of cerebral air embolism. Cerebrovasc Dis 2007;23:459-462.

384. Yeh T, Austin EH, Sehic A, Edmonds HL: Rapid recognition and treatment of cerebral air embolism: The role of neuroimaging. J Thorac Cardiovasc Surg 2003;126:589-591.

385. Lefkovitz NW, Roessman U, Kori S: Major cerebral infarction from tumor embolus. Stroke 1986;17:555-557.

386. Banerjee AK, Chopra JS: Cerebral embolism from a thyroid carcinoma. Arch Neurol 1972;27:186-187.

387. Kase CS, White R, Vinson TL, Eichelberger RP: Shotgun pellet embolus to the middle cerebral artery. Neurology 1981;31:458-461.

388. Yaari R, Ahmadi J, Chang GY: Cerebral shotgun pellet embolism. Neurology 2000;54:1487.

389. Duncan I, Fourie PA: Embolization of a bullet in the internal carotid artery. Am J Roentgenol 2002;178:1572-1573.

390. Langenbach M, Leopold H-C, Hennerici M: Neck trauma with embolization of the middle cerebral artery by a metal splinter. Neurology 1990;40:552-553.

391. Dato GMA, Arsianian A, Di Marzio P, et al: Posttraumatic and iatrogenic foreign bodies in the heart: Report of fourteen cases and review of the literature. J Thorac Cardiovasc Surg 2003;126:408-414.

392. Crie JS, Hajar R, Folger G: Umbilical catheter masquerading at echocardiography as a left atrial mass. Clin Cardiol 1989;12:728-730.

393. Mattox KL, Beall AC, Ennix CL, DeBakey ME: Intravascular migratory bullets. Am J Surg 1979;137:192-195.

393a. Kase CS, White R, Vinson TL, Eichelberger RP: Shotgun pellet embolism to the middle cerebral artery. Neurology 1981;31:458-461.

394. Caplan LR, Thomas C, Banks G: Central nervous system complications of "Ts and blues" addiction. Neurology 1982;32:623-628.

395. Aplan LR, Hier DB, Banks G: Stroke and drug abuse. Curr Concepts Cerebrovasc Dis (Stroke) 1982;27:9-13.

396. Atlee W: Talc and cornstarch emboli in the eyes of drug abusers. JAMA 1972;219:49-51.

397. Mizutami T, Lewis R, Gonatas N: Medial medullary syndrome in a drug abuser. Arch Neurol 1980;37:425-428.

398. Chillar RK, Jackson AL, Alaan L: Hemiplegia after intracarotid injection of methylphenidate. Arch Neurol 1982;39:598-599.

Hypoxic-Ischemic Encephalopathy, Cardiac Arrests, and Cardiac Encephalopathy

10

The brain is particularly vulnerable to any decrease in its blood, oxygen, or fuel supply. Patients with hypotension or hypoxia often present to their physicians or the emergency room because of cerebral dysfunction. Most often, decreased brain perfusion is caused by arrhythmia or pump failure, which in turn is often caused by an acute myocardial infarction. Shock and hypovolemia also decrease whole-brain perfusion. Because circulatory failure usually leads to hypoventilation, and hypoxia soon causes diminished cardiac function, hypoxia and hypoperfusion are usually combined. The general term *hypoxic-ischemic encephalopathy* reflects the dual nature of the central-nervous-system stress. Pulmonary embolism is another acute disorder that causes hypotension and diminished blood oxygenation. In some patients, decreased cerebral perfusion is caused by acute blood loss or hypovolemia.

CLINICAL FINDINGS

A global decrease in perfusion causes generalized nonfocal brain dysfunction. Dizziness, lightheadedness, confusion, and difficulty in concentrating are common. Focal symptoms and signs, such as hemiplegia, hemianopia, and aphasia, are rarely caused by circulatory failure but are usual findings in the other categories of ischemic stroke. At times, prior strokes or vascular occlusions do lead to asymmetries on neurologic examination. Examination of a patient with globally decreased cerebral perfusion usually shows an ill-appearing person with sweating, tachycardia, hypotension (especially postural), and physical examination or electrocardiographic signs of cardiac dysfunction. The two common circumstances in which neurologists might see patients with brain hypoperfusion resulting from systemic causes are (1) acute central nervous system symptoms in the absence of a known incident of circulatory failure, and (2) after known cardiac arrest, hypotension, or cardiac surgery. In the first circumstance, the major problem is diagnosis. When there is a known cardiac arrest, the consulting physician usually asks the neurologist about the prognosis of the brain injury.

Patient 1

LB, a 63-year-old man, suddenly became agitated and restless and seemed confused. He entered the hospital 2 days before for abdominal pain, had no neurologic symptoms or abnormalities, and had routine gastrointestinal x-rays. A psychiatrist who was called to examine and calm the patient requested neurologic consultation because of concern about an organic cause for the behavioral change. Neurologic examination showed an agitated, restless man. He did not know his whereabouts, nor could he give any account of the previous few days. He recalled none of the three objects told to him 3 minutes before, and could not even remember that he had been given objects to recall. He spoke normally and could repeat and understand spoken language. He could write but not read. He also could not identify objects in his environment by sight and saw only parts of pictures shown to him. When the same objects were placed in his hands, he correctly named them. There were no abnormalities of motor, reflex, or somatosensory function. Gait was normal but he held his hands outstretched when he walked, as if feeling for objects and walls.

This patient had abnormalities in three major spheres—memory, vision, and behavior. These findings indicate bilateral dysfunction of the posterior portions of the cerebral hemispheres. Embolization to the rostral basilar artery, causing bilateral temporo-occipital lobe infarcts in the posterior cerebral artery (PCA) territory, could cause these findings. Alternatively, an unrecognized episode of prolonged hypotension might have led to hypoperfusion in the posterior border zone between the middle cerebral artery (MCA) and PCA territories. Distal-field infarction most often affects the posterior hemispheres, possibly because they are the regions farthest from the heart.[1] Figures 2-6 and 2-7C illustrate the concept of border-zone vulnerability to systemic hypoperfusion.

Lesions in the posterior watershed (between the MCA and PCA) often disconnect the preserved calcarine visual cortex in the occipital

375

lobe from the more anterior centers that control eye movements. A visual problem first described by an ophthalmologist, called Balint's syndrome, often results.[1-4] Patients act as if they cannot see, but sometimes surprisingly they notice small objects. The features of Balint's syndrome follow:

1. Asimultagnosia: Patients see things piecemeal; they do not see all the objects in their field of vision at one time and may notice only parts of objects. To test for this problem, physicians should ask patients to count the number of people or objects in a picture or on a table, ask patients to read a paragraph aloud to determine whether they omit words or phrases, and show patients multiple objects held up together for verbal identification.
2. Optical ataxia: Patients cannot coordinate hand and eye movements and point erratically at objects. Physicians should test for optical ataxia by asking patients to touch the noses of people in a picture or to touch the crossing point of several Xs on a page. Physicians should ask patients to trace, first with one hand and then the other, a complex drawing constructed by the examiner.
3. Apraxia of gaze: Patients are unable to gaze directly where desired. Physicians should ask patients to look at an object held to the side, look at the examiner's nose, and then repeat the same task. Physicians should also note how patients explore a picture.

Visual abnormalities can be more severe in either the left or right visual field. Balint's original cases were probably caused by systemic hypoperfusion, the most common mechanism of bilateral parieto-occipital damage. PCA infarction also can lead to Balint's syndrome. Occasionally, patients with Alzheimer's or Creutzfeldt-Jakob disease or a degenerative condition dubbed *posterior cortical atrophy* by Benson[5] have features of Balint's syndrome, but the findings develop gradually and insidiously rather than abruptly. Memory dysfunction and agitation can also be caused by bilateral PCA-territory infarcts or border-zone ischemia. These conditions are discussed in Chapter 7.

When hypotension is more severe, lesions can spread to the anterior border zones between the anterior cerebral artery (ACA) and MCA and may extend like a triangle toward the ventricle (Fig. 10-1).[6,7] The areas of the motor homunculus most affected are those related to the shoulder, arm, and thigh. The face territory in the central portion of the MCA territory and the foot region in the center of the ACA supply are spared. The distribution of weakness has been likened by Mohr to a "man in a barrel."[1,8]

Among a prospective series of 34 patients with coma presumably caused by an episode of systemic hypotension, 11 had the man-in-the-barrel syndrome.[8] They moved neither arm but moved both legs spontaneously or in response to pain. The frontal eye fields are also affected, so that roving eye movements and hyperactive passive head movements (doll's eye reflexes) result. At times, perhaps because of previously asymmetric occlusive disease of extracranial and intracranial arteries, the signs can be quite asymmetric with unilateral or asymmetric arm paralysis and conjugate-eye deviation toward the side of the larger lesion. Stupor results from extensive bilateral border-zone ischemia.

> LB was sedated and a computed tomography (CT) scan was ordered. The scan showed small but definite approximately symmetric hypodensities in the posterior parietal regions with sparing of the medial calcarine cortex and temporal lobes. An electrocardiogram showed evidence of acute myocardial infarction and multifocal, frequent, premature ventricular contractions.

CT confirmed that the lesions were between the PCA and MCA territories, supporting the diagnosis of border-zone infarction. This led to more cardiac testing, which showed an unsuspected myocardial infarction and a potentially serious arrhythmia. In retrospect, after further questioning by the patient's physician, the acute abdominal pain was probably caused by coronary artery disease. The diagnosis of border-zone ischemia leads to a different array of diagnostic tests than those that apply to infarction in the center of a vascular territory. I have also occasionally seen demented patients whose neurologic examination and CT scans indicated border-zone infarcts caused by repeated, unrecognized episodes of hypotension or globally decreased cerebral perfusion.

LB had a relatively slight insult and recuperated well with time. The nature of the insult and its reversibility should be emphasized. In general, it is unwise to push the patient back to work too quickly or self-confidence may be lost. Many patients are not restored mentally for months after their cardiac events, but gradually regain their usual intellectual vigor over time. Time and reassurance are needed.

Patient 2

A 45-year-old previously well man, AR, collapsed at work, clutching his chest in pain. Paramedics found him pulseless minutes later and administered cardiopulmonary resuscitation (CPR) on the way to the hospital. Pulse and blood pressure were restored, but the patient

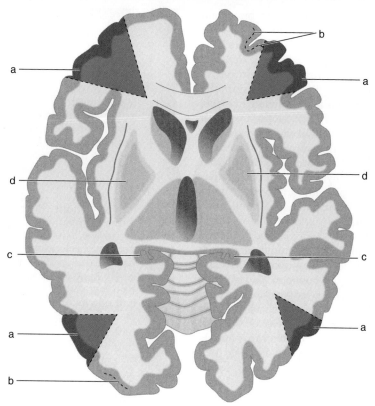

Figure 10-1. Drawing of a horizontal section of the cerebrum showing common patterns of hypoxic-ischemic brain damage. **a,** Border-zone infarct between anterior and middle cerebral arteries and between middle and posterior cerebral arteries. **b,** Zones of laminar necrosis within the cerebral cortex. **c,** Hippocampal necrosis. **d,** Necrosis of nerve cells within the globus pallidus and putamen. (Adapted from Caplan LR, Hurst JW, Chimowitz MI: Clinical Neurocardiology. New York: Marcel Dekker, 1999.)

lay comatose. A neurologist examined the patient the next morning, 18 hours after the arrest. The patient was sleepy but could be momentarily aroused by shouting or pinching. He would appropriately flick off painful stimuli but did not speak, obey oral commands, or answer queries. There were spontaneous restless limb movements. Blinking, swallowing, and tongue-protrusion movements were seen. Pupillary, corneal, and doll's eye reflexes were normal. Plantar responses were extensor, but there was no abnormal limb posturing.

In this patient, the neurologist knew that the abnormal neurologic state was caused by cardiac arrest. Was the central nervous system insult likely to be lethal? What would be the quality of survival? Should orders not to resuscitate be given? This scenario is frequent in hospital practice today. Successful CPR, once rare, has become commonplace. Advances in technique, widespread teaching of medical, paramedical, and lay volunteer personnel, and the availability of special mobile equipment and facilities in some communities have saved many lives.[9-11] The heart is often

able to recover from ischemia, but the brain has often been irreversibly damaged by the ischemic-anoxic insult of circulatory failure. New technology can prolong life indefinitely in a vegetative state, at great emotional, physical, and economic cost to the community and family. Physicians involved with CPR must be familiar with prognostic indicators for cerebral recovery after cardiac arrest and should consider their own ethical and moral values in applying this knowledge.

PATHOLOGY

Signs of brain dysfunction secondary to hypoxic-ischemic insults can best be remembered by visualizing the brain regions most vulnerable to circulatory failure and their pathology. The location and severity of the pathology depends on the patient's age; the completeness of the circulatory arrest; serologic factors, such as the blood sugar and pH; and the relative admixture of hypoxia and ischemia.

Severe prolonged hypoxic-ischemic insults cause necrosis of the cerebral and cerebellar cortex, cerebral edema, and injury to brainstem nuclei. The most vulnerable neurons are those in the cerebral cortex, especially in the middle lamina of the cortex; pyramidal neurons in the CA1 zone of the hippocampus; neurons in portions of the amygdaloid nucleus; Purkinje cells in the cerebellar cortex; neurons in the caudate nucleus, putamen, and globus pallidus; motor nuclei in the brainstem; and neurons in the anterior, dorsomedial, and pulvinar thalamic nuclei.[11,12]

The pattern and distribution of injury also depends on the anatomy of the arterial circulation. Border zones show more injury than brain areas in the heart of the major feeding brain arteries. Selective vulnerability, arterial anatomy, and differential responses to hypoxia and ischemia explain the various patterns of brain damage seen in patients with cardiac arrest and severe hypoxia (Figure 10-2). The most common patterns are listed in Table 10-1. Acknowledgment of the anatomic patterns helps clinicians recognize the clinical syndromes and also the use of some of the investigations used in evaluating patients with hypoxic-ischemic encephalopathy.

CLINICAL ABNORMALITIES AND SYNDROMES

Brainstem and Bihemispheral Coma

Consciousness is maintained by continuous stimulation of the cerebral hemispheres by neurons within the brainstem tegmentum. Coma develops after damage to the bilateral medial portions of

Table 10-1.	**Patterns of Hypoxic-Ischemic Injury and Their Causes**

1. Diffuse cerebral cortical injury, often with laminar necrosis of the middle cortical layers, cardiac arrest, or prolonged hypotension
2. Ischemic damage to border-zone regions, especially between the middle and posterior cerebral artery territories, and between the anterior and middle cerebral artery territories, cardiac arrest, or prolonged hypotension
3. Necrosis of hippocampal neurons, especially in the CA1 zone, cardiac arrest, or prolonged hypotension
4. Necrosis of basal ganglia and thalamic neurons; delayed necrosis of the basal ganglia and cerebral white matter; severe hypoxia, especially strangulation, hanging, carbon monoxide poisoning, and drowning
5. Necrosis of Purkinje cells in the cerebellum, prolonged ischemia
6. Necrosis of brainstem motor and tegmental nuclei, especially cranial nerve nuclei, inferior colliculus, vestibular nuclei, and superior olive; sudden severe hypotension in infants, children, and young adults

Modified from Caplan LR: Cardiac arrest and other hypoxic ischemic insults. In Caplan LR, Hurst JW, Chimowitz MI: Clinical Neurocardiology. New York: Marcel Dekker, 1999.

the brainstem tegmentum in the pons and midbrain or when there is severe damage to the bilateral cerebral hemispheres. All patients who have had cardiac arrest have an initial period of coma. When comatose patients are first examined, there are two different patterns of findings depending on the presence or absence of brainstem reflexes. In patients with severe prolonged hypoperfusion-anoxic insults, the pupils are dilated, corneal reflexes are absent, and the eyes remain midline and do not move horizontally or vertically to doll's eye reflex or to ice-water irrigation of the ear canals. Some patients have no spontaneous respirations and must be ventilated mechanically. Spontaneous limb movements, except for low-level decorticate or decerebrate movements, are absent. This state is usually referred to as *brainstem coma* because it indicates injury to brainstem tegmental nuclei. When this state is prolonged, death invariably follows.

Infants, young children, and occasionally adults have selective necrosis of their brainstem tegmental nuclei.[13,14] These patients have loss of

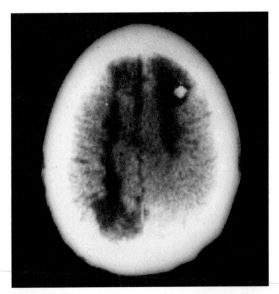

Figure 10-2. CT scan from a patient with prolonged cardiac arrest showing infarction along border-zone regions.

reflex eye movements; facial, pharyngeal, and tongue weakness; and loss of the gag reflex. They usually have stiff, immobile limbs and only automatic and autonomic responses to environmental stimuli. Control of respirations is often lost, and the pulse and blood pressures may fluctuate widely. This state invariably proves fatal. Imaging may show no cerebral hemispheral abnormalities, and the brainstem may even appear normal on gross inspection at necropsy. Microscopic examination shows selective necrosis of brainstem nuclei.

Some patients with brainstem coma regain normal brainstem reflexes and spontaneous respirations and enter a state called *bihemispheral coma.* Other patients have bihemispheral coma when first examined neurologically and have not gone through a stage of brainstem coma. Patients with bihemispheral coma are unresponsive to noise, voice, or bright light. There may be some spontaneous movements of all limbs. The pupils are normal or constricted and react to light. The eyes usually remain in the midline, move from side to side, or are deviated upward. Passive movements readily elicit horizontal eye movements. Often, doll's eye movements are hyperactive, indicating lack of cerebral inhibition of the vestibulo-ocular reflex. Vertical eye movements can usually be elicited by flexing and extending the neck. In patients with forced upward eye deviation, it may be difficult to get the eyes to move fully downward on vertical doll's eyes maneuvers. The gag reflex is usually present. Some patients with bihemispheral coma have their mouths open, and some keep their jaws tightly clenched and "bulldog" down on tubes or sticks placed in their mouths, making it difficult to see the pharynx or perform the gag reflex. Watching these patients from the foot of the bed shows that they often spontaneously blink, yawn, sneeze, cough, hiccup, protrude their tongue, lick their lips, sigh, and swallow. These spontaneous mouth, face, and tongue movements are mediated through brainstem structures and indicate that the brainstem is functioning.[15] Coma is caused by loss of the normal functions of both cerebral hemispheres.

Spontaneous limb movements and responses to pinch in the limbs vary considerably.[15] Patients who have dysfunction of the corticospinal tracts often have preserved adduction and flexion movements of the shoulders, arms, and wrists. When pinched on either the flexor or extensor surface of the arm, forearm, or hand, they flex and adduct the arm and shoulder irrespective of the site of stimulation. The flexion response brings the arm into stimuli on the flexor surface. Spontaneous or reactive extension, abducting movements of the arm or forearm, preserved movements of individual fingers, and limb withdrawal from pinch appropriate to the site of stimulation (flexion or adduction when pinched on the extensor surface, and extension or abduction when pinched on the flexor surface, movements that move the upper limb away from the stimulus) show that the corticospinal tracts are preserved and functioning. Similarly, loss of corticospinal tract function leads to extension and adduction of the lower limbs. Flexion and adduction movements of the lower limbs that occur spontaneously or in response to pinch usually indicate corticospinal tract preservation. The ability to remove or react to pinch with either the same or contralateral arm indicates that the stimulus has been perceived. Use of the arm contralateral to the pinch to ward off the noxious stimulus almost always indicates weakness of the stimulated arm. Major asymmetries of motor or sensory function usually mean asymmetric brain damage.

Patients with bihemispheral coma may remain in a vegetative state poorly responsive to environmental stimuli or they can become more alert and responsive. A number of clinical patterns of dysfunction can ensue from the bihemispheral coma stage.

As stupor lightens, agitation, restlessness, confusion, and even delirium supervene. An examination performed after the patient awakens often uncovers features of Balint's syndrome, as described in the first patient. Other patients have a selective difficulty with memory and are unable to recall recent happenings or form new lasting memories. This amnesic state clinically resembles Korsakoff's syndrome and is caused by selective vulnerability of the hippocampus and adjacent medial temporal lobe structures to hypoxic-ischemic insults.[11,12,16-19] Active memory testing is required to identify and quantify the memory loss. Physicians should give patients a 10-fact story, three objects, or three pictures, emphasizing that they will later be asked to recall the information. Patients should be asked to repeat the items to be certain that they have been registered. Later, patients should be asked to recite the items to be recalled, grading the performance (i.e., as three out of five objects after 5 minutes). Passive memory testing—asking patients what happened that morning or what they ate during their last meal—is less reliable than active memory testing.

The cerebral cortex often undergoes selective damage to the middle lamina, sparing the deeper and more superficial cortical layers.[12,20,21] This laminar necrosis frequently causes seizures. Seizures may follow severe or moderate laminar injury and may take the form of multifocal myoclonic jerks, twitches, or frank grand mal seizures.

Myoclonic jerks are often exaggerated or provoked by moving or stimulating a limb. Seizures caused by diffuse hypoxic-ischemic injury are relatively resistant to treatment. Care should be taken to avoid overdosing with anticonvulsants, thus compounding the patient's stupor. If seizures create respiratory compromise, cause myoglobinuria, or release of high levels of muscle enzymes, the use of agents that paralyze muscles and mechanical ventilation may be necessary. Repetitive generalized myoclonus, lasting longer than 30 minutes, carries a poor prognosis in patients who survive a cardiac arrest.[22-24] In one series of 11 such patients, none regained consciousness after resuscitation and all remained comatose until death.[22] Each of these patients had extensive hypoxic-ischemic damage to the cerebral cortex, especially the hippocampus and calcarine cortices. The basal ganglia, thalamus, cerebellum, and brainstem nuclei were all severely damaged.[22]

Severe laminar necrosis can be associated with extensive loss of cortical functions, so that patients survive in a persistent vegetative state with little meaningful response to the environment but preserved brainstem function. These patients appear awake. They have sleep-wake cycles with eyes open, but make no response to stimulation or to the environment.[21,25] Necropsy examinations of 10 patients with the persistent vegetative state showed extensive cortical necrosis, often laminar in distribution, and multiple microinfarcts.[21]

Prolonged partial ischemia, especially in the young, can cause damage to the basal ganglia, particularly the globus pallidus and thalamus. Strangulation and carbon monoxide poisoning produce a similar insult, in which hypoxia antedates and overshadows circulatory compromise.[26] Rigidity, decorticate posturing, and flexion of all limbs result. Although the eyes are open and fixate, patients are often mute and usually do not respond to environmental stimuli. Patients with mutism and rigidity after cardiac arrest have a poor prognosis for recovery.

Although hypoxic-ischemic cerebellar damage is often found at necropsy, clinical signs of cerebellar dysfunction are rare and are usually overshadowed by cerebral abnormalities. After cardiac arrest, some patients have spontaneous arrhythmic fine or coarse muscle jerking, markedly exaggerated when the limbs are used. This disorder of movements, usually called *action myoclonus* or *the Lance-Adams syndrome* after the physicians who originally described it, is often accompanied by gait ataxia.[27] The movement disorder can progress, even without further ischemic stress. Some patients, especially those with pre-existing occlusive disease of the vertebral arteries, may have prominent ataxia caused by border-zone cerebellar infarcts, mostly between the main supply of the three major circumferential cerebellar arteries.

Plum and colleagues described delayed progressive deterioration after a single hypoxic insult.[28] Three of the five patients reported deteriorated after exposure to noxious gases and had predominately hypoxic injuries. The other two patients worsened after surgery and both had hypotension and anoxia. The patients were all comatose when first examined after the insult but awakened within 24 hours and resumed relatively normal activities and functions for 4 to 10 days. These patients then developed cognitive and behavioral abnormalities characterized mostly by apathy, irritability, agitation, restlessness, and confusion. Walking then became clumsy and the limbs became rigid and stiff. Outcome varied from full recovery to severe disability to death. Necropsy in the two patients that died showed extensive white matter demyelination in the cerebral hemispheres. One patient also had cystic necrosis in the medial globus pallidus bilaterally.

Subsequent reports confirmed the existence of a leukoencephalopathy, often with basal ganglionic damage that may follow hypoxic-ischemic events.[29,30] The white matter damage involves diffuse injury to the white matter, which ranges from patchy demyelination to hemorrhagic white matter necrosis. Most reported patients have been young, and the insult has most often been predominantly hypoxic (e.g., carbon monoxide intoxication, strangulation, drowning, and gas inhalation). When initially examined after the insult, the patients were in coma, often with loss of muscle tone, quadriparesis, or involuntary movements of the limbs. Most patients who developed severe limb dysfunction with rigidity, abnormal movements, and dystonia never improved after the initial hypoxic-ischemic event, but some have had delayed deterioration, as was first reported by Plum et al.[28] The dystonic rigid state is associated with severe damage to deep subcortical basal ganglionic and white matter tracts, usually with relative preservation of the cerebral cortex. The pathologic substrate of this syndrome presents a sharp contrast to the cerebral cortex necrosis with usual preservation of subcortical structures found in patients with the persistent vegetative state.

In two reports, two patients with delayed hypoxic leukoencephalopathy have shown a reduction of arylsulfatase-A activity to less than 50% of normal.[31,32] Although this degree of reduction does not ordinarily cause symptoms, hypoxia could cause tissue acidosis, which might potentiate myelin damage. Arylsulfatase-A is a lysosomal enzyme active in the lipid metabolism of myelin. In the presence of local tissue acidosis, this enzyme deficiency could make patients vulnerable to demyelination. Another reported patient, a woman who required resuscitation after hysterectomy surgery for menorrhagia, was comatose for 2 days. She then awakened, functioned normally for two weeks, and then developed a severe leukoencephalopathy but had normal arylsulfatase-A activity.[32a] Delayed leukoencephalopathy has also been reported after heroin inhalation.[32b] Proton magnetic resonance spectroscopy of the white matter lesions helped to characterize the white matter abnormalities in three cases,[32,32a,32b] and might be useful in evaluating other patients with hypoxic-ischemic encephalopathies. Progressive worsening is rare after cardiac arrest, although it has been described. The mechanism of progressive loss of function after single self-limited insults is uncertain.

Occasionally, patients recover from coma without obvious cerebral damage but instead have paraplegia related to hypoxic-ischemic damage to the spinal cord.[33,34] The most vulnerable spinal regions are the upper and lower thoracic and lumbar spinal cord segments. The cervical cord is usually not involved, so that the arms are normal despite severe weakness of the lower limbs. The localization of the spinal cord ischemic necrosis relates to the anatomy of the arterial supply of the spinal cord. Although arteries from each side feed into the paired posterior spinal arteries at each spinal segment, the segmental arteries that supply the single unpaired midline anterior spinal artery originate at variable levels, and one supply artery can be mostly responsible for nourishing four or five segments. The vascular anatomy is detailed further in Chapter 15. The largest and most well-known artery, the artery of Adamkiewicz, originates anywhere between the ninth thoracic and second lumbar segment and supplies the lumbar spinal cord and conus medullaris. The upper and lower thoracic regions are border-zone areas between the supply of major anterior feeding arteries. The spinal damage involves mostly the anterior portion of the spinal cord, which is fed by the anterior spinal artery. The anterior horn motor neurons and the pyramidal tracts are included, but usually the posterior columns are spared. The resulting syndrome is usually a flaccid paralysis of both lower limbs. Spasticity often develops later. Control of urination and defecation is often lost and there may be a sensory level to pain and temperature on the trunk. Position and vibration sense and touch are usually preserved. Atrophy and fasciculations often develop in the thighs and legs. Spinal cord infarction is a rare but important result of cardiac arrest or prolonged systemic hypotension. In some patients, the cerebral findings are prominent and it is not recognized.

Prognosis

Often, the most important consideration in patients with potentially severe hypoxic-ischemic insults is prediction of outcome. What findings allow physicians to predict the likelihood of survival and the presence, nature, and severity of residual neurologic abnormalities? Investigators have struggled to find reliable prognosticators since the 1970s.[35-47] Table 10-2 lists the various clinical indicators that have been studied and analyzed. Persistence or absence of clinical findings has different prognostic use during the first hours, day, week, and after the first month. Unfortunately, although clinicians and investigator have striven for objective imaging, electrophysiologic, and biomarkers that would aid in prognosis, from a practical view, in most patients the laboratory and imaging results have not proven very helpful, and clinicians must rely predominantly on the clinical neurologic findings, and their changes over time.

Survival after cardiac arrest depends on three major factors: (1) the severity of the cardiac disease and the duration of the hypoxic-ischemic cardiac injury, (2) the extent and reversibility of brainstem damage, and (3) cardiopulmonary infectious complications that occur in the hospital. The heart may be even more vulnerable than the brain to hypoxia and ischemia. After severe

Table 10-2.	Clinical Prognosticators in Patients Examined after Hypoxic-Ischemic Events

1. Depth and duration of coma
2. Brainstem reflexes
   a. Pupillary light reflex
   b. Corneal reflex
   c. Oculovestibular responses
3. Spontaneous respirations and requirement for a ventilator
4. Motor responses to stimuli
5. Eye positions and movements
6. Vocal responses
7. Ability to follow commands
8. Seizures, myoclonus, and other involuntary movements

From Caplan LR: Cardiac arrest and other hypoxic ischemic insults. In Caplan LR, Hurst JW, Chimowitz MI: Clinical Neurocardiology. New York: Marcel Dekker, 1999.

10

anoxia of 4 minutes duration or longer, arrhythmias and asystole often develop, causing decreased cardiac output and decreased brain perfusion. The brainstem nuclei control automatic and autonomic functions, including control of cardiovascular functions and respirations. Survival is rare after severe damage to the bilateral brainstem tegmentum. Pulmonary embolism, congestive heart failure, recurrent cardiac arrhythmias and cardiac arrests, pneumonia, and urinary tract sepsis are common and often serious complications in patients after cardiac arrest, especially in those patients who remain in coma or states of reduced consciousness.

The nature and severity of persistent neurologic signs depends on the severity and location of the cerebral, cerebellar, and spinal damage. Prediction of the nature and severity of persistent neurologic deficits can only be assessed when brainstem coma has cleared and the patient is in bihemispheral coma or has awakened.

During the first minutes and hours after cardiac arrest or other hypoxic-ischemic insults, the most important signs of prognostic importance are the depth and duration of the coma, brainstem functions, and reflexes.[37-44] Persistent brainstem dysfunction causes deep, prolonged coma, an absence of brainstem reflex functions, and poor control of respirations. Patients with irreversible, severe bilateral medial tegmental brainstem damage do not survive. Testing of brainstem reflex functions is important in all comatose patients. Clinicians should note the rate, depth, and regularity of respirations and the need for mechanical ventilation. Some spontaneous movements, such as blinking, yawning, coughing, sneezing, gagging, and swallowing, use brainstem reflex functions. The presence of these movements indicates preserved lower brainstem function.[15]

In the Snyder et al series, all patients who at 3 hours after cardiopulmonary arrest had no corneal reflexes or absent pupillary light reflexes died.[39,40] By 6 hours, no survivors had absence of the three brainstem reflexes studied (pupillary light response, corneal reflex, and reflex eye movements. By 24 to 48 hours, only 3 of 25 survivors (12%) had any brainstem reflex abnormality. In another series, 52 of 210 patients (25%) with hypoxic-ischemic coma had absent pupillary light reflex when first examined, and none of the 52 patients had a final outcome better than severe disability.[38]

Pupillary size during the initial hours after the insult is another useful prognostic indicator.[46] The pupils dilate and responsiveness to light are lost within a few minutes of cardiac arrest. Pupillary dilatation throughout resuscitation indicates a poor prognosis. Drugs, especially catecholamines and atropine, can affect pupillary size, so clinicians should be cautious about using pupillary size as a prognostic sign in patients who have received drugs that affect pupillary diameter. Persistent dilation of the pupils is an ominous sign.

The depth of coma is another important indicator during the first hours after cardiac arrest. Deep coma usually means extensive brainstem dysfunction or important injury to the cerebral hemispheres bilaterally. In most adults when the hypoxic-ischemic insult is severe enough to injure the brainstem and cause deep coma and loss of brainstem reflexes, the cerebral hemispheres are even more severely damaged because structures in the cerebrum are more vulnerable to hypoxia than brainstem nuclei.

During the early hours, analysis of spontaneous movements of the limbs and motor responses of the limbs to sensory stimuli are useful in prognosis. The absence of limb movement, even after pinching, is an unfavorable prognostic sign. The presence of only automatic decorticate (flexion of the upper limbs and extension of the lower limbs) or decerebrate (extension of the upper and lower limbs) responses to painful stimuli also is an unfavorable sign for survival and good recovery. Spontaneous varied limb movements and normal withdrawal of limbs to pain is a favorable sign.

Some patients have frequent myoclonic movements during the first hours after resuscitation. Sudden jerks of the limbs, face, jaw, and eyelids are common. The jerks are often bilateral and synchronous and can be accompanied by upward movement of the eyes and twitching of the eyelids. The jerks are often precipitated by touch, tracheal suctioning, insertion of catheters, and noise. The jerks can also be precipitated by a loud clap. Frequent myoclonic jerks predict death or at best a persistent vegetative state.

Roine analyzed the prognostic importance of seizures among 155 patients who survived out-of-hospital cardiac arrest in Helsinki.[35] Seizures during the first 24 hours were not helpful prognostically. Fifty-three percent of patients who had seizures during the first day survived, compared with 70% of survivors who had no first-day seizures. Seizures after the first day were associated with a poor outcome, however, because only three of 15 patients (20%) with seizures after the first day recovered consciousness, and only one patient (7%) lived for 1 year. Status epilepticus at any time after cardiac arrest was a dire sign because all nine patients with epileptic status died.

In patients who survive the first 24 hours, prognostic indicators are somewhat different during the next few days. Absence of the normal brainstem pupillary, corneal, oculovestibular, and pharyngeal reflexes at 24 hours indicates a poor prognosis. Persistent brainstem dysfunction means brainstem and severe hemispheral damage because the hemispheres are almost always more damaged than the brainstem. Most patients who eventually survive the acute hypoxic-ischemic insult have bihemispheral coma or have become alert by 24 hours. The duration and depth of coma is probably the most important prognostic indicator during the first days. Prolonged bihemispheral coma is a poor prognostic indicator. In one series, day 2 was the most common time for patients to emerge from coma, and most patients who survived awakened by the end of day 2. Only 2 of the 27 patients (7%) in deep coma through day 2 survived.[39] In another series, no patient in postanoxic coma after the third day survived.[42] In another series, 5 of 12 patients (42%) with good outcome remained in coma for 2 or more days, but all but 1 of the 12 patients awakened and reached their best level of function within the first week after resuscitation.[47]

Eye opening, eye movements, and motor responses are also useful prognostic indicators during the first few days. By the end of the first day, the absence of spontaneous eye opening indicates a poor prognosis. Most patients who have a good recovery begin to open their eyes and have at least intermittent visual fixation movements. The presence of eye opening, however, does not always indicate a good outcome. In one large series, spontaneous eye opening often occurred by 48 hours in patients with both good and bad outcomes. Persistent roving eye movements without visual fixation usually mean severe bilateral cerebral hemispheral damage and indicate a poor outcome. Sustained up-gaze also carries a poor prognosis.[48]

The absence of withdrawal limb movements when painful stimuli are given is also a poor prognostic sign, as is persistence of obligatory reflex decorticate or decerebrate posturing. Most patients who have a good recovery begin to obey commands during the first few days. The most reliable way of judging prognosis is to perform careful repeated neurologic examinations within the first hours and days after the insult.

Clinicians are often involved in declaring brain death after cardiac arrest. The following criteria are often used as indicators of brain death, an irreversible state in which there is no precedent for meaningful survival.[49-51] Physicians in some states within the USA and other countries can declare death if criteria for brain death are met, despite persistence of cardiac function. However, the issue of when an individual is dead has very important religious, economic, and political implications and rules vary considerably even between different hospitals in the same region.

1. Coma with loss of cerebral reactivity
2. Absence of spontaneous respiration
3. Loss of brainstem reflexes (pupillary, corneal, oculovestibular, and oculocephalic)
4. Electrocerebral silence (so-called flat electroencephalogram [EEG]) for longer than 12 hours (in the absence of hypothermia or sedative drugs)

Often, the local rules require a time duration for persistent loss of brainstem reflexes including respiratory drive, most often 24 hours. The requirement for electrocerebral silence by EEG is variable. Absence of blood flow in the cranium is another criteria sometime applied.

> In AR, blood sugar was 150 mg/dl on admission. At 1 hour after arrest, the pH was 7.32. CT was normal. EEG showed diffuse delta and theta slowing, but the background changed when the patient was pinched and light was shown in the face. By day 3, he had awakened and spoke normally but had a severe amnesic syndrome.

The level of blood sugar at the time of arrest is one factor that affects recovery. Myers and Yamaguchi showed that young monkeys given infusions of glucose before induced cardiac arrest had more cerebral damage than similarly studied animals infused with saline.[52] Others have corroborated these findings in adult animals and showed that more severe damage also results when glucose is given after the ischemic insult.[53] The damage may be caused by production of lactate, which can injure brain tissue. Systemic lactic acidosis can clearly compound the cerebral damage. Poor neurologic recovery after cardiac arrest was linked to higher blood-sugar levels (300 mg/dL) in one human study.[54] High blood-sugar levels also contribute to a poor outcome in patients with embolic brain infarcts and intracerebral hemorrhage and after thrombolysis. Theoretically, high blood calcium levels might also have a deleterious effect.

EEGs of patients in coma after cardiac arrest are usually abnormal and contain diffuse slowing in the theta and delta ranges, as well as periodic phenomena and epileptiform discharges. In the most severe injuries, the EEG may be flat-electrocerebral silence. Severe slowing or low amplitude of the background activity has a bad prognosis, especially if documented in EEGs 12 or 24 hours apart.

Some patients in deep coma from hypoxic-ischemic injury have preserved alpha activity.

Alpha coma activity differs from normal rhythms as follows[55,56]:

1. It is usually faster (9 to 12 cycles/second), compared with the usual (8 to 10 cycles/second) alpha.
2. It is more frontal, central, and parietal, as compared with the usual occipital location.
3. It is usually temporary.
4. It does not respond to auditory, photic, or tactile stimuli.

Evoked-response testing may also help determine the severity of cerebral injury. The bilateral absence of somatosensory evoked potentials predicts that the patient with hypoxic/ischemic coma will not survive.[56a,57,58] The N20 and N70 responses are particularly useful for prognosis. The absence of the N20 response is predictive of death or a vegetative state. In one study, only one of 21 patients with loss of the N20 component of the somatosensory evoked potential survived, compared with survival of 11 of 26 patients in whom the N20 response was present.[58] Five patients that had retained N70 responses recovered awareness in this study.[58]

Brain imaging has often not been helpful during the first days after cardiac arrest, but few studies of CT or magnetic resonance imaging (MRI) have been performed during the acute period after cardiac arrest.[59-63] Many patients are too unstable to be transported to MRI scanners. Kjos et al studied early CT findings in 10 patients.[59] Nine patients had some evidence of diffuse cerebral edema, and six patients had poor discrimination between the grey and white matter. Watershed cerebral and cerebellar infarcts and bilateral basal ganglia and thalamic hypodensities are also found in some patients. Diffuse mass effect with obliteration of basal cisterns has been described but is rare.[60] In some patients, brain edema and discrete infarcts are seen after several days.

Roine analyzed MRI findings among 155 patients resuscitated after out-of-hospital cardiac arrest and compared the findings with 88 controls.[61] Brain infarcts were more common after cardiac arrest but the difference was significant only for deep infarcts. Twenty-five percent of patients had cortical infarcts, 14% had cerebral watershed infarcts, 21% had deep cerebral infarcts, and 4% had deep watershed infarcts. The number of infarcts and multiple infarcts were more common in the resuscitated group. Two patients had diffuse hypointensity of the cerebral white matter. Severe edema on MRI or CT scans was a dire prognostic sign. Repeated MRI examinations during the course of patients with severe neurologic deficits may show high-signal

intensity cortical lesions compatible with laminar necrosis[62] or restricted diffusion in the splenium of the corpus callosum.[63]

Single-photon emission CT (SPECT) can show changes in cerebral blood flow after cardiac arrest, but the changes are quite nonspecific.[64] Usually, the decreased perfusion is most severe frontally. In one study, regional cerebral blood flow was almost invariably abnormal after cardiac arrest.[35] Regional blood flow improved over time in some patients but often remained abnormal. No consistent correlation was found between blood flow and outcome.

The brains of patients considered brain dead are usually soft and necrotic at necropsy. Angiography before death reveals an absence of intracranial circulation. Brain swelling is extensive, as to block antegrade flow of blood into the cranium. Absence of blood flow into the intracranial arteries is not compatible with survival. The transcranial Doppler (TCD) system has been used since the early 1990s to evaluate patients for the determination of brain death.[65-67]

TREATMENT

Little is known about optimal treatment of patients to minimize cerebral damage after cardiac arrest, although many experimental and clinical studies deal with this problem. Surprisingly, at the time of this writing no neuroprotectant drug had undergone randomized trials in this group of patients. Certainly, it is important to maintain good cardiac output and ventilation and prevent complications of the stuporous state, such as aspiration, pneumonia, and urosepsis. Recent studies have shown that hypothermia can be effective, but the use of hypothermia requires experience.

Hypothermia

When many of these treatments are combined in the experimental animal, brain damage is reduced, although evidence that any single treatment is effective is scant.[71] Much more work is needed to answer the important question of how to optimally treat patients with brain dysfunction after cardiac arrest.

Cardiac Encephalopathy

Patients with diverse heart diseases often develop abnormal states of alertness and cognitive and behavioral abnormalities, especially those in congestive heart failure.[72,73] The causes of brain dysfunction in patients with congestive heart failure are multifactorial. Systemic venous pressure is increased leading to increased pressure in the dural venous sinuses and veins within the cranial cavity. Increased intracranial venous pressure decreases absorption of cerebrospinal fluid (CSF) and so an increased amount of fluid may accumulate in the cisterns around the brain, in the subarachnoid spaces, and sometimes within the cerebral ventricles. The CSF pressure may be elevated when measured by lumbar puncture. Brain edema may result from the increased venous pressure and increased amounts of CSF.

Maintenance of an effective arteriovenous pressure difference is required to adequately perfuse the brain. Arterial pressure and cerebral blood flow must be maintained and even augmented in patients with elevated intracranial venous pressures. Cardiac decompensation can limit the ability of the heart and systemic circulation to increase cerebral blood flow and create an effective arteriovenous pressure difference to maintain adequate brain perfusion.

Left heart failure is often associated with fluid accumulation and venous distention in the lungs and the development of pleural effusions. Hypoxia related to pulmonary dysfunction and hypoventilation reduces the oxygen content of the blood that reaches neurons in the brain. Dysfunction of other organs especially the liver and kidneys, and electrolyte, blood volume, acid-base abnormalities, and drug side effects also can compound the cardiac encephalopathy.

Neurological abnormalities most often occur when cardiac failure is most severe and the clinical signs are indistinguishable from those found in patients with renal failure and CO_2 narcosis or in other metabolic encephalopathies. These abnormalities include decreased state of alertness and consciousness, a generalized decrease in all intellectual functions, variability from minute to minute and from hour to hour in neurologic signs, asterixis (a metabolic "flap"), and diffuse slowing of rhythms on EEGs.

A somewhat different clinical picture, similar to that found in patients with hydrocephalus, occasionally develops in patients with congestive heart failure. This syndrome can develop during treatment of congestive failure and may occur even after cardiac compensation when the patient is recovering from heart failure. The major feature of this syndrome is abulia. Abulic patients have severely reduced spontaneous behavior. They seem content to sit or lie about without doing much. They show little or no interest in television, reading, listening to the radio, conversations, or any other activity. The quantity of spontaneous initiated speech is reduced. When asked questions or urged to perform tasks, abulic patients often fail to respond or do so only after a relatively long interval. When the examiner repeats questions or directions, patients often say that they had heard the request the first time, but just couldn't get started to reply or act. Responses when they are forthcoming are generally short, laconic, and terse. Patients don't persist with familiar tasks, such as naming 10 zoo animals or 10 articles of clothing, and counting backward from 20 to 1. Intellectual functions including memory, language, and ability to draw and copy are usually preserved, although these functions take longer than usual to perform and require frequent prodding to complete. The patients remain alert despite their inactivity and slowness in contrast to other encephalopathies that are invariably accompanied by drowsiness and later stupor. Friends and family describe abulic patients as "bumps on a log" or "couch potatoes."

> A 67-year-old woman entered the hospital in severe congestive heart failure. She was known to have severe aortic and mitral valve disease and had lower extremity edema, ascites, and pleural effusions. She was vigorously treated with diuretics, bed rest, and thoracentesis and her congestive heart failure greatly improved. As her heart failure improved, her husband and family noted a marked personality change. Usually outgoing, friendly, and talkative, now she became very quiet, uninterested, apathetic, and inert. She denied any feelings of discouragement or depression. She seemed not to heed questions. Her replies were usually one or two words—yes, no, or single-word—that were usually correct. Her motor, sensory, visual, and reflex examinations were normal except that she had bilateral Babinski signs. Cranial CT scan was read as showing "cerebral atrophy" because of increased CSF in the sulci. After lumbar punctures that removed CSF, she returned to her former self and her plantar responses became flexor.[72,73]

This abulic syndrome associated with congestive heart failure is most likely caused by retention of CSF within the intracranial cavity. Pericardial, pleural, and peritoneal effusions are quite common and well known in patients with congestive heart failure. Effusions within the cranial cavity probably have the same explanation as pleural and peritoneal effusions. The meninges are connective tissue structures very similar in structure and function to the pleura, pericardium, and peritoneum. CSF effusions can develop similarly to pleural effusions. Increased venous pressure leads to decreased absorption of CSF at the same time that production of CSF continues unchanged. The amount of CSF increases and fluid accumulates in the cisterns around the brain, in the subarachnoid space, and sometimes in the ventricles. Compensation and correction of congestive heart failure does not always result in full reabsorption of pleural and pericardial effusions and ascites. The pressure in the intracranial venous sinuses and neck and cranial veins that drain the head may normalize sufficiently to prevent further CSF effusions but not enough to allow absorption and clearing of the effusions already present. Similarly thoracentesis and abdominocentesis may be needed to remove persistent pleural fluid and ascites even after treatment with diuretics and cardiac drugs.

CT scans in patients with the hydrocephalic, abulic syndrome are often read as showing "brain atrophy." Radiologists see increased CSF between cerebral and cerebellar gyri and interpret the widening of the sulci as indicating loss of brain tissue. Of course increased quantity of intracranial CSF can expand the sulci and cause an increased amount of fluid outside the brain (so-called "external hydrocephalus") as well as some enlargement of the ventricular system ("internal hydrocephalus"). Usually there is no major enlargement of the cerebral ventricles. Lumbar puncture in patients with the abulic syndrome, may be followed by clinical improvement and normalization of the "brain atrophy" shown by CT. Sulci become smaller and the gyri widen. CT scans may take time to normalize after lumbar puncture and after treatment of congestive heart failure.

Some reports of patients with, severe heart disease, syncope, and congestive heart failure have noted a high frequency of cognitive abnormalities and strokes.[72-78] The most detailed information about cognitive functions in patients with severe heart disease comes from studies of patients considered for cardiac transplantation.[77,78] Neuropsychological tests are often included as part of the routine battery of testing before transplantation, and these tests are sometimes repeated after transplantation. Schall and colleagues studied 54 patients, among whom 20 had idiopathic myocardiopathies and 25 had ischemic cardiomyopathies.[77] The mean left ventricular ejection fraction in these patients was 20%, and the mean cardiac index was 2.6 L/minute/m[2]. The most consistent impairments were in tests of memory and visual and tactile perception; 56% of patients were moderately impaired on logical memory tests and this increased to 61% when 30-minute delays were introduced into the memory testing.[77] Bornstein et al studied 62 patients (mean age 44.7 years) who were evaluated for cardiac transplantation.[78] Forty-five percent of these patients had dilated cardiomyopathies and 40% had ischemic cardiomyopathies. The patients were impaired on 50% of the neuropsychological measures; 58% of patients met the authors' prespecified criteria for overall impairment, which was that 45% or more of the cognitive test scores fell into an impaired range. Impaired intellectual functioning correlated with elevated right atrial pressure. Better performance correlated with higher stroke volume, stroke volume index, and cardiac index. Eleven of these patients were retested (seven who had transplantation and four who did not) on average 36 months after the initial test battery. The transplant patients generally showed improvement and those patients who did not have transplantation usually had lower scores than before.[78] The authors considered that elevated right atrial pressure was probably a marker for biventricular failure and low cardiac output and that the cognitive deficits might relate to chronically reduced brain blood flow.[78]

The syndromes of cardiac encephalopathy are under-recognized and are virtually unknown to cardiologists. Congestive heart failure is, however, becoming more widely recognized as an important risk factor for cognitive dysfunction.[79]

References

1. Mohr JP: Neurological complications of cardiac valvular disease and cardiac surgery including systemic hypotension. In Vinken P, Bruyn G (eds): Handbook of Clinical Neurology, vol 38. Neurological Manifestations of Systemic Disease. Amsterdam: North Holland Publishing, 1979, pp 143-171.
2. Balint R: Seelenlahmung des Schauens, optische Ataxie, raumliche Storung der Aufmerksamkeit. Z Psychiatr Neurol 1909;25:51-81.
3. Tyler HR: Cerebral Disturbance of Vision in Neuro-Ophthalmology, vol 4. St. Louis: Mosby, 1968.
4. Hecaen H, Ajuriaguerra J: Balint's syndrome and its minor forms. Brain 1954;77:373-400.
5. Benson DF, Davis RJ, Snyder BD: Posterior cortical atrophy. Arch Neurol 1988;45:789-793.
6. Zulch K: On the circulatory disturbances in the borderline zones of the cerebral and spinal vessels. In Greenfield JG, Russell D (eds): Proceedings of the Second International Congress on Neuropathology, vol 8. Amsterdam: Excerpta Medica, 1955, pp 894-895.
7. Romanul F, Abramowicz A: Changes in brain and pial vessels in arterial border zones. Arch Neurol 1974;11:40-65.
8. Sage JI, Van Uitest RL: Man-in-the-barrel syndrome. Neurology 1986;36:1102-1103.
9. Copley D, Mantel J, Rogers W, et al: Improved outcome for prehospital cardiopulmonary collapse with resuscitation by bystanders. Circulation 1977;56:901-905.
10. Lund I, Skulberg A: Cardiopulmonary resuscitation by lay people. Lancet 1975;2:702-704.
11. Caplan LR: Cardiac arrest and other hypoxic ischemic insults. In Caplan LR, Hurst JW,

Chimowitz M (eds): Clinical Neurocardiology. New York: Marcel Dekker, 1999, pp 1-34.

12. Adams JH, Brierley JB, Connor RCR, Treip CS: The effects of systemic hypotension upon the human brain: Clinical and neuropathological observations in 11 cases. Brain 1966;89: 235-268.

13. Gilles F: Hypotensive brainstem necrosis. Arch Pathol 1969;88:32-41.

14. Roland EH, Hill A, Norman MG, et al: Selective brainstem injury in an asphyxiated newborn. Ann Neurol 1988;23:89-92.

15. Fisher CM: The neurological examination of the comatose patient. Acta Neurol Scand 1969;45(suppl 36):5-56.

16. Caronna J, Finkelstein S: Neurologic syndrome after cardiac arrest. Stroke 1978;9:517-520.

17. Volpe B, Hirst W: The characterization of an amnesic syndrome following hypoxic-ischemic injury. Arch Neurol 1983;40:436-440.

18. Cummings J, Tomiyasu U, Reed S, et al: Amnesia with hippocampal lesion after cardiopulmonary arrest. Neurology 1984;34:679-681.

19. Petito C, Feldmann E, Pulsinelli W, Plum F: Delayed hippocampal damage in humans following cardiorespiratory arrest. Neurology 1987;37: 1281-1286.

20. Brierley JB, Adams JH, Graham D, et al: Neocortical death after cardiac arrest: A clinical, neurophysiological, and neuropathological report of two cases. Lancet 1971;2:560-565.

21. Dougherty J, Rawlinson D, Levy D, et al: Hypoxic-ischemic brain injury and the vegetative state: Clinical and neuropathologic correlation. Neurology 1981;31:991-997.

22. Young GB, Gilbert JJ, Zochodne DW: The significance of myoclonic status epilepticus in postanoxic coma. Neurology 1990;40: 1843-1848.

23. Wijdicks EFM, Parisi JE, Sharbrough FW: Prognostic value of myoclonic status in comatose survivors of cardiac arrest. Ann Neurol 1994;35:239-243.

24. Krumholz A, Stern BJ, Weiss HD: Outcome from coma after cardiopulmonary resuscitation. Relation to seizures and myoclonus. Neurology 1988;38: 401-405.

25. Jennett B, Plum F: Persistent vegetative state after brain damage: A syndrome in search of a name. Lancet 1972;1:734-737.

26. Dooling E, Richardson E: Delayed encephalopathy after strangling. Arch Neurol 1976;33:196-199.

27. Lance J, Adams R: The syndrome of intention and action myoclonus as a sequel to hypoxic encephalopathy. Brain 1963;86:111-133.

28. Plum F, Posner JB, Hain R: Delayed neurologic deterioration after anoxia. Arch Intern Med 1962;110:56-67.

29. Ginsberg MD, Hedley-White T, Richardson EP: Hypoxic-ischemic leukoencephalopathy in man. Arch Neurol 1976;33:5-14.

30. Hori A, Hirose G, Kataoka K, et al: Delayed postanoxic encephalopathy after strangulation. Arch Neurol 1991;48:871-874.

31. Weinberger LM, Schmidley JW, Schafer IA, Raghaven S: Delayed postanoxic demyelination and arylsulfatase—A pseudodeficiency. Neurology 1994;44:152-154.

32. Gottfried JA, Mayer SA, Shungu DC, et al: Delayed posthypoxic demyelination: Association with arylsulfatase—A deficiency and lactic acidosis on proton MR spectroscopy. Neurology 1997;49:1400-1404.

32a. Chen-Plotkin AC, Pau KT, Schmahmann JD: Delayed leukoencephalopathy after hypoxic-ischemic injury. Arch Neurol 2008;65:144-145.

32b. Kriegstein AR, Shungu DC, Miller WS et al: Leukoencephalopathy and brain raised lactate from heroin vapor inhalation ("chasing the dragon"). Neurology 1999;53:1765-1773.

33. Caronna J, Finkelstein S: Neurologic syndromes after cardiac arrest. Stroke 1978;9:517-520.

34. Silver JR, Buxton PH: Spinal stroke. Brain 1974;97:539-550.

35. Roine RO: Neurological Outcome of Out-of-Hospital Cardiac Arrest [dissertation]. University of Helsinki, 1993.

36. Earnest MP, Breckinridge JC, Yarnell PR, Oliva PB: Quality of survival after out-of-hospital cardiac arrest: Predictive value of early neurologic evaluation. Neurology 1979;29:56-60.

37. Wijdicks E: Neurological complications of cardiac arrest. In Wijdicks EFM (ed): Neurology of Critical Illness. Philadelphia: FA Davis, 1995, pp 86-103.

38. Levy DE, Caronna JJ, Singer BH, et al: Predicting outcome from hypoxic-ischemic coma. JAMA 1985;253:1420-1426.

39. Snyder BD, Loewenson RB, Gumnit RJ, et al: Neurologic prognosis after cardiopulmonary arrest: II. Level of consciousness. Neurology 1980;30:52-58.

40. Snyder BD, Gumnit RJ, Leppik IE, et al: Neurologic prognosis after cardiopulmonary arrest: IV. Brainstem reflexes. Neurology 1981;31: 1092-1097.

41. Bates D, Caronna J, Cartlidge NEF, et al: A prospective study of nontraumatic coma: Methods and results in 310 patients. Ann Neurol 1977;2:211-220.

42. Bell JA, Hodgson HJF: Coma after cardiac arrest. Brain 1974;97:361-372.

43. Longstreth WT, Diehr P, Inui TS: Prediction of awakening after out-of-hospital cardiac arrest. N Engl J Med 1983;308:1378-1382.

44. Shewmon DA, DeGiorgio CM: Early prognosis in anoxic coma: Reliability and rationale. Neurol Clin 1989;7:823-843.

45. Plum F: Vulnerability of the brain and heart after cardiac arrest. N Engl J Med 1991;324: 1278-1280.

46. Steen-Hansen JE, Hansen NN, Vaagenes P, Schreiner B: Pupil size and light reactivity during cardiopulmonary resuscitation. A clinical study. Crit Care Med 1988;16:69-70.

47. Bassetti C, Bomio F, Mathis J, Hess CW: Early prognosis in coma after cardiac arrest: A prospective clinical, electrophysiological,

10

and biochemical study of 60 patients. J Neurol Neurosurg Psychiatry 1996;61: 610-615.

48. Keane JR: Sustained upgaze in coma. Ann Neurol 1981;9:409-412.

49. Ad Hoc Committee of the Harvard Medical School: A definition of irreversible coma. Report of the Ad Hoc Committee of the Harvard Medical School to examine the definition of brain death. JAMA 1968;205:337-340.

50. Walker A: An appraisal of the criteria of cerebral death. JAMA 1977;237:982-986.

51. Shemie SD, Pollack MM, Morioka M, Bonner S: Diagnosis of brain death in children. Lancet Neurol 2007;6:87-92.

52. Myers C, Yamaguchi S: Nervous system effects of cardiac arrest in monkeys. Arch Neurol 1977;34:65-74.

53. Plum F: What causes infarction in ischemic brain? Neurology 1983;33:222-233.

54. Longstreth W, Inui T: High blood glucose level on hospital admission and poor neurological recovery after cardiac arrest. Ann Neurol 1984;15:59-63.

55. Westmoreland B, Klass D, Sharbrough F, et al: Alpha coma. Arch Neurol 1975;32:713-718.

56. Chokroverty S: "Alpha-like" rhythms in electro-encephalograms in coma after cardiac arrest. Neurology 1975;25:655-663.

56a. Chen R, Bolton CF, Young B: Prediction of outcome in patients with anoxic coma: A clinical and electrophysiological study. Crit Care Med 1996;24:672-678.

57. Kaplan PW: Electrophysiological prognostication and brain injury from cardiac arrest. Semin Neurol 2006;26:403-412.

58. Young GB, Doig G, Ragazzoni A: Anoxic-ischemic encephalopathy: Clinical and electrophysiological associations with outcome. Neurocrit Care 2005;2:159-164.

59. Kjos BO, Brandt-Zawadzki M, Young RG: Early CT findings of global central nervous system hypoperfusion. AJNR Am J Neuroradiol 1983;4:1043-1048.

60. Morimoto Y, Kemmotsu O, Kitami K, et al: Acute brain swelling after out-of-hospital cardiac arrest: Pathogenesis and outcome. Crit Care Med 1993;21:104-110.

61. Roine RO, Raininko R, Erkinjuntti T, et al: Magnetic resonance imaging findings associated with cardiac arrest. Stroke 1993;24:1005-1014.

62. Sawada H, Udaka F, Seriu N, et al: MRI demonstration of cortical laminar necrosis and delayed white matter injury in anoxic encephalopathy. Neuroradiology 1990;32:319-321.

63. Bianchi MT, Sims JR: Restricted diffusion in the splenium of the corpus callosum after cardiac arrest. Open Neuroimag J 2008;2:1-4.

64. Roine RO, Launes J, Nikkinen P, et al: Regional cerebral blood flow after human cardiac arrest. Arch Neurol 1991;48:625-629.

65. Caplan LR, Brass LM, DeWitt LD, et al: Transcranial Doppler ultrasound: Present status. Neurology 1990;40:696-700.

66. Kirkham F, Levin S, Padayachee T, et al: Transcranial pulsed Doppler ultrasound findings in brainstem death. J Neurol Neurosurg Psychiatry 1987;50:1504-1513.

67. Ropper A, Kehne S, Wechsler L: Transcranial Doppler in brain death. Neurology 1987;37: 1733-1735.

68. McIntyre LA, Fergusson DA, Hebert PC, et al: Prolonged therapeutic hypothermia after traumatic brain injury in adults: A systematic review. JAMA 2003;289:2992-2999.

69. Greer DM: Hypothermia for cardiac arrest. Curr Neurol Neurosci Rep 2006;6:518-524.

70. Sanders AB: Therapeutic hypothermia after cardiac arrest. Curr Opin Crit Care 2006;12: 213-217.

71. Giswold S, Safar P, Rao G, et al: Multifaceted therapy after global brain ischemia in monkeys. Stroke 1984;15:803-812.

72. Caplan LR: Cardiac encephalopathy and congestive heart failure: A hypothesis about the relationship. Neurology 2006;66:99-101.

73. Caplan LR: Encephalopathies and neurological effects of drugs used in cardiac patients. In Caplan LR, Hurst JW, Chimowitz MI (eds): Clinical Neurocardiology. New York: Marcel Dekker, 1999, pp 186-225.

74. Appelros P: Heart failure and stroke. Stroke 2006;37:1637.

75. Zuccala G, Cattel C, Manes-Gravina, et al: Left ventricular dysfunction: A clue to cognitive impairment in older patients with heart failure. J Neurol Neurosurg Psychiatry 1997;63:509-512.

76. Garcia CA, Tweedy JR, Blass JP: Underdiagnosis of cognitive impairment in a rehabilitation setting. J Am Geriatr Soc 1984;32:339-342.

77. Schall RR, Petrucci RJ, Brozena SC, et al: Cognitive function in patients with symptomatic dilated cardiomyopathy before and after cardiac transplantation. J Am Coll Cardiol 1989;14:1666-1672.

78. Bornstein RA, Starling RC, Myerowitz P, Haas GJ: Neuropsychological function in patients with end-stage heart failure before and after cardiac transplantation. Acta Neurol Scand 1995;91: 260-265.

79. Sangha SS, Uber PA, Park MH, et al: Difficult cases in heart failure: The challenge of neurocognitive dysfunction in severe heart failure. Congest Heart Fail 2002;8:232-234.

Nonatherosclerotic Vasculopathies

11

Many different nonatherosclerotic vascular diseases cause brain ischemia. Some of these conditions also cause ocular ischemia and intracranial hemorrhage. Some have been well characterized, whereas information about pathogenesis and clinical features for others is meager. Herein, I discuss the most frequent and important conditions. Some are also discussed in other chapters. The topic is so diverse that I can only include brief descriptions with reference citations. *Uncommon Causes of Stroke*, 2nd edition, offers much more detailed descriptions of many of these conditions.[1]

ARTERIAL DISSECTIONS

Dissection of extracranial arteries was once considered rare. Reports of Fisher, Ojemann, and colleagues in the 1970s clarified the clinical and radiologic features in patients with dissection of the internal carotid artery (ICA).[2,3] Increased awareness of the clinical symptoms and signs, and the advent of safe and rapid non-invasive vascular imaging has led to more frequent diagnosis of arterial dissections of brain-supplying arteries.[4,5] The extracranial ICA is the most commonly affected artery and is usually involved in its pharyngeal and distal extracranial segments well above the ICA origin. This location is unusual for atherosclerosis, which almost invariably affects the internal carotid origin or the carotid siphon. Dissections of the extracranial vertebral artery (ECVA) affect the vessel in its distal segment between its emergence from the vertebral column and its dural penetration, or in the first segment of the artery above the vertebral artery (VA) origin but before entrance into the transverse foramina.[4-8] The pharyngeal ICA and the first and third segments of the ECVA are more mobile and less firmly anchored than the origins and intracranial penetration sites of these arteries. Dissections often involve loops and redundant portions of the extracranial arteries.[9]

Most dissections involve some trauma, stretch, or mechanical stress. Trauma may be severe but can be trivial (e.g., twisting the neck to avoid a falling tree branch, lunging for a Ping-Pong ball, or turning the neck abruptly while backing up a car or skiing). Many examples of so-called spontaneous dissection are triggered by minor trauma that is forgotten or deemed inconsequential by the patient. Congenital or acquired abnormalities of the connective tissue elements in the media or elastica of the arteries and edema of the arterial wall can promote dissection. Marfan's syndrome, cystic medial necrosis, fibromuscular dysplasia, Ehlers-Danlos type 4 syndrome, Loeys-Dietz syndrome, and migraine are disorders found more often than expected in patients with arterial dissections.[4,5] Ultrastructural connective tissue abnormalities of collagen and extracellular matrix are sometimes found in the skin of patients with extracranial arterial dissections.[10] Plasma levels of matrix metalloproteinase-2 (MMP-2) are higher in patients with cervical artery dissections than controls especially in patients with recurrent dissections.[10a]

A tear within the arterial wall leads to bleeding. Usually, blood dissects within the media along the longitudinal course of the artery. Dissection in the plane between the media and adventitia sometimes causes aneurysmal out-pouching of the artery. Dissections also produce an intimal tear, allowing the intramural hematoma to reenter the lumen (Fig. 11-1). The expanded arterial wall may encroach on the lumen. Thrombus is often present within the lumen as a result of reentry of the intramural hematoma or because of stasis of blood flow caused by luminal compromise. The intramural expansion probably also stimulates the endothelium to release factors promoting thrombosis. The luminal clot is usually only loosely adherent to the intima and can readily embolize distally. In the weeks and months after dissection, the intramural blood is absorbed, and the lumen usually returns to its normal size. Aneurysmal pouches may remain as a mark of the healed lesion.

Often in carotid artery dissection, the most impressive feature is pain. Ipsilateral throbbing headache and sharp pain locally in the neck, jaw, pharynx, or face are often noted, separating dissection from ordinary atherosclerotic occlusion.[4,5,11-14] The sympathetic fibers traveling along the wall of the ICA are usually disturbed, leading to an ipsilateral partial Horner's syndrome characterized by ptosis and meiosis. Facial sweat function is preserved because the sympathetic innervation of the sweat glands travels along the external carotid artery (ECA).

Transient ischemic attacks (TIAs) are common and may involve the ipsilateral eye and brain. The

11

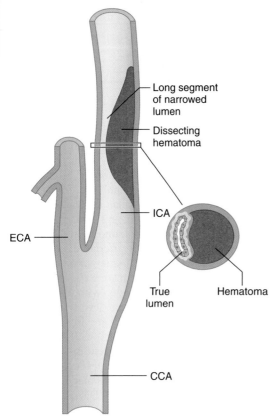

Figure 11-1. Cartoon showing dissection of the internal carotid artery. The inset is a cross-section view showing the hematoma and the luminal compromise. CCA, common carotid artery; ECA, external carotid artery; ICA, internal carotid artery.

spells often occur in rapid succession over hours or a few days leading Fisher to coin the term *carotid allegro*.[2] Some patients with ICA dissection have visual scintillations and bright sparkles resembling migraine, even though many have had no personal or family history of migraine. Some patients hear a pulsatile noise in the head or ear. TIAs are probably caused by luminal compromise with distal hypoperfusion, but most patients with severe strokes have evidence of embolization of clot to the middle cerebral artery (MCA) from thrombus at the site of the dissection. When the ICA dissection extends to the carotid siphon, ischemic optic neuropathy can develop as a result of decreased perfusion of arteries supplying the optic nerve.[15] If a stroke develops, it usually occurs soon after the ICA dissection but may occur during the days and weeks after the event. Late stroke is rare but has been reported after traumatic ICA dissection.[16] At times, dissections cause sequential symptoms during days to weeks. Pain may first develop in the neck and persist for days and subside. The pain may recur days or even weeks later and be accompanied by ischemic attacks or strokes.

Undoubtedly, the initial tear extended and more intramural bleeding developed when the symptoms worsened. At times, both carotid arteries and even the VAs are dissected at the same time.

Ultrasound testing can suggest the presence of dissection. B-mode ultrasound can show tapering of the ICA lumen beginning well above the ICA origin, an irregular membrane crossing the lumen, and even demonstration of true and false lumens.[17,17a] Continuous wave (CW) Doppler can show a typical pattern characterized by a high-amplitude signal with markedly reduced systolic Doppler frequencies and alternating flow directions over the region of luminal narrowing.[18] This Doppler signal probably results from abnormal vessel wall pulsations and some bidirectional movement of the blood column. Duplex scans of the VAs in the neck can also suggest dissection.[19] Typical findings are increased arterial diameter, decreased pulsatility, intravascular abnormal echoes, and hemodynamic evidence of decreased flow. Color Doppler flow imaging can also show the regions of dissection within the neck. Diminished flow in the high neck at the level of the atlas detected by CW Doppler and decreased flow in the intracranial VA shown by transcranial Doppler (TCD) suggest the presence of distal ECVA dissections. In patients with extracranial ICA dissections, TCD may show diminished intracranial velocities in the ICA siphon and MCA. When this occurs in young patients without risk factors for atherosclerosis or embolism with normal ICA bifurcations in the neck, the diagnosis of dissection is likely.

Diagnosis of arterial dissection has traditionally been made by standard catheter angiography. Figure 11-2 is a cartoon that illustrates various

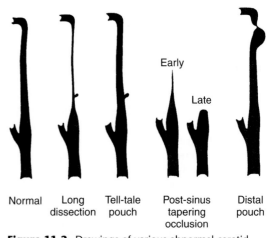

Figure 11-2. Drawings of various abnormal carotid arteriograms in patients with carotid-artery dissection. (From Fisher CM, Ojemann RG, Robertson GH: Spontaneous dissection of cervicocerebral arteries, Can J Neurol Sci 1978;5:9-19, with permission.)

arteriographic features of carotid dissections. Figure 11-3 is a montage of angiograms in patients with extracranial ICA dissections. The most common angiographic finding is a string sign (see Fig. 11-3A), consisting of a long, narrow column of contrast material that begins distal to the carotid bifurcation and can extend to the base of the skull.[2,3] There may also be total occlusion of the ICA. This occlusion differs from the typical atherosclerotic occlusion; ICA

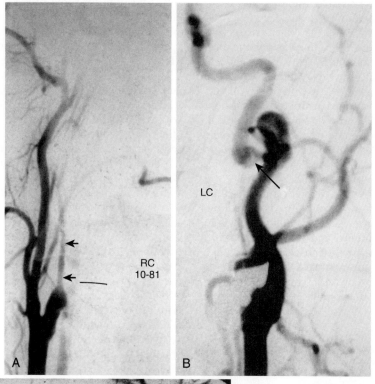

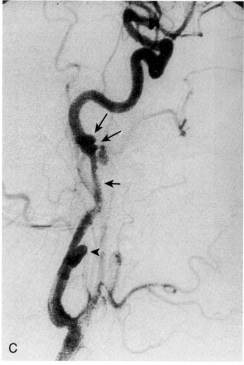

Figure 11-3. Montage of carotid artery angiograms in patients with extracranial ICA dissections. **A,** Abrupt change in diameter of the internal carotid artery with a long string-like narrowing *(small black arrows)*. **B,** Aneurysmal dilatation of a tortuous carotid artery with an acute dissection. The *large black arrow* points to a region of narrowing. **C,** Long carotid-artery dissection with regions of narrowing and aneurysmal pouches. The *arrowhead* points to an aneurysmal dilatation at the proximal end of the dissection. The *lower black arrow* points to a region of narrowing of the artery and the *double black arrows* point to an irregular aneurysmal dilatation more distally in the pharyngeal portion of the artery.

11

occlusions caused by dissection usually begin more than 2 cm distal to the origin of the ICA, spare the carotid sinus, and have a gradually tapering segment that ends in the occlusion. There may also be localized aneurysmal sacs or outpouchings both proximal and distal along a narrowed, normal, or unusually dilated portion of the artery (see Figs. 11-3B and C and 6-10). Computed tomography (CT) and magnetic resonance imaging (MRI) taken as axial cross-sections through the area of dissection can show the intramural bleeding and mural expansion and can confirm the diagnosis of dissection. Figure 11-4 is an MRI cross-section that shows a bilateral traumatic ICA dissection. Figure 6-9C also shows a fat-saturated MRI examination of a carotid artery dissection. Magnetic resonance angiography (MRA) (Fig. 6-9A and B) and computed tomography angiography (CTA) can also show typical abnormalities in patients with dissections.

ICA dissection, especially with pharyngeal aneurysm formation, can also lead to dysfunction of the lower cranial nerves at the skull base. Dysgeusia, Horner's syndrome, and weakness and atrophy of the tongue are the most common cranial-nerve signs. Tongue weakness and atrophy are caused by compression and ischemia of the hypoglossal nerve as it lies adjacent to the carotid

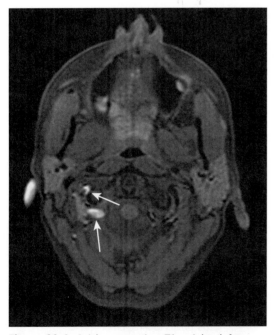

Figure 11-4. Axial cross-section, T1-weighted, fat-saturated image of a patient with an extracranial ICA dissection. The white hyperintensity is seen at two sites as the artery curves (white arrows). The dark flow void represents the arterial lumen and the high-intensity bright areas represent intramural hematoma.

sheath. At times, the IX, X, XI, and XII cranial nerves are involved.

ECVA dissections were first recognized in patients who had neck trauma or chiropractic manipulation.[11,20-22] VA injuries have also been reported in patients who manipulate their own necks[23,24] or have maintained their necks in a fixed position for some time.[22,25-28] ECVA dissections also occur after surgery and resuscitation presumably because of sustained neck postures in patients who are anesthetized or unresponsive.[29] These lesions most often involve the distal extracranial (third segment) of the VA. Figure 11-5 is a montage of angiograms in patients with ECVA dissections. Spontaneous ECVA dissections clinically and radiologically mimic those related to trauma.[5-8] Pain in the posterior neck or occiput and generalized headache are common.

Pain often precedes neurologic symptoms by hours, days, and, rarely, weeks. Some patients with ECVA dissections have only neck pain and do not develop neurologic symptoms or signs. TIAs most often include dizziness, diplopia, veering, staggering, and dysarthria. TIAs are less common in ECVA dissections than ICA dissections. Infarcts usually cause signs that begin suddenly. The most common patterns of ischemic brain damage are cerebellar infarction in posterior inferior cerebellar artery (PICA) distribution and lateral medullary infarction. As in extracranial ICA dissections, infarcts are invariably explained by embolization of fresh thrombus to the ICVA. Occasionally, dissections extend or begin intracranially. Sometimes, emboli reach the superior cerebellar arteries (SCAs), main basilar artery, or posterior cerebral arteries (PCAs). ECVA dissections can also cause cervical root pain.[30,31] Aneurysmal dilatation of the ECVA adjacent to nerve roots causes the radicular pain and can lead to radicular distribution motor, sensory, and reflex abnormalities.[30,31] Occasionally, spinal cord infarction results because of hypoperfusion in the supply zones of arteries from the ECVA that nourish the cervical spinal cord.[31,32]

Many patients with extracranial ICA and VA dissections have headache, pain, and TIAs without lasting neurologic deficits. Intracranial dissection is less common but has been considered more serious and almost invariably associated with severe deficits or death unless the dissection had a limited extent.

Intracranial dissections can cause infarction, subarachnoid bleeding, or mass effects.[5,22,33-38] When the dissections are between the media and the intima, luminal narrowing and local hypoperfusion usually occur and lead to infarction in the regions of supply. In the anterior circulation, the supraclinoid ICA and mainstem MCA are most

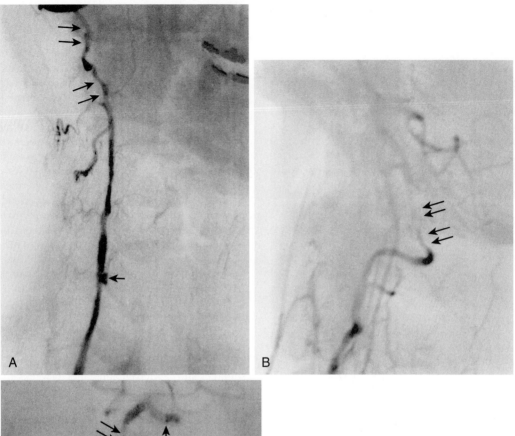

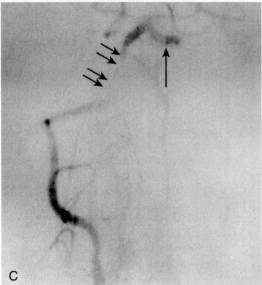

Figure 11-5. A montage of ECVA dissections. **A,** Vertebral angiogram-lateral view. A long vertebral artery dissection showing regions of irregular narrowing *(top arrows)* and an aneurysmal pouch *(lower arrow)*. **B,** Vertebral angiogram, lateral view. Dissection in the distal extracranial vertebral artery with narrowing and near occlusion of the artery *(black arrows)*. Flow above the dissection is severely compromised. **C,** Vertebral angiogram, anteroposterior view. The distal ECVA is narrowed and flow is compromised *(small black arrows)*. Dye refluxes into the contralateral ICVA *(long black arrow at right of figure)*.

often involved.[33,35,37] Figure 11-6 is an arteriogram of an intracranial ICA dissection that extends into the MCA and anterior cerebral artery (ACA). In the posterior circulation, the intracranial vertebral arteries (ICVAs) and basilar artery are most often affected.[5,22,34] The PCAs are occasionally involved.[38] Intracranial dissections were considered in the past to always be devastating or fatal, but modern technology has led to increased recognition of patients with intracranial dissections who have only minor signs. When dissections extend between the media and the adventitia, aneurysms and tears through the adventitia may lead to subarachnoid hemorrhage (SAH), which can be repeated. At times, dissections lead to prominent aneurysmal masses, which can present as space-taking lesions that compress adjacent cranial nerves or brain parenchyma.

Occasionally, patients have chronic dissections with aneurysms and multifocal regions of dissection of various ages.[5,22,34] These patients usually have abnormal arterial media and elastic

11

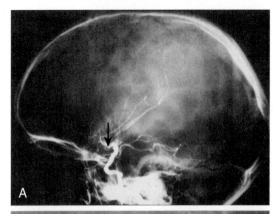

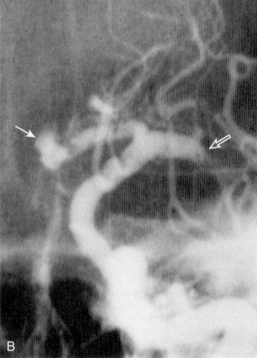

Figure 11-6. Intracranial ICA dissection in a child. **A,** Carotid angiogram, lateral view. The *black arrow* points to the dissection within the intracranial ICA. **B,** A magnified close-up view shows the dissection. The *closed white arrow* on the left shows that the MCA is occluded and the *open arrow* on the right of the picture points to an occluded anterior cerebral artery.

membranes and the arteries show healing intramural hematomas and tears of different ages. I have cared for two such patients, one with recurrent SAH and the other with recurrent posterior-circulation TIAs and strokes.[34] In the latter patient, thrombus was visible within each bilateral ICVA-dissecting aneurysm, and symptoms stopped after treatment with warfarin and aspirin combined. Some patients with chronic or recurrent dissections have fibromuscular dysplasia.[38a] When intracranial arteries are

involved, hemorrhage and local mass effect can be prominent.

Most extracranial dissections heal spontaneously with time. Their location high in the neck usually makes surgical repair difficult or impossible. When complete occlusion has occurred, the arteries often do not recanalize and remain occluded. Arteries that retain some residual lumen invariably heal and normalize. Intracranial dissections have been repaired surgically in patients with SAH, although the incidence of spontaneous healing and recurrent bleeding is unknown. Although there have been no controlled trials of medical therapy, I am impressed by many anecdotal reports[38b] and my own positive experience with anticoagulants. Prevention of embolization of thrombus at or shortly after the dissection should prevent stroke. Anticoagulants have not seemed to increase the extent of the dissections, which is a major theoretical concern. Because the risk of embolization is only during the acute period, I use heparin followed by warfarin. I try to maximize cerebral blood flow (CBF) during the acute period to augment collateral circulation. Healing of dissections can be monitored using MRI, MRA,[39] CTA,[40] and ultrasound. I stop anticoagulants after 6 weeks in patients with dissected arteries that remain occluded. I continue anticoagulants in patients with patent arteries until luminal stenosis improves to the point that flow is not significantly obstructed. I monitor the patient using ultrasound or MRA. When arterial blood flow is improved, I switch to drugs that modify platelet function, such as aspirin, clopidogrel, or modified-release dipyridamole. Engelter et al reviewed the experience with various antithrombotic drugs as of 2007.[41]

Stents have also been used to treat patients who have ICA dissections in the neck.[42-44] I believe that the indications for such stenting are very limited. When dissected arteries are open they almost invariably heal and become widely patent with time. The only indications for angioplasty and stenting are as part of an intra-arterial approach to lysing MCA intra-arterial emboli arising from ICA dissections when the ICA is occluded or nearly occluded,[43] and in patients with continued hypoperfusion, a rare occurrence.[44]

Dissections within the anterior circulation are also discussed in Chapter 6 and posterior circulation dissections are also covered in Chapter 7.

FIBROMUSCULAR DYSPLASIA

First recognized in the renal arteries, fibromuscular dysplasia is known to affect many other systemic arteries, including extracranial and cerebral arteries.[45,46] It is a nonatheromatous multifocal condition that can involve any or all of the three layers of the arterial wall. In the cerebral circulation, it is reported in only 0.6% of nonselected consecutive cerebral arteriograms.[47,48] No data exist on its true incidence in patients evaluated for stroke. This blood vessel abnormality is most often described in middle-aged women.[48] Bilateral ICA involvement is common (86%); abnormalities usually involve the pharyngeal portion of the artery and extend from the level of C1 proximally 7 to 8 cm, with sparing of the carotid bifurcation and the intracranial carotid artery. Twenty percent of patients have coexistent ECVA fibromuscular disease.[48]

The most common form of fibromuscular dysplasia affects the media. Constricting bands composed of fibrous dysplastic tissue and proliferating smooth-muscle cells in the media alternate with areas of luminal dilatation related to medial thinning and disruption of the elastic membrane.[49,50] These abnormalities produce the characteristic string-of-beads appearance on arteriography (Fig. 11-7). Hypertrophy of fibrous tissues in the adventitia or intima can cause segmental areas of stenosis. Occasionally, patients have band-like shelves or diaphragms within greatly enlarged carotid bulbs in the neck; superimposed thrombi sometimes develop in these "megabulbs."[51] Some patients with fibrous septa have had typical string-of-beads abnormalities in the pharyngeal carotid arteries on angiography but some have not had other obvious changes characteristic of fibromuscular dysplasia.[51] Fibromuscular dysplasia is probably not a single disease but may be a general term for a variety of different conditions that affect the arterial walls.

Although most fibromuscular dysplasia vascular lesions are asymptomatic, this vascular abnormality can cause brain ischemia. Fibromuscular dysplasia can be accompanied by aneurysms of the extracranial and intracranial arteries.[45,52] In one series of 37 patients with fibromuscular dysplasia, 19 patients had a total of 25 aneurysms.[52] The diagnosis of fibromuscular dysplasia is occasionally made at the time of evaluating SAH. Fibromuscular dysplasia also predisposes patients to arterial dissections with related stroke syndromes. In other patients, fibromuscular dysplasia affecting an artery appropriate to explain the brain imaging and clinical findings is the only abnormality uncovered. The lumen is not often severely compromised. The mechanism of the distal ischemia in this circumstance is unknown. Functional changes in vessel contraction (vasoconstriction) could lead to distal hypoperfusion. In one of my patients, a shelf in the distal ICA in the neck was seen on one angiographic run and not seen on a later run. Vasoconstriction can cause reversible constrictions.

Altered blood flow with stasis could lead to thrombus formation and distal intra-arterial embolism. Any medium-sized muscular intracranial artery can be affected. The most prominent clinical features are TIAs and strokes of minor or moderate severity. Fatal or severe strokes are unusual. Headache, syncope, and Horner's syndrome are also frequent accompanying symptoms.

Most research and clinical interest have been directed at atherosclerotic disease of the intima and subintima of arteries. Little is known about the other portions of the arterial wall. Clearly, disease of the artery walls can lead to altered contractility, dilatation with aneurysm formation, and tears with intramural hematomas. The disorder called *fibromuscular dysplasia* is pathologically heterogenous and may occur as a result of various etiologies that share abnormalities of connective tissue. The collagen, elastic tissue, and extracellular matrix can be involved. Knowledge of these disorders of vascular connective tissue is rudimentary.

Angioplasty, often with stenting, has been used to dilatate arteries harboring fibromuscular dysplasia lesions.[53,54] In a series of patients with stroke presumably caused by fibromuscular dysplasia, the recurrence rate is quite low even without therapy.[49] Insufficient data are available to warrant rational therapeutic suggestions. I usually prescribe antiplatelet aggregating agents but rarely use anticoagulants or recommend surgical repair or mechanical dilation of the arteries. I often prescribe calcium channel blockers to prevent vasoconstriction. If the patient is hypertensive, the renal arteries should be studied. When fibromuscular dysplasia is found on angiography, CTA, MRA, or standard arteriography is warranted to exclude associated intracranial aneurysms.

HERITABLE DISORDERS OF CONNECTIVE TISSUE

Disorders of connective tissue are a group of hereditary disorders that are usually recognizable in childhood and involve the skin, vascular system, and skeletal tissues. The full spectrum of these disorders is still unraveling and little in-depth analysis has been made of the neurological and cerebrovascular features.

Pseudoxanthoma elasticum (PXE), also referred to as Gronblad-Strandberg disease, has an estimated prevalence of approximately 1 in 160,000 and has both autosomal dominant and recessive hereditary patterns.[55,56] The genetic defect has now been mapped to the ABCC6 gene on chromosome 16p13.1.[57,58] The ABCC6 gene belongs to the ABC (ATP-binding cassette) transmembrane

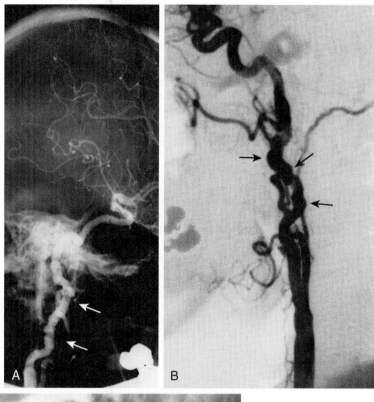

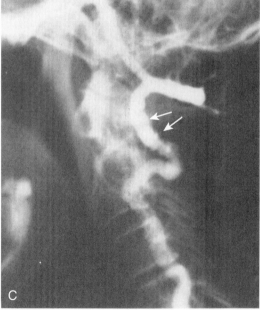

Figure 11-7. Fibromuscular dysplasia. **A,** Carotid arteriogram, lateral view, showing typical sausage-like, string-of-beads effect *(white arrows).* **B,** Carotid angiogram, subtraction lateral view. Contractile areas are shown with *black arrows.* **C,** Vertebral artery angiogram, lateral view. FMD changes involving the distal extracranial vertebral artery *(white arrows).*

transporter family of proteins. Genetic studies have identified about 60 mutations as well as large deletions in the gene.[58] The most easily recognized abnormalities are skin changes.[57-60] The skin of the face, neck, axilla, antecubital, inguinal, and periumbilical regions first becomes thickened and grooved. Yellowish papules and plaques are seen in these areas and also on the mucosa of the lips, palate, buccal area, vagina, and rectum. Later, the skin becomes lax and redundant. Angioid streaks, which are reddish-brown or gray, radiate from the optic disk and are usually wider than veins. Figure 11-8 is a fundus photograph that shows angioid streaks in a patient with PXE.

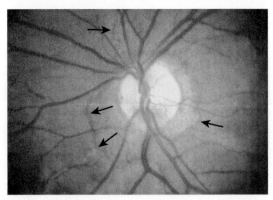

Figure 11-8. Angioid streaks *(small black arrows)* in the retina in a patient with pseudoxanthoma elasticum. (Courtesy of Dr Thomas Hedges III.)

Another fundoscopic finding seen in some patients with pseudoxanthoma elasticum is a speckled, yellowish mottling of the posterior pole of the retina temporal to the macula. This appearance has been dubbed "peau d'orange" because it resembles the skin of an orange.

The abnormality of connective and elastic tissue causes tortuosity of vessels, premature vascular calcification, intimal thickening, microaneurysms, and fusiform aneurysms. Gastrointestinal bleeding is common and is a result of the vascular changes.[59] Premature occlusive vascular disease affects the coronary, peripheral limb, retinal, and cerebral arteries. Degenerative vascular changes begin with fragmentation and calcification of the internal elastic lamina and are followed by extensive intimal and medial calcification.[59] Cardiac manifestations relate to premature coronary artery disease, and endocardial abnormalities. Coronary artery disease with resulting angina pectoris, myocardial infarction, and sudden death are common and may occur at quite a young age.[56,57] Some patients have an ischemic cardiomyopathy. Histologic examination of coronary artery specimens in patients with PXE show loss of elastic tissue, fragmentation of the internal elastic membrane, and calcifications between the intima and media.[57] Abnormalities in the elastic tissue of the endocardium can produce thickened mitral valves, mitral annular calcification, and mitral stenosis in patients with PXE. The abnormal mitral valve can show fragmentation, coiling, and disruption of collagen bundles.

The arteries of the aortic arch and intracranial arteries are involved. Some patients with PXE show tortuosity and ectasia of the neck arteries on angiography. One patient had occlusion of both ICAs at the skull base and a carotid-cavernous fistula.[61] Hypertension and mitral valve prolapse (MVP) are common,[56] and SAH and intracerebral hemorrhage (ICH) occur. The cerebrovascular lesions most often consist of lacunar infarcts and white matter ischemia of the microangiopathic Binswanger type. Cortical infarcts are less common. Many of the cerebrovascular complications relate to the hypertension that often accompanies PXE.

Ehlers-Danlos syndrome describes a group of clinically and genetically heterogeneous conditions that share defects in collagen.[62] The skin is hyperextensible and easily bruised, and the joints show hypermobility and excessive scarring after an injury. Over 80% of Ehlers-Danlos syndrome patients have types I, II, or III, but most individuals with cerebrovascular complications have type IV, which occurs in 1 in 50,000 to 500,000 individuals.[63] Cardiac and cerebrovascular lesions are common and include mitral and tricuspid valve prolapse, septal defects, and dilatation of the aortic root and pulmonary arteries.[64] The most important and frequent cerebrovascular complications are carotid-cavernous fistulas, and arterial dissections.[62,65,66,66a]

Extracranial and intracranial aneurysms have also been reported, including several individuals with multiple intracranial aneurysms.[67,68] The ICA is the most common site of aneurysm formation, typically in the cavernous sinus or just as it emerges from the sinus. Rupture of various systemic and cerebral vessels leads to frequent bleeding and SAH. Angiography and angioplasty have a high rate of complications and extreme caution should be exercised in choosing these procedures in Ehlers-Danlos syndrome patients.[62] Surgery is also difficult because the arteries are friable and difficult to suture.

Marfan's syndrome is a hereditary disorder that is probably more common than other hereditary disorders and occurs in approximately 4 to 6 per 100,000 individuals.[69] The condition is inherited as a dominant trait, being sporadic in less than one quarter of individuals. A gene defect is located in the long arm of chromosome 15, in which a mutation in the FBN1 gene that encodes fibrillin-1 was first reported in 1991.[70,71] Since then, more than 600 mutations were identified, most of them causing Marfanoid or fragments of the Marfan's syndrome phenotype.[70]

Marfan's syndrome is a connective tissue disorder associated with extensive and generalized malformation of organs and systems.[69] The skeleton is disproportionately arranged and unstable, the eyes often have lens dislocations and are myopic; a cystic disease of the lungs can be present.[70] Defective formation of cardiac valves and blood vessels underlies the more serious occurrences in Marfan's syndrome. The vascular abnormalities relate to abnormal collagen and elastin. The phenotype of long limbs, pectus chest deformity, arachnodactyly, and joint laxity is easily recognizable. Subluxation of the lens occurs in more than one half of the patients, and ophthalmologic examination is helpful in diagnosis. The diameter of the aortic root is invariably enlarged, and aortic regurgitation and mitral valve prolapse are common. Aortic aneurysms and dissections are very frequent clinical problems in patients with Marfan's syndrome.

Most of the cerebrovascular events in patients with Marfan syndrome relate to the cardiac and aortic manifestations of the condition. A few patients with carotid and vertebral artery dissections have been reported.[72,73] Whether or not there is also a predisposition for intracranial aneurysms in Marfan syndrome patients has been debated with some data favoring a relationship,[74] and others arguing that the frequency is no higher than in the general population.[75] There does not appear to be an excess frequency of SAH in patients with Marfan syndrome.[76]

The Loeys-Dietz syndrome is an autosomal dominantly inherited syndrome consisting of various bony and connective tissue abnormalities and a predilection for aortic and arterial aneurysms and dissections.[76a,b,c] Like Marfan's syndrome there are often long limbs and fingers and lax joints. Widely spaced eyes, cleft palate or bifid uvula, scoliosis, and indented or protruding chest wall are other common features. Gradual weakening and stretching of the dura mater can cause nerve root irritation and leg pains. Congenital heart abnormalities especially patent ductis arteriosis and atrial septal defects are also often found. This condition is caused by a mutation in the genes encoding transforming growth factor beta receptor (TGFBR 1 or TGFBR 2).

DILATATIVE ARTERIOPATHY (DOLICHOECTASIA)

Patients with dilatative arteriopathy have elongated, ectatic, tortuous intracranial arteries. Dilatation can be so severe that portions of the artery become a fusiform aneurysm. Approximately one patient in eight who has brain imaging has some increase in the length and diameter of intracranial arteries.[77-79] This abnormality can be found in children and often involves multiple arteries.[77,80-84] Hereditary factors probably play an important role, especially in the young. In one reported family, three brothers had large fusiform basilar artery aneurysms and alpha-glucosidase deficiency.[82] In an 11-year-old girl who died from a ruptured dolichoectatic basilar artery aneurysm, necropsy showed that the artery had large gaps in the internal elastic lamina with only short segments of elastica remaining in some regions.[81]

Pathologic examination in other young patients with dolichoectasia has shown deficiencies in the muscularis and internal elastic lamina with irregular thickness of the media, multiple gaps in the internal elastica, and regions of fibrosis. At times, the intima is thickened, and there is severe elastic tissue degeneration and an increase in the vasa vasorum. Dolichoectasia is also prominent in children with Fabry disease, sickle cell disease, and AIDS, and it occurs in patients with Ehlers-Danlos syndrome.[77] Patients with dilatative arteriopathy also have a high frequency of enlarged aortic diameters and lacunar infarcts due to penetrating artery disease.[84-86]

The most frequent location is in the posterior fossa where the basilar artery or one or both VAs are involved.[87-91] Figure 11-9A shows a montage of dye-contrast cerebral arteriograms of six patients with vertebrobasilar dolichoectatic arteries. Figure 11-9B and C shows ectatic basilar arteries with poor antegrade blood flow. The dolichoectatic anomaly is often recognized on CT as curvilinear, calcified channels that usually cross the cerebellopontine angle.[87,89] The MCAs are also often involved, and some patients have dolichoectatic abnormalities in both circulations.

Extensive atherosclerotic plaques, often with calcification, encroachment on the lumen, and thrombus formation, are frequently found at necropsy. On microscopic examination, there are often fibrotic changes in the vessel wall with reduced muscularis and attenuated, fragmented, or absent elastica.[92] Clinically, the most common symptoms are caused by brain ischemia. Mass effect with compression or displacement of cranial nerves or brain parenchyma is also common. The aneurysmally dilatated arteries can compress the medullary pyramids[93] and cerebral peduncles and may indent and deform the basis pontis. Some patients have had hydrocephalus, possibly related to the effects of the dolichoectatic aneurysms on the third ventricle.

Ischemia is most often found in the distribution of penetrating arteries to the brainstem and basal ganglia. Ischemia is related to the effects of the disease in the parent arteries on the branches. Plaques or clot may obliterate or obscure the orifices of branches or can embolize into the branches. Angiography may show thrombi within dolichoectatic aneurysms.[87,94] In other patients, distortion and elongation of the branches may reduce blood flow without obliteration of the branch ostia or lumens. Occasionally, clot within the aneurysms can embolize to the larger distal branches.[87,94,95] Rupture of these aneurysms with resulting subarachnoid bleeding is unusual but does occur.[87,92,94]

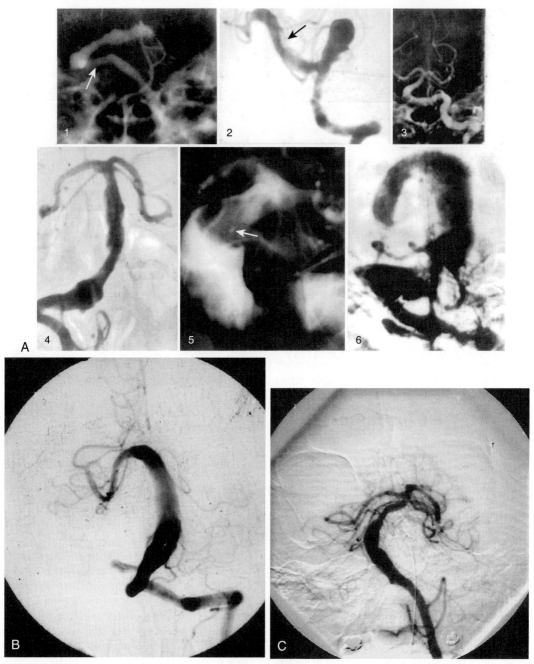

Figure 11-9. Dolichoectatic vertebrobasilar arteries. **A,** Montage of vertebrobasilar fusiform aneurysms in six patients. Patient 1 *(upper left)* has marked tortuosity and ectasia of the basilar artery with a proximal atheromatous stenosis *(white arrow)*; patient 2 has a filling defect *(black arrow)* representing thrombus in the midbasilar artery; patient 3 has a very tortuous left vertebral and basilar artery; patient 4 shows irregular plaques in a dilatated basilar artery; patient 5 has a markedly dilatated basilar artery with a filling defect *(white arrow)* representing thrombus. The apparent lower filling defect is an artifact representing an aerated sinus. Patient 6 has a very dilatated ectatic artery with poor filling of the distal segment and nonfilling of the PCAs because of reduced antegrade flow. **B,** Vertebral angiogram, anteroposterior view. The basilar artery is extremely dilatated and the distal portion and its branches are poorly opacified. **C,** Very irregular ectatic basilar artery with extensive atheromatous plaques. The branches of the rostral basilar artery are not well opacified because of reduced antegrade blood flow. (**A,** From Pessin MS, Chimowitz MI, Levine SR, et al: Stroke in patients with fusiform vertebrobasilar aneurysms. Neurology 1989;39:16-21.)

CT, MRI, and MRA[96] usually suffice to identify the aneurysmally dilated ectatic arteries and may suggest the presence of clot within the vessels. TCD is helpful in diagnosis and may show reduced mean-flow velocities with relatively preserved peak-flow velocities.[97] Blood flow may be to and fro within the dilatated artery, causing reduced antegrade flow. The reduced antegrade flow may lead to poor opacification on MRA, falsely suggesting occlusion of the dolichoectatic artery. CTA and standard angiography are able to image the artery in this circumstance. In patients with recurrent ischemia and thrombi within the dolichoectatic arteries, warfarin may prevent strokes. Intravenous thrombolytic agents also have been used in patients with large thrombi within dolichoectatic arteries.[94] Agents that modify platelet function have not been studied in patients with dilatative arteriopathy. The vascular abnormality often increases with time and there is a relatively high frequency of strokes despite present therapy.[97a]

CEREBRAL AMYLOID ANGIOPATHY

Cerebral amyloid angiopathy (CAA), also called congophilic angiopathy, is also discussed in Chapter 13 because the major clinical feature is recurrent lobar ICH. The disorder is characterized by thickening of the walls of small- and medium-sized arteries by an amorphous eosinophilic-staining material with a smudged appearance on light microscopy.[98,99] The walls of some amyloid-laden vessels appear to be split (Fig. 11-10A). The material within the vessel wall shows a yellow-green birefringence when stained with Congo red and viewed under a polarizing microscope—hence the term *congophilic*. Figure 11-10B is a photomicrograph of the cerebral cortex stained for beta-amyloid in a patient with CAA. The abnormalities usually involve many arteries, especially those in the leptomeninges and cortex of the cerebral lobes. The brainstem, basal gray nuclei, hippocampi, and subcortical white matter are spared.[98] The amyloid deposition is most prevalent in the parietal and occipital lobes, but ICH is also often frontal and central, and can be cerebellar.[99-104] Affected arteries, especially those in the leptomeninges, have a distinctive double-barrel lumen with amyloid found in the outer or inner media.[98]

The most common clinical syndromes recognized are ICH, usually multiple and subcortical lobar, and SAH.[98-104] MRI T2* susceptibility-weighted echo-planar images often show multiple, small, old hemorrhages in patients with CAA who present with a stroke. These small accumulations of hemosiderin-laden cells are usually referred to as "microbleeds." These microbleeds are

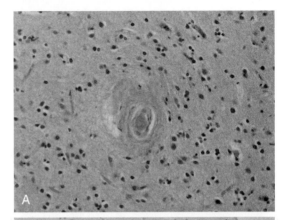

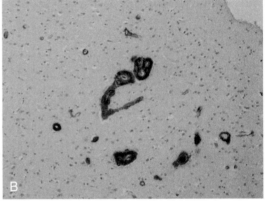

Figure 11-10. A, Photomicrograph of the cerebral cortex, hematoxylin-eosin stain showing splitting of the amyloid-laden wall of a small artery. **B,** Photomicrograph of the cerebral cortex immunostained for beta-amyloid with a hematoxylin counterstain. Amyloid is seen in many small vessels. (Courtesy of Dr Steven Greenberg.)

common and their amount and location does predict a risk of further brain hemorrhage.[105,106] Figure 11-11A shows an echo-planar image of a patient with a recent amyloid angiopathy-related brain hemorrhage, as well as multiple old regions of bleeding. The smaller regions of susceptibility have often been labeled "microbleeds." Figure 11-11B shows an echo-planar image of a man who presented with transient aphasia whose images show many cortical microbleeds.

Senile plaques containing amyloid and Alzheimer's changes are also prevalent in brains of patients harboring CAA. Many patients with CAA are demented or develop intellectual deterioration with time caused by multiple strokes and Alzheimer's pathology.[99] Both APOE2 and APOE4 play a role in facilitating the deposition of Aβ amyloid in cerebral blood vessels. and APOEε2 seems to increase the likelihood of ICH in patients with cerebral amyloid angiopathy.[107,108] ICH is especially common in APOE2 carriers after head trauma or use of antithrombotic agents.[109]

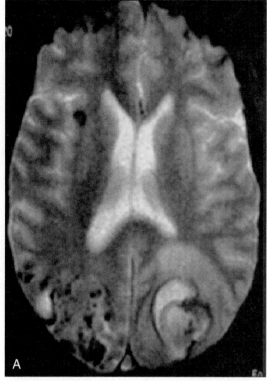

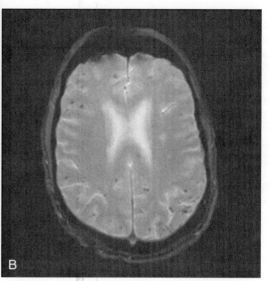

Figure 11-11. A, Gradient-echo MRI images of a man with a recent left occipital-parietal intracerebral hemorrhage. Multiple old hemorrhages *(black regions)* are shown. **B,** Gradient-echo MRI images of a 68-year-old man who presented with transient aphasia. Images show many lobar microbleeds diagnostic of cerebral amyloid angiopathy. (**A,** Courtesy of Drs Charlotte Cordonnier and Didier Leys, and published in *Uncommon Causes of Stroke*, 2nd ed. Cambridge: Cambridge University Press, 2008; **B,** courtesy of Dr Steven Greenberg.)

Early studies also noted that scattered small infarcts were also prevalent in brains of patients with amyloid-related ICH.[101-103] TIAs can occur.[110] Some patients with CAA have multiple infarcts and a prominent leukoencephalopathy with periventricular, subcortical, and corona radiata lucency on CT and signal abnormalities on MRI.[104,111-114] The clinical picture is that of Binswanger's disease. In fact, CAA may be an important, often unrecognized, cause of this chronic ischemic microangiopathy.

The cause of CAA is unknown. Familial CAA has been identified, especially in Icelandic, Dutch, and German families, and is usually inherited as an autosomal-dominant trait with high penetrance.[99] The Icelandic variety has been attributed to abnormal metabolism of a gamma-trace protein.[99,115,116]

At times, there are prominent inflammatory changes in relation to the amyloid-staining arteries, and there have been reports of patients who had CAA and granulomatous arteritis (or the CAA evoked a granulomatous reaction in these patients).[98,117-119]

Although it was once considered that drainage of CAA-related hematomas might be hazardous, data show that surgical results are not different from other causes of ICH.[120,121] Reducing the systemic blood pressure to the lowest levels tolerated is a strategy often used to reduce the frequency of ICH. Advances in recognition and understanding the pathogenesis of CAA should lead to more specific therapeutic strategies.[122]

VASCULITIS AND OTHER POSSIBLY INFLAMMATORY VASCULAR DISORDERS

Arteritis is mentioned as a cause of stroke in the differential diagnosis of nearly every medical student, non-neurologist, and some neurologists. Although often considered, documented arteritis is a rare cause of stroke. Most often, central nervous system (CNS) vasculitis presents as an encephalopathy with headache, seizures, decreased alertness, and cognitive and behavioral abnormalities, often with multifocal signs. Recognition of those rare instances in which arteritis is caused by a specific microbial infection is critical for effective treatment. Patients with allergic

11

hypersensitivity and systemic vasculitis may respond to corticosteroids or other treatments used to control systemic autoimmune diseases.

ARTERITIS CAUSED BY INFECTIONS

Bacterial and Fungal Infections

In patients with acute bacterial meningitis (e.g., pneumococcal or meningococcal), the pial arteries and veins are often surrounded by pus. Vascular occlusions and strokes may complicate the clinical picture, which is invariably dominated by headache, fever, stiff neck, and decreased alertness. Brain infarction develops in about 15% to 20% of adults with bacterial meningitis, typically pneumococcal meningitis.[123,124,124a] Occasionally spinal cord and brainstem infarction occur during meningococcal meningitis.[125,126]

Listeria monocytogenes may produce a characteristic inflammatory disorder involving predominantly the medulla and pontine tegmentum.[127-130] Multiple, lower cranial-nerve palsies and vestibular and oculomotor signs develop. Figure 11-12 shows MRI scans from a patient with *Listeria* rhombencephalitis treated with penicillin.[130] At times, the onset of symptoms is abrupt and subsequent necropsy shows an arteritis with multiple infarcts as well as focal encephalitis. The cerebrospinal fluid (CSF) shows a pleocytosis.[127-130] Occasionally, patients with *cat-scratch disease*,[131] a disorder known to be caused by *Bartonella henselae*, have presented

with an acute focal neurologic deficit associated with intracranial stenoses and arteritis.[132]

In patients with *syphilis*, the spirochete probably invades cerebral arteries at the time of the meningitis of secondary lues. Meningovascular syphilis results and is characterized by apoplectic attacks of hemiplegia, headache, seizures, and CSF pleocytosis.[133] Arteries may appear stenotic on vascular imaging.[134,135] The serology is always positive in patients with meningovascular syphilis. The spinal arterial circulation can also be affected. All forms of syphilis are more common and severe in patients with acquired immunodeficiency syndrome (AIDS).[133,136]

Lyme borreliosis mimics syphilis in many ways. Meningitis, multiple cranial-nerve palsies, and root- and peripheral-nerve syndromes predominate.[137-140] Strokes have been described but rarely.[141-143] Strokes are much less common than peripheral nerve and root sensory symptoms and the syndrome of headache, fatigue, and difficulty concentrating. The CSF is invariably abnormal and specific antibodies to *Borrelia* are present in the blood and CSF.[143]

Chronic basal meningitis, usually caused by tuberculosis[144-148] or particular fungi (i.e., *Cryptococcus*, *Histoplasma*, and *Coccidioides*),[149-151] is often complicated by inflammation of the arteries within the exudate. The proximal MCA and arteries in the posterior perforated substance are most often involved. The exudate surrounds the

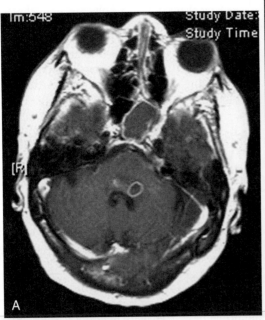
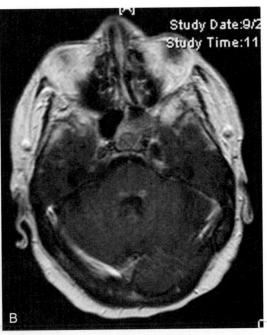

Figure 11-12. *Listeria* rhombencephalitis. **A,** T1-weighted MRI after gadolinium enhancement showing ring-enhancing lesions in the pons adjacent to the floor of the IVth ventricle. **B,** T1-weighted, gadolinium-enhanced MRI taken a month later after penicillin treatment. (From Silvestri N, Ajani Z, Savitz S, Caplan LR: A 73-year-old woman with an acute illness causing fever and cranial nerve abnormalities. Rev Neurol Dis 2006;3:29-30, 35-37. Figures reprinted with permission from MedReviews LLC. All rights reserved.)

arteries, producing thickening and inflammation of the walls of the arteries, usually called Heubner's arteritis. Infarcts in the basal ganglia and midbrain result and can develop even after sterilization of the microbial agent. Other fungi, especially *Aspergillus*[152,153] and *Mucor*,[154] cause a necrotizing arteritis with regions of brain infarction and necrosis. *Mucor* is usually spread from the paranasal sinuses,[154] and *Aspergillus* reaches the cerebral circulation by hematogenous spread usually without meningitis.[152,153] *Aspergillus* infections are especially common in patients who take corticosteroids or who are immunosuppressed, and *Mucor* is common in patients with diabetic ketoacidosis and those in renal failure.

Viral Infections

Viruses may be responsible for many cases of vasculitis that are considered idiopathic. Hepatitis-B surface antigen, immunoglobulin, and complement are found in the vessel walls of patients with polyarteritis nodosa who have hepatitis-B antigenemia.[155] The varicella-zoster virus is also known to directly invade CNS vessels, sometimes without causing much visible inflammatory reaction.[156,157] Viruses can cause vasculitis by direct invasion or by triggering an immune response to components of vessels.[157] Alternatively, immune-complex deposition can injure arteries and cause inflammation. Evidence of herpes varicella-zoster virus (HZV) infection by polymerase chain reaction (PCR) analysis of biopsy or necropsy material may be found in patients with the typical clinical findings of polyarteritis nodosa.[157]

HZV is the most well known and best documented of the viral arteritides. The most common clinical syndrome is delayed brain infarction, usually causing hemiplegia contralateral to herpes zoster ophthalmicus.[158-160] The symptoms begin days to weeks (range 6 to 18 weeks)[158,159,160a] after onset of the painful rash. Infarcts are usually hemispheral and cause hemiparesis, hemisensory loss, and aphasia, or right-hemispheric types of cognitive and behavioral changes. Usually, the infarct is ipsilateral to the rash. However, HVZ angiopathy can occur without a rash.[160a] Angiography has shown occlusion of the carotid siphon, MCA, or ACA, and sometimes stenosis of these arteries.[158-160] Small arteries are also very often involved and may become occluded.[160a] At times, TIAs may precede the stroke but most often the onset is abrupt and the neurologic signs develop immediately. Some patients have an accompanying encephalitis. Recurrent ischemia and multiple infarcts have been reported. The mortality has been estimated at approximately 25%. This mortality rate is higher than comparable-sized infarcts caused by atherosclerosis.[159] The CSF usually shows a slight pleocytosis and immunoglobulins (Ig) and IgG indices may be elevated.[158,159] Rarely, the rash involves other divisions of the Vth nerve (maxillary or mandibular) and can occur in the back of the neck and upper cervical dermatomes.[161-163] The PCA and vertebrobasilar territory are occasionally involved.[161-163]

Postvaricella arteriopathy and brain infarction have now been studied extensively in children.[164-167] The course and progression of the arteriopathy was studied in 27 children who had serial vascular imaging.[167] They had chickenpox at age 1 to 10.4 (median 4.4 years) and had their first episode of brain ischemia 4 to 47 weeks later (median 17 weeks).[167] Arterial imaging abnormalities most often involved the supraclinoid ICA, the M1 and M2 segments of the MCA, and the A1 segment of the ACA. Single regions of focal ring-like stenosis and gradual longer segments of stenosis and multifocal narrowings were found. Brain infarcts were predominantly deep in the basal ganglia, internal capsule, and thalamus. In some patients stenosis was maximal on initial studies, but often later progressed to involve previously uninvolved arteries. The vascular abnormalities improved or completely regressed during follow-up during 6 to 79 months. Brain ischemic episodes recurred, either acutely or during the 1 to 33 weeks after symptom onset, often with progression of abnormalities on vascular imaging.

At necropsy, patients with HZV arteritis may show inflamed necrotic arteries, granulomatous changes,[156-158] or occluded arteries with scant inflammation. Doyle and colleagues were able to demonstrate virions that were characteristic of HZV in the nuclei and cytoplasm of smooth-muscle cells in the involved arteries.[160] Amplification of HZV viral DNA by PCR was obtained in the left anterior, middle, and posterior cerebral arteries of a patient who developed left-cerebral hemisphere infarction after left herpes zoster opthalmicus.[168] Presumably, the virus spread from the infected gasserian ganglion through trigeminovascular connections to the proximal portions of the ipsilateral MCA and ACA.[168] Trigeminovascular projections also go from V1 to the SCA, and the upper cervical ganglia probably project to the ICVAs, basilar artery, and the anterior inferior cerebellar artery (AICA) and SCA.[169] Spread to the intima can activate the endothelium to release factors promoting thrombosis. As in other virus diseases, inflammation is not always visible under the microscope.

Patients with human immunodeficiency virus infection have an increased frequency of stroke.[170-174] The mechanisms of stroke in AIDS patients vary. Some strokes are caused by hypercoagulability provoked by chronic infection, concomitant drug abuse, and infection with agents that can cause arteritis, such as fungi.[170-174] Children with AIDS may have a dilatative arteriopathy with fusiform aneurysms involving the intracranial arteries.[175] SAH may develop.

Kawasaki disease is an acute disorder occurring predominantly in children that is posited to be caused by an as yet unidentified infectious agent.[176] It causes vasculopathies mostly in the form of coronary artery aneurysm and the aorta. The carotid arteries are sometimes also often involved.[176-178]

Parasitic Infections

Cysticercosis may be associated with endarteritis and strokes.[179-187] Cysticercosis is caused by infection with the larvae (cysticerci) of *Taenia solium*, the pork tapeworm. Paracytic cysts containing cysticerci lodge within brain parenchyma in the subarachnoid space and within the brain

ventricles. Stroke occurs predominantly in the subarachnoid form of the disease.[179-184] Meningitic inflammation can spread to the major basal intracranial arteries, leading to an endarteritis and brain infarction. Subcortical small infarcts and large cortical-subcortical infarcts may occur. The most common vessels involved are the MCAs, PCAs, and the ACAs, but the basilar artery may also be affected.[184,185] Figure 11-13 shows a severe instance of subarachnoid cysticercosis that compromises the MCAs bilaterally. In one study, among 28 patients with subarachnoid cysticercosis who had cerebral angiography, 15 patients (53%) had angiographic evidence of arteritits.[184] A clinical stroke syndrome was present in 12 of these patients, and 8 patients had brain infarcts on MRI.[185] When patients with arterial narrowing caused by cysticercosis are followed sequentially using TCD, sometimes the stenosis improves with time.[186] Precipitation of brain infarction after praziquantel therapy has also been reported.[187] Destruction of

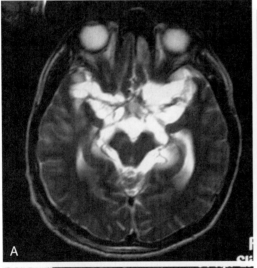
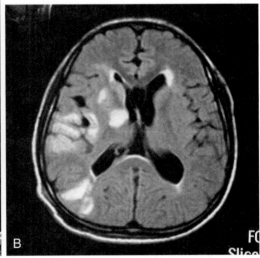
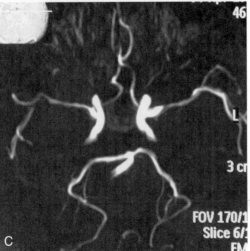

Figure 11-13. Cerebral infarction in patient with cysticercotic angiitis. **A,** T2-weighted MRI show huge subarachnoid racemose cysts in the sylvian fissures engulfing both middle cerebral arteries. **B,** MRI FLAIR scan shows recent infarction in the territory of the right middle cerebral artery. **C,** MRA shows stenosis of the MCAs bilaterally. (Courtesy of Dr Julio Lama, Guayaquil, Ecuador; from Del Bruto OH: Stroke and vasculitis in patients with cysticercosis. In Caplan LR [ed]: Uncommon Causes of Stroke, 2nd ed. Cambridge: Cambridge University Press, 2008, pp 53-58, with permission.)

the cysticercotic cysts within the subarachnoid space may cause an inflammatory response, which can cause or exacerbate an endarteritis.[179,187]

Plasmodium falciparum is the most frequent parasitic infection of the CNS. Cerebral malaria is characterized by coma and convulsions after a prodromal period of fever and headache.[188] Parasitized red blood cells distend capillaries and venules and lead to intracranial hypertension, brain edema, and petechial hemorrhages throughout the brain. Subarachnoid hemorrhage has also been reported.[189] In children, convulsions and hemiparesis are relatively common. Angiography and TCD in children with hemiparesis often shows focal stenosis of the basal intracranial arteries.[190,191]

Trypanosoma cruzi infection causes a disorder called *Chagas disease*, which is common in Brazil, Paraguay, and other parts of South America.[192] *T. cruzi* parasites are transmitted to humans by large bedbugs that deposit feces on the mucous membranes or scraped skin while they bite. When individuals rub the bite wound, the parasites enter the bloodstream. Cardiac involvement (cardiac dilatations, arrhythmias, and conduction abnormalities) is present in over 90% of patients. Intestinal (megaesophagus, megacolon) involvement is also common. The clinical presentation is that of a dilatated cardiomyopathy. The cardiac disorder is caused by involvement of the autonomic nervous system innervation of the heart rather than direct attack by the parasites. Strokes are relatively common in patients with Chagas disease and are mainly due to embolism from the heart.[192-196]

SYSTEMIC VASCULITIDES, INCLUDING COLLAGEN VASCULAR DISEASES

Systemic vasculitis syndromes can be conveniently divided into polyarteritis nodosa, allergic angiitis and granulomatosis (Churg-Strauss syndrome), hypersensitivity vasculitis, Wegener's granulomatosis, and overlap syndromes sharing features of other subtypes.[155,197-203] All of these syndromes have in common multisystem involvement.

Polyarteritis nodosa (PAN) affects small- and medium-sized arteries, especially at branch points.[201-205] Infiltration of polymorphonuclear leukocytes and monocytes is followed by intimal proliferation, fibrinoid necrosis, and thrombosis of arteries. The most common neurologic signs probably relate to mononeuritis multiplex. CNS involvement occurs in 20% to 40% of patients and the onset occurs usually after systemic symptoms and signs and neuropathy.[198,204,205] Some patients have a diffuse encephalopathy and others have focal or multifocal

abnormalities. Occasionally, hemispheral, spinal cord, cerebellar and brainstem infarcts occur. When strokes occur, it is usually late in the illness. Hypertension is common in patients with PAN, and is responsible for many of the ischemic infarcts and hemorrhages. I have not seen or known of a report of PAN presenting initially as a stroke syndrome.

Patients with *Churg-Strauss syndrome* invariably have pulmonary involvement, including asthma, and eosinophilia.[198,206-209] A history of previous allergic disorders usually exists. The lesions tend to involve smaller vessels, especially capillaries and venules.[198,206-211] Encephalopathy and peripheral neuritis are common, but strokes are extremely rare.

The *hypersensitivity vasculitides* are a group of disorders in which the cause is usually known and a major finding is a rash, often with palpable purpuric skin lesions, especially on the legs. Some are drug induced, postinfectious, or related to known foreign antigens (e.g., serum sickness). Mixed cryoglobulinemia and Henoch-Schönlein purpura are other forms of hypersensitivity vasculitis. Neurologic involvement is not prominent in patients with the various hypersensitivity vasculitis syndromes, and when it occurs, neuropathies, plexopathies, and encephalopathies predominate.[198,211] Strokes occur but rarely and most often are explained by bleeding related to systemic purpura.[212-214]

Wegener's granulomatosis is a necrotizing, often fatal, granulomatous vasculitis that involves chiefly the lungs, sinuses, upper respiratory tract, and kidneys.[198,215] Orbital involvement, palsies of extraocular muscles, and retinal and optic nerve ischemia are often reported.[216-219] Brain infarcts and cerebral arteritis are occasionally described.[220,221] The diagnosis can be made by biopsy and by detection of antineutrophilic cytoplasmic antibody and is treatable with cyclophosphamide and other immune suppressants.[222]

Nervous system findings are quite common in patients with *systemic lupus erythematosus (SLE)*.[223,224] Headaches that often share features with migraine, seizures, psychosis with decreased cognition, chorea, and mononeuropathies and polyneuropathies are important features of SLE.[223] The usual assumption has been that vasculitis underlies these diverse neurologic syndromes. Necropsy and clinical studies, however, indicate that true arteritis is not a common cause of the CNS findings.[225,226] In a necropsy study, Johnson and Richardson found scant evidence of inflammation of brain arteries.[225]

Sudden-onset neurologic signs do occur in patients with SLE and can be a prominent clinical feature. MRI often shows discrete focal lesions in patients with SLE usually in the absence of a clinical history of stroke.[226,227] The infarcts are of diverse causes. Small vessel vasculopathy with small deep infarcts and hemorrhages are usually caused by hypertension, which accompanies the renal disease of SLE. Cortical and cortical-subcortical infarcts are most often caused by abnormalities of coagulation and cardiac-origin embolism. Angiography often shows occlusion of intracranial artery branches.[228]

Hematologic abnormalities are extremely common in SLE. The presence of lupus anticoagulant (LA) and antiphospholipid antibodies often correlates with clinical hypercoagulability, characterized by miscarriages, recurrent thrombophlebitis, and strokes.[229] Thrombocytopenia and other platelet abnormalities are also common, as is reduced prostacyclin activity.[230] In a 1988 clinicopathologic study of 50 patients dying with SLE, a syndrome clinically resembling thrombotic thrombocytopenic purpura (TTP) developed in 14 patients (28%).[226] Seven of these 14 patients had platelet-thrombi occluding their capillaries and arteries, segmental subendothelial hyalin deposits, and arteriolar microaneurysms at necropsy—findings typical for TTP.[226] In this same study, vasculitis was not seen in the brain or spinal cord in any of the 50 patients.

Echocardiography in patients with SLE shows a high frequency of valvular disease, especially Libman-Sacks endocarditis.[231] Other heart lesions are also common. In their clinicopathologic study, Devinsky et al found that 25 of 50 patients had cardiac lesions that were potential sources of brain emboli.[226] These included Libman-Sacks vegetations (8 patients), acute and chronic mitral valvulitis (12), marantic endocarditis (2), and bacterial endocarditis (1). Two patients had mural thrombi—one in the left atrium and one in the left ventricle.[226] Endocarditis in SLE is discussed in more detail in Chapter 9. Myocarditis is also a feature of SLE. Evaluation of patients with SLE who have focal neurologic signs or focal lesions on MRI should include thorough hematologic and cardiac evaluation.

Thrombotic thrombocytopenic purpura (TTP) is characterized clinically by fever, renal failure, thrombocytopenia, and microangiopathic hemolytic anemia.[232-235] Abnormalities of the metabolic pathway of von Willebrand factor (vWF), particularly of its cleaving protease, are thought to be important in the pathogenesis of TTP.[232] Platelet-rich thrombi fill arterioles and capillaries, causing microinfarcts within the brain. Transient focal neurologic signs, which improve quickly, and a more diffuse encephalopathy are common clinical features. Some reports note that neurologic deficits occasionally persist, and occlusions of large intracranial arteries and their branches are sometimes

found.[232,236,237] Brain hemorrhages have also been reported.[238] Some patients with TTP develop an encephalopathy associated with headache, seizures, and visual loss, accompanied by reversible brain-imaging abnormalities predominantly located in the posterior portions of the cerebral hemispheres.[238] This reversible posterior leukoencephalopathy syndrome is related to altered renal function and probably represents a "capillary leak" syndrome that is potentially reversible.[239] Modern neuroimaging might show in the future that strokes are rather common in TTP, but are usually minor and nondisabling. Some drugs, including ticlopidine and clopidogrel, are reported to cause TTP.[240-242] Plasma exchange can be an effective treatment, so this condition is important to recognize.[243]

Severe *rheumatoid arthritis (RA)* can be complicated by neuropathies, meningitis, and rheumatoid dural nodules. True arteritis with fibrinoid necrosis is occasionally seen and can cause an encephalopathy or multifocal small infarcts.[198,244-247] In patients with active RA, levels of fibrinogen, fibrinogen turnover, and fibrin degradation products are increased.[244-248] Also, high titers of circulating rheumatoid factor can cause a hyperviscosity syndrome.[249] Undoubtedly, these serologic changes contribute to brain infarcts in patients with RA.

Patients with *Sjögren's syndrome* often have a neuropathy, especially involving the trigeminal nerves.[250] These patients also often have cognitive and behavioral abnormalities.[251,252] In a neuroimaging study of 38 patients with Sjögren's syndrome, 8 patients had focal neurologic deficits—most often hemiparesis, aphasia, and ataxia, as well as other cognitive and behavioral abnormalities.[252] MRI in this study showed CNS abnormalities in 75% of patients, most often in the white matter. Occasionally, discrete cortical lesions were seen that resembled infarcts.[252] Vasculitis has been found at necropsy in patients with Sjögren's syndrome, but many of the lesions clinically and on MRI resemble multiple sclerosis, and are likely due to demyelination rather than brain infarcts.[252,253]

Headache is common in patients with *systemic sclerosis (scleroderma)*. Occasionally, brain infarcts and SAH are reported.[254-256] Hypertension is common in scleroderma, and some of the neurovascular symptoms are probably caused by high blood pressure and reversible vasoconstriction.

SARCOIDOSIS

Sarcoidosis causes a variety of CNS manifestations, including intraparenchymatous granulomas, meningitis, and myelopathy.[257-259] Sarcoidosis occasionally causes a cerebral vasculitis almost invariably accompanied by a CSF pleocytosis. Retinal inflammatory changes are also often present.[260-263] The cerebrovascular abnormalities probably represent spread of inflammatory cells from the meninges through Virchow-Robin spaces to the smaller pial vessels. Veins are predominantly affected, so the vascular lesion is probably most accurately classified as a phlebitis or venulitis.[264] Periphlebitis can be noted on ophthalmoscopic examination of the fundus. The retinal lesions are characterized by a yellowish-white focal or diffuse sheathing of retinal veins. Figure 11-14 shows fundus photographs that illustrate the periphlebitis. Hard exudates, sometimes termed *taches de bougie* because of their resemblance to candle-wax drippings, are often related to the periphlebitis and can leave white chorioretinal scars.[261,265]

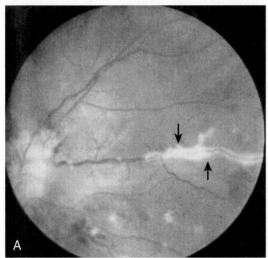

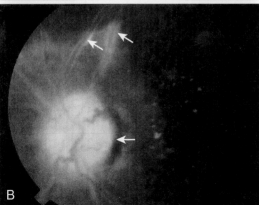

Figure 11-14. Retinal fundus photographs of patients with sarcoidosis illustrating periphlebitis. **A,** Extensive focal perivenous sheathing *(black arrows).* **B,** Perivenous sheathing is prominent, involving the veins at the top of the fundus photograph *(small white arrows).* The optic disc is pale and atrophic. (**A,** From Forbes CD, Jackson WF: A Colour Atlas and Text of Clinical Medicine. London: Wolfe Medical Publications, 1993, with permission; **B,** courtesy of Dr Larry Frohman, University of New Jersey School of Medicine.)

TIAs, strokes, and evidence of meningeal, hypothalamic, and pituitary dysfunction are the clinical features of angiitic neurosarcoidosis, a disorder that can also affect the spinal cord, peripheral nervous system, and muscle. The periphlebitis and meningitis often respond to corticosteroids when given in substantial doses and over long periods (e.g., 60 mg of prednisone daily for 3 to 6 months or more). Immunosuppressant drugs, such as immuran, cyclosporine, and methotrexate, have been used with success in some patients.

GIANT CELL (TEMPORAL) ARTERITIS

Giant cell arteritis usually affects elderly men and women.[266-268] Although the branches of the ECA, especially the superficial temporal and occipital arteries, are most frequently involved, the ICA, ECVA, subclavian, coronary, femoral, and even intracranial arteries can be affected.[267-270] Blindness is caused by granulomatous arteritis in the arteries supplying the optic nerve and retina.[266,268] The lesions most often causing strokes are located in the distal extracranial ICAs as they enter the carotid siphon and in the distal ECVAs.[270,271] Rarely, patients have been described with encephalopathy and multifocal neurologic signs who have the findings of temporal arteritis in pial and brain arteries.[272] Occasional patients present with multi-infarct dementia.[273]

Temporal arteritis usually presents as a systemic illness. Patients often develop headaches that differ from past headaches. Headaches are not pulsatile and are accompanied by aching in the proximal muscles, low-grade fever, weight loss, malaise, fatigue, and jaw claudication. Jaw claudication results from ischemia of the masseter muscles supplied by branches of the ECAs. The superficial temporal arteries may be tender, cord-like, and nonpulsatile, and the scalp may be diffusely tender. The best-known and most feared complication is vision loss. An ischemic optic neuropathy results from occlusion of the posterior ciliary arteries. Additionally, occlusion of the central retinal artery can lead to an ischemic retina. If vision loss occurs, it is usually severe. Involvement of one eye is often followed by involvement of the other.[267,268]

Laboratory findings that may be of help are an elevated erythrocyte sedimentation rate, elevated CRP, elevated fibrinogen levels, slight anemia, and an elevated leukocyte count.[267] Temporal arteritis may be present with a normal erythrocyte sedimentation rate. Color duplex ultrasonography of the superficial temporal arteries and their major branches may show stenoses, occlusions, or a diagnostic hypoechoic halo around the perfused lumen of the arteries.[274] Biopsy of the temporal

11

artery is the most secure manner to make the diagnosis. Angiography with opacification of the ECA branches and the intracranial circulation can be suggestive. If possible, I choose to biopsy a smaller scalp branch of the superficial temporal artery. It is best to biopsy a segment of artery identified as abnormal by palpation, ultrasonography, or angiography. A long segment of the artery is taken to avoid possible skip lesions, but the major portion of this artery is preserved. It is important to look for the general features of temporal arteritis in elderly patients with stroke. Stroke, however, is rarely the first manifestation of temporal arteritis.

Treatment with prednisone (60 to 80 mg/day) is begun before biopsy in patients with clinically probable temporal arteritis. In such patients, rapid relief of headache and other systemic symptoms usually occurs. Steroids are tapered by titrating the dose against the symptoms and the erythrocyte sedimentation rate. Treatment does not reverse established central or ocular ischemia but helps prevent further involvement of blood vessels.

ISOLATED CENTRAL NERVOUS SYSTEM ANGIITIS

In some patients, arteritis is limited to the CNS. This syndrome of isolated CNS angiitis, also called granulomatous angiitis and giant cell granulomatous angiitis of the CNS, is rare and can be difficult to diagnose.[275,275a] Any age can be affected (mean age is approximately 49 years) and males predominate (nearly 2 to 1).[275,276] The disorder can be acute, with symptoms developing within a few weeks, or it can evolve during a period of months to years.[276,277] Usually, the clinical picture is that of a diffuse or multifocal encephalopathy.[275-279] Cognitive and behavioral changes are found in more than 60% of patients and headache, asymmetric motor signs, somnolence, and seizures are common findings.[276-279] Occasionally, TIAs or sudden strokes are described.[275-277] A myelopathy may also be present.[276,277] Focal signs may occur at onset, but more often step-like worsening punctuates the course of a progressive multifocal encephalopathy. The erythrocyte sedimentation rate is elevated in approximately two thirds of patients, but other serologic and systemic tests are not helpful.[276] The CSF usually has a slight-to-moderate pleocytosis, and the CSF protein is usually high (80%), often higher than 100 mg/dL.[276]

CT and MRI may show small or large focal lesions, usually infarcts, but small hematomas and hemorrhagic infarcts have also been noted.[276,281] In approximately one half of the patients, angiography is abnormal and shows segmental narrowing and sausage-shaped dilatation of arteries ("beading").[276,281,282] In some patients, however, angiography is completely normal or shows nonspecific abnormalities.[280,281] Segmental vascular narrowing is also found in patients who abuse drugs and in reversible vasoconstriction syndromes, so this angiographic finding is not specific for arteritis. In fact, segmental vasoconstriction is many times more common than isolated CNS angiitis. Figure 11-18 shows a patient who had a reversible vasoconstriction syndrome and illustrates vascular narrowing and dilatation that is often misdiagnosed by radiologists as representing an arteritis.

Biopsy or necropsy shows a segmental, necrotizing granulomatous vasculitis affecting mostly the leptomeningeal, cortical, and spinal vessels. Any size artery or vein can be involved, but usually vessels 200 to 500 μm in diameter are most affected. In some patients, granulomatous changes have been predominantly venular.[276,277] The intima and adventitia of arteries are infiltrated with lymphocytes, giant cells, and granulomas. Granulomas can extend into the adjacent brain parenchyma. Specific diagnosis is important because treatment with prednisone and immunosuppressant agents, such as cyclophosphamide, may allow recovery from a disease that is nearly always fatal when untreated.[275,276,279] Biopsy should be pursued in patients with multifocal lesions and encephalopathy, especially if they have a CSF pleocytosis and a high-protein content. Moore urges biopsy of the nondominant hemisphere, especially the tip of the temporal lobe, choosing tissue that contains a longitudinally oriented surface vessel.[279]

TAKAYASU'S ARTERITIS

Often called *pulseless disease*, Takayasu's arteritis was originally described in young Japanese girls and women.[283,284] The condition is well known in other countries, but is still uncommon in North America.[285] Although girls and women are predominantly infected, often at young ages, in India middle aged men develop a similar clinical picture.[286] Some patients have a prodromal phase of malaise, fever, and night sweats, and laboratory analysis reveals anemia and an increased sedimentation rate. Later, severe occlusive disease of the aortic arch and its branches develops, often leading to absent neck and limb pulses.[284-288]

Surprisingly, strokes or focal neurologic signs are not the predominant clinical feature. Headache, dizziness, syncope, and visual blurring are more common. In some patients, neurologic function is well preserved despite striking radiologic signs of occlusion of vessels at their origin from the aortic arch.[289] Occlusions, stenosis, luminal irregularities, and ectasia or aneurysm formation are found. The most common sites of involvement are the midportion of the left CCA, left and right subclavian arteries, and the midportion of the innominate artery.[289-292] The inflammatory process involves the media and adventitia, which are infiltrated with plasma cells, lymphocytes, and histiocytes.[290-293] During the inflammatory stage, elastic fibers and smooth muscle cells are destroyed. After the inflammatory stage subsides, fibrosis replaces the damaged portions of the arterial intima, media, and adventitia.[293] The intracranial arteries,[294] heart, and heart valves are sometimes involved.[286,295]

Diagnosis of Takayasu's arteritis can often be made by ultrasonography. Duplex scans invariably show bilateral involvement in the proximal portions of the CCAs, consisting of long segments of concentric thickening of the arterial walls.[296] The subclavian artery lesions are also readily shown by ultrasonography.[296] Ultrasound can also be used to monitor the lesions and their response to treatment.

Arm and leg claudication is commonly related to the subclavian, aortic, and iliofemoral disease. Hypertension is present in more than one half of the patients and may be difficult to control. The chronic proximal occlusive disease often leads to retinal microaneurysms and arteriovenous anastomoses. Vision loss can result from the chronic eye ischemia.[297] The proximal occlusive disease leads to extensive collateral circulation. Hypertension and increased flow through collateral channels can cause SAHs and ICHs similar to that found in the moyamoya syndrome. Corticosteroids, immunosuppressive therapy, angioplasty, and surgical bypass treatment[293,298] have all been used. Corticosteroids (prednisone 30 mg/day initially, then tapered to 5 to 10 mg/day maintenance) may prevent or diminish vascular complications.[283,293,299]

BEHÇET'S DISEASE

Behçet's disease is a relapsing, remitting illness first described by a Turkish dermatologist who recognized the triad of oral ulcers, genital ulcers, and uveitis.[300,301] The disease is most often found in Turkey, Saudi Arabia, Mediterranean countries, and Japan but does occur in North America, Europe, and worldwide. Behçet's disease is important for neurologists to recognize. The predominant clinical systemic findings are aphthous ulcers in the mouth and genital tissues, uveitis, synovitis, other skin findings (e.g., folliculitis and erythema nodosum), ulcerative lesions in the bowel mucosa (especially the colon), and thrombophlebitis.[302-304] The disorder affects mostly young adults in their 20s. The male-to-female ratio ranges from 2:1 to

4:1.[301-306] Neurologic involvement probably occurs in approximately 6% to 10% of patients. Among a large series containing 323 patients with Behçet's disease followed in a clinic in Turkey, only 46 patients were referred because of headache and neurologic signs and only 17 patients (5.3%) had neurologic abnormalities.[302]

The most common neurologic syndromes are (1) a meningitic form, in which headache is the major symptom; (2) an encephalitic form, with gradually evolving multifocal signs; (3) strokes, characterized by relatively acute-onset focal signs; and (4) headache, with papilledema caused by dural sinus thrombosis.[297,302-309] Characteristically, the neurologic signs occur during attacks with remissions between, a course that closely mimics multiple sclerosis. CT and MRI show that the most frequent sites of involvement are the pons and midbrain, followed by the basal ganglia and thalamus. The lesions most often are small foci that have high signals on T2-weighted MRI images and are isointense or hypointense on T1-weighted images.[305,306] Some lesions are large. The brainstem lesions often do not conform to arterial territories and are larger than those found in arteritis.[303] The spinal cord is also frequently involved clinically and by MRI. The lesions often contain hemosiderin, and the distribution in gray and white matter separates the lesions from those found in multiple sclerosis. Usually, angiography does not show arterial abnormalities.

The CSF is almost always abnormal, including pleocytosis, high-protein content, and increased levels of immunoglobulins, that are produced intrathecally.[313] The CSF pressure is sometimes elevated. The levels of oligoclonal bands of IgA and IgM correlate well with neurologic disease activity and are useful to follow. At necropsy, there often is a diffuse meningoencephalitis with perivascular lymphocytic cuffing predominantly around veins, venules, and capillaries, with occasional arterial involvement.[306,309] The dural sinuses and large veins may be occluded.[300,307,310,312] Thromboses of leg veins and even the vena cava are important systemic features, and the pathology is predominantly venous. The brain shows areas of necrosis, demyelination, and scarring, especially in the rostral brainstem, internal capsule, and basal ganglia, as well as in the spinal cord. The lesions probably represent focal hemorrhagic venous infarcts and areas of encephalitic change. Corticosteroids may suppress ocular and brain symptoms.[307]

COGAN'S SYNDROME

Cogan described a syndrome of interstitial keratitis with vestibulo-auditory dysfunction.[314] The condition is probably an autoimmune vasculitic disorder that affects young adults. The earliest symptoms are photophobia, reduced vision, and redness of the eyes.[315-317] An interstitial keratitis is found on ophthalmologic examination, occasionally with uveitis. Blindness can result from corneal opacification. Tinnitus, reduced hearing, vertigo, and ataxia appear before, during, or after eye abnormalities.[315,317] Microscopic study shows a vasculitis of small- and medium-sized arteries. Some patients have fever, and the aortic valve and bowel may be involved.[315,316] The aorta is occasionally involved, causing aortitis and aortic aneurysm formation.[315,318] Some patients have an accompanying meningo-encephalitis,[315] intracranial vascular regions of constriction and dilatation and ectasia have been reported but are quite rare in Cogan's syndrome.[315,319]

EALES'S DISEASE

Eales described an ocular disorder characterized by abnormal retinal vessels and recurrent vitreous hemorrhages.[320,321] The condition that Eales described is probably not a specific disease entity, but is a retinopathy found in a variety of vascular retinal conditions.[321,322] Eales-type retinopathy affects mostly young men and is most common in the Middle East and India. Visual symptoms include specks, floaters, cobwebs, curtains, and blurred vision.[323] The visual symptoms are caused by retinal periphlebitis, nonperfusion of retinal capillaries, and vitreous hemorrhages.[321-323] Some patients have extensive retinal revascularization and fibrovascular proliferation.[321]

Ophthalmologic examination shows prominent sheathing of veins and arteries, flame-shaped retinal hemorrhages, and vitreous hemorrhages. Although the symptoms usually begin in one eye, both eyes are invariably involved. The macular arteries are relatively spared, so that central vision is often preserved.[323] A vasculitis affecting both retinal arteries and veins causes the eye findings. Sometimes, the uvea is also involved.

CNS involvement has been described in the form of meningitis, focal infarcts, and vascular occlusions.[321,325-328] In one patient, a left cerebral infarct was caused by MCA occlusion.[325] Spinal cord involvement has also been reported.[327] Usually, there are no systemic symptoms or characteristic laboratory abnormalities, although the CSF may show a pleocytosis.[325] Diagnosis is made on the basis of the characteristic ophthalmoscopic abnormalities.

MICROANGIOPATHY OF THE BRAIN, EAR, AND RETINA

An unusual, but distinct, occlusive vascular disorder was called microangiopathy of the brain and retina by Susac and colleagues.[329-332] Although this condition (also called Susac's syndrome and retino-cochleo-cerebral vasculopathy[333]) resembles granulomatous angiitis in some ways, there are important differences. In microangiopathy of the brain and retina, there is always obliteration of large retinal arteries, causing gradual, severe, bilateral visual loss.[329-336] The retinal vascular abnormalities are easily seen through the ophthalmoscope. Some retinal arteries are amputated, whereas others are severely narrowed or attenuated and light streaking characterizes their thickened arterial walls. Figure 11-15 shows photographs of the ocular fundus in a patient with this condition. Tinnitus and hearing loss are also prominent.

The most important clinical neurologic signs are cognitive and behavioral abnormalities, bilateral

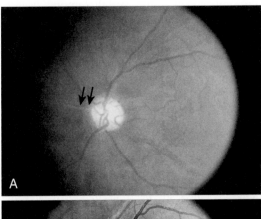
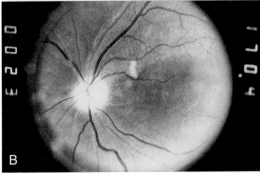

Figure 11-15. Retinal fundus photographs of a patient with microangiopathy of the brain and retina. **A,** *Small black arrows* point to a white occluded retinal artery. The other arteries are also attenuated. The larger vessels are veins. The optic disc is very pale and atrophic. **B,** The other eye shows many occluded and attenuated retinal arteries. Fluffy exudates and pale regions of retina are also shown. The optic disc is chalky white. The patient was blind because of the retinal arterial disease. (Courtesy of Dr Thomas Hedges III.)

motor weakness with pyramidal signs, and cerebellar dysfunction. MRI often shows small increased signal foci on T2-weighted brain imaging, located in both grey and white matter but usually sparing the corpus callosum.[332] The condition affects mostly young women in their second to fourth decade and it usually progresses stepwise or gradually. The CSF protein is high, sometimes more than 1 g/dL, but usually there is no major pleocytosis. Brain biopsy has shown obliteration of small arteries without prominent inflammation or granulomas, as well as multiple microinfarcts.[329-336] Some patients with this condition have improved at least temporarily after corticosteroids and immunosuppressive therapy.[336]

OTHER OCULOCEREBRAL ARTERIOPATHIES

Acute posterior, multifocal, placoid-pigment epitheliopathy was first described by J Donald Gass as an ophthalmologic syndrome rather than a specific entity, that was characterized by "multiple cream-colored placoid lesions" located in the posterior pole at the level of the pigment epithelium and choroids.[337-339] It is an acute chorioretinal condition that usually develops in young adults often after a flu-like febrile illness.[337-341] Both eyes are usually affected simultaneously but sometimes sequentially. Symptoms include visual blurring, distortion, and scotomas. The optic fundus shows multiple, well-circumscribed, gray-white flat lesions at the level of the retinal pigment epithelium. Vision usually returns to normal after several weeks. Occasionally, however, patients develop progressive disease with significant loss of vision.[341] A choroidal vasculitis is the posited cause. Headache, CSF pleocytosis, optic neuritis, and strokes have been reported.[337-344] Cerebral angiography sometimes shows an arteritis.[341] In one patient, brain histopathology showed focal granulomatous inflammation of medium-sized arteries.[345]

Vogt-Koyanagi-Harada syndrome is an important differential diagnostic consideration in patients with ocular inflammatory lesions. The disorder is often called uveo-meningo-encephalitis. Patients with this syndrome may have premature whitening of the hair and eyelashes, alopecia, vitiligo, iridocyclitis, choroiditis, and loss of hearing.[346] They may also have meningeal signs and a CSF pleocytosis.[346-349] An inflammatory adhesive arachnoiditis develops and explains many of the symptoms. Fluorescein angiography shows leakage from retinal vessels. Papilledema and increased intracranial pressure can occur. Some patients have had prominent neurologic signs but whether these were a manifestation of vascular inflammation is not clear. The clinical findings are similar to Behçet's disease except for the absence of dermatologic abnormalities. Usually, the disorder remits after 6 to 12 months, but there may be recurrences.

I have seen a number of patients during the years with ocular inflammatory disorders with vascular abnormalities that involve the iris, aqueous and vitreous humors and the retina who also have had CSF pleocytosis, headache, neurologic signs, and MRI lesions that could represent infarcts. These patients did not have illnesses that correspond to the commonly recognized oculocerebral vasculopathies. Many other arteriopathies probably exist that have a predilection for the eye and nervous system, among other organ involvement.

SNEDDON'S SYNDROME

Sneddon's syndrome is characterized by a chronic skin lesion, livedo reticularis, and recurrent strokes. This syndrome is often found in young patients without risk factors for stroke.[350-354] The most important and diagnostic clinical feature is livedo reticularis, a bluish-gray mottling of the skin that usually involves the trunk and all limbs (Fig. 11-16). The cutaneous findings are obvious by simply looking at the skin with the patient undressed. A cold environment makes the skin abnormality more obvious. I have seen several patients with Sneddon's syndrome who had undergone multiple invasive tests but apparently had never been examined without clothes. Usually, the hands and feet are cold and peripheral pulses are reduced. Hand angiography may show dramatic occlusions of digital arteries with areas of narrowing and dilatation.[354] Skin biopsy may show distinctive abnormalities. Small- to medium-sized arteries at the border between the dermis and subcutis show early inflammatory lesions followed by subendothelial proliferation and later, fibrosis.[354]

I have also seen many patients with irregular grayish areas of irregular mottling of the skin especially in the thighs and proximal arms and trunk whose findings would not qualify for livedo reticularis who have had otherwise unexplained penetrating artery-related brain infarcts. Others have had migraine. I wonder if their skin vascular abnormalities could be a window into a more generalized endotheliopathy or vascular contractile disorder that includes the blood vessels in the brain.

The neurologic findings in patients with Sneddon's syndrome are explained by multiple acute-onset strokes. CT and MRI often show multiple infarcts in the cerebral cortex and white matter.[350,352-354] Cerebral angiography often shows

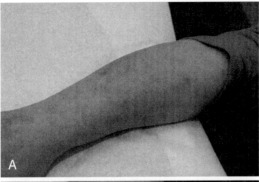

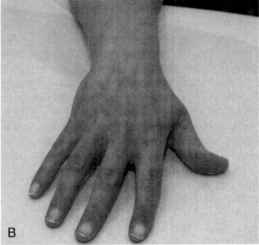

Figure 11-16. Photographs of the hand and arm of a patient with Sneddon's syndrome showing livedo reticularis.

branch occlusions of intracranial arteries.[351,355] At times, the disorder is familial.[356] Some patients with Sneddon's syndrome have antiphospholipid antibodies.[350,357] Valvular cardiac abnormalities are also relatively common in patients with Sneddon's syndrome, and some of the brain infarcts may be caused by cardiac-origin embolism.[352,356,357]

The skin vasculature may provide a clue to the small vessels within the eye and brain. It is essential to examine stroke patients undressed to ensure inspection of the trunk and extremities for skin abnormalities.

KOHLMEIER-DEGOS SYNDROME

Kohlmeier-Degos syndrome, also called malignant atrophic papulosis, is a vascular occlusive disorder with characteristic skin changes.[358,359] The condition can begin at any age and has been described in children.[359] The skin lesions begin as small, yellow-pink raised lesions, usually on the trunk and arms.[358-361] The central part of the skin lesions becomes atrophic and looks porcelain-white, flat,

and depressed, and each lesion is surrounded by a raised pink zone, often with telangiectasis.[360] Small- and medium-sized arteries in the skin undergo a progressive fibrosis with infarcts of the skin.[358-362] Skin biopsy shows fibrous proliferation between the intima and internal elastica with rare inflammatory changes.[360-362] The bowel is also commonly involved, causing ulcers, decreased motility, bowel dilatation, and, often, perforation.[358-362] Although the vessels in other visceral organs are often involved at necropsy, systemic symptoms are usually limited to the skin and gut.

CNS symptoms occur in approximately one fifth of patients with Kohlmeier-Degos syndrome.[360] Strokes do occur. Brain imaging shows infarcts and small hemorrhages. Angiography may show occlusion and beading of distal branches of intracranial arteries.[360] Neuropathologic examination shows hyalinization or fibrous proliferation between the endothelium and internal elastic membrane, often with superimposed thrombosis.[358-362] Inflammatory abnormalities are slight or absent. Occasionally, SAH and dural sinus thrombosis are present.[360,362] At times, strokes precede skin and bowel involvement. Kohlmeier-Degos's disease is often fatal, but some patients may have remissions.[362]

VASCULOPATHY IN DRUG ABUSERS

Drug abuse has become an important cause of stroke in adolescents and young adults. ICH caused by drugs is considered in Chapter 13 and is most often caused by amphetamines and cocaine.[363] Ischemic stroke usually relates to one of five different situations: (1) heroin addiction, (2) amphetamine abuse, (3) abuse of drugs synthesized for oral use, (4) infection as a complication of an addictive lifestyle, and (5) cocaine use.

Heroin Addiction

In heroin addicts, strokes are most often ischemic and may be cerebral or spinal. Stroke frequently follows the reintroduction of intravenous heroin after a period of abstention.[364-368] Brain ischemia may directly follow the heroin injection but is more often delayed by 6 to 24 hours. Heroin addicts also often have serologic and systemic abnormalities, including eosinophilia, elevated immune globulins and gamma globulins, false-positive serology, Coombs-positive hemolysis, and lymph-node hypertrophy.[367] Increased binding of serum globulins by morphine has been found in rabbits with implanted morphine pellets. In some narcotic addicts, morphine also binds gamma globulins.[369] Illicitly available heroin is often adulterated with a host of fillers and foreign substances. These observations make it likely that immune-complex deposition or other hyperimmune mechanisms underlie the strokes in patients who are chronically exposed to many recurrently introduced antigens.[367] Definitive immunologic or pathologic studies of strokes in heroin addicts are wanting.

Amphetamine Use

A number of amphetamine-like substances are used or abused, including dextroamphetamine, methamphetamine, methylphenidate, ephedrine, pseudoephedrine, and phenylpropanolamine.[364] Stimulation is the commonest reason for abuse, while weight-loss preparations and cold remedies also often have contained amphetamine-like substances. Brain hemorrhages are more common after methamphetamine abuse than brain ischemia. Infarcts are sometimes seen at necropsy but a clinical ischemic stroke is unusual. Hemorrhages usually develop soon after amphetamine use and are caused by the sudden elevation in blood pressure induced by the surge of catecholamines.[363] Hypertension is likely an idiosynchratic reaction to phenylpropanolamine in some individuals.

In some patients with amphetamine abuse, necrotizing angiitis has been shown pathologically. The lesions resemble polyarteritis nodosa and can affect the brain and other viscera.[370] In experimental animals[371] and humans[372] who have taken amphetamines orally or intravenously, angiography shows segmental changes in intracerebral vessels with prominent beading. Patients with SAH or ICH after amphetamine abuse have a relatively low frequency of harboring aneurysms and vascular malformations that are the source of intracranial bleeding.[363]

Abuse of Drugs Synthesized for Oral Use

A different pattern of disease affects patients who inject intravenous drugs that have been designed for oral use; methylphenidate (Ritalin) and pentazocine (Talwin) with pyribenzamine are the best-documented drugs. These compounds contain talc, microcrystalline cellulose, and other fillers that are used to maintain the chemicals in pill form. Addicts mash the pills, dissolve them in tap water, and inject them intravenously or even directly into the carotid artery.[373] Particles of drugs and fillers still remain in the fluid injected and are trapped by the lung arterioles and small arteries, causing an obliterative arteritis.[373,374] Pulmonary arteriovenous shunts develop and passage through these shunts is probably responsible for crystals that reach the brain and eyes of addicts.[373-375] Strokes and seizures usually follow quickly after intravenous injection. Deep, small cerebral arteries, such as the lenticulostriate[373] and anterior spinal arteries, are most often affected.[376]

Infection as a Complication of an Addictive Lifestyle

Drug abusers seldom follow strict sterile precautions. Hepatitis, AIDS, infective endocarditis, and fungal infections are common complications of their habit and lifestyle. Endocarditis can cause embolic strokes. Fungal infections, especially *Nocardia* and *Aspergillus*, can cause focal necrotic infarcts or brain abscesses.[149,151,152]

Cocaine Use

Cocaine use has become the most common cause of drug-related strokes. Cocaine use is rampant. In a 1990 study among 214 patients aged 15 to 44 years admitted to the San Francisco General Hospital during a 10-year period, 34% were drug users and cocaine was the predominant drug used.[377] Cocaine is snorted or injected as cocaine hydrochloride or is smoked as the free-base alkaloidal form, usually called crack cocaine.[364,368,378-380] Crack cocaine is made by mixing aqueous cocaine hydrochloride with ammonia and sometimes baking soda. The free-base cocaine is usually smoked after the cocaine has become alkalinized and precipitated. Crack cocaine induces a more rapid increase in blood levels than cocaine hydrochloride and produces a more rapid high than does snorted or injected cocaine hydrochloride. Its use is associated with a higher frequency of brain infarcts.[364,368,381] The strokes usually begin shortly after cocaine use, irrespective of the portal of entry (snorted, inhaled, or injected). Brain infarcts have a predilection for the brainstem.[382] Spinal cord infarcts also have been reported to develop soon after cocaine use.[383] The mechanism of ischemia is unknown but vasoconstriction related to cocaine itself or its metabolites is the major posited mechanism. Bowel and myocardial ischemia and an eosinophilic myocarditis are also found after chronic cocaine abuse.[364,384] Many patients drink alcohol while using cocaine. There appears to be a synergism between cocaine and ethanol.[364,385] Cocaine is metabolized in the presence of ethanol to cocaethylene, which binds more powerfully than cocaine itself to monoamine transporter proteins.[364,385]

Vasoconstriction, increased platelet aggregation, and apparent vasculitis are posited as potential causes of stroke in cocaine users. Arterial constrictions (predominantly MCAs and PCAs (focal and diffuse) were found on MRA studies taken 20 minutes after intravenous cocaine administration in healthy subjects who had used cocaine previously but were not addicts.[385]

11

Cocaine use is also associated with SAHs and ICHs.[363,364] For unclear reasons, there is a higher incidence of aneurysms and vascular malformations in cocaine-related hemorrhages than in hemorrhages after amphetamines.[363,387] Angiography should be performed unless the cocaine-related hemorrhage is in a characteristic location for hypertensive ICH. Cocaine also enhances vasospasm after aneurysmal SAH.[364] Cocaine users can also develop a picture that resembles hypertensive encephalopathy with multiple hemorrhages and brain edema. Figure 11-17 is a brain specimen that illustrates hypertensive encephalopathy with hemorrhages after cocaine use.

MIGRAINE AND VASOCONSTRICTION SYNDROMES

Vascular headaches are among the most common disorders treated by physicians and neurologists. Migraine is prevalent at all ages, including young children and the elderly. Although migraine most likely begins with a discharge within the brain, vasoconstriction is an important part of the migraine syndrome.[388-390] A genetic tendency for

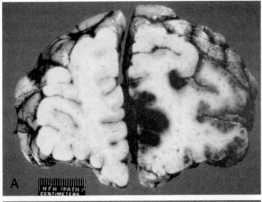

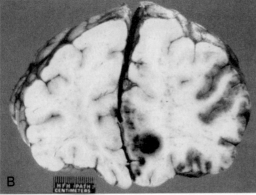

Figure 11-17. Brain specimens at necropsy in a patient who died after crack cocaine use. Multiple brain hemorrhages and brain edema are shown. (Courtesy of Dr Steven Levine.)

migraine also predisposes patients to a number of neurologic syndromes in which reversible vasoconstriction plays an important role.[388-390] During migraine attacks, angiography, CBF studies, and TCD have clearly documented changes in intracranial vessel diameter, flow velocities, and CBF.[390] Reversible vasoconstriction has been shown to be an important cause of ischemia, especially in the coronary circulation and in the brain after subarachnoid bleeding. Migraine is a clinical diagnosis usually applied when there is a past history and family history of pulsating, usually unilateral headaches, with or without characteristic visual, somatosensory, or other migraine accompaniments and followed by nausea and vomiting. Although vasoconstriction and vasodilatation have been shown to occur during migraine attacks, not all vasoconstriction occurs in patients with migraine.

Neuroimaging in patients with migraine shows a more frequent-than-expected incidence of infarcts.[388,391] Migraine-related strokes have been the subject of a number of reports and case series.[388,390,392-395] Retrospective and prospective studies report an increased risk of ischemic stroke especially among migraineurs with aura.[396,397] A meta-analysis of several observational studies showed a twofold risk of ischemic stroke in patients with migraine and a threefold risk if migraine was accompanied with aura.[398] Stroke is especially common in young women who have migraine with aura for 12 or more years.[399]

Infarction can be caused by prolonged intense vasoconstriction,[388,389,400] causing permanent ischemia or thrombosis of arteries. Intense vasoconstriction can impede flow, promoting thrombosis; platelets are activated during migraine, and the vasoconstrictive process itself may stimulate the endothelium to release factors that promote thrombosis. My own investigations on stroke within the PCA and basilar-artery territories in patients with migraine show that some patients develop thrombi within the basilar artery and the PCA.[390,394,401]

Migrainous accompaniments can precede, accompany, or follow headache and can occur in the absence of headache. Transient vasoconstriction accounts for many examples of temporary spells of neurologic dysfunction in the elderly,[402-404] including transient global amnesia.[388,390,405,406] Fisher[402,403] and I[390] have attempted to separate migraine accompaniments from atherosclerotic ischemia by analyzing the clinical features (Table 11-1). To complicate matters, atherosclerotic lesions in the coronary arteries of humans and in the extracranial and retinal arteries of experimental animals seem to predispose them to superimposed vasoconstriction. Thus, vasoconstriction can complicate atherostenosis. TCD shows promise in

Table 11-1.   Migraine Accompaniments versus Atherosclerotic Ischemia

Migraine	Atherosclerotic Ischemia
Sensory modalities involved sequentially (e.g., vision, tactile, speech)	Modalities involved together (e.g., visual, somatosensory, and aphasic abnormalities noted at same time)
Within each modality, first symptoms are "positive" (e.g., visual brightness, shining, somatosensory paresthesias)	Usually negative symptoms (e.g., loss of vision, numbness)
Symptoms gradually progress within each modality; vision loss gradually affects field; paresthesias move from one finger to hand to body—often takes 20 minutes to travel fully	Visual field or body involved at once without spread
Within each modality, positive followed by negative (e.g., brightness leaves scotoma in its wake; paresthesias followed by numbness)	Usually negative effects only
One modality clears before the next is involved	Modalities are involved simultaneously
Headache most often follows after neurologic symptoms have cleared	Headache accompanies persistent deficits or is absent
Attacks usually last 15 to 30 minutes (average, 20 minutes)	Attacks last usually about 1 to 2 minutes, often 5 minutes
Different attacks involve different sides and vascular territories	Attacks always involve the same vascular territory
Spells may occur over years and often begin in the 20- to 40-years of age span	Attacks occur during a span usually limited to days, weeks, or months; most patients are >50 years of age
Stroke risk factors often absent	Stroke risk factors present
Women predominate over men	Men predominate over women except after the menopausal years

identification of vasoconstriction by showing high velocities that change with time and various pharmacologic treatments.

Call, Fleming, and colleagues called attention to a syndrome that they called reversible cerebral segmental vasoconstriction.[389,407] The syndrome most often affects young women, especially during the puerperium, but also occurs at menopause and is found at all ages. When it occurs after childbirth, the syndrome has been called postpartum angiopathy.[408] The onset is often with a so-called thunderclap severe headache.[409,409a] Some patients have developed this syndrome after carotid endarterectomy.[410] The use of serotonin reuptake inhibitors prescribed for depression and cannabis, especially when smoked in a binge, can provoke the syndrome.[409a]

Recurrent headache, focal neurologic signs, and occasionally seizures are the predominant symptoms. Vasoconstriction involves many large, medium, and small-sized cerebral arteries. The clinical findings include severe headache, decreased alertness, seizures, and changing multifocal neurologic signs. Brain edema and death can occur. Brain imaging may show focal subarachnoid blood on the surface of the brain,[409a,410a] and in adjacent sulci and small regions of abnormality on FLAIR-MRI imaging representing small infarcts. Angiography shows sausage-shaped focal regions of vasodilatation and multifocal regions of vascular narrowing. Figure 11-18 shows angiographic abnormalities in a patient with this syndrome. TCD shows high velocities in many intracranial arteries. At times the initial vascular imaging studies are normal and only become abnormal after a few days or a week.[409a] Corticosteroids, calcium channel blockers, anticonvulsants, and treatments for increased intracranial pressure have been used to treat this disorder. Many of the patients have had a history of migraine.

Two other important clinical syndromes that include migraine-like headache and neurologic signs are the Bartleson and SMART syndromes.[388] Bartleson's syndrome (also referred to as a pseudomigraine syndrome with pleocytosis) is characterized by attacks resembling migrainous auras that occur in a flurry and are accompanied by prominent headache and cerebrospinal fluid pleocytosis.[411,412] The CSF contains a lymphocytic predominant pleocytosis (>100 cells) and an elevated protein content. Many patients have recurrent aphasia sometimes associated with visual

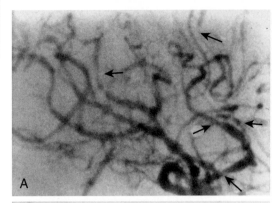

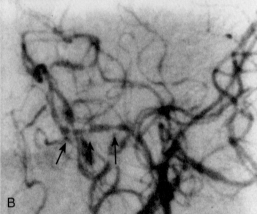

Figure 11-18. Carotid artery angiograms, intracranial magnified views from a patient with a reversible vaso-constriction syndrome. The *black arrows* point to focal regions of narrowing of arterial branches. Sausage-like dilatations are also present.

blurring or scotomata and with right limb sensory or motor dysfunction. Right hemisphere attacks also occur. The attacks are relatively stereotyped in individual patients and always involve either the left or right cerebral hemisphere in each attack. The attacks last between 15 minutes and an hour. Attacks may occur more than once a day and cluster during a period of 3 to 6 weeks. The condition may represent a primary migraine disorder with an inflammatory etiology but other possibilities include a viral meningovascular infection or some other undefined aseptic meningitis. The clinical course of Bartleson's syndrome is typically self-limited, and lasts usually from 4 to 12 weeks. Calcium-channel blockers are effective in my experience.

Stroke-like migraine attacks after radiation therapy (SMART) is a relatively new syndrome in which stroke-like migraine attacks occur as a late consequence of brain irradiation.[388,413,414] Attacks may begin years after radiation. The migraine-like events consist of prolonged, but reversible, neurologic dysfunction that may persist

for several weeks. Headaches are often but not always preceded by aura. MRI may show diffuse cortical enhancement that resolves. No pattern to date has been found that associates the dose of radiation, tumor type, or specific chemotherapeutic agents with the occurrence of this syndrome.[388,413,414]

ICH occasionally complicates a severe migraine attack.[388,415-417] Intense vasoconstriction leads to ischemia of a local brain region with edema and ischemia of the small vessels perfused by the constricted artery. When vasoconstriction abates, blood flow to the region is augmented and the reperfusion can cause hemorrhage from the damaged arteries and arterioles.[388,415-417] The mechanism is the same as that found in hemorrhage after carotid endarterectomy and in reperfusion after brain embolization.[417]

I am convinced that vasoconstriction accounts for many more strokes than is currently recognized or appreciated. Surveys of strokes in the young attribute many infarcts to migraine. I take seriously the risk of stroke in patients with prolonged classic migraine attacks, especially if the deficits last for hours or more after the attack. In these patients and in those with migraine-related infarcts, I use prophylactic agents (most often calcium channel blockers, topiramate, cyproheptadine, or methysergide), along with agents that modify platelet function and coagulation. Aspirin is used most often, but I sometimes use warfarin in patients with prior infarcts and thrombosis of cerebral arteries.

ECLAMPSIA

Eclampsia is a very important, serious, often life- and brain-threatening disorder of pregnancy and the early postpartum period that, like the Call-Fleming syndrome, includes cerebral vasoconstriction.[408,418] Preeclampsia is characterized by increased blood pressure over the usual base-line value and often proteinuria, hyperreflexia, and restlessness. If a seizure then occurs, the condition is called eclampsia. Severe preeclampsia and eclampsia can develop during the first 10 days after delivery.

Although magnesium sulfate has been shown to prevent seizures it is not a very effective agent to reduce the hypertension and the blood pressure must be reduced. Brain hemorrhage, brain infarction, renal and liver failure and the HELLP syndrome (hemolysis, elevated liver function tests, and low platelets) are important complications of inadequately treated preeclampsia and eclampsia. Vascular imaging testing in patients with eclampsia often shows reversible vasoconstriction identical to that found in nonpregnant women with the Call-Fleming syndrome discussed and illustrated above.[408,419,420]

One complication of eclampsia is the *reversible posterior leukoencephalopathy syndrome*.[421-425] The syndrome is characterized by agitation and restlessness, confusion, seizures, and visual dysfunction that includes visual hallucinations and cortical blindness. Brain imaging most often shows white matter hyperintensities maximal in the occipital and posterior temporal white matter but sparing the paramedian occipital striate regions. Figure 11-19 shows a CT scan and MRI scans in a patient with the reversible posterior leukoencephalopathy syndrome. This syndrome is likely a capillary leak syndrome related to endothelial dysfunction and increased body fluid volumes. Many different conditions including preeclampsia and eclampsia are associated with the syndrome including: hypertensive encephalopathy, immunosuppressive drugs including cyclosporine and

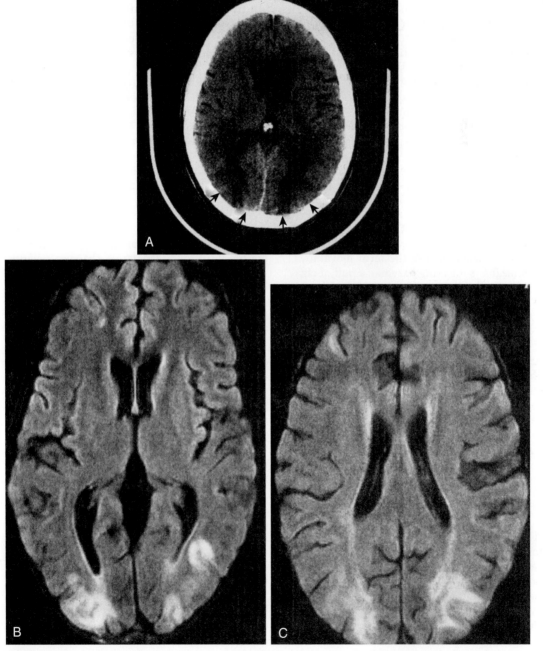

Figure 11-19. Reversible posterior leukoencephalopathy. **A,** CT scan showing hypodensity in the occipital lobes. **B** and **C,** T2-weighted MRI scans of same patient showing bilateral occipital temporal hyperintensities.

tacrolinus, pheochromocytoma, acute glomerulo-nephritis, and acute endocrinopathies. Many are accompanied by increased blood pressure, proteinuria, and tissue edema. Experience has shown that the cortex as well as white matter are often involved, that the abnormalities can be frontal, brainstem, cerebellar, and diffuse and are not always limited to the posterior cerebral hemispheres, and in some patients irreversible tissue damage develops, especially if the blood pressure elevations and edema are not treated rapidly and effectively.[425]

MOYAMOYA SYNDROME

Moyamoya, although sometimes referred to as a disease, is probably better thought of as a syndrome defined by a characteristic angiographic appearance.[426] The intracranial ICAs undergo progressive tapering and progressive occlusion at their intracranial bifurcations (the so-called T-portion of the ICAs). Basal penetrating branches of the ICAs, ACAs, and MCAs enlarge to provide collateral circulation. These vessels form large prominent anastomosing channels, basal telangiectasias, which appear on angiograms as a cloud of smoke. These arteries are especially prominent because of the paucity of MCA sylvian branches. The appearance of these basal telangiectasias led Japanese clinicians to use the term moyamoya, which means "something hazy like a puff of cigarette smoke drifting in the air."[426-428] Although first described in Japan,[428] the condition has been reported worldwide.[426,429,430]

Necropsy studies, although few, have shown severe vascular occlusive abnormalities characterized by endothelial hyperplasia and fibrosis, with intimal thickening and abnormalities of the internal elastic lamina.[431] In contrast, the intracerebral perforating arteries show microaneurysm formation, lipohyalinosis, focal fibrin deposition, and thinning of the elastic laminas and arterial walls.[432] These changes in the perforating arteries are probably the result of greatly increased flow through these small vessels.[426-428,432] The vessels do not show inflammatory abnormalities.

In 1991, Ikeda studied the extracranial arteries of 13 Japanese patients with spontaneous occlusions of the circle of Willis at necropsy who met the research definition of moyamoya syndrome.[433] Extracranial arteries showed the same intimal lesions as the intracranial arteries. Characteristically, the proximal pulmonary arteries had fibrous nodular intimal thickening without inflammatory abnormalities.[433] Moyamoya vascular abnormalities have been found in a variety of situations, including sickle cell disease, neurofibromatosis,

Takayasu's disease, Down's syndrome, atherosclerosis, and fibromuscular dysplasia, and can be found in young women, especially those who smoke cigarettes and take oral contraceptives.[431] A variety of different conditions can probably cause intimal changes, which lead to fibrosis and luminal narrowing.

Moyamoya syndrome is approximately 50 times more common in girls and women than in boys and men.[434] Clinically, the disorder has a bimodal distribution, presenting most often in children younger than 15 years and in adults in their third to fifth decades of life. Children usually present with transient episodes of hemiparesis or other focal neurologic signs often precipitated by physical exercise or hyperventilation. Several of my own young patients have had intermittent choreoathetosis. Other patients have sudden-onset deficits, such as hemiplegia, or the gradual development of intellectual deterioration. Headaches and seizures are common.[426-428] These symptoms are often accompanied by CT and MRI evidence of infarction and CBF studies that show regions of hypoperfusion. The abnormal vasculature is often visible on MRI.

Adults, in contrast, usually present with brain hemorrhages, typically in the thalamus, basal ganglia, or deep white matter. These hemorrhages are the result of degenerative changes (aneurysmal dilatation and thinning) in the anastomotic basal vessels that are overtaxed and cannot accommodate the volume of blood needed for perfusion. At times, the hemorrhages are subarachnoid and intraventricular. Some patients with moyamoya syndrome develop aneurysms involving arteries of the circle of Willis, especially the anterior cerebral anterior communicating artery region and the basilar artery.[435] Angiography shows progressive changes that may be asymmetric initially but always involve the intracranial ICAs bilaterally and usually also involve the proximal portions of the MCAs and ACAs. As the intracranial arteries narrow, collaterals develop involving the basal penetrating arteries, orbital vessels (so-called ethmoidal moyamoya), and vessels over the vault derived from transdural anastomoses from the meningeal and superficial temporal arteries.[426-428] Later, the telangiectasias may regress and become less prominent. Suzuki and others have staged the severity of disease by the angiographic findings.[427,428]

Some patients with moyamoya syndrome stabilize clinically, often after they have developed disabilities. The best treatment is not known.[428a] A variety of different surgical revascularization procedures have been used. These usually involve anastomosing the superficial temporal artery to the MCA or placing the superficial temporal and middle meningeal arteries adjacent to the pia, or placing vascularized connective tissue elements and muscle on the surface of the pia matter.[434,436-438] The surgical revascularization created is often called synangiosis. Angiography after surgical revascularization shows improved collateral blood flow.[436-438] It is hoped that revascularization might prevent further ischemia and hemorrhage, but no systematic trials have investigated the effectiveness of revascularization procedures.

HEMATOLOGIC DISORDERS, INCLUDING ABNORMALITIES OF COAGULATION, VISCOSITY, AND SERUM CONSTITUENTS

Since the 1980s, knowledge of blood constituents and their function in the coagulation process has dramatically advanced. Brain ischemia and hemorrhage can develop as a direct result of hematologic abnormalities rather than from primary diseases of the blood vessels.[439,440] In other patients with endothelial lesions in the aorta, heart, and blood vessels, activation of coagulation functions causes thrombi to form on the abnormal endothelial surfaces and often precipitates strokes. In turn, occlusion of arteries increases coagulation factors. The endothelia, blood vessels, and circulating blood are so intricately interwoven that it is often difficult to know which changes are primary and cause the disorder and which are secondary to the occlusive vascular process. I have discussed most of the hematologic conditions in Chapters 4 and 5 regarding laboratory diagnosis and treatment. Only a brief cataloging of these disorders is presented here.

Cellular Abnormalities

Abnormalities in the formed cellular constituents of the blood may be quantitative or qualitative. Polycythemia has long been known to increase blood viscosity, decrease CBF, and increase thrombosis. Severe anemia is also associated with increased coagulability and can predispose to venous sinus thrombosis.

Sickle cell disease and sickle cell hemoglobin C disease are examples of qualitative red blood cell abnormalities that affect blood flow. Sickle cell disease is associated with occlusive changes in large intracranial arteries and small penetrating vessels.[441-444] Subcortical, cortical, and borderzone infarcts are often found on CT and MRI. Angiography has shown intracranial occlusions of the major basal arteries. The walls of intracranial arteries are thickened, and intimal and subintimal proliferation occurs. Arteries may become dilatated and ectatic even in childhood.[445] Occasionally, veins and dural sinuses may thrombose.[446] TCD offers a noninvasive method for detecting velocity changes related to intracranial large artery narrowing and allows monitoring of patients with sickle cell disease.[441,442,447,448] Blood transfusions for children whose TCD blood-flow velocities in the ICAs or MCAs or both exceed 200 cm per second have been shown in a trial to prevent stroke from developing.[448]

Paroxysmal nocturnal hemoglobinuria (PNH) is characterized by a qualitative abnormality of red blood cells that leads to hemolysis and life-threatening thrombotic episodes.[449-451] This condition is known to be caused by a mutation in hematopoietic stem cells that leads to clones of blood cells that are deficient in surface proteins that are normally attached to cell membranes. Neutropenia and thrombocytopenia are also common. The incidence of thrombosis reaches about 30% by 8 years after diagnosis and increases to nearly 50% after 15 years.[450,451] Cerebrovascular events are an important contributor to morbidity and mortality. The cranial veins and arteries are the second most important site of thrombosis secondary only to hepatic vein thromboses.[450,451] Cerebral venous and dural sinus thromboses are the most common clinical neurologic manifestations. Systemic and intracranial hemorrhages can result from the thrombocytopenia, which may be severe.

Increased platelet counts, especially those higher than 1 million, are also associated with hypercoagulability. The thrombocytosis can be primary, so-called essential *thrombocythemia*, and can be associated with other myeloproliferation, or, less often, can be secondary to systemic disease. Essential thrombocythemia is associated with strokes and digital occlusions.[452-456] The lack of correlation between the platelet count and the thrombotic complications has led to the assumption that there are also qualitative abnormalities of platelet function.[439,452-454] In some patients, increased coagulability has been attributed to increased adhesion and aggregation of platelets (so-called sticky platelets) in the absence of thrombocytosis.[453,454,457-459] Thrombocytopenia caused by a variety of different conditions can lead to important brain and systemic bleeding.

Leukemia is complicated occasionally by brain hemorrhages and microinfarcts. When the white blood cell count is high (increased leukocrit), the white blood cells can pack capillaries, leading to microinfarcts and vascular rupture with small brain hemorrhages. Larger brain hemorrhages and SAHs are most often related to thrombocytopenia caused by replacement of the bone marrow with leukocyte precursors.

Serologic Abnormalities: Hypercoagulability and Bleeding

Normally, natural inhibitors of coagulation circulate to discourage spontaneous blood clotting. The best known of these inhibitors, antithrombin III and proteins C and S, can be deficient on a hereditary basis or be reduced by disease.[439,440,460] Congenital deficiency of antithrombin III may be quantitative or qualitative and is most often an autosomal-dominant condition.[439,460,461] Reduced synthesis of antithrombin III, as in patients with liver disease or renal loss in the nephrotic syndrome, can lead to acquired deficiencies. Inherited deficiencies of proteins C and S can also contribute to or cause increased coagulability.[439,440,460,462] An inherited coagulation deficit referred to as resistance to activated protein C was described by Dutch investigators from Leiden, and is the most common cause of abnormal protein C activity.[463,464] In most instances, resistance to activated protein C is caused by a point mutation in the gene that encodes for coagulation factor V.[464] The presence of this mutation, called factor V Leiden, is accompanied by a threefold to fivefold increase in the frequency of venous thromboembolism in the lower extremities[463] and an increased frequency of cerebral venous and dural sinus thrombosis. Factor V Leiden is the most common genetic disorder that leads to hypercoagulability.

The second most common genetic mutation that leads to a prothrombic state is a mutation in the gene encoding prothrombin.[466] This mutation involves a transition from guanine to adenine at position 20210 in the sequence of the 3' untranslated region of the prothrombin gene.[466] The frequency of cerebral and peripheral venous thrombosis is greatly increased in carriers of the prothrombin gene mutation, especially if they also take oral contraceptive pills.[466-468] Genetic analysis is warranted in patients with unexplained hypercoagulability, especially those with cerebral venous thrombosis and recurrent peripheral venous thromboembolism. Most often, clotting is venous, but arterial occlusions have also been described.

Systemic and inherited conditions can alter the levels of the serine protease coagulation factors. The best known of these disorders is hemophilia, which causes bleeding into the joints, skin, and cranium. In 1989, my colleagues and I measured factor VIII levels in a large number of patients with brain ischemia.[469] Some patients have chronically increased concentrations of factor VIII, with frequent episodes of venous thrombosis, spontaneous abortion, and strokes.[470] In others, factor VIII levels are high, probably as an epiphenomenon to the initial thromboembolic event.

Some patients with infectious and inflammatory diseases, such as Crohn's disease and ulcerative colitis, have increased factor VIII levels as a result of serologic changes induced by the primary disease.[471-474] Venous dural sinus occlusions, thrombophlebitis, and arterial occlusions may result. Hematologic changes in inflammatory bowel disease are complex because elevated levels of factors V and VIII, reduced levels of antithrombin III, and quantitative and qualitative platelet abnormalities have all been described.[471,473]

Studies have also shown that infections of various types are often present in the days and weeks before stroke onset.[475,476] Infections and various inflammatory disorders provoke an increase in acute phase reactants and white blood cells, fibrinogen, and coagulation factors V, VII, and VIII, which induce thrombosis in patients with preexisting endothelial lesions.[477,478]

Cancers are also often associated with hypercoagulability.[479-481] My colleagues and I studied patients with mucinous adenocarcinomas who had venous occlusions, large artery thrombi, and multiple small artery occlusions.[482] Mucin was seen inside and directly outside of small vessels, presumably contributing to the hypercoagulability evident clinically. In some situations (e.g., during pregnancy, the puerperium, or use of oral contraceptives), the mechanism of hypercoagulability is not fully known.

The advent of thrombolytic and fibrinolytic treatment, especially with recombinant tissue plasminogen activator, has led to more detailed study of the body's normal fibrinolytic activity and abnormalities of the fibrinolytic system.[483-485] Plasminogen deficiencies, dysfibrinogenemias, and abnormalities of tissue plasminogen activator and its inhibitors can cause an increased tendency toward both venous and arterial thrombosis.[483,486-489] Increased thrombosis is caused by a deficiency of plasminogen or increased inhibition of plasminogen activator by plasminogen inhibitior (PAI-1).[486-489] Thrombin and fibrinolytic activity can be monitored during acute stroke by measuring a number of substances.[483,490,491] For example, the levels of fibrinopeptide A correlate with thrombin activity, and the levels of cross-linked D-dimer, a breakdown product of fibrin polymer, are a useful index of fibrinolytic activity.[490,491]

Bleeding can also result from serological abnormalities. Acquired hemophilia is a condition seen most often in the elderly in which factor VIII autoantibodies, usually of the IgG type develop and can cause life-threatening bleeding.[492,493]

Acquired hemophilia may develop after pregnancy and after a variety of illnesses including cancer and collagen vascular disease. Patients show a prolonged aPTT that is not normalized by mixing their plasma with normal plasma because an inhibitor is preventing thromboplastin generation. Excess fibrinolytic activity can also cause bleeding and is most common after thrombolysis for myocardial or brain ischemia.

Von Willebrand disease is another condition that can occasionally be associated with intracranial as well as systemic bleeding. The condition is caused by a deficiency or altered function of von Willebrand factor, a plasma glycoprotein that is involved in platelet adherence and adhesion and that stabilizes blood coagulation factor VIII.[493a,b,c] The disease has autosomal dominant and recessive inheritance. The von Willebrand-factor gene is located on chromosome 12. Bleeding is related to impaired platelet functions or reduced concentrations of factor VIII. Bleeding is often heavily menstrual or after wounds or surgeries.

Immunologic Abnormalities

Attention has been drawn to the presence of circulating antibodies that react to various hematologic and vascular components. Acquired hemophilia was mentioned as an example. The best known and most common of these autoantibodies are the lupus anticoagulant (LA) and anticardiolipin antibodies. These substances react against phospholipids. Phospholipids are ubiquitous components of vascular structures and various blood constituents.

The presence of LA or anticardiolipins has been referred to as the antiphospholipid antibody (APLA) syndrome.[494] The LA (a misnomer because it is associated with increased coagulability, not bleeding) is a phospholipid antibody that interferes with the formation of the prothrombin activator.[494-496] In the laboratory, there is a prolonged activated partial thromboplastin time that does not correct when normal plasma is added, indicating the presence of an inhibitor of clotting rather than a deficiency of a needed component.[494-497] Some patients with LA have SLE but most do not.

When antiphospholipids of the IgG, IgM, or IgA classes are found in the absence of a known systemic illness, the disorder is referred to as a primary APLA syndrome.[494,496-502] Clinically, these patients have an increased incidence of spontaneous abortions, thrombophlebitis, pulmonary embolism, and large- and small-artery occlusions. In addition to the presence of LA or anticardiolipins or both, laboratory abnormalities include positive VDRL, thrombocytopenia, and antinuclear antibodies. Some patients have mitral and aortic valve abnormalities and ocular ischemia.[494,496,501,502] The cardiac lesions are identical to those described as Libman-Sacks and involve the valves as well as the endothelium of the heart. The mechanism of increased coagulability and valvular changes is not known, but these probably relate to immune-related endothelial and valve-surface injuries.[503-505] Patients with high-positive IgG and APLA have a high incidence of subsequent vascular occlusive lesions.[506,507] Anti-beta 2-glycoprotein I and antiphosphatidylserine antibodies seem to be better predictive of the tendency to thrombosis than other measured antibodies.[504,505] Antiphosphatidylserine antibodies form complexes with prothrombin.[505] Angiography in patients with APLA syndrome shows a high frequency of intracranial occlusive disease, atypical extracranial occlusive arterial disease, and venous and dural sinus occlusions.[508] Some patients with APLA have a Binswanger type leukoencephalopathy.

Disseminated intravascular coagulation (DIC) is a disorder that affects cellular and serologic factors.[509-513] When a primary disorder leads to local or diffuse clotting, the coagulation cascade may be activated with generation of excess intravascular thrombin. The coagulation system then is further activated, fibrin is deposited into the microcirculation, hemostatic elements have a shortened survival, and the fibrinolytic system is activated.[509] The most common disorders inciting DIC are infections, obstetric and vascular emergencies, and cancer.[510,511] Head trauma, SAH, brain tumors, and vascular malformations can also cause DIC.[510,512,513] The laboratory findings include thrombocytopenia, reduced fibrinogen levels, prolongation of prothrombin time and partial thromboplastin time, and increased levels of fibrin split products. DIC can be associated with nonbacterial thrombotic endocarditis, especially in patients with cancer.[479,482,510,512,513] Neurologic findings are frequent and include an encephalopathy with multifocal signs and frank thrombotic and embolic infarcts. Bleeding can also occur.

Blood flow, especially in the brain microcirculation, depends heavily on the viscosity of the blood. *Blood viscosity* is most affected by the erythrocyte content of the blood and serum fibrinogen level.[514-516] Polycythemia and hyperfibrinogenemia can increase whole-blood viscosity and decrease CBF, especially in patients with cerebrovascular disease. High fibrinogen levels are an important risk factor for stroke and other large artery occlusive disease.[517] Less often, increased viscosity is caused by high levels of globulins (e.g., in Waldenström's macroglobulinemia or in other disorders with abnormal proteins or cryoglobulins, such as multiple myeloma).[518] Rarely, high levels of serum lipids cause significant hyperviscosity.[514,519]

Clinically, patients with hyperviscosity syndromes have an encephalopathy characterized by somnolence, stupor, headache, seizures, ataxia, and decreased vision.[514,518] A clue to the presence of hyperviscosity is the ophthalmoscopic appearance of the retina. Retinal veins are dilatated and tortuous and may show segmentations in the blood columns within retinal vessels. Serum viscosity is measured relative to water; the average normal level is approximately 1.8. Serum viscosity of 5 or 6 is usually associated with encephalopathy but lower levels may be important in patients with hypertensive microvasculopathy and atherosclerotic disease.

NEOPLASTIC CONDITIONS

Lymphomatoid granulomatosis is an angiocentric lymphoproliferative condition predominantly affecting the lungs in which granulomatous nodules can involve brain arteries and veins and produce stroke-like deficits.[520-522] Lymphomatoid granulomatosis has recently been found to be caused by an Epstein-Barr viral infection of B lymphocytes and is classified as an Epstein-Barr virus–associated form of lymphoproliferative disease.[522] The lung and brain regions of necrosis are presumably related to infarction caused by the cellular vascular infiltrate ("angiitis"). The most common extrapulmonary findings are in the skin and nervous system—each accounting for about a third of patients. The skin lesions usually consist of a raised erythematous rash and occasionally skin nodules, especially on the trunk. CNS lesions are more common than cranial or peripheral neuropathies and usually consist of focal and multifocal brain mass lesions.[520-523]

Lymphomas can present as a solely intravascular tumor. This entity, now called *intravascular lymphoma*, was previously called neoplastic angioendotheliosis.[524-529] Large pleomorphic mononuclear cells proliferate within the lumens of capillaries, venules, arterioles, and small arteries. The neoplastic intraluminal cells usually have a B-cell phenotype although they may rarely be of T-cell or NK-cell origin.[524] The neoplastic cells occlude small arteries, leading to multiple microinfarcts. The disorder can be systemic, producing erythematous skin plaques and patches, subcutaneous nodules, high sedimentation rates, fever, and renal failure. The disorder can affect the spinal cord.[530] Headache, multifocal neurologic signs, and a progressive course are typical. The brain lesions on MRI vary and range between white matter hyperintensity to large areas of signal abnormalities. Meningeal enhancement can occur and is explained by microinfarcts within the meninges or slow flow through meningeal blood vessels. Angiography is usually normal because the blood vessels involved are too small to be seen during angiograms.

Hodgkin's disease in the meninges often causes occlusions of meningeal arteries and veins, with hemorrhagic infarction in the underlying cerebral cortex. I have already commented in this chapter on leukemic blockage of small arteries and on the coagulopathies associated with cancer, especially of the mucinous adenocarcinoma type.

SOME GENETIC DISORDERS THAT CAUSE STROKES

Many of the conditions already discussed in this chapter, such as hereditary disorders of connective tissue and the hereditofamilial cerebral amyloid angiopathies, are known to be genetically determined. Many others are probably influenced by genetic predispositions. Dyslipoproteinemias, hemoglobinopathies, diabetes, hypertension, and atherosclerosis are strongly governed by genetic factors. I close this chapter by briefly discussing a few other disorders with mendelian etiologies. Knowledge of the genetic factors in stroke is growing rapidly.[531-535]

The *MELAS syndrome* (mitochondrial myopathy, encephalopathy, lactic acidosis, and stroke-like episodes) is one form of mitochondrial encephalomyopathy.[536-538] Seizures, headaches, and intellectual deterioration are most prominent clinically.[536-541] Short stature and sensorineural deafness are also common features.[538] Constipation is common before and at onset of neurologic symptoms. Affected patients often have acute-onset episodes of visual deterioration, hemiparesis, and ataxia, often with seizures. Lactic and pyruvic acid levels in the blood are often high and muscle biopsy may show ragged red fibers.[536-539] CT and MRI show discrete multifocal abnormalities that are most often in the parieto-occipital and temporal lobes.[540-544] These lesions affect the cortex and underlying white matter. These lesions are caused by ischemia, but the arteries supplying these zones are normal. They are probably explained by the metabolic abnormality characterized by decreased cytochrome oxidase activity within mitochondria, leading to energy failure. Basal-ganglia calcifications are also prominent. The disorder is caused by a maternal mutation in mitochondrial DNA.[533,536] Other mitochondrial disorders may also be associated with white matter abnormalities on MRI that resemble infarcts.

Strokes, renal failure, painful dysesthesias, and cutaneous angiokeratomas characterize *Fabry disease*. The disorder is a sex-linked lysosomal storage disease. Most clinical cases involve homozygous men. Occasionally, heterozygous women are affected.[545-551] The diagnosis is suggested by finding the characteristic tiny, pinhead-size, dark-reddish purple non-pruritic papules that are located predominantly along the inner thighs, perineum, and near the umbilicus in a so-called bathing trunk distribution (Fig. 11-20). Because of a deficiency of a lysosomal enzyme (alpha-galactosidase), trihexosyl

ceramide (a sphingolipid) accumulates and causes a diffuse vasculopathy.[545-550] The disease is often manifest in adolescent boys who have severe lower extremity pain especially during and after exercise and syncope related to a small fiber and autonomic neuropathy. Sweating is also diminished or absent, so that heat and exercise intolerance are common. The myocardium is also often involved, and the condition presents in some patients as a cardiomyopathy. Deafness is also common and may begin abruptly.

Multiple vascular occlusions and strokes are common. Strokes tend to be lacunar related to penetrating artery disease. Some patients have had dolichoectatic dilatated intracranial arteries.[545,546] Some strokes are cardioembolic related to the cardiomyopathy sometimes found in patients with Fabry disease. Angiography often shows occlusion of branch arteries. The endothelium is infiltrated with the sphingolipid. Death is most often caused by renal failure unless dialysis is performed. Regular infusions of recombinant alpha-galactosidase A is able to clear endothelial deposits of globotriaosylceramide in the kidneys, skin, and endomyocardium and to reduce pain from autonomic neuropathy.[550,551] Young individuals with Fabry disease and enzyme deficiency should receive infusions of the enzyme.[551]

Cerebral autosomal dominant arteriopathy with subcortical infarcts and leukoencephaly (*CADASIL*) is an important familial condition characterized by headache, multiple lacunar infarcts, and extensive white matter abnormalities of the Binswanger type.[552-557] The small arteries within the brain are thickened by eosinophilic, periodic acid-Schiff–positive granular deposits, which have not been characterized fully biochemically.[552,557] The substance within the arteries differs from amyloid. Skin biopsy, especially using electron microscopy, shows the same material within skin arteries. The clinical findings are strokes, progressive gait disorder, and frontal lobe-type subcortical dementia.[552-557] Mood disorders, especially depression, are also common. Headache is a prominent symptom in some patients and in relatives of patients with this leukoencephalopathy.

The MRI shows characteristic lesions.[552,558] White matter hyperintensities are sometimes found before clinical symptoms develop. The white matter abnormalities are common in the anterior temporal lobes, a location rare in hypertensive Binswanger leukoencephalopathy. CADASIL is caused by a mutation of the notch 3 gene on chromosome 19.[552,560] A somewhat similar microangiopathic familial disorder has also been described in Japan. This condition affects predominantly young men and is characterized by a Binswanger-type leukoencephalopathy,

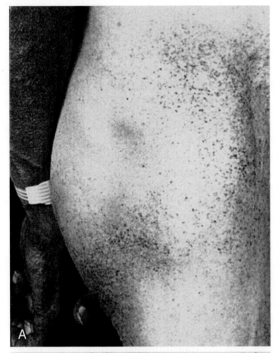

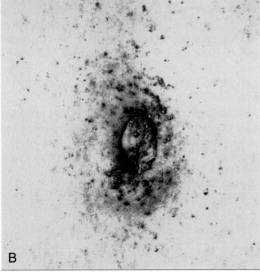

Figure 11-20. Angiokeratomas in Fabry disease.
A, Photo of the buttocks showing typical small lesions.
B, Periumbilical angiokeratomas. (Courtesy of Dr Edward Kaye.)

alopecia, and prominent back pain.[560] The small arteries are infiltrated by fibrous intimal proliferation and severe hyalinosis, with splitting of the intima and internal elastic membrane.[560] There are likely other genetically determined microangiopathies that involve deposition of different biochemical materials into cerebral and systemic arteries that differ genetically from CADASIL.

Menkes disease (trichopoliodystrophy or kinky-hair disease) is an X-linked recessive condition in which mitochondrial dysfunction is caused by impaired intestinal absorption of copper.[561,564] The basic genetic defect is a mutation in *ATP7A*, a gene mapped to the long arm of the X-chromosome (Xq12-q13) that encodes a highly evolutionarily conserved P-type ATP protein (ATP7A) essential for the translocation of metal cations across cellular membranes.[561,563,564] The delivery of copper to cells requires transporters, one of which is deficient in patients with Menkes disease. The deficiency of copper leads to subnormal cytochrome oxidase function within mitochondria and widespread energy failure. The copper content of cultured fibroblasts, myotubes, and lymphocytes derived from patients with Menkes disease is several times greater than control cells.[561] The hair is abnormal and is course, stiff, and easily broken. Hypotonia, hypothermia, seizures, and failure to thrive are common.[561,562,565,566] Ragged red fibers may be seen on muscle biopsy. Electron microscopic studies of the brain can show abnormal mitochondria. MRI studies of the brain show rapidly developing cerebral atrophy and often small deep and cortical infarcts. Subdural hematomas are also common.[561] At necropsy, the brain contains multiple microinfarcts and intracranial branch arteries are often occluded. Most patients die in early childhood. Neonatal diagnosis is now possible and the early diagnosis provides an opportunity for early life copper supplementation.[566a] Copper supplementation, using daily injections of copper-histidine, is the most promising treatment. Parenterally administered copper corrects the hepatic copper deficiency and restores serum copper and ceruloplasmin levels to normal.[561,566a]

Patients with *neurofibromatosis type 1 (NF1)* are known to develop renal and systemic artery and cerebrovascular abnormalities. NF1 is due to a mutation on chromosome 17q11.2, the gene product being neurofibromin (a GTPase-activating enzyme). Café au lait spots, peripheral neurofibromas, and Lisch nodules are the commonest clinical manifestations of NF1.[567] Aneurysms and arterial stenoses occur. Both ischemic stroke and subarachnoid hemorrhage are described.[567-570] Aneurysms can develop both in the neck and intracranially. The most frequent intracranial aneurysms site is within the ICAs as they emerge from the cavernous sinus just after the origins of the ophthalmic arteries.[567-570] A moyamoya picture can result from multiple occlusions of basal arteries (Fig. 11-21). Hypertension may be caused by renal artery occlusion or pheochromocytomas, which occur at increased frequency in patients with this genetic condition.

Homocystinuria is probably the most common genetic disease that affects the brain vasculature and leads to premature atherosclerosis and strokes.[571,572] Severe hyperhomocystinemia and homocystinuria is a genetic disorder first described in children and known to be associated with premature strokes, mental retardation, and a Marfan-like syndrome. Lesser degrees of hyperhomocystinemia are associated with premature atherosclerosis.

Classic homocystinuria is caused by a hereditary deficiency of the enzyme cystathione-beta-synthase, an enzyme that is required for the conversion of methionine-derived homocysteine to cystathione. In humans, approximately 15 to 20 mmol/L of homocysteine is formed each day by demethylation of the amino acid methionine.[572] Homocysteine is subsequently metabolized by one of two pathways, either remethylation or transulfuration. In the remethylation process, homcysteine is remethylated to methionine in a reaction catalyzed by methionine synthase.[572] Vitamin B_{12} is an essential cofactor for methionine synthase, and N5-methyl-tetrahydrofolate is the methyl donor in this reaction. N5,N10-methylene-tetrahydrofolate reductase functions as the catalyst in this remethylation reaction.[572,573] Homocysteine can also be transulfurated when homocysteine condenses with serine to form cystathione, a reaction catalyzed by the vitamin B_6-dependent enzyme cystathione beta-synthase[572-574]. Cystathione is then hydrolyzed to cysteine, which in turn can be incorporated into glutathione or further metabolized to sulfate and excreted in the urine.[572,573,575]

Cystathione-beta-synthase deficiency is the most common genetic cause of severe hyperhomocystinemia. The homozygous form of this disorder is called congenital homocystinuria and is associated with plasma homocystine concentrations of up to 400 (mol/L during the fasting state.[572,573] This genetic disorder is rare (5 in 1 million births). Affected individuals have ectopic lenses, skeletal deformities, a Marfan-like habitus, and severe premature atherosclerosis. Typically, a clinical thromboembolic event in the form of strokes or myocardial infarcts occur before age 30 years.[576] A homozygous deficiency of N5,N10-methylene-tetrahydrofolate reductase, the enzyme involved in the B_{12}-dependent remethylation of homocysteine, can also cause severe hyperhomocystinemia. Patients with this metabolic defect have an even worse prognosis than those with cystathione-beta-synthase deficiency.[572,573]

Less severe forms of hyperhomocystinemia occur in heterozygotes with these enzyme deficiencies. Deficiencies in the cofactors folate and vitamins B$_{12}$ and B$_6$, which are required for homocysteine metabolism, can also cause an elevated homocysteine level. In patients with nutritional deficiencies in these vitamin cofactors, prescribing these substances can reduce homocysteine levels. Increased levels of homocysteine also occur in patients being treated with methotrexate, theophylline, and phenytoin and in patientswith (1) renal insufficiency; (2) hyperthyroidism; (3) breast, pancreatic, and ovarian can0cers; (4) lymphatic leukemia; and (5) pernicious anemia.[572,573] Cigarette smoking has also been associated with elevated homocysteine levels, presumably because of interference with the synthesis of pyridoxal phosphate.[577]

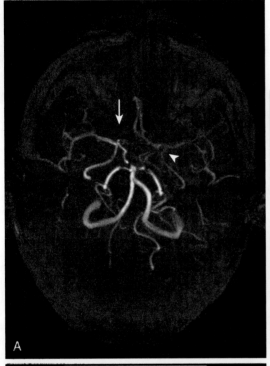

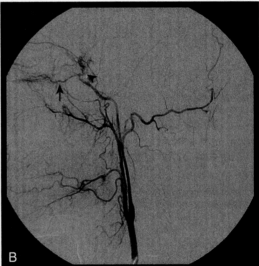

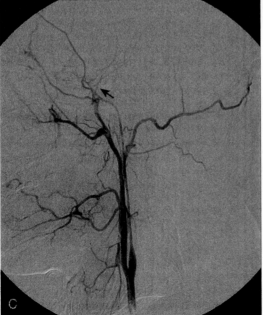

Figure 11-21. A 23-year-old woman with moyamoya syndrome. **A,** MR angiography shows occlusion of the distal right internal carotid artery with dilatated lenticulostriate collaterals *(puff of smoke, arrow)* with a small left internal carotid artery that is occluded in the cavernous portion *(arrowhead).* There is poor flow in the left middle cerebral artery via collaterals. **B,** Catheter digital-subtraction, right-common-carotid artery angiogram shows a large, right ophthalmic artery *(arrow)*, occlusion of the terminal internal carotid artery with dilatated lenticulostriate collaterals *(arrowhead).* **C,** Left common-carotid angiogram shows a small, collapsed, left internal carotid artery with distal occlusion *(arrow)* and no filling of the left middle and anterior cerebral arteries.

Elevated levels of homocysteine have been unequivocally related to strokes, premature atherosclerosis, myocardial infarction, and venous thromboembolism.[572,573,578,579] Evidence from more than 20 case-controlled studies that included more than 2000 individuals has validated the relationship between elevated homocysteine levels and accelerated atherosclerosis.[572,573] Patients with increased levels of homocysteine have more severe carotid artery disease than individuals with normal levels.[580] Experimental evidence shows that increased homocysteine levels injure the vascular endothelium. This injury leads to platelet activation and the formation of thrombi.[581,582] Homocysteine also stimulates vascular smooth muscle cells to proliferate.[583] I have seen several adult males in their 40s who have had repeated lacunar strokes and white matter hyperintensities who have had very high homocysteine levels (>40) and no other stroke risk factors.

Progeria (Hutchinson-Gilford progeria syndrome) is a rare condition characterized by premature ageing beginning in very early life and ending in premature death.[584,584a] Clinical manifestations involve the skin and appendages, joints, and blood vessels causing coronary and cerebrovascular disease during youth.[584] Progeric individuals have a characteristic facial and body appearance readily recognized during the first decade of life. Progeria can result from mutations of the LMNA gene coding for the nuclear membrane protein lamin A and from abnormal DNA repair. Progeria is most often caused by a mutation of the LMNA gene on chromosome 1q.[584-586] The LMNA gene encodes lamin A and C, filamentous structural proteins found in the nuclear lamina. In progeria, the LMNA mutation results in the accumulation of a lipid-modified (farnesylated) prelamin A (*progerin*), impairing nuclear membrane function.[584] Vascular occlusive large artery lesions in the neck and intracranially can appear in the first decade and mirror lesions found in atherosclerotic adults.

Hereditary hemorrhagic telangiectasia (Osler-Weber-Rendu disease) is a disorder characterized by frequent nosebleeds, cutaneous and visceral telangiectasia with gastrointestinal bleeds, brain vascular malformations, and pulmonary arteriovenous fistulas (Fig. 11-22).[587-590] Mutations on two genes, endoglin and activin receptor-like kinase 1, located on chromosomes 9 and 12, respectively, that encode proteins expressed predominantly on vascular endothelial cells relate to the vascular abnormalities.[587,589] The telangiectasias are composed of dilatated post-capillary venules. With time venules become

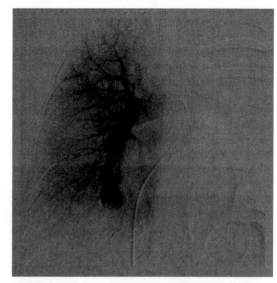

Figure 11-22. A pulmonary angiogram in a patient with hereditary hemorrhagic telangiectasia that shows a pulmonary arteriovenous fistula. This was the cause of a paradoxical embolus to the brain.

more dilatated and convoluted and are characterized by excessive layers of smooth muscle without elastic fibers.[587,589] Arterioles can also dilatate and communicate directly with venules without intervening capillaries. Hereditary hemorrhagic telangiectasia patients often have brain arteriovenous malformations and arteriovenous fistulas. The largest arteriovenous malformations occur in the lungs, liver, and brain. Paradoxical brain embolism can develop in patients with these pulmonary fistulas. Examination of patients with hereditary hemorrhagic telangiectasia nearly always shows telangiectasias on the lips, nasal mucosa, and mucosal surfaces in the mouth.

The *COL4A1 mutation syndrome* has recently been characterized as a familial syndrome of fragile blood vessels with a susceptibility to intracranial hemorrhage.[591-594] Different mutations in the COL4A1 gene that encodes the alpha 1 chain of type IV collagen are implicated. Type IV collagen is an essential component of basement membranes. In mice, COL4A1 mutants have frequent perinatal hemorrhages and have structurally abnormal basement membranes in brain, eyes, and kidneys.[591,592]

Infantile hemiparesis with porencephaly and perinatal hemorrhages are probably related to brain hemorrhages in utero or perinatally. The clinical picture is characterized by a susceptibility to intracerebral and subarachnoid hemorrhages after trauma and during anticoagulation. The retinal blood vessels are tortuous and white matter hyperintensities are common. The COL4A1 mutation syndrome shares with CADACIL a predilection for involvement of small intracranial blood vessels but the tendency for hemorrhage and vascular fragility is unique.[591-594]

References

1. Caplan LR (ed): Uncommon Causes of Stroke, 2nd ed. Cambridge: Cambridge University Press, 2008.

Arterial Dissections

2. Ojemann RG, Fisher CM, Rich JC: Spontaneous dissecting aneurysms of the internal carotid artery. Stroke 1972;3:434-440.
3. Fisher CM, Ojemann RG, Roberson GH: Spontaneous dissection of cervicocerebral arteries. Can J Neurol Sci 1978;5:9-19.
4. Baumgartner RW, Bogousslavsky J, Caso V, Paciaroni M (eds): Handbook on Cerebral Artery Dissection. Basel: Karger, 2005.
5. Caplan LR: Dissections of brain-supplying arteries. Nat Clin Pract Neurol 2008;4:34-42.
6. Caplan LR, Zarins C, Hemmatti M: Spontaneous dissection of the extracranial vertebral artery. Stroke 1985;16:1030-1038.
7. Mokri B, Houser OW, Sandok BA, Piepgras DG: Spontaneous dissection of the vertebral arteries. Neurology 1988;38:880-885.
8. Caplan LR, Tettenborn B: Vertebrobasilar occlusive disease: Review of selected aspects: I. Spontaneous dissection of extracranial and intracranial posterior circulation arteries. Cerebrovasc Dis 1992;2:256-265.
9. Barbour PJ, Castaldo JE, Rae-Grant AD, et al: Internal carotid artery redundancy is significantly associated with dissection. Stroke 1994;25:1201-1206.
10. Brandt T, Hausser I, Orberk E, et al: Ultrastructural connective tissue abnormalities in patients with spontaneous cervicocerebral artery dissections. Ann Neurol 1998;44:281-285.
10a. Guillon B, Peynet J, Bertrand M et al: Do extracellular-matrix-regulating enzymes play a role in cervical artery dissections? Cerebrovasc Dis 2007;23:299-303.
11. Hart RG, Easton JD: Dissection of cervical and cerebral arteries. In Barnett HJM (ed): Neurologic Clinics, vol 1. Philadelphia: Saunders, 1983, pp 155-182.
12. Friedman WA, Day AL, Quisling RG, et al: Cervical carotid dissecting aneurysms. Neurosurgery 1980;7:207-214.
13. Silbert PL, Mokri B, Schievink WI: Headache and neck pain in spontaneous internal carotid and vertebral artery dissection. Neurology 1995;45:1517-1522.
14. Bogousslavsky J, Despland PA, Regli F: Spontaneous carotid dissection with acute stroke. Arch Neurol 1987;44:137-140.
15. Biousse V, Schaison M, Touboul P-J, et al: Ischemic optic neuropathy associated with internal carotid artery dissection. Arch Neurol 1998;55:715-719.
16. Pozzali E, Giuliani G, Poppi M, Faenza A: Blunt traumatic carotid dissection with delayed symptoms. Stroke 1989;20:412-416.
17. Sturzenegger M: Ultrasound findings in spontaneous carotid artery dissection: The value of duplex sonography. Arch Neurol 1991;48:1057-1063.
17a. Alecu C, Fortrat JO, Ducrocq X, et al: Duplex scanning diagnosis of internal carotid artery dissections. Cerebrovasc Dis 2007;23:441-447.
18. Hennerici M, Steinke W, Rautenberg W: High-resistance Doppler flow pattern in extracranial ICA dissection. Arch Neurol 1989;46:670-672.
19. Touboul PJ, Mas JL, Bousser MG, Laplane D: Duplex scanning in extracranial vertebral artery dissection. Stroke 1987;18:116-121.
20. Krueger BR, Okazaki H: Vertebral-basilar distribution infarction following chiropractic cervical manipulation. Mayo Clin Proc 1980;55:322-332.
21. Sherman DG, Hart RG, Easton JD: Abrupt change in head position and cerebral infarction. Stroke 1981;12:2-6.
22. Caplan LR: Posterior Circulation Disease. Clinical Findings, Diagnosis, and Management. Boston: Blackwell, 1996.
23. Cook JW, Sanstead JK: Wallenberg's syndrome following self-induced manipulation. Neurology 1991;41:1695-1696.
24. Rothrock JF, Hesselink JR, Teacher TM: Vertebral artery occlusion and stroke from cervical self-manipulation. Neurology 1991;41:1696-1697.
25. Tramo MJ, Hainline B, Petito F, et al: Vertebral artery injury and cerebellar stroke while swimming: Case report. Stroke 1985;16:1039-1042.
26. Hope EE, Bodensteiner JB, Barnes P: Cerebral infarction related to neck position in an adolescent. Pediatrics 1983;72:335-337.
27. Bostrom K, Liliequist B: Primary dissecting aneurysm of the extracranial part of the internal carotid and vertebral arteries. Neurology 1967;17:179-186.
28. Grossman FI, Davis KR: Positional occlusion of the vertebral artery: A rare cause of embolic stroke. Neuroradiology 1982;23:227-230.
29. Tettenborn B, Caplan LR, Sloan MA, et al: Postoperative brainstem and cerebellar infarcts. Neurology 1993;43:471-477.
30. Giroud M, Gras P, Dumas R, Becker F: Spontaneous vertebral artery dissection initially revealed by a pain in one upper arm. Stroke 1993;24:480-481.
31. Dubard T, Pouchot J, Lamy C, et al: Upper limb peripheral motor deficits due to extracranial vertebral artery dissection. Cerebrovasc Dis 1994;4:88-91.

32. Goldsmith P, Rowe D, Jager R, Kapoor R: Focal vertebral artery dissection causing Brown-Séquard syndrome. J Neurol Neurosurg Psychiatry 1998;64:416-417.

33. Yonas H, Agamanolis D, Takaoka Y, White RJ: Dissecting intracranial aneurysms. Surg Neurol 1977;8:407-415.

34. Caplan LR, Baquis G, Pessin MS, et al: Dissection of the intracranial vertebral artery. Neurology 1988;38:868-879.

35. Anson J, Crowell RM: Cervicocranial arterial dissection. Neurosurg 1991;29:89-96.

36. O'Connell B, Towfighi J, Brennan R, et al: Dissecting aneurysms of head and neck. Neurology 1985;35:993-997.

37. Chaves C, Estol C, Esnaola MM, et al: Spontaneous intracranial internal carotid artery dissection. Arch Neurol 2002;59: 977-981.

38. Caplan LR, Estol CJ, Massaro AR: Dissection of the posterior cerebral arteries. Arch Neurol 2005;62:1138-1143.

38a. de Bray JM, Marc G, Pautot G, et al: Fibromuscular dysplasia may herald symptomatic recurrence of cervical artery dissection. Cerebrovasc Dis 2007;23:448-452.

38b. Schievink WI: The treatment of spontaneous carotid and vertebral artery dissections. Curr Opin Carotid 2000;15:316-321.

39. Kasner SE, Hankins LL, Bratina P, Morganstern LB: Magnetic resonance angiography demonstrates vascular healing of carotid and vertebral artery dissections. Stroke 1997;28: 1993-1997.

40. Leclerc X, Lucas C, Godefroy O, et al: Helical CT for the follow-up of cervical internal carotid artery dissections. AJNR Am J Neuroradiol 1998;19:831-837.

41. Engelter ST, Brandt T, Debette S, et al: Antiplatelets versus anticoagulation in cervical artery dissection. Cervical Artery Dissection in Ischemic Stroke Patients (CADISP) Study Group. Stroke 2007;38:2605-2611.

42. Kadkhodayan Y, Jeck DT, Moran CJ, et al: Angioplasty and stenting in carotid artery dissection with or without associated pseudoaneurysm. AJNR Am J Neuroradiol 2005;26: 2328-2335.

43. Lavallee PC, Mazighi M, Saint-Maurice J-P, et al: Stent-assisted endovascular thrombolysis versus intravenous thrombolysis in internal carotid artery dissection with tandem internal carotid and middle cerebral artery occlusion. Stroke 2007;38:2270-2274.

43a. Ansari SA, Thompson BG, Gemmete JJ, Gandhi D: Endovascular treatment of distal cervical and intracranial dissections with the neuroform stent. Neurosurgery 2008;62: 636-646.

44. Janjua N, Qureshi AI, Kirmani J, Pullicino P: Stent-supported angioplasty for acute stroke caused by carotid dissection. Neurocrit Care 2006;4:47-53.

Fibromuscular Dysplasia

45. Caplan LR: Fibromuscular dysplasia. In Uncommon Causes of Stroke, 2nd ed. Caplan LR (ed): Cambridge: Cambridge University Press, 2008, pp 491-495.

46. Slovut DP, Olin JW: Fibromuscular dysplasia. N Engl J Med 2004;350:1862-1871.

47. So EL, Toole JF, Dalal P, et al: Cephalic fibromuscular dysplasia in 32 patients. Arch Neurol 1981;38:619-622.

48. Corrin LS, Sandok BA, Houser OW: Cerebral ischemic events in patients with carotid artery fibromuscular dysplasia. Arch Neurol 1981;38:616-618.

49. Sandok BA: Fibromuscular dysplasia of the internal carotid artery. Neurol Clin 1983;1:17-26.

50. Luscher TF, Lie JT, Stanson AW, et al: Arterial fibromuscular dysplasia. Mayo Clin Proc 1987;62:931-952.

51. Kubis N, von Langsdorrff D, Petitjean C, et al: Thrombotic carotid megabulb: Fibromuscular dysplasia, septae, and ischemic stroke. Neurology 1999;52:883-886.

52. Mettinger K, Ericson K: Fibromuscular dysplasia and the brain. Stroke 1982;13:46-52.

53. Finsterer J, Strassegger J, Haymerle A, Hagmuller G: Bilateral stenting and asymptomatic internal carotid artery stenosis due to fibromuscular dysplasia. J Neurol Neurosurg Psychiatry 2000;69:683-686.

54. Assadian A, Senekowitsch C, Assadian O, et al: Combined open and endovascular stent grafting of internal carotid artery fibromuscular dysplasia: Long-term results. Eur J Vasc Endovasc Surg 2005;29:345-349.

Heritables Disorders of Connective Tissue

Pseudoxanthoma Elasticum

55. Pessin MS, Chung C-S: Eales disease and Gröenblad-Strandberg disease (pseudoxanthoma elasticum). In Bogousslavsky J, Caplan LR (eds): Stroke Syndromes. Cambridge: Cambridge University Press, 1995, pp 443-447.

56. Lebwohl MG, Distefano D, Prioleau PG, et al: Pseudoxanthoma elasticum and mitral-valve prolapse. N Engl J Med 1982;307: 228-231.

57. Caplan LR, Chung C-S: Pseudoxanthoma elasticum. In Caplan LR (ed): Uncommon Causes of Stroke, 2nd ed. Cambridge: Cambridge University Press, 2008, pp 135-138.

58. Laube S, Moss C: Pseudoxanthoma elasticum. Arch Dis Child 2005;90:754-756.

59. Strole WE, Margolis R: Case records of the Massachusetts General Hospital: Case 10-1983. N Engl J Med 1983;308:579-585.

60. Altman LK, Fialkow PJ, Parker F, et al: Pseudoxanthoma elasticum: An underdiagnosed genetically heterogenous disorder with protean manifestations. Arch Intern Med 1974;134: 1048-1054.

61. Rios-Montenegro E, Behrens MM, Hoyt WF: Pseudoxanthoma elasticum: Association with bilateral carotid rete mirabile and unilateral carotid-cavernous sinus fistula. Arch Neurol 1972;26:151-155.

EHLERS-DANLOS SYNDROME

62. Roach ES: Ehlers-Danlos syndrome. In Caplan LR (ed): Uncommon Causes of Stroke, 2nd ed. Cambridge: Cambridge University Press, 2008, pp 139-144.
63. Byers PH: Ehlers-Danlos syndrome type IV: A genetic disorder in many guises. J Invest Dermatol 1995;105:311-313.
64. Leier CV, Call TD, Fulkerson PK, Wooley CF: The spectrum of cardiac defects in the Ehlers-Danlos syndrome types I and III. Ann Intern Med 1980;92:171-178.
65. Pretorius ME, Butler IJ: Neurologic manifestations of Ehlers-Danlos syndrome. Neurology 1983;33:1087-1089.
66. Lach B, Nair SG, Russell NA, Benoit BG: Spontaneous carotid-cavernous fistula and multiple arterial dissections in type IV Ehlers-Danlos syndrome. J Neurosurg 1987;66:462-467.
66a. Sareli AE, Janssen WJ, Sterman D, et al: What's the connection? N Engl J Med 2008;358:626-632.
67. North KN, Whiteman DAH, Pepin MG, Byers PH: Cerebrovascular complications in Ehlers-Danlos syndrome type IV. Ann Neurol 1995;38:960-964.
68. Schievink WI, Limburg M, Oorthuys JW, et al: Cerebrovascular disease in Ehlers-Danlos syndrome type IV. Stroke 1990;21:626-632.

MARFAN SYNDROME

69. Schievink WI, Parisi JE, Piepgras DG, Michels VV: Intracranial aneurysms in Marfan's syndrome: An autopsy study. Neurosurgery 1997;41:866-870.
70. Conway JE, Hutchins GM, Tamargo RJ: Marfan syndrome is not associated with intracranial aneurysms. Stroke 1999;30:1632-1636.
71. Pyeritz RE: The Marfan syndrome. Annu Rev Med 2000;51:481-510.
72. Cunha L: Marfan's syndrome. In Caplan LR (ed): Uncommon Causes of Stroke, 2nd ed. Cambridge: Cambridge University Press, 2008, pp 131-134.
73. Kainulainen K, Pulkkinen L, Savolainen A, et al: Location on chromosome 15 of the gene defect causing Marfan syndrome. N Engl J Med 1990;323:935-939.
74. Schievink WI, Björnsson J, Piepgras DG: Coexistence of fibromuscular dysplasia and cystic medial necrosis in a patient with Marfan's syndrome and bilateral carotid artery dissections. Stroke 1994;12:2492-2496.
75. Youl BD, Coutellier A, Dubois B, et al: Three cases of spontaneous extracranial vertebral artery dissection. Stroke 1990;4:618-625.
76. van den Berg JS, Limburg M, Hennekam RC: Is Marfan syndrome associated with symptomatic intracranial aneurysms? Stroke 1996;27:10-12.

LOEYS-DIETZ SYNDROME

76a. Loeys BL, Chen J, Neptune ER, et al: A syndrome of altered cardiovascular, craniofacial, neurocognitive and skeletal development caused by mutations in TGFBR1 or TGFBR2. Nat Genet 2005;37:275-281.
76b. Loeys BL, Schwarze U, Holm T, et al: Aneurysm syndromes caused by mutations in the TGF-beta receptor. N Engl J Med 2006;355:788-798.
76c. LeMaire SA, Pannu H, Tran-Fadulu V, et al: Severe aortic and arterial aneurysms associated with TGFBR2 mutation. Nat Clin Pract Cardiovasc Med 2007;4:167-171.

Dilatative Arteriopathy (Dolichoectasia)

77. Savitz S, Caplan LR: Dilatative arteriopathy (dolichoectasia). In Caplan LR (ed): Uncommon Causes of Stroke, 2nd ed. Cambridge: Cambridge University Press, 2008, pp 479-482.
78. Smoker WR, Price MJ, Keyes WD, et al: High-resolution computed tomography of the basilar artery: 1. Normal size and position. AJNR Am J Neuroradiol 1986;7:55-60.
79. Pico F, Labreuche J, Cohen A, et al: Intracranial arterial dolichoectasia is associated with enlarged descending thoracic aorta. Neurology 2004;63:2016-2021.
80. Read D, Esiri MM: Fusiform basilar artery aneurysm in a child. Neurology 1979;29:1045-1049.
81. Hirsch CS, Roessmann U: Arterial dysplasia with ruptured basilar artery aneurysm: Report of a case. Hum Pathol 1975;6:749-758.
82. Makos MM, McComb RD, Hart MN, Bennett DR: Alpha-glucosidase deficiency and basilar artery aneurysm: Report of a sibship. Ann Neurol 1987;22:629-633.
83. Schwartz A, Rautenberg W, Hennerici M: Dolichoectatic intracranial arteries: Review of selected aspects. Cerebrovasc Dis 1993;3:273-279.
84. Caplan LR: Dilatative arteriopathy (dolichoectasia): What is known and not known. Ann Neurol 2005;57:469-471.
85. Pico F, Labreuche J, Touboul PJ, Amarenco P: Intracranial arterial dolichoectasia and its relation with atherosclerosis and stroke subtype. Neurology 2003;61:1736-1742.
86. Pico F, Labreuche J, Touboul PJ, et al: Intracranial arterial dolichoectasia and small-vessel disease in stroke patients. Ann Neurol 2005;57:472-479.
87. Pessin MS, Chimowitz MI, Levine SR, et al: Stroke in patients with fusiform vertebrobasilar aneurysms. Neurology 1989;39:16-21.
88. Moseley IF, Holland IM: Ectasia of the basilar artery: The breadth of the clinical spectrum and the diagnostic value of computed tomography. Neuroradiology 1979;18:83-91.
89. Little JR, St Louis P, Weinstein M, et al: Giant fusiform aneurysms of the cerebral arteries. Stroke 1981;12:183-188.
90. Echiverri HC, Rubino FA, Gupta SR, Gujrati M: Fusiform aneurysm of the vertebrobasilar arterial system. Stroke 1989;20:1741-1747.

91. Nishizaki T, Tamaki N, Takeda N, et al: Dolicho-ectatic basilar artery: A review of 23 cases. Stroke 1986;17:1277-1281.

92. Shokunbi MT, Vinters HV, Kaufmann JC: Fusiform intracranial aneurysms: Clinicopathologic features. Surg Neurol 1988;29:263-270.

93. Savitz SI, Ronthal M, Caplan LR: Vertebral artery compression of the medulla. Arch Neurol 2006;63:234-241.

94. DeGeorgia M, Belden J, Pao L, et al: Thrombus in vertebrobasilar dolichoectatic artery treated with intravenous urokinase. Cerebrovasc Dis 1999;9:28-33.

95. Cohen MM, Hemalatha CP, D'Addario RT, Goldman HW: Embolism from a fusiform middle cerebral artery aneurysm. Stroke 1980;11: 158-161.

96. Aichner FT, Felber SR, Birhamer GG, Posch A: Magnetic resonance imaging and magnetic resonance angiography of vertebrobasilar dolichoectasia. Cerebrovasc Dis 1993;3: 280-284.

97. Hennerici M, Rautenberg W, Schwartz A: Transcranial Doppler ultrasound for the assessment of intracranial arterial flow velocity: II. Evaluation of intracranial arterial disease. Surg Neurol 1987;27:523-532.

97a. Passero S, Rossi S: Natural history of vertebrobasilar dolichoectasia. Neurology 2008;70:66-72.

Cerebral Amyloid Angiopathy

98. Vinters HV: Cerebral amyloid angiopathy: A critical review. Stroke 1987;18:311-324.

99. Cordonnier C, Leys D: Cerebral amyloid angiopathies. In Caplan LR (ed): Uncommon Causes of Stroke, 2nd ed. Cambridge: Cambridge University Press, 2008, pp 455-464.

100. Vinters HV, Gilbert JJ: Cerebral amyloid angiopathy: Incidence and complications in the aging brain: II. The distribution of amyloid vascular changes. Stroke 1983;14:924-928.

101. Okazaki H, Reagan TJ, Campbell RJ: Clinico-pathological studies of primary cerebral amyloid angiopathy. Mayo Clin Proc 1979;54:22-31.

102. Cosgrove G, Leblanc R, Meagher-Villemure K, et al: Cerebral amyloid angiopathy. Neurology 1985;34:625-631.

103. Gilbert JJ, Vinters HV: Cerebral amyloid angiopathy: Incidence and complications in the aging brain: I. Cerebral hemorrhage. Stroke 1983;14:915-923.

104. Kase CS: Cerebral amyloid angiopathy. In Kase CS, Caplan LR (eds): Intracerebral Hemorrhage. Boston: Butterworth-Heinemann, 1994, pp 179-200.

105. Greenberg SM, Eng JA, Ning M, et al: Hemorrhage burden predicts recurrent intracerebral hemorrhage after lobar hemorrhage. Stroke 2004;35:1415-1420.

106. Greenberg SM, Finklestein SP, Schaefer PW: Petechial hemorrhages accompanying lobar hemorrhage: Detection by gradient-echo MRI. Neurology 1996;46:1751-1754.

107. Greenberg SM, Hyman BT: Cerebral amyloid angiopathy and apolipoprotein E: Bad news for the good allele? Ann Neurol 1997;41:701-702.

108. O'Donnell HC, Rosand J, Knudsen KA, et al: Apolipoprotein E genotype and the risk of recurrent lobar intracerebral hemorrhage. N Engl J Med 2000;342:240-245.

109. McCarron MO, Nicoll JA, Ironside JW, et al: Cerebral amyloid angiopathy-related hemorrhage. I. Interaction of APOE epsilon2 with putative clinical risk factors. Stroke 1999;30:1643-1646.

110. Smith DB, Hitchcock M, Philpott PJ: Cerebral amyloid angiopathy presenting as transient ischemic attacks: Case report. J Neurosurg 1985;63:963-964.

111. Gray F, Dubas F, Roullet E, Escourolle R: Leukoencephalopathy in diffuse hemorrhagic cerebral amyloid angiopathy. Ann Neurol 1985;18:54-59.

112. Loes DJ, Biller J, Yuh WTC, et al: Leukoencephalopathy in cerebral amyloid angiopathy: MR imaging in four cases. AJNR Am J Neuroradiol 1990;11:485-488.

113. DeWitt LD, Louis DN: Case records of the Massachusetts General Hospital: Case 27-1991. N Engl J Med 1991;325:42-54.

114. Greenberg SM, Vonsattel JPG, Stakes JW, et al: The clinical spectrum of cerebral amyloid angiopathy: Presentations without lobar hemorrhage. Neurology 1993;43:2073-2079.

115. Grubb A, Jensson O, Gudmundsson G, et al: Abnormal metabolism of Y-trace alkaline microprotein: The basic defect in hereditary cerebral hemorrhage with amyloidosis. N Engl J Med 1984;311:1547-1549.

116. Stefansson K, Antel JP, Ojer J, et al: Autosomal dominant cerebrovascular amyloidosis: Properties of peripheral blood lymphocytes. Ann Neurol 1980;7:436-440.

117. Fountain NB, Eberhard DA: Primary angiitis of the central nervous system associated with cerebral amyloid angiopathy: Report of two cases and review of the literature. Neurology 1996;46:190-197.

118. Caplan LR: Case records of the Massachusetts General Hospital. Case 10-2000. N Engl J Med 2000;342:957-964.

119. Eng JA, Frosch MP, Choi K, et al: Clinical manifestations of cerebral amyloid angiopathy-related inflammation. Ann Neurol 2004;55:250-256.

120. Greene GM, Godersky JC, Biller J, et al: Surgical experience with intracerebral hemorrhage secondary to cerebral amyloid angiopathy. Stroke 1990;21:170.

121. Izumihara A, Ishihara T, Iwamoto N, et al: Postoperative outcome of 37 patients with lobar intracerebral hemorrhage related to cerebral amyloid angiopathy. Stroke 1999;30:29-33.

122. Greenberg SM: Cerebral amyloid angiopathy. Prospects for clinical diagnosis and treatment. Neurology 1998;51:690-694.

Infection-related arteritis

BACTERIAL (PNEUMOCOCCAL & MENINGOCOCCAL) MENINGITIS

123. van de Beek D, de Gans J, Spanjaard L, et al: Clinical features and prognostic factors in adults with bacterial meningitis. N Engl J Med 2004;351:1849-1859.
124. van de Beek D, de Gans J, Tunkel AR, et al: Community-acquired bacterial meningitis in adults. N Engl J Med 2006;354:44-53.
124a. Bentley P, Quadri F, Wild EJ, et al: Vasculitic presentation of staphylococcal meningitis. Arch Neurol 2007;64:1788-1789.
125. O'Farrell R, Thornton J, Brennan P, et al: Spinal cord infarction and tetraplegia—Rare complications of meningococcal meningitis. Br J Anesth 2000;84:514-517.
126. van de Beek D, Patel R, Wijdicks EFM: Meningococcal meningitis with brainstem infarction. Arch Neurol 2007;64:1350-1351.

Listeria monocytogenes

127. Weinstein AJ, Schianone WA, Furlan AJ: *Listeria* rhomboencephalitis. Arch Neurol 1982;39:514-516.
128. Brown RH, Sobel RA: Case records of the Massachusetts General Hospital. N Engl J Med 1989;321:739-750.
129. Frayne J, Gates P: *Listeria* rhomboencephalitis. Clin Exp Neurol 1987;24:175-179.
130. Silvestri N, Ajani Z, Savitz S, Caplan LR: A 73-year-old woman with an acute illness causing fever and cranial nerve abnormalities. Rev Neurol Dis 2006;3:29-30,35-37.

Cat-Scratch Disease

131. Windsor JJ: Cat-scratch disease: Epidemiology, aetiology and treatment. Br J Biomed Sci 2001;58:101-110.
132. Selby G, Walker GL: Cerebral arteritis in cat-scratch disease. Neurology 1979;29:1413-1418.

Syphilis

133. Davis LE, Graham GD: Neurosyphilis and stroke. In Caplan LR (ed): Uncommon Causes of Stroke, 2nd ed. Cambridge: Cambridge University Press, 2008, pp 35-40.
134. Flint AC, Liberato BB, Anziska Y, et al: Meningovascular syphilis as a cause of basilar artery stenosis. Neurology 2005;64:391-392.
135. Gaa J, Weidauer S, Sitzer M, et al: Cerebral vasculitis due to treponema pallidum infection: MRI and MRA findings. Eur Radiol 2004;14:746-747.
136. Golden MR, Marra CM, Holmes KK: Update on syphilis: Resurgence of an old problem. JAMA 2003;290:1510-1514.

Lyme Disease

137. Rahn DW, Malawista SE: Lyme disease: Recommendations for diagnosis and treatment. Ann Intern Med 1991;114:472-481.
138. Steere AC, Sikand VK: The presenting manifestations of Lyme disease and the outcomes of treatment. N Engl J Med 2003;348:2472-2474.
139. Halperin JJ, Luft BJ, Anand AK, et al: Lyme neuroboreliosis: Central nervous system manifestations. Neurology 1989;39:753-759.
140. Pachner AR, Duray P, Steere AC: Cerebral nervous system manifestations of Lyme disease. Arch Neurol 1989;46:790-795.
141. Uldry PA, Regli F, Bogousslavsky J: Cerebral angiopathy and recurrent strokes following Borrelia burgdorferi infection. J Neurol Neurosurg Psychiatry 1987;50:1703-1704.
142. Schmiedel J, Gahn G, von Kummer R, Reichmann H: Cerebral vasculitis with multiple infarcts caused by lyme disease. Cerebrovasc Dis 2004;17:79-81.
143. Halperin JJ: Stroke in Lyme disease. In Caplan LR (ed): Uncommon Causes of Stroke, 2nd ed. Cambridge: Cambridge University Press, 2008, pp 59-66.

Tuberculosis

144. Katrak SM: Vasculitis and stroke due to tuberculosis. In Caplan LR (ed): Uncommon Causes of Stroke, 2nd ed. Cambridge: Cambridge University Press, 2008, pp 41-46.
145. Leiguarda R, Berthier M, Starkstein S, et al: Ischemic infarction in 25 children with tuberculous meningitis. Stroke 1988;19:200-204.
146. Katrak SM, Shembalkar PK, Bijwe SR, Bhandarkar LD: The clinical, radiological and pathological profile of tuberculous meningitis in patients with and without human deficiency virus infection. J Neurol Sci 2000;181:118-126.
147. Bernaerts A, Vanhoenacker FM, Parizel PM et al: Tuberculosis of the central nervous system: overview of neuroradiological findings. Eur Radiol 2003;13:1876-1890.
148. Chan KH, Cheung RT, Lee R, et al: Cerebral infarcts complicating tuberculous meningitis. Cerebrovasc Dis 2005;19:391-395.

Fungal Infections

149. Hier DB, Caplan LR: Stroke due to fungal infections. In Caplan LR (ed): Uncommon Causes of Stroke, 2nd ed. Cambridge: Cambridge University Press, 2008, pp 47-52.
150. Kobayashi RM, Coil M, Niwayama G, Trauner D: Cerebral vasculitis in coccidioidal meningitis. Ann Neurol 1977;1:281-284.
151. Walsh TJ, Hier DB, Caplan LR: Fungal infection of the central nervous system: Comparative analysis of the risk factors and clinical signs in 57 patients. Neurology 1985;35:1654-1657.
152. Walsh TJ, Hier DB, Caplan LR: Aspergillosis of the central nervous system: Clinicopathological analysis of 17 patients. Ann Neurol 1985;18:574-582.

11

153. Kleinschmidt-DeMasters BK: Central nervous system aspergillosis: A 20 year retrospective series. Hum Pathol 2002;33:116-124.

154. Rangel-Guerra R, Martinez HR, Saenz C, et al: Rhinocerebral and systemic mucormycosis. Clinical experience in 36 cases. J Neurol Sci 1996;143:19-30.

Virus-Related Vasculitis

155. Moore PM, Cupps TR: Neurologic complications of vasculitis. Ann Neurol 1983;14:155-167.

156. Bischof M, Baumgartner RW: Varicella-zoster and other virus-related cerebral vasculopathy. In Caplan LR (ed): Uncommon Causes of Stroke, 2nd ed. Cambridge: Cambridge University Press, 2008, pp 17-26.

157. Gilden DH, Kleinschmidt-DeMasters BK, Wellish M, et al: Varicella-zoster virus, a cause of waxing and waning vasculitis: The New England Journal of Medicine case 5-1995 revisited. Neurology 1996;47:1441-1446.

158. Bourdette DN, Rosenberg NL, Yatsu FM: Herpes zoster ophthalmicus and delayed ipsilateral cerebral infarction. Neurology 1983;33:1428-1432.

159. Hilt DC, Buchholz D, Krumholz A, et al: Herpes zoster ophthalmicus and delayed contralateral hemiparesis caused by cerebral angiitis: Diagnosis and management approaches. Ann Neurol 1983;14:543-553.

160. Doyle PW, Gibson G, Dolman C: Herpes zoster ophthalmicus with contralateral hemiplegia: Identification of cause. Ann Neurol 1983;14:84-85.

160a. Nagel MA, Cohrs RJ, Mahalingam R, et al: The varicella zoster virus vasculopathies. Clinical, CSF, imaging and virologic features. Neurology 2008;70:853-860.

161. Powers JM: Herpes zoster maxillaris with delayed occipital infarction. J Clin Neuroophthalmol 1986;2:113-115.

162. Snow BJ, Simcock JP: Brainstem infarction following cervical herpes zoster. Neurology 1988;38:1331.

163. Ross MH, Abend WK, Schwartz RB, Samuels MA: A case of C2 herpes zoster with delayed bilateral pontine infarction. Neurology 1991;41:1685-1686.

164. Caekebeke JFV, Peters ACB, Vandvik B, et al: Cerebral vasculopathy associated with primary varicella infection. Arch Neurol 1990;47:1033-1035.

165. Askalan R, Laughlin S, Mayank S, et al: Chickenpox and stroke in childhood: A study of frequency and causation. Stroke 2001;32:1257-1262.

166. Hausler MG, Ramaekers VT, Reul J, et al: Early and late onset manifestations of cerebral vasculitis related to varicella zoster. Neuropediatrics 1998;29:202-207.

167. Lanthier S, Armstrong D, Domi T, deVeber G: Post-varicella arteriopathy of childhood. Neurology 2005;64:660-663.

168. Melanson M, Chalk C, Georgevich L, et al: Varicella-zoster virus DNA in CSF and arteries in delayed contralateral hemiplegia: Evidence for viral invasion of cerebral arteries. Neurology 1996;47:569-570.

169. Saito K, Moskowitz MA: Contributions from the upper cervical dorsal roots and trigeminal ganglia to the feline circle of Willis. Stroke 1989;20:524-526.

Human Immunodeficiency Virus

170. Pinto AN: AIDS and cerebrovascular disease. Stroke 1996;27:538-543.

171. Gillams AR, Allen E, Hrieb K, et al: Cerebral infarction in patients with AIDS. AJNR Am J Neuroradiol 1997;18:1581-1585.

172. Cole John W, Pinto AN, Hebel JR, et al: Acquired immunodeficiency syndrome and the risk of stroke. Stroke 2004;35:51-56.

173. Berger JR: AIDS and stroke risk. Lancet Neurol 2004;3:206-207.

174. Fritz V, Bryer A: Stroke in persons infected with HIV. In Caplan LR (ed): Uncommon Causes of Stroke, 2nd ed. Cambridge: Cambridge University Press, 2008, pp 93-100.

175. Dubrovsky T, Curless R, Scott G, et al: Cerebral aneurysmal arteriopathy in childhood IDS. Neurology 1998;51:560-565.

Kawasaki Disease

176. Lipton J, Rivkin MJ: Kawasaki disease: Cerebrovascular and neurologic complications. In Caplan LR (ed): Uncommon Causes of Stroke, 2nd ed. Cambridge: Cambridge University Press, 2008, pp 81-86.

177. Amano S, Hazama F, Hamashima Y: Pathology of Kawasaki disease: II. Distribution and incidence of the vascular lesions. Jpn Circ J 1979;43: 741-748.

178. Amano S, Hazama F, Kubagawa H, et al: General pathology of Kawasaki disease. On the morphological alterations corresponding to the clinical manifestations. Acta Pathol Jpn 1980;30:681-694.

Cysticercosis

179. Del Bruto OH: Stroke and vasculitis in patients with cysticercosis. In Caplan LR (ed): Uncommon Causes of Stroke, 2nd ed. Cambridge: Cambridge University Press, 2008, pp 53-58.

180. García HH, Del Brutto OH: Neurocysticercosis: Updated concepts about an old disease. Lancet Neurol 2005;4:653-661.

181. Escobar A, Weidenheim KM: The pathology of neurocysticercosis. In Singh G, Prabhakar S (eds): Taenia solium cysticercosis. From basic to clinical science. Oxon, UK: CAB International;2002: 289-305.

182. Caplan LR: How to manage patients with neurocysticercosis. Eur Neurol 1997;37:124-131.

183. Rodriguez-Carbajal J, del Brutto OH, Penagos P, et al: Occlusion of the middle cerebral artery due to cysticercotic angiitis. Stroke 1989;20:1095-1099.

184. Monteiro L, Almeida-Pinto J, Leite I, et al: Cerebral cysticercus arteritis: Five angiographic cases. Cerebrovasc Dis 1994;4:125-133.

185. Barinagarrementaria F, Cantu C: Frequency of cerebral arteritis in subarachnoid cysticercosis. An angiographic study. Stroke 1998;29:123-125.

186. Cantu C, Villarreal J, Soto JL, Barinagarrementaria F: Cerebral cysticercotic arteriits: Detection and follow-up by transcranial Doppler. Cerebrovasc Dis 1998;8:2-7.

187. Bang OY, Heo JH, Choi SA, Kim DI: Large cerebral infarction during praziquantel therapy in neurocysticercosis. Stroke 1997;28:211-213.

Malaria

188. Newton CR, Warrell DA: Neurological manifestations of falciparum malaria. Ann Neurol 1998;43:695-702.

189. Gall C, Spuler A, Fraunberger P: Subarachnoid hemorrhage in a patient with cerebral malaria. N Engl J Med 1999 341:611-613.

190. Omanga U, Ntihinyurwa M, Shako D, Mashako M: Les hemiplegies au cours de l'acces pernicieux a *Plasmodium falciparum* de l'enfant. Ann Pediatr (Paris) 1983;30:294-296.

191. Newton CR, Marsh K, Peshu N, Kirkham FJ: Perturbations of cerebral hemodynamics in Kenyan children with cerebral malaria. Pediatr Neurol 1996;15:41-49.

Chagas Disease

192. Massaro AR: Cerebrovascular problems in Chagas disease. In Caplan LR (ed): Uncommon Causes of Stroke, 2nd ed. Cambridge: Cambridge University Press, 2008, pp 87-92.

193. Carod-Artal FJ, Vargas AP, Melo M, Horan TA: American trypanosomiasis (Chagas' disease): An unrecognised cause of stroke. J Neurol Neurosurg Psychiatry 2003;74:516-518.

194. Carod-Artal FJ, Vargas AP, Horan TA, Nunes LG: Chagasic cardiomyopathy is independently associated with ischemic stroke in Chagas disease. Stroke 2005;36:965-970.

195. Leon-Sarmiento FE, Mendoza E, Torres-Hillera M, et al: Trypanosoma cruzi-associated cerebrovascular disease: A case-control study in Eastern Colombia. J Neurol Sci 2004;217:61-64.

196. Oliveira-Filho J, Viana LC, Vieira de Melo RM, et al: Chagas disease is an independent risk factor for stroke: Baseline characteristics of a Chagas disease cohort. Stroke 2005;36:2015-2017.

Systemic Vasculitis including Collagen Vascular Diseases

197. Fauci AS, Haynes BF, Katz P: The spectrum of vasculitis: Clinical, pathologic, immunologic and therapeutic considerations. Ann Intern Med 1978;89:660-676.

198. Moore PM, Richardson B: Neurology of the vasculitides and connective tissue disease. J Neurol Neurosurg Psychiatry 1998;65:10-22.

199. Scott DG: Classification and treatment of systemic vasculitis. Br J Rheumatol 1988;27:251-257.

200. Moore PM, Fauci AS: Neurologic manifestations of systemic vasculitis: A retrospective and prospective study of the clinico-pathologic features and responses to therapy in 25 patients. Am J Med 1981;71:517-524.

201. Kissel JT, Rammohan KW: Pathology and therapy of nervous system vasculitis. Clin Neuropharmacol 1991;14:28-48.

202. Moore PM, Richardson B: Neurology of the vasculitides and connective tissue diseases. J Neurol Neurosurg Psychiatry 1998;65:10-22.

203. Villringer A, Moore PM: Vasculitides and other nonatherosclerotic vasculopathies of the nervous system. In Brandt T, Caplan LR, Dichgans J, et al (eds): Neurological Disorders. San Diego: Academic Press, 1996, pp 305-327.

Polyarteritis Nodosa

204. Reichhart MD, Meuli R, Bogousslavsky J: Microscopic polyangiitis (MPA) and polyarteritis nodosa (PAN). In Caplan LR (ed): Uncommon Causes of Stroke, 2nd ed. Cambridge: Cambridge University Press, 2008, pp 311-330.

205. Caplan LR, Hedley-White ET: Case records of the Massachusetts General Hospital: Case 5-1995. N Engl J Med 1995;332:452-459.

Churg-Strauss Syndrome and Hypersensitivity Vasculitis

206. Mehdirrata M, Caplan LR: Churg-Strauss syndrome. In Caplan LR (ed): Uncommon Causes of Stroke, 2nd ed. Cambridge: Cambridge University Press, 2008, pp 331-334.

207. Churg J, Strauss L: Allergic granulomatosis, allergic angiitis, and periarteritis nodosa. Am J Pathol 1951;27:277-301.

208. Chumbley LC, Harrison EG, DeRemee RA: Allergic granulomatosis and angiitis (Churg-Strauss syndrome): Report and analysis of 30 cases. Mayo Clin Proc 1977;52:477-484.

209. Sehgal M, Swanson JW, DeRemee RA, Colby TV: Neurologic manifestations of Churg-Strauss syndrome. Mayo Clin Proc 1995;70:337-341.

210. Hauser SL, Shahani B, Hedley-White ET: Case records of the Massachusetts General Hospital: Case 38-1990. N Engl J Med 1990;323:812-822.

211. Jennette JC, Falk RJ: Small-vessel vasculitis. N Engl J Med 1997;337:1512-1523.

212. Savitz S, Caplan LR: Cerebrovascular complications of Henoch-Schoenlein purpura. In Caplan LR (ed): Uncommon Causes of Stroke, 2nd ed. Cambridge: Cambridge University Press, 2008, pp 309-310.

213. Chiaretti A, Caresta E, Piastra M, et al: Cerebral hemorrhage in Henoch-Schoenlein syndrome. Childs Nerv Syst 2002;18:365-367.

214. Eun SH, Kim SJ, Cho DS, et al: Cerebral vasculitis in Henoch-Schoenlein purpura: MRI and MRA

11

findings, treated with plasmapharesis alone. Pediatr Int 2003;45:484-487.

Wegener's Granulomatosis

215. Fauci AS, Haynes BF, Katz P, Wolff SM: Wegener's granulomatosis: Prospective clinical and therapeutic experience with 85 patients for 21 years. Ann Intern Med 1983;98:76-85.
216. Haynes BF, Fishman ML, Fauci AS, Wolff SM: The ocular manifestations of Wegener's granulomatosis: Fifteen years' experience and review of the literature. Am J Med 1977;63:131-141.
217. Lapresle J, Lasjaunias P: Cranial nerve ischemic arterial syndromes. Brain 1985;109:207-215.
218. Palaic M, Yeadon C, Moore S, Cashman N: Wegener's granulomatosis mimicking temporal arteritis. Neurology 1991;41:1694-1695.
219. Frohman LP, Lama P: Annual review of systemic diseases: 1995-1996, part 1. J Neuroophthalmol 1998;18:67-79.
220. Satoh J, Miyasaka N, Yamada T, et al: Extensive cerebral infarction due to involvement of both anterior cerebral arteries by Wegener's granulomatosis. Ann Rheum Dis 1988;47:606-611.
221. Provenzale JM, Allen NB: Wegener granulomatosis: CT and MR findings. AJNR Am J Neuroradiol 1996;17:785-792.
222. Nölle B, Specks U, Lüdemann J, et al: Anticytoplasmic autoantibodies: Their immunodiagnostic value in Wegener's granulomatosis. Ann Intern Med 1989;111:28-40.

Systemic Lupus Erythematosus

223. Feinglass EJ, Arnett SC, Dorsch CA, et al: Neuropsychiatric manifestations of systemic lupus erythematosus: Diagnosis, clinical spectrum, and relationship to other features of the disease. Medicine (Baltimore) 1976;55:323-339.
224. Futrell N: Systemic lupus erythematosis. In Caplan LR (ed): Uncommon Causes of Stroke, 2nd ed. Cambridge: Cambridge University Press, 2008, pp 335-342.
225. Johnson RT, Richardson EP: The neurological manifestations of systemic lupus erythematosus: A clinical-pathological study of 24 cases and review of the literature. Medicine (Baltimore) 1968;47:337-369.
226. Devinsky O, Petito C, Alonso D: Clinical and neuropathological findings in systemic lupus erythematosus: The role of vasculitis, heart emboli, and thrombotic thrombocytopenic purpura. Ann Neurol 1988;23:380-384.
227. Alsen AM, Gabrulsen TO, McCune WJ: MR imaging of systemic lupus erythematosus involving the brain. AJNR Am J Neuroradiol 1985;6:197-201.
228. Trevor RF, Sondheimer FK, Fessel WJ, et al: Angiographic demonstration of major cerebral vessel occlusion in systemic lupus erythematosus. Neuroradiology 1972;4:202-207.
229. Hart R, Miller V, Coull B, et al: Cerebral infarction associated with lupus anticoagulants: Preliminary report. Stroke 1984;15:114-118.

230. McVerry BA, Machin SJ, Parry H, et al: Reduced prostacycline activity in systemic lupus erythematosus. Ann Rheum Dis 1980;39:524-525.
231. Galve E, Candell-Riera J, Pigrau C, et al: Prevalence, morphological types, and evaluation of cardiac valvular disease in systemic lupus erythematosus. N Engl J Med 1988;319:817-823.

Thrombotic Thrombocytopenic Purpura

232. Moncayo-Gaete J: Thrombotic thrombocytopenic purpura. In Caplan LR (ed): Uncommon Causes of Stroke, 2nd ed. Cambridge: Cambridge University Press, 2008, pp 301-308.
233. Petitt RM: Thrombotic thrombocytopenic purpura: A thirty year review. Semin Thromb Hemost 1980;6:350-355.
234. Kwaan HC: Clinicopathological features of thrombotic thrombocytopenic purpura. Semin Hematol 1987;24:71-81.
235. Silverstein A: Thrombotic thrombocytopenic purpura: The initial neurological manifestations. Arch Neurol 1968;18:358-362.
236. Rinkel G, Wijdicks E, Hene RJ: Stroke in relapsing thrombotic thrombocytopenic purpura. Stroke 1991;22:1087-1088.
237. Kelly PJ, McDonald CT, Neill GO, et al: Middle cerebral artery main stem thrombosis in two siblings with familial thrombocytopenic purpura. Neurology 1998;50:1157-1160.
238. Bakshi R, Shaikh ZA, Bates VE, Kinkel PR: Thrombotic thrombocytopenic purpura: Brain CT and MRI findings in 12 patients. Neurology 1999;52:1285-1288.
239. Hinchey J, Chaves C, Apignani B, et al: A reversible posterior leukoencephalopathy syndrome. N Engl J Med 1996;334:494-500.
240. Bennett CL, Weinberg PD, Rozenberg-Ben-Dror K, et al: Thrombotic thrombocytopenic purpura associated with ticlopidine. A review of 60 cases. Ann Intern Med 1998;128, 541-544.
241. Bennett CL, Connors JM, Carwile JM, et al: Thrombotic thrombocytopenic purpura associated with clopidogrel. N Engl J Med 2000;342:1773-1777.
242. Zakarija A, Bennett C: Drug-induced thrombotic microangiopathy. Semin Thromb Hemost 2005;31:681-690.
243. Shepard KV, Bukowski RM: The treatment of thrombotic thrombocytopenic purpura with exchange transfusions, plasma infusions and plasma exchange. Semin Hematol 1987;24:178-193.

Rheumatoid Arthritis

244. Rubens E, Savitz S: Rheumatoid arthritis and cerebrovascular disease. In Caplan LR (ed): Uncommon Causes of Stroke, 2nd ed. Cambridge: Cambridge University Press, 2008, pp 343-346.
245. Ramos M, Mandybur TI: Cerebral vasculitis in rheumatoid arthritis. Arch Neurol 1975;32:271-275.
246. Watson P: Intracranial hemorrhage with vasculitis in rheumatoid arthritis. Arch Neurol 1979;36:58.

247. Watson P, Fekete J, Dick J: Central nervous system vasculitis in rheumatoid arthritis. Can J Neurol Sci 1977;4:269-271.
248. Takeda Y: Studies of the metabolism and distribution of fibrinogen in patients with rheumatoid arthritis. J Lab Clin Med 1967;69:624-633.
249. Jasin HE, LoSpalluto J, Ziff M: Rheumatoid hyperviscosity syndrome. Am J Med 1970;49:484-493.

Sjögren's Syndrome

250. Alexander EL, Provost TT, Stevens MB, Alexander GE: Neurologic complications of primary Sjögren's syndrome. Medicine (Baltimore) 1982;61:247-257.
251. Alexander GE, Provost TT, Stevens MB, Alexander EL: Sjögren syndrome: Central nervous system manifestations. Neurology 1981;31:1391-1396.
252. Alexander EL, Beall S, Gordon B, et al: Magnetic resonance imaging of cerebral lesions in patients with the Sjögren syndrome. Ann Intern Med 1988;108:815-823.
253. Alexander EL, Malinow K, Lijewski JE, et al: Primary Sjögren syndrome with central nervous system disease mimicking multiple sclerosis. Ann Intern Med 1986;104:323-330.

Scleroderma

254. Rubens E: Scleroderma. In Caplan LR (ed): Uncommon Causes of Stroke, 2nd ed. Cambridge: Cambridge University Press, 2008, pp 429-431.
255. Estey E, Lieberman A, Pinto R, et al: Cerebral arteritis in scleroderma. Stroke 1979;10:595-597.
256. Pathak R, Gabor AJ: Scleroderma and central nervous system vasculitis. Stroke 1991;22:410-413.

Sarcoidosis

257. Olugemo O, Stern BJ: Stroke and neurosarcoidosis. In Caplan LR (ed): Uncommon Causes of Stroke, 2nd ed. Cambridge: Cambridge University Press, 2008, pp 75-80.
258. Newman LS, Rose CS, Maier LA: Sarcoidosis. N Engl J Med 1997;336:1224-1234.
259. Scott TF: Neurosarcoidosis: Progress and clinical aspects. Neurology 1993;43:8-12.
260. Stern BJ, Krumholz A, Johns C, et al: Sarcoidosis and its neurological manifestations. Arch Neurol 1985;42:909-917.
261. Caplan LR, Corbett J, Goodwin J, et al: Neuro-ophthalmological signs in the angiitic form of neurosarcoidosis. Neurology 1983;33:1130-1135.
262. Meyer J, Foley J, Campagna-Pinto D: Granulomatous angiitis of the meninges in sarcoidosis. Arch Neurol Psychiatry 1953;69:587-600.
263. Alajouanine T, Bertrand J, Degos R, et al: Sarcoidose ganglionaire, cutanee et oculaire, avec atteinte secondaire diffuse, peripherique et centrale du système nerveux. Rev Neurol (Paris) 1958;99:421-447.

264. Urich H: Neurosarcoidosis or granulomatous angiitis: A problem of definition. Mt Sinai J Med 1977;44:718-725.
265. Karmi A: Ophthalmic changes in sarcoidosis. Acta Ophthalmol 1979;141(suppl):1-94.

Giant Cell (Temporal) Arteritis

266. Thevathasan AW, Davis SM: Temporal arteritis. In Caplan LR (ed): Uncommon Causes of Stroke, 2nd ed. Cambridge: Cambridge University Press, 2008, pp 9-16.
267. Melson MR, Weyland CM, Newman NJ, Biousse V: The diagnosis of giant cell arteritis. Rev Neurol Dis 2007;4:128-142.
268. Goodwin J: Temporal arteritis. In Vinken P, Bruyn G (eds): Handbook of Clinical Neurology, vol 39, part 2. Amsterdam: North Holland, 1980, pp 313-342.
269. Klein RG, Hunder GG, Stanson AW, et al: Large artery involvement in giant cell arteritis. Ann Intern Med 1975;83:806-812.
270. Wilkinson I, Russel R: Arteries of the head and neck in giant cell arteritis. Arch Neurol 1972;27:378-391.
271. Thielen KR, Wijdicks EFM, Nichols DA: Giant cell (temporal) arteritis: Involvement of the vertebral and internal carotid arteries. Mayo Clin Proc 1998;73:444-446.
272. Enzmann D, Scott WR: Intracranial involvement of giant-cell arteritis. Neurology 1977;27:794-797.
273. Casselli RJ: Giant cell (temporal) arteritis: A treatable cause of multi-infarct dementia. Neurology 1990;40:753-755.
274. Schmidt WA, Kraft HE, Vorpahl K, et al: Color Duplex ultrasonography in the diagnosis of temporal arteritis. N Engl J Med 1997;337:1336-1342.

Angiitis Limited to the Central Nervous System

275. Zuber M: Isolated angiitis of the central nervous system. In Caplan LR (ed): Uncommon Causes of Stroke, 2nd ed. Cambridge: Cambridge University Press, 2008, pp 1-8.
275a. Salvarani C, Brown RD, Calamia KT, et al: Primary central nervous system vasculitis: of 101 patients. Ann Neurol 2007;62:442-451.
276. Hankey GJ: Isolated angiitis/angiopathy of the central nervous system. Cerebrovasc Dis 1991;1:2-15.
277. Kolodny EH, Rebeiz JJ, Caviness VS, Richardson EP: Granulomatous angiitis of the central nervous system. Arch Neurol 1968;19:510-524.
278. Vollmer TL, Guarnaccia J, Harrington W, et al: Idiopathic granulomatous angiitis of the central nervous system. Diagnostic challenges. Arch Neurol 1993;50:925-930.
279. Moore PM: Diagnosis and management of isolated angiitis of the central nervous system. Neurology 1989;39:167-173.
280. Burger PC, Burch JG, Vogel FS: Granulomatous angiitis: An unusual etiology of stroke. Stroke 1977;8:29-35.

281. Harris KG, Tran DD, Sickels WJ, et al: Diagnosing intracranial vasculitis: The role of MR and angiography. AJNR Am J Neuroradiol 1994;15:317-330.

282. Alhalabi M, Moore PM: Serial angiography in isolated angiitis of the central nervous system. Neurology 1994;44:1221-1226.

Takayasu's Disease

283. Shinohara Y: Takayasu disease. In Caplan LR (ed): Uncommon Causes of Stroke, 2nd ed. Cambridge: Cambridge University Press, 2008, pp 27-32.

284. Shimizuki K, Sano K: Pulseless disease. J Neuropathol Clin Neurol 1951;1:37-47.

285. Ask-Upmark E: On the pulseless disease outside of Japan. Acta Med Scand 1954;149:161-178.

286. Subramanyan R, Joy J, Balakrishnan KG: Natural history of aortoarteritis (Takayasu's disease). Circulation 1989;80:429-437.

287. Lupi-Herrera E, Sanchez-Torres G, Marcushamer J, et al: Takayasu's arteritis: Clinical study of 107 cases. Am Heart J 1977;93:94-103.

288. Ishikawa K: Natural history and classification of occlusive thromboaortopathy (Takayasu's disease). Circulation 1978;57:27-35.

289. Sano K, Alga T, Saito I: Angiography in pulseless disease. Radiology 1970;94:69-74.

290. Hall S, Barr W, Lee JT, et al: Takayasu arteritis: A study of 32 North American patients. Medicine (Baltimore) 1985;54:89-99.

291. Hargraves RW, Spetzler RF: Takayasu's arteritis: Case report. Barrow Neurol Inst Q 1991;7:20-23.

292. Kerr GS, Hallahan CW, Giordano J, et al: Takayasu arteritis. Ann Intern Med 1994;120:919-929.

293. Naritomi H: Takayasu's arteritis. In Bogousslavsky J, Caplan LR (eds): Stroke Syndromes. Cambridge: Cambridge University Press, 1995, pp 437-442.

294. Klos K, Flemming KD, Petty GW, Luthra HS: Takayasu's arteritis with arteriographic evidence of intracranial vessel involvement. Neurology 2003;60:1550-1551.

295. Talwar KK, Kumar K, Chopra P, et al: Cardiac involvement in nonspecific aortoarteritis (Takayasu's arteritis). Am Heart J 1991;122:1666-1670.

296. Sun Y, Yip P-K, Jeng J-S, et al: Ultrasonographic study and long-term follow-up of Takayasu's arteritis. Stroke 1996;27:2178-2182.

297. Ishikawa K, Uyama M, Asayama K: Occlusive thromboaortopathy (Takayasu's disease): Cervical occlusive stenosis, retinal artery pressure, retinal microaneurysms and prognosis. Stroke 1983;14:730-735.

298. Takagi A, Tada Y, Sato O, et al: Surgical treatment for Takayasu's arteritis: A long-term follow-up study. J Cardiovasc Surg 1989;30:553-558.

299. Fraga A, Mintz G, Valle L, Flores-Izquierdo G: Takayasu's arteritis: Frequency of systemic manifestations (study of 22 patients) and favorable response to maintenance steroid therapy with adrenocorticosteroids (12 patients). Arthritis Rheum 1972;15:617-624.

Behçet's Disease

300. Kumral E: Behçet's disease. In Caplan LR (ed): Uncommon Causes of Stroke, 2nd ed. Cambridge: Cambridge University Press, 2008, pp 67-74.

301. Chajek T, Fainaro M: Behçet's disease: Report of 41 cases and a review of the literature. Medicine (Baltimore) 1975;54:179-195.

302. Shimizu T, Ehrlich GE, Inaba G, et al: Behçet's disease (Behçet's syndrome). Semin Arthritis Rheum 1979;8:223-260.

303. Wechsler B, Davatchi F, Mizushima Y, et al: Criteria for diagnosis of Behçet's disease. Lancet 1990;335:1078-1080.

304. International Study Group for Behçet's Disease: Evaluation of diagnostic ("classification") criteria in Behçet's disease: Towards internationally agreed criteria. Br J Rheum 1992;31:299-308.

305. Serdaroglu P, Yazici H, Ozdemir C, et al: Neurologic involvement in Behçet's syndrome: A prospective study. Arch Neurol 1989;46:265-269.

306. Herskovitz S, Lipton RB, Lantos G: Neuro-Behçet's disease: CT and clinical correlates. Neurology 1988;38:1714-1720.

307. Bousser M-G, Wechsler B: Behçet's disease. In Bogousslavsky J, Caplan LR (eds): Stroke Syndromes. Cambridge: Cambridge University Press, 1995, pp 460-465.

308. Al Kawi MZ, Bohlega S, Banna M: MRI findings in neuro-Behçet's disease. Neurology 1991;41:405-408.

309. Banna M, El-Ramahi K: Neurologic involvement in Behçet's disease: Imaging findings in 16 patients. AJNR Am J Neuroradiol 1991;12:791-796.

310. Pamir MN, Kansu T, Erbengi A, Zileli T: Papilledema in Behçet's syndrome. Arch Neurol 1981;38:643-645.

311. Bousser MG, Chiras J, Bories J, Castaigne P: Cerebral venous thrombosis: A review of 38 cases. Stroke 1985;16:199-213.

312. Wechsler B, Vidailhet M, Piette JC, et al: Cerebral venous thrombosis in Behçet's disease: Clinical study and long-term follow-up of 25 cases. Neurology 1992;42:614-618.

313. Sharief MK, Hentges R, Thomas E: Significance of CSF immunoglobulins in monitoring neurologic disease in Behçet's disease. Neurology 1991;41:1398-1401.

Cogan's Syndrome

314. Cogan DG: Syndrome of nonsyphilitic interstitial keratitis and vestibulo-auditory symptoms. Arch Ophthalmol 1945;33:144-149.

315. Calvetti O, Biousse V: Cogan's syndrome. In Caplan LR (ed): Uncommon Causes of Stroke, 2nd ed. Cambridge: Cambridge University Press, 2008, pp 259-262.

316. Cheson BD, Bluming AZ, Alroy J: Cogan's syndrome: A systemic vasculitis. Am J Med 1976;60:549-555.

317. Peeters GJ, Pinckers AJ, Cremers CW, Hoefnagels WH: Atypical Cogan's syndrome: An autoimmune disease. Ann Otol Rhinol Laryngol 1986;95: 173-175.

318. Romain PL, Aretz HT: Case records of the Massachusetts General Hospital: Case 6-1999. N Engl J Med 1999;340:635-641.

319. Albayram MS, Wityk R, Yousem DM, Zinreich SJ: The cerebral angiographic findings in Cogan syndrome. AJNR Am J Neuroradiol 2001;22:751-754.

Eales's Disease

320. Eales H: Case of retinal hemorrhage, associated with epistaxis and constipation. Birmingham Med Rev 1880;9:262-273.

321. Biousse V: Eales retinopathy. In Caplan LR (ed): Uncommon Causes of Stroke, 2nd ed. Cambridge: Cambridge University Press, 2008, pp 235-236.

322. Biswas J, Sharma T, Gopal L, et al: Eales disease—An update. Surv Ophthalmol 2002;47:197-214.

323. Miller NR: Walsh and Hoyt's Clinical Neuroophthalmology, vol 4, 4th ed. Baltimore: Williams & Wilkins, 1991.

324. Raizman MB, Haas JJ: Case records of the Massachusetts General Hospital: Case 4-1998. N Engl J Med 1998;338:313-319.

325. Gordon MF, Coyle PK, Golub B: Eales disease presenting as stroke in the young adult. Ann Neurol 1988;24:264-266.

326. Herson RN, Squier M: Retinal perivasculitis with neurological involvement. J Neurol Sci 1978;36:111-117.

327. Singhal BS, Dastur DK: Eales disease with neurological involvement. J Neurol Sci 1976;27:312-321,323-345.

328. White RH: The etiology and neurological complications of retinal vasculitis. Brain 1961;84:262-273.

Microangiopathy of the Brain, Ear, and Retina (Susac's syndrome)

329. Susac J, Hardman J, Selhorst J: Microangiopathy of the brain and retina. Neurology 1979;29: 313-316.

330. Susac JO: Susac's syndrome: The triad of microangiopathy of the brain and retina with hearing loss in young women. Neurology 1994;44:591-593.

331. Papo T, Biousse V, Lehoang P, et al: Susac syndrome. Medicine (Baltimore) 1998;77:3-11.

332. Henriques I, Bogousslavsky J, Caplan LR: Microangiopathy of the retina, inner ear, and brain: Susac's syndrome. In Caplan LR (ed): Uncommon Causes of Stroke, 2nd ed. Cambridge: Cambridge University Press, 2008, pp 247-254.

333. Petty G, Engel A, Younge BR, et al: Retinocochleocerebral vasculopathy. Medicine (Baltimore) 1998;77:122-140.

334. Coppeto J, Currie J, Monteiro M, et al: A syndrome of arterial-occlusive retinopathy and encephalopathy. Am J Ophthalmol 1984;98: 189-202.

335. Swanson R, Mario L, Monteiro M, et al: A microangiopathic syndrome of encephalopathy, hearing loss and retinal artery occlusion. Neurology 1985;35(suppl 1):145.

336. Bogousslavsky J, Gaio JM, Caplan LR, et al: Encephalopathy, deafness, and blindness in young women: A distinct retino-cochleo-cerebral arteriolopathy. J Neurol Neurosurg Psychiatry 1989;52:43-46.

Acute Posterior Multifocal Placoid Pigment Epitheliopathy

337. Reichhart M: Acute posterior multifocal placoid pigment epitheliopathy (APMPPE). In Caplan LR (ed): Uncommon Causes of Stroke, 2nd ed. Cambridge: Cambridge University Press, 2008, pp 237-246.

338. Gass JDM: Acute posterior multifocal placoid pigment epitheliopathy. Arch Ophthalmol 1968;80:177-185.

339. Gass JD: Acute posterior multifocal placoid pigment epitheliopathy. Retina 2003;23: 177-185.

340. Jones NP: Acute posterior multifocal placoid pigment epitheliopathy. Br J Ophthalmol 1995;79:384-389.

341. Comu S, Verstraeten T, Rinkoff JS, Busis NA: Neurological manifestations of acute posterior multifocal placoid pigment epitheliopathy. Stroke 1996;27:996-1001.

342. Smith CH, Savino PJ, Beck RW, et al: Acute posterior multifocal placoid pigment epitheliopathy and cerebral vasculitis. Arch Neurol 1983;40:48-50.

343. Weinstein JM, Bresnick GH, Bell CL, et al: Acute posterior multifocal placoid pigment epitheliopathy with cerebral vasculitis. J Clin Neuroophthalmol 1988;8:195-201.

344. Bewermeyer H, Nelles G, Huber M, et al: Pontine infarction in acute posterior multifocal placoid pigment epitheliopathy. J Neurol 1993;241:22-26.

345. Wilson CA, Choromokos EA, Sheppard R: Acute posterior multifocal placoid pigment epitheliopathy and cerebral vasculitis. Arch Ophthalmol 1988;106:796-800.

Vogt-Koyanagi-Harada Syndrome

346. Manor RS: Vogt-Koyanagi-Harada syndrome and related diseases. In Vinken P, Bruyn G, Klawans H (eds): Handbook of Clinical Neurology, vol 34, part 2. Amsterdam: North Holland, 1978, pp 513-544.

347. Andreoli CM, Foster CS: Vogt-Koyanagi-Harada disease. Int Ophthalmol Clin 2006;46:111-122.

348. Kato Y, Kurimura M, Yahata Y, et al: Vogt-Koyanagi-Harada's disease presenting polymorphonuclear pleocytosis in the cerebrospinal fluid at the early active stage. Intern Med 2006;45:779-781.

11

349. Khoury T, Gonzalez-Fernandez F, Munschauer 3rd FE, Ostrow P: A 47-year-old man with sudden onset of blindness, pleocytosis, and temporary hearing loss. Vogt-Koyanagi-Harada syndrome (Uveomeningoencephalitic syndrome). Arch Pathol Lab Med 2006;130: 1070-1072.

Sneddon's Syndrome

350. De Reuck JL, De Bleecker JL: Sneddon's syndrome. In Caplan LR (ed): Uncommon Causes of Stroke, 2nd ed. Cambridge: Cambridge University Press, 2008, pp 405-412.
351. Sneddon B: Cerebro-vascular lesions and livedo reticularis. Br J Dermatol 1965;77: 180-185.
352. Tourbah A, Piette JC, Iba-Zizen MT, et al: The natural course of cerebral lesions in Sneddon syndrome. Arch Neurol 1997;54:53-60.
353. Thomas DJ, Kirby JD, Britton KE, Galton DJ: Livedo reticularis and neurological lesions. Br J Dermatol 1982;106:711-712.
354. Rebollo M, Val JF, Garijo F, et al: Livedo reticularis and cerebrovascular lesions (Sneddon's syndrome). Brain 1983;106:965-979.
355. Stockhammer G, Felber SR, Zelger B, et al: Sneddon syndrome: Diagnosis by skin biopsy and MRI in 17 patients. Stroke 1993;24: 685-690.
356. Pettee AD, Wasserman BA, Adams NL, et al: Familial Sneddon's syndrome: Clinical, hematologic, and radiographic findings in two brothers. Neurology 1994;44:399-405.
357. Levine SR, Langer SL, Albers JW, Welch KMA: Sneddon's syndrome: An antiphospholipid antibody syndrome? Neurology 1988;38:798-800.

Kohlmeier-Degos Syndrome

358. Cornett O, Rosenbaum DH: Kohlmeier-Degos disease (malignant atrophic papulosis). In Caplan LR (ed): Uncommon Causes of Stroke, 2nd ed. Cambridge: Cambridge University Press, 2008, pp 377-380.
359. Caviness Jr VS, Sagar P, Israel EJ, et al: Case 38-2006: A 5-year-old boy with headache and abdominal pain. N Engl J Med 2006;355: 2575-2584.
360. Petit WA, Soso MJ, Higman H: Degos disease: neurologic complications and cerebral angiography. Neurology 1982;32:1305-1309.
361. Strole WE, Clark WH, Isselbacher KJ: Progressive arterial occlusive disease (Kohlmeier-Degos). N Engl J Med 1967;276:195-201.
362. Subbiah P, Wijdicks E, Muenter M, et al: Skin lesion with a fatal neurologic outcome (Degos' disease). Neurology 1996;46:636-640.

Strokes and Vasculopathy in Drug Abusers

363. Caplan LR: Drugs. In Kase CS, Caplan LR (eds): Intracerebral Hemorrhage. Boston: Butterworth-Heinemann, 1994, pp 201-220.
364. Brust JC: Stroke and substance abuse. In Caplan LR (ed): Uncommon Causes of Stroke,

2nd ed. Cambridge: Cambridge University Press, 2008, pp 365-370.
365. Brust J, Richter R: Stroke associated with addiction to heroin. J Neurol Neurosurg Psychiatry 1978;39:194-199.
366. Woods B, Strewler G: Hemiparesis occurring six hours after intravenous heroin injection. Neurology 1972;22:863-866.
367. Caplan LR, Hier DB, Banks G: Current concepts in cerebrovascular disease-stroke: Stroke and drug abuse. Stroke 1982;13:869-872.
368. Brust JC: Stroke and drugs. In Vinker P, Bruyn G, Klawans H (eds): Handbook of Clinical Neurology, vol 11. Amsterdam: Elsevier, 1989, pp 517-531.
369. Pearson J, Richter R: Addiction to opiates: Neurologic aspects. In Vinken P, Bruyn G (eds): Handbook of Clinical Neurology, vol 37. Amsterdam: North Holland, 1979, pp 365-400.
370. Citron B, Halpern M, McCarron M, et al: Necrotizing angiitis associated with drug abuse. N Engl J Med 1970;283:1003-1011.
371. Rumbaugh C, Bergeron R, Gang H, et al: Cerebral vascular changes secondary to amphetamine abuse in the experimental animal. Radiology 1971;101:345-351.
372. Rumbaugh C, Bergeron R, Gang H, et al: Cerebral angiographic changes in the drug abuse patient. Radiology 1971;101:335-344.
373. Caplan LR, Thomas C, Banks G: Central nervous system complications of "T's and Blues" addiction. Neurology 1982;32:623-628.
374. Szwed JJ: Pulmonary angiothrombosis caused by "blue velvet" addiction. Ann Intern Med 1970;73:771-774.
375. Atlee W: Talc and cornstarch emboli in the eyes of drug abusers. JAMA 1972;219:49-51.
376. Mizutami T, Lewis R, Gonatas N: Medial medullary syndrome in a drug abuser. Arch Neurol 1980;37:425-428.
377. Kaku D, Lowenstein DH: Emergence of recreational drug abuse as a major risk factor for stroke in young adults. Ann Intern Med 1990;133:821-827.
378. Levine SR, Welch KM: Cocaine and stroke: Current concepts of cardiovascular disease. Stroke 1988;19:779-783.
379. Daras M, Tuchman AJ, Marks S: Central nervous system infarction related to cocaine abuse. Stroke 1991;22:1320-1325.
380. Levine SR, Washington JM, Jefferson ME, et al: "Crack" cocaine-associated stroke. Neurology 1987;37:1849-1853.
381. Levine SR, Brust JC, Futrell N, et al: A comparative study of the cerebrovascular complications of cocaine-alkaloidal versus hydrochloride—a review. Neurology 1991;41:1173-1177.
382. Rowley HA, Lowenstein DH, Rowbotham MC, Simon RP: Thalamomesencephalic strokes after cocaine abuse. Neurology 1989;39:428-430.
383. Di Lazzaro, V, Restuccia D, Oliviero A, et al: Ischaemic myelopathy associated with cocaine: Clinical, neurophysiological, and neuroradiological

features. J Neurol Neurosurg Psychiatry 1997;63:531-533.

384. Isner JM, Estes NA, Thompson PD, et al: Acute cardiac events temporally related to cocaine. N Engl J Med 1986;315:1438-1443.

385. Brust JCM: Neurological Aspects of Substance Abuse, 2nd ed. Boston: Butterworth-Heinemann, 2004.

386. Kaufman MJ, Levin JM, Ross MH, et al: Cocaine-induced cerebral vasoconstriction detected in humans with magnetic resonance angiography. JAMA 1998;279:376-380.

387. Nolte KB, Brass LM, Fletterick CF: Intracranial hemorrhage associated with cocaine abuse: A prospective study. Neurology 1996;46: 1291-1296.

Migraine and Vasoconstriction Syndromes

388. Savitz S, Caplan LR: Migraine and migraine-like conditions. In Caplan LR (ed): Uncommon Causes of Stroke, 2nd ed. Cambridge: Cambridge University Press, 2008, pp 529-531.

389. Singhal AB, Koroshetz WF, Caplan LR: Reversible cerebral vasoconstriction syndromes. In Caplan LR (ed): Uncommon Causes of Stroke, 2nd ed. Cambridge: Cambridge University Press, 2008, pp 505-514.

390. Caplan LR: Migraine in Posterior Circulation Disease: Diagnosis, Clinical Findings, and Management. Boston: Blackwell, 1996.

391. Kruit MC, van Buchem MA, Hofman PA, et al: Migraine as a risk factor for subclinical brain lesions. JAMA 2004;291:427-434.

392. Rothrock JF, Walicke P, Swendon M, et al: Migrainous stroke. Arch Neurol 1988;45:63-67.

393. Bogousslavsky J, Regli F, Van Melle G, et al: Migraine stroke. Neurology 1988;38:223-227.

394. Caplan LR: Migraine and vertebrobasilar ischemia. Neurology 1991;41:55-61.

395. Rothrock J, North J, Madden K, et al: Migraine and migrainous stroke: Risk factors and prognosis. Neurology 1993;43:2473-2476.

396. Henrich JB, Horwitz RI: A controlled study of ischemic stroke risk in migraine patients. J Clin Epidemiol 1989;42:773-780.

397. Stang PE, Carson AP, Rose KM, et al: Headache, cerebrovascular symptoms, and stroke: The Atherosclerosis Risk in Communities Study. Neurology 2005;64:1573-1577.

398. Etminan M, Takkouche B, Isorna FC, Samii A: Risk of ischaemic stroke in people with migraine: Systematic review and meta-analysis of observational studies. BMJ 2005;330:63.

399. Donaghy M, Chang CL, Poulter N: European Collaborators of The World Health Organisation Collaborative Study of Cardiovascular Disease and Steroid Hormone Contraception: Duration, frequency, recency, and type of migraine and the risk of ischaemic stroke in women of childbearing age. J Neurol Neurosurg Psychiatry 2002;73:747-750.

400. Solomon S, Lipton RB, Harris PY: Arterial stenosis in migraine: Spasm or arteriopathy? Headache 1990;30:52-61.

401. Pessin MS, Lathi ES, Cohen MB, et al: Clinical features and mechanisms of occipital infarction in the posterior cerebral artery territory. Ann Neurol 1987;21:290-299.

402. Fisher CM: Late-life migraine accompaniments as a cause of unexplained transient ischemic attacks. Can J Neurol Sci 1980;7:9-17.

403. Fisher CM: Late-life migraine accompaniments: Further experience. Stroke 1986;17:1033-1042.

404. Wijman CAC, Wolf PA, Kase CS, et al: Migrainous visual accompaniments are not rare in late life. The Framingham Study. Stroke 1998;29:1539-1543.

405. Caplan LR, Chedru F, Lhermitte F, Mayman C: Transient global amnesia and migraine. Neurology 1981;31:1167-1170.

406. Caplan LR: Transient global amnesia: Characteristic features and overview. In Markowitsch HJ (ed): Transient Global Amnesia and Related Disorders. Toronto: Hogrife and Huber, 1990, pp 15-27.

407. Call GK, Fleming MC, Sealfon S, et al: Reversible cerebral segmental vasoconstriction. Stroke 1988;19:1159-1170.

408. Bogousslavsky J, Despland PA, Regli F, Dubuis PY: Postpartum cerebral angiopathy: Reversible vasoconstriction assessed by transcranial Doppler ultrasound. Eur Neurol 1989;29: 102-105.

409. Chen S-P, Fuh J-L, Lirng J-F, et al: Recurrent primary thunderclap headache and benign CNS angiopathy. Neurology 2006;67:2164-2169.

409a. Ducros A, Boukobza M, Porcher R, et al: The clinical and radiological spectrum of reversible cerebral vasoconstriction syndrome. A prospective series of 67 patients. Brain 2007;130: 3091-3101.

410. Lopez-Valdes E, Chang H-M, Pessin MS, Caplan LR: Cerebral vasoconstriction after carotid surgery. Neurology 1997;49:303-304.

410a. Moustafa RR, Allen CMC, Baron J-C: Call-Fleming syndrome associated with subarachnoid haemorrhage: Three new cases. J Neurol Neurosurg Psychiatry 2008;79:602-605.

411. Bartleson JD, Swanson JW, Whisnant JP: A migrainous syndrome with cerebrospinal fluid pleocytosis. Neurology 1981;31:1257-1262.

412. Gomez-Aranda F, Canadillas F, Marti-Masso JF, et al: Pseudomigraine with temporary neurological symptoms and lymphocytic pleocytosis. A report of 50 cases. Brain 1997;120:1105-1113.

413. Black DF, Bartleson JD, Bell ML, Lachner DH: SMART: Stroke-like migraine attacks after radiation therapy. Cephalgia 2006;26:1137-1142.

414. Pruitt A, Dalmau J, Detre J, et al: Episodic neurologic dysfunction with migraine and reversible imaging findings after radiation. Neurology 2006;67:676-678.

415. Cole AJ, Aube M: Migraine with vasospasm and delayed intracerebral hemorrhage. Arch Neurol 1990;47:53-56.

416. Gautier JC, Majdalani A, Juillard JB, et al: Hemorragies cerebrales au cours de la migraine. Rev Neurol (Paris) 1993;149:407-410.

417. Caplan LR: Intracerebral hemorrhage revisited. Neurology 1988;38:624-627.

Eclampsia

418. Digre K, Varner M, Caplan LR: Eclampsia and stroke during pregnancy and the puerperium. In Caplan LR (ed): Uncommon Causes of Stroke, 2nd ed. Cambridge: Cambridge University Press, 2008, pp 515-528.

419. Hoffmann M, Keiseb J, Moodley J, Corr P: Appropriate neurological evaluation and multimodality magnetic resonance imaging in eclampsia. Acta Neurol Scand 2002;106:159-167.

420. Neudecker S, Stock K, Krasnianski M: Call-Fleming postpartum angiopathy in the puerperium: A reversible cerebral vasoconstriction syndrome. Obstet Gynecol 2006;107:446-449.

Reversible Posterior Leukoencephalopathy Syndrome

421. Duncan R, Hadley D, Bone I, et al: Blindness in eclampsia: CT and MR imaging. J Neurol Neurosurg Psychiatry 1998;52:899-902.

422. Easton JD, Mas J-L, Lamy C, et al: Severe preeclampsia/eclampsia: hypertensive encephalopathy of pregnancy? Cerebrovasc Dis 1998;8:53-58.

423. Hinchey J, Chaves C, Appignani B, et al: A reversible posterior leukoencephalopathy syndrome. N Engl J Med 1996;334:494-500.

424. Schwartz RB, Feske SK, Polak JF, et al: Preeclampsia-eclampsia: Clinical and neuroradiographic correlates and insights into the pathogenesis of hypertensive encephalopathy. Radiology 2000;217:371-376.

425. Hinchey JA: Reversible leukoencephalopathy syndrome: what have we learned in the past 10 years. Arch Neurol 2008;65:175-176.

Moyamoya Syndrome

426. Adams H, Davis P, Hennerici M: Moyamoya. In Caplan LR (ed): Uncommon Causes of Stroke, 2nd ed. Cambridge: Cambridge University Press, 2008, pp 465-478.

427. Suzuki J, Kodama N: Moyamoya disease—A review. Stroke 1983;14:104-109.

428. Suzuki J: Moyamoya Disease. Berlin: Springer, 1986.

428a. Kuroda S, Hashimoto N, Yoshimoto T, et al: Radiological findings, clinical course, and outcome in aymptomatic moyamoya disease. Stroke 2007;38:1430-1435.

429. Chiu D, Shedden P, Bratina P, Grotta JC: Clinical features of moyamoya disease in the United States. Stroke 1998;29:1347-1351.

430. Taveras JM: Multiple progressive intracranial arterial occlusions: A syndrome of children and young adults. AJR Am J Roentgenol 1969;106:235-268.

431. Bruno A, Adams HOP, Bilbe J, et al: Cerebral infarction due to moyamoya disease in young adults. Stroke 1988;19:826-833.

432. Mauro AJ, Johnson ES, Chikos PM, Alvord EC: Lipohyalinosis and miliary microaneurysms causing cerebral hemorrhage in a patient with moyamoya. A clinicopathological study. Stroke 1980;11:405-412.

433. Ikeda E: Systemic vascular changes in spontaneous occlusion of the circle of Willis Stroke 1991;22:1358-1362.

434. Ueki K, Meyer FB, Mellinger JF: Moyamoya disease: The disorder and surgical treatment. Mayo Clin Proc 1994;69:749-757.

435. Herreman F, Nathal E, Yasui N, Yonekawa Y: Intracranial aneurysms in moyamoya disease: Report of ten cases and review of the literature. Cerebrovasc Dis 1994;4:329-336.

436. Robertson RL, Burrows PE, Barnes PD, et al: Angiographic changes after pial synangiosis in childhood moyamoya disease. AJNR Am J Neuroradiol 1997;18:837-845.

437. Houkin K, Kamiyama H, Abe H, et al: Surgical therapy for adult moyamoya disease. Can surgical revascularization prevent the recurrence of intracerebral hemorrhage? Stroke 1996;27:1342-1346.

438. Smith ER, Scott RM: Surgical management of moyamoya syndrome. Skull Base 2005;15:15-26.

Hematological Disorders and Stroke

439. Hart RG, Kanter MC: Hematologic disorders and ischemic stroke: A selective review. Stroke 1990;21:1111-1121.

440. Markus HS, Hambley H: Neurology and the blood: haematological abnormalities in ischaemic stroke. J Neurol Neurosurg Psychiatry 1998;64:150-159.

Sickle Cell Disease

441. Adams RJ: Big strokes in small persons. Arch Neurol 2007;64:1567-1574.

442. Switzer JA, Hess DC, Nichols FT, Adams RJ: Pathophysiology and treatment of stroke in sickle-cell disease: Present and future. Lancet 2006;5:501-512.

443. Rothman SM, Fulling KH, Nelson JS: Sickle cell anemia and central nervous system infarction: A neuropathological study. Ann Neurol 1986;20:684-690.

444. Adams RJ, Nichols FT, McKie V, et al: Cerebral infarction in sickle cell anemia: mechanisms based on CT and MRI. Neurology 1988;38:1012-1017.

445. Steen RG, Langston JW, Ogg RJ, et al: Ectasia of the basilar artery in children with sickle cell disease: Relationship to hematocrit and psychometric measures. J Stroke Cerebrovasc Dis 1998;7:32-43.

446. Oguz M, Aksungur EH, Soyupak SK, Yildirim AU: Vein of Galen and sinus thrombosis with bilateral thalamic infarcts in sickle cell anemia: CT follow-up and angiographic demonstration. Neuroradiology 1994;36:155-156.

447. Adams RJ: TCD in sickle-cell disease: An important and useful test. Pediatr Radiol 2005;35:229-234.

448. Adams RJ, McKie VC, Hsu L, et al: Prevention of a first stroke by transfusions in children with sickle cell anemia and abnormal results on transcranial Doppler ultrasonography. N Engl J Med 1998;339:5-11.

Paroxysmal Nocturnal Hemoglobinuria

449. Hillmen P, Lewis SM, Bessler M, et al: Natural history of paroxysmal nocturnal hemoglobinuria. N Engl J Med 1995;333:1253-1258.

450. Ziakas PD, Poulou LS, Rokas GI, et al: Thrombosis in paroxysmal nocturnal hemoglobinuria: Sites, risks, outcome. An overview. J Thromb Haemost 2007;5:642-645.

451. Poulou LS, Vakrinos G, Pomoni A, et al: Stroke in paroxysmal nocturnal haemoglobinuria: Patterns of disease and outcome. Thromb Haemost 2007;98:699-701.

Platelet Disorders

452. Murphy S, Iland H, Rosenthal D, Laszlo J: Essential thrombocythemia: An interim report from the Polycythemia Vera Study Group. Semin Hematol 1986;23:177-182.

453. Jabaily J, Iland HJ, Laszlo J, et al: Neurologic manifestations of essential thrombocythemia. Ann Intern Med 1983;99:513-518.

454. Hehlmann R, Jahn M, Baumann B, Kopcke W: Essential thrombocythemia. Clinical characteristics and course of 61 cases. Cancer 1988;61:2487-2496.

455. Arboix A, Besses C, Acin P, et al: Ischemic stroke as the first manifestation of essential thrombocythemia. Stroke 1995;26:1463-1466.

456. Ogata J, Yonemura K, Kimura Y, et al: Cerebral infarction associated with thrombocythemia: An autopsy case study. Cerebrovasc Dis 2005;19:201-205.

457. Wu K: Platelet hyperaggregability and thrombosis in patients with thrombocythemia. Ann Intern Med 1978;88:7-11.

458. Al-Mefty O, Marano G, Rajaraman S, et al: Transient ischemic attacks due to increased platelet aggregation and adhesiveness. J Neurosurg 1979;50:449-453.

459. Trip MD, Cats VM, van Capelle FJL, Vreeken J: Platelet hyperreactivity and prognosis in survivors of myocardial infarction. N Engl J Med 1990;322:1549-1554.

Coagulopathies

460. Védy D, Schapira M, Angelillo-Scherrer A: Bleeding disorders and thrombophilia. In Caplan LR (ed): Uncommon Causes of Stroke, 2nd ed. Cambridge: Cambridge University Press, 2008, pp 283-300.

461. Thaler E, Lechner K: Antithrombin III deficiency and thromboembolism. Clin Haematol 1981;10:369-390.

462. Camerlingo M, Finazzi G, Casto L, et al: Inherited protein C deficiency and nonhemorrhagic arterial stroke in young adults. Neurology 1991;41:1371-1373.

463. Dahlback B, Carlsson M, Svensson PJ: Familial thrombophilia due to a previously unrecognized mechanism characterized by poor anticoagulant response to activated protein C: Prediction of a cofactor to activated protein C. Proc Natl Acad Sci U S A 1993;90:1004-1008.

464. Zoller B, Dahlback B: Linkage between inherited resistance to activated protein C and factor V gene mutation in venous thrombosis. Lancet 1994;343:1536-1538.

465. Ridker PM, Miletich JP, Stampfer MJ, et al: Factor V Leiden and risks of recurrent idiopathic venous thromboembolism. Circulation 1997;95:1777-1782.

466. Poort SR, Rosendaal FR, Reitsma PH, Bertina RM: A common genetic variation in the 3' untranslated region of the prothrombin gene is associated with elevated prothrombin levels and an increase in venous thrombosis. Blood 1996;88:3698-3703.

467. Huberfeld G, Kubis N, Lot G, et al: G20210A Prothrombin gene mutation in two siblings with cerebral venous thrombosis. Neurology 1998;51:316-317.

468. Martinelli I, Sacchi E, Landi G, et al: High risk of cerebral-vein thrombosis in carriers of a prothrombin-gene mutation and in users of oral contraceptives. N Engl J Med 1998;338:1793-1797.

469. Estol C, Pessin MS, DeWitt LD, Caplan LR: Stroke and increased factor VIII activity. Neurology 1989;39(suppl 1):1159.

470. Kosik KS, Furie B: Thrombotic stroke associated with elevated factor VIII. Arch Neurol 1980;8:435-437.

471. De Georgia MA, Rose DZ: Stroke in patients who have inflammatory bowel disease. In Caplan LR (ed): Uncommon Causes of Stroke, 2nd ed. Cambridge: Cambridge University Press, 2008, pp 381-386.

472. Talbot RW, Heppell J, Dozois RR, Beart RW: Vascular complications of inflammatory bowel disease. Mayo Clin Proc 1986;61:140-145.

473. Johns DR: Cerebrovascular complications of inflammatory bowel disease. Am J Gastroenterol 1991;86:367-370.

474. Sigsbee B, Rottenberg DA: Sagittal sinus thrombosis as a complication of regional enteritis. Ann Neurol 1978;3:450-452.

475. Grau A, Buggle F, Heindl S, et al: Recent infection as a risk factor for cerebrovascular ischemia. Stroke 1995;26:373-379.

476. Syrjanen J, Valtonen VV, Iivanainen M, et al: Preceding infection as an important risk factor for ischaemic brain infarction in young and middle aged patients. BMJ 1988;296:1156-1160.

477. Grau A, Buggle F, Steichen-Wiehn C, et al: Clinical and histochemical analysis in infection-associated stroke. Stroke 1995;26:1520-1526.

478. Grau A: Infection, inflammation, and cerebro-vascular ischemia. Neurology 1997;49(suppl 4): S47-S51.

479. Leira R, Davalos A, Castillo J: Cancer and paraneoplastic strokes. In Caplan LR (ed): Uncommon Causes of Stroke, 2nd ed. Cambridge: Cambridge University Press, 2008, pp 371-376.

480. Sack GH, Levin J, Bell WR: Trousseau's syndrome and other manifestations of chronic disseminated coagulopathy in patients with neoplasms. Medicine (Baltimore) 1977;56:1-37.

481. Graus F, Rodgers LR, Posner JB: Cerebrovascular complications in patients with cancer. Medicine (Baltimore) 1985;64:16-35.

482. Amico L, Caplan LR, Thomas C: Cerebrovascular complications of mucinous cancers. Neurology 1989;39:523-526.

483. Hajjar K, Francis CW: Fibrinolysis and thrombolysis. In Lichtman MA, Beutler E, Kipps TJ, Seligsohn U, Kaushansky K, Prchal JT (eds): Williams Hematology, 7th ed. New York: McGraw-Hill, 2006, pp 2089-2115.

484. Sloane MA: Thrombolysis and stroke-past and future. Arch Neurol 1986;44:748-768.

485. Del Zoppo GH, Zeumer H, Harker LA: Thrombolytic therapy in stroke: Possibilities and hazards. Stroke 1986;17:595-607.

486. Francis RB: Clinical disorders of fibrinolysis. Blut 1989;59:1-14.

487. Nilsson IM, Ljungner H, Tengborn L: Two different mechanisms in patients with venous thrombosis and defective fibrinolysis: Low concentrations of plasminogen activator or increased concentration of plasminogen activator inhibitor. BMJ 1985;290:1453-1456.

488. Collen D, Lijnen HR: The fibrinolytic system in man. Crit Rev Oncol Hematol 1986;4:249-301.

489. Nagayama T, Shinohara Y, Nagayama M, et al: Congenitally abnormal plasminogen in juvenile ischemic cerebrovascular disease. Stroke 1993;24:2104-2107.

490. Hunt FA, Rylatt DB, Hart R, Bundesen PG: Serum cross-linked fibrin (XDP) and fibrinogen/fibrin degradation products (FDP) in disorders associated with activation of the coagulation or fibrinolytic systems. Br J Haematol 1985;60:715-722.

491. Feinberg WM, Bruck DC, Ring ME, Corrigan JJ: Hemostatic markers in acute stroke. Stroke 1989;20:582-587.

492. Delgado J, Jimenez-Yuste V, Hernandez-Navarro F, Villar A: Acquired hemophilia. Review and meta-analysis focused on therapy and prognostic factors. Br J Haematol 2003;121:21-35.

493. Johansen RF, Sorensen B, Ingerslev J: Acquired haemophilia: Dynamic whole blood coagulation utilized to guide haemostatic therapy. Haemophilia 2006;12:190-197.

493a. Ruggeri ZM, Zimmerman TS: von Willebrand factor and von Willebrand disease. Blood 1987;70:895-904.

493b. Wilde JT: Von Willebrand disease. Clin Med 2007;7:629-632.

493c. Nurden P, Nurden AT: Congenital disorders associated with platelet dysfunctions. Thromb Haemost 2008;99:253-263.

Antiphospholipid Antibodies

494. Roldan J, Brey RL: Antiphospholipid antibody syndrome. In Caplan LR (ed): Uncommon Causes of Stroke, 2nd ed. Cambridge: Cambridge University Press, 2008, pp 263-274.

495. Levine SR, Welch KMA: Cerebrovascular ischemia associated with lupus anticoagulant. Stroke 1987;18:257-263.

496. DeWitt LD, Caplan LR: Antiphospholipid antibodies and stroke. AJNR Am J Neuroradiol 1991;12:454-456.

497. Cervera R, Piette JC, Font J, et al: Antiphospholipid syndrome: Clinical and immunologic manifestations and patterns of disease expression in a cohort of 1,000 patients. Arthritis Rheum 2002;46:1019-1027.

498. Coull BM, Goodnight SH: Antiphospholipid antibodies, prethrombotic states, and stroke. Stroke 1990;21:1370-1374.

499. Levine SR, Kim S, Deegan MI, Welch KMA: Ischemic stroke associated with anticardiolipin antibodies. Stroke 1987;18:1101-1106.

500. Montalban J, Codina A, Ordi J, et al: Antiphospholipid antibodies in cerebral ischemia. Stroke 1991;22:750-753.

501. Pope JM, Canny CL, Bell DA: Cerebral ischemic events associated with endocarditis, retinal vascular disease, and lupus anticoagulant. Am J Med 1991;90:299-309.

502. Antiphospholipid Antibodies in Stroke Study (APASS) Group: Clinical and laboratory findings in patients with antiphospholipid antibodies and cerebral ischemia. Stroke 1990;21:1268-1273.

503. Lopez LR, Dier KJ, Lopez D, et al: Anti-beta 2-glycoprotein I and antiphosphatidylserine antibodies are predictors of arterial thrombosis in patients with antiphospholipid syndrome. Am J Clin Pathol 2004;121: 142-149.

504. Atsumi T, Ieko M, Bertolaccini ML, et al: Association of autoantibodies against the phosphatidylserine-prothrombin complex with manifestations of the antiphospholipid syndrome and with the presense of lupus anticoagulant. Arthritis Rheum 2000;43:1982-1993.

505. Feldmann E, Levine SR: Cerebrovascular disease with antiphospholipid antibodies: Immune mechanisms, significance, and therapeutic options. Ann Neurol 1995;37(suppl 1): S114-S130.

506. Levine SR, Salowich-Palm L, Sawaya KL, et al: IgG anticardiolipin antibody titer >40 GPL and the risk of subsequent thrombo-occlusive events and death. A prospective cohort study. Stroke 1997;28:1660-1665.

507. Verro P, Levine SR, Tietjen GE: Cerebrovascular ischemic events with high positive anticardiolipin antibodies. Stroke 1998;29:2245-2253.
508. Provenzale JM, Barboriak DP, Allen NB, Ortel TL: Antiphospholipid antibodies: Findings at arteriography. AJNR Am J Neuroradiol 1998;19:611-616.

Disseminated Intravascular Coagulation

509. Bick RL: Disseminated intravascular coagulation and related syndromes: A clinical review. Semin Thromb Hemost 1988;14:299-338.
510. Wen PY, Sobel RA: Case records of the Massachusetts General Hospital: Case 36-1991. N Engl J Med 1991;325:714-726.
511. Colman RW, Rubin RN: Disseminated intravascular coagulation due to malignancy. Semin Oncol 1990;17:172-186.
512. Schwartzman RJ, Hill JB: Neurologic complications of disseminated intravascular coagulation. Neurology 1982;32:791-797.
513. Schwartzman RJ, Kumar M: Disseminated intravascular disease. In Caplan LR (ed): Uncommon Causes of Stroke, 2nd ed. Cambridge: Cambridge University Press, 2008, pp 275-282.

Hyperviscosity

514. Dashe J: Hyperviscosity and stroke. In Caplan LR (ed): Uncommon Causes of Stroke, 2nd ed. Cambridge: Cambridge University Press, 2008, pp 347-356.
515. Grotta J, Ackerman R, Correia J, et al: Whole blood viscosity parameters and cerebral blood flow. Stroke 1982;13:296-301.
516. Coull BM, Beamer N, de Garmo P, et al: Chronic blood hyperviscosity in subjects with acute stroke, transient ischemic attack, and risk factors for stroke. Stroke 1991;22:162-168.
517. Ernst E, Resch KL: Fibrinogen as a cardiovascular risk factor: A meta-analysis and review of the literature. Ann Intern Med 1993;118:956-963.
518. Fahey JL, Barth WF, Solomon A: Serum hyperviscosity syndrome. JAMA 1965;192:464-467.
519. Rosenson RS, Baker AL, Chow M, Hay R: Hyperviscosity syndrome in a hypercholesterolemic patient with primary biliary cirrhosis. Gastroenterology 1990;98:1351-1357.

Neoplastic Conditions

LYMPHOMATOID GRANULOMATOSIS

520. Fauci A, Haynes BF, Costa J, et al: Lymphatoid granulomatosis: Prospective clinical and therapeutic experience over 10 years. N Engl J Med 1982;306:68-74.
521. Hogan PJ, Greenberg MK, McCarty GE: Neurologic complications of lymphomatoid granulomatosis. Neurology 1981;31:619-620.
522. Hochberg EP, Gilman MD, Hasserjian RP: Case records of the Massachusetts General Hospital. Case 17-2006—a 34-year-old man with cavitary lung lesions. N Engl J Med 2006;354:2485-2493.
523. Mizuno T, Takanashi Y, Onodera H, et al: A case of lymphomatoid granulomatosis/angiocentric immunoproliferative lesion with long clinical course and diffuse brain involvement. J Neuro Sci 2003;213:67-76.

INTRAVASCULAR LYMPHOMA

524. Rubens EO: Intravascular lymphoma. In Caplan LR (ed): Uncommon Causes of Stroke, 2nd ed. Cambridge: Cambridge University Press, 2008, pp 533-537.
525. Petito CK, Gottlieb GJ, Dougherty JH, Petito FA: Neoplastic angioendotheliosis: Ultrastructural study and review of the literature. Ann Neurol 1978;3:393-399.
526. Beal MF, Fisher CM: Neoplastic angioendotheliosis. J Neurol Sci 1982;53:359-375.
527. Reinglass JL, Miller J, Wissman S: Central nervous system angioendotheliosis. Stroke 1977;8:218-221.
528. Raroque HG, Mandler RN, Griffey MS, et al: Neoplastic angioendotheliomatosis. Arch Neurol 1990;47:929-930.
529. Glass J, Hochberg FH, Miller DC: Intravascular lymphomatosis—A systemic disease with neurologic manifestations. Cancer 1993;71:3156-3164.
530. Hamada K, Hamada T, Satoh M, et al: Two cases of neoplastic angioendotheliomatosis presenting with myelopathy. Neurology 1991;41:1139-1140.

Genetic Disorders

531. Natowicz M, Kelley RI: Mendelian etiologies of stroke. Ann Neurol 1987;22:175-192.
532. Albert M: Genetics of Cerebrovascular Disease. Armonk, NY: Futura, 1999.
533. Alberts MJ: Genetics of cerebrovascular disease. Stroke 2004;35:342-344.
534. Meschia JF, Worrall BB: New advances in identifying genetic anomalies in stroke-prone probands. Curr Neurol Neurosci Rep 2004;4:420-426.
535. Hoy A, Leininger-Muller B, Poirier O, et al: Myeloperoxidase polymorphisms in brain infarction. Association with infarct size and functional outcome. Atherosclerosis 2003;167:223-230.

MELAS and Other Mitochondrial Disorders

536. Hirt L: MELAS and other mitochondrial disorders. In Caplan LR (ed): Uncommon Causes of Stroke, 2nd ed. Cambridge: Cambridge University Press, 2008, pp 149-154.
537. Pavlakis SG, Phillips PC, DiMauro S, et al: Mitochondrial myopathy, encephalopathy, lactic acidosis, and stroke-like episodes: A distinctive clinical syndrome. Ann Neurol 1984;16:481-488.
538. Morgan-Hughes JA: Mitochondrial diseases. In Engel AG, Franzini-Armstrong C (eds): Myology, vol 2, 2nd ed. New York: McGraw-Hill, 1994, pp 1610-1660.

539. Kuriyama M, Umezaki H, Fukuda Y, et al: Mitochondrial encephalomyopathy with lactate-pyruvate elevation and brain infarctions. Neurology 1984;34:72-77.

540. Allard JC, Tilak C, Carter AP: CT and MR of MELAS syndrome. AJNR Am J Neuroradiol 1988;9:1234-1238.

541. Koo B, Becker LE, Chuang S, et al: Mitochondrial encephalomyopathy, lactic acidosis, stroke like episodes (MELAS): Clinical, radiological, and genetic observations. Ann Neurol 1993;34:25-32.

542. Matthews PM, Tampieri D, Berkovic SF, et al: Magnetic resonance imaging shows specific abnormalities in the MELAS syndrome. Neurology 1991;41:1043-1046.

543. Clark JM, Marks MP, Adalsteinsson E, et al: MELAS: Clinical and pathological correlations with MRI, xenon/CT, and MR spectroscopy. Neurology 1996;46:223-227.

544. Sue CM, Crimmins DS, Soo YS, et al: Neuroradiological features of six kindreds with MELAS tRNALeu A3243G point mutation: Implications for pathogenesis. J Neurol Neurosurg Psychiatry 1998;65:233-240.

Fabry's Disease

545. Mitsias P, Levine SR: Cerebrovascular complications of Fabry's disease. Ann Neurol 1996;40:8-17.

546. Mitsias P, Papamitsakis NIH, Amory CF, Levine SR: Cerebrovascular complications of Fabry disease. In Caplan LR (ed): Uncommon Causes of Stroke, 2nd ed. Cambridge: Cambridge University Press, 2008, pp 123-130.

547. Brady RO, Gal AE, Bradley RM, et al: Enzymatic defect in Fabry's disease: Ceramide trihexosidase deficiency. N Engl J Med 1967;276:1163-1167.

548. Dawson DM, Miller DC: Case records of the Massachusetts General Hospital: Case 2-1984. N Engl J Med 1984;310:106-114.

549. Kint JA: Fabry's disease: Alpha-galactosidase deficiency. Science 1970;167:1268-1269.

550. Eng CM, Guffon N, Wilcox WR, et al: Safety and efficacy of recombinant human alpha-galactosidase A—Replacement therapy in Fabry's disease. N Engl J Med 2001;5: 345:9-16.

551. Desnick RJ, Brady R, Barranger J, et al: Fabry disease, an under-recognized multi-systemic disorder: Expert recommendations for diagnosis, management, and enzyme replacement therapy. Ann Intern Med 2003;138:338-346.

CADASIL

552. Chabriat H, Bousser M-G: Cerebral autosomal dominant arteriopathy with subcortical infarcts and leukoencephalopathy (CADASIL). In Caplan LR (ed): Uncommon Causes of Stroke, 2nd ed. Cambridge: Cambridge University Press, 2008, pp 115-122.

553. Tournier-Lasserve E, Iba-Zizen M-T, Romero N, Bousser M-G: Autosomal dominant syndrome with stroke-like episodes and leukoencephalopathy. Stroke 1991;22:1297-1302.

554. Mas JL, Dilouya A, de Recondo J: A familial disorder with subcortical ischemic strokes, dementia, and leukoencephalopathy. Neurology 1992;42:1015-1019.

555. Hutchinson M, O'Riordan J, Javed M, et al: Familial hemiplegic migraine and autosomal dominant arteriopathy with leukoencephalopathy (CADASIL). Ann Neurol 1995;38:817-824.

556. Ragno M, Tournier-Lasserve E, Fiori MG, et al: An Italian kindred with cerebral autosmal dominant arteriopathy with subcortical infarcts and leukoencephalopathy (CADASIL). Ann Neurol 1995;38:231-236.

557. Dichgans M, Mayer M, Uttner I, et al: The phenotypic spectrum of CADASIL: Clinical findings in 102 cases. Ann Neurol 1998;44:731-739.

558. Chabriat H, Levy C, Taillia H, et al: Patterns of MRI lesions in CADASIL. Neurology 1998;51:452-457.

559. Joutel A, Corpechot C, Ducros A, et al: Notch 3 mutations in CADASIL, a hereditary adult-onset condition causing stroke and dementia. Nature 1996;383:707-710.

560. Fukutake T, Hirayama K: Familial young-adult-onset arteriosclerotic leukoencephalopathy with alopecia and lumbago without arterial hypertension. Eur Neurol 1995;35:69-79.

Menkes' Disease

561. Menkes J: Menkes disease (kinky hair disease). In Caplan LR (ed): Uncommon Causes of Stroke, 2nd ed. Cambridge: Cambridge University Press, 2008, pp 225-230.

562. Menkes J, Alter M, Steigleder G, et al: A sex-linked recessive disorder with retardation of growth, peculiar hair and focal cerebral and cerebellar degeneration. Pediatrics 1962;29:764-779.

563. Moller JV, Juul B, Le Maire M: Structural organization, ion transport, and energy transduction of P-type ATP-ases. Biochem Biophys Acta 1996;1286:1-51.

564. Moller LB, Tumer Z, Lund C, et al: Similar splice-site mutations of the ATP7A gene lead to different phenotypes: Classical Menkes disease or occipital horn syndrome. Am J Hum Genet 2000;66:1211-1220.

565. Iannaccone ST, Rosenberg RN: Menkes disease. In Berg B (ed): Principles of Child Neurology. New York: McGraw-Hill, 1995, pp 473-475.

566. Morgello S, Peterson HD, Kahn LJ, Laufer H: Menkes kinky hair disease with "ragged red fibers." Dev Med Child Neurol 1988;30:812-816.

566a. Kaler S, Holmes CS, Goldstein DS, et al: Neonatal diagnosis and treatment of Menkes disease. N Engl J Med 2008;358:605-614.

Neurofibromatosis

567. Nedeltchev N, Mattle HP: Cerebrovascular manifestations of neurofibromatosis. In Caplan LR (ed): Uncommon Causes of Stroke, 2nd ed. Cambridge: Cambridge University Press, 2008, pp 221-224.
568. Taboada D, Alonso A, Moreno J: Occlusion of the cerebral arteries in Recklinghausen's disease. Neuroradiology 1979;18:281-284.
569. Levinsohn PM, Mikhael MA, Rothman SM: Cerebrovascular changes in neurofibromatosis. Dev Med Child Neurol 1978;20:789-793.
570. Rizzo JF, Lessell S: Cerebrovascular abnormalities in neurofibromatosis type l. Neurology 1994;44: 1000-1002.

Homocystinuria and Homocysteinemia

571. Boers GH, Smals AG, Trijbels FJ, et al: Heterozygosity for homocystinuria in premature peripheral and cerebral occlusive disease. N Engl J Med 1985;313:709-715.
572. Welch GN, Loscalzo J: Homocysteine and atherothrombosis. N Engl J Med 1998;338:1042-1050.
573. Caplan LR, Hurst JW: Homocysteinemia and homocystinuria. In Caplan LR, Hurst JW, Chimowitz M (eds): Clinical Neurocardiology. New York: Marcel Dekker, 1999, pp 431-432.
574. Ueland PM, Refsum H, Stabler SP, et al: Total homocysteine in plasma or serum: methods and clinical applications. Clin Chem 1993;39: 1764-1769.
575. Finkelstein JD, Martin JJ, Harris BJ: Methionine metabolism in mammals: The methionine-sparing effect of cystine. J Biol Chem 1988;263:11750-11754.
576. Mudd SH, Skovby F, Levy HL, et al: The natural history of homocystinuria due to cystathione-beta-synthase deficiency. Am J Hum Genet 1985;37:1-31.
577. Vermaak WJ, Ubbink JB, Barnard HC, et al: Vitamin B6 nutrition status and cigarette smoking. Am J Clin Nutr 1990;51:1058-1061.
578. Clarke R, Daly L, Robinson K, et al: Hyperhomocysteinemia: An independent risk factor for vascular disease. N Engl J Med 1991;324: 1149-1155.
579. Evers S, Koch H-G, Grotemeyer K-H, et al: Features, symptoms, and neurophysiological findings in stroke associated with hyperhomocysteinemia. Arch Neurol 1997;54:1276-1282.
580. Selhub J, Jacques PF, Bostom AG, et al: Association between plasma homocysteine concentrations and extracranial carotid-artery stenosis. N Engl J Med 1995;332:286-291.
581. Harker LA, Slichter SJ, Scott CR: Homocystinemia: Vascular injury and arterial thrombosis. N Engl J Med 1974;291:537-543.
582. Harker LA, Ross R, Slichter SJ, Scott CR: Homocystine-induced arteriosclerosis: The role of endothelial cell injury and platelet response in its genesis. J Clin Invest 1976;58:731-741.

583. Tsai J-C, Perrella MA, Yoshizumi M, et al: Promotion of vascular smooth muscle cell growth by homocysteine: A link to atherosclerosis. Proc Natl Acad Sci U S A 1994;91:6369-6373.

Progeria

584. Roach ES, Anselm I, Rosman NP, Caplan LR: Progeria. In Caplan LR (ed): Uncommon Causes of Stroke, 2nd ed. Cambridge: Cambridge University Press, 2008, pp 145-148.
584a. Merideth MA, Gordon LB, Clauss S, et al: Phenotype and course of Hutchinson-Gilford progeria syndrome. N Engl J Med 2008;358:592-604.
585. Delgado Luengo W, Rojas Martinez A, Ortiz Lopez R, et al: Del(1)(q23) in a patient with Hutchinson-Gilford progeria. Am J Med Genet 2002;113:298-301.
586. McClintock D, Gordon LB, Djabali K: Hutchinson-Gilford progeria mutant lamin A primarily targets human vascular cells as detected by an anti-lamin A G608G antibody. Proc Natl Acad Sci U S A 2006;103:2154-2159.

Hereditary Hemorrhagic Telangiectasia

587. Zuber M: Hereditary hemorrhagic telangiectasia (Osler-Weber-Rendu disease). In Caplan LR (ed): Uncommon Causes of Stroke, 2nd ed. Cambridge: Cambridge University Press, 2008, pp 109-114.
588. Osler W: On a family form of recurring epistaxis, associated with multiple telengiectases of the skin and mucous membranes. John Hopkins Hosp Bull 1901;12:333-337.
589. Peery WH: Clinical spectrum of hereditary haemorrhagic telangiectasia (Osler-Weber-Rendu disease). Am J Med 1987;82: 989-997.
590. Guttmacher AE, Marchuk DA, White RI: Hereditary hemorrhagic telangiectasia. N Engl J Med 1995;333:918-924.

COL4A1 Mutation Syndrome

591. Gould DB, Phalan FC, Breedveld GJ, et al: Mutations in Col4a1 cause perinatal cerebral hemorrhage and porencephaly. Science 2005;308:1167-1171.
592. Gould DB, Phalan FC, van Mil SE, et al: Role of COL4A1 in small vessel disease and hemorrhagic stroke. N Engl J Med 2006;354:1489-1496.
593. Vahedi K, Boukobza M, Massin P, et al: Clinical and brain MRI follow-up study of a family with COL4A1 mutation. Neurology 2007;69:1564-1568.
594. Meschia JF, Rosand J: Fragile vessels. Handle with care. Neurology 2007;69:1560-1561.

12

Subarachnoid Hemorrhage, Aneurysms, and Vascular Malformations

Intracranial hemorrhages involve the brain parenchyma or subarachnoid space, or both. Approximately 20% of all strokes are hemorrhagic, with subarachnoid hemorrhage (SAH) and intracerebral hemorrhage (ICH) accounting for about 10%. SAH occurs when a blood vessel near the brain surface leaks, causing extravasation of blood into the subarachnoid space. SAH is most often caused by rupture of a saccular aneurysm or hemorrhage from an arteriovenous malformation (AVM). Less common causes include head injury, use of illicit drugs, especially amphetamines and cocaine, amyloid angiopathy, rupture of an artery near the pial surface due to hypertension, dural venous sinus thrombosis, and bleeding disorders.

Symptoms depend on the rapidity and duration of the bleeding and the volume of blood. Rupture of an arterial aneurysm causes the abrupt introduction of blood under arterial pressure into the subarachnoid space. This abruptly increases intracranial pressure and leads to transient cessation of activity, severe headache, and vomiting. Slower leakage of blood does not increase intracranial pressure as rapidly. Blood in the subarachnoid space acts as a meningeal irritant and incites headache, photophobia, and stiff neck. Confusion, restlessness, and transient or persistent decreased levels of consciousness are common in patients with SAH and are caused by the increased intracranial pressure, and meningeal irritation.

ANEURYSMS

Ruptured saccular aneurysms are a common and serious medical problem. According to necropsy and angiography series, approximately 5% to 6% of individuals have intracranial aneurysms.[1,2] The prevalence of aneurysms is low during the first two decades of life and increases steadily after the third decade.[1] The frequency of SAH from ruptured saccular aneurysms is relatively low, estimated at between 6 to 11 per 100,000 persons per year, or about 1 per 10,000.[3-8] The relatively low rupture-to-prevalence rate shows that most aneurysms do not rupture. Much research has tackled identification of those aneurysms most

likely to rupture and treating them before a first SAH. Overall, ruptured aneurysms are more common in women. Although ruptured aneurysms are more common in men younger than 40 years, women prevail after age 40.[9,10] The average age at rupture is approximately 50 years.[4]

Once an aneurysm ruptures, death or severe long-term disability often results. Among 100 typical patients with SAH caused by ruptured aneurysms, it is estimated that 33 will die before receiving medical attention. Another 20 will die while in the hospital or will remain incapacitated from the original hemorrhage. Seventeen patients who survive the initial hemorrhage will deteriorate later, with eight patients recovering and nine patients left with severe neurologic sequelae.[11] Only 30 of the original 100 patients will do well, surviving without major disability. If the ruptured aneurysm remains surgically untreated and the patient does not have recurrent hemorrhage during the first 6 months, approximately 3% of the remaining patients will rebleed each year.[12] Even among patients admitted to the hospital in good condition, the prognosis is poor. In one series, 29% of these patients died and only 55% made a good recovery at 90 days.[13] A delay often occurs in referring patients with SAH to neurologic and neurosurgical centers for treatment. In one series among 150 consecutive patients with aneurysmal SAH, only 36% were referred within 48 hours.[14] The median time to referral was 3.6 days. Tragically, delayed diagnosis by physicians and logistic and policy issues accounted for more than 70% of the delays.[14]

Dolichoectatic aneurysms and dissecting aneurysms can also rupture, causing SAH. These lesions are discussed and illustrated in Chapter 11.

Locations, Familial Occurrence, and Pathogenesis

Saccular aneurysms typically form at arterial bifurcations (see Fig. 2-34). Aneurysms are especially likely to form at bifurcations that have a hypoplastic small branch and bifurcations with a sharp acute angle.[14a] Approximately 90% of aneurysms involve anterior circulation arteries.[4,15]

Common sites in the anterior circulation include (1) the junction between the anterior communicating artery (AComA) and the anterior cerebral artery (ACA); (2) bifurcation of the middle cerebral artery (MCA); and (3) the internal carotid artery (ICA) junction with the ophthalmic artery, posterior communicating artery (PComA), anterior choroidal artery (AChA), and MCAs.[4] In the posterior circulation, the apex of the basilar artery and the intracranial vertebral artery, especially at the origins of the posterior inferior cerebellar arteries (PICAs), are the most common sites.[4,15]

Multiple aneurysms are present in approximately 14% to 24% of patients and are more common in women.[2,5,16] In patients with multiple aneurysms, two are present in 77%, three in 15%, and four or more in 8%.[5] Saccular aneurysms are known to be more common in patients with polycystic kidney disease, coarctation of the aorta, fibromuscular dysplasia, pseudoxanthoma elasticum, and Marfan's syndrome.

The familial occurrence of intracranial aneurysms is well known.[17-19] Approximately 7% to 20% of patients with a ruptured aneurysm have a first or second degree relative with an intracranial aneurysm, and, among first degree relatives of a patient who has had a ruptured aneurysm, the risk of having a ruptured intracranial aneurysm is approximately four times higher than in the general population.[2,5,17-19] Late teenage and adult first-degree relatives in families where two or more first-degree relatives have been shown to have a cerebral aneurysm should be screened with MRA or CTA for the presence of aneurysms. Since aneurysms can develop later, they probably should later be screened again, although the optimal interval between screenings is not clear. Preliminary studies are beginning to show some genetic associations in patients with familial and sporadic saccular aneurysms.[20-23,23a,23b] Variations in or near the proteoglycan versican gene likely play a role in susceptibility to intracranial aneurysm formation.[23a]

No completely satisfactory explanation of the origin, growth, and rupture of saccular aneurysms exists. Intracerebral arteries are normally composed of an outer collagenous adventitia, a prominent muscular media, an internal elastic lamina, and an intima lined by endothelial cells. An external elastic lamina does not exist. Intracranial arteries are more susceptible than extracranial arteries to aneurysm formation because intracranially, the arterial walls are thin, there is less elastin, an external elastic lamina is not present, and arteries that are located within the subarachnoid space lack surrounding supporting tissue. Various theories cite congenital and genetic abnormalities that cause defects in the arterial media, hypertensive and atherosclerotic degenerative changes in the vessel walls, inflammatory proliferative arteritis, and focal degeneration of the internal elastic lamina. Some investigators emphasize that aneurysms form because of congenital defects in the media of arteries. The most common defect in the arterial media is a localized loss of muscular elements. These focal deficits are often located at arterial bifurcations. Some patients with intracranial aneurysms have reduced production of type III collagen.[24]

Ferguson proposed a theory of aneurysm development and growth that I find plausible and attractive.[25] He suggested that cerebral aneurysms result from mechanically induced degeneration of arteries. Maximal hemodynamic stress occurs at the apices and bifurcations of arteries. Imbalance between the strength of an artery at a particular bifurcation and the hemodynamic stresses applied to it causes degeneration of the internal elastic lamina and aneurysmal outpouching. Turbulent flow in and around aneurysms produces vibration in vessel walls, further weakening the vessel's structural integrity and allowing aneurysm growth.[25] The observation that aneurysms tend to form at sites of increased flow-feeding AVMs and in arteries that provide collateral blood flow supports the contention that increased pressure and flow contribute to aneurysm formation. Stress on the vessel wall increases as aneurysms become thinner, the radius of the aneurysm enlarges, or the intraaneurysmal pressure increases because of elevated blood pressure. When the wall stress exceeds the wall strength, aneurysms rupture.

Aneurysms may rupture at any time, but especially when blood pressure or blood flow is increased. Rupture often occurs during strenuous activity, such as weight lifting, exercise, coition, defecation, and heavy work. Many aneurysms, however, leak during relatively inactive periods. One third of the aneurysms in the Cooperative Study of Intracranial Aneurysms and Subarachnoid Hemorrhage ruptured while patients were asleep, and another one third ruptured during ordinary daily activities.[10,11,26] Size plays a major role; up to a point, the larger the aneurysm, the more likely it is to rupture. In different autopsy series, the critical size for rupture has varied from 7 to 10 mm.[27-29] Aneurysms larger than 10 mm in diameter are more likely to rupture during follow-up than smaller aneurysms.[2]

Aneurysms larger than 2.5 cm in size are usually referred to as giant aneurysms. The notion that they rarely rupture and produce SAH is not correct. Drake reported that 33% of giant aneurysms present with bleeding and another

10% have a history of remote hemorrhage.[30] Giant aneurysms often contain thrombi within their arterial lumens.

Once an intracranial aneurysm has ruptured, the course is often stormy and the outcome poor. It is estimated that among the 28,000 patients with ruptured aneurysms each year in the United States and Canada, 7000 are misdiagnosed, never referred, or referred too late for definitive therapy.[14,31] The greatest impact improving morbidity and mortality from SAH is not through the efforts of neurologists or neurosurgeons, but rather through early recognition of SAH by primary care physicians and emergency room physicians.[32,33] Diagnosed early, these patients can be referred while still relatively intact to centers with appropriate neurologic, neurosurgical, neuroradiologic, and neuroanesthetic capabilities. Neurologic-neurosurgical intensive care units are especially important for definitive treatment of patients with ruptured aneurysms and their complications.

Clinical Findings

A 32-year-old woman, PN, came to the emergency ward because of a headache that had been unremitting for 48 hours. She had migraine headaches as an adolescent. One month ago, she awakened at night with moderately severe headache and vomiting. After the headache persisted for 3 days, she consulted her physician, who diagnosed her with the flu. Although she had no fever, she felt too ill to do her daily chores and stayed in bed for a week, after which the headache gradually cleared. Two days ago, she developed a severe headache that came on suddenly. She was taking heavy trash cans out for garbage collection when the pain struck her in the left temple and top of the head and quickly radiated to her neck and back. Her knees buckled with the pain and she vomited. She stumbled into the house and was in bed and rather sleepy when her husband returned from work and insisted that she go to the hospital.

Headache

Intracranial saccular aneurysms often present with a warning leak or so-called sentinel hemorrhage—a minute rent in the aneurysm results in bleeding that lasts only seconds, spilling blood into the subarachnoid space under high pressure. The patient has sudden, severe headaches, often occipital or nuchal in location, and constant. The headache usually resolves in 48 hours but can last longer. It is best distinguished from migraine by its rapidity of onset and longer duration. Only seconds elapse before it reaches maximum intensity. Vomiting and cessation of activity (e.g., the knees buckling in patient PN) and decrease in alertness often accompany the headache. Migraine headaches, on the other hand, are usually more throbbing and build in intensity over minutes or hours. Nausea and vomiting usually develop after migraine headache has been present for a while. Sentinel headaches usually last from days to a week, during which time patients are seldom able to continue normal activities. Sentinel hemorrhages are often misdiagnosed as migraine, flu, hypertensive encephalopathy, aseptic meningitis, cervical neck strain, or even gastroenteritis.[32,33] Headache, restlessness, and vomiting are often falsely attributed to food poisoning or an acute gastrointestinal disorder.

In patient PN, the headache she had 1 month before her episode was probably a warning leak. The duration was too long for migraine, and inability to carry out daily activities should have alerted her physician to evaluate her further. In the Michael Reese Stroke Registry and the University of Illinois Stroke Registry, 31% of patients with SAH had sentinel headaches.[34] In the Danish Aneurysm Study, a warning leak was present in 166 of 1076 patients (15.4%).[35] In 99 of the 166 patients (54%) with warning leaks, the headache episode was evaluated by a doctor but misdiagnosed.[35] Ostergaard estimated that as many as 50% to 60% of patients with SAH have headache or other warning signs before presenting with major bleeds.[36] In patients with headaches of acute onset, the index of suspicion for SAH should be high and the threshold for lumbar puncture (LP) low.[32,33] In patients with sudden, severe headache without focal neurologic signs, the only absolute contraindications to LP are no back or needle. If series of LPs for headache contain only taps positive for blood, then too few LPs are being performed, and sentinel hemorrhages are being missed.

PN's headache that began 2 days before her episode is typical of that found in SAH. Sudden onset with rapid radiation, especially to the neck and back or sciatic region, suggests meningeal irritation. The focal asymmetric headache is a fairly reliable sign that the bleeding lesion was on the left side—the site of the head pain.

Neurologic Symptoms and Signs

Examination of PN in the emergency room showed a restless but sleepy woman with a stiff neck. The left eyelid drooped. When the lid was lifted, the left eye rested down and out. The left pupil was dilated and unreactive to light. Plantar responses were bilaterally extensor.

Aneurysms may present by compressing adjacent brain tissue or cranial nerves. Giant aneurysms are particularly likely to cause focal symptoms and signs related to mass effect. Giant middle cerebral artery (MCA) aneurysms can cause seizures, hemiparesis, or dysphasia. The third nerve can be compressed by aneurysms that occur at the intracranial internal carotid artery (ICA) and posterior communicating artery (PCA) junction (often referred to as *posterior communicating artery aneurysms* (PComA) or by superior cerebellar artery (SCA) aneurysms. A giant SCA aneurysm can cause contralateral hemiplegia (Weber's syndrome) by compressing the pyramidal tracts in the midbrain. Figure 12-1 shows a large aneurysm compressing the cerebral peduncle on one side. An isolated sixth-nerve paresis can be caused by mass effect. In the cavernous sinus, an aneurysm may compress the sixth, fourth, or third cranial nerves, producing ophthalmoplegia. Basilar bifurcation aneurysms that point forward can mimic pituitary tumors and cause visual field defects and hypopituitarism. Basilar bifurcation aneurysms that point vertically can cause an amnesic syndrome combined with third-nerve paresis, bulbar signs, and quadriparesis.[15,37] In PN, the right third-nerve palsy suggested a right PComA aneurysm.

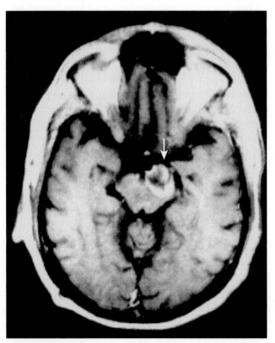

Figure 12-1. MRI shows a large aneurysm *(large white arrow)* compressing the cerebral peduncle on one side associated with a third nerve palsy and contralateral hemiparesis (Weber's syndrome). (From Winn WR, Richardson AE, Jane JA: The long-term prognosis in untreated cerebral aneurysms: I. The incidence of late hemorrhage in cerebral aneurysms—A ten year evaluation of 364 patients. Ann Neurol 1977;1: 358-370, with permission.)

Occasionally, aneurysms present with transient neurologic deficits. These transient ischemic attacks may be secondary to ischemia or seizures. Stewart and colleagues reported short, recurrent, stereotyped episodes in three patients with ischemia and in a fourth patient with transient spells secondary to partial complex seizures.[38] Cranial CT scans, LP, and electroencephalograms were normal. No cardiac source of embolism could be identified. Cerebral arteriography showed aneurysms in appropriate locations to explain the symptoms in all cases. Thrombi may form within aneurysms, dislodge, and then embolize distally, causing stroke. Fisher and colleagues reported seven patients who had episodes of transient focal brain ischemia.[39] All had saccular aneurysms in arteries that would explain the symptoms and no other embolic source. Thrombosis within the aneurismal sac had embolized distally. Sutherland et al confirmed this thromboembolic hypothesis, by showing deposition of platelets within giant aneurysms.[40] In three of the six patients in their series with active platelet deposition, episodes of recurrent transient neurologic dysfunction occurred. Identification of aneurysms presenting in this manner is another indication for performing vascular imaging in patients with recurrent transient neurologic deficits, particularly those in whom no cardiac source has been identified and in patients younger than 45 years of age. Magnetic resonance imaging (MRI) scans also often show heterogeneous signals, indicating thrombi within aneurysms. In Figure 12.2A and B, MRI scans show heterogeneous signals, indicating thrombus within a large basilar artery aneurysm that compressed the pons. Figure 12-3 is an angiogram that shows a filling defect caused by thrombus within an aneurysm.

Patients with SAH usually report sudden-onset constant headaches that reach maximal intensity within seconds. Nausea, vomiting, stiff neck, and transient loss of consciousness are common accompaniments. The patient is often quite agitated and restless. The headache is of such note that the patient is sometimes later able to describe in minute detail the circumstances surrounding the episode. SAH is rarely present without headache. Occasionally, I have cared for patients in whom the initial manifestation of the subarachnoid bleed was neck pain or backache with sciatic radiation. Patients may not report headache if they have confusion, lethargy, aphasia, or amnesia for the event.

Transient loss of consciousness is caused by the sudden increase of intracranial pressure (ICP) that occurs as arterial blood suddenly enters the subarachnoid space. The increased ICP, dissection of blood into the optic-nerve sheath, and

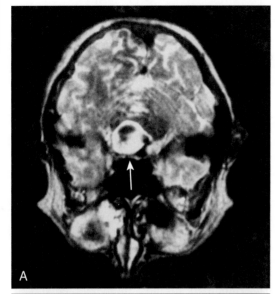

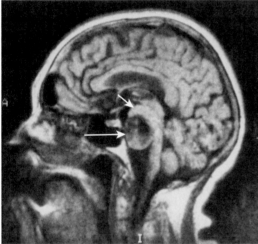

Figure 12-2. A, T2-weighted MRI; *white arrow* points to large basilar artery aneurism containing heterogeneous signals representing thrombus formation. **B,** Sagittal MRI showing aneurysm with clot *(large white arrow)* compressing the pons *(small white arrow).*

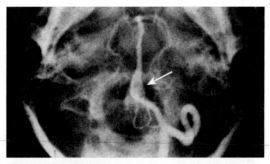

Figure 12-3. Vertebral arteriogram, intracranial Towns view; *arrow* points to a filling defect in a dissecting aneurysm, representing thrombus.

increased pressure in central retinal veins can cause retinal hemorrhages, usually subhyaloid in location. These hemorrhages appear as large red masses of blood spreading outward from the optic disk into the retina. Papilledema may develop later. Unilateral or bilateral sixth-nerve paresis is also common, and is a reflection of increased ICP. Some focal signs that suggest the sites of aneurysmal rupture have already been mentioned. Additional signs are noted in Table 12-1.

Because aneurysms that have previously bled may become adherent to the adjacent brain, recurrent rupture is often characterized by intracerebral and subarachnoid bleeding, so-called meningocerebral hemorrhage.

The patient's clinical state has traditionally been graded according to the scale of Hunt and Hess (Table 12-2),[42] which is useful for predicting short- and long-term prognosis.[43] In general, the higher the grade, the worse the prognosis. I classified patient PN's status as Hunt and Hess grade II. Other scales have traditionally been used to grade comatose patients. The most commonly used is the Glasgow Coma Scale.[44,45] This scale was designed for prognosticating recovery in patients with severe head injury but has since been widely used to evaluate any patient with reduced consciousness. It included grading eye opening and best motor and verbal responses (Table 12-3). More recently, Mayo Clinic physicians devised a new scale that includes eye movements, brainstem reflexes, aspects of motor behavior, and respiration and entitle their scale the Four Score scale[46] (Table 12-4). This scale is likely more useful for neurologists than the Glasgow Coma Scale in grading coma of different etiologies. Since these scales are in relatively wide use, neurologists should become familiar with them.

Diagnostic Testing

Cranial CT in PN was suboptimal because of motion. Diffuse opacification of the cortical gyri occurred, and blood was visible in the basal cisterns. LP revealed bloody fluid with an opening

Table 12-1.	**Focal Signs in Patients with Aneurysmal Rupture**

1. Leg weakness, confusion, and bilateral Babinski's signs in patients with anterior communicating artery (AComA) aneurysms[41]
2. Homonymous hemianopia in PCA aneurysms
3. Aphasia, hemiparesis, and anosognosia in MCA aneurysms
4. Monocular visual disturbances in ophthalmic artery aneurysms

Table 12-2. Hunt and Hess Classification of Subarachnoid Hemorrhage

Grade I: Asymptomatic or minimal headache and slight nuchal rigidity

Grade II: Moderate to severe headache, nuchal rigidity, no neurologic deficit other than cranial nerve palsy

Grade III: Drowsiness, confusion, or mild focal deficit

Grade IV: Stupor, moderate to severe hemiparesis, possible early decerebrate rigidity and vegetative disturbance

Grade V: Deep coma, decerebrate rigidity, moribund appearance

From Hunt W, Hess R: Surgical risk as related to time of intervention in the repair of intracranial aneurysms. J Neurosurg 1968;28:14-20.

pressure of 420 mm Hg. She was placed at bed rest and observed carefully.

Computed Tomography

Cranial CT is most often the first diagnostic test in the evaluation of patients with suspected SAH. CT often verifies the presence of blood in the subarachnoid space and shows associated intraparenchymal blood. The location of the blood often suggests the etiology and the site of the aneurysm

Table 12-3. Glasgow Coma Scale

Eyes open

Spontaneous	4
To sound	3
To pain	2
Never	1

Best verbal response

Oriented	5
Confused conversation	4
Inappropriate words	3
Incomprehensible sounds	2
None	1

Best motor response

Obeys commands	6
Localize pain	5
Flexion (withdrawal)	4
Flexion (abnormal)	3
Extension	2
None	1
Total	**3 to 15**

Table 12-4. Four Score Scale

Eye response

4. Eyelids open or opened; tracking or blinking to command
3. Eyelids open but not tracking
2. Eyelids closed but open to loud voice
1. Eyelids closed but open to pain
0. Eyelids remain closed with pain

Motor response

4. Thumbs up, fist or peace sign to command
3. Localizes to pain
2. Flexion response to pain
1. Extensor posturing
0. No response to pain or myoclonic status epilepticus

Brainstem reflexes

4. Pupil and corneal reflexes present
3. One pupil wide and fixed
2. Pupil or corneal reflexes absent
1. Both pupil and corneal reflexes absent
0. Absent pupil. Corneal, and cough reflex

Respiration

4. Not intubated; regular breathing pattern
3. Not intubated; Cheyne-Stokes breathing
2. Not intubated: irregular breathing pattern
1. Breathes above ventilator rate
0. Breathes at ventilator rate or apnea

Total 0 to 16

that bled. In patients with anterior communicating artery (AComA) aneurysms blood often pools in the subfrontal region at the base of the brain and extends into the frontal interhemispheric fissure and the pericallosal cistern.[41,47-49] Often there is an accompanying frontal lobe hematoma or a midline hematoma that extends through the lamina terminalis into the septum pellucidum. The bleeding often extends into the lateral ventricles.[41,47-49] A temporal-lobe hematoma or collection of blood in the sylvian fissure predominantly on one side suggests a MCA aneurysm. Figure 12-4 is a CT scan that shows blood in the subarachnoid space and basal cisterns with the major collection occurring in the left sylvian fissure region. This patient has a large ruptured left MCA aneurysm.

Blood localized mostly in the perimesencephalic and prepontine cisterns with little in the supratentorial regions suggests a perimesencephalic (pre-truncal) hemorrhage usually not caused by bleeding from an aneurysm.[50-53] The presence of subarachnoid blood localized to the convexity sulci and fissures on one side is also not indicative of aneurysmal bleeding but suggests an unusual cause such as dural sinus or venous occlusion, or focal arterial disease.[54,55]

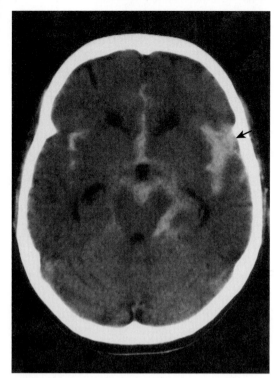

Figure 12-4. CT scan showing blood in the subarachnoid space and basal cisterns. The most blood is pooled in the left sylvian fissure *(small black arrow)*. This patient had an aneurysm of the left MCA that is shown in Figure 12-7b.

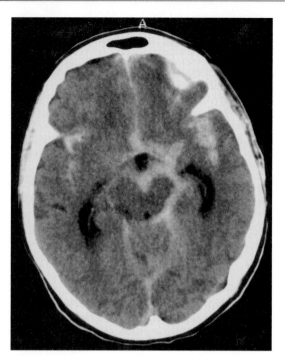

Figure 12-5. CT scan showing blood in the subarachnoid space, predominantly in the basal cisterns. There is more blood on the left side.

Large aneurysms (>10 mm) are occasionally also shown. In a contrast-infused CT scan, aneurysms appear as small, round densities on arteries located along the circle of Willis. Giant aneurysms can also be shown as contrast-enhancing masses. The amount of blood helps predict the likelihood of subsequent vasoconstriction.[56-59] CT may show a dilated ventricular system with hydrocephalus caused by disturbance of cerebrospinal fluid (CSF) dynamics by blood clogging the basal cisterns and pacchionian granulations.

A normal CT scan does not exclude SAH; a normal scan occurs if the hemorrhage is small, especially if the scan is delayed 24 to 72 hours.[33,60] Computed tomography angiography (CTA) can most often image intracranial aneurysms on the arteries of the circle of Willis.[61-63] In PN, SAH was confirmed by CT (Fig. 12-5); the amount of blood was moderate and most of the blood was located in the basal cisterns, with more on the left side.

Magnetic Resonance Imaging

MRI is probably less sensitive than CT in showing acute subarachnoid blood. Vascular malformations, especially cavernous angiomas, however,

are seen clearly on MRI as well-circumscribed structures with heterogeneous signals. Magnetic resonance angiography (MRA) is proving quite accurate in imaging aneurysms and showing the relationship of the aneurysm to adjacent brain structures. In one series, aneurysms as small as 3 to 4 mm were usually reliably detected by MRA, but some lesions (3 among 21 aneurysms) were missed.[64] Some arteries and aneurysms were not well imaged, and details were often insufficient for surgeons to define the neck and the extent of the aneurysms. Others have shown an acceptable aneurysm detection rate for MRA especially when contrast enhancement is performed.[65,66] At present, CTA and MRA are best used as screening tests for asymptomatic aneurysms in patients with a familial history of aneurysms or known risk factors such as polycystic kidney disease and fibromuscular arterial dysplasia. These techniques reliably show large aneurysms. They often do not show sufficient detail to guide surgical or interventional management of aneurysms that are shown.

Lumbar Puncture

I advocate LP as a very important diagnostic step, especially if CT is normal and clinical suspicion of SAH is still present.[33,67,68] The usual spinal fluid findings are noted in Table 12-5.

Table 12-5.	**Common Spinal Fluid Findings in Patients with Subarachnoid Hemorrhage**

1. Large numbers of red blood cells, without clearing of cells, between the first and last tubes
2. A faint pink color of supernatant fluid if examined within 4 to 5 hours of hemorrhage
3. A deep yellow (xanthochromic) color of the centrifuged supernatant fluid, secondary to breakdown of heme pigments; hemoglobin is first formed and is later transformed to bilirubin
4. Elevated protein
5. Pleocytosis, usually mononuclear
6. Increased pressure
7. Normal glucose

The opening and closing pressures should be measured and noted. Some advocate waiting at least 6 and preferably 12 hours after headache onset to perform a lumbar puncture.[69] The rationale is that it takes that long for bilirubin to form and color the fluid yellow. Spinal fluid obtained after 72 hours may show only an elevated pressure, xanthochromia, and increased protein content. Spectrophotometry, by quantifying the amounts of hemoglobin and bilirubin, provides information regarding the approximate age of the hemorrhage.[67,70] However, spectrophotometric analysis of CSF shows only moderate specificity for the demonstration of subarachnoid hemorrhage.[71]

Controversy exists as to the advisability of LP in confirmed SAH. Some argue that sudden lowering of pressure may provoke bleeding. I advocate LP, even in CT-confirmed SAH. The initial LP gives a baseline pressure and quantification of the number of red blood cells. This information may be useful later if the patient deteriorates and a second hemorrhage is suspected. The level of CSF pressure is an important parameter to follow. Spinal tap also helps remove blood and CSF. Also, by lowering CSF pressure, spinal tap often relieves headache. Subsequent LPs help document the pressure and blood contents. Surgical complications are more common when the CSF pressure is greater than 180 mm Hg at the time of surgical treatment of aneurysms.

Digital Subtraction Cerebral Angiography

PN gradually became more alert and her headache waned. By the third hospital day (5 days after onset of SAH), the plantar responses were

flexor. Angiography showed an 8-mm by 12-mm large irregular aneurysm at the junction of the left ICA and PComA (Fig. 12-6). No important focal or generalized vascular narrowing existed. On the next day, repeat LP showed an opening pressure of 160 mm Hg and no fresh blood. Surgical clipping of the aneurysm was accomplished on the following day.

Cerebral angiography remains the definitive method of showing intracranial aneurysms. Arterial digital subtraction angiography is the preferred technique, allowing excellent arterial opacification and rapid filming with less dye. The increased use of interventional management of aneurysms has changed the approach to the timing of angiography. Since interventions are often performed emergently soon after SAH, early and definitive imaging of aneurysms and other etiologies is important in guiding treatment decisions and should be performed as soon as possible. Figure 12-7 shows angiograms of aneurysms at the most common sites.

Because aneurysms may be multiple, all four intracranial arteries should be studied, with anteroposterior, lateral, and oblique views if needed. Table 12-6 lists observations concerning identification of the aneurysm that most likely bled multiple aneurysms are identified. At times, despite well-documented SAH, no aneurysm is identified angiographically. In general, the prognosis of these patients is better than when an aneurysm is shown, but the etiologies of such bleeds are diverse.[72,73]

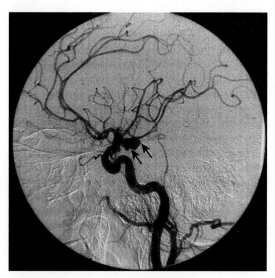

Figure 12-6. Large left PComA aneurysm *(small black arrows)*, 8 × 12 mm in size. (Courtesy of Galen Henderson, MD, and Rafael Linas, MD.)

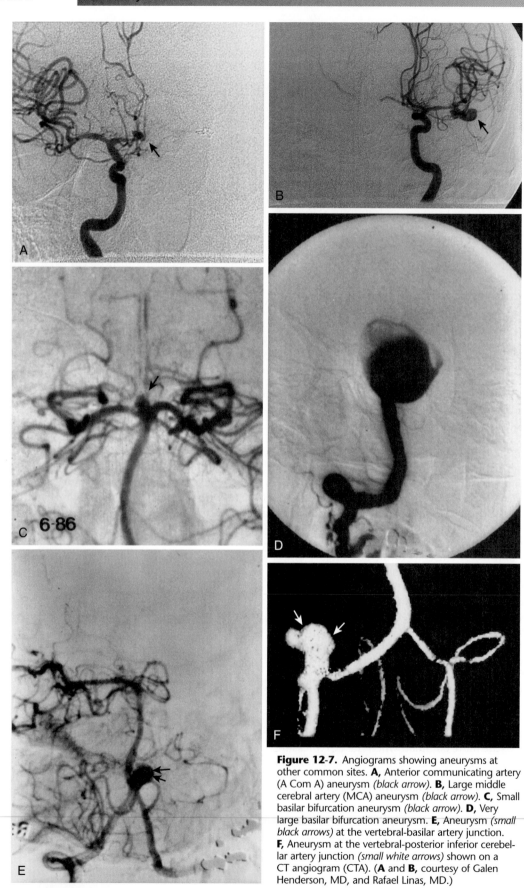

Figure 12-7. Angiograms showing aneurysms at other common sites. **A,** Anterior communicating artery (A Com A) aneurysm *(black arrow)*. **B,** Large middle cerebral artery (MCA) aneurysm *(black arrow)*. **C,** Small basilar bifurcation aneurysm *(black arrow)*. **D,** Very large basilar bifurcation aneurysm. **E,** Aneurysm *(small black arrows)* at the vertebral-basilar artery junction. **F,** Aneurysm at the vertebral-posterior inferior cerebellar artery junction *(small white arrows)* shown on a CT angiogram (CTA). (**A** and **B,** courtesy of Galen Henderson, MD, and Rafael Linas, MD.)

Table 12-6.	Identifying Aneurysm That Most Likely Bled When Multiple Aneurysms Are Present

1. Largest aneurysm
2. Most irregularly shaped aneurysm
3. Aneurysm with the most associated focal spasm,
4. Aneurysm in the vascular territory, explaining the focal signs
5. Aneurysm that best correlates with the collection of blood on computed tomography

Other Diagnostic Techniques

Transcranial Doppler (TCD) is a useful technology for detecting AVMs[74-77] and monitoring the intracranial circulation for vasoconstriction.[74,78-81] Serial TCD measurements of flow velocities in the basal arteries after moderate- and large-volume SAHs often show an increase in velocities during days 3 to 10 and maximum velocities between days 11 and 20. Time-averaged maximum velocities in the MCA greater than 140 cm per second accurately predict vascular narrowing at angiography. Velocities greater than 200 cm per second predict severe vasoconstriction.[74,79] Doppler-measured velocities in the MCA have an inverse relationship to vascular diameter.

Single-photon emission computed tomography (SPECT) is also a useful test for monitoring the presence of vasoconstriction because of its ability to show regions of decreased cerebral blood flow. Regional hypoperfusion correlates well with vasoconstriction and delayed brain infarcts in patients with SAH.[81,82] Xenon-enhanced CT scanning can also show and quantify regional blood flows.[83,84] Diffusion and perfusion MR scanning has the added capability of showing zones of infarction as well as underperfused regions.[85,86] These techniques and CT perfusion scanning are all potentially effective in monitoring SAH patients.

Differential Diagnosis

Van Gijn and colleagues noted that a high proportion of patients with SAHs located predominantly in the perimesencephalic cisterns by CT had normal cerebral angiography.[50,51,72] Newer-generation CT scans and MRI have shown that these hemorrhages are often centered around the prepontine cistern. Because these hemorrhages are concentrated around the brainstem, Schievink, Wijdicks, and colleagues suggest that they be called pretruncal subarachnoid hemorrhages (truncus cerebri is another term for the brainstem), rather than perimesencephalic hemorrhages.[52,87] The clinical course in patients with pretruncal hemorrhage is different from aneurysmal SAH because few patients die, rebleed acutely, or develop delayed cerebral infarction or hydrocephalus.[52,88] The outcome is much more benign than in patients with aneurysms shown by angiography. The etiology of these hemorrhages around the brainstem is unknown, but a venous or capillary leak is often posited. In one patient with a pretruncal hemorrhage, a capillary telangiectasia was shown in the ventral pons by MRI.[89] Because SAH resulting from rupture of a posterior circulation aneurysm can also cause bleeding centered around the brainstem, an angiogram is always warranted in such patients. If the initial angiogram is technically adequate and negative, however, a repeat angiogram has a low yield of showing an aneurysm.

Patients with SAH and normal angiography have a variety of different etiologies.[72] I have seen a number of patients who had hemorrhage into the caudate nucleus with extension into the ventricular system, which simulates SAH clinically but CT or MRI would show the caudate and intraventricular blood.[90] AVMs may also involve the subependymal region and may bleed directly into the ventricles and CSF. Before the era of CT scans, these intraventricular hemorrhages and other brain hemorrhages may have accounted for some examples of SAH with normal arteriography. Cerebral amyloid angiopathy is an important, oft-neglected cause of bleeding into the subarachnoid space. Amyloid laden arteries are common along the pial surface of the brain. The differential diagnosis of subarachnoid blood is listed in Table 12-7.

The possibility of an erroneous diagnosis of SAH should also be considered. Other conditions, such as tumor, infection, or traumatic LP, can mimic SAH. If the clinical picture is characterized by back pain, radicular signs, or myelopathic signs, I order a spinal MRI and perform studies seeking a spinal aneurysm, AVM, or spinal dural fistula (see Chapter 15). In situations in which vasoconstriction is prominent but no aneurysm is seen, I repeat angiography to better visualize the intracranial arteries after the clinical state improves.

Complications of Aneurysmal Subarachnoid Hemorrhage and Their Management

Management of patients with SAH is one of the most difficult problems in clinical medicine. The complications are myriad and management trends change almost yearly. Table 12-8 lists common complications of SAH during the acute

Table 12-7.   Entities to Be Considered in Differential Diagnosis of Subarachnoid Hemorrhage When No Aneurysm Has Been Found

1. Subarachnoid hemorrhage secondary to occult trauma
2. Blood dyscrasias and sickle cell disease
3. Nonvisualized arteriovenous malformations or an unseen small aneurysm
4. Thrombosis of a ruptured aneurysm
5. Leakage from a small nonaneurysmal artery on the brain surface[91]
6. Dural arteriovenous malformations[72,92]
7. Spinal arteriovenous malformations
8. Cerebral venous and dural sinus occlusions[93,94]
9. Intracranial arterial dissections
10. Cerebral amyloid angiopathy[95]
11. Cocaine abuse
12. Pituitary apoplexy
13. Vasculitis (especially polyarteritis nodosa and Wegener's granulomatosis[96,97])

and later periods. For ease of recall, I think of the "nine H's."

Rebleeding

The most feared complication in patients with SAH is recurrent aneurysmal rupture. The initial bleed and rehemorrhage are major causes of death in patients with aneurysmal SAH. In one study that had a 45% (36/80) mortality, 64% (23/36) of deaths were attributable to the initial SAH and eight of the remaining 13 deaths were caused by recurrent hemorrhages.[98] The mortality rate in patients who rebled has been cited as about 50%.[99,100]

Table 12-8.   Complications of Subarachnoid Hemorrhage (Nine H's)

Early
  Hypertension (intracranial)
  Hypertension (systemic)
  Heart failure and arrhythmia
  Hematoma
Delayed
  Hemorrhage (rebleed)
  Hypoperfusion (vasospasm)
  Hydrocephalus
  Hypovolemia
  Hyponatremia

Rebleeding is heralded by sudden, abrupt, severe headache. Rebleeds tend to be both intraparenchymal and subarachnoid. The frequency of bleeding into the brain is higher than in the original aneurysm rupture. Signs include meningismus, focal neurologic abnormalities associated with intraparenchymal hemorrhage, and often rapid development of coma. Among aneurysms that rebled, approximately 20% do so in the first 2 weeks, 30% by the end of the first month, and 40% by the end of 6 months. Beyond 6 months, rerupture occurs at a rate of approximately 3% per year.[6,10] No infallible rules predict which patients will have recurrent hemorrhages.

Efforts are directed to reduce those factors that may promote rebleeding. Patients are placed at bed rest with minimal stimuli. Pain is controlled with analgesics. Sedatives are used. Patients are kept from straining at stool by regular use of laxatives and stool softeners. These measures are attempts to avoid elevations in blood pressure, which could increase intra-aneurysmal pressure and increase the risk of rebleeding. Blood pressure is monitored and medications are used to lower pressures when they are in the greater than 160/100 range. When feasible, early obliteration of the aneurysm by surgery or intravascular interventional measures is the best way to prevent a second bleed.

Delayed Cerebral Ischemia (Vasoconstriction)

Second only to rebleeding as a cause of significant morbidity and mortality is vasoconstriction. Vasoconstriction is defined as abnormal narrowing of intracranial arteries. The narrowing of intracranial arteries found in patients with SAH has customarily been called *vasospasm*. Purists argue that vasoconstriction is a more accurate designation because it is a structural term that does not imply duration or mechanism, whereas spasm usually refers to functional reversible changes. The narrowing of arteries often persists, and chronic morphologic changes develop in both experimental animals[101] and humans[102,103] with SAH. Therefore, vasospasm is an inaccurate designation.

The pathogenesis of vasoconstriction is not fully clarified but is probably related to the release of substances into the CSF from the subarachnoid blood and the interaction of these substances within the arteries in the subarachnoid space. Erythrocytes and their subsequent hemolysis are necessary for vasospasm to develop.[104,105] The most likely putative substance is oxyhemoglobin, which affects the function of platelet-derived growth factor, released from platelets adherent to the arterial wall; endothelial factors, especially endothelial-derived relaxing factor, and components of the coagulation cascade, especially thrombin, plasmin, and fibrinogen.[105] An abnormal contraction or failure of relaxation of the arterial smooth muscle occurs.

Patients who die from SAH with vasoconstriction less than 3 weeks after the initial hemorrhage show necrosis of the media, whereas patients who live longer than 3 weeks show marked concentric intimal thickening, subendothelial fibrosis, and medial atrophy.[105-109] The adventitia shows adherent clot with inflammatory cell infiltrates and degeneration of perivascular nerve terminals.[105] The media shows smooth muscle contraction with varying degrees of fibrosis and necrosis. The intima develops longitudinal furrows and endothelial cells often desquamate, necrose, and have abnormalities of intercellular tight junctions.[105]

SAH probably induces vasoconstriction that is then followed by arterial wall necrosis. Vasoconstriction usually has its onset 3 to 5 days after the hemorrhage. The peak timing for vasoconstriction is 5 to 9 days. Most vasospasm resolves after the second week.[105,110-112] Vasoconstriction also occurs postoperatively, probably because of the handling of arteries and, at times, is caused by intraoperative bleeding. Vasoconstriction has been detected arteriographically in 30% to 70% of SAH patients.[113] Approximately two thirds of patients undergoing angiography during the second week after SAH show vasoconstriction.[105] Angiographic diagnosis is based on the narrowed appearance of the intracranial arteries. Severe vasoconstriction is associated with a lumen smaller than 0.5 μm with delayed forward flow and evidence of collateral artery blood flow from anastomotic circulation. Some arteries are diffusely narrowed, whereas others show focal constrictions. CTA and MRA have also been used to show vasoconstriction and accompanying brain infarction. Among patients with subarachnoid hemorrhage, CTA and digital subtraction angiography have a very high correlation. The absence of vasoconstriction on CTA has a negative predictive value of 95%.[113a] Decreased blood flow as imaged by CT perfusion studies is also helpful in predicting the development of brain infarction.[113b] Increased blood-flow velocities detected by TCD correlate well with angiographically documented vasoconstriction.[74,77,114] Only approximately one half of the patients with arteriographically demonstrable vasoconstriction are symptomatic.

Early signs of vasoconstriction include tachycardia, hypertension, electroencephalographic (EEG) abnormalities, and decreased level of consciousness.[115] Some patients, especially those with diffuse vasoconstriction, develop signs of diffuse brain dysfunction, including headache, stupor, and confusion. Focal neurologic signs often accompany these global signs and depend on the artery involved. Often, the most severe vasoconstriction is in the artery harboring the aneurysm or lying within the surrounding blood clot. Occasionally, maximal vasoconstriction occurs at a distance from the aneurysm. Patients with MCA vasoconstriction develop hemiparesis, hemisensory loss, aphasia, anosognosia, and confusion. With ACA vasoconstriction, there may be weakness in one or both lower extremities, abulia, and apraxia. PCA-territory ischemia causes hemianopia and hemisensory loss. CT scans and MRI protocols of the brain provide confirmatory data, ruling out intraparenchymal hemorrhage and hydrocephalus as a cause of the delayed deterioration. Focal hypodensity representing infarction is often seen. SPECT, xenon-enhanced CT scans, CT perfusion studies, and perfusion MRI may provide images of regions of decreased perfusion of brain supplied by the constricted arteries. There is likely to be genetic variability in the development of vasoconstriction and of delayed brain ischemia. A meta-analysis showed that patients with an E4 allele in the APOE genotype have a higher risk of delayed ischemia and poor outcome after subarachnoid hemorrhage.[115a]

The clinical, laboratory and neuroimaging findings that correlate with the development of significant vasoconstriction are noted in Table 12-9. The ideal treatment of vasoconstriction is prevention. Prevention has taken various directions, including early surgery, volume expansion, clot removal or lysis, and prophylactic drug regimens.[105] Blood can be washed from the subarachnoid space during early surgery, and some authors report a low incidence of symptomatic vasospasm in those patients in whom postoperative CT scans showed removal of blood.[116,117] Another approach has

Table 12-9.	**Findings That Correlate with Development of Cerebral Vasoconstriction after Subarachnoid Hemorrhage**

1. Thick blood clots localized in subarachnoid cisterns and amount of subarachnoid blood[5,56-60]
2. Arterial lumen size smaller than 0.5 mm, with low distal perfusion
3. Aneurysms located on circle of Willis
4. Decreased level of consciousness[58,114]
5. Intraventricular blood[58]
6. Elevated levels of brain natriuretic peptide[115]

been to use urokinase or tissue plasminogen-activator to lyse CSF clots after aneurysm clipping.[118-119] Placement of nicardipine prolonged-release implants within the basal cisterns in contact with the exposed blood vessels among 32 SAH patients decreased angiographic vasospasm (73% in control patients and 7% in those with implants) and delayed cerebral ischemia (47% controls vs 14% of those with implants) in one randomized, double-blind study.[120]

During the past decade, the most effective and established treatment used in patients with vaso-constriction is the use of "triple-H therapy," which consists of hypervolemia, hypertension (often induced pharmacologically), and hemodilution, usually accomplished by volume expansion with colloids or crystalloids without concomitant blood transfusions.[121-123] Elevation of arterial pressure pharmacologically is only advisable after aneurysms are clipped or when patients are hypotensive. Volume expansion, induced hypervolemia, hypertension, and hemodilution have no known effects on the vascular narrowing but help maintain CBF above ischemic thresholds by increasing cardiac output and improving blood rheology.[121-125] Aggressive volume expansion requires intensive care, and substantial risk of complications exists.[105] Many neurologists and neurosurgeons advocate avoidance of hypotension, hyponatremia, hypovolemia, and administration of at least 3 liters of fluid a day rather than aggressive volume expansion.[105] When this therapy fails to reverse the clinical syndrome, endovascular angioplasty (mechanical dilatation of the arteries in spasm by balloons) and/or intra-arterial infusions of vasodilators such as calcium channel blockers or papaverine have now been established as very effective treatments.[5,69,100]

The results of preliminary British[126] and American[127] trials reported during the early 1980s suggested that nimodipine, a calcium channel blocker, might decrease the incidence and severity of vasoconstriction and could improve outcome. Potential mechanisms of action of nimodipine, nicardipine, and other calcium channel blockers include a decrease in vasoconstriction, improved blood flow by dilation of collateral arteries, neuronal protection by decreasing entry of calcium into cells, and improvement of blood rheology.[105] A number of trials have shown that nimodipine does improve outcome and decreases the frequency of delayed cerebral infarction. A systematic review of 10 trials (including 2756 patients) of calcium channel blockers in patients with SAH reported a 33% relative risk reduction in the frequency of ischemic neurologic deficits and a 20% relative risk reduction in the development of infarcts on CT scans.[128] The relative risk

reduction of poor outcome (death or dependence) was 16% and 10% for death alone.[128] Administration of nimodipine, nicardipine, and other calcium channel-blocking agents can cause decreased blood pressure and renal function, especially when the drugs are given intravenously, so that blood pressure, urinary output, and renal function must be carefully monitored. Nimodipine is the drug of choice and is given 15 to 30 g/kg per hour intravenously or 30 to 90 mg enterally every 4 hours. More experience is needed concerning implantation of calcium-channel drugs into the CSF in sustained-release forms. Recently milrinone, a phosphodiesterase inhibitor, was shown in a preliminary study to be a potentially safe and effective treatment for cerebral vasoconstriction after SAH.[128a]

Since 1989, patients with vasoconstriction shown angiographically who have accompanying neurologic symptoms and/or signs, have been treated by interventional radiologists with transluminal angioplasty using various catheter devices.[129-132] The technology is still evolving and changes frequently. Intra-arterial papaverine (a vasodilator) or a calcium-channel blocker is often used as an adjunct to angioplasty.

It seems prudent to prevent hypovolemia by liberal use of fluids orally and intravenously in patients with SAH. Nimodipine is given intravenously or enterally for the first 10 days. In those with vasoconstriction shown angiographically, volume expansion and maintenance of blood pressure should be pursued. This is best supervised in an intensive care unit, and, usually, measurement of pulmonary wedge pressures are needed during aggressive volume expansion. ICP monitoring is also often helpful in following the effects of osmotic diuretics, steroids, and fluid removal on ICP and CBF. TCD is used to monitor blood-flow velocities in the basal arteries and hemispheric blood flow. Diffusion- and perfusion-weighted MRI is also helpful in detecting and quantifying vasoconstriction-related regions of hypoperfusion. Small, often multiple regions of ischemia shown by diffusion-weighted imaging are surrounded by larger regions of decreased perfusion.[86] Angioplasty performed by a trained and experienced interventionist is used when available in patients with symptomatic vasospasm who have not responded to medical therapy. Surgery or intra-arterial aneurysm ablation should be performed as early as possible when patients are in good condition.[5,119,133]

Hydrocephalus

In addition to rebleeding and vasospasm, other complications can lead to deterioration of patients with ruptured aneurysms. Acute hydrocephalus is caused by alteration in normal CSF dynamics. CSF flow is blocked by blood in the cisterns around the brainstem and reabsorption is impaired when blood attaches to the pacchionian granulations. The syndrome can be recognized by increasing headache, lethargy, incontinence, and decreased spontaneity. Diagnosis is readily confirmed by noncontrast CT scans. In a large study of the timing of aneurysm surgery, the authors analyzed factors that predicted hydrocephalus among 3521 patients with SAH admitted within 3 days of bleeding.[134] The factors that increased the likelihood of hydrocephalus were older age, hypertension (by history, admission blood pressure, and postoperative measures), thick local or diffuse blood on CT, intraventricular hemorrhage, use of antifibrinolytic drugs, and reduced level of consciousness.[134] Often, repeat LPs are adequate to treat ventricular enlargement, which often becomes obvious early after SAH. A few patients will need ventricular drainage using a catheter inserted into a lateral ventricle. In the months to years that follow SAH, normal-pressure hydrocephalus may develop as the arachnoid becomes fibrotic and adhesions prevent normal CSF flow.

Cardiac and Pulmonary Abnormalities

Cardiopulmonary complications occur often in patients with SAH. Careful surveillance for arrhythmias, heart failure, and myocardial infarction is required. I monitor cardiac rhythm, obtain baseline and follow-up electrocardiograms (ECGs) and cardiac enzymes, and carefully watch for clinical signs of congestive heart failure. SAHs can be accompanied by ECG abnormalities,[135-138] enzyme elevations mimicking myocardial infarction,[138,139] regional left ventricular wall motion abnormalities,[139a] and arrhythmias.[138,140-143] The most striking ECG changes are so-called waterfall T waves, which are seen across the endocardium. ECG abnormalities include alterations in QRS configuration, Q-T interval prolongation, T-wave abnormalities, and S-T segment elevation or depression.[135-138]

Subendocardial hemorrhages and myofibrillary degeneration have been noted at necropsy in patients dying after SAH and other strokes.[137,144,145] Left ventricular wall motion abnormalities are also common, especially in patients with large SAHs.[145a] The pathologic abnormalities of cardiac muscle cells has usually been referred to as myocytolysis. Striations within myocardial muscle cells are lost, and the cytoplasm often becomes hyalinized. Measurements show that some enzymes are lost from the muscle cells. The number of muscle cells decrease, but the sarcolemma, stroma, and nuclei usually remain. Lipofuchsin is found within myofibrils. Often, there is a coagulative type of myocytolysis in which cardiac muscle cells die in a hypercontracted state with early myofibrillar damage and anomalous irregular cross-band formation.[137] This type of pathologic change has also been called myofibrillar degeneration and contraction band necrosis. Early calcium entry with calcifications are seen in regions of myocytolysis.[137,144,145]

Elevated circulating serum catecholamines or sympathetic discharges that originate from the hypothalamus and affect the myocardium may be responsible for these myocardial cell abnormalities.[137,144] Cardiac lesions probably represent excitotoxin-induced injury. Although ECG changes are common, myocardial infarction is rare.

Cardiac abnormalities are occasionally accompanied by clinical and necropsy evidence of pulmonary edema.[137,146,147] In one series of 178 fatal SAHs, 71% had necropsy evidence of pulmonary edema, recognized clinically in only 31%.[147] Pulmonary edema is neurogenic in origin. It is characterized by rapid onset, high protein in the edema fluid, and acutely elevated ICP. Weir suggested that pulmonary edema is caused by an acute rise in ICP, which triggers a massive autonomic discharge that results in increased cerebral perfusion and accumulation of fluid within the lungs and hypoxemia.[147] Treatment is directed at lowering ICP and eliminating excess fluid. Intubation, controlled ventilation, positive end-expiratory pressure, osmotic and loop diuretics, and drainage of spinal fluid may be needed.

Fluid, Electrolyte, and Endocrine Abnormalities

Less common, but still an important cause of neurologic worsening, are fluid and electrolyte abnormalities.[148,149] Slight sodium and potassium shifts without clinical consequence occurred among 25% in one series of aneurysm patients.[148] Sodium levels were in the range of 130 to 135 mEq/L. Potassium levels were in the range of 4.5-5 mEq/L. In another 14% of patients, more severe abnormalities included five patients with diabetes insipidus, two abnormalities of thirst regulation, one instance of inappropriate secretion of antidiuretic hormone, and nine patients with serious sodium and potassium shifts.[148] In these patients, the serum sodium was less than 130 mEq/L and the potassium was greater than 5 mEq/L. Hyponatremia is associated with a poor prognosis. Hydrocortisone given intravenously after surgery at a rate of 1200 mg/day overcomes excess naturesis and prevents hyponatremia.[149a] Water and electrolyte disturbances are most frequent with aneurysms of the AComA.

In postmortem studies, severe fluid and electrolyte abnormalities are associated with hemorrhage or ischemic changes in the hypothalamus.[149] In the past, hyponatremia has been attributed to inappropriate secretion of antidiuretic hormone, but in 1991, it was shown that the plasma concentration of atrial natriuretic factor is elevated and higher in patients with suprasellar and intraventricular blood.[115,150,151]

Neuroendocrine dysfunction can also follow SAH.[151a] In one study among 21 patients screened, 9 (43%) had deficiency of at least one pituitary axis hormone.[152] In another analysis of pituitary function, 14 of 30 (47%) of patients screened 12 to 24 months after aneurismal SAH had isolated or combined deficiencies of neuroendocrine hormones.[153] Growth hormone deficiency was most common followed by low adrenocorticotrophin (ACTH) values. Weight gain often accompanied the growth hormone abnormalities. Aneurysms of the AComA most often were followed by neuroendocrine dysfunction.[152,153] Hypoperfusion to the hypothalamic-pituitary blood supply is the posited mechanism that led to the endocrine abnormalities.

Peerless identified 30 additional, less common causes of neurologic deterioration after SAH, including enlargement of the aneurysm, seizures, pulmonary emboli, infection, medication side effects, renal failure, and hepatic failure.[154]

Other Treatment Considerations

Blood Pressure Control

Care must be taken in managing blood pressure. Elevated ICP causes an increase in venous pressure inside the cranium. To perfuse the brain, an arteriovenous pressure gradient must be maintained for systemic blood pressure to rise. Both too-high and too-low blood pressure can have adverse effects. Patients whose mean arterial pressure exceeds 130 mm Hg or is lower than 70 mm Hg have poorer outcomes than comparable patients with blood pressures between those two values.[155] If the blood pressure is not excessively high, I do not routinely lower it, especially if vasoconstriction is present. If the blood pressure is excessive (i.e., above 160/100 mm Hg), I do attempt to reduce it while carefully monitoring the patient's level of alertness and neurologic signs to ensure that hypoperfusion does not develop as the pressure is lowered. If blood pressure remains excessive, I prescribe hydrochlorothiazide, low doses of propranolol, labetalol, or angiotensin-converting enzyme inhibitors, such as captopril or enalapril, or sodium nitroprusside. Sodium nitroprusside has rapid and easily titratable effects.[156] Nimodipine and nicardipine

also lower blood pressure when used to treat or prophylax against vasoconstriction. No absolute levels of blood pressure to aim for exist; rather, the patient's clinical state should be observed to ensure that blood flow and cerebral perfusion are adequate.

Antifibrinolytic Agents

Antifibrinolytic agents have been used in patients with SAH to prevent rebleeding.[157,158] The most frequently used antifibrinolytic drug was aminocaproic acid (Amicar), which was usually given in a dose of 24 g per day intravenously for 3 days, followed by oral administration for 3 weeks or until surgery. Kassell and colleagues reviewed the experience of the Cooperative Study of Intracranial Aneurysms and Subarachnoid Hemorrhage with respect to antifibrinolytic drugs.[159] Although Amicar decreased the rate of rebleeding, it did not improve morbidity or mortality. Vasoconstriction, thrombophlebitis with pulmonary embolism, and hydrocephalus were more common in patients given antifibrinolytic agents.[159] Although they may be useful in selected patients with high potential for rebleeding, antifibrinolytic agents have too many adverse effects to be recommended for general use in patients with SAH.

Obliteration of Aneurysms by Surgery or Intra-Arterial Interventions

Obliteration of aneurysms is essential to prevent rebleeding. All agree that aneurysms should be ablated as soon as feasible after rupture. Debate, however, still surrounds the optimal means—surgical clipping or coiling through an intra-arterial approach.

During intracranial surgery, the patient is anesthetized using hypotensive anesthesia. The brain is made slack by using dehydrating agents and controlled removal of CSF, and the neurosurgeon uses a dissecting microscope to approach the aneurysm. Ideally, the aneurysm is clipped at its origin from the parent artery at its neck. If this is not possible, the aneurysm may be trapped between two clips and wrapped in supportive material, or the feeding arteries may be obliterated. During operations to obliterate aneurysms, rebleeding and ischemic infarction may occur. Infarction is secondary to arterial injury during retraction of the brain or from injury to penetrating arteries as aneurysms are approached and treated. Amnesic syndromes are common after surgery for AComA aneurysms, particularly if the aneurysms are trapped rather than ligated at their neck.[160,161] Trapping leads to disruption of the perforators that originate from the ACA and AComA, with resultant ischemia in the area of the anterior wall of the third ventricle and the orbital frontal lobes and basal forebrain nuclei.[160,161] Similar clinical deficits are often caused by vasoconstriction in patients with ruptured AComA aneurysms. Similarly, surgery on basilar artery bifurcation aneurysms can be followed by infarction in the paramedian midbrain and thalamus, causing a "top of the basilar syndrome."

Surgery sometimes was delayed until 10 to 14 days after the hemorrhage. This technically difficult surgery is easier to perform as the brain edema resolves and the clot and blood in the subarachnoid space are diminished. Rebleeding at the time of surgery is also minimized, because the clot in the aneurysm is better organized. Early surgery may afford a better outcome with regard to vasoconstriction. If a clot can be removed from the subarachnoid space at the time of surgery, vasoconstriction may be less likely to occur. If it does occur because the aneurysm has been clipped, more aggressive medical treatment can be given.

Although endovascular treatment of aneurysms has been known for more than 3 decades, it is only recently that the frequency of interventional intra-arterial treatment has equaled and even surpassed that of direct surgical management. Fedor Serbinenko, a Russian neurosurgeon was the first to popularize endovascular treatment of aneurysms. He used catheters with detachable latex balloons.[162] Guido Guglielmi and colleagues in 1991 reported their experience using a technique that involved electrolytic detachable platinum coils.[163,164] These coils (by custom named Guglielmi detachable coils [GDCs]) were introduced into aneurysms through a microcatheter and detached from a stainless-steel microguidewire by an electrical current.[163-165] The techniques of coil embolization have improved since then. By mid-2002, about 10,000 patients had had coiling used to obliterate aneurysms through an endovascular approach. About 1500 patients or more each month have endovascular treatment of their aneurysms.[165,166]

An international study, the International Subarachnoid Aneurysm Trial (ISAT) compared clipping versus coiling of aneurysms.[167,168] Patients were included in the study if they had a SAH due to a ruptured aneurysm that was considered suitable for both neurosurgical clipping and endovascular treatment. The study group consisted of 1070 patients randomized to the surgical group and 1063 to coiling. These patients were derived from an initial 9559 patients with aneurismal SAH, among whom 9% refused participation and 69% were excluded because their aneurysm was deemed unsuited to either coiling or surgery.[168] Among aneurysms randomized, 95% were in the anterior circulation and 90% were smaller than 10 μm. At one year after treatment, 30.9% of the neurosurgical group were dead or dependent versus 23.5% of the endovascular treated group.[167] Rebleeding was slightly more common in the endovascular treated patients (7 vs 2), and seizures were more frequent in the surgical group (44 vs 27 discharge to 1-year period).[167]

Of course treatment outcomes depend heavily on the experience and skill of the individual performing the endovascular or surgical procedure, as well as patient selection. For both surgery and endovascular occlusion, larger aneurysm size is associated with an increased rate of complications and of incomplete occlusion. The size of the neck of an aneurysm has been a predictor of complete occlusion by coiling. A neck diameter of less than 5 mm and a ratio of neck diameter to largest aneurysm dimension of less than 0.5 are associated with better outcomes after coiling.[165,169]

Intravascular stents are occasionally used to exclude aneurysms from the circulation and to ensure patency of parent arteries.[169a-d] When aneurysms have a wide neck, coils placed within an aneurysm can readily escape into the circulation. Neuroform stents and other stents designed to navigate tortuous intracranial vessels are now increasingly used in the treatment of wide necked aneurysms. A stent is placed within the parent artery on the luminal side covering the neck of the aneurysm. A microcatheter is introduced through the cells of the stent into the aneurysm. Coils are then inserted through the microcatheter into the aneurysm, after which the microcatheter is removed. The stent prevents the coils from prolapsing into the parent artery. Covered stents are being developed that will completely exclude aneurysms from the parent vessel and lead to thrombosis of the aneurysm. Figure 12-8 shows a large cavernous carotid artery aneurysm that was treated with stent assisted coiling.

Location of the aneurysm is also very important. MCA aneurysms are somewhat difficult to coil and surgical results in treating these aneurysms is better than at other loci.[165] Posterior circulation aneurysms have a relatively high surgical morbidity and mortality and are best treated with coiling when feasible.[165] Cavernous carotid artery aneurysms rarely cause SAH or severe neurologic morbidity,[170] are very difficult to treat surgically, and are best treated by coiling.

All other considerations being equal, there is a general consensus that if an aneurysm is suitable for endovascular treatment, this approach is preferred over craniotomy with neurosurgical management.

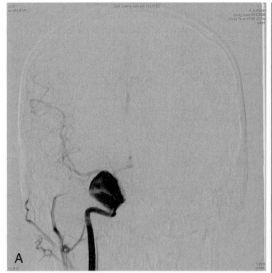

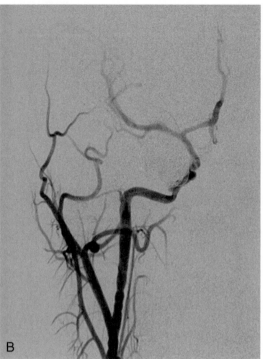

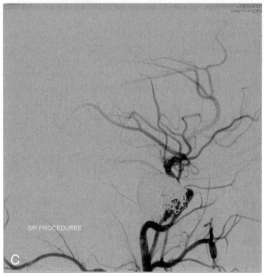

Figure 12-8. Carotid artery angiograms. **A,** Antero-posterior view showing a large petrous carotid artery aneurysm. Anteroposterior (**B**) and lateral (**C**) view after coiling. A catheter was first placed in the aneurysm. A stent was then deployed internal to the catheter. Coils were then introduced into the aneurysm through the catheter. After coiling, the stent was removed. The stent covered the large neck of the aneurysm preventing the coils from entering the parent artery. (Courtesy of Ajith Thomas, MD.)

Mycotic Aneurysms

Patients with bacterial endocarditis often develop cerebral aneurysms caused by bacterial emboliza-tion to the vasa vasorum of intracranial arteries. These so-called mycotic aneurysms usually do not develop in the basal arteries of the circle of Willis but favor branch arteries. Mycotic aneu-rysms are often multiple. Identical aneurysms develop in patients with cardiac myxomas.

These aneurysms may be identified after subarachnoid hemorrhage but many are found during evaluations for meningitis, embolic brain infarction, and encephalopathy in patients with infective endocarditis.[171] Some aneurysms iden-tified by angiography resolve after effective antibiotic treatment.[171,172] In one series, 20 of 28 mycotic aneurysms were followed angio-graphically.[171] Ten aneurysms became smaller or

disappeared, 10 were unchanged or enlarged—one with a fatal rupture. Seven mycotic aneu-rysms ruptured, resulting in two deaths and two with aphasia or cognitive impairment.[171] The authors suggested that single accessible aneu-rysms in medically stable patients be obliterated and that vascular imaging should be performed after medical treatment in patients in whom mycotic aneurysms had been shown earlier.[171]

Treatment of Unruptured Aneurysms

Management of patients with unruptured aneu-rysms presents a challenging problem in benefit versus risk analysis.[28,29,173] Unruptured aneu-rysms are discovered as part of the evaluation of another ruptured aneurysm, during investigation of a mass lesion, or during evaluation of another neurologic problem, such as ischemic vascular disease. Large aneurysms, symptoms, location within the posterior circulation, female sex, and age over 60 years increase the likelihood of aneurysm rupture.[173a]

Unruptured aneurysms that are not compressing neural structures have been estimated to bleed at a rate of 2% to 3% per year.[174] Aneurysms that cause neurologic symptoms rupture at a higher rate, with 15% bleeding within 6 months of onset of symptoms.[29] The operative mortality in patients with aneurysms and normal neurologic function is quite low (≤1.6%).[175] Mortality after endovascular coiling of neurologically intact patients is even lower. One series compared outcomes of coiling and clipping of unruptured aneurysms. Among 130 patients—68 treated surgically and 62 endovascularly—more treated surgically than by endovascular management had a change in Rankin scale of 2 or more (25% vs 8%).[173] Therefore, I recommend endovascular treatment or surgical therapy in selected patients with unruptured aneurysms.

The rate of aneurysm rupture is related to size. The International Study of Unruptured Intracranial Aneurysms showed that aneurysms of 10 mm or larger ruptured much more often than smaller aneurysms.[2] In other studies, the critical size for aneurysmal rupture has been 7 to 10 mm, 9 mm, and 8 mm.[27] Surgery on unruptured aneurysms has relatively high morbidity and mortality that are highly dependent on age. In a meta-analysis that included 2460 patients (in 61 studies), the mortality of surgery was 2.6%, and the permanent morbidity was 10.9%.[176] In a study of 1172 patients operated on for newly diagnosed unruptured intracranial aneurysms, the combined surgery-related morbidity and mortality at 1 year was 6.5% for patients younger than 45 years, 14.4% for those between 45 and 64 years, and 32% for those older than 64 years.[2] I concur with Kassell and Drake that the data support the idea that aneurysms 5 to 10 mm in size bleed more often than smaller lesions,[31] and aneurysms larger than 10 mm probably rupture at an even higher rate.[2] In good-risk young patients, aneurysms larger than 5 mm should most often be obliterated. An endovascular approach is preferred in posterior fossa aneurysms and in others that are suitable for coiling. Some unruptured aneurysms are likely more suitably treated surgically by neurosurgeons with extensive experience with aneurysm surgery. Lesions smaller than 5 mm should be followed up using vascular imaging. If these smaller aneurysms show growth, then endovascular or surgical therapy can be considered. CTA and MRA allow recognition and monitoring of unruptured aneurysms because patients can be studied noninvasively as outpatients. The decision with regard to surgery or interventional obliteration of unruptured aneurysms is complex, especially in older patients, and many factors must be carefully considered in each patient. Blood pressure control is important in patients with unruptured aneurysms.

Once a cerebral aneurysm has ruptured, the course is stormy, and the prognosis may be grim, even in the best of hands. To make a major impact on the morbidity and mortality of cerebral aneurysms, there must be early recognition of this serious disease, so that appropriate therapy can be undertaken while the patient is still in good condition. I stress the need for a high index of suspicion of SAH and a low threshold for use of LP and vascular imaging in suspected cases.

VASCULAR MALFORMATIONS

AVMs are the second most common cause of non-traumatic SAH. AVMs are one tenth as common as aneurysms. In 1980, it was estimated that about 1000 new cases were identified every year in the United States.[177] Others have estimated the AVM detection rate at 1.1[178] and 1.27[179] per 100,000 person-years. Cerebral aneurysms have a peak incidence of rupture beyond age 30 years: AVMs, however, rupture more commonly in the second and third decades of life.[180] Hemorrhage from an AVM is most often intraparenchymal and rarely just subarachnoid.

Classification and Distribution

Vascular malformations, often also called angiomas, usually arise from the failure of normal development of embryonic vascular networks. Some malformations, such as some arteriovenous fistulas, especially dural AVMs, and some cavernous angiomas are acquired during life. Because dural arteriovenous fistulas represent different clinical problems, they are discussed separately at the end of this chapter. McCormick wrote extensively about his experience with vascular malformations and classified them into five subtypes based on the predominant vasculature.[15,181-185]

Arteriovenous Malformations

AVMs contain arteries, arterialized veins, and veins. The size of the component vessels varies greatly, but the largest vessels are always venous. Sometimes the arterial supply is small and "cryptic." These lesions contain no recognizable normal capillary bed[184]; abnormal gliotic parenchyma usually is found between the component vessels. The small arteries within the malformation often have a deficient muscularis.[186] Thrombosis and inflammation are often found within AVMs. Arteriograms usually show shunting directly from the arteries to the venous components of the malformations. Figure 12-9 is a cartoon that illustrates the appearance of an unruptured AVM.

A subtype of AVMs dubbed "cerebral proliferative angiopathy" has recently been described.[186a] The distinctive feature of this condition is a large nidus made up of densely enhancing vascular spaces intermingled with normal parenchyma associated with a small volume of blood shunting to the venous drainage. These occur predominantly in young women who present with headaches, seizures, and ischemic symptoms and a low frequency of hemorrhage.[186a] Angiogenesis may be a prominent feature of these large lesions.

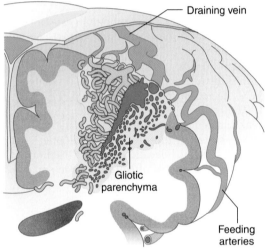

Figure 12-9. Cartoon illustration of an unruptured, parietal-lobe arteriovenous malformation.

Venous Angiomas

The most common type of vascular malformation found in the brain at necropsy is venous angiomas, which are composed of anomalous veins; there is no direct arterial input. These lesions are now most appropriately referred to as developmental venous anomalies (DVAs), rather than angiomas. They are composed of a group of anomalous veins usually separated by morphologically normal brain parenchyma. One or more large central draining veins are usually conspicuous and may be dilated into a varix or varices. The walls of the veins can become thick and hyalinized. These angiomas do not opacify during the arterial phase of cerebral angiography. Figure 12-10 illustrates a DVA. Figure 12-11 shows the lesion in a brain specimen, and Figure 12-12 is an MRI that shows a DVA.

Cavernous Angiomas

Cavernous angiomas consist of a relatively compact mass of sinusoidal vessels close together without intervening brain parenchyma. The lesions are well encapsulated, especially those that are superficial and large. Hyalinization and thickening of the component vessels, especially on the periphery of the angiomas, is common. These angiomas are not visualized well, if at all, on angiography because they have no direct arterial input. Cavernous malformations occur in a sporadic, nonhereditary form, in patients who tend to have a single isolated lesion, and in a familial form characterized by the presence of multiple lesions.[187-190] In the familial form, the number of lesions found increases with age. The familial

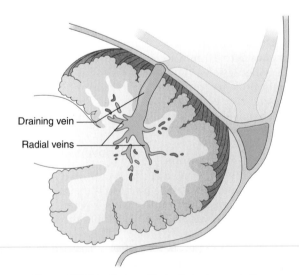

Figure 12-10. Cartoon illustration of a cerebellar developmental venous anomaly (venous angioma).

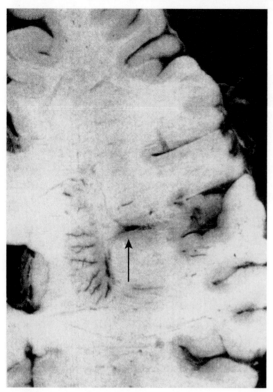

Figure 12-11. Brain specimen showing a venous malformation located mostly in the cerebral periventricular white matter. A radial array of dilated medullary veins drain into a dilated central vein *(arrow)*, which then drains toward the cerebral cortex. (From Johnson PC, Wachser TM, Golfinos J, Spetzler RF: Definition and pathologic features from Awad IA, Barrow DL (eds): Cavernous Malformations. Park Ridge, Ill: American Association of Neurological Surgeons, 1993, pp 1-11, with permission.)

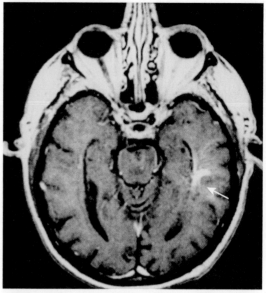

Figure 12-12. MRI showing a developmental venous anomaly located in temporal lobe. The *white arrow* points to an abnormal venous structure. (From Caplan LR: Subarachnoid hemorrhage, aneurysms, and vascular malformations. In Caplan LR: Posterior Circulation Disease: Clinical Findings, Diagnosis, and Management. Boston: Blackwell, 1996, pp 633-685, with permission.)

form has been noted to occur with greater frequency in Hispanics. Mutations in the Krev interaction trapped 1 (KRIT1) gene have been identified as underlying the familial form of cerebral cavernous malformations.[190,190a] The KRIT1 protein, the product of the KRIT-1 gene, is found in vascular endothelium, astrocytes, and pyramidal cells in adult brains.[190] Figure 12-13 shows a cartoon that illustrates the gross appearance of a cavernous angioma in the brain. Figures 12-14, 12-15, and 12-16 show cavernous angiomas in the temporal lobe, pons, and lateral ventricles.

Patients with DVAs have a much higher-than-expected co-occurrence of cavernous angiomas, especially in the posterior fossa.[190] These two congenital lesions often occur close together, so that these lesions probably share etiologic features during their development.[190-192] Cavernous angiomas are also known to develop after cranial irradiation.

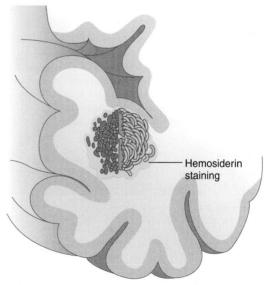

Hemosiderin staining

Figure 12-13. Cartoon illustration of an unruptured cavernous malformation. There is no smooth muscle or intervening brain parenchyma within the interstices of the thin-walled vascular channels. Surrounding hemosiderin indicates prior bleeding.

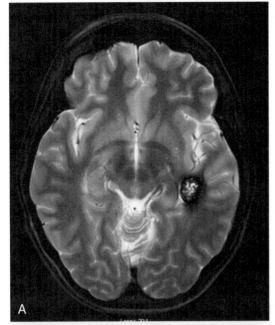

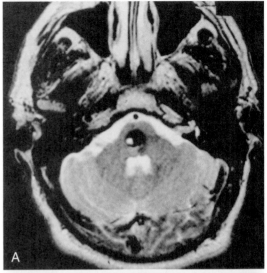

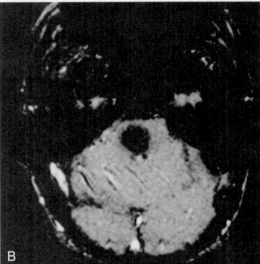

Figure 12-15. Cavernous angioma in the pons.
(**A**) T2-weighted axial section shows white eccentric density surrounded by a dark hemosiderin ring.
(**B**) Gradient-echo MRI section shows the hemosiderin ring around the lesion quite well. (From Caplan LR: Subarachnoid hemorrhage, aneurysms, and vascular malformations. In Caplan LR: Posterior Circulation Disease: Clinical Findings, Diagnosis, and Management. Boston: Blackwell, 1996, pp 633-685, with permission.)

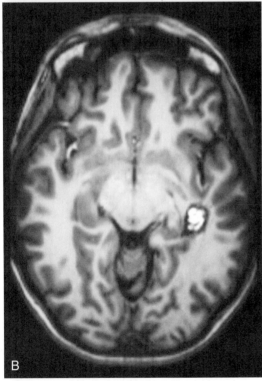

Figure 12-14. Temporal-lobe cavernous angioma shown in gradient echo (**A**) and T1-weigthed MRI (**B**) images. (Courtesy of Robert Hamill, MD.)

Telangiectases

Telangiectases (also called *telangiectasias*) are small lesions in which the component capillaries are separated from each other by normal brain parenchyma. They appear as small, pink, spongy

areas most often located in the pons. These lesions are not shown by angiography.

Pathogenesis of Arteriovenous Malformations

AVMs are composed of clusters of abnormal vessels comprised of arteries and veins of varying size. The arteries within the cluster are large, thin-walled vessels with poorly developed internal elastic lamina and media, whereas the

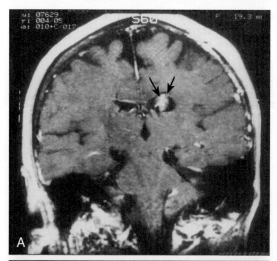

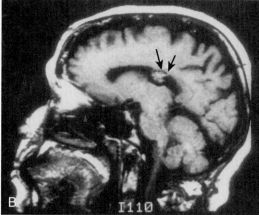

Figure 12-16. T2-weighted MRI images showing an intraventricular cavernoma. The lesion appears as a white hyperintensity *(small black arrows)* within the lateral ventricle.

arteries feeding this abnormality have hypertrophy of the media and endothelial thickening.[181] The hypertrophic media and endothelial thickening sometimes lead to thrombosis of feeding arteries. Deep AVMs are usually fed by penetrating arteries and drain into the deep venous system, whereas superficial cortical malformations usually drain into cortical veins.[186] In some patients, the afferent vessels of the malformation can become stenotic and even occluded.[193,194] Some patients with AVMs have more diffuse occlusive arterial disease, despite the fact that they do not have atherosclerotic risk factors.[194] Blood circulates rapidly through the central core of AVMs and is quickly shunted into large, dilatated, draining veins. The increased flow can promote the formation of aneurysms, and, occasionally, aneurysms are found associated with AVMs, especially along major feeding arteries.[195,196] The aneurysms and afferent vascular stenoses are related to altered

vascular hemodynamic factors involving the inflow channels. Occlusive changes can also be found in the draining venous channels and contribute to changes in pressures and flow within the malformations.[197,198]

Location of Malformations

Any part of the brain and spinal cord can harbor a vascular malformation. Cavernous angiomas and AVMs are often larger than the other types of malformations and more commonly cause symptoms. Telangiectases are usually asymptomatic but can be a source of repeated small bleeds. Some extensive malformations extend from the cortical surface to abut on the ventricular surface. Cavernous angiomas may be limited to the brain, spinal cord, subarachnoid space, or dura, or they may involve more than one of these regions. Table 12-10 shows the locations of cavernous

Table 12-10. **Distribution of Cavernous Angiomas**

Distribution	Number	Percent
Supratentorial	455	74
Lobar	256	41
Frontal lobe	99	
Temporal lobe	68	
Parietal lobe	72	
Occipital lobe	16	
Deep	31	5
Basal ganglia	22	
Thalamus	7	
Hypothalamus	2	
Ventricular	20	3
Lateral ventricles	13	
Paraventricular	2	
Third ventricle	5	
Extra-axial	4	0.5
Infratentorial	163	26
Cerebellum	28	4.5
Brainstem	82	13
Midbrain	20	
Pons	43	
Medulla	13	
Pontomedullary	6	
Fourth ventricle	3	0.5
Cerebellopontine angle	6	1
Spinal cord	2	0.3
Unspecified	58	9

Data from Caplan LR: Subarachnoid hemorrhage, aneurysms, and vascular malformations. In Caplan LR: Posterior Circulation Disease: Clinical Findings, Diagnosis, and Management. Boston: Blackwell Science, 1996, pp 633-685.

12

angiomas in one large series.[15,199] Bleeding from cavernous angiomas is predominantly into brain parenchyma, but angiomas that abut on the ventricular or meningeal surface may also leak into the CSF.

AVMs can be predominantly within brain parenchyma or within the subarachnoid space, but most AVMs have parenchymatous and subarachnoid components, so bleeding can be intracerebral, subarachnoid, or meningocerebral. Table 12-11 shows the location of AVMs in three large series of patients.[15,200-203] The blood supply of large AVMs is usually extensive, originating from the anterior and posterior intracranial circulations, as well as from extracranial components.

AVMs are believed to arise in early fetal life as a result of the failure of primitive vessels to differentiate into normal arteries, veins, and capillaries. Despite their congenital origin, AVMs rarely produce symptoms during the first decade of life. The asymptomatic nature of lesions in early life is probably related to their small size and the inherent plasticity of the developing brain, which allows the function of one area of the brain to be assumed by another. AVMs often enlarge as individuals age. The feeding arteries and draining veins grow, and additional vasculature is recruited. Malformations may enlarge for multiple reasons. Hook suggested that undifferentiated arteries and veins might not easily tolerate arterial pressure and therefore would enlarge.[204]

Small recurrent ICHs cause loss of brain substance as clot and necrotic brain are reabsorbed. The decrease in supporting tissue around malformations might allow growth of the vascular anomaly.[205] Decreased strength of supporting tissue may also be caused by pulsation of arteries, which can damage the surrounding brain.

Clinical Symptoms and Signs

As vascular malformations enlarge, symptoms are related to a number of mechanisms. Consider the following patient:

> At 15 years of age, AG began to have spells in which she saw sparkling lights off to her left. Some spells were followed by loss of consciousness and a generalized seizure. By age 21 years, she noted progressive loss of vision toward her left. Four years later during the first trimester of her first pregnancy while shopping, she fell to the ground with a severe headache, nausea, vomiting, and a stiff neck. Examination showed a left homonymous hemianopia.

The most frequent and dramatic presentation of vascular malformations is bleeding. Prior to modern brain imaging, intracerebral hemorrhage was the event that led to diagnosis of AVMs in about 50% of patients.[204] Currently about two thirds of AVMs are diagnosed before they have bled.[179] The immediate cause of bleeding in AVMs is not known, but probably relates to fragility of the abnormal vessels. Vessels on the cortical or ventricular surfaces are more prone to rupture, because they lack the support offered by the surrounding brain parenchyma. A first hemorrhage from an AVM usually occurs between the ages of 20 and 40 years of age.[205a]

Symptoms and signs depend on the location of the hemorrhage. With CSF extension of blood, there are signs of meningeal irritation similar to those accompanying aneurysmal rupture. Not all ruptures are symptomatic. Frequently, patients

Location of Arteriovenous Malformations	Perret and Nishioka[138] n (%)	Crawford et al[139] n (%)	Graf et al[140] n (%)
Frontal lobe	102 (23)	85 (21)	33 (25)
Temporal lobe	82 (18)	41 (10)	25 (19)
Parietal lobe	122 (27)	145 (36)	41 (30)
Occipital lobe	23 (5)	69 (17)	7 (5)
Brainstem	11 (2)		5 (4)
Cerebellum	21 (4)	36[a] (9)	6 (4.5)
Basal ganglia		27	14 (10)
Other	92 (20)		3 (2.5)
Total	453	403	134

Table 12-11.   Location of Arteriovenous Malformations Diagnosed during Life

[a]Brainstem and cerebellar lesions grouped together.

Data from Caplan LR: Subarachnoid hemorrhage, aneurysms, and vascular malformations. In Caplan LR (ed): Posterior Circulation Disease: Clinical Findings, Diagnosis, and Management. Boston: Blackwell Science, 1996, pp 633-685.

with no clinical history of hemorrhage show evidence of bleeding at surgery or necropsy. In one surgical series, 6 of 55 patients with AVMs had evidence of hemorrhage without recognized symptoms.[177]

In the years before the hemorrhage, AG had partial seizures with secondary generalization and progressive neurologic signs. Seizures are the presenting feature in 15% to 53% of AVM patients.[179,206] Most are grand mal but partial and partial complex seizures are also common. Supratentorial cavernous angiomas often present because of seizures.

Progressive neurologic symptoms occur in only about 8% to 11% of AVM patients.[179,207] In the past, progression has often been explained by "stealing" of blood away from normal tissue, but this mechanism has been difficult to establish. Venous hypertension and increased mass effect of the nidus of the AVM and occult bleedings are alternate explanations.[179,207]

Chronic headaches are also a frequent complaint in patients with AVMs. The headaches may be throbbing in nature, sometimes closely mimicking classic migraine. No good rules exist to distinguish ordinary migraine from migrainous headaches related to vascular malformations. Migraine-like accompaniments that are always stereotyped and occur on the same side or headaches always localized to the same side should lead doctors to suspect the possibility of an AVM. Even patients with unruptured AVMs can have increased ICP and papilledema.[208] The increased pressure may contribute to headaches.

In the brainstem, AVMs and cavernous angiomas may present with serious bleeding or gradually progressive neurologic deficits. Depending on location, there may be cranial nerve, cerebellar, pyramidal, or sensory dysfunction. Some have a fluctuating course of neurologic dysfunction, which may simulate multiple sclerosis.[15,190,209,210] Distinction between these two processes is now easily accomplished with modern brain imaging. With cavernous angiomas, the neurologic dysfunction can be localized to one site, most often in the pons. CT or MRI usually shows a typical cavernoma as the site of prior bleeding.

AVMs rarely present with hydrocephalus. In such cases, the mass of blood vessels can compress the ventricular system, disrupting the normal flow of CSF. Aneurysms of the vein of Galen are the most common cause of this rare presentation. Prior small bleeds can also block absorption of CSF, leading to hydrocephalus. Rarely, patients with large AVMs can present because of a bruit that is audible to the patient or doctor. In children, large AVMs can produce enough shunting of blood to cause high-output congestive heart failure.

In the spinal cord, vascular malformations typically present with back pain, myelopathic symptoms, and root dysfunction. These lesions are discussed in Chapter 15. Because headache so often accompanies spinal AVM rupture, cerebral sources of hemorrhage are often sought, and the spinal origin can be missed. In one series, 80% of patients with spinal malformations had intracranial symptoms, including headache, mental status changes, loss of consciousness, papilledema, decreased vision, nystagmus, diplopia, seizures, sixth nerve paresis, and oculomotor paresis.[211]

Diagnosis and Imaging Findings

The diagnosis of vascular malformations can often be suspected clinically. Common features are noted in Table 12-12.

Brain imaging in nearly all patients shows vascular malformations. MRI is able to define the lesions better than CT. Plain unenhanced CT scans can show serpiginous channels; these vessels are enhanced after intravenous contrast administration.[213] Brain atrophy and dilatation of ventricles adjacent to malformations may exist. Small calcifications may be seen within malformations. Sometimes, frank cysts are also found adjacent to AVMs.[214] If there has been a recent hemorrhage, these recent findings may be obscured by the intraparenchymal, subarachnoid, and intraventricular blood. Cavernomas are often missed on CT scans unless there has been recent bleeding. Developmental venous anomalies are seldom identifiable on CT scanning.

MRI has vastly improved the diagnosis of vascular malformations. AVMs usually appear as a region of honeycomb-like spaces with flow voids that contrast with the surrounding brain tissue on

Table 12-12.	**Common Presenting Features in Patients with Arteriovenous Malformations**

1. History of a seizure disorder or progressive neurologic deficit
2. Throbbing headaches or migraine-like auras, or both, always localized to one side of the cranium
3. A patient in the second or third decade of life
4. Subarachnoid hemorrhage in a pregnant woman. Arteriovenous malformations may enlarge or bleed during pregnancy
5. Clinical signs and symptoms of intraparenchymal and subarachnoid blood
6. Cranial bruit

T1-weighted and T2-weighted images. MRI gives useful information about the localization and topographic relationships between AVM vessels, nidus, and nervous structures, as well as showing past hemorrhage.[215-217] MRA gives some information about the arterial and venous components but is not as definitive as catheter angiography.

Cavernous angiomas usually appear as well-circumscribed, well-defined lesions, with a central core of mixed heterogeneous signal intensity surrounded by a rim of signal void.[190,218-221] Figures 12-14 and 12-15A and B are MRIs that show this appearance. The heterogeneous center is caused by blood and blood metabolites in various stages of evolution, and the dark rim is caused by hemosiderin.

The typical MRI appearance of DVAs is a linear or globular hypointense region on T1-weighted images and hypo- or hyper-intensity on T2-weighted images.[222-224] DVAs can usually be seen to join deep and/or superficial veins.[224] Figure 12-12 illustrates the MRI findings in a patient with a DVA. Recent hemorrhages in all types of malformations have the same imaging characteristics as other causes of ICH. MRI can also be helpful by showing hemosiderin resulting from old hemorrhage in the lesions and adjacent meninges.

TCD is also useful in the initial diagnosis and monitoring of AVMs.[74-78] The increased flow to the AVMs is associated with increased flow velocities in arteries feeding the malformations. At times, musical-type murmurs can be heard, and unusual unmodulated high- or middle-frequency bands are seen on the Doppler spectrum.[74] Abnormal collateralization and steal effects can be found with reduction of mean and peak flow velocities in some arteries.[74] Changes in velocities can be monitored during therapeutic embolization and after surgical or radiation therapy.[78] Vasomotor reactivity to CO_2 inhalation also gives information about AVMs. Relatively normal vasomotor reactivity in arteries ipsilateral to AVMs suggests a high-pressure AVM with a high risk of bleeding, whereas abnormal vasomotor reactivity in ipsilateral and contralateral arteries is most often found in low-pressure AVMs that show hemodynamically-induced neurologic signs.[225]

A detailed angiogram is needed to identify all possible arterial feeders when surgery is considered in patients. Angiographic features typical of AVMs include (1) large feeding arteries; (2) a central tangle of vessels; (3) enlarged, tortuous draining veins; and (4) rapid arterial-to-venous shunting of blood. Some angiographic findings, such as large size, presence of multiple feeding arteries, and drainage into peripheral cortical veins, correlate with the development of progressive neurologic signs that have been attributed by

some to stealing of blood from normal vessels to the malformations.[226] Arteriography is occasionally normal in patients in whom clinical suspicion of an AVM is high. The explanations for this are noted in Table 12-13.

Prognosis

Features that have been identified that seem to predict bleeding from a known AVM are noted in Table 12-14.[179,227-229] AVMs that have already bled have a higher risk of bleeding than those that have not as yet bled.[179] In the short term, the prognosis of ruptured AVMs is much better than that of aneurysms. The rebleeding rate is low—only about 6% during the first year[230]—and vasoconstriction occurs only rarely. Mortality from the first hemorrhage is relatively low (1.5% to 9%).[179] In the long term, however, the prognosis of AVMs is not as good. Estimates of recurrent hemorrhage during subsequent years vary from 1% in 4 to 7 years[205] to 2% per year after the first year.[230] With repeated hemorrhages, the morbidity and mortality rates increase.[226]

Table 12-13.	**Normal Angiography in Patients with Hemorrhages That Clinically Suggest Arteriovenous Malformation as Cause**

1. Spontaneous thrombosis of the malformation may have occurred, representing a self-cure.
2. With rupture, obliteration of the malformation may have occurred, representing another cure.
3. Malformation may be a cavernous angioma or developmental venous anomaly, without a direct arterial feeder, and therefore not visualized on angiography.
4. The bleeding could arise from a spinal-origin aneurysm or malformation.

Table 12-14.	**Features That Correlate with Risk of Bleeding in Arteriovenous Malformations[179,227-229]**

Small arteriovenous malformation size
Deep venous drainage
Deep location of arteriovenous malformation
Location not in border-zone region
Presence of arterial aneurysm

With each recurrent hemorrhage, the chances of additional hemorrhages increase.[205] In one large series of 137 patients with AVMs treated conservatively between 1942 and 1967, 10% died from AVMs, 24% were disabled, and only 40% were well at the time of the 1970 report[230]; 7 years later, only 19% of the initial group were well.[231,232] Because AVMs tend to occur in younger patients, the probability that recurrent hemorrhage with disability or death will occur is substantial. The authors of one study estimated that almost 50% of patients with recurrent hemorrhage will have some deterioration in working capacity or become an invalid during the 20 to 40 years after the first hemorrhage.[233] One study noted a better outcome for patients with hemorrhage from AVMs than prior reports. Among 119 AVM patients followed at Columbia Presbyterian Medical Center, 115 had a bleed as the presenting diagnostic event, and 27 of these patients had subsequent hemorrhages.[234] Four other patients had symptoms other than hemorrhage that prompted diagnosis, but had subsequent bleeds during follow-up. The incident hemorrhage resulted in no clinical deficit in 47%, and another 37% were independent in daily activities. During follow-up, 20 of 27 patients (74%) with more than one hemorrhage were still normal or independent.[234]

Parietal, central, and infratentorial malformations may be more likely to bleed than frontal, temporal, or occipital malformations.[232] Morbidity from hemorrhages depends on the location of the malformation. Occurrence in an "eloquent" brain region poses a higher risk for morbidity from a bleed, but also from surgical intervention. High arterial input pressures and restriction of venous outflow to only deep venous drainage are risk factors that increase the likelihood of hemorrhage in AVMs.[235]

Patients who present with seizures alone have a better prognosis than those that present with hemorrhage. Only a 25% chance exists of a clinically symptomatic hemorrhage in 15 years.[233] In one long-term series of patients with seizures, there was only a 12% mortality and an additional 16% overall disability.[230] A more conservative approach, prescribing only anticonvulsant therapy for patients with seizures alone, is reasonable. Seizures can be well controlled by anticonvulsants, and surgical removal of malformations often does not improve seizure control.[236] Patients presenting with progressive neurologic deficits have a poor prognosis, but these patients also often have the largest malformations, which are difficult to treat.[226]

Data are not available regarding long-term prognosis in patients with asymptomatic AVMs. These lesions are usually discovered during the evaluation of other problems. Aminoff has argued convincingly for conservative management of most unruptured AVMs.[236] AVMs that have not bled may have a better prognosis than those lesions that have already bled.

The most common presentation of cavernous angiomas is seizures, which occur in approximately one half of the patients.[237] Focal deficits and hemorrhages are the next most common presentations. Although almost all cavernous malformations show some surrounding blood on MRI or when examined pathologically, clinically significant hemorrhage is not as common. Hemorrhage is more common in patients who have already bled than in patients whose lesions have never bled. Robinson and colleagues prospectively followed 76 cavernomas detected by MRI among 66 patients.[238] Only one hemorrhage occurred during a 26-month period, for a rate of 0.7% per lesion per year.[238] In another study, follow-up information was available for 122 patients with cavernous malformations.[239] Multiple lesions were present in one-fifth of patients. Cavernomas were located in the brainstem (35%), basal ganglia and thalamus (17%), and cerebral hemispheres (48%). In retrospect, one half of the patients had one bleed, 7% had two hemorrhages, and 2% had had three bleeds.[239] The retrospective annual hemorrhage rate was 1.3%. Prospective follow-up of these patients for an average of 34 months showed a prospective annual rate of hemorrhage of only 0.6% for those lesions that had never previously bled. Patients with prior bleeds had a 4.5% per year rate of recurrent hemorrhage.[239] In this study, location of the cavernomas did not affect the rate of bleeding.[239] Hemorrhages are more common in women, especially if they are pregnant.[240] Hemorrhages are often difficult to document clinically or on MRI because part of the natural history of cavernous angiomas is slow oozing of blood into surrounding brain tissue, forming a hemosiderin-laden ring around the angioma.[240]

Moran et al performed a systematic review of the literature and analyzed the findings among supratentorial cavernous angiomas.[241] Figure 12-17 from this report diagrams the clinical manifestations among 296 patients and shows overlapping of symptoms. Seizures were by far the most common presentation, followed by hemorrhage and focal neurologic deficits.[241] After diagnosis, only six patients developed a hemorrhage during a mean 5.6 years of follow-up, yielding a hemorrhage rate of 0.7% per year.[241]

Prognosis for Developmental Venous Anomalies

In the large majority of patients, venous malformations have a benign course.[242-244] Garner et al observed 100 patients with DVAs, only one of

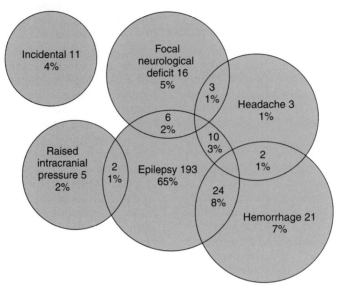

Figure 12-17 The clinical findings among 296 patients with supratentorial cavernous malformations. (From Moran NF, Fish DR, Kitchen N, et al: Supratentorial cavernous haemangiomas and epilepsy: A review of the literature and case series. J Neurol Neurosurg Psychiatry 1999;66:561-568, with permission.)

which was associated with hemorrhage.[242] Naff et al followed 92 patients with DVAs for an average of 4.2 years.[244] The most common locations of the lesions were the frontal lobes (56%) and the cerebellum (27%). The most frequent presenting symptoms were headache (51%), focal neurologic deficits (40%), and seizures (30%). The prevalence of headache and seizures decreased over time, even without treatment. Only two patients developed a symptomatic hemorrhage during follow-up, giving an annual risk of hemorrhage of 0.15%.[244] Occasional patients with DVAs have recurrent brain edema or ischemia in regions drained by the anomalous veins.

Treatment of Vascular Malformations

A 33-year-old, right-handed school teacher, BC, had occasional left-sided throbbing headaches while in college. At age 27 years, he had his first epileptic seizure, which began with a warm feeling in his right lip and tongue. The feeling rapidly spread to his hand, and then he lost consciousness. At age 33 years while shoveling snow, he developed a severe diffuse headache and vomited. On examination, he was restless and complained of headache, but had no abnormal neurologic signs except a right extensor plantar response. LP showed blood-tinged CSF at a pressure of 210 mm Hg. CT showed a thin layer of subarachnoid blood, and contrast injection opacified a large sylvian

group of tortuous veins. Angiography revealed a large parasylvian central AVM fed primarily from the left MCA.

How should this patient be treated? In this case, the diagnosis of AVM is certain. The prodromal history of headaches and seizures was typical. The present bleed was subarachnoid, arising from the surface of the lesion. No intraparenchymatous hematoma was evident, either clinically or by CT. In this patient, surgery or embolization carries the risk of aphasia or right hemiparesis, each possibly disabling. Because there were no important neurologic signs, I chose to watch the patient during the next years to see the natural history of the lesion. If he had presented with an intracerebral hematoma and had aphasia and right hemiplegia, the situation would have been quite different and surgery might have been indicated.

Four therapeutic options are available that can be used in combination or alone to treat vascular malformations: (1) surgery; (2) interventional radiology, including embolization; (3) radiotherapy; and (4) a strictly medical approach. Interventional radiologic treatment is only used for AVMs because the other lesions do not have important arterial feeders. Because venous anomalies are developmental abnormalities with a benign natural history, and resection carries a substantial risk of venous infarction, hemorrhage, and brain edema, lesions should be managed only medically.[244]

Surgery

A surgical approach is the oldest method of treatment. Initially, neurosurgeons ligated the major feeding arteries to the malformation. This method of treatment has been largely abandoned because of its failure to obliterate the lesion and the hazards inherent in the procedure. Stroke often occurs as blood flow to normal brain is interrupted. Malformations continue to draw blood from nonligated, deep, inaccessible vessels.

Direct surgical excision of lesions has been improved with the use of the operating microscope. Lesions are meticulously approached, avoiding critical cerebral vessels and vital neurologic structures. Operations may be performed using local anesthesia and evoked response monitoring, so that the exact location of vital areas can be accurately determined. Dissection is done, if possible, in the gliotic plane that surrounds the tangle of vessels, so that malformations can be removed en bloc.

Surgical excision can be carried out in most appropriate patients with a relatively low morbidity and mortality by very experienced and skilled neurosurgeons.[231,232] Castel and Kantor reviewed the results among 2425 AVM patients who had surgery.[179,245] Among these patients, postoperative mortality was 3.3% and postoperative permanent morbidity varied from 1.5% to 18.7% in different series.[245]

The major complications of surgical excision are loss of normal brain tissue, with additional loss of neurologic function and bleeding. A phenomenon unique to obliteration of AVMs is so-called breakthrough phenomenon.[246] This term is used to describe massive brain swelling and ICH occurring postoperatively that is caused by redirection of the large volume of blood that previously flowed into the malformation into the small vessels surrounding the malformation. These vessels are unable to handle the large volume of blood, and cerebral edema or hemorrhage can result.[246]

The advent of microsurgical techniques also makes it possible to remove deep-seated cavernous angiomas, including those in the brainstem. Surgical treatment of cavernomas is appropriate only for lesions that have caused intractable seizures and serious neurologic signs or have re-bled.[190]

Some cavernomas can be shelled out by experienced neurosurgeons who take advantage of the plane between the lesions and the normal brain.[190]

Endovascular Treatment

Embolization of AVMs can be performed alone, before surgery, or at the time of surgery. Initially, small pellets were used to fill the abnormal vessels within the central nidus. Because flow to malformations is increased, pellets released into feeding arteries tend to travel to the malformations. There, they occlude the lumens of vessels, it is hoped, in sufficient quantity to thrombose the vascular malformation. The particle embolization technique, however, has many problems. Emboli rarely enter arteries with acute or right angles. Furthermore, as vessels within malformations become occluded, flow to the malformations equals the flow to the normal brain and particles stray into the normal circulation, causing ischemia.

Since the early 1980s, calibrated-leak balloon catheters have been advanced into feeding arteries close to the malformation. Various kinds of "glues," rapidly setting tissue adhesives, such as isobutyl-2-cyanoacrylate, can then be administered.[248,249] These adhesives form clots in the segments of the lesion irrigated predominantly by that artery. Several feeding arteries are then injected. This technique often reduced the size of the lesion, but rarely obliterated the abnormality.

Embolization can also be done at the time of surgery when materials can be injected into cannulated blood vessels. Complications of this technique, in addition to postembolization hemorrhage related to altered blood flow, include hemorrhage or ischemic stroke induced by the balloon catheter, gluing of the balloon catheter complex in place by the tissue adhesive, or occlusion of normal arteries by the plastic material. In addition, some substances, such as bucrylate, can be toxic to tissues and cause angionecrosis and escape into the extravascular spaces.[250]

Endovascular techniques are especially important in treating lesions that are not surgically accessible and as an adjunct to surgical removal. Newer imaging technology has clearly facilitated the use of various interventional techniques.

Radiotherapy

Attempts have been made to use radiotherapy to obliterate AVMs. High energy from conventional x-rays, gamma rays, or protons induces subendothelial deposition of collagen and hyaline substances, which narrow the lumen of small vessels and shrink the nidus of the malformation by progressive occlusion of vessels during the months after treatment. Newer techniques focus the radiation beam on small regions. An example is the so-called gamma knife, a system that uses a cobalt source to generate highly collimated gamma rays that converge on a focal point.[251] Modified linear accelerators can deliver radiation to a defined volume of tissue with good accuracy. Radiation necrosis occurs in approximately 9% of patients.[251] Approximately 40% of AVMs are obliterated in 1 year, 84% after 2 years, and 97% after 3 years.[252] Small volume, deep location, and plexiform angioarchitecture correlate with successful obliteration of AVMs by radiotherapy.[252,253] The major disadvantage of radiation treatment of AVMs is that it may take months to years after treatment until the AVM is obliterated.[179] During this time the AVM is at risk of hemorrhage.

In a review of 3854 patients who had AVMs treated by radiotherapy, the average rate of permanent neurologic deficits in these 16 series was about 6%.[179,254] Complications include radionecrosis of normal brain, hydrocephalus, immediate posttherapy seizures, loss of body temperature regulation, and possibly long-term cognitive-function deficits. Further data are needed before the frequency of these complications and the therapeutic use of focused radiotherapy in patients with AVMs is known. Focused radiotherapy is probably best reserved for small deep lesions not easily amenable to surgery that have bled.

Because cavernous angiomas have only been well defined since the advent of MRI, there is less information about the use of radiotherapy in treating cavernomas as compared to AVMs. Gamma knife radiosurgery aiming the treatment precisely at the lesions using a stereotaxic three-dimensional frame has made it possible to treat small, deep lesions in the brainstem, basal ganglia, and thalamus with preliminary success.[255]

Medical Treatment

The most conservative therapeutic option for AVMs is a medical approach. Blood pressure is strictly controlled within the normal range. Anticoagulants and platelet-antiaggregant drugs are avoided. Because the rate of hemorrhage in pregnant women with AVMs is relatively high, I discuss the risk of pregnancy with fertile women and suggest appropriate contraception if desired.

Arteriovenous vascular malformations, if left untreated, are often hazardous. No one therapeutic option is entirely successful or without risk. Treatment of these malformations is often complicated by numerous feeding arteries, extensive size, or location within the brain parenchyma in areas vital to normal neurologic function. Decisions regarding therapy must consider these factors.[255a] Also important is the age of the patient and mode of presentation. These two factors are major determinants of the natural history of the disease.

For the most common mode of presentation-hemorrhage in patients with AVMs, I recommend an aggressive approach, including surgery or surgery combined with embolization if the following criteria are met:

1. The patient is relatively young (younger than 55 years and has a life expectancy of more than 15 years).
2. Recovery of neurologic function after the hemorrhage is moderately good, so that a reasonable lifestyle can be anticipated.
3. The malformation is superficial in location and does not extensively involve vital neural structures—so-called eloquent brain.

Because the rate of early rebleeding is low, I wait until the patient is in good medical condition before suggesting surgery. Because surgery can cause neurologic signs, the presence of a remaining neurologic deficit related to the bleeding is a factor favoring surgery, whereas postbleed return to complete normality argues against surgery.

I adopt a more conservative approach, using embolization and radiotherapy if available, or strictly medical management if the following criteria are met:

1. The patient is older than 60 years, and life expectancy is less than 10 years.
2. The deficit from the initial hemorrhage is severe.
3. The malformation is extensive and deep within the dominant hemisphere, in the brainstem or other vital eloquent areas.

I use these same criteria for patients who present with progressive neurologic deficits. I treat patients who present with seizures medically. Anticonvulsants are given to control the seizures, blood pressure is regulated, and anticoagulants and platelet antiaggregating drugs are avoided. If seizures remain intractable despite medical therapy, a more aggressive plan using surgical excision might be considered.

In asymptomatic patients, including those with only headache, I follow a conservative medical approach. Because the natural history of asymptomatic lesions is unknown, it is unwise to undertake therapy that may be more hazardous than the lesion itself. Furthermore, initial hemorrhages are rarely fatal; if a hemorrhage does occur, the opportunity for more aggressive therapy is then available.

DURAL ARTERIOVENOUS FISTULAS

Dural arteriovenous malformations (DAVMs) are lesions that contain abnormal arteriovenous shunts within the leaflets of the dura mater, usually within or near the walls of dural venous sinuses.[15,256] Figure 12-18 shows angiograms in a patient who has a DAVM with filling from arterial branches of the MCAs and external carotid arteries that drain into the superior sagittal sinus and

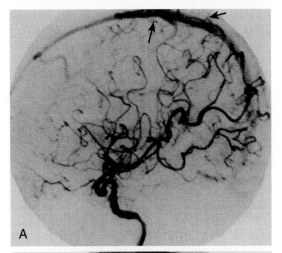

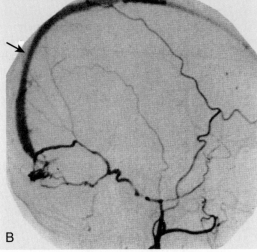

Figure 12-18. Dural arteriovenous malformation of the superior sagittal sinus and torcula. **A,** Internal carotid artery angiogram. Lateral view shows that multiple branches of the MCA drain directly into the superior sagittal sinus *(black arrows).* **B,** External carotid injection shows that internal maxillary branches also fill the sagittal sinus *(black arrow).* (From Dion J: Dural arteriovenous malformations: Definition, classification, and diagnostic imaging. In Awad IA, Barrow DL (eds): Dural Arteriovenous Malformations. Park Ridge, Ill: American Association of Neurological Surgeons, 1993, pp 1-19, with permission.)

torcula herophili. DAVMs have different etiologies, pathophysiologies, and clinical symptoms when compared with parenchymal and pial AVMs. DAVMs represent 10% to 15% of all AVMs.

DAVMs may drain only into dural sinuses or there may be prominent drainage into the cortical and deep venous systems. DAVMs with prominent cortical venous drainage have a higher incidence of bleeding than those without.[257,258] The cause of most of the complications and symptoms and signs in patients with DAVMs is thought to be venous hypertension.[259,260] The two major mechanisms of

increased pressure within the venous drainage system are (1) increased blood flow through draining veins (e.g., related to increased arterial inputs); and (2) restriction or obstruction of the draining system, causing an increase in pressure in the tributary veins. Venous hypertension probably promotes cortical venous drainage and increases the risk of brain hemorrhage.

Some DAVMs are probably congenital, especially those that involve the vein of Galen. Retention of an embryonic median porencephalic vein, which normally drains the choroid plexus of the fetus, is the explanation usually given for vein of Galen malformations.[261] When this vein persists, it becomes the sac for the aneurysmally enlarged vein of Galen. These lesions should probably be classified as AVMs rather than true DAVMs. Most DAVMs are probably acquired.[15,260] Well-documented instances exist of adult patients who had normal angiograms and later, angiography showed that DAVMs had formed, proving these lesions were acquired in these patients.[262] Trauma is undoubtedly an important cause in some patients. Hormonal factors may also be important because female hormones are known to influence placental and uterine vascular growth and increase angiomas at many body sites. Dural sinus thrombosis, an important cause of DAVMS, is more common in women. Approximately twice as many women as men have the most common form of DAVM with drainage into the lateral sinuses.[263,264] DAVMs may first become symptomatic during pregnancy. Some DAVMs regress after delivery. Occlusion of a dural sinus is an important cause of DAVMs.[263,263a] Houser and colleagues reported two patients in whom dural sinus thrombosis was documented years before development of DAVMs.[263] One patient had previous angiography because of transient bilateral limb weakness that showed sigmoid sinus occlusion but no fistula; a year later after the development of pulsatile tinnitus, a repeat angiogram showed a DAVM of the transverse sinus adjacent to the occluded sigmoid sinus. Another patient with a history of thrombophlebitis and thromboembolism developed headache, drowsiness, leg weakness, and papilledema. Angiography showed a transverse sinus occlusion. When he developed an increase in his symptoms, a repeat angiogram 2.5 years later showed a transverse sinus DAVM.[263] Thrombosis or stenosis within the draining dural sinus often causes enlargement of the DAVMs and augments venous hypertension. Trauma is a very important cause of dural fistula formation, especially in patients with carotid-cavernous fistulas.[263a,263b] Several reports document progressive obstruction and occlusion of dural sinuses in patients known to have DAVMs.[15,265]

The clinical problems that develop in patients with DAVMs, such as headaches, papilledema, hydrocephalus, and hemorrhages, are probably explained by venous hypertension.[265] The focal symptoms and signs that develop depend heavily on the location of the DAVMs and whether the lesions are solely dural or have a prominent drainage pattern into the brain's cortical and deep veins.[266] Hemorrhages are most often intraparenchymatous or subdural, but occasionally are subarachnoid. First hemorrhages from DAVMs have an approximate 30% mortality rate. An especially high mortality and severe disabling morbidity rate occurs in patients with hemorrhages from DAVMs who are taking anticoagulants. Venous infarcts, which are often hemorrhagic, and brain edema can also result from the venous hypertension. Seizures, headache, and signs of increased intracranial pressure develop, often with papilledema. Brain edema is an important sequel in some patients with DAVMs, especially those with venous hypertension and dural sinus occlusions.[15,267]

Pulsatile tinnitus is another frequent and annoying symptom. Some patients only have headaches, either generalized or localized to the side of the DAVM. I have seen several patients with DAVMs who had positionally sensitive headache with worsening in the supine position and improvement when sitting or standing.[15] The erect position may have allowed better venous drainage toward the heart.

The most common location of DAVMs is in relation to the lateral sinuses, involving the transverse or sigmoid portion of the lateral sinus. Lateral sinus malformations account for five eighths of DAVMs.[15,268] Potential feeding arteries to these lateral sinus fistulas include (1) external carotid artery branches, such as the occipital, middle meningeal, accessory meningeal, and ascending pharyngeal arteries; (2) dural branches of the ICA, especially the meningohypophyseal trunk (the artery of Bernasconi and Casaneri); and (3) dural branches of the vertebral arteries, such as posterior meningeal, cerebellar falcine, and cervical muscular anastomotic arteries. Venous drainage of lateral sinus DAVMs can be into a normal transverse or sigmoid sinus, or the wall of the sinus may be irregular and partially or completely thrombosed.

Cavernous sinus fistulae are the next most common lesion and are found in approximately one eighth of patients with DAVMs.[268] These lesions are characterized by abnormal shunting of blood from the internal or external carotid arteries into the cavernous sinus. Blood often drains into the orbital veins, causing increased venous pressure in the eye and orbital contents leading to proptosis, chemosis caused by conjunctival edema,

scleral injection, conjunctival hemorrhages, glaucoma, and papilledema.[263b,269,270] These lesions can drain into the petrosal veins and sinuses and the basal vein of Rosenthal, and cause venous hypertension within the brainstem.[271,272] Trauma and rupture of infraclinoid carotid artery aneurysms into the cavernous sinus are important causes of these fistulae.

Tentorial-incisural DAVMs account for approximately one twelfth of all DAVMs.[273] Less common locations include the cerebral convexity-sagittal sinus region, orbital-anterior falx region, sylvian-middle fossa region, and those that drain into the torcula herophili. Some DAVMs drain into deep structures, such as the vein of Galen, straight sinus, or dural venous structures in the posterior falx region. The vein of Galen is an unusual structure, both anatomically and embryologically. It is a bridge between the subarachnoid venous system and the dural straight sinus. The vein of Galen can be the site of shunting or can be recruited into the venous drainage pattern in cases of high-flow lesions or when distal outlets are stenosed or thrombosed. The two distinct types of vein of Galen malformations follow[261]:

1. A congenital lesion that develops in utero in which the arterial input is into a persistent medial prosencephalic vein, which can become aneurysmally dilatated. These patients present with congestive heart failure. These lesions are probably true AVMs and the dural sinuses are patent.
2. A DAVM in which the shunt is into the wall of the vein of Galen. These are acquired in adulthood usually in relation to dural sinus occlusions in a similar fashion to other DAVMs. True vein-of-Galen DAVMs presenting in adulthood are supplied from the middle meningeal and vertebral artery, PCA, and meningohypophyseal artery branches. Occasionally, a vein-of-Galen aneurysm can be associated with DAVMs.

DAVMs are difficult to diagnose without angiography. In my experience, the angiographic results often come as a surprise and were not suspected from the clinical or imaging data. CT does not show the DAVM but can show related abnormalities, such as hemorrhages, thrombosed sinuses, hydrocephalus, and dilated pial veins or varices. Contrast enhancement aids recognition of the abnormal veins and thrombosed sinuses. Similarly, MRI may show the abnormal veins and sinuses, suggesting the diagnosis, but does not show the arterial input. Although MRI and MRA can undoubtedly be helpful in suggesting the diagnosis, catheter angiography using high-resolution digital arterial subtraction angiography is still needed to identify the arterial feeders and draining venous patterns.

The natural history of DAVMs is variable. Some close spontaneously. In others, symptoms are slight and include mostly headache and pulsatile tinnitus. The nature of the venous drainage pattern is considered by many to be important in predicting the prognosis.[15] Drainage into subarachnoid and parenchymal veins with retrograde flow away from the lesion seems to correlate with dural sinus outflow obstruction and venous hypertension.[199] This predicts an aggressive course, often with brain hemorrhages, intraventricular hemorrhages, subdural hemorrhages, and SAHs.[268]

Endovascular treatment of DAVMs has been limited, although technology is rapidly changing.[274,275] The plethora of arterial feeders from multiple major arterial systems, and the small size of many of the feeders, especially pial arteries, limit the effectiveness of embolization strategies. Transvenous endovascular treatment is promising. In some patients, a combined approach using transarterial embolization, transvenous ablation, and microneurosurgery has been effective.[275]

Surgical treatment of DAVMs is often quite difficult. Mullan emphasized that surgeons should attempt to obliterate the fistulous communication, which appears as "multiple watering can spouts into the sinus lumen."[276] Some fistulas drain into an isolated vein in the wall of a dural sinus. Effective obliteration involves occluding the vein flush with the external wall of the sinus.[276] Obliteration or ligation of feeders often does not result in effective ablation of the DAVMs because new feeders are recruited. Packing the sinus in the region of the fistula is usually effective but is difficult and requires considerable surgical experience. The high flow in DAVMs makes blood loss and a bloody surgical field important problems in effective ablation. A conservative nonsurgical approach to DAVMs is probably best in fistulas that do not have prominent leptomeningeal venous drainage or variceal or aneurysmal abnormalities within the draining venous system.[277] Clinical observation, repeat neuroimaging, and angiography are advised for those patients not treated surgically.[277]

Modern neuroimaging technology greatly facilitates diagnosis and should allow physicians to learn more about the natural history of DAVMs and other craniocerebral vascular malformations. Modern technology facilitates logical treatment.

References

1. Rinkel GJE, Djibuti M, Algra A, van Gijn J: Prevalence and risk of rupture of intracranial aneurysms. A systematic review. Stroke 1998;29:251-256.

2. The International Study of Unruptured Intracranial Aneurysms Investigators: Unruptured intracranial aneurysms—Risk of rupture and risks of surgical intervention. N Engl J Med 1998;339:1725-1733.

3. Mayberg MR, Batjer HH, Dacey R, et al: Guidelines for the management of aneurysmal subarachnoid hemorrhage. A statement for healthcare professionals from a special writing group of the Stroke Council, American Heart Association. Stroke 1994;25:2315-2328.

4. Weir B: Aneurysms Affecting the Central Nervous System. Baltimore: Williams & Wilkins, 1987.

5. Kaibara T, Heros RC: Aneurysms. In Caplan LR (ed): Uncommon Causes of Stroke, 2nd ed. Cambridge: Cambridge University Press, 2008, pp 171-179.

6. Parkarinen S: Incidence, etiology, and prognosis of primary subarachnoid hemorrhage: A study based on 589 cases diagnosed in a defined urban population during a defined period. Acta Neurol Scand 1967;43(suppl 29):1-128.

7. Phillips LH, Whisnant JP, O'Fallan W, et al: The unchanging pattern of subarachnoid hemorrhage in a community. Neurology 1980;30:1034-1040.

8. Ingall TJ, Whisnant JP, Wiebers DO, O'Fallon WM: Has there been a decline in subarachnoid hemorrhage mortality? Stroke 1989;20:718-724.

9. Garraway WM, Whisnant JP, Furlan AJ, et al: The declining incidence of stroke. N Engl J Med 1979;300:449-452.

10. Locksley HB: Report of the Cooperative Study of Intracranial Aneurysms and Subarachnoid Hemorrhage. Sec V, part I: Natural history of subarachnoid hemorrhage, intracranial aneurysms, and arteriovenous malformation-based on 6,368 cases in the cooperative study. J Neurosurg 1966;25:219-239.

11. Locksley HB: Report of the Cooperative Study of Intracranial Aneurysms and Subarachnoid Hemorrhage. Sec V, part II: Natural history of subarachnoid hemorrhage, intracranial aneurysms, and arteriovenous malformation. J Neurosurg 1966;25:321-368.

12. Heros RC, Kistler JP: Intracranial arterial aneurysms—an update. Stroke 1983;14:628-631.

13. Winn WR, Richardson AE, Jane JA: The long-term prognosis in untreated cerebral aneurysms: I. The incidence of late hemorrhage in cerebral aneurysms—a ten-year evaluation of 364 patients. Ann Neurol 1977;1:358-370.

14. Kassell NF, Kongable GL, Torner JC, et al: Delay in referral of patients with ruptured aneurysms to neurosurgical attention. Stroke 1985;16:587-590.

14a. Bor ASE, Velthuis BK, Majoie CB, Rinkel GJE: Configuration of intracranial arteries and development of aneurysms. Neurology 2008;70:700-705.

15. Caplan LR: Subarachnoid hemorrhage, aneurysms, and vascular malformations. In Caplan LR (ed): Posterior Circulation Disease: Clinical Findings, Diagnosis, and Management. Boston: Blackwell, 1996, pp 633-685.

16. Suzuki J, Onuma T, Yoshimoto T: Results of early operations on cerebral aneurysms. Surg Neurol 1979;11:407-412.

17. Bromberg JE, Rinkel GJ, Algra A, et al: Familial subarachnoid hemorrhage: Distinctive features and patterns of inheritance. Ann Neurol 1995;38:929-934.

18. Raaymakers TW, Rinkel GJ, Ramos LM: Initial and follow-up screening for aneurysms in families with familial subarachnoid hemorrhage. Neurology 1998;51:1125-1130.

19. Schievink WI, Schaid DJ, Rogers HM, et al: On the inheritance of intracranial aneurysms. Stroke 1994;25:2028-2037.

20. Ruigrok YM, Rinkel GJE, Wijmenga C: Genetics of intracranial aneurysms. Lancet Neurology 2005;4:179-189.

21. Ruigrok YM, Seitz U, Wolterink S, et al: Association of polymorphisms and pairwise haplotypes in the elastin gene in Dutch patients with subarachnoid hemorrhage from non-familial aneurysms. Stroke 2004;35:2064-2068.

22. Ruigrok YM, Rinkel GJE: Genetics of intracranial aneurysms. Stroke 2008;39:1049-1055.

23. Nahed BV, Bydon M, Ozturk AK, et al: Genetics of intracranial aneurysms. Neurosurgery 2007;60:213-225.

23a. Ruigrok YM, Rinkel GJE, Wijmenga C: The Versican gene and the risk of intracranial aneurysms. Stroke 2006;37:2372-2374.

23b. Ruigrok YM, Wijmenga C, Rinkel GJE, et al: Genomewide linkage in a large dutch family with intracranial aneurysms. Stroke 2008;39:1096-1102.

24. van den Berg JSP, Limburg M, Pais G, et al: Some patients with intracranial aneurysms have a reduced type III/type I collagen ratio. Neurology 1997;49:1546-1551.

25. Ferguson GG: Physical factors in the initiation, growth, and rupture of human intracranial saccular aneurysms. J Neurosurg 1972;37:666-677.

26. Adams HP, Kassell N, Torner JC, et al: Early management of aneurysmal subarachnoid hemorrhage. J Neurosurg 1981;54:141-145.

27. Ferguson GG, Peerless SJ, Drake CG: Natural history of intracranial aneurysms. N Engl J Med 1981;305:99.

28. Caplan LR: Should intracranial aneurysms be treated before they rupture? N Engl J Med 1998;339:1774-1775.

29. Wiebers DO, Whisnant JP, O'Fallon WM: The natural history of unruptured intracranial aneurysms. N Engl J Med 1981;304:696-698.

30. Drake CG: Giant intracranial aneurysm: Experience with surgical treatment in 174 patients. In Carmel PW PW (ed): Clinical Neurosurgery. Baltimore: Williams & Wilkins, 1979, pp 12-95.

31. Kassell N, Drake CG: Review of the management of saccular aneurysms. In Barnett HJM (ed): Neurological Clinics, vol 1. Philadelphia: Saunders, 1983, pp 73-86.

32. Adams HP, Jergenson DD, Kassell NF, Sahs AL: Pitfalls in the recognition of subarachnoid hemorrhage. JAMA 1980;244:794-796.

33. Edlow JA, Caplan LR:. Avoiding pitfalls in the diagnosis of subarachnoid hemorrhage. N Engl J Med 2000;342:29-36.

34. Gorelick PB, Hier DB, Caplan LR, Langenberg P: Headache in acute cerebrovascular disease. Neurology 1986;36:1445-1450.

35. Hauerberg J, Andersen BB, Eskesen V, et al: Importance of the recognition of a warning leak as a sign of a ruptured intracranial aneurysm. Acta Neurol Scand 1971;83:61-64.

36. Ostergaard JR: Warning leak in subarachnoid haemorrhage. BMJ 1990;301:190-191.

37. Drake CG: The treatment of aneurysms of the posterior circulation. In Carmel PW (ed): Clinical Neurosurgery. Baltimore: Williams & Wilkins, 1979, pp 96-144.

38. Stewart RM, Samsom D, Diehl J, et al: Unruptured cerebral aneurysms presenting as recurrent transient neurological deficits. Neurology 1980;30:47-51.

39. Fisher M, Davidson RI, Marcus EM: Transient focal cerebral ischemia as a presenting manifestation of unruptured cerebral aneurysms. Ann Neurol 1980;8:367-372.

40. Sutherland GR, King ME, Peerless SJ, et al: Platelet interaction within giant intracranial aneurysms. J Neurosurg 1982;56:53-61.

41. Weisberg LA: Ruptured aneurysms of anterior cerebral or anterior communicating arteries. Neurology 1985;35:1562-1566.

42. Hunt WE, Hess RM: Surgical risk as related to time of intervention in the repair of intracranial aneurysms. J Neurosurg 1968;28:14-20.

43. Alvord EC, Loeser JD, Bailey WL, et al: Subarachnoid hemorrhage due to ruptured aneurysm: A simple method of estimating prognosis. Arch Neurol 1972;27:273-284.

44. Teasdale G, Jennett B: Assessment of coma and impaired consciousness. A practical scale. Lancet 1974;2:81-84.

45. Teasdale G, Jennett B: Assessment and prognosis of coma after head injury. Acta Neurochir (Wien) 1976;34:45-55.

46. Wijdicks EFM: Clinical scales for comatose patients: The Glasgow Coma Scale in historical context and the new Four Score. Rev Neurol Dis 2006;3:109-117.

47. Weisberg L: Computed tomography in aneurysmal subarachnoid hemorrhage. Neurology 1979;29:802-808.

48. Liliequist B, Lindquist M: Computer tomography in the evaluation of subarachnoid hemorrhage. Acta Radiol Diagn (Stockh) 1980;21:327-331.

49. van der Jagt M, Hasan D, Bijvoet HWC, et al: Validity of prediction of the site of ruptured intracranial aneurysm with CT. Neurology 1999;52:34-39.

50. Van Gijn J, van Dongen KJ, Vermeulen M, et al: Perimesencephalic hemorrhage: A nonaneurysmal and benign form of subarachnoid hemorrhage. Neurology 1985;35:483-487.

51. Rinkel GJ, Wijdicks E, Vermeulen M, et al: The clinical course of perimesencephalic nonaneurysmal subarachnoid hemorrhage. Ann Neurol 1991;29:463-468.

52. Schievink WI, Wijdicks EFM: Pretruncal subarachnoid hemorrhage: An anatomically

correct description of the perimesencephalic subarachnoid hemorrhage. Stroke 1997; 28:2572.

53. Kershenovich A, Rappaport ZH, Maimon S: Brain computed tomography angiographic scans as the sole diagnostic examination for excluding aneurysms in patients with perimesencephalic subarachnoid hemorrhage. Neurosurgery 2006;59:798-801.

54. Patel KC, Finelli PF: Non-aneurysmal convexity subarachnoid hemorrhage. Neurocrit Care 2006;4:229-233.

55. Spitzer C, Mull M, Rohde V, Kosinski CM: Non-traumatic cortical subarachnoid haemorrhage: Diagnostic work-up and aetiological background. Neuroradiology 2005;47:525-531.

56. Fisher CM, Kistler JP, Davis JM: Relation of cerebral vasospasm to subarachnoid hemorrhage visualized by computed tomographic scanning. Neurosurgery 1980;6:1-9.

57. Kistler JP, Crowell RM, Davis KR, et al: The relation of cerebral vasospasm to the extent and location of subarachnoid blood visualized by CT scan: A prospective study. Neurology 1983;33:424-437.

58. Hijdra A, van Gijn J, Nagelkerke N, et al: Prediction of delayed cerebral ischemia, rebleeding, and outcome after aneurysmal subarachnoid hemorrhage. Stroke 1988;19: 1250-1256.

59. Brouwers PJ, Dippel DW, Vermeulen M, et al: Amount of blood on computed tomography as an independent predictor after aneurysm rupture. Stroke 1993;24:809-814.

60. Sherlock M, Agha A, Thompson CJ: Aneurysmal subarachnoid hemorrhage. N Engl J Med 2006; 354:1755-1757.

61. Alberico RA, Patel M, Casey S, et al: Evaluation of the circle of Willis with three-dimensional CT angiography in patients with suspected intracranial aneurysms. AJNR Am J Neuroradiol 1995;16:1571-1578.

62. Jayaraman MV, Mayo-Smith WW, Tung GA, et al: Detection of intracranial aneurysms: multi-detector row CT angiography compared with DSA. Radiology 2004;230:510-518.

63. Yoon DY, Lim KJ, Choi CS, et al: Detection and characterization of intracranial aneurysms with 16-channel multidetector row CT angiography: A prospective comparison of volume-rendered images and digital subtraction angiography. AJNR Am J Neuroradiol 2007;28:60-67.

64. Ross J, Masaryk T, Modic M, et al: Intracranial aneurysms: Evaluation by MR angiography. AJNR Am J Neuroradiol 1990;11:449-456.

65. Okahara M, Kiyosue H, Yamashita M, et al: Diagnostic accuracy of magnetic resonance angiography for cerebral aneurysms in correlation with 3D-digital subtraction angiographic images: A study of 133 aneurysms. Stroke 2002;33: 1803-1808.

66. Unlu E, Cakir B, Gocer B, et al: The role of contrast-enhanced MR angiography in the assessment of recently ruptured intracranial aneurysms: A comparative study. Neuroradiology 2005;47:780-791.

67. Caplan LR, Flamm ES, Mohr JP, et al: Lumbar puncture and stroke. Stroke 1987;18:540A-544A.

68. Edlow JA: Diagnosis of subarachnoid hemorrhage. Neurocrit Care 2005;2(2):99-109.

69. Van Gign J, Kerr RS, Rinkel GJE: Subarachnoid haemorrhage. Lancet 2007;369:306-318.

70. Van der Meulen JP: Cerebrospinal fluid xanthochromia: An objective index. Neurology 1966;16:170-178.

71. Perry JJ, Sivilotti ML, Stiell IG, et al: Should spectrophotometry be used to identify xanthochromia in the cerebrospinal fluid of alert patients suspected of having subarachnoid hemorrhage? Stroke 2006;37:2467-2472.

72. Hayward RS: Subarachnoid hemorrhage of unknown etiology. J Neurol Neurosurg Psychiatry 1977;40:926-931.

73. Rinkel GJE, van Gijn J, Wijdicks EFM: Subarachnoid hemorrhage without detectable aneurysm: A review of the causes. Stroke 1993;24:1403-1409.

74. Caplan LR, Brass LM, DeWitt LD, et al: Transcranial Doppler ultrasound: Present status. Neurology 1990;40:696-700.

75. Sloan MA, Alexandrov AV, Tegeler CH, et al: Assessment: Transcranial Doppler ultrasonography: Report of the Therapeutics and Technology Assessment. Subcommittee of the American Academy of Neurology. Neurology 2004;62:1468-1481.

76. Lindegaard K, Grolemund P, Aaslid R, Normes H: Evaluation of cerebral AVMs using transcranial Doppler ultrasound. J Neurosurg 1986;65:335-344.

77. Schwartz A, Hennerici M: Noninvasive transcranial Doppler ultrasound in intracranial angiomas. Neurology 1986;36:626-635.

78. Petty GW, Massaro AR, Tatemichi TK, et al: Transcranial Doppler ultrasonographic changes after treatment for arteriovenous malformations. Stroke 1990;21:260-266.

79. Harders AG, Gilsbach JM: Time course of blood velocity changes related to vasospasm in the circle of Willis measured by transcranial Doppler ultrasound. J Neurosurg 1987;66: 718-728.

80. Sloan MA, Haley EC, Kassell NF, et al: Sensitivity and specificity of transcranial Doppler ultrasonography in the diagnosis of vasospasm following subarachnoid hemorrhage. Neurology 1989;391:1514-1518.

81. Sekhar L, Wechsler L, Yonas H, et al: Value of transcranial Doppler examination in the diagnosis of cerebral vasospasm after subarachnoid hemorrhage. Neurosurgery 1988;22:813-821.

82. Davis SM, Andrews JT, Lichtenstein M, et al: Correlations between cerebral arterial velocities, blood flow, and delayed ischemia after subarachnoid hemorrhage. Stroke 1992;23:492-497.

83. Davis S, Andrews J, Lichtenstein M, et al: A single-photon emission computed tomography study of hyperperfusion after subarachnoid hemorrhage. Stroke 1990;21:252-259.

84. Chieregato A, Sabia G, Tanfani A, et al: Xenon-CT and transcranial Doppler in poor-grade or complicated aneurysmatic subarachnoid hemorrhage patients undergoing aggressive management of intracranial hypertension. Intensive Care Med 2006;32:1143-1150.

85. Hillman J, Sturnegk P, Yonas H, et al: Bedside monitoring of CBF with xenon-CT and a mobile scanner: A novel method in neurointensive care. Br J Neurosurg 2005;19:395-401.

86. Rordorf G, Koroshetz WJ, Copen WA, et al: Diffusion- and perfusion-weighted imaging in vasospasm after subarachnoid hemorrhage. Stroke 1999;30:599-605.

87. Condette-Auliac S, Bracard S, Anxionnat R, et al: Vasospasm after subarachnoid hemorrhage: Interest in diffusion-weighted MR imaging. Stroke 2001;32:1818-1824.

88. Wijdicks EFM, Schievink W, Miller GM. Pretruncal subarachnoid hemorrhage. Mayo Clin Proc 1998;73:745-752.

89. Rinkel GJ, Wijdicks E, Vermeulen M, et al: Outcome in perimesencephalic (nonaneurysmal) subarachnoid hemorrhage: A follow-up study in 37 patients. Neurology 1990;40:1130-1132.

90. Wijdicks EFM, Schievink WI: Perimesencephalic nonaneurysmal subarachnoid hemorrhage: First hint of a cause? Neurology 1997;49:634-636.

91. Stein RW, Kase CS, Hier DB, et al: Caudate hemorrhage. Neurology 1984;34:1549-1554.

92. Hochberg F, Fisher CM, Roberson G: Subarachnoid hemorrhage caused by rupture of a small superficial artery. Neurology 1974;24:309-311.

93. Lasjaunias P, Chiu M, ter Brugge K, et al: Neurological manifestations of intracranial dural arteriovenous malformations. J Neurosurg 1986;64:724-730.

94. Chang R, Friedman DP: Isolated cortical venous thrombosis presenting as subarachnoid hemorrhage: A report of three cases. AJNR Am J Neuroradiol 2004;25:1676-1679.

95. Oppenheim C, Domigo V, Gauvrit JY, et al: Subarachnoid hemorrhage as the initial presentation of dural sinus thrombosis. AJNR Am J Neuroradiol 2005;26:614-617.

96. Ohshima T, Endo T, Nukui H, et al: Cerebral amyloid angiopathy as a cause of subarachnoid hemorrhage. Stroke 1990;21:480-483.

97. Thompson B, Burns A: Subarachnoid hemorrhages in vasculitis. Am J Kidney Dis 2003;42:582-585.

98. Fomin S, Patel S, Alcasid N, et al: Recurrent subarachnoid hemorrhage in a 17 year old with Wegener granulomatosis. J Clin Rheumatol 2006;12:212-213.

99. Broderick JP, Brott TG, Duldner JE, et al: Initial and recurrent bleeding are the major causes of death following subarachnoid hemorrhage. Stroke 1994;25:1342-1347.

100. Suarez JI, Tarr RW, Selman WR: Aneurysmal subarachnoid hemorrhage. N Engl J Med 2006;354:387-396.

101. Bambidakis NC, Selman WR: Subarachnoid hemorrhage. In Suarez JL (ed): Critical Care Neurology and Neurosurgery. Towata, NJ: Humana Press, 2004, pp 365-377.

102. Clower BR, Smith RR, Haining JL, Lockard J: Constrictive endarteropathy following experimental subarachnoid hemorrhage. Stroke 1981;12:501-508.

103. Smith RR, Clower BR, Grotendorst GM, et al: Arterial wall changes in early human vasospasm. Neurosurgery 1985;16:171-176.

104. Yamamoto Y, Smith RR, Bernanke DH: Accelerated nonmuscle contraction after subarachnoid hemorrhage: Culture and characterization of myofibroblasts from human cerebral arteries in vasospasm. Neurosurgery 1992;30:337-345.

105. Macdonald RL, Weir BKA: A review of hemoglobin and the pathogenesis of cerebral vasospasm. Stroke 1991;22:971-982.

106. Macdonald RL: Cerebral Vasospasm. In Welch KMA, Caplan LR, Reis DJ, et al: (eds): Primer on Cerebrovascular Diseases. San Diego: Academic Press, 1997, pp 490-497.

107. Hughes JT, Schianchi PM: Cerebral artery spasm: A histological study at necropsy of the blood vessels in cases of subarachnoid hemorrhage. J Neurosurg 1978;48:515-525.

108. Conway LW, McDonald LW: Structural changes of the intradural arteries following subarachnoid hemorrhage. J Neurosurg 1972;37:715-723.

109. Wellum GR, Peterson JW, Zervas NT: The relevance of in vivo smooth muscle experiments to cerebral vasospasm. Stroke 1985;16:573-581.

110. Kassell NF, Sasaki T, Colohan AR, Nazar G: Cerebral vasospasm following aneurysmal subarachnoid hemorrhage. Stroke 1985;16: 562-572.

111. Kwak R, Niizuma H, Ohi J, et al: Angiography study of cerebral vasospasm following rupture of intracranial aneurysms: I. Time of the appearance. Surg Neurol 1979;11:257-262.

112. Weir B, Grace M, Hansen J, et al: Time course of vasospasm in man. J Neurosurg 1978;48:173-178.

113. Heros RC, Zervas NT, Varsos V: Cerebral vasospasm after subarachnoid hemorrhage: An update. Ann Neurol 1983;14:599-608.

113a. Chaudhary SR, Ko N, Dillon W, et al: Prospective evaluation of multidetector-row CT angiography for the diagnosis of vasospasm following subarachnoid hemorrhage: A comparison with digital subtraction angiography. Cerebrovasc Dis 2008;25:144-150.

113b. Pham M, Johnson A, Bartsch AJ, et al: CT perfusion predicts secondary cerebral infarction after aneurismal subarachnoid hemorrhage. Neurology 2007;69:762-765.

114. Sviri GE, Feinsod M, Soustiel JF: Brain natriuretic peptide and cerebral vasospasm in subarachnoid hemorrhage: Clinical and TCD correlations. Stroke 2000;31:118-122.

115. Hop JW, Rinkel GJE, Algra A, van Gijn J: Initial loss of consciousness and risk of delayed

cerebral ischemia after subarachnoid hemorrhage. Stroke 1999;30:2268-2271.

115a. Lanterna LA, Ruigrok Y, Alexander S, et al: Meta-analysis of APOE genotype and subarachnoid hemorrhage. Neurology 2007;69:766-775.

116. Mizukami M, Kawase T, Usami T, et al: Prevention of vasospasm by early operation with removal of subarachnoid blood. Neurosurgery 1982;10:301-307.

117. Taneda M: Effect of early operation for ruptured aneurysm in prevention of delayed ischemic symptoms. J Neurosurg 1982;5:622-628.

118. Findlay JM, Kassell NF, Weir BKA, et al: A randomized trial of intraoperative, intracisternal tissue plasminogen activator for prevention of vasospasm. Neurosurgery 1995;37:168-178.

119. Sasaki T, Kodama N, Kawakami M, et al: Urokinase cisternal irrigation therapy of symptomatic vasospasm after aneurismal subarachnoid hemorrhage. Stroke 2000;31:1256-1262.

120. Barth M, Capelle H-H, Weidauer S, et al: Effect of nicardipine prolonged-release implants on cerebral vasospasm and clinical outcome after severe aneurismal subarachnoid hemorrhage. A prospective randomized double-blind phase II study. Stroke 2007;38:330-336.

121. Macdonald RL: Cerebral vasospasm. Neurosurg Q 1995;5:73-97.

122. Kassell NF, Peerless SJ, Durward QJ, et al: Treatment of ischemic deficits from vasospasm with hypervolemia and induced arterial hypertension. Neurosurgery 1982;11:337-343.

123. Solomon RA, Fink ME, Lennihan L: Prophylactic volume expansion therapy for the prevention of delayed cerebral ischemia after early aneurysm surgery. Arch Neurol 1988;45:325-332.

124. Solomon RA, Post KD, McMurty JG: Depression of circulating blood volume in patients after subarachnoid hemorrhage: Implications for the management of symptomatic vasospasm. Neurosurgery 1984;15:354-361.

125. Wood JH, Simeone FA, Kron RE, et al: Rheological aspects of experimental hypervolemic hemodilation with low molecular weight dextran. Neurosurgery 1982;11:739-753.

126. Pickard JD, Murray GD, Illingworth R, et al: Effect of oral nimodipine in cerebral infarction and outcome after subarachnoid hemorrhage: British Aneurysm Nimodipine trial. BMJ 1981;298:636-642.

127. Allen GS: Cerebral arterial spasm: A controlled trial of nimodipine in subarachnoid hemorrhage patients—the nimodipine cerebral arterial spasm study group. Stroke 1983;14:122.

128. Feigin VL, Rinkel GJE, Algra A, et al: Calcium antagonists in patients with aneurysmal subarachnoid hemorrhage. A systematic review. Neurology 1998;50:876-883.

128a. Fraticelli AT, Cholley BP, Losser M-R, et al: Milrinone for the treatment of cerebral vasospasm after aneurismal subarachnoid hemorrhage. Stroke 2008;39:893-898.

129. Higashida RT, Halbach VV, Cahan LD, et al: Transluminal angioplasty for treatment of intracranial arterial vasospasm. J Neurosurg 1989;71:648-653.

130. Hoh BL, Ogilvy CS: Endovascular treatment of cerebral vasospasm: Transluminal balloon angioplasty, intra-arterial papaverine, and intra-arterial nicardipine. Neurosurg Clin N Am 2005;16:501-516,

131. Brisman JL, Eskridge JM, Newell DW: Neurointerventional treatment of vasospasm. Neurol Res 2006;28:769-776.

132. Newell DW, Eskridge JM, Mayberg M, et al: Angioplasty for the treatment of symptomatic vasospasm following subarachnoid hemorrhage. J Neurosurg 1989;91:654-660.

133. Leroux PD, Winn HR: Timing of surgery and special features of ruptured anterior circulation aneurysms. In Welch KMA, Caplan LR, Reis DJ, et al (eds): Primer on Cerebrovascular Diseases. San Diego: Academic Press, 1997, pp 450-454.

134. Graff-Radford NR, Torner J, Adams HP, Kassell NF: Factors associated with hydrocephalus after subarachnoid hemorrhage. Arch Neurol 1989;46:744-752.

135. Samuels MA: Electrocardiographic manifestations of neurologic disease. Semin Neurol 1984;4:453-460.

136. Brouwers PJ, Wijdicks EF, Hasan D, et al: Serial electrocardiographic recording in aneurysmal subarachnoid hemorrhage. Stroke 1989;20:1162-1167.

137. Caplan LR, Hurst JW: Cardiac and cardiovascular findings in patients with nervous system diseases. In Caplan LR, Hurst JW, Chimowitz MI (eds): Clinical Neurocardiology. New York: Marcel Dekker, 1999, pp 298-312.

138. Provencio JJ: Subarachnoid hemorrhage: A model for heart-brain interactions. Cleveland Clin J Med 2007;74(suppl 1):S86-S90.

139. Fabinyi G, Hunt D, McKinley L: Myocardial creatine kinase isoenzyme in serum after subarachnoid hemorrhage. J Neurol Neurosurg Psychiatry 1977;40:818-820.

139a. Kothavale A, Banki NM, Kopelnik A, et al: Predictors of left ventricular regional wall motion abnormalities after subarachnoid hemorrhage. Neurocrit Care 2006;4:199-205.

140. Norris JW, Frogatt GM, Hachinski VC: Cardiac arrythmias in acute stroke. Stroke 1978;9:392-396.

141. Oppenheimer SM, Cechetto DF, Hachinski VC: Cerebrogenic cardiac arrythmias. Cerebral electrocardiographic influences and their role in sudden death. Arch Neurol 1990;47:513-519.

142. Di Pasquale G, Pinelli G, Andreoli A, et al: Holter detection of cardiac arrythmias in intracranial subarachnoid hemorrhage. Am J Cardiol 1987;59:596-600.

143. Di Pasquale G, Pinelli G, Andreoli A, et al: Torsade de pointes and ventricular flutter-fibrillation following spontaneous cerebral subarachnoid hemorrhage. Int J Cardiol 1988;18:163-172.

144. Kolin A, Norris JW: Myocardial damage from acute cerebral lesions. Stroke 1984;15:990-993.

145. Samuels M: "Voodoo" death revisited: The modern lessons of neurocardiology. Neurologist 1997;3:293-304.

145a. Kothvale A, Banki N, Kopelnik A, et al: Predictors of left ventricular regional wall motion abnormalities after subarachnoid hemorrhage. Neurocrit Care 2006;4:199-205.

146. Ciongoli AK, Poser CM: Pulmonary edema secondary to subarachnoid hemorrhage. Neurology 1972;22:867-870.

147. Weir BK: Pulmonary edema following fatal aneurysmal rupture. J Neurosurg 1978;49:502-507.

148. Landolt AM, Yasargil MG, Krayenbuhl H: Disturbances of the serum electrolytes after surgery of intracranial arterial aneurysm. J Neurosurg 1972;37:210-218.

149. Takaku A, Shindo K, Tanaki S, et al: Fluid and electrolyte disturbances in patients with intracranial aneurysms. Surg Neurol 1979;11:349-356.

149a. Katayama Y, Haraoka J, Hirabayashi H, et al: A randomized controlled trial of hydrocortisone against hyponatremia in patients with aneurismal subarachnoid hemorrhage. Stroke 2007;38:2373-2375.

150. Diringer MN, Lim JS, Kirsch JR, Hawley DF: Suprasellar and intraventricular blood predict elevated plasma atrial natriuretic factor in subarachnoid hemorrhage. Stroke 1991;22:572-581.

151. Wijdicks EFM, Ropper AH, Hunnicutt EJ, et al: Atrial natriuretic factor and salt wasting after aneurysmal subarchnoid hemorrhage. Stroke 1991;22:1519-1524.

151a. Schneider HJ, Kreitschmann-Andermahr I, Ghiko E, et al: Hypothalamopituitary dysfunction following traumatic brain injury and aneurismal subarachnoid hemorrhage. A systemic review. JAMA 2007;298:1429-1438.

152. Kreitschmann-Andermahr I, Hoff C, Niggemeier S, et al: Pituitary deficiency following aneurismal subarachnoid haemorrhage. J Neurol Neurosurg Psychiatry 2003;74:1133-1135.

153. Dimopoulou I, Kouyialis AT, Tzanella M, et al: High incidence of neuroendocrine dysfunction in long-term survivors of aneurismal subarachnoid hemorrhage. Stroke 2004;35:2884-2489.

154. Peerless SJ: Pre- and postoperative management of cerebral aneurysm. Clin Neurosurg 1979;26:209-231.

155. Claasen J, Vu A, Kreiter KT, et al: Effect of acute physiologic derangements on outcome after subarachnoid hemorrhage. Crit Care Med 2004;32:832-838.

156. Calhoun DA, Oparil S: Treatment of hypertensive crises. N Engl J Med 1990;323:1177-1183.

157. Adams HP: Current status of antifibrinolytic therapy for treatment of patients with aneurysmal subarachnoid hemorrhage. Stroke 1982;13:256-259.

158. Ramirez-Laseppas M: Antifibrinolytic therapy in subarachnoid hemorrhage caused by ruptured intracranial aneurysm. Neurology 1981;31:316-322.

159. Kassell N, Torner D, Adams H: Antifibrinolytic therapy in the acute period following aneurysmal subarachnoid hemorrhage. J Neurosurg 1984;61:225-230.

160. Garde A: Amnesia after operations on aneurysms of the anterior communicating artery. Surg Neurol 1982;18:46-49.

161. Damasio AR, Graff-Radford N, Eslinger P, et al: Amnesia following basal forebrain lesions. Arch Neurol 1985;42:263-271.

162. Serbinenko FA: Balloon catheterization and occlusion of major cerebral vessels. J Neurosurg 1974;41:125-145.

163. Guglielmi G, Vinuela F, Sepetka I, Macellari V: Electrothrombosis of saccular aneurysms via endovascular approach, part 1: Electrochemical basis, technique, and experimental results. J Neurosurg 1991;75:1-7.

164. Guglielmi G, Vinuela F, Dion J, Duckwiler G: Electrothrombosis of saccular aneurysms via endovascular approach, part 2: Preliminary clinical experience. J Neurosurg 1991;75:8-14.

165. Johnston SC, Higashida RT, Barrow DL, Caplan LR, et al: Recommendations for the endovascular treatment of intracranial aneurysms. A statement for health care professionals from the Committee on Cerebrovascular Imaging of the American Heart Association Council on Cardiovascular Radiology. Stroke 2002;33:2536-2544.

166. Hopkins LN, Lanzino G, Guterman LR: Treating nervous system vascular disorders through a "needle stick": Origins, evolution, and future of endovascular therapy. Neurosurgery 2001;48:463-475.

167. Molyneux AJ, Kerr RSC, Yu L-M, et al: International Subarachnoid Aneurysm Trial (ISAT) of neurosurgical clipping versus endovascular coiling in 2143 patients with ruptured intracranial aneurysms: A randomized comparison of effects on survival, dependency, seizures, rebleeding, subgroups, and aneurysm occlusion. Lancet 2005;366:809-817.

168. Britz GW: ISAT trial: Coiling or clipping for intracranial aneurysms? Lancet 2005;366:783-785.

169. Debrun GM, Aletich VA, Kehrli P, et al: Selection of cerebral aneurysms for treatment using Guglielmi detachable coils: The preliminary University of Illinois at Chicago experience. Neurosurgery 1998;43:1281-1295.

169a. Lanzino G, Wakhloo AK, Fessler RD, et al: Efficacy and current limitations of intravascular stents for intracranial internal carotid, vertebral, and basilar artery aneurysms. J Neurosurg 1999;91:538-546.

169b. Greenberg E, Katz JM, Janardhan V, et al: Treatment of a giant vertebrobasilar artery aneurysm using stent grafts. Case report. J Neurosurg 2007;107:165-168.

169c. Katsaridis V, Papagiannaki C, Violaris C: Placement of a Neuroform2 stent into the parent vessel by navigating it along the inner wall of the aneurysm sac: A technical case report. Neuroradiology 2007;49:57-59.

169d. Pero G, Denegri F, Valvassori L, et al: Treatment of a middle cerebral artery giant aneurysm using a covered stent. Case report. J Neurosurg 2006;104:965-968.

170. Kupersmith MJ, Stiebel-Kalish H, Huna-Baron R, et al: Cavernous carotid aneurysms rarely cause subarachnoid hemorrhage or major neurological morbidity. J Stroke Cerebrovasc Dis 2002;11:9-14.

171. Brust JCM, Dickinson PCT, Hughes JEO, Holtzman RNN: The diagnosis and treatment of cerebral mycotic aneurysms. Ann Neurol 1990;27:238-246.

172. Moskowitz MA, Rosenbaum AE, Tyler HR: Angiographically monitored resolution of cerebral mycotic aneurysms. Neurology 1974;24:1103-1108.

173. Johnston SC, Wilson CB, Halbach VV, et al: Endovascular and surgical treatment of unruptured cerebral aneurysms: Comparison of risks. Ann Neurol 2000;48:11-19.

173a. Wermer MJH, van der Schaaf IC, Algra A, Rinkel GJE: Risk of rupture of unruptured intracranial aneurysms in relation to patient and aneurysm characteristics. An updated meta-analysis. Stroke 2007;38:1404-1410.

174. Winn HR, Berga SL, Richardson AE, et al: Long-term evaluation of patients with cerebral aneurysms. Ann Neurol 1981;10:106.

175. Sundt TM, Whisnant JP: Subarachnoid hemorrhage from intracranial aneurysm. N Engl J Med 1978;299:116-122.

176. Raaymakers TWM, Rinkel GJE, Limburg M, Algra A: Mortality and morbidity of surgery for unruptured intracranial aneurysms. A meta-analysis. Stroke 1998;29:1531-1538.

177. Stein BM, Wolpert SM: Arteriovenous malformations of the brain: I. Current concepts and treatment. Arch Neurol 1980;37:1-5.

178. Brown RD, Wiebers DO, Torner JC: Frequency of intracranial hemorrhage as a presenting symptom and subtype analysis: A population-based study of intracranial vascular malformations in Olmstead County, Minnesota. J Neurosurg 1996;85:29-32.

179. Hartmann A, Mast H, Choi JH, et al: Treatment of arteriovenous malformations of the brain. Curr Neurol Neurosci Rep 2007;7:28-34.

180. Tonnis W, Schiefer W, Walter W: Signs and symptoms of supratentorial arteriovenous aneurysms. J Neurosurg 1953;15:471-480.

181. McCormick WF: The pathology of vascular ("arteriovenous") malformations. J Neurosurg 1966;24:807-816.

182. McCormick WF: Pathology of vascular malformations of the brain. In Wilson CB, Stein BM (eds): Intracranial Arteriovenous Malformations: Current Neurosurgical Practice. Baltimore: Williams & Wilkins, 1984, pp 44-63.

183. McCormick WF, Boulter TR: Vascular malformations ("angiomas") of the dura mater. J Neurosurg 1966:309-311.

184. McCormick WF: The pathology of angiomas. In Fein JM, Flamm ES (eds): Cerebrovascular Surgery, vol IV. New York: Springer, 1985, pp 1073-1095.

185. McCormick WF, Hardman JM, Boulter TR: Vascular malformations ("angiomas") of the brain, with special reference to those occurring in the posterior fossa. J Neurosurg 1968;28:241-251.

186. The Arteriovenous Malformations Study Group: Arteriovenous malformations of the brain in adults. N Engl J Med 1999;340:1812-1818.

186a. Lasjaunias PL, Landrieu P, Rodesch G, et al: Cerebral proliferative angiopathy. Clinical and angiographic description of an entity different from cerebral AVMs. Stroke 2008;39:878-885.

187. Rigamonti D, Hadley MN, Drayer BP, et al: Cerebral cavernous malformations: Incidence and familial occurrence. N Engl J Med 1988;319:343-347.

188. Savoiardo M, Strada L, Passerini A: Intracranial cavernous hemangiomas: Neuroradiologic review of 36 operated cases. AJNR Am J Neuroradiol 1983;4:945-950.

189. Mason I, Aase JM, Orrison WW, et al: Familial cavernous angiomas of the brain in an Hispanic family. Neurology 1988;38:324-326.

190. Metellus P, Kharkar S, Lin D, et al: Cavernous angiomas and developmental venous anomalies. In Caplan LR (ed): I Uncommon Causes, 2nd ed. Cambridge: Cambridge University Press, 2008, pp 189-219.

190a. Denier C, Labauge P, Brunereau L, et al: Clinical features of cerebral cavernous malformations patients with KRIT1 mutations. Ann Neurol 2004;55:213-220.

191. Wilms G, Bleus E, Demaerel P, et al: Simultaneous occurrence of deveopmental venous anomalies and cavernous angiomas. AJNR Am J Neuroradiol 1994;15:1247-1254.

192. Abe T, Singer RJ, Marks MP, et al: Coexistence of occult vascular malformations and developmental venous anomalies in the central nervous system: MR evaluation. AJNR Am J Neuroradiol 1998;19:51-57.

193. Omojola M, Fox A, Vinuela F, Debrun G: Stenosis of afferent vessels of intracranial arteriovenous malformations. AJNR Am J Neuroradiol 1985;6:791-793.

194. Mawad ME, Hilal SK, Michelson J, et al: Occlusive vascular disease associated with cerebral arteriovenous malformations. Radiology 1984;153:401-408.

12

195. Marks MP, Lane B, Steinberg GK, Snipes GJ: Intranidal aneurysms in cerebral arteriovenous malformations: Evaluation and endovascular treatment. Radiology 1992;183:355-360.

196. Kondziolka D, Nixon BJ, Lasjaunias P, et al: Cerebral arteriovenous malformations with associated arterial aneurysms: Hemodynamic and therapeutic considerations. Can J Neurol Sci 1988;15:130-134.

197. Miyasaka Y, Yada K, Ohwada T, et al: An analysis of the venous drainage system as an actor in hemorrhage from arteriovenous malformations. J Neurosurg 1992;76:239-243.

198. Vinuela F, Nombela L, Roach MR, et al: Stenotic and occlusive disease of the draining venous system of deep brain AVMs. J Neurosurg 1985;63:180-184.

199. Hsu FPK, Rigamonti D, Huhn SL: Epidemiology of cavernous malformations. In Awad IA, Barrows DL (eds): Cavernous Malformations. Park Ridge, IL: American Association of Neurological Surgeons, 1993, pp 13-23.

200. Kase CS: Aneurysms and vascular malformations. In Kase CS, Caplan LR (eds): Intracerebral Hemorrhage. Boston: Butterworth-Heinemann, 1995, pp 153-178.

201. Perret G, Nishioka H: Report on the Cooperative Study of Intracranial Aneurysms and Subarachnoid Hemorrhage. Section VI. Arteriovenous malformations. An analysis of 545 cases of cranio-cerebral arteriovenous malformations and fistulae reported to the Cooperative Study. J Neurosurg 1966;25:467-490.

202. Crawford PM, West CR, Chadwick DW, et al: Arteriovenous malformations of the brain: Natural history in unoperated patients. J Neurol Neurosurg Psychiatry 1986; 49:1-10.

203. Graf CJ, Perret GE, Torner JC: Bleeding from cerebral arteriovenous malformations as part of their natural history. J Neurosurg 1983;58: 331-337.

204. Hook C, Johanson C: Intracranial arteriovenous aneurysms: A follow-up study with particular attention to their growth. Arch Neurol Psych 1958;80:39-54.

205. Patterson JH, McKissock W: A clinical survey of intracranial angiomas with special reference to their mode of progression and surgical treatment: A report of 110 cases. Brain 1965;79:233-266.

205a. Friedlander RM: Arteriovenous malformations of the brain. N Engl J Med 2007;356: 2704-2712.

206. Hofmeister C, Stapf C, Hartman A, et al: Demographic, morphological, and clinical characteristics of 1289 patients with brain arteriovenous malformation. Stroke 2000;31:1307-1310.

207. Mast H, Mohr JP, Osipov A, et al: "Steal" is an unestablished mechanism for the clinical presentation of cerebral arteriovenous malformations. Stroke 1995;26:1215-1220.

208. Chimowitz MI, Little JR, Awad IA, et al: Intracranial hypertension associated with unruptured cerebral arteriovenous malformations. Ann Neurol 1990;27:474-479.

209. DeJong RN, Hicks SP: Vascular malformation of the brainstem: Report of a case with long duration and fluctuating course. Neurology 1980;30:995-997.

210. Stahl SM, Johnson KP, Malamud N: The clinical and pathological spectrum of brainstem vascular malformations. Arch Neurol 1980;37:25-29.

211. Caroscio JT, Brannan T, Budabin M, et al: Subarachnoid hemorrhage secondary to spinal arteriovenous malformation and aneurysm. Arch Neurol 1980;37:101-103.

212. Robinson JC, Hall CS, Sedzimir CB: Arteriovenous malformations, aneurysms, and pregnancy. J Neurosurg 1974;41:63-70.

213. Jensen H, Klinge H, Lemke J, et al: Computerized tomography in vascular malformations of the brain. Neurosurg Rev 1980;3:119-127.

214. Daniels D, Houghton V, Williams A, et al: Arteriovenous malformation simulating a cyst on computed tomography. Radiology 1979;133: 393-394.

215. Kaibara T, Heros RC: Arteriovenous malformations of the brain. In Caplan LR (ed): Uncommon Causes of Stroke, 2nd ed. Cambridge: Cambridge University Press, 2008.

216. Leblanc R, Levesque M, Comair Y, Ethier R: Magnetic resonance imaging of cerebral arteriovenous malformations. Neurosurgery 1987;21:15-20.

217. Smith HJ, Strother CM, Kikuchi Y, et al: MR imaging in the management of supratentorial intracranial AVMs. AJR Am J Roentgen 1988;150:1143-1153,

218. Rigamonti D, Drayer B, Johnson PC, et al: The MRI appearance of cavernous malformations (angiomas). J Neurosurg 1987;67:518-524.

219. Gomori JM, Grossman RI, Hackney DB, et al: Variable appearances of subacute intracranial hematomas on high-field spin-echo MR. AJR Am J Roentgen 1988;150:171-178.

220. Requena I, Arias M, Lopez-Iber L: Cavernomas of the cerebral nervous system in clinical and neuroimaging manifestations in 47 patients. J Neurol Neurosurg Psychiatry 1991;54:590-594.

221. Perl J, Ross JS: Diagnostic imaging of cavernous malformations. In Awad IA, Barrow DL (eds): Cavernous Malformations. Park Ridge, IL: American Association of Neurological Surgeons, 1993, pp 37-48.

222. Hardjasudarma M: Cavernous and venous angiomas of the central nervous system. Neuroimaging and clinical controversies. J Neuroimaging 1991;1:191-196.

223. Rigamonti D, Spetzler RF, Drayer BP, et al: Appearance of venous malformations on magnetic resonance imaging. J Neurosurg 1988;69:535-539.

224. Lee C, Pennington MA, Kenney CM: MR evaluation of developmental venous anomalies:

medullary venous anatomy of venous angiomas. AJNR Am J Neuroradiol 1996;17:61-70.

225. Diehl RR, Henkes H, Nahser H-C, et al: Blood flow velocity and vasomotor reactivity in patients with arteriovenous malformations. A transcranial Doppler study. Stroke 1994;25:1574-1580.

226. Marks M, Lane B, Steinberg G, Chang P: Vascular characteristics of intracerebral arteriovenous malformations in patients with clinical steal. AJNR 1991;12:489-496.

227. Stapf C, Mohr JP, Sciacca RR, et al: Incident hemorrhage risk of brain arteriovenous malformations located in the arterial borderzones. Stroke 2000;31:2365-2368.

228. Mast H, Young WL, Koennecke HC, et al: Risk of spontaneous hemorrhage after diagnosis of cerebral arteriovenous malformation. Lancet 1997;350:1065-1068.

229. Mansmann U, Meisel J, Brock M, et al: Factors associated with intracranial hemorrhage in cases of cerebral arteriovenous malformations. Neurosurgery 2000;46:272-279.

230. Drake CG: Arteriovenous malformations of the brain: The options for management. N Engl J Med 1983;309:308-310.

231. Heros RC, Tu Y-K: Is surgical therapy needed for unruptured arteriovenous malformations? Neurology 1987;37:279-286.

232. Drake CG: Cerebral arteriovenous malformations: Considerations for and experience with surgical treatment in 166 cases. Clin Neurosurg 1979;26:145-208.

233. Forster DMC, Steiner L, Hakanson S: Arteriovenous malformations of the brain: A long-term clinical study. J Neurosurg 1972;37:562-570.

234. Hartmann A, Mast H, Mohr JP, et al: Morbidity of intracranial hemorrhage in patients with cerebral arteriovenous malformation. Stroke 1998;29:931-934.

235. Duong DH, Young WL, Vang MC, et al: Feeding artery pressure and venous drainage pattern are primary determinants of hemorrhage from arteriovenous malformations. Stroke 1998;29:1167-1176.

236. Aminoff MJ: Treatment of unruptured cerebral arteriovenous malformations. Neurology 1987;37:815-819.

237. Barrow DL: Classification and natural history of cerebral vascular malformations: Arteriovenous, cavernous, and venous. J Stroke Cerebrovasc Dis 1997;6:264-267.

238. Robinson JR, Awad IA, Little JR: Natural history of the cavernous angioma. J Neurosurg 1991;75:709-714.

239. Kondziolka D, Lundsford LD, Kestle JRW: The natural history of cerebral cavernous malformations. J Neurosurg 1995;83:820-824.

240. Robinson JR, Awad IA: Clinical spectrum and natural course. In Awad IA, Barrows DL (eds): Cavernous Malformations. Park Ridge, IL: American Association of Neurological Surgeons, 1993, pp 25-36.

241. Moran NF, Fish DR, Kitchen N, et al: Supratentorial cavernous haemangiomas and epilepsy: A review of the literature and case series. J Neurol Neurosurg Psychiatry 1999;66:561-568.

242. Garner TB, Curling OD Jr, Kelly DL Jr, et al: The natural history of intracranial venous angiomas. J Neurosurg 1991;75:715-722.

243. Rigamonti D, Spetzler RF, Medina M, et al: Cerebral venous malformations. J Neurosurg 1990;73:560-564.

244. Naff NJ, Wemmer J, Hoenig-Rigamonti K, Rigamonti DR: A longitudinal study of patients with venous malformations: Documentation of a negligible hemorrhage risk and benign natural history. Neurology 1998;50:1709-1714.

245. Castel JP, Kantor G: Postoperative morbidity and mortality after microsurgical exclusion of cerebral arteriovenous malformations. Current data and analysis of recent literature. Neurochiurgie 47:369-383.

246. Spetzler RF, Wilson CB, Weinstein P, et al: Normal perfusion pressure breakthrough theory. Clin Neurosurg 1978;25:651-672.

247. Fournier D, TerBrugge KG, Willinsky R, et al: Endovascular treatment of intracerebral arteriovenous malformations: Experience in 49 cases. J Neurosurg 1991;75:228-233.

248. Vinuela F, Fox AJ, Debrun G, et al: Progressive thrombosis of brain arteriovenous malformations after embolization with isobutyl-2-cyanoacrylate. AJNR Am J Neuroradiol 1983;4:959-966.

249. The N-BCA Trialists: N-butyl cyanoacrylate embolization of cerebral arteriovenous malformations: Results of a prospective, multi-center trial. AJNR Am J Neuroradiol 2002;23:748-755.

250. Vinters HV, Lundie MJ, Kaufmann JC: Long-term pathological follow-up of cerebral arteriovenous malformations treated by embolization with buccylate. N Engl J Med 1986;314:477-483.

251. Lunsford LD, Flickinger J, Coffey RJ: Stereotactic gamma knife radiosurgery. Initial North American experience in 207 patients. Arch Neurol 1990;47:169-175.

252. Heros R, Korosue K: Radiation treatment of cerebral arteriovenous malformations. N Engl J Med 1990;323:127-129.

253. Meder JF, Oppenheim C, Blustajn J, et al: Cerebral arteriovenous malformations: The value of radiologic parameters in predicting response to radiosurgery. AJNR Am J Neuroradiol 1997;18:1473-1483.

254. Hartmann A, Marx P, Schilling A, et al: Neurologic complications following radiosurgical treatment of brain arteriovenous malformations. Cerebrovasc Dis 2002;13:50.

255. Coffey RJ, Lunsford LD: Radiosurgery of cavernous malformations and other angiographically occult vascular malformations. In Awad IA, Barrow DL (eds): Cavernous Malformations. Park Ridge, IL: American Association of Neurological Surgeons, 1993, pp 187-200.

255a. Ogilvy CS, Stieg PE, Awad I, et al: Recommendations for the management of intracranial arteriovenous malformations. A statement for healthcare professionals from a special writing group of the Stroke Council, American Stroke Association. Circulation 2001;103:2644-2657.

256. Dion J: Dural arteriovenous malformations: Definition, classification, and diagnostic imaging. In Awad IA, Barrow DL (eds): Dural Arteriovenous Malformations. Park Ridge, IL: American Association of Neurological Surgeons, 1993, pp 1-19.

257. Castaigne P, Bories J, Brunet P, et al: Les fistules arterio-veineuse meningees pures a drainage veineux cortical. Rev Neurol (Paris) 1976;132:169-181.

258. Gaston A, Chiras J, Bourbotte G, et al: Meningeal arteriovenous fistulae draining into cortical veins: 31 cases. J Neuroradiol 1984;11:161-177.

259. Bederson JB: Pathophysiology and animal models of dural arteriovenous malformations. In Awad IA, Barrow DL (eds): Dural Arteriovenous Malformations. Park Ridge, IL: American Association of Neurological Surgeons, 1993, pp 23-33.

260. Friedman AH: Etiologic factors in intracranial dural arteriovenous malformations. In Awad IA, Barrow DL (eds): Dural Arteriovenous Malformations. Park Ridge, IL: American Association of Neurological Surgeons, 1993, pp 35-47.

261. Raybaud CA, Hald JK, Strother CM, et al: Aneurysms of the vein of Galen. Angiographic study and morphogenetic considerations. Neurochirurgie 1987;33:302-314.

262. Hansen JH, Segaard I: Spontaneous regression of an extra- and intracranial arteriovenous malformation: Case report. J Neurosurg 1976;45:338-341.

263. Houser OW, Campbell JK, Campbell RJ: Arteriovenous malformation affecting the transverse dural venous sinus: An acquired lesion. Mayo Clin Proc 1979;54:651-661.

263a. Chung SJ, Kim JS, Kim JC, et al: Intracranial dural arteriovenous fistulas: Analysis of 60 patients. Cerebrovasc Dis 2002;13:79-88.

263b. Feiner L, Bennett J, Volpe NJ: Cavernous sinus fistulas: Carotid cavernous fistulas and dural arteriovenous malformations. Curr Neurol Neurosci Rep 2003;3:415-420.

264. Fermand M, Reizine D, Melki JP, et al: Long term follow-up of 43 pure dural arteriovenous fistulae (AVF) of the lateral sinus. Neuroradiology 1987;29:348-353.

265. Lasjaunias PL, Rodesch G: Lesion types, hemodynamics, and clinical spectrum. In Awad IA, Barrow DL (eds): Dural Arteriovenous Malformations. Park Ridge, IL: American Association of Neurological Surgeons, 1993, pp 49-79.

266. Awad IA, Little JR, Akrawi WP, et al: Intracranial dural arteriovenous malformations: Factors predisposing to an aggressive neurological course. J Neurosurg 1990;72:839-850.

267. Zeidman SM, Monsein LH, Arosarena O, et al: Reversability of white matter changes and dementia after treatment of dural fistulas. AJNR Am J Neuroradiol 1995;16:1080-1083.

268. Awad IA: Dural arteriovenous malformations with aggressive clinical course. In Awad IA, Barrow DL (eds): Dural Arteriovenous Malformations. Park Ridge, IL: American Association of Neurological Surgeons, 1993, pp 93-104.

269. Wecht DA, Awad IA: Carotid cavernous and other dural arteriovenous fistulas. In Welch KMA, Caplan LR, Reis DJ, et al (eds): Primer on Cerebrovascular Diseases. San Diego: Academic Press, 1997, pp 541-548.

270. Purdy PD: Management of Carotid Cavernous Fistula. In Batjer HH, Caplan LR, Friberg L, et al (eds): Cerebrovascular Disease. Philadelphia: Lippincott-Raven, 1997, pp 1159-1168.

271. Takahashi S, Tomura N, Watarai J, et al: Dural arterioveinous fistula of the cavernous sinus with venous congestion of the brain stem: Report of two cases. AJNR Am J Neuroradiol 1999;20:886-888.

272. Halbach VV, Higashida RT, Hieshima GB, et al: Treatment of dural fistulas involving the deep cerebral venous system. AJNR Am J Neuroradiol 1989;10:393-399.

273. Awad IA: Tentorial incisura and brain stem dural arteriovenous malformations. In Awad IA, Barrow DL (eds): Dural Arteriovenous Malformations. Park Ridge, IL: American Association of Neurological Surgeons, 1993, pp 131-146.

274. Halbach VV, Higashida RT, Hieshima GB, et al: Transvenous embolization of dural fistulas involving the transverse and sigmoid sinuses. AJNR Am J Neuroradiol 1989;10:385-392.

275. Barnwell S: Endovascular therapy of dural arteriovenous malformations. In Awad IA, Barrow DL (eds): Dural Arteriovenous Malformations. Park Ridge, IL: American Association of Neurological Surgeons, 1993, pp 193-211.

276. Mullan S: Surgical therapy: Indications and general principles. In Awad IA, Barrow DL (eds): Dural Arteriovenous Malformations. Park Ridge, IL: American Association of Neurological Surgeons, 1993, pp 213-229.

277. Awad IA, Barrow DL: Conceptual overview and management strategies. In Awad IA, Barrow DL (eds): Dural Arteriovenous Malformations. Park Ridge, IL: American Association of Neurological Surgeons, 1993, pp 131-241.

Intracerebral Hemorrhage 13

Bleeding into the substance of the brain was recognized as a cause of stroke by Morgagni in 1761.[1] Cheyne wrote a treatise on apoplexy and coma in 1812, in which he included examples of intracerebral hemorrhage (ICH).[2] Clinicians of the 19th and 20th centuries considered ICH invariably lethal. Postmortem examples were usually studied because the tests available could not identify ICH during life. Clinicians correlated the clinical findings with the size and location of hemorrhages found in brains at necropsy. Gowers[3] and Osler,[4] writing at the turn of the 20th century, included long and detailed chapters on the usual locations of ICH, and accompanying clinical signs and symptoms in their respective textbooks. In 1935, Aring and Merritt[5] correlated the clinical and pathologic findings of 245 patients with stroke who came to necropsy at the Boston City Hospital. Aring and Merritt emphasized the features that separated hemorrhage from infarction. The major teachings emanating from these works are summarized in the following general rules:

1. ICH occurred at a younger age than brain infarction.
2. The major cause of ICH was hypertension, often severe.
3. Symptoms of ICH began abruptly.
4. Loss of consciousness was a nearly constant feature.
5. Headache always accompanied ICH, and was usually severe.
6. The most common locations for ICH were the putamen, internal capsule, thalamus, pons, and cerebellum.
7. ICH was invariably fatal or devastating, with few, if any, intact survivors.

This work, however, was published long before computed tomography (CT) scanning. Aring and Merritt's teachings evolved from correlation with fatal cases. Technology did not exist to diagnose less severe hemorrhages during life, especially if the lesions did not communicate with the cerebrospinal fluid (CSF). CT and MRI now allow accurate localization of small- and medium-sized hemorrhages. Brain imaging not only shows clinicians whether a lesion is a hemorrhage, but also accurately shows the location, size, spread within

the brain, drainage into the ventricles and spaces around the brain, and presence of edema and mass effect. Magnetic resonance imaging (MRI), by its capability of showing the presence of hemosiderin, can help define the age of hemorrhages and can identify old regions of prior bleeding. Old infarcts and hemorrhages can look similar on CT. When the subject of ICH is reviewed in light of results with newer imaging techniques, the old rules are found to apply to larger hemorrhages, which is only a small fraction of ICHs. I begin this chapter by reviewing the general rules and findings applicable to ICH at any site. I then review the etiologies of ICH and the findings in hemorrhages at their common locations in the brain.

INCIDENCE AND EPIDEMIOLOGY

Approximately 10% of strokes are caused by ICH.[6-10] Populations that have a high frequency of hypertension, such as African Americans and individuals of Chinese, Japanese, Korean, and Thai ancestry, have higher frequencies of ICH. ICH affects a wide age range, with many examples in the seventh, eighth, and ninth decades of life. Figure 13-1 displays the age and sex distribution of ICH in the Harvard Stroke Registry (HSR).[11] Although it is probably accurate to say that a higher percentage of strokes in patients younger than 40 years are hemorrhagic, ICH is also common during the later years of life.

CLINICAL COURSE AND ACCOMPANYING SYMPTOMS

JT, a 44-year-old, African-American schoolteacher, rushed to arrive at an important job interview. While being stressfully interrogated, he noted tingling in his left hand that gradually spread to his arm. He excused himself to go to the washroom, and then noted a similar feeling in his left leg. As he washed his hands, he realized that his left hand and arm were clumsy and weak. He tripped on his left foot as he walked back. The interviewer was alarmed by slurring of words and a droop of the left face, which he noticed when JT returned.

An ambulance was called. JT began to feel a headache over his right scalp. After 10 minutes,

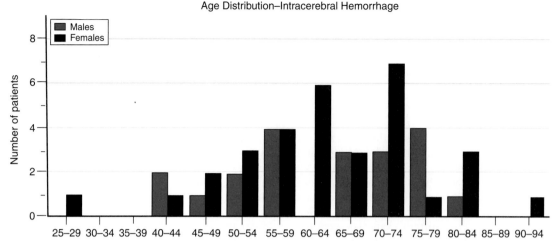

Figure 13-1. Age distribution in patients with intracerebral hemorrhage (from the Harvard Stroke Registry). (Data from Caplan LR, Mohr JP: Intracerebral hemorrhage: An update. Geriatrics 1978;33:42-52.)

the emergency team arrived. JT could no longer move his left arm and leg, but seemed unaware and unconcerned with his handicap. He now had a severe headache and was sleepy. While being placed on a stretcher, he began to vomit. He had no history of hypertension or drug use. Blood pressure was 175/110 mm Hg when he was first examined by the emergency personnel.

The course of illness in this patient was the gradual accumulation of focal neurologic signs, during a period of approximately 20 minutes. As the neurologic symptoms and disability worsened, headache, decreased alertness, and vomiting developed.

ICH develops gradually. Bleeding into the brain tissues from small, deep, penetrating vessels is usually under arteriolar or capillary pressure. This situation contrasts with subarachnoid hemorrhage (SAH), in which arteries on the brain surface leak blood under systemic arterial pressure. Symptoms in patients with SAH begin instantaneously and consist of headache, loss of concentration and alertness, and vomiting. These symptoms are caused by sudden increase in intracranial pressure (ICP), resulting from blood rapidly disseminating through the CSF around the brain substance. In contrast, ICH develops gradually during minutes or sometimes hours.

Fisher examined serial sections of ICH studied at necropsy.[12] At the center of the lesions was a large mass of blood. At the periphery were many of what he called fibrin globes, representing little caps of fibrinous material that plugged small vessels, which had broken and leaked during life. As ICH develops, pressure within the central core increases and compresses small vessels at the periphery of the hematoma. These peripheral arterioles and capillaries in turn break, and blood

escapes, enlarging the lesion. The hematoma grows like a snowball rolling downhill, accumulating more snow on its outer circumference as it rolls. ICP increases as the lesion enlarges, and tissue pressure around the lesion also mounts. Finally, an equilibrium is reached between the pressure within the hematoma and surrounding pressure, and bleeding stops. If the hematoma reaches the ventricle or brain surface, it may communicate with the CSF, discharge part of its contents at the same time, and, in doing so, decompress the pressure within the lesion.

Visualizing the pathology of the lesion and its development helps predict the pace of the symptoms. Bleeding is directly into brain parenchyma, rather than the CSF, as occurs in SAH. The brain is devoid of pain fibers, so the initial release of blood does not cause headaches. Instead, blood disrupts the function of that particular local brain region. If the hematoma began in the left putamen, the patient might note right-limb weakness. As the hemorrhage grows during the next few minutes, the weakness becomes more severe. Sensory symptoms, loss of speech, and conjugate eye deviation to the side of the hemorrhage might ensue. In JT, the combination of sensory (tingling) and motor symptoms in the left side of his face, and left arm and leg, suggests a process in the deep structures of the right cerebral hemisphere, affecting the internal capsule region. If the hemorrhage grew to a size that increased ICP and distorted adjacent meningeal structures, the patient would develop headache, vomiting, and reduced alertness. In JT, headaches, sleepiness, and vomiting started and evolved after he became hemiplegic and his lesion expanded. If the hematoma continued to grow, coma and death might result from compression of vital brainstem centers.

Sometimes, clinical symptoms and signs evolve over a period of days, rather than minutes or hours. Studies of patients with acute ICHs using sequential CT studies show that hematomas relatively often expand dramatically during hours.[13-16] Repeat CT may show dramatic enlargement of hematoma mass and ventricular drainage, developing within hours after the first CT scan. Invariably, clinical worsening was also present and was an indication for repeat scanning in some patients. In one study, 41 out of 204 patients with ICH had expansion of ICHs on repeat CT scans.[16] Expansion in this study was most often detected during the first 6 hours, but 5 out of 33 hematomas (15%) expanded between 6- and 12-hour scans, and 2 out of 34 hematomas (6%) enlarged between 12- and 24-hour scans.[16] Patients with ICH who have a bleeding diathesis are especially prone to hematomas that expand gradually and enlarge over periods of days.[17-19]

Analysis of the course of illness in 54 well-documented patients with ICH studied in the HSR showed that 37 had gradual development of symptoms during a period of minutes or a few hours.[11] In the 17 remaining patients, progression of symptoms did not seem to develop after patients were first found by others. In many of this latter group, an accurate account of the earliest development of symptoms was not available because of aphasia, lack of awareness of the deficit, or stupor. A smooth, gradual worsening of function during minutes, followed by headache and vomiting, was the rule in larger lesions. Some patients who had stabilized during the first 24 to 48 hours later developed progressively decreased alertness and increasing focal signs within 48 to 72 hours, probably caused by the development of edema around the hematomas.

I find quite memorable an early description of the gradual evolution of symptoms in a fatal case of ICH.[20] This patient, seen in 1937, developed and evolved his hematoma while entirely under observation. He was sent to the hospital because of "malignant hypertension." While his history was taken, he noted weakness and dizziness. He reported that he noted numbness and tingling of the hands just before he left the admitting area during the time his heart was examined. He became extremely restless and apprehensive while his history was taken. He complained of inability to hear, difficulty in swallowing, and dyspnea. The patient was placed on the examining table, and his blood pressure was found to be 245 systolic and 170 diastolic. Under the eyes of several examiners, complete bilateral palsy of the sixth nerve developed; both pupils dilated, and the corneal reflexes disappeared. The patient was still able to talk, but with a typical bulbar speech, and he appeared almost completely deaf. His left leg became paretic, and rapid clonic

movements were observed. Babinski's sign was present bilaterally. Within an hour, the patient was completely stuporous and his blood pressure had risen to 280 systolic and 170 diastolic. The author commented that this rapidly progressive chain of events was most unpleasant to witness and produced a depressing effect on the nurses and physicians.[20]

I had a similar experience during my first week as a medical intern at the Boston City Hospital. An elderly hypertensive Chinese man came to the emergency room with slight weakness of his right limbs. He spoke normally. He was placed on the danger list, and a porter and I pushed his stretcher through the underground hospital tunnels toward the ward. As we pushed the stretcher, his right limbs became weaker, and he stopped talking. Soon, his eyes and head deviated to the left, and I could not rouse him. By the time we reached the ward, he was comatose and decerebrate. He died within hours.

Like Kornyey and his colleagues,[20] I felt helpless watching brain function inexorably vanish. When a detailed history is possible, nearly all patients with ICH have had a gradual evolution of symptoms and signs—some more rapidly evolving than others.[21]

Headache

Headache was not an invariable symptom in the 60 HSR patients with ICH. Headache was described in only 17 patients (28%) near the outset of neurologic symptoms.[11] Another seven patients (12%) noted headache later. Twenty-four patients (40%) had no headache at any time during their ICH. The 12 stuporous or comatose patients (20%) could not provide data regarding headache.[11] Headache was much more frequent with larger lesions, and was often absent or minimal in patients with small lesions.

Among 289 patients with ICH studied at one Portuguese hospital, 165 patients (57%) had a headache near the onset of their ICHs.[22] Headache was most common in patients with lobar and cerebellar hematomas, locations near the meningeal surface, and was common in patients with meningeal signs.[22] Patients with small, deep hematomas often never develop headache during their course of illness. In many patients, headache occurs as the hematoma enlarges and is accompanied by vomiting and decreased alertness.[21]

Decreased Level of Consciousness

Loss of consciousness accompanies only large hematomas and those found in the brainstem. Diminished alertness in patients with ICH is

13

caused by mass effect and increased ICP, or direct involvement of the brainstem reticular activating system. In the HSR, 30 of 60 patients were alert when first seen. Fourteen patients (23%) were lethargic, and 16 patients (27%) were stuporous or comatose.[11] In the Stroke Data Bank patients with ICH, decreased level of consciousness was the most important adverse prognostic sign. Decreased level of consciousness has been found to be an important prognostic sign in nearly all series of ICH patients.[21,23-25] In the Stroke Data Bank, all patients with ICH who had severely reduced levels of consciousness died.[23] Early reduction of consciousness is not an invariable accompaniment of ICH. When it occurs, however, it has an ominous prognosis. The sleepiness that developed in JT was a serious finding and should have triggered urgent evaluation and treatment when he arrived at the hospital.

Vomiting

JT started to vomit while he was taken to the hospital, and continued to vomit in the emergency room. Vomiting is an especially important sign in patients with ICH. In ICH and SAH, vomiting is usually caused by ICP or local distortion of the fourth ventricle. Few patients with ischemic lesions within the cerebral hemispheres vomit, but nearly one half of patients with hemispheral hemorrhages vomit. In the posterior circulation, vomiting usually reflects dysfunction of the vestibular nuclei, or the so-called vomiting center, in the floor of the fourth ventricle.[26] Vomiting occurs in approximately one third of patients with occlusive posterior circulation disease. Vomiting also occurs in more than one half of patients with posterior circulation hemorrhages. Patients with cerebellar hemorrhage almost always vomit early in their clinical course.

Seizures

Seizures are not common during the acute phase of a stroke, but are slightly more frequent in ICH than other stroke types, except embolism.[8,21] Among three series of patients with spontaneous nontraumatic ICH, 12.5%,[27] 15.4%,[28] and 17%[29] of patients had seizures during their early course. Lobar hemorrhages, slit-like hemorrhages situated near the gray-white junction of the cortex, and putaminal hemorrhages that undercut the cerebral cortex are especially epileptogenic.[30] Electrographic seizure discharges are often found by continuous EEG monitoring in patients with subcortical, large, and expanding hemorrhages.[30a]

Other Symptoms and Signs

Neck stiffness is uncommon in putaminal hemorrhage,[22] but is often found in patients with caudate, thalamic, and cerebellar hemorrhages.[30-32] Fever is relatively common, but is often related to infectious complications, such as pulmonary and urinary tract infections. Subhyaloid retinal hemorrhages, common in SAH, are rare in ICH, unless the hematoma has developed rapidly and is large.[33] Cardiac arrhythmias and pulmonary edema develop in some patients with ICH, and are usually attributed to changes in ICP and catecholamine release, a similar pathogenesis to that used to explain cardiac findings in patients with SAH.[21]

ETIOLOGIES

Although aneurysms and vascular malformations are important causes of ICH, I discuss these vascular lesions in Chapter 12 and do not repeat the discussions here.

Hypertension

The most common cause of ICH is hypertension, but the blood pressure does not need to be elevated to malignant ranges. Many patients present to the hospital with ICH and have no prior history of hypertension but have high blood pressure on admission. In this circumstance, it is difficult to know how much, if any, of the blood pressure elevation is secondary to raised ICP (the Cushing response), and what the level of blood pressure was before the bleed.

When hypertension first develops, the small arteries and capillaries are exposed to a high head of pressure and can leak. This situation is comparable to the hemodynamics found in patients with mitral valve stenosis. Left atrial failure develops because of mitral valve obstruction. The left atrial failure causes increased pressure in the pulmonary veins. To perfuse the lungs, pulmonary artery pressure rises to maintain an arteriovenous pressure gradient. The pulmonary capillaries and arterioles are exposed to the increased head of pressure and break, causing hemoptysis. Later, small arteries and arterioles hypertrophy, protecting the capillary bed from high central pressure. Hemoptysis becomes less frequent when arterioles hypertrophy, but the heart bears the brunt of the increased arterial resistance. In this instance, right heart failure may develop. Similarly, increased arterial pressure, early in the course of development of systemic hypertension, causes arteriolar and capillary rupture. Later in the course of hypertension, degenerative changes in the form of lipohyalinosis and miliary Charcot-Bouchard aneurysms develop, caused by long-standing blood pressure elevations. ICH occurs when these and related degenerative abnormalities cause arterial and arteriolar rupture. The occurrence of ICH is biphasic, with patients presenting both at the onset of hypertension and later, after developing considerable wear and tear on penetrating brain arteries.[34,35]

Some hypertensive hemorrhages arise from degenerative changes, such as fibrinoid degeneration and microaneurysms that develop in patients with hypertension. Cole and Yates examined the brains of 100 hypertensive patients and 100 normotensive controls.[36] All 13 patients with ICH had microaneurysms and were hypertensive. Among 63 patients with microaneurysms, 46 patients had hypertension recognized during life. The age distribution of microaneurysms was also interesting. Among 21 hypertensive patients younger than 50 years, only two patients had microaneurysms, whereas 71% of hypertensive patients in the 65- to 69-year age range had microaneurysms.[36]

Rosenblum analyzed the morphology of aneurysms and their parent vessels.[37] Some arteries had early aneurysmal dilatations, whereas others had sclerosed aneurysms with flask-shaped collections of collagen joined to a small artery by a narrow neck. Microaneurysms are often surrounded by hemosiderin-laden macrophages, indicating previous leakage. The lesions are most common in penetrating arteries that supply the basal ganglia, thalamus, pons and cerebellum, and arteries supplying the gray-white matter cortical junctions of the hemispheres. Figure 13-2 shows a section through a microaneurysm that

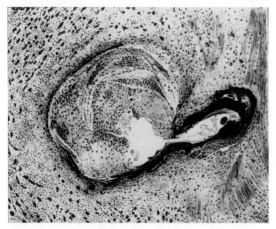

Figure 13-2. Section of a pontine aneurysm stained with hematoxylin and eosin and Sudan III. The sac is partially occluded by organizing blood clot. Recent hemorrhage is seen around the aneurysm. (From Green FHK: Miliary aneurysms in the brain. J Pathol Bacteriol 1930;33:71-77.)

was found associated with a hemorrhage in the pons. The same arteries that bear microaneurysms also contain foci of lipohyalinosis and fibrinoid degeneration, which explains the dictum that ischemic lacunes have the same relative distribution as hypertensive ICH.

Fisher described the results from examination of serial sections of patients with ICH. Fibrin globes, meshes of platelets encircled by a thin layer of fibrin, protruded from ruptured sites and clearly marked vessels that had bled.[12] A relationship between iris aneurysms and cerebral microaneurysms exists because rabbits with experimentally induced hypertension develop iris aneurysms approximately proportional to their development of cerebral microaneurysms.[38] Studies from Japan regarding surgical specimens of acute ICH show that penetrating arteries frequently break, but often not in relation to microaneurysms.[39,40] Degenerative lipohyalinotic changes were present in the broken and adjacent arteries. Degenerative changes caused by aging and hypertension can predispose to ICH, but microaneurysms may not often be the bleeding lesion.[35,39,40]

Considerable evidence has accumulated that shows acute changes in blood pressure and blood flow can precipitate rupture of penetrating arteries in the absence of prior hypertension.[34,35] In a large necropsy study of patients who died from ICH, Bakemuka used heart weights to estimate the frequency of hypertension; only 46% of fatal cases of spontaneous ICH had moderate to severe chronic hypertension or left ventricular hypertrophy.[41] Brott and colleagues reviewed the records of 154 patients with spontaneous ICH in Cincinnati, Ohio, during 1 year, to determine the frequency of past recognized hypertension.[42] Only 45% had a history of hypertension; another 12% without a history of hypertension had left ventricular hypertrophy. The authors judged that approximately 50% of cases were not attributable to chronic hypertension.[42]

In these two series,[41,42] the location of the hemorrhages, increased blood pressure on admission, and absence of other etiologies makes it highly probable that these hematomas were, in fact, satisfactorily classified as hypertensive ICH. Probably, hypertension was acute and led to bleeding from unprotected capillaries and arterioles. My own observations and those of others have documented ICH in situations in which blood pressure probably increased abruptly.[34,35]

My first experience with patients who had acute hypertension-related ICH was with patients who developed ICH after exposure to severe cold weather.[43] While outdoors in temperatures below −10° F, three patients developed putaminal,

13

thalamic, and cerebellar hematomas, respectively. One patient was in the midst of alcohol withdrawal, one was removing ice from his car window, and the third patient was waiting in line to pay rent. All had increased blood pressure on admission, but their pressures normalized soon thereafter. Immersion in cold is known to be a strong sympathetic nervous system stimulus. Formerly, the cold-pressor test (immersion of hands in ice water) was used clinically to induce transient hypertension, a phenomenon said to be more common in patients with essential hypertension.[44] Sympathetic stimulation caused by alcohol withdrawal and stress may have added to the effects of cold exposure in these patients.

Dental procedures,[45,46] surgery directly involving or placing traction on the trigeminal nerve,[47,48] and stimulation of the trigeminal nerve[49] have also been associated with ICH. In one patient known to have been previously normotensive, dental pain after irrigation of the mouth was followed immediately by a fatal temporal lobe hemorrhage.[45] Blood pressure was elevated acutely. Necropsy showed no evidence of hypertensive vascular damage in any organ and no other cause of brain hemorrhage.[45] In a series of patients operated on intracranially for trigeminal neuralgia, hematomas developed at locations typical for hypertensive ICH.[47] Other procedures involving manipulation of the trigeminal nerve for treatment of trigeminal neuralgia have also been complicated by ICH.[35,49] Monitoring of blood pressure and heart rate during trigeminal stimulation often shows important fluctuations in blood pressure and pulse rate.[50,51] The blood vessels of the brains of animals and humans have important trigeminal innervation.[52,53]

ICH also develops after the use of illicit drugs, especially cocaine and methamphetamine, which are known to have sympatheticomimetic effects. I discuss drug-induced ICH in more detail later in this chapter because of its growing frequency as an important cause of stroke and ICH. Patients have also developed ICH after sudden augmentation of cerebral blood flow, either locally to one hemisphere, as in the circumstance of ICH after carotid endarterectomy,[54-56] or systemically, after correction of congenital heart defects or cardiac transplantation in the young.[57,58] ICH has also been reported to develop during recovery from migraine.[34,59] Intense vasoconstriction leads to diminished flow and, perhaps, ischemia to local blood vessels. Reperfusion then leads to ICH in the zone of prior vascular damage. A similar mechanism probably underlies most examples of hemorrhagic infarction caused by brain embolism.[60] This mechanism of brain hemorrhage is discussed in detail in Chapter 9.

Probably more important than the unusual circumstances just cited are events of everyday life that can raise blood pressure. Wilson was quite aware of this concept. He wrote in his neurology text, "Emotional experience, joy, anger, fear, or apprehension may disturb the action of the heart, trivial though the incident may be—an address at a public meeting, trouble with a cook, and so on."[61]

> A patient of mine, LF, presented a vivid example of the possible interrelationship between daily activities and stresses, and the triggering of ICH. He was a retired university professor who came to ask my opinion about what he called a "strange stroke" he had a few years previously. Because he never had high blood pressure before or after the stroke, he was puzzled that his physicians attributed his condition to a hypertensive ICH. The events of his day are as follows:
>
> LF had an active teaching day, with more than the usual responsibilities. He hurried to finish his work so he could be on time for an engagement that night. His wife had symphony tickets. They planned to go with a couple (whom he considered to be unpleasant bores) to hear Mahler (whom he found tedious). He arrived late at the restaurant, and had a hurried and unpleasant meal. The two couples had to run to the symphony hall nearby to arrive in time to be seated, and they rushed to their seats in front. As he hustled toward his seat, he recalled thinking how wonderful it would have been to remain at work. He got to his seat in a sweat and noticed a gradually developing left hemiparesis.

I reviewed LF's CT and hospital records. A typical small right putaminal hemorrhage was present. His blood pressure was transiently elevated on arrival in the emergency room, but soon normalized. Acute fluctuations in blood pressure and flow and chronic degenerative changes are important in the etiology of so-called hypertensive ICH. In either case, bleeding is into the territories of penetrating arteries. It is not known whether the size, location, and clinical picture in these two types of hypertensive ICH differ.[35]

In the case of JT, he was hypertensive when first examined, but had no history of hypertension. Could the stressful interview have contributed to an acute blood pressure rise, or had he developed hypertension recently? His blood pressure stayed elevated during hospitalization, and he required antihypertensive treatment at the time of hospital discharge.

Older patients, often in their 70s or 80s, may present with ICH. Is this because of degenerative changes in these patients' arterial system? Does ICH occur because of coexistent amyloid angiopathy, which is recognized with increasing frequency when sought in elderly patients with lobar hemorrhages? Older patients seem to develop ICH at relatively lower blood pressures than younger patients. Probably because of atrophy, symptoms of increased ICP, such as headache, vomiting, and reduced alertness, are less common in older patients, even with sizable lesions. This observation makes differentiation between hemorrhage and infarction more difficult in geriatric patients.

Because hemorrhages arise from deep penetrating arteries, they primarily affect brain regions supplied by these vessels. The most common locations for hypertensive ICH in various series are: putamental-lateral ganglionic (25%-40%), thalamic (15%-30%), lobar (10%-30%), caudate (5%-10%), pontive (5%-10%), cerebellar (5%-10%), and intraventricular (0%-5%). In postmortem analyses, an increasing number of patients dying of lobar brain hemorrhages are found to have an unsuspected amyloid angiopathy. Rupture of fragile amyloid-encased arteries could be enhanced by raised arterial pressure.

Bleeding Diathesis

A variety of coagulopathies can lead to bleeding into the brain substance, sometimes accompanied by systemic bleeding. Anticoagulation with heparin or warfarin accounts for an all-too-high percentage of this type of ICH.[62,63] Considering the large number of patients treated with anticoagulants, the number that develop ICH is small. Among a series of 1626 patients treated with long-term anticoagulants, 30 had ICH, of which two-thirds were fatal.[62] The occurrence of anticoagulant-related ICH seems to be increasing.[63] The most consistent risk factor for intracranial or systemic bleeding was prolongation of the prothrombin time beyond the therapeutic range. Some hemorrhages occur even when the international normalized ratio is in the therapeutic range.[17,18] As with other etiologies of ICH, hypertension aggravates the tendency to bleed intracranially. The three features that characterize anticoagulant-induced ICH as distinct from other causes are as follows:

1. Hemorrhage often develops gradually and insidiously during many hours, or even days; 6 of 14 patients with anticoagulant-related ICH in one series had an insidious clinical course).[17,19]
2. The cerebellum and cerebral lobes are involved more frequently than in hypertensive ICH.[17,18,64]
3. A high morbidity and mortality rate exist (15 of 24 patients died),[17,18] and only patients with smaller hematomas (less than 30-cc volume) had a favorable chance for survival;

only 1 of 24 patients with ICH had bleeding elsewhere.

Anticoagulant-related ICH is a particularly difficult situation to treat because many patients take warfarin to prevent ischemic stroke. Patients with prosthetic heart valves, rheumatic mitral stenosis, or atrial fibrillation have a high risk for cerebral emboli without warfarin therapy. Especially when the indication for anticoagulants is strong and the early presenting symptoms are slight, treating physicians might be inclined to continue anticoagulant therapy. Treating physicians may not reverse the hypoprothrombinemia with vitamin K, activated factor VIIa, or fresh frozen plasma.[19] In my experience, this tactic is a mistake because many anticoagulant-related hemorrhages insidiously progress. Because of their size and location in the surgically accessible cerebellum and cerebral lobes, many eventually require life-saving surgery.

The initial clinical diagnosis may also be difficult in the group on warfarin for stroke prophylaxis because the first reaction to the neurologic symptoms is to predict that the patient had an ischemic stroke despite the treatment. I have found these two axioms useful:

1. If a patient on anticoagulants develops neurologic symptoms, the cause is anticoagulant-related hemorrhage until proven otherwise.
2. If anticoagulant hemorrhage is verified, immediately give vitamin K, factor VIIa, or fresh frozen plasma.

Pursue all measures aggressively to stop the bleeding. Although no formal prospective studies clarify the optimal time for restarting anticoagulants after ICH in patients who require long-term treatment, a retrospective analysis found that after 10 to 14 days, recurrent ICH did not develop.[65] The decision on if and when to restart anticoagulants depends on the risk of embolization from the donor source (atrial fibrillation, prosthetic heart valves, etc.) and the risk of further intracranial bleeding. Studies seem to show that the risk of embolization while anticoagulants are stopped is less than predicted and the risk of hemorrhage if anticoagulants are reintroduced is also less than expected.[66,67] I suggest waiting a week or 10 days, timing that seems practical, and reinitiating anticoagulation with heparin rather than coumadin. When the indication for anticoagulation is relative or questionable, it is probably best to discontinue anticoagulants, perhaps using platelet antiaggregants instead.

Leukemia, hemophilia, thrombocytopenia, von Willebrand disease, and disseminated intravascular coagulation are other important causes of ICH,

13

although it is unusual in these disorders for bleeding to be confined only to the brain. Patients given recombinant tissue plasminogen activator to treat coronary artery thrombosis sometime develop ICH, most often in the cerebral lobes or cerebellum.[68] The frequency is rather low, but the brain hematomas are usually devastating or fatal.[68] ICH also occurs after recombinant tissue plasminogen activator infusion to treat occlusive cerebrovascular lesions. In this circumstance, hematomas usually begin within the region of brain infarction.

Drugs

A variety of commonly abused substances are known to cause ICH.[69,70] Alert clinicians should always think of the possibility of drug-related hemorrhage in young patients, in whom other causes of ICH, except trauma and arteriovenous malformations (AVMs), are rare. Perhaps best known are amphetamine ("speed") hemorrhages. Hemorrhage often develops within a few minutes of drug use. The most frequent presenting symptoms are headache, confusion, and seizures.[69-71] Despite large-volume ICHs, few focal signs are present in such patients. This phenomenon is perhaps explained by the frequent coexistence of brain edema, infarcts, and a diffuse vasculopathy, in addition to the focal ICH. In some patients, acute hypertension follows amphetamine use and can potentiate ICH. When first examined by physicians, most patients with amphetamine hemorrhage do not have signs of sympathetic overactivity, such as hypertension, tachycardia, or fever.[69-72]

Citron et al studied 14 drug abusers, almost all admitting use of methamphetamine, among other drugs.[73] At necropsy, a fibrinoid necrosis of the media and intima of small- and medium-sized arteries existed, resembling polyarteritis nodosa.[73] Rumbaugh and colleagues studied the angiographic features of a group of methamphetamine abusers and noted beaded arteries with segmental constriction and dilatation of intracranial arteries.[74] In monkeys given intravenous amphetamines, angiography showed similar changes as found in human patients. Necropsy showed small brain hemorrhages, zones of infarction, microaneurysms, and a vasculitis similar to that described by Citron.[75]

I reviewed 30 reported, well-documented examples of intracranial hemorrhage after amphetamine use.[69] Twenty-four patients were known drug abusers; some patients also used other drugs, and many often used alcohol. Amphetamine, methamphetamine, and dextroamphetamine were the most frequently used drugs. Seventeen individuals (57%) took oral amphetamines, 12 (40%) administered the drug intravenously, and one person inhaled amphetamine nasally. Amphetamine (14% of patients) and methamphetamine use were more often responsible for hemorrhage than dextroamphetamine (4%) use in causing intracranial bleeding. The dose used was often unknown or unstated, but hemorrhage followed doses as small as 20 mg of oral amphetamine.[69,72] Age among the 22 men and eight women ranged from 19 to 51 years, with an average age of 25.4 years.[69] In 23 individuals, the bleeding was intracerebral and most often lobar. In contrast to cocaine-related hemorrhage, only 1 of the 30 individuals (3%) had an underlying vascular lesion in the form of an aneurysm or AVM.[69,76] Amphetamine-related hemorrhage can be serious; seven patients with hemorrhage died (23%), and nine required surgical drainage (30%).[69] A potent solid form of d-methamphetamine base that can be smoked is now peddled in the streets (known as *ice*). This form is more potent and rapid acting. The ice-amphetamine relation has the potential to prove similar to the crack-cocaine-hydrochloride relationship in terms of complications and potency.

Angiography has often shown striking abnormalities in chronic amphetamine users and other patients with amphetamine-related ICH. Most common are segmental areas of constriction, irregularity, and occasionally fusiform dilatation.[69,72,77,78] The focal vascular abnormalities usually emphasize superficial cortical arterial branches and are often referred to as *beading*. At times, the changes disappear on subsequent angiography.[77] Unfortunately, these arteriographic changes have often been falsely attributed to arteritis. Beading and areas of vasoconstriction and dilatation is a non-specific sign and more often than not is not due to arteritis.[79] Amphetamines are known to be potent vasoconstrictors. Vasoconstriction can become chronic and produce chronic morphologic changes in the media of involved arteries. Segmental changes and beading in some amphetamine users is probably caused by pharmacologic effects of the drugs used, and does not represent a true arteritis.

Since the early 1980s, cocaine has become a very important cause of stroke and drug-related ICH. Cocaine hydrochloride is usually snorted nasally. Some addicts use crack cocaine, a substance made by mixing aqueous cocaine hydrochloride with ammonia and sometimes baking soda. Crack cocaine is smoked or inhaled after the cocaine is mixed in the alkaline solution and is precipitated as alkaloidal cocaine. Crack cocaine is absorbed quickly, reaching the brain in less than 10 seconds.[69] Cocaine hydrochloride can be taken in a variety of ways—orally, vaginally, rectally, sublingually, nasally, and by subcutaneous, intramuscular, or intravenous injection. Cardiovascular effects begin immediately after use and consist of an increase in pulse, blood pressure, temperature, and metabolism. The pressor effects of cocaine are similar to those of amphetamine and are probably mediated through a peripheral catecholamine mechanism.[69,70,80,81]

In a 1994 text, I reviewed 45 examples of cocaine-related ICH.[69] The series included 28 men and 17 women, with ages ranging from 22 to 57 years (average age, 33.6 years). Headache, focal neurologic signs, and sudden loss of consciousness were the most frequent symptoms and usually began immediately or shortly after the episode of drug use.[69,81] Concurrent use of alcohol was common. ICH followed use of cocaine by any route. Fifteen individuals used crack, 14 snorted cocaine nasally, and 11 injected the drug intravenously. The acute mortality was relatively high (14 out of 45, 31%).[69]

The most common location of cocaine-related ICH was lobar (57%). In others, the bleeding often involved deep structures known to be frequent sites of hypertensive ICH. These included one caudate, three thalamic, and eight putaminal hematomas. Of great interest and importance was the frequent presence of an underlying vascular lesion. Twelve patients had AVMs, three had aneurysms, and one had a glioma with recurrent hemorrhage.[69] Similarly, among 31 patients who developed SAH after cocaine use, 15 (48%) had aneurysms. Among 29 patients with adequate angiographic or necropsy study, or both, 25 (86%) had aneurysms.[69] Cocaine-related ICH has a high mortality and high frequency of underlying aneurysms and AVMs. Clearly, cocaine-related intracranial bleeding is an indication for angiography, especially when the bleeding is subarachnoid or lobar. Underlying vascular lesions are less common when the ICH is deep. Most authors have attributed cocaine-related hemorrhage to the sympatheticomimetic effects of the drug. In some reported cases, the blood pressure is high after admission (i.e., 210 to 240 systolic and 110 to 140 diastolic).[69] Some patients have had a hypertensive encephalopathy with multiple ICHs and brain edema. An example of these changes is shown in Figure 11-17.

Another drug known to have sympatheticomimetic capabilities is phencyclidine, known as PCP or angel dust, which has also been occasionally implicated as a cause of ICH,[82,83] and hypertensive encephalopathy.[84] Two other hallucinogens, lysergic acid diethylamide (known as LSD) and mescaline, are also known to raise blood pressure and cause vasoconstriction. To my knowledge, however, no reports document ICH after use of these drugs.

More controversial is the issue of ICH after use of amphetamine-like drugs that are mostly used as anorexic agents to lose weight, and were an ingredient in some cold remedies. These drugs are usually sold over the counter as diet suppressants or stimulants. The most commonly cited agent is phenylpropanolamine (PPA), which is often combined with an antihistamine and caffeine. PPA is primarily a partial alpha-adrenergic agonist and has little, if any, beta-adrenergic agonist activity.[85] PPA was used by individuals who developed ICH, but the numbers are relatively small, considering the frequency of use. Among 19 patients, only four were men.[69] Ten of the 19 patients were younger than 30 years. In some, the PPA compounds were taken in high doses in suicidal attempts. Two patients had SAH only, and 17 patients had ICH (two of which were multiple).[86,87] Twelve PPA-related hematomas were lobar, seven were putaminal-capsular, and two were thalamic.[69] Blood pressures recorded on initial examination were usually within the normal range, but some were high (i.e., 210/130 mm Hg, 160/104 mm Hg, and 210/110 mm Hg). PPA-related hemorrhages have been most often described after use for weight control and the dosage was often higher than suggested. PPA ingestion in the usual amounts elevates blood pressure by only a few millimeters. In some individuals, there may be an idiosyncratic reaction with more severe blood pressure rises. There are very few cases of hemorrhage after use of cold remedies, but PPA has been removed from cold remedies in many countries.

Segmental vascular changes on angiography, similar to those found after amphetamine use, have been described.[88] In one patient, the angiographic changes cleared after abstinence from PPA for 1 month.[88] In four patients, histologic analysis of tissue removed at surgical drainage of hematomas was available. Three patients had no indication of vascular lesion on light microscopy, but the fourth patient did have a necrotizing vasculitis.[89]

Examples of putative PPA-related hemorrhages are difficult to evaluate. In some cases, use of diet pills was surely incidental, and in other patients, other multiple drugs and risk factors coexisted.[69] In several patients, ICH occurred a few weeks postpartum, a time of vulnerability for spontaneous vascular complications. Although PPA has been shown to be associated with ICH in experimental animals and humans,[69,85-91] reactions to PPA compounds are often idiosyncratic. A risk of ICH clearly exists for those who use PPA in a higher-than-suggested dose. Prior hypertension; additional use of alcohol, coffee, or caffeine; concomitant use of monoamine oxidase inhibitors; and use during the postpartum period increase the risk of hemorrhage after PPA ingestion.

Occasionally, ICH develops after the intravenous use of drugs that are manufactured for oral consumption, such as pentazocine and pyribenzamine ("T's and blues") or methylphenidate.[69,92] Talc, methylcellulose crystals, and cornstarch obliterate the lung arterioles, allowing the injected particles to reach the systemic circulation after intravenous use. The damage to brain arterioles then predisposes users to develop ICH.[92]

Occasional examples of intracerebral hemorrhage have been described after the use of phosphodiesterase inhibitors (sildenafil [Viagra], vardenafil [Levitra], and tadalafil [Cialis]) prescribed to enhance erectile function in men.[92a-d] It is not clear if the intracerebral hemorrhages in these patients was explained by increased blood pressure during sexual intercourse, or by the phosphodiesterase inhibitors alone, or a combination of the agents and circulatory changes accompanying sexual activity.

Cerebral Amyloid Angiopathy

Congophilic or cerebral amyloid angiopathy (CAA) was recognized by Zenkevich as a potential cause of ICH,[93] but Jellinger is probably most responsible for bringing this disorder to the attention of the neurologic community.[94,95] I discuss this condition in Chapter 11.

Awareness of CAA has led to wider use of special stains and recognition that an ever-increasing percentage of ICH, especially in the elderly, is related to CAA. The disorder usually affects small arteries and arterioles in the leptomeninges and cerebral cortex; involved arteries are thickened by an acellular hyaline material that stains positively with periodic acid-Schiff stains, and has an apple-green birefringence with polarized Congo red stain.[96] Figure 11-10 shows a brain section that contains amyloid-staining arterioles. Sometimes, the vessel wall seems to be reduplicated or split. CAA predominantly affects persons older than 65 years and increases in frequency in the eighth and ninth decades[96]; in some series of patients, a striking female predilection exists.[97-99] At necropsy, most patients have senile plaques, and many patients have been diagnosed clinically with Alzheimer's disease.

Amyloid-laden arteries are most often found in the occipital and parietal regions, less often in the other cerebral lobes; rarely, if ever, are these arteries found in the deep basal gray matter or brainstem. They are occasionally found in the cerebellum. Hemorrhages may be quite large and are often multiple.[98-101] Some patients have recurrent ICH or SAH in different lobar sites, a finding in an elderly person that is virtually diagnostic of CAA. At necropsy, small scattered cerebral infarcts and Alzheimer's-related changes are found, along with evidence of old slit-like lobar hemorrhages. Echo planar MRI scans often show many small old hemorrhages, usually referred to as microbleeds.[102-105] Microbleeds are associated with white matter abnormalities and are likely predictive of future hemorrhages in patients with cerebral amyloid angiopathy.[101-104] Some patients have a Binswanger-like picture, with chronic white matter gliosis and atrophy. Like anticoagulant-related hemorrhages, CAA-related hemorrhages may develop insidiously. Perhaps because of coexisting atrophy, pressure symptoms, such as headache and vomiting, are less frequent than in younger patients with hypertensive or AVM-related hemorrhages.

Trauma

Trauma is an important cause of intracerebral bleeding. In some patients, a traumatic etiology is not clear from the history. I have seen several patients who were rendered aphasic or stuporous by head blows delivered by others and who could give no history of the trauma; assailants and others did not disclose their complicity. In other patients, retrograde amnesia developed after the head injury, and patients had no recollection of a fall or other injury. A search for superficial head bruises or lacerations is worthwhile when the etiology of ICH is not obvious. Traumatic ICH is most often accompanied by contusions in the basal frontal and temporal lobes, which may be multiple.[106] Occasionally, a late or delayed hemorrhage, referred to as a *spät hemorrhage*, develops into an area of traumatic brain edema when the local swelling subsides.[106,107]

Other Causes and the Frequency of Various Etiologies

Brain tumors[108] and vasculitis and vasculopathies of various types[109] are occasionally complicated by ICH. Rare patients with a mutation in a gene that encodes type IV collagen alpha 1 chain (COL4A1) have genetically influenced intracerebral and subdural hemorrhages that develop especially after trauma, dilated perivascular spaces and a diffuse leukoencephalopathy.[109a,b] Dural sinus and cerebral venous thrombosis is another important cause of ICH and is discussed in Chapter 16. Table 13-1 lists the frequencies of common etiologies among six large series of ICH patients.[110-117] Table 13-2 shows the frequency of various causes of ICH in a series of 200 Mexican patients younger

Table 13-1. Causes of Intracerebral Hemorrhage in Large Series of Patients

	Russell[101] n (%)	Mutlu[102] n (%)	McCormick[103] n (%)	Schutz[104] n (%)	Jellinger[105] n (%)	Weisbeg[106] n (%)	Qureshi[107] n (%)
Hypertension	232 (50)	135 (60)	37 (26)	140 (56)	80 (47)	197 (66)	311 (77)
Vascular malformations, including aneurysms	117 (25)	50 (22)	35 (24)	30 (12)	53 (31)	28 (9)	11 (3)
Bleeding disorder, including thrombolysis/anticoagulation	36 (8)	30 (13)	28 (20)	21 (8)	5 (3)	14 (5)	8 (2)
Tumor	9 (2)	2 (1)	13 (9)	8 (3)	12 (7)	5 (2)	—
Arteritis	13 (3)	2 (1)	5 (3)	2 (1)	2 (1)	—	—
Other	38 (8)	6 (3)	14 (10)	—	13 (8)	2 (1)	—
Unknown	16 (4)	—	12 (8)	49 (20)	5 (3)	50 (17)	73 (18)
Totals	461	225	144	250	170	296	403

Data from Caplan LR, Kase CS: Mechanisms of Intracerebral Hemorrhage. In Kase CS, Caplan LR (eds): Intracerebral Hemorrhage. Boston: Butterworth-Heinemann, 1994, pp 95-98.

Table 13-2. Frequency of Location of Intracerebral Hemorrhage by Cause in Patients <40 Years Old

Cause	Lobar n = 110	Ganglionic n = 43	Brainstem n = 26	Cerebellum n = 10	Intraventricular n = 8	Mixed n = 3
Hypertension, n = 22	2	16	3	0	0	1
Arteriovenous malformation, n = 67	45	7	6	6	3	0
Cavernous angioma, n = 32	15	3	11	2	1	0
Cerebral venous thrombosis, n = 10	9	1	0	0	0	0
Drugs, n = 7	3	4	0	0	0	0
Toxemia, n = 7	3	4	0	0	0	0
Other, n = 14	9	1	0	1	2	1
Unknown, n = 41	24	7	6	1	2	1

Data from Ruiz-Sandoval JL, Cantu C, Barinagarrementeria F: Intracerebral hemorrhage in young people: Analysis of risk factors, locations, causes, and prognosis. Stroke 1999;30:537-541; and Kase CS: Intracranial Tumors. In Kase CS, Caplan LR (eds): Intracerebral Hemorrhage. Boston: Butterworth-Heinemann 1994, pp 243-261.

than 40 years. This table illustrates the locations of hemorrhages in patients with these etiologies.[118]

SIGNS AND SYMPTOMS OF INTRACEREBRAL HEMORRHAGE AT COMMON LOCATIONS

Just as there are physicians who believe that the introduction of chest x-rays made the stethoscope obsolete, some doctors believe that detailed knowledge of the findings on neurologic examination of patients with central nervous system lesions is no longer necessary since the advent of CT and MRI scans. Because hemorrhages are so well imaged by CT, why bother to learn the physical findings? In the future, physicians will probably not have an inexpensive pocket or portable CT or MRI to replace the examination of patients. Prognosis and treatment of ICH often depend on the locale of the hemorrhage. Particular locations (i.e., cerebral lobes, right putamen, and cerebellum) are relatively accessible to surgical drainage, whereas others (i.e., thalami and brainstem) are not accessible. Clinical distinction between ICH and superficial cerebral infarction caused by large vessel occlusive disease or cerebral embolism depends on localization of the lesion to deep (ICH) or superficial (infarct) location. Knowledge of findings in patients with hemorrhages at various locations teaches clinicians to search for tumors, abscesses, demyelinating lesions, and other disorders in the same locations in other patients. Historically, hemorrhages in the cerebellum, thalami, and caudate nucleus were recognized before cerebellar, thalamic, or caudate infarction. Awareness of the clinical syndromes associated with ICH in these locations made it possible to later recognize infarcts in these regions. For these and many other reasons, it is still important for clinicians to know the common clinical syndromes in ICH and be able to localize clinically the lesion in most patients with intracranial hemorrhages.[119]

Keys to localization of ICH follow:

1. Motor signs—quadriparesis, hemiparesis, or no paresis
2. Pupillary function—asymmetry, size, and light reaction
3. Extraocular movements—supranuclear, nuclear, internuclear gaze palsies
4. Gait abnormalities, especially ataxia

Figure 13-3 and Table 13-3 summarize the usual abnormalities of these functions in patients with hemorrhages at the most common locations of ICH.

Hemorrhages of the Lateral Basal Ganglia, Putamen, and Internal Capsule

The most common location of hypertensive ICH is the lateral basal ganglionic capsular region.[120,121] These lesions are usually referred to as putaminal hemorrhage because they most often begin in the putamen. The usual findings include contralateral hemiparesis, contralateral hemisensory loss, and conjugate deviation of the eyes toward the side of the hematoma. The pupils are generally normal and gait is hemiparetic. Patients with a left putaminal hemorrhage usually have a nonfluent aphasia with relative preservation of ability to repeat spoken language. Right-sided lesions are associated with left visual neglect, motor impersistence, and constructional dyspraxia. These abnormalities of higher cortical function are probably caused by disconnection and undercutting of cortical zones, and are usually more transient than in patients with cortical infarcts of equal size. Some patients develop ipsilateral adventitious movements that the family or observers call "tremor"; these movements are probably caused by involvement of ipsilateral descending projections of the extrapyramidal system.

In patients with large putaminal hemorrhages, stupor increases as the lesion enlarges; the ipsilateral pupil at first becomes smaller, and later, larger than the opposite pupil; the ipsilateral plantar response becomes extensor; and a bilateral horizontal gaze palsy develops. The presence of any of these signs—ipsilateral Babinski's sign, abnormal ipsilateral pupil, or ipsilateral gaze paresis—has a grim prognosis.[11,23,120] These additional findings are caused by midline shift or compression of the rostral brainstem by the expanding hematoma. Figure 13-4 shows necropsy brain specimens of large putaminal hemorrhages.

The findings described above are those found in patients with large hematomas, which involve the medial and most anterior portions of the posterior putamen, and the anterior two thirds of the posterior limb of the internal capsule.[120-123] This location is the most common site for putaminal hemorrhage because it is supplied by the largest of the lateral lenticulostriate arteries. Some lesions affect the anterior limb of the internal capsule and anterior putamen and

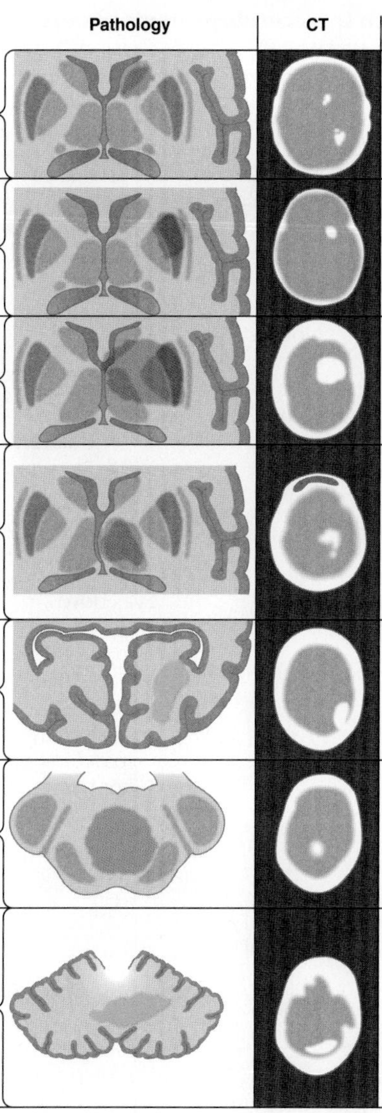

	Pathology	CT	Pupils	Eye movements	Motor and sensory deficits	Other
Caudate nucleus (blood in ventricle)			Sometimes ipsilaterally constricted	Conjugate deviation to side of lesion, slight ptosis	Contralateral hemiparesis, often transient	Headache, confusion
Putamen (small hemorrhage)			Normal	Conjugate deviation to side of lesion	Contralateral hemiparesis and hemisensory loss	Aphasia (if lesion on left side)
Putamen (large hemorrhage)			In presence of herniation, pupil dilated on side of lesion	Conjugate deviation to side of lesion	Contralateral hemiparesis and hemisensory loss	Decreased consciousness
Thalamus			Constricted, poorly reactive to light bilateraly	Both lids retracted. Eyes positioned downward and medially. Cannot look upward	Slight contralateral hemiparesis, but greater hemisensory loss	Aphasia (if lesion on left side)
Occipital lobar white matter			Normal	Normal	Mild, transient hemiparesis	Contralateral hemianopsia
Pons			Constricted, reactive to light	No horizontal movements. Vertical movements preserved	Quadriplegia	Coma
Cerebellum			Slight constriction on side of lesion	Slight deviation to opposite side. Movements toward side of lesion impaired, or sixth cranial nerve palsy	Ipsilateral limb ataxia. No hemiparesis	Gait ataxia, vomiting

Figure 13-3. Clinical manifestations related to site in intracerebral hemorrhage.

produce a less severe, more transient hemiparesis without sensory abnormalities.[120-122] When hematomas are in the posterior third of the internal capsule and far posterior extreme of the putamen, sensory abnormalities predominate, with little or no hemiparesis. An inferior quadrantanopia or hemianopia may be present. Patients with lesions in the far posterior left putamen may have fluent Wernicke-like aphasia because of undercutting of the temporal lobe or extension of the lesion into the temporal isthmus, giving the hematoma a hockey stick-like configuration. Figure 13-5 shows the anatomic distribution of lesions within the lateral basal ganglionic region on horizontal brain section.

The most common and largest lesions affecting the anterior part of the posterior limb of the internal capsule are often referred to as the middle type, whereas the others are termed anterior or posterior types of putaminal hematomas.[120,121] Lateral ganglionic hemorrhages occur in the distribution of the various medial and lateral lenticulostriate arteries. Figure 13-6 shows various typical putaminal hematomas.

Putaminal hemorrhages vary greatly in size. In one series of 24 patients, the smallest hematoma volume was 20 mm^2, whereas the largest was 225 mm^2.[30] Patients with small hematomas, as shown in Figures 13.6A and 13.7, have a good outcome. Larger hemorrhages are more

13

Table 13-3. Neurologic Findings in Patients with Intracerebral Hemorrhage at Common Sites

Locale	Motor Weakness	Sensory Loss	Hemianopia	Pupils	Eye Movements	Other
Caudate	Hemiparesis	−	−	Normal	−Normal or transient conjugate gaze palsy contralateral	Confusion
Putamen						
Small	Hemiparesis ++	+	−	Normal	−	−
Large	Hemiparesis ++++	++	++	± Ipsilateral fixed, dilated	Conjugate palsy contralateral	L: aphasia R: left–sided neglect, con-struc-tional apraxia
Thalamus	Hemiparesis +	+++	±	Small, nonreactive	Eyes down, or down and in; vertical gaze palsy; conjugate gaze palsy ipsilateral or contralateral; pseudo VI nerve palsy	Confusion L: apha-sia
Lobar	Hemiparesis ±					Abular
Frontal		−	−	Normal	−	L: aplasia
Parietal		+++	++	Normal	−	R: Left–sided neglect, con-struc-tional apraxia
Temporal	−	−	++	Normal	−	L: aphasia, agitation
Occipital	− or tran-sient	− or tran-sient	++++	Normal	−	−
Pontine (me-dial basil) (lateral tegmental)	Quadripa-resis ++++	±	−	Small reaction	Bilateral horizontal conjugate gaze palsy, bobbing	Hyperven-tilation
Cerebellar	− or tran-sient	Contralateral hemisen-sory +++	−	Ipsilateral small reaction	1 − {½} syndrome	Limb ataxia
	−	−	−	Small reaction	Ipsilateral sixth nerve palsy of ipsilateral conjugate gaze palsy	Gait ataxia

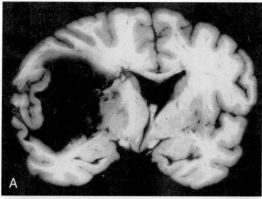

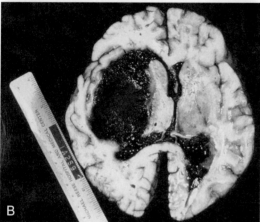

Figure 13-4. Large putaminal hemorrhages. **A,** A coronal section of the brain at necropsy showing a large hemorrhage on the left of the figure. The insular cortex is displaced laterally and the basal ganglia are displaced medially. The hemorrhage has drained into the lateral ventricles. The midline is shifted to the right. **B,** Axial section (in usual CT plane) of the brain at necropsy showing a very large putaminal hemorrhage that displaces the midline and drains into the lateral ventricles. (From Kase CS, Caplan LR: Putaminal hemorrhage. In Kase CS, Caplan LR (eds): Intracerebral Hemorrhage. Boston: Butterworth-Heinemann, 1994, pp 309-327 with permission.)

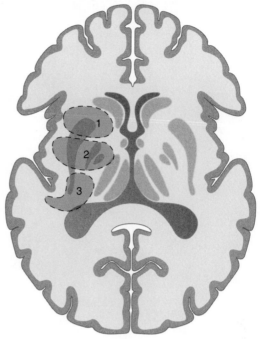

Figure 13-5. Artist's cartoon drawing of an axial brain section showing, using circles, the loci of putaminal hemorrhages: (1) anterior type involving anterior putamen and anterior limb of the internal capsule, (2) middle type involving the capsular genu and the globus pallidus and middle portion of the putamen, and (3) posterior type involving the far posterior limb of the internal capsule and often affecting the optic radiations and spreading into the temporal lobe isthmus.

likely to rupture into the ventricle, and have a much higher mortality than small putaminal hematomas.[30,120,121,124] Most often, bleeding extends along the anteroposterior axis of the brain, but some lesions are globoid, and others extend laterally toward the cortical surface along white matter tracts.[30,120,121] Analysis of CT scans at the level of the body of the lateral ventricles can help prognosticate the likelihood of recovery from hemiplegia.[122] When the hematoma occupies CT sections containing the bodies of the lateral ventricles, then the middle type of hematoma is usually present and hemiplegia is likely to persist. When this region is free of bleeding, hemiparesis is more

often absent, slight, or transient.[122] The multiple planes shown in MRI imaging make it easier to visualize the location, spread, and size of hematomas. T2*-weighted (susceptibility) images show hemorrhages best.

Cerebral angiography may be helpful in studying patients with putaminal hemorrhage. Using microangiography, Mizukami and colleagues studied 60 postmortem specimens from patients with ICH.[125] They identified the source of bleeding as lateral lenticulostriate arteries, analyzed the postmortem displacement of these vessels, and correlated their findings with the angiographic anatomy in 100 other patients with autopsy or surgically confirmed ICH.[125] In large putaminal hemorrhages, the most lateral lenticulostriate arteries are displaced medially, increasing the distance between the most lateral lenticulostriate arteries and the insular artery. Anterior and posterior lesions have different patterns of displacement of lenticulostriate arteries.[125]

Since the mid-1980s, positron emission tomography and single-photon emission computed tomography have yielded insights into the

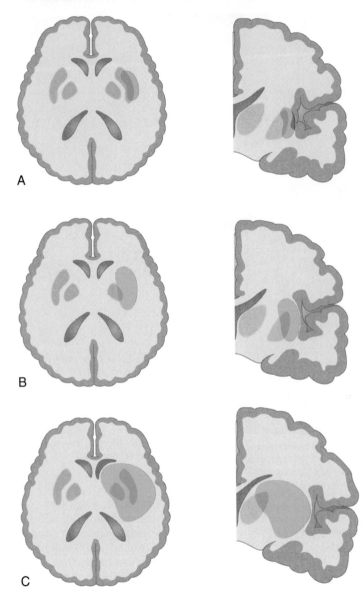

Figure 13-6. Examples of putaminal hemorrhage. **A,** Hemorrhage within the boundaries of the putamen. **B,** Encroachment on the internal capsule. **C,** Hematoma compressing lateral ventricle.

clinical findings in patients with putaminal hemorrhage.[126] Anterior lesions show depression of frontal lobe function ipsilaterally, whereas posterior lesions more often affect the temporal and parietal lobes. The pattern of cortical depression in left cerebral hematomas helps predict aphasia type and recovery.[126]

Caudate Hemorrhage

Hemorrhage into the caudate nucleus accounts for approximately 7% of ICH.[121,127-129] Hematomas at this site frequently discharge quickly into the adjacent lateral ventricle, or may spread laterally toward the internal capsule or inferiorly toward the hypothalamus. Early ventricular dilatation by blood probably accounts for the most common symptoms of caudate hemorrhage—headache, vomiting, decreased alertness, and stiff neck.[127-130] Figure 13-8 is a CT scan showing a caudate hemorrhage that emptied into the adjacent lateral ventricle. Some patients also are confused, disoriented, and have poor memory.[127-130] The larger parenchymatous hematomas cause a contralateral hemiparesis, conjugate deviation of the eyes to the side of the lesion, conjugate gaze palsy to the opposite side, and an ipsilateral

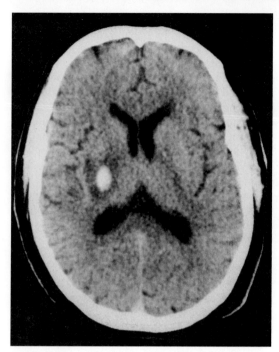

Figure 13-7. CT showing a small left putaminal hemorrhage.

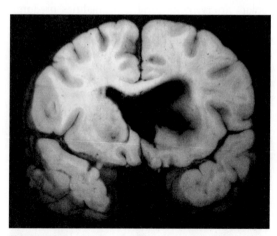

Figure 13-8. Necropsy brain specimen showing a caudate hemorrhage that extended into the adjacent lateral ventricle. (From Caplan LR: Caudate hemorrhage. In Kase CS, Caplan LR (eds): Intracerebral Hemorrhage. Boston: Butterworth-Heinemann, 1994, pp 329-340, with permission.)

small pupil or Horner's syndrome.[121,127,129] Sensory findings are usually absent or minimal. The usual cause of caudate hemorrhage is hypertension, but AVMs are also common, especially in the young. Caudate hematomas have a better prognosis than comparable-sized putaminal hemorrhages.

Symptoms and signs of caudate hemorrhage closely mimic SAH, but the CT appearance of blood in the caudate and lateral ventricles is distinctive.

Thalamic Hemorrhage

Neurologic signs in patients with thalamic hemorrhages differ greatly depending on the size, location within the thalamus of the hematoma, and dissection into and pressure effects on the third ventricle and adjacent brain structures.[131,132] The largest hemorrhages are located in the ventrolateral and posteromedial portions of the thalamus in the territories of the thalamogeniculate and thalamic-subthalamic arteries.[132] Other hemorrhages are located anteriorly in the territory of the tuberothalamic (polar) arteries and dorsally in the territory of the lateral posterior choroidal arteries.[132]

Most thalamic hematomas are posterior to the pyramidal-tract fibers in the internal capsule, so that contralateral sensory abnormalities are usually more prominent than contralateral hemiparesis. Some large thalamic hematomas dissect laterally and rostrally and involve the anterior portion of the posterior limb of the internal capsule, causing a hemiplegia. Sometimes, limbs contralateral to hematomas are slightly ataxic or have choreic movements. The contralateral hand may rest in a fisted or dystonic posture. The key neurologic findings that separate thalamic from caudate or putaminal hemorrhages are the eye signs. Patients with caudate or putaminal hemorrhages have conjugate deviation of the eyes toward the side of the lesion and paresis of conjugate gaze to the opposite side. The characteristic oculomotor abnormalities in patients with thalamic hematomas are as follows:

1. Paralysis of upward gaze, often with one or both eyes resting downward
2. Hyperconvergence of one or both eyes,[33,131-133] with a combination of these findings giving patients the appearance of peering downward and inward at the tops of their noses
3. Ocular skewing, in which one eye rests below the other, with this divergence in vertical eye position remaining constant in gaze in all directions
4. Eyes gazing the wrong way resting toward the opposite side[33,131]
5. Disconjugate gaze, with limited abduction of one or both eyes (so-called pseudo sixth-nerve paresis[131,134]), failure of ocular abduction caused by visual fixation of the adducted eye, and increased convergence vectors neutralizing abduction-not caused by involvement of the sixth nerve[134]

These oculomotor abnormalities are caused by direct extension of the hematoma to the

13

diencephalic-mesencephalic junction or compression of the quadrigeminal plate region by the thalamic hematoma. In thalamic hemorrhage, the pupils are usually small and react poorly to light because of interruption of the afferent limb of the pupillary reflex arc.

Patients with large left thalamic hemorrhages often have an unusual aphasia.[131,135-137] After beginning a conversation almost normally, patients may lapse into a remarkable fluent aphasia, with many jargon or nonexistent words and poor communication of ideas. In contrast to patients with Wernicke's aphasia, comprehension of spoken language is good. Patients with thalamic ICH may repeat and duplicate words or syllables at the ends of words in spoken and written language. Paraphasic errors and poor naming are also common. Patients with right thalamic hematomas often have left visual neglect, anosognosia, and visual-spatial abnormalities.[130,138]

Decreased levels of alertness and hypersomnolence are common at the onset of thalamic hemorrhage because of involvement of the rostral reticular activating system. The prognosis for recovery from thalamic hemorrhages is not as good as caudate or putaminal hemorrhages of comparable size, but coma is not as dire a prognostic sign in thalamic lesions as it is in other supratentorial sites. Also, unlike putaminal hemorrhage, the severity of the deficit and mortality do not correlate with ventricular extension in patients with thalamic

hematomas.[139] Figure 13-9 shows a CT scan from a patient with an anterior-thalamic hematoma, which spread into the ventricles. She made an excellent recovery. Figure 13-10 shows a necropsy specimen of a patient with an anterior thalamic hemorrhage who died of a medical complication. Thalamic hemorrhages are not accessible surgically unless they extend far laterally. Most studies have not differentiated medial from lateral or posterior thalamic hematomas, although lesions at these various sites yield different clinical syndromes and have different prognoses for recovery.[131,132]

Since the mid-1980s, it is possible to distinguish syndromes related to small discrete hemorrhages in the thalamus using MRI and CT.[132,140,141] Posterolateral thalamic hematomas in the territory of the thalamogeniculate arteries are the most common and largest type of thalamic hematomas. These lesions often spill out of the thalamus laterally and may cause motor paralysis by involving the internal capsule. Sensorimotor signs predominate, and pupillary and eye-movement abnormalities are slight or absent, unless the hematoma is quite large and spreads to or compresses the medial thalamus.[131,132] Anterior or anterolateral thalamic hematomas are in the distribution of the tuberothalamic (polar) artery; behavioral abnormalities predominate, especially apathy and abulia.[131,132] Posteromedial hematomas are in the distribution of the thalamic-subthalamic thalamoperforating arteries; abnormalities of consciousness, pupillary function, and vertical gaze predominate. These hematomas often spread to the third ventricle and can compress the diencephalic-mesencephalic junction and obstruct the third ventricle, causing hydrocephalus.[132,142,143] Oculomotor abnormalities found in patients with posteromedial hematomas may improve after ventricular drainage, indicating these abnormalities were caused by downward pressure

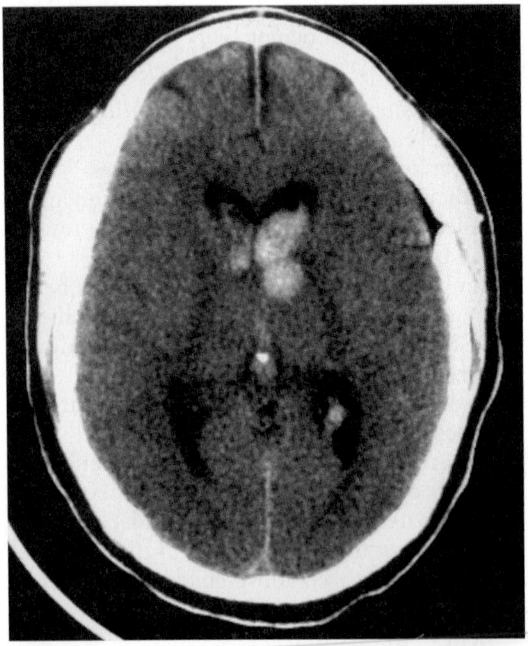

Figure 13-9. CT showing a small left anterior thalamic hematoma, which drained into the lateral ventricles. Blood casts are seen within the ventricle.

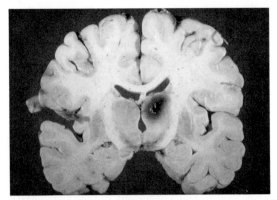

Figure 13-10. Necropsy specimen showing a small anterior thalamic hemorrhage. (From Caplan LR: Thalamic hemorrhage. In Kase CS, Caplan LR (eds): Intracerebral Hemorrhage. Boston: Butterworth-Heinemann, 1994, pp 341-362, with permission.)

on the midbrain.[142,143] Far posterior and dorsal lesions mostly involve the pulvinar in the distribution of the posterior choroidal arteries; slight sensorimotor signs may be found but are usually transient, and aphasia and behavioral abnormalities are common.[132] Figure 13-11 shows MRIs of a large thalamic hematoma that likely originated in the pulvinar region in a patient with a prior brain hemorrhage.

Lobar Hemorrhages

ICH may develop beneath the region of the gray-white junction of the cerebral cortex. These subcortical hemorrhages usually spread in a linear direction along white matter pathways. When the hematomas absorb, linear cavities remain, giving the lesions the name "slit hemorrhage." Figure 13-12 is a GRE MRI image that shows a typical old "slit"-shaped lateral ganglionic hemorrhage. The lesions undercut cortex and often do not obey the strict divisions of cerebral lobes; hence, the term lobar hemorrhage actually is inaccurate. Nonetheless, I use this term because of its widespread acceptance.

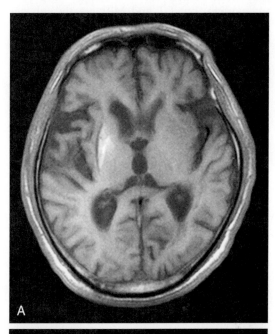

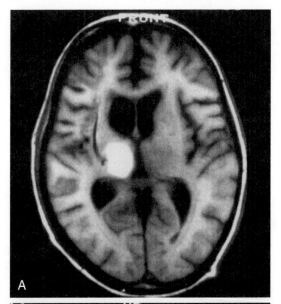

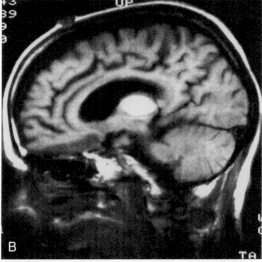

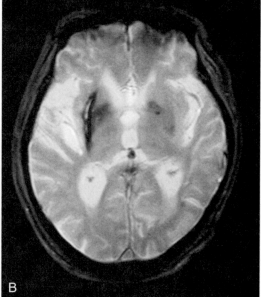

Figure 13-11. MRI T2-weighted axial (**A**) and sagittal (**B**) sections, showing a large thalamic hematoma located in the pulvinar. A cavity related to an old slit putaminal hemorrhage is also in **A**.

Figure 13-12. MRI scans showing an old linear "slit" hemorrhage involving the right putamen. **A**, T1-weighted MRI scan. **B**, GRE MRI scan.

Undercutting of the cortex can be epileptogenic, causing repeated focal seizures of limited duration.[144-146]

Subcortical hemorrhages are important to diagnose because the symptoms and signs are often erroneously attributed to cerebral infarction. Inappropriate therapy might be prescribed unless brain imaging shows the hematomas. Also, if subcortical hemorrhages are large, they are relatively superficial and are more accessible to surgical drainage than deeper hematomas. In the past, subcortical hemorrhages were rarely diagnosed antemortem, but CT and MRI greatly enhance recognition of these lesions. Many lobar hemorrhages are caused by AVMs, cavernous angiomas, and amyloid angiopathy, each of which has a predilection for cortical and subcortical regions. Hypertension is also an important cause of lobar hematomas. The parietal and occipital lobes are affected more often than the frontal and parietal regions. Symptoms and signs depend on the lobes affected, as follows[144-146]:

1. Frontal hematomas: Far anterior lesions usually cause abulia. Patients appear apathetic and have reduced spontaneity, prolonged latency in responding, and short, terse replies. If the lesions extend deeply or toward the precentral gyrus, conjugate eye deviation toward the side of the hematoma and contralateral hemiparesis are found. Figure 13-13 is a CT scan that shows a large frontal lobar hematoma.

2. Paracentral hematomas: Lesions near the central sulcus produce contralateral motor and sensory signs, sometimes with aphasia if the lesion is in the left hemisphere.

3. Parietal hemorrhages: Parietal hemorrhages are usually accompanied by contralateral hemisensory loss, with neglect of the contralateral visual field. The limbs contralateral to the hemorrhage are often uncoordinated. Aphasia and disorders of reading, writing, and arithmetic functions are present when the lesions involve the left inferior parietal lobule. Patients with right inferior parietal hematomas have defective drawing and copying and may have difficulty with visual-spatial functions.

4. Occipital hematomas: Occipital hemorrhages cause a severe contralateral hemianopia, often with slight contralateral hemisensory or motor signs and visual neglect.

5. Temporal-lobe lesions: Temporal-lobe lesions often cause agitation and delirium. Wernicke-type aphasia accompanies left temporal lesions. Temporal-lobe hematomas are particularly likely to swell and may cause herniation without preceding hemiparesis. Figure 13-14 is a CT scan that shows a large temporal lobe lobar hemorrhage. Brainstem compression may develop insidiously, with deepening stupor. An ipsilaterally dilated pupil follows.

Lobar hematomas are usually smaller in volume than deep lesions and have a lower mortality rate.[144-146] The functional outcome in patients with lobar ICH is also generally better than other forms of ICH. The exception to good outcome is the occurrence of lobar hemorrhage in patients taking anticoagulants. Anticoagulant hemorrhages have a predilection for the cerebral lobes and the cerebellum, and often gradually increase in size. The diagnosis of lobar hemorrhage is often quite difficult without CT or MRI. Because of the higher incidence of vascular malformations and other bleeding lesions in patients with lobar hematomas, angiography is often indicated, especially in patients who are young and not hypertensive.[147]

Primary Intraventricular Hemorrhages

Most intraventricular bleeding occurs when parenchymal hemorrhages develop adjacent to the ventricular system and empty directly into a ventricle.[147a] Caudate and thalamic hemorrhages are the most common sites for direct ventricular drainage. In some patients, the principal locus of bleeding is within the ventricular cavities.[148-150]

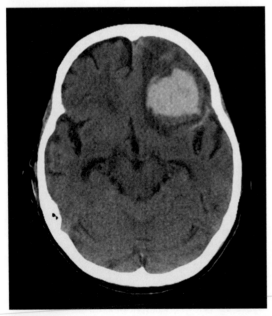

Figure 13-13. CT scan showing a large left frontal hematoma.

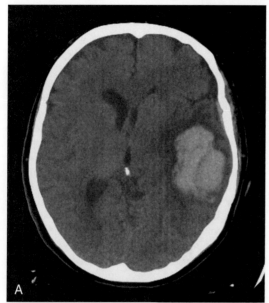

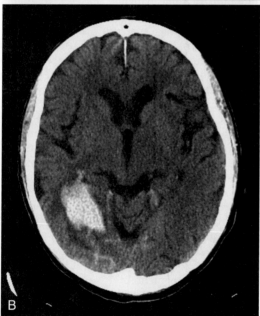

Figure 13-14. A, CT scan showing a large left temporal lobe hemorrhage with compression of the ipsilateral lateral ventricle. **B,** CT scan showing a smaller right temporal lobe hemorrhage.

Ventricular bleeding usually arises from small subependymal AVMs or cavernous angiomas or from hemorrhage into the caudate nucleus or thalamus just adjacent to the ventricles. Primary intraventricular hemorrhage is especially common in premature newborns in whom bleeding arises from the germinal matrix adjacent to the cerebral ventricles. The clinical syndrome closely mimics SAH, with sudden headache, stiff neck, vomiting, and lethargy. At times, bilateral, usually symmetric hyper-reflexia and extensor plantar responses occur. Also at times, the bleeding is primarily into one lateral ventricle, and asymmetric focal signs may predominate. Decreased consciousness is almost an invariable sign. CT shows blood distending the lateral ventricles and third ventricle and some blood density within the subarachnoid space. In childhood, the most common cause is an AVM, which can destroy itself as it ruptures. Small angiomas may arise in the choroid plexus[148] (see Fig. 12-16). In adults, most intraventricular hemorrhages are caused by ventricular spread of primary hypertensive bleeds into periventricular structures.[148-150] Intraventricular hemorrhage, both primary and secondary to drainage of supratentorial brain parenchymatous hemorrhages, has received increased attention recently because of the advent of hemostatic and thrombolytic treatments and stereotactic drainage techniques that are used to limit and remove blood from the ventricles.[151-153,153a] Figure 13-15 is a necropsy specimen showing a primary intraventricular hemorrhage.

Pontine Hemorrhage

Primary brainstem hemorrhages are located most often in the pons. Midbrain and medullary hemorrhages are rare and, when present, are usually caused by blood dyscrasias and vascular malformations.[154] Raised ICP, especially if it develops quickly, frequently causes secondary lesions, so-called Düret hemorrhages, in the median or paramedian zones of the thalamus, midbrain, and

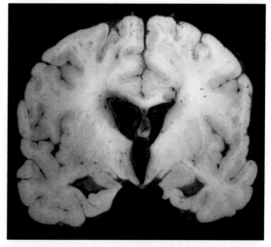

Figure 13-15. Necropsy specimen showing a primary intraventricular hemorrhage. (From Caplan LR: Intraventricular hemorrhage. In Kase CS, Caplan LR (eds): Intracerebral Hemorrhage. Boston: Butterworth-Heinemann, 1994, pp 383-401, with permission.)

13

pons caused by stretching of paramedian vascular structures.[106,154-156]

Primary pontine hemorrhages usually begin in the center of the pons at the tegmental-basal junction. Figure 13-16 is a sagittal section of a large pontine hematoma found at necropsy. These hematomas grow quickly and assume a round or oval shape, usually destroying the center of the tegmentum and base of the pons. Blood may dissect rostrally into the midbrain, but rarely extends caudally into the medulla. Hematomas frequently dissect into the fourth ventricle. Figure 13-17 shows a large paramedian pontine hematoma. These large pontine hemorrhages arise from the larger median pontine penetrating vessels that originate from the basilar artery. Figure 2-21 shows various pontine penetrating arteries. Bleeding from these arteries causes various syndromes,

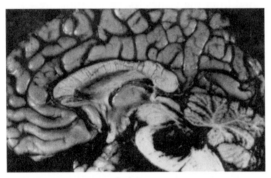

Figure 13-16. Sagittal section through the pons at necropsy showing a large hematoma. (From Caplan LR: Pontine hemorrhage. In In Kase CS, Caplan LR (eds): Intracerebral Hemorrhage. Boston: Butterworth-Heinemann, 1994, pp 403-423, with permission.)

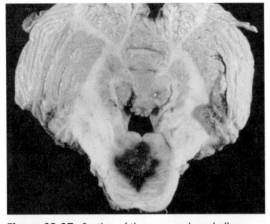

Figure 13-17. Section of the pons and cerebellum at necropsy showing a large paramedian pontine hematoma. (From Caplan LR: Pontine hemorrhage. In Kase CS, Caplan LR (eds): Intracerebral Hemorrhage. Boston: Butterworth-Heinemann, 1994, pp 403-423, with permission.)

depending on the location and size of the pontine hematomas.

Signs accompanying large medial pontine hematomas include (1) quadriparesis, often with limb stiffness and rigidity; (2) coma; (3) absent horizontal eye movements; (4) small but reactive pupils; and (5) rapid or irregular respirations.[155,157,158] Headache and vomiting occasionally occur. Some pontine hemorrhages develop gradually,[20] and early findings may be asymmetric. A hemiparesis is common early in the course. Deafness, dysarthria, facial numbness, asymmetric facial or limb weakness, and dizziness occasionally precede the development of coma. Some patients have twitching, shivering, or spasmodic movements of the limbs, usually culminating in decerebrate rigidity. These adventitious movements are often misinterpreted as convulsive seizures. Vertical reflex eye movements are preserved unless the lesion extends rostrally into the midbrain. In some patients, the eyes spontaneously and repeatedly bob downward.[155] Very large pontine hemorrhages are invariably fatal, but not usually instantaneously. Death usually occurs 24 to 48 hours after onset. Survival for 7 to 10 days, however, is not rare. Some patients with large medial pontine hematomas survive with quadriplegia. Hyperthermia is sometimes noted.

MRI allows documentation of three other types of pontine hemorrhage (lateral tegmental pontine hematomas,[155,159-165] small basal hematomas,[155,159,166-170] and small medial tegmental bleeds).[159,171-173] These sites correspond to the usual distribution of penetrating pontine arteries (see Fig. 2-21B). In Silverstein's series of 50 necropsy-proven pontine hemorrhages found during autopsy at the Philadelphia General Hospital, 28 were massive central hematomas. Eleven were located in the lateral basis pontis, and 11 were tegmental.[158] Nakajima reported 24 patients with pontine hematomas who came to necropsy; among these, 21 patients had large central hematomas, two had bilateral tegmental lesions, and one had a unilateral basal-tegmental hematoma.[159] Series of cases involving pontine hematomas identified by neuroimaging scans contain a higher frequency of unilateral basal, tegmental, and basal-tegmental lesions than prior autopsy series.

Lateral basal hematomas can cause pure motor hemiparesis,[166,167] ataxic hemiparesis,[168,169] or dysarthria-clumsy hand syndrome,[170] thus mimicking the findings in lacunar infarction involving the pons. Lateral basal lesions can spread into the adjacent lateral tegmentum, causing unilateral cranial nerve signs and contralateral hemiparesis. Lateral tegmental hematomas arise from penetrating vessels that course from lateral to medial after branching from the lateral circumferential pontine arteries (see Fig. 2-21B artery labelled C). These lesions involve the rostral pons. Findings on neurologic examination are those of a predominantly unilateral tegmental lesion.

Most distinctive and diagnostic of lateral tegmental pontine hematomas are the oculomotor abnormalities, which include ipsilateral conjugate gaze paresis, ipsilateral internuclear ophthalmoplegia, or a combination of ipsilateral internuclear ophthalmoplegia and gaze palsy (a "one and one-half syndrome"[33,155,160]), in which the only preserved eye motion is abduction of the contralateral eye. Because the sensory lemniscus (joining of the medial lemniscus and spinothalamic tracts) is lateral tegmental, accompanying loss of pinprick, temperature, and position sense on the opposite side of the body is common. Limb and truncal ataxia are usually present and may be bilateral or predominantly ipsilateral. Unilateral facial numbness or weakness, ipsilateral miosis, and transient deafness may also be present. When contralateral hemiparesis occurs, it is usually slight and transient. Patients with small pontine hematomas generally survive with slight to moderate clinical neurologic deficits. Small tegmental hematomas may cause only sensory abnormalities, involving the contralateral limbs and trunk (a pure sensory stroke syndrome)[162,163] or sensory findings limited to the ipsilateral face,[164,165] or ipsilateral sixth nerve or lateral gaze paresis.[171-173]

Cerebellar Hemorrhages

Hemorrhage into the cerebellum probably accounts for approximately 10% of ICH, approximating the relative percentage of weight of the cerebellum in reference to the entire brain. Anticoagulant usage and bleeding diatheses account for a disproportionate percentage of cases of cerebellar hemorrhage. In a recent Japanese series, 38 of 327 (12%) consecutive ICHs were cerebellar and 75% of the cerebellar hemorrhages developed in patients on warfarin therapy.[64] Although the frequency of cerebellar hemorrhage is low, establishing the diagnosis is important because of the potentially serious outcome if not treated and the contrasting relatively good prognosis after surgical treatment.

Cerebellar hemorrhage usually originates in the region of the dentate nucleus, arising from distal branches of the posterior inferior cerebellar artery and the superior cerebellar artery. Hematomas collect around the dentate and spread into the cerebellar hemispheral white matter, frequently extending into the fourth ventricle. The adjacent brainstem is seldom directly involved, but is compressed from above by the lesion. Occasional cerebellar hemorrhages arise in the vermis in medial branches of the posterior inferior cerebellar artery or the superior cerebellar artery. Figure 13-18 is a necropsy specimen that shows a large cerebellar hemorrhage that is compressing the fourth ventricle.

The most consistent symptom is inability to walk.[174-177] Some patients even have difficulty remaining in a sitting or standing position, often leaning or tilting toward the side of the hematoma. Patients have been known to crawl, slide, or bump on their bottom to get to the bathroom or telephone. Vomiting is also frequent, occurring in 68 (92%) of 72 patients from several series.[153] Headache is also common, usually affecting the occiput, neck, or frontal region. Dysarthria, hiccups, and tinnitus occur, but are less frequent. Loss of consciousness at onset is distinctly unusual, but by the time these patients reach the hospital, approximately one third are obtunded.[174-177]

Neurologic signs include (1) an ipsilateral abducens or gaze palsy toward the side of the hematoma; (2) small pupils, with the ipsilateral pupil slightly smaller; (3) rebound overshoot of the rapidly elevated ipsilateral arm; and (4) gait ataxia. Hemiparesis rarely occurs in patients with cerebellar hemorrhage, but cerebellar lesions do produce an apparent asthenia or slowness of the affected limbs.[153,174-177] Inferior extremity reflexes are usually symmetrically exaggerated, but plantar responses are flexor. Knee jerks are typically pendular with an increased span of leg movement. Classic cerebellar-type incoordination of

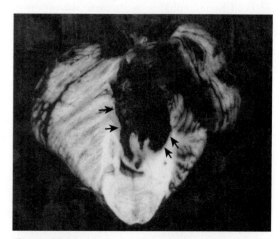

Figure 13-18. Necropsy section of the pons and cerebellum showing a large cerebellar hemorrhage *(small black arrows)*. The fourth ventricle is compressed and distorted from above. (From Caplan LR: Posterior Circulation Disease: Clinical Findings, Diagnosis, and Management. Boston: Blackwell Science, 1996, with permission.)

the arm on finger-to-nose or toe-to-object testing and frank intention tremor are uncommon. In my experience with patients with cerebellar infarction and hemorrhage, the single most useful cerebellar sign is elicited when the patient is asked to raise both arms together rapidly, then to brake the ascent quickly. Next, the patient is directed to drop the arms quickly, again braking the descent before the hands hit the bed or table. The arm on the side of the cerebellar lesion lags behind the other arm and overshoots the endpoint.

Patients with large cerebellar hematomas often have brainstem compression. They develop increasing stupor, lateral gaze palsy toward the side of the hematoma, and bilateral extensor plantar responses. Among those patients not comatose on admission in one series, only 20% had a smooth, uneventful recovery.[174] Eighty percent deteriorated to coma, with 25% of these becoming comatose within 3 hours after onset.[174] In the series of Fisher et al,[175] only 2 of 18 patients had a benign course. The other 16 patients developed coma, usually within a few hours. Because the hematoma usually affects the caudal cerebellum, the medulla is the portion of the brainstem compressed. Thus, vasomotor disturbances and respiratory arrest may develop. Untreated patients with cerebellar hemorrhage who become comatose invariably die of brainstem compression. CT and MRI not only document the size, locale, and position of the hematoma, but also give considerable information about posterior-fossa pressure. An expanding lesion obliterates the cerebellopontine angle and ambient cisterns, and displaces the fourth ventricle toward the opposite side. Usually, the fourth ventricle compression leads to hydrocephalus, with early dilatation of the temporal horns of the lateral ventricles.

Occasionally, patients with cerebellar hemorrhage have a more indolent course, presenting with symptoms and signs of hydrocephalus. Abulia, dementia, slow-stepped shuffling gait, and incontinence are the characteristic signs of hydrocephalus. The patient and family may fail to emphasize the preceding symptoms of dizziness, headache, and vomiting that had been interpreted as influenza or other viral illness. Other patients have laterally placed cerebellar hematomas that compress the cerebellopontine angle structures. These patients develop dysfunction of the fifth, sixth, seventh, and eighth cranial nerves, in addition to ataxia.

Hemorrhage into the vermis, with headache, vomiting, and sudden coma, is more rare.[177] These large medially placed vermal hemorrhages quickly compress the fourth ventricle and create pressure on the bilateral pontine tegmentum. At times, vermal hemorrhages are smaller and present with dizziness and gait ataxia. Figure 13-19 shows a small vermian hemorrhage.

Because the course of cerebellar hematomas is unpredictable and large lesions frequently cause coma and death, it is probably wise to drain lesions that are 3 cm or larger, especially if a decrease in level of alertness develops.[177,178] Some patients have been successfully treated by medical decompression (steroids and osmotic diuretic agents) or ventricular drainage.[177,179] Ventricular shunts do not treat brainstem compression and have been followed by delayed deterioration.[180] Ventricular drainage can create a vacuum effect that accentuates herniation of the cerebellum upward through the tentorial notch, to compress the rostral brainstem.[181] Prognosis depends very much on the size of the hematoma and whether the patient has developed stupor or coma before treatment.[182] The outlook for patients with small cerebellar hematomas is excellent. Even patients with large cerebellar hematomas do well if surgically decompressed before they develop reduced consciousness.[174-177,182]

DIAGNOSIS, PROGNOSIS, AND TREATMENT

Diagnosis

Accurate bedside diagnosis of ICH rests on the presence of an appropriate ecologic background, such as hypertension or bleeding diathesis; the nonfluctuating, usually gradually progressive course over minutes or hours; accompanying

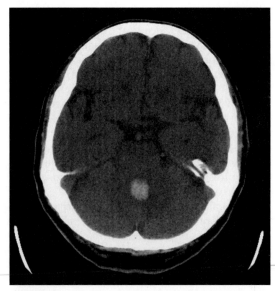

Figure 13-19. CT scan showing vermal cerebellar hemorrhage.

symptoms, such as headache and vomiting; and neurologic signs compatible with a deep lesion. CT has proven to be an excellent instrument for the diagnosis of ICH. Blood provides dense contrast, even acutely. One reported patient with ICH had an abrupt increase in symptoms while in the CT scanner.[183] The initial films had shown a small, round hyperdensity in the lentiform nucleus. A second film of the same area showed a much larger, hyperdense, irregular zone extending laterally from the putamen to the insula.[183] Others have also described enlargement of hematomas on sequential CT scans.[13-17]

Findings on CT and MRI scans can help determine the age of the hematoma.[184] Hematomas are at first regular and smooth. During the first 48 hours, large hematomas may show fluid blood levels, indicating that the hematoma is partially liquid and has not solidified.[185] During the first 72 hours or longer, edema produces a hypodense area around the lesion and considerable mass effect is noted.[186-188] From 3 to 20 days after bleeding, the dense area becomes smaller, beginning at the periphery. The border develops an irregular contour, which is enhanced with the use of contrast.[184,186-188] Reduction of edema and mass effect also occurs during this period. Intraventricular blood has usually disappeared by 5 weeks.[189] The absorption coefficient of the hematoma decreases gradually, and the lesion develops a lucent appearance, with absorption characteristics resembling edema fluid or CSF. By 9 weeks, mass effect and enhancement are usually gone, and a local circumscribed region of slight hypodensity remains.[189]

On MRI scans, the zone of altered attenuation or abnormal metabolism is usually much larger than the hypodensity seen on CT. MRI is also effective in imaging acute hematomas,[190-192] and is more useful than CT in recognizing hemorrhage in chronic lesions. In Chapter 4, I discuss MRI findings in hematomas in some detail. Table 4-1 tabulates the findings depending on various MR imaging techniques. Acute hematomas are isointense or hypointense on T1-weighted scans, sometimes with a darker hypointense rim, and they are bright and hyperintense on T2-weighted images.[187] Figure 13-11 shows a large acute hematoma in the thalamus, imaged by T2-weighted MRI. Later, the center of the hematoma appears dark on T2 and is surrounded by a bright rim. Chronic hematomas are bright on T2-weighted images.

Angiography is generally unnecessary unless the lesion is in an unusual locus or the patient has no risk factors for hemorrhage, such as hypertension or bleeding diathesis. Catheter subtraction angiography is used to show AVMs or aneurysms that might have caused ICH. Angiography can also suggest the likelihood of hematoma enlargement. Extravasation of contrast during angiography correlates well with subsequent enlargement of the hematoma and poorer outcome.[193] MR and CT angiography can be used in a similar fashion. Extravasation of contrast (gadolinium during MRI[194] and of contrast medium during CTA[195]) predicts subsequent enlargement of a hematoma.

Prognosis

The three most important predictors of outcome after ICH are size of hemorrhage, location of bleeding, and state of consciousness of the patient at presentation.[23-25,196] Hemorrhage expansion also indicates a worse prognosis when the hematoma attains a large size. Size and locale of the lesion on brain imaging scans renders very useful prognostic information. In putaminal hemorrhages, lesions larger than 140 mm^2 in one slice have a poorer outcome.[30] In thalamic hemorrhage, lesions larger than 3.3 cm in maximal diameter have a poor prognosis,[31] as do cerebellar lesions larger than 3 cm.[197] In six additional studies, large-volume hematomas were associated with a poor outcome.[23,24,139,198-200] Pulse pressure, admission blood pressure, and level of consciousness, as measured by the Glasgow Coma Scale, are also important prognostic variables.[23,25,199,201] High systolic, mean blood pressure, and pulse pressure correlate with poor outcome. The presence of hydrocephalus in patients with supratentorial hemorrhages is also an adverse prognostic sign.[200]

During the acute phase of ICH, the mass effect of the developing hematoma presents a much greater risk of death than does a comparable-sized brain infarct. In the case of ICH, something extra (blood) has been added to the intracranial contents. In brain infarction, the already existing contents (brain tissue) are ischemic, but an acute mass has not been added. Later, infarcts and hematomas become edematous, increasing ICP. In the chronic phase, if the patient with ICH has survived, the prognosis for recovery is actually much better than brain infarcts of similar size and location. Hematomas have dissected and separated the cerebral cortex and other brain parts, but usually the surrounding cortex is preserved. In contrast, infarcts leave dead, nonfunctioning cortex when they heal. Unlike SAH, recurrence of ICH during the acute illness is rare. These simple facts dictate the approach to ICH treatment-that is, aggressively try to limit the expanding hematoma to prevent death and late morbidity. In patients with ICH, the concern is control of acute mass effect, whereas in SAH, the goal is to prevent rebleeding and arterial vasoconstriction.

Treatment

13

Careful medical management of patients with ICH may be lifesaving and is important, even in those patients who later have surgical drainage of their hematomas. Increased ICP causes decreased responsiveness and hypoventilation; in turn, hypoventilation causes a low arterial oxygen tension and high carbon dioxide tension, which lead to vasodilatation and further increase in ICP. Maintenance of a good airway and mechanical hyperventilation can reverse this process and quickly lower ICP. Control of systemic blood pressure helps stop intracranial bleeding, but must be done cautiously. In some patients with ICH, systemic blood pressure is further increased to ensure adequate perfusion of the brain. Increased ICP causes increased venous pressure, so elevated arterial pressure is needed to overcome the increased venous pressure to perfuse the tissues. Overzealous lowering of blood pressure can lead to underperfusion and clinical deterioration. Blood pressure should be lowered quickly, but not to hypotensive levels. Patients must be watched carefully during the treatment. Guidelines from the Stroke Council of the American Heart Association recommend maintaining the mean arterial pressure below 130 mm Hg.[202]

So-called medical decompression with corticosteroids, mannitol, hypertonic saline, or glycerol is widely used in patients with ICH. Because edema develops around a hematoma and adds to mass effect, reduction of the surrounding edema is an important therapeutic goal. The perihematomal edema volume peaks during the third or fourth day after bleeding. The release of iron-containing breakdown products of hemoglobin likely contribute to the development of edema.[202a]

Elevation of the head of the bed, hyperventilation, temperature control, and ventricular drainage have also been used to control increased ICP.[203] Few data exist, however, about the effectiveness of these strategies. Concern exists that hypertonic agents could diffuse into the ICH and cause a secondary increase in volume of the hematoma because of ingress of fluid. Langfitt noted that mannitol and forced hyperventilation were effective in reducing ICP in a group of patients with ICH.[204] Poungvarin et al studied the usefulness of dexamethasone treatment in patients with supratentorial ICH in a double-blind randomized trial. They found that it did not improve mortality, and infections and diabetic complications were more often found in the corticosteroid-treated group.[205]

When considering surgery and other therapies, hematomas, in practice, can be divided into the following three main groups:

1. Massive, rapidly developing lesions that effectively kill or devastate patients before they reach the hospital. For these lesions, little can or should be done.
2. Small hematomas, from which the patient will make an excellent spontaneous recovery. Treatment consists of controlling the etiologic factors, such as hypertension, to prevent recurrences.
3. Medium-sized hemorrhages (hematoma volumes between the two extremes) with developing mass effect after the patient reaches the hospital. Within this third group, medical measures and surgery are most helpful.

Because hematomas represent the development of so-called benign masses, the logical treatment for life-threatening lesions is surgical drainage. The factors outlined in the following should be considered in deciding on surgical therapy.

Size

Hematomas larger than 3 cm in their widest diameter have a higher mortality and a more delayed recovery rate than smaller lesions. Thus, the larger the lesion on CT, the more logical its drainage would be.

Location

Some hematomas are more accessible surgically, such as those in the cerebellum and cerebral lobes. Although putaminal hemorrhages can be drained through the sylvian fissures and insular cortex, large left basal-ganglionic hemorrhages usually leave patients aphasic and dependent. Thus, treatment should be less aggressive than for right-sided lesions. Cerebellar ICH can cause respiratory arrest without preceding gradual deterioration of neurologic function or alertness, and surgical removal of a portion of the cerebellum often leaves no important residual handicap. For these reasons, the threshold for recommending surgery for cerebellar hematomas is lower than other lesions of comparable size. Cerebellar, lobar, and right putaminal hemorrhages are most accessible to surgical drainage.

Mass Effect and Drainage Pattern

Size of the hematoma does not, by itself, solely determine mass effect. Older patients may have sufficient preexisting atrophy to be able to accommodate a sizable hematoma without a critical rise in ICP or shift in intracranial compartments. Some lesions have a great deal of surrounding edema, whereas others have relatively little. Hydrocephalus can add to the increased mass effect. Does the hematoma compress the third or lateral ventricle? Has a shift of the midline occurred? Is uncal herniation present? In posterior fossa ICH, has displacement of the fourth ventricle been found? Are the ambient, cerebellopontine, and other cisterns effaced? Does the lesion drain into the ventricles or superficially into the subarachnoid space? Entry into the CSF may spontaneously decompress the lesion. Surgical drainage would be indicated more strongly for lesions with greater mass effect and no spontaneous decompression.

Etiology

Even after surgical drainage, hematomas caused by amyloid angiopathy may tend to bleed because of the fragility of the blood vessels.[206] Similarly, hemorrhages in patients with anticoagulant-related or other bleeding disorders also continue to bleed unless the coagulopathy is reversed before surgery. Although anticoagulant-related hemorrhage patients usually do worse than those with other etiologies, some patients have good outcomes after surgical drainage despite large size and midline shifts.[207] When operating on hematomas caused by vascular malformations, ideally, surgeons like to remove the malformations while also draining the hematoma. The threshold for surgical treatment should be most favorable for vascular malformations, moderately so for accessible lesions caused by hypertension, and least favorable for CAA or ICH caused by a bleeding diathesis.

Timing

During the first 24 to 36 hours, hematomas are still at least partly liquid and can be more easily drained. Later, hematomas solidify and become more difficult to drain. Unfortunately the present CT and MRI technologies do not reliably show the liquidity of hematomas unless there is a fluid level within the lesion. Clinicians posited that very early surgery, within 4 hours after symptom onset, might allow drainage of liquid blood and lead to better outcomes than surgery after 12 hours. A planned study to test this hypothesis was stopped prematurely after 11 patients in the 4-hour arm had surgery.[208] Median time to surgery was 180 minutes; median hematoma volume was 40 mL; median baseline NIH Stroke Scale score was 19. Postoperative rebleeding occurred in four patients, three of whom died. Rebleeding occurred in 40% of the patients treated within 4 hours, compared with 12% of the patients treated within 12 hours and those that re-bled had a higher mortality.[208]

Clearly, too early surgery can promote rebleeding, which adversely affected outcome. The ideal time to operate is unknown. After 7 to 10 days, blood begins to be absorbed, and the lesion becomes softer again. Ideally, drainage should occur either early or after 7 to 10 days for technical reasons. In general, if the patient has survived the first week, improvement occurs as edema subsides. Thus, little argument for late drainage exists except for concurrent removal of a vascular malformation. Some have wondered whether late surgery (1 to 2 weeks) would speed recovery, but this argument is unsupported by data.

Clinical Course

Perhaps the most important factor to consider is whether the patient is improving, stable, or worsening. Patients who deteriorate and show a decrease in level of consciousness to severe lethargy or stupor have a poor outlook for recovery.[23,25,196] In patients with putaminal hemorrhage, other poor prognostic signs include the development of ipsilateral pupillary dilation, an ipsilateral extensor plantar response, or an ipsilateral conjugate gaze paresis. These signs are indicative of midline shift or early brainstem compression. In patients with cerebellar hemorrhage, development of bilateral extensor plantar responses is a poor prognostic sign.[175] In deteriorating patients with accessible lesions, surgery should not be delayed if medical decompression is not quickly beneficial.

The effectiveness of surgical decompression of ICHs is controversial and has been extensively studies and debated.[25,202,208-215,215a] The largest randomized trial to date, the STICH trial (International Surgical Trial in Intracerebral Haemorrhage), failed to show a definite superiority of either medical or surgical treatment.[212,214] In the STICH trial, 1033 patients from 83 medical centers in 27 countries were randomized to have surgery within 24 hours of randomization or to initial conservative nonsurgical treatment. Among those randomized to early surgery, 26% had a favorable outcome compared with 24% randomized to initial conservative treatment (odds ratio 0.89 [95% confidence interval 0.66 to 1.19], $P = 0.414$). Deep and lobar hemorrhages in this analysis were considered together. Among the 530 patients randomized to initial conservative treatment, 140 patients crossed over and had surgery, complicating the analysis and interpretation of the results.[215] The investigators concluded that overall "patients with spontaneous supratentorial intracerebral hemorrhage in neurosurgical units show no overall benefit from early surgery when compared with initial conservative treatment."[214] The STICH trial[215] and other studies[203] showed

13

that intraventricular bleeding and hydrocephalus adversely affected outcomes.

Lobar and cerebellar hematomas are probably most amenable to surgical decompression. Fleming and colleagues analyzed the Mayo Clinic experience regarding patients with lobar hematomas that deteriorated after hospital admission.[216] Decreased consciousness (Glasgow Coma Scale score of <14) was the most important single predictor of deterioration. Large hematoma volume (>60 mL), midline shift, effacement of the contralateral perimesencephalic and ambient cisterns, and dilatation of the contralateral temporal horn of the lateral ventricle were the other predictive features.[216] Patients who deteriorate during the first 12 hours usually have enlargement of hematoma on follow-up CT scans. Those that deteriorate after the first day usually do so because of brain edema around the hematoma.

During the last two decades, surgeons have explored stereotactic drainage of hematomas with and without thrombolytic agent softening of the hematomas.[217-225] Stereotactic techniques have been used more often in Asian countries than in the west. Drainage is performed through a small burr hole and no cortisectomy is involved. Stereotactic surgery has been performed with and without a stereotactic frame and with and without administration of a thrombolytic agent directly into the intracerebral clot. The results show promise and are likely to prove superior in the hands of experienced surgeons to direct surgical drainage. Endoscopic drainage of blood is another promising technique.[153a,226] Drainage of subacute hemorrhages, by reducing intracranial pressure can improve alertness and reduce the frequency and severity of medical complications that often develop in stuporous patients.[224]

Since intraventricular blood, especially a large amount, adversely effects outcome, clinicians have posited that more aggressive drainage of the ventricular blood might improve outcomes in patients with brain hemorrhages that included the cerebral ventricles.[203,227] A preliminary trial showed that intraventricular thrombolysis with urokinase was able to speed the resolution of intraventricular blood clots, compared with treatment with ventricular drainage alone.[227]

I believe that in the foreseeable future, more aggressive drainage of intracerebral and intraventricular hematomas using advanced stereotactic and endoscopic techniques and thrombolytic agents to liquefy clots will result in improved outcomes for patients with intracerebral hematomas.

Recently, clinicians and investigators have attempted to limit hematoma expansion by administering recombinant activated factor VII (rFVIIa) to patients (even those patients who do not have a known coagulopathy) early in the course of intracerebral bleeding.[228-234] A randomized trial of rF-VIIa showed some effectiveness but also some risk related to the induced hypercoagulability.[230] In this trial, 399 patients with CT confirmed intracerebral hematomas were randomly assigned within three hours after onset to receive placebo (96 patients) or 40 μg of rFVIIa per kilogram (108 patients), 80 μg/kg (92 patients), or 160 μg/kg (103 patients) within 1 hour after the initial CT scan. The primary outcome measure was the percent change in the volume of the intracerebral hemorrhage measured at 24 hours. Hematoma volume increased more in the placebo group than in the rFVIIa groups. The mean increase was 29% in the placebo group, contrasted with 16%, 14%, and 11% in the those given 40 μg, 80 μg, and 160 μg of rFVIIa/kg, respectively (P = 0.01 for the comparison of the three rFVIIa groups with the placebo group). Growth in the volume of intracerebral hemorrhage was reduced by 3.3 mL, 4.5 mL, and 5.8 mL in the three treatment groups, compared with the placebo group (P = 0.01). Sixty-nine percent of placebo-treated patients died or were severely disabled compared with 55%, 49%, and 54% of patients given 40, 80, and 160 μg of rFVIIa, respectively (P = 0.004 for the comparison of the three rFVIIa groups with the placebo group). Mortality at 90 days was 29% for placebo-treated patients, and 18% in the three rFVIIa groups combined (P = 0.02). Serious thromboembolic adverse events, mainly myocardial or cerebral infarction, occurred in 7% of rFVIIa-treated patients, compared with 2% of those given placebo (P = 0.12).[230-232] Expansion of hematoma volume was shown to be an important determinant of morbidity and mortality.[231]

In another report, elevated troponin occurred in 20% and myocardial infarction in 10% of 20 ICH patients treated with rFVIIa compared with troponin elevation in 3% and myocardial infarction in 1% of 110 ICH patients who received standard medical management.[232] In patients with preexisting severe vascular occlusive disease involving the coronary or peripheral arteries, or past venous thromboembolism, the administration of rFVIIa poses a risk of myocardial infarction or venous occlusion with pulmonary embolism.

A second confirmatory trial of the utility of rFVIIa in patients with acute intracerebral hematomas enrolled 841 patients.[233,234] Treatment with 80 μg of rFVIIa significantly reduced hematoma volume compared to 20 μg of rFVIIa and placebo but there was no significant difference in the proportion of patients with poor outcome. Arterial thromboembolic events were more common in the 80-μg rFVIIa-treated group.[233,234] In this study, there were more intraventricular hemorrhages at baseline in the 80-μg treatment group compared to the placebo group (41% vs 29%), and the mortality rate and Rankin scores were lower in the placebo group in this trial compared to the earlier trial. Although there still may be a group of patients with intracerebral hemorrhages that can benefit from rFVIIa, the conclusion of these trials is that reduction in volume of hematoma, in general, does not exert a major effect on outcome.[234]

A CT scan in JT showed a large, deep putaminal hemorrhage, with spread to the thalamus and lateral ventricles. At this time, he was comatose; had bilateral horizontal gaze palsies; dilated, unreactive pupils; and bilateral extensor plantar reflexes. I judged that nothing could or should be done to reverse his mortal bleed.

Much must be learned regarding therapy for patients with ICH. The technological revolution has made diagnosis easy. More well-designed studies of different modes of treatment in patients with lesions of various etiologies, sizes, locations, and varying levels of consciousness are needed.

References

1. Morgagni GB: De sedibus, et causis morborum per anatomen indagatis libri quinque. Vienna: Typographica Remondiana, 1761.
2. Cheyne J: Cases of apoplexy and lethargy with observations on comatose patients. London: Thomas Underwood, 1812.
3. Gowers W: A Manual of Diseases of the Nervous System, vol 2, 2nd ed. London: J & A Churchill, 1892.
4. Osler W: The Principles and Practices of Medicine, 5th ed. New York: Appleton, 1903.
5. Aring C, Merritt H: Differential diagnosis between cerebral hemorrhage and cerebral thrombosis: Clinical and pathological study of 245 cases. Arch Intern Med 1935;56:435-456.
6. Kunitz S, Gross C, Heyman A, et al: The Pilot Stroke Data Bank: Definition, design, and data. Stroke 1984;15:740-746.
7. Caplan LR, Hier DB, D'Cruz I: Cerebral embolism in the Michael Reese Stroke Registry. Stroke 1983;14:530-540.
8. Mohr JP, Caplan LR, Melski J, et al: The Harvard Cooperative Stroke Registry: A prospective registry. Neurology 1978;28:754-762.
9. Whisnant J, Fitzgibbons J, Kurland L, et al: Natural history of stroke in Rochester, Minnesota, 1945-1954. Stroke 1971;2:11-22.
10. Matsumoto N, Whisnant J, Kurland L, et al: Natural history of stroke in Rochester, Minnesota, 1955-1969. Stroke 1973;4:20-29.
11. Caplan LR, Mohr JP: Intracerebral hemorrhage: An update. Geriatrics 1978;33:42-52.
12. Fisher CM: Pathological observations in hypertensive cerebral hemorrhages. J Neuropathol Exp Neurol 1971;30:536-550.
13. Kelly R, Bryer JR, Scheinberg P, Stokes IV: Active bleeding in hypertensive intracerebral hemorrhage: Computed tomography. Neurology 1982; 32:852-856.
14. Broderick JP, Brott TG, Tomsick T, et al: Ultra-early evaluation of intracerebral hemorrhage. J Neurosurg 1990;72:195-199.
15. Fujii Y, Tanaka R, Takeuchi S, et al: Hematoma enlargement in spontaneous intracerebral hemorrhage. J Neurosurg 1994;80:51-57.
16. Kazui S, Naritomi H, Yamamoto H, et al: Enlargement of spontaneous intracerebral hemorrhage: Incidence and time course. Stroke 1996;27: 1783-1787.
17. Kase C, Robinson K, Stein R, et al: Anticoagulant-related intracerebral hemorrhage. Neurology 1985;35:943-948.
18. Kase CS: Bleeding disorders. In Kase CS, Caplan LR (eds): Intracerebral Hemorrhage. Boston: Butterworth-Heinemann, 1994, pp 117-151.
19. Aguilar MI, Hart RG, Kase CS, et al: Treatment of warfarin-associated intracerebral hemorrhage: Literature review and expert opinion. Mayo Clin Proc 2007;82:82-92.
20. Kornyey S: Rapidly fatal pontile hemorrhage: Clinical and anatomic report. Arch Neurol Psychiatry 1939;41:793-799.
21. Caplan LR: General Symptoms and Signs. In Kase CS, Caplan LR (eds): Intracerebral Hemorrhage. Boston: Butterworth-Heinemann, 1994, pp 31-43.
22. Mello TP, Pinto AN, Ferro JM: Headache in intracerebral hematomas. Neurology 1996;47: 494-500.
23. Tuhrim S, Dambrosia JM, Price TR, et al: Prediction of intracerebral hemorrhage survival. Ann Neurol 1988;24:258-263.
24. Broderick JP, Brott TG, Duldner JE, et al: Volume of intracerebral hemorrhage. Stroke 1993;24: 987-993.
25. Kase CS, Crowell RM: Prognosis and treatment of patients with intracerebral hemorrhage. In Kase CS, Caplan LR (eds): Intracerebral Hemorrhage. Boston: Butterworth-Heinemann, 1994, pp 467-489.
26. Borison H, Wang S: Physiology and pharmacology of vomiting. Pharmacol Rev 1953;5:193-230.
27. Faught E, Peties D, Bartolucci A, et al: Seizures after primary intracerebral hemorrhage. Neurology 1989;39:1089-1093.
28. Kilpatrick CJ, Davis SM, Tress BM, et al: Epileptic seizures in acute strokes. Arch Neurol 1990;47:157-160.
29. Berger AR, Lipton RB, Lesser ML, et al: Early seizures following intracerebral hemorrhage. Neurology 1988;38:1363-1365.
30. Hier DB, Davis K, Richardson EP, et al: Hypertensive putaminal hemorrhage. Arch Neurol 1977;1:152-159.
30a. Classen J, Jette N, Chum F, et al: Electrographic seizures and periodic discharges after intracerebral hemorrhage. Neurology 2007;69: 1356-1365.

13

31. Walshe T, Davis K, Fisher CM: Thalamic hemorrhage, a computed tomographic-clinical correlation. Neurology 1977;29:217-222.

32. Hier DB, Babcock DJ, Foulkes MA, et al: Influence of site on course of intracerebral hemorrhage. J Stroke Cerebrovasc Dis 1993;3:65-74.

33. Fisher CM: Some neuro-ophthalmological observations. J Neurol Neurosurg Psychiatry 1967;30:383-392.

34. Caplan LR: Intracerebral hemorrhage revisited. Neurology 1988;38:624-627.

35. Caplan LR: Hypertensive intracerebral hemorrhage. In Kase CS, Caplan LR (eds): Intracerebral Hemorrhage. Boston: Butterworth-Heinemann, 1994, pp 99-116.

36. Cole F, Yates P: Intracerebral microaneurysms and small cerebrovascular lesions. Brain 1967;90:759-768.

37. Rosenblum WI: Miliary aneurysms and "fibrinoid" degeneration of cerebral blood vessels. Hum Pathol 1977;8:133-139.

38. Santos-Buch CA, Goodhue W, Ewald B: Concurrence of iris aneurysms and cerebral hemorrhage in hypertensive rabbits. Arch Neurol 1976;33:96-103.

39. Takebayashi S, Kaneko M: Electron microscopic studies of ruptured arteries in hypertensive intracerebral hemorrhage. Stroke 1983;14:28-36.

40. Takebayashi S, Sakata N, Kawamura K: Re-evaluation of miliary aneurysms in hypertensive brain: Recanalization of small hemorrhage. Stroke 1990;21(suppl 1):59-60.

41. Bakemuka M: Primary intracerebral hemorrhage and heart weight: A clinicopathologic case-control review of 218 patients. Stroke 1987;18:531-536.

42. Brott T, Thalinger K, Hertzberg V: Hypertension as a risk factor for spontaneous intracerebral hemorrhage. Stroke 1986;17:1078-1083.

43. Caplan LR, Neely S, Gorelick PB: Cold-related intracerebral hemorrhage. Arch Neurol 1984;41:227.

44. Hines F, Brown G: A standard test for measuring the variability of blood pressure: Its significance as an index of the prehypertensive state. Ann Intern Med 1933;7:209-217.

45. Barbas N, Caplan LR, Baquis G, et al: Dental chair intracerebral hemorrhage. Neurology 1987;37:511-512.

46. Cawley CM, Rigamonti D, Trommer B: Dental chair apoplexy. South Med J 1991;84:907-909.

47. Haines S, Maroon J, Janetta P: Supratentorial intracerebral hemorrhage following posterior fossa surgery. J Neurosurgery 1978;49:881-886.

48. Waga S, Shimosaka S, Sakakura M: Intracerebral hemorrhage remote from the site of the initial neurosurgical procedure. Neurosurgery 1983;13:662-665.

49. Sweet WH, Poletti CE: Complications of standard treatment for trigeminal neuralgia: Need for mechanism for prompt reporting of complications (abstract). Poster presentation #82, Annual Meeting of the American Association of Neurological Surgeons, Denver, Colorado, 1986, p 243.

50. Sweet WH, Poletti CE, Roberts JT: Dangerous rises in blood pressure upon heating of trigeminal rootlets: Increased bleeding times in patients with trigeminal neuralgia. Neurosurgery 1985;17:843-844.

51. Kehler CH, Brodsky JB, Samuels SI, et al: Blood pressure response during percutaneous rhizotomy for trigeminal neuralgia. Neurosurgery 1982;10:200-202.

52. Norregaard TV, Moskowitz MA: Substance P and sensory innervation of intracranial and extracranial feline cephalic arteries. Brain 1985;108:517-533.

53. Moskowitz MA: The neurobiology of vascular head pain. Ann Neurol 1984;16:157-168.

54. Caplan LR, Skillman J, Ojemann R, Fields W: Intracerebral hemorrhage following carotid endarterectomy: A hypertensive complication. Stroke 1978;9:457-460.

55. Bruetman MF, Fields WS, Crawford ES, DeBakey ME: Cerebral hemorrhage in carotid artery surgery. Arch Neurol 1963;9:458-467.

56. Wylie EJ, Hein MF, Adams JE: Intracerebral hemorrhage following surgical revascularization for treatment of acute strokes. J Neurosurg 1964;21:212-215.

57. Humphreys RP, Hoffman JH, Mustard WT, et al: Cerebral hemorrhage following heart surgery. J Neurosurg 1975;43:671-675.

58. Sila CA: Spectrum of neurologic events following cardiac transplantation. Stroke 1989;20:1586-1589.

59. Cole A, Aube M: Migraine with vasospasm and delayed intracerebral hemorrhage. Arch Neurol 1990;47:53-56.

60. Fisher CM, Adams RD: Observations on brain embolism with special reference to hemorrhagic infarction. In Furlan A (ed): The Heart and Stroke. London: Springer, 1987, pp 17-36.

61. Wilson SAK, Bruce AN: Neurology, 2nd ed. London: Butterworth, 1955.

62. Askey JM: Hemorrhage during long-term anticoagulant drug therapy: Intracranial hemorrhage. Calif Med 1966;104:6-10.

63. Flaherty ML, Kissela B, Woo D, Kleindorfer D: The increasing incidence of anticoagulant-associated intracerebral hemorrhage. Neurology 2007;68:116-121.

64. Toyoda K, Okada S, Inoue T, et al: Antithrombotic therapy and predilection for cerebellar hemorrhage. Cerebrovasc Dis 2007;23:109-116.

65. Babikian V, Kase CS, Pessin MS, et al: Intracerebral hemorrhage in stroke patients anticoagulated with heparin. Stroke 1989;20:1500-1503.

66. Hacke W: The dilemma of reinstituting anticoagulation for patients with cardioembolic sources and intracranial hemorrhage: How wide is the strait between Skylla and Karybdis? Arch Neurol 2000;57:1682-1684.

67. Phan TG, Koh M, Wijdicks EF: Safety of discontinuation of anticoagulation in patients with intracranial hemorrhage at high thromboembolic risk. Arch Neurol 2000;57: 1710-1713.

68. Kase CS, Pessin MS, Zivin JA, et al: Intracranial hemorrhage after coronary thrombolysis with tissue plasminogen activator. Am J Med 1992;92: 384-390.

69. Caplan LR: Drugs. In Kase CS, Caplan LR (eds): Intracerebral Hemorrhage. Boston: Butterworth-Heinemann, 1994, pp 201-220.

70. Brust JC: Stroke and substance abuse. In Caplan LR (ed): Uncommon Causes of Stroke, 2nd ed. Cambridge: Cambridge University Press, 2008, pp 365-369.

71. Caplan LR, Hier DB, Banks G: Stroke and drug abuse. Curr Concepts Cerebrovasc Dis (Stroke) 1982;17:9-14.

72. Harrington H, Heller HA, Dawson D, et al: Intracerebral hemorrhage and oral amphetamine. Arch Neurol 1983;40:503-507.

73. Citron B, Halpern M, McCarron M, et al: Necrotizing angiitis associated with drug abuse. N Engl J Med 1970;283:1003-1011.

74. Rumbaugh C, Bergeron R, Fang H, et al: Cerebral angiographic changes in the drug abuse patient. Radiology 1971;101:335-344.

75. Rumbaugh C, Bergeron R, Scanlon R, et al: Cerebral vascular changes secondary to amphetamine abuse in the experimental animal. Radiology 1971;101:345-351.

76. Lukes SA: Intracerebral hemorrhage from an arteriovenous malformation after amphetamine injection. Arch Neurol 1983;40:60-61.

77. Cahill D, Knipp HJ, Mosser J: Intracranial hemorrhage with amphetamine usage. Neurology 1981;31:1058-1059.

78. Yu YJ, Cooper DR, Wellenstein DE, Block B: Cerebral and intracerebral hemorrhage associated with methamphetamine abuse: Case report. J Neurosurg 1983;58:109-111.

79. Schmidley JW: Central Nervous System Angiitis. Oxford: Butterworth-Heinemann, 2000.

80. Levine SR, Welch KMA: Cocaine and stroke. Stroke 1988;19:779-783.

81. Levine SR, Brust JCM, Futrell N, et al: Cerebrovascular complications of alkaloid cocaine. N Engl J Med 1990;323:699-704.

82. Eastman J, Cohen S: Hypertensive crisis and death associated with phencyclidine poisoning. JAMA 1975;231:1270-1271.

83. Bessen H: Intracranial hemorrhage associated with phencyclidine abuse. JAMA 1982;248: 585-586.

84. Stratton M, Witherspoon J, Kirtley T: Hypertensive crisis and phencyclidine abuse. Va Med 1978;105: 569-572.

85. Lasagna L: Phenylpropanolamine: A Review. New York: Wiley, 1988.

86. Kikta DG, Devereux MW, Chandar K: Intracranial hemorrhage due to phenylpropanolamine. Stroke 1985;16:510-512.

87. Kase CS, Foster TE, Reed JE, et al: Intracerebral hemorrhage and phenylpropanolamine use. Neurology 1987;37:399-404.

88. McDowell JR, Leblanc H: Phenylpropanolamine and cerebral hemorrhage. West J Med 1985;142: 688-691.

89. Glick R, Hoying J, Cerullo L, Perlman S: Phenylpropanolamine: An over-the-counter drug causing cerebral nervous system vasculitis and intracerebral hemorrhage. Neurosurgery 1987; 20:969-974.

90. Mueller S, Muller J, Asdell S: Cerebral hemorrhage associated with phenylpropanolamine in combination with caffeine. Stroke 1984;15: 119-123.

91. Mueller S: Neurologic complications of phenylpropanolamine use. Neurology 1983;33: 650-652.

92. Caplan LR, Thomas C, Banks G: Central nervous system complications of addiction to T's and blues. Neurology 1982;32:623-628.

92a. Buxton N, Flannery T, Wild D, Bassi S: Sildenafil (Viagra) induced spontaneous intracerebral hemorrhage. Br J Neurosurgery 2001;15:347-349.

92b. McGee HT, Egan RA, Clark WM: Visual field defect and intracerebral hemorrhage associated with use of vardenafil (Levitra). Neurology 2005;64:1095-1096.

92c. Monastero R, Pipia C, Camarda LK, Camarda R: Intracerebral hemorrhage associated with sildenafil citrate. J Neurol 2001;248:141-142.

92d. Gazzeri R, Neroni M, Galarza M, Esposito S: Intracerebral hemorrhage associated with use of tadalafil (Cialis). Neurology 2008;70: 1289-1290.

93. Zenkevich GS: Role of congophilic angiopathy in the genesis of subarachnoid-parenchymatous hemorrhages in middle-aged and elderly persons. Zh Nevropatol Psikhiatr 1978;78:52-57.

94. Jellinger K: Cerebral hemorrhage in amyloid angiopathy. Ann Neurol 1977;1:604.

95. Jellinger K: Cerebrovascular amyloidosis with cerebral hemorrhage. J Neurol 1977;214:195-206.

96. Vinters H, Gilbert J: Cerebral amyloid angiopathy: Incidence and complications in the aging brain: II. The distribution of amyloid vascular changes. Stroke 1983;14:923-928.

97. Lee S, Stemmerman G: Congophilic angiopathy and cerebral hemorrhage. Arch Pathol Lab Med 1978;102:317-321.

98. Gilbert J, Vinters H: Cerebral amyloid angiopathy: Incidence and complications in the aging brain: I. Cerebral hemorrhage. Stroke 1983;14: 915-923.

99. Kase CS: Cerebral amyloid angiopathy. In Kase CS, Caplan LR (eds): Intracerebral Hemorrhage. Boston: Butterworth-Heinemann, 1994, pp 179-200.

100. Gilles C, Brucher J, Khoubesserian P, et al: Cerebral amyloid angiopathy as a cause of multiple intracerebral hemorrhages. Neurology 1984;34:730-735.

101. Finelli P, Kessimian N, Bernstein P: Cerebral amyloid angiopathy manifesting as recurrent intracerebral hemorrhage. Arch Neurol 1984; 41:330-333.

102. Chen YW, Gurol ME, Rosand J, et al: Progression of white matter lesions and hemorrhages in cerebral amyloid angiopathy. Neurology 2006; 67:83-87.

103. Imaizumi T, Honma T, Horita Y, et al: Hematoma size in deep intracerebral hemorrhage and its correlation with dot-like hemosiderin spots on gradient echo T2*-weighted MRI. J Neuroimaging 2006;16:236-242.

104. Imaizumi T, Horita Y, Hashimoto Y, Niwa J: Dotlike hemosiderin spots on T2*-weighted magnetic resonance imaging as a predictor of stroke recurrence: A prospective study. J Neurosurg 2004;101:915-920.

105. Maia LF, Vasconcelos C, Seixas S, et al: Lobar brain hemorrhages and white matter changes: Clinical, radiological and laboratorial profiles. Cerebrovasc Dis 2006;22:155-161.

106. Caplan LR: Head trauma and related intracerebral hemorrhage. In Kase CS, Caplan LR (eds): Intracerebral Hemorrhage. Boston: Butterworth-Heinemann, 1994, pp 221-241.

107. Alvarez-Sabin J, Turon A, Lozano-Sanchez M, et al: Delayed posttraumatic hemorrrhage, "spat-apoplexie." Stroke 1995;26:1531-1535.

108. Kase CS: Intracranial tumors. In Kase CS, Caplan LR (eds): Intracerebral Hemorrhage. Boston: Butterworth-Heinemann, 1994, pp 243-261.

109. Kase CS: Vasculitis and other angiopathies. In Kase CS, Caplan LR (eds): Intracerebral Hemorrhage. Boston: Butterworth-Heinemann, 1994, pp 263-303.

109a. Vahedi K, Boukobza M, Massin P, et al: Clinical and brain MRI follow-up study of a family with COL4A1 mutation. Neurology 2007;69: 1564-1568.

109b. Meschia JF, Rosand J: Fragile vessels. Handle with care. Neurology 2007;69:1560-1561.

110. Caplan LR, Kase CS: Mechanisms of intracerebral hemorrhage. In Kase CS, Caplan LR (eds): Intracerebral Hemorrhage. Boston: Butterworth-Heinemann, 1994, pp 95-98.

111. Russell DS: The pathology of spontaneous intracranial hemorrhages. Proc R Soc Med 1954;47:689-693.

112. Mutlu N, Berry RG, Alpers BJ: Massive cerebral hemorrhage: Clinical and pathological correlations. Arch Neurol 1963;8:74-91.

113. McCormick WF, Rosenfield DB: Massive brain hemorrhage: A review of 144 cases and an examination of their causes. Stroke 1973;4: 946-954.

114. Schutz H: Spontane intrazerebrale hamatome: Pathophysologie, klinik, und therapie. Heidelberg: Springer, 1988.

115. Jellinger K: Zur atiologie und pathogenese der spontanen intrazerebralen blutung. Therapiewoche 1972;22:1440-1450.

116. Weisberg LA: Computerized tomography in intracranial hemorrhage. Arch Neurol 1979;36: 422-426.

117. Qureshi AI, Suri MAK, Safdar K, et al: Intracerebral hemorrhage in blacks. Risk factors, subtypes, and outcome. Stroke 1997;28:961-964.

118. Ruiz-Sandoval JL, Cantu C, Barinagarrementeria F: Intracerebral hemorrhage in young people: Analysis of risk factors, locations, causes, and prognosis. Stroke 1999;30:537-541.

119. Fisher CM: Clinical syndromes in cerebral hemorrhage in pathogenesis and treatment of cerebrovascular disease. In Fields W (ed): Proceedings of the Annual Meeting of the Houston Neurological Society. Springfield, IL: Thomas, 1961, pp 318-342.

120. Caplan LR: Putaminal hemorrhage. In Kase CS, Caplan LR (eds): Intracerebral Hemorrhage. Boston: Butterworth-Heinemann, 1994, pp 309-327.

121. Chung C-S, Caplan LR, Yamamoto Y, et al: Striatocapsular haemorrhage. Brain 2000;123:1850-1862.

122. Koba T, Yokoyama T, Kaneko M: Correlation between the location of hematoma and its clinical symptoms in the lateral type of hypertensive intracerebral hemorrhage. Stroke 1977;8:676-680.

123. Mizukami M, Nishijuma M, Kin H: Computed tomographic findings of good prognosis for hemiplegia in hypertensive putaminal hemorrhage. Stroke 1981;12:648-652.

124. Stein R, Caplan LR, Hier DB: Intracerebral hemorrhage: Role of blood pressure, location, and size of lesions. Ann Neurol 1983;14:132-133.

125. Mizukami M, Kin H, Araki G, et al: Surgical treatment of primary intracerebral hemorrhage: I. New angiographical classification. Stroke 1976;7:30-36.

126. Metter EJ, Jackson C, Kempler D, et al: Left hemisphere intracerebral hemorrhages studied by (F-18)-fluorodeoxyglucose PET. Neurology 1986;36:1155-1162.

127. Stein R, Kase C, Hier DB, et al: Caudate hemorrhage. Neurology 1984;34:1549-1554.

128. Weisberg L: Caudate hemorrhage. Arch Neurol 1984;41:971-974.

129. Caplan LR: Caudate hemorrhage. In Kase CS, Caplan LR (eds): Intracerebral Hemorrhage. Boston: Butterworth-Heinemann, 1994, pp 329-340.

130. Pedrazzi P, Bogousslavsky J, Regli F: Hematomes limites a la tete du Noyau Caude. Rev Neurol 1990;146:12:726-738.

131. Caplan LR: Thalamic hemorrhage. In Kase CS, Caplan LR (eds): Intracerebral Hemorrhage. Boston: Butterworth-Heinemann, 1994, pp 341-362.

132. Chung CS, Caplan LR, Han W, et al: Thalamic haemorrhage. Brain 1996;119:1873-1886.

133. Barraquer-Bordas L, Illa I, Escartin A, et al: Thalamic hemorrhage: A study of 23 patients with diagnosis by computed tomography. Stroke 1981;12:524-527.

134. Caplan LR: "Top of the basilar" syndrome: selected clinical aspects. Neurology 1980;30:72-79.

135. Mohr JP, Walters W, Duncan G: Thalamic hemorrhage and aphasia. Brain Lang 1975;2:3-17.

136. Ciemins V: Localized thalamic hemorrhage: A cause of aphasia. Neurology 1970;20:776-782.

137. Samarel A, Wright T, Sergay S, et al: Thalamic hemorrhage with speech disorder. Trans Am Neurol Assoc 1975;101:283-285.

138. Watson R, Heilman K: Thalamic neglect. Neurology 1979;29:690-694.

139. Young WB, Lee KP, Pessin MS, et al: Prognostic significance of ventricular blood in supratentorial hemorrhage: A volumetric study. Neurology 1990;40:616-619.

140. Kawahara N, Sato K, Muraki M, et al: CT classification of small thalamic hemorrhages and their clinical implications. Neurology 1986;35:165-172.

141. Ikeda K, Yamashima T, Uno E, et al: Clinical manifestations of small thalamic hemorrhages. Brain Nerve 1985;37:171-179.

142. Gilner L, Avin B: A reversible ocular manifestation of thalamic hemorrhage: A case report. Arch Neurol 1977;34:715-716.

143. Waga S, Okada M, Yamamoto Y: Reversibility of Parinaud syndrome in thalamic hemorrhage. Neurology 1979;29:407-409.

144. Kase C, Williams J, Wyatt D, et al: Lobar intracerebral hematomas: Clinical and CT analysis of 22 cases. Neurology 1982;32:1146-1150.

145. Ropper A, Davis K: Lobar cerebral hemorrhages: Acute clinical syndromes in 26 cases. Ann Neurol 1980;8:141-147.

146. Kase CS: Lobar hemorrhage. In Kase CS, Caplan LR (eds): Intracerebral Hemorrhage. Boston: Butterworth-Heinemann, 1994, pp 363-382.

147. Zhu XL, Chan MSY, Poon WS: Spontaneous intracranial hemorrhage: which patients need diagnostic cerebral angiography. A prospective study of 296 cases and review of the literature. Stroke 1997;28:1406-1409.

147a. Hallevi H, Albright KC, Aronowski J, et al: Intraventricular hemorrhage. Anatomic relationships and clinical implications. Neurology 2008;70:848-852.

148. Caplan LR: Primary intraventricular hemorrhage. In Kase CS, Caplan LR (eds): Intracerebral Hemorrhage. Boston: Butterworth-Heinemann, 1994, pp 383-401.

149. Butler A, Partain R, Netsky M: Primary intraventricular hemorrhage in adults. Surg Neurol 1977;8:143-149.

150. Little JR, Blomquist G, Ethier R: Intraventricular hemorrhage in adults. Surg Neurol 1977;8:143-149.

151. Naff NJ, Hanley DF, Keyl PM, et al: Intraventricular thrombolysis speeds blood clot resolution: Results of a pilot, prospective, randomized, double-blind, controlled trial. Neurosurgery 2004;54:577-584.

152. Steiner T, Diringer MN, Schneider D, et al: Dynamics of intraventricular hemorrhage in patients with spontaneous intracerebral hemorrhage: Risk factors, clinical impact, and effect of hemostatic therapy with recombinant activated factor VII. Neurosurgery 2006;59:767-773.

153. Bhattathiri PS, Gregson B, Prasad KS, Mendelow AD: Intraventricular hemorrhage and hydrocephalus after spontaneous intracerebral hemorrhage: Results from the STICH trial. Acta Neurochir Suppl 2006;96:65-68.

153a. Zhang Z, Li X, Liu Y, et al: Application of neuroendoscopy in the treatment of intraventricular hemorrhage. Cerebrovasc Dis 2007;24:91-96.

154. Kase C, Caplan LR: Parenchymatous posterior fossa hemorrhage. In Barnett HJM, Mohr JP, Stein B, Yatsu F (eds): Stroke: Pathophysiology, Diagnosis and Management. New York: Churchill Livingstone, 1985, pp 621-641.

155. Caplan LR: Pontine hemorrhage. In Kase CS, Caplan LR (eds): Intracerebral Hemorrhage. Boston: Butterworth-Heinemann, 1994, pp 403-423.

156. Caplan LR, Zervas N: Survival with permanent midbrain dysfunction after surgical treatment of traumatic subdural hematoma: The clinical picture of a Düret hemorrhage. Ann Neurol 1977;1:587-589.

157. Steegman T: Primary pontile hemorrhage. J Nerv Ment Dis 1951;114:35-65.

158. Silverstein A: Primary pontine hemorrhage. In Vinken P, Bruyn G (eds): Handbook of Clinical Neurology, vol 12, part 2. Vascular Diseases of the Nervous System. Amsterdam: North Holland, 1972, pp 37-53.

159. Nakajima K: Clinicopathological study of pontine hemorrhage. Stroke 1983;14:485-493.

160. Caplan LR, Goodwin J: Lateral tegmental brainstem hemorrhage. Neurology 1982;32:252-260.

161. Kase C, Maulsby G, Mohr JP: Partial pontine hematomas. Neurology 1980;30:652-655.

162. Graveleau P, DeCroix JP, Samson Y, et al: Deficit sensitive isole d'un hemicorps par hematome du pont. Rev Neurol (Paris) 1986;142:788-790.

163. Araga S, Fukada M, Kagimoto H, et al: Pure sensory stroke due to pontine hemorrhage. J Neurol 1987;235:116-117.

164. Holtzman RNN, Zablozki V, Yang WC, et al: Lateral pontine tegmental hemorrhage presenting as isolated trigeminal sensory neuropathy. Neurology 1987;37:704-706.

165. Veerapen R: Spontaneous lateral pontine hemorrhage with associated trigeminal nerve root hematoma. Neurosurgery 1989;25:451-454.

166. Gobernado J, de Molina A, Gineno A: Pure motor hemiplegia due to hemorrhage in the lower pons. Arch Neurol 1980;37:393.

167. Kameyama S, Tanaka R, Tsuchida T: Pure motor hemiplegia due to pontine hemorrhage. Stroke 1989;20:1288.

168. Schnapper R: Pontine hemorrhage presenting as ataxic hemiparesis. Stroke 1982;13:518-519.

169. Kobatake K, Shinohara Y: Ataxic hemiparesis in patients with primary pontine hemorrhage. Stroke 1983;14:762-764.

170. Tuhrim S, Yang WC, Rubinowitz H, et al: Primary pontine hemorrhage and the dysarthria-clumsy hand syndrome. Neurology 1982;32:1027-1028.

171. Lhermitte F, Pages M: Abducens nucleus syndrome due to pontine haemorrhage. Cerebrovasc Dis 2006;22:284-285.

172. Sherman SC, Saadatmand B: Pontine hemorrhage and isolated abducens nerve palsy. Am J Emerg Med 2007;25:104-105.

173. Watanabe A, Kobashi T: Lateral gaze disturbance due to cerebral microbleed in the medial lemniscus in the mid-pontine region: A case report. Neuroradiology 2005;47:908-911.

174. Brennan R, Berglund R: Acute cerebellar hemorrhage: Analysis of clinical findings and outcome in 12 cases. Neurology 1977;27:527-532.

175. Fisher CM, Picard E, Polak A, et al: Acute hypertensive cerebellar hemorrhage: Diagnosis and surgical treatment. J Nerv Ment Dis 1965;140:38-57.

176. Ott K, Kase C, Ojemann R, et al: Cerebellar hemorrhage: Diagnosis and treatment. Arch Neurol 1974;31:160-167.

177. Kase CS: Cerebellar hemorrhage. In Kase CS, Caplan LR (eds): Intracerebral Hemorrhage. Boston: Butterworth-Heinemann, 1994, pp 425-443.

178. Ojemann R, Heros R: Spontaneous brain hemorrhage. Stroke 1983;14:468-474.

179. Shenkin H, Zavala M: Cerebellar strokes: mortality, surgical indications and results of ventricular damage. Lancet 1982;2:429-432.

180. Richardson AE: Spontaneous Cerebellar Hemorrhage. In Vinken P, Bruyn G (eds): Handbook of Clinical Neurology. Amsterdam: North Holland, 1972, pp 54-67.

181. Ecker A: Upward transtentorial herniation of the brainstem and cerebellum due to tumor of the posterior fossa. J Neurosurg 1948;5:51-61.

182. Dolderer S, Kallenberg K, Aschoff A, et al: Long-term outcome after spontaneous cerebellar haemorrhage. Eur Neurol 2004;52:112-119.

183. Longo M, Fiumara F, Pandolfo I, et al: CT observation of an ongoing intracerebral hemorrhage. J Comput Assist Tomogr 1983;7:362-363.

184. Tarr RW: Intraparenchymal hemorrhage. In Babikian VL, Wechsler LR, Higashida RT (eds): Imaging Cerebrovascular Disease Philadelphia: Butterworth-Heinemann, 2003, pp 225-239.

185. Zilkha A: Intraparenchymal fluid-blood level: A CT sign of recent intracerebral hemorrhage. J Comput Assist Tomogr 1983;7:301-305.

186. Pineda A: Computed tomography in intracerebral hemorrhage. Surg Neurol 1977;8:55-58.

187. Dul K, Drayer B: CT and MR imaging of intracerebral hemorrhage. In Kase CS, Caplan LR (eds): Intracerebral Hemorrhage. Boston: Butterworth-Heinemann, 1994, pp 73-93.

188. Scott W, New P, Davis K, et al: Computerized axial tomography of intracerebral and intraventricular hemorrhage. Radiology 1974;112:73-80.

189. Herald S, Kummer R, Jaeger C: Follow-up of spontaneous intracerebral hemorrhage by computed tomography. J Neurology 1982;228:267-276.

190. Schellinger PD, Jansen O, Fiebach JB, et al: A standardized MRI protocol. Comparison with CT in hyperacute intracerebral hemorrhage. Stroke 1999;30:765-768.

191. Linfante I, Llinas RH, Caplan LR, Warach S: MRI features of intracerebral hemorrhage within 2 hours from symptom onset. Stroke 1999;30:2263-2267.

192. Kidwell CS, Chalela JA, Saver JL, et al: Comparison of MRI and CT for detection of acute intracerebral hemorrhage. JAMA 2004;292:1823-1830.

193. Yasui T, Kishi H, Komiyama M, et al: Very poor prognosis in cases with extravasation of the contrast medium during angiography. Surg Neurol 1996;45:560-564.

194. Murai Y, Ikeda Y, Teramoto A, Tsuji Y: Magnetic resonance imaging documented extravasation as an indicator of acute hypertensive intracerebral hemorrhage. J Neurosurg 1988;88:650-655.

195. Goldstein JN, Fazen LE, Snider R, et al: Contrast extravasation on CT angiography predicts hematoma expansion in intracerebral hemorrhage. Neurology 2007;68:889-894.

196. Ruiz-Sandoval JL, Chiquete E, Romero-Vargas S, et al: Grading scale for prediction of outcome in primary intracerebral hemorrhages. Stroke 2007;38:1641-1644.

197. Little J, Blomquist G, Ethier R: Cerebellar hemorrhage in adults: Diagnosis by computerized tomography. J Neurosurg 1978;48:575-579.

198. Radberg JA, Olsson JE, Radberg CT: Prognostic parameters in spontaneous intracerebral hematomas with special reference to anticoagulant treatment. Stroke 1991;22:571-576.

199. Terayama Y, Tanahashi N, Fukuuchi Y, Gotoh F: Prognostic value of admission blood pressure in patients with intracerebral hemorrhage. Keio Cooperative Stroke Study. Stroke 1997;28:1185-1188.

200. Diringer MN, Edwards DF, Zazulia A: Hydrocephalus: A previously unrecognized predictor of poor outcome from supratentorial intracerebral hemorrhage. Stroke 1998;29:1352-1357.

201. Dandapani B, Suzuki S, Kelley RE, et al: Relation between blood pressure and outcome in intracerebral hemorrhage. Stroke 1995;26:21-24.

202. Broderick JP, Adams HP, Barsan W, et al: Guidelines for the management of spontaneous intracerebral hemorrhage: A statement for healthcare professionals from a special writing group of the Stroke Council, American Heart Association. Stroke 1999;30:905-915.

202a. Mehdiratta M, Kumar S, Hackney D, et al: Association between serum ferritin level and perihematoma edema volume in patients with spontaneous intracerebral hemorrhage. Stroke 2008;39:1165-1170.

203. Hanley DF, Syed SJ: Current acute care of intracerebral hemorrhage. Rev Neurol Dis 2007;4:10-18.

204. Langfitt T: Conservative care of intracranial hemorrhage. In Thompson R, Green J (eds): Advances in Neurology, vol 11. Stroke. New York: Raven, 1977, pp 169-180.

205. Poungvarin N, Bhoopat W, Viriyavejakul A, et al: Effects of dexamethasone in primary supratentorial intracerebral hemorrhage. N Engl J Med 1987;316:1229-1233.

206. Tyler K, Poletti C, Heros R: Cerebral amyloid angiopathy with multiple intracerebral hemorrhages. Neurosurgery 1982;577:286-289.

207. Rabinstein AA, Wijdicks EFM: Determinants of outcome in anticoagulation-associated cerebral hematoma requiring emergency evacuation. Arch Neurol 2007;64:203-206.

208. Morgenstern LB, Demchuk AM, Kim DH, et al: Rebleeding leads to poor outcome in ultra-early craniotomy for intracerebral hemorrhage. Neurology 2001;56:1294-1299.

209. Batjer HH, Reisch JS, Allen BC, et al: Failure of surgery to improve outcome in hypertensive putaminal hemorrhage. A prospective randomized trial. Arch Neurol 1990;47:1103-1106.

210. Morganstern LB, Frankowski RF, Shedden P, et al: Surgical treatment for intracerebral hemorrhage (STICH). A single-center randomized clinical trial. Neurology 1998;51:1359-1363.

211. Hankey GJ: Surgery for primary intracerebral hemorrhage: Is it safe and effective? A systematic review of case series and randomized trials. Stroke 1997;28:2126-2132.

212. Rabinstein AA, Wijdicks EFM: Surgery for intracerebral hematoma: The search for the elusive right candidate. Rev Neurol Dis 2006;3:163-172.

213. Prasad K, Browman G, Srivastava A, Menon G: Surgery in primary supratentorial intracerebral hematoma: A meta-analysis of randomized trials. Acta Neurol Scand 1997;95:103-110.

214. Mendelow AD, Gregson BA, Fernandes HM, et al: Early surgery versus initial conservative treatment in patients with spontaneous supratentorial intracerebral haematomas in the International Surgical Trial in Intracerebral Haemorrhage (STICH): A randomised trial. Lancet 2005;365:387-397.

215. Prasad KS, Gregson BA, Bhattathiri PS, et al.; The significance of crossovers after randomization in the STICH trial. Acta Neurochir Suppl 2006;96:61-64.

215a. Broderick J, Connolly S, Feldmann, et al: Guidelines for the management of spontaneous intracerebral hemorrhage in adults, 2007 update: A guideline from the American Heart Association/American Stroke Association Stroke Council, High Blood Pressure Research Council and the Quality of Care and Outcomes in Research Interdisciplinary Working Group. Stroke 2007;38:2001-2023.

216. Fleming KD, Wijdicks EFM, St Louis EK, Li H: Predicting deterioration on patients with lobar haemorrhages. J Neurol Neurosurg Psychiatry 1999;66:600-605.

217. Kandel EL, Peresadov VV: Stereotactic evacuation of spontaneous intracerebral hematomas. J Neurosurg 1985;62:206-213.

218. Nizuma H, Suzuki J: Stereotactic aspiration of putaminal hemorrhage using a double track aspiration technique. Neurosurgery 1988;22:432-436.

219. Nguyen JP, Decq P, Brugieres P, et al: A technique for stereotactic aspiration of deep intracerebral hematomas under computed tomographic control using a new device. Neurosurgery 1992;31:330-335.

220. Mohadjer M, Eggert R, May J, Mayfrank L: CT-guided stereotactic fibrinolysis of spontaneous and hypertensive cerebellar hemorrhage: Long-term results. J Neurosurg 1990;73:217-222.

221. Schaller C, Rhode V, Meyer B, Hassler W: Stereotactic puncture and lysis of spontaneous intracerebral hemorrhage using recombinant tissue-plasminogen activator (rtPA) after stereotactic aspiration: Initial results. Neurosurgery 1995;36:328-335.

222. Shields CB, Friedman WA: The role of stereotactic technology in the management of intracerebral hemorrhage. Neurosurg Clin North Am 1992;3:685-702.

223. Niizuma H, Shimizu Y, Yonemitsu T, et al: Results of stereotactic aspiration in 175 cases of putaminal hemorrhage. Neurosurgery 1989;24:814-819.

224. Marquardt G, Wolff R, Sager A, et al: Subacute stereotactic aspiration of haematomas within the basal ganglia reduces occurrence of complications in the course of haemorrhagic stroke in noncomatose patients. Cerebrovasc Dis 2003;15:252-257.

225. Thiex R, Rohde V, Rohde I, et al: Frame-based and frameless stereotactic hematoma puncture and subsequent fibrinolytic therapy for the treatment of spontaneous intracerebral hemorrhage. J Neurol 2004;251:1443-1450.

226. Cho DY, Chen CC, Chang CS, et al: Endoscopic surgery for spontaneous basal ganglia hemorrhage: Comparing endoscopic surgery, stereotactic aspiration, and craniotomy in noncomatose patients. Surg Neurol 2006;65:547-556.

227. Naff NJ, Hanley DF, Keyl PM, et al: Intraventricular thrombolysis speeds blood clot resolution: Results of a pilot, prospective, randomized, double-blind, controlled trial. Neurosurgery 2004;54:577-584.

228. Mayer SA: Ultra-early hemostatic therapy for intracerebral hemorrhage. Stroke 2003;34:224-229.

229. Mayer SA, Brun NC, Broderick J, et al: Europe/AustralAsia NovoSeven ICH Trial Investigators. Safety and feasibility of recombinant factor VIIa for acute intracerebral hemorrhage. Stroke 2005;36:74-79.

230. Mayer SA, Brun NC, Begtrup K, et al: Recombinant Activated Factor VII Intracerebral Hemorrhage Trial Investigators. Recombinant activated factor VII for acute intracerebral hemorrhage. N Engl J Med 2005;352:777-785.

231. Davis SM, Broderick J, Hennerici M: Recombinant Activated Factor VII Intracerebral Hemorrhage Trial Investigators. Hematoma growth is a determinant of mortality and poor outcome after intracerebral hemorrhage. Neurology 2006 Apr 25;66(8):1175-1181

232. Sugg RM, Gonzales NR, Matherne DE, et al: Myocardial injury in patients with intracerebral hemorrhage treated with recombinant factor VIIa. Neurology 2006;67:1053-1055.

233. Mayer SA, Brun NC, Begtrup K, et al: Efficacy and safety of recombinant activated factor VII for acute intracerebral hemorrhage. N Engl J Med 2008;358:2127-2137.

234. Tuhrim S: Intracerebral hemorrhage—Improving outcome by reducing volume. N Engl J Med 2008;358:2174-2176.

Stroke in Children and Young Adults 14

Strokes are not especially common in the young, but when they occur, clinical features and evaluation strategies are rather different from adult patients in the usual stroke age group (50 to 85 years). In this chapter, I briefly outline some of the key differences, and review the differential diagnoses of strokes in the young. I do not repeat descriptions of stroke syndromes and vascular disorders covered in more depth elsewhere in this book. Chapter 11 includes discussions of many of the conditions that cause stroke in the young.

GENERAL FEATURES AND DIFFERENCES FROM STROKES AND CEREBROVASCULAR DISEASE IN GERIATRIC-AGE PATIENTS

Heterogeneity

Causes of stroke in the young are more heterogeneous than in the older population. The differential diagnosis list includes many genetic, congenital, metabolic, and systemic disorders that are rarely encountered in mature adult populations. Also, more often than in adults, the cause of childhood stroke remains obscure, even after thorough evaluation.

Etiologic Variations Associated with Age

Causes of stroke differ considerably with age. For example, the differential diagnosis of stroke in a young baby is quite different from that in a 40-year-old adult, yet both are often referred to as stroke in the young. Three convenient groups can be distinguished: perinatal and neonatal, children (ages 1 to 15 years), and adolescents and young adults (ages 15 to 40 years). Each of these groups has different frequencies of various stroke etiologies. Causes also vary considerably, depending on geographic, socioeconomic, and environmental factors. For instance, tuberculous meningitis is an important cause of stroke in India,[1,2] and neurocysticercosis is an important cause of stroke in Mexico and parts of Central and South America.[3,4] These causes of stroke, however, are much less common in the United States.

Prevalence of Hemorrhagic Stroke

Hemorrhagic strokes, including subarachnoid hemorrhage (SAH) and intracerebral hemorrhage (ICH), are relatively more common in the young. In the geriatric years, the ischemic to hemorrhagic stroke ratio is approximately 4 to 1 (80% of strokes are ischemic), whereas in the young, the ratio is close to 1.0 to 1.5 (60% are hemorrhagic).[5,6] Accurate comparative statistics are hard to gather because hemorrhagic strokes are often cared for on neurosurgical units, and ischemic strokes are usually admitted to pediatric and adult neurology units.

Prevalence of Particular Etiologies of Stroke

Migraine, trauma (including dissection), and cardiac disease are especially important etiologies in children and young adults. A relatively new category, *vasculopathy*, is prevalent in children and probably represents a special predilection for vasoreactivity provoked by various conditions in this age group. Drugs and systemic, genetic, and hematologic causes are also important in children and young adults. Occlusion of dural venous sinuses and cerebral veins is a more important cause of stroke in the young than in mature adults.

Locations of Lesions

Brain and vascular location of lesions are somewhat different in the young. Brain infarcts tend to be more often limited to deep regions of the cerebral hemispheres, especially the striatocapsular region. Vascular-occlusive lesions are more often intracranial, affecting especially the supraclinoid internal carotid artery (ICA), proximal middle cerebral artery (MCA), and basilar artery. Extracranial occlusive disease is much less common. When the occlusive process affects the MCA before the lenticulostriate branches, the striatum and internal capsule are often involved. Because of the absence of extensive vascular disease, collateral circulation over the convexity is usually good, accounting for sparing of the MCA cortical territory.[7,8] Similarly, proximal posterior cerebral artery occlusion before the thalamogeniculate branches usually leads to thalamic infarcts, with sparing of the temporal and occipital lobes.[9,10] Vascular malformations are more often periventricular or intraventricular than in adults.

Clinical Presentations and Features

In youths, the clinical presentations and features of stroke are also different. For instance, apoplectic sudden onset is the rule. Transient ischemic attacks are unusual. Seizures are common and are often the presenting feature. Brain edema and increased intracranial pressure are also common. Less reserve space in the cranium exists because of the absence of brain atrophy relative to geriatric patients. Aphasias in childhood are most often nonfluent, regardless of brain lesion location.[11] In children, agitation and general confusion are often described, but specific disorders of higher cognitive function are harder to recognize and are less well characterized than in adults. Abnormalities of posture and movement, such as dystonias, chorea, and athetosis, are more frequent features and sequelae of stroke than in adults.[12] These extrapyramidal disorders probably reflect the predominance of striatocapsular ischemia. In young children with ischemic damage to the basal ganglia and thalamus, these basal gray-matter tissues become hypermyelinated, giving them a marbled appearance, referred to as status marmoratus.[13]

Prognosis

In youths, the outlook for recovery is better than in adults with comparable lesions. The absence of generalized vascular disease and presence of good collateral circulation often minimizes the eventual brain damage, making the ultimate infarct smaller than in adults. Also, the developing brain shows more plasticity. Undamaged areas can frequently assume the functions of damaged regions. As a result, focal disorders of cognition and aphasia often improve, leaving no major speech deficit, although general intellectual function may be less than that expected before the stroke. Although the prognosis is better than in the geriatric age group, strokes in the young are far from benign. Among 1040 children with arterial ischemic strokes in the Canadian Pediatric Ischemic Stroke Registry, neurologic deficits were found in 61% of children who had neonatal strokes and neurologic deficits and recurrent strokes were common in older children.[14] A 1994 study of the prognosis of strokes in patients aged 15 to 45 years showed that most stroke survivors had emotional, social, or physical impairments that adversely affected employment and reduced their quality of life.[15]

STROKES IN NEONATES

Hypoxic-ischemic and metabolic injuries are relatively common in neonates. The causes of neonatal brain injury are extremely varied; laboratory and imaging advances are still identifying new etiologies.[16,16a] The neonatal brain is especially vulnerable to oxidative damage related to a high concentration of unsaturated fatty acids, free radicals, high rate of oxygen consumption, and low concentration of antioxidants.[16,16b] Many of the lesions in premature infants are located in the periventricular white matter. Ischemic cerebral white matter is quite susceptible to free-radical mediated injury to immature oligodendrocytes.[16b] Hypoxia and ischemia are most often attributable to (1) intrauterine asphyxia; (2) birth-related problems, such as umbilical cord prolapse, forceps delivery, and breech presentation; (3) uterine and placental abruption; (4) respiratory insufficiency after birth, caused by aspirated meconium; (5) recurrent apnea; (6) hyaline-membrane disease in premature infants; and (7) severe congenital heart disease, with left-to-right shunts in premature and full-term neonates.[17-20] In preterm infants, fetal heart-rate abnormalities, hypoglycemia, and twin-to-twin transfusion syndrome are other conditions that predispose to arterial strokes.[20a] Twin-to-twin transfusion syndrome is due to monochorionic implantation with vascular interconnections or intrauterine death of a co-twin, explaining redistribution of thromboplastic material and potential emboli.[20a]

Cerebral blood flow is lower in preterm than term newborns (20 mL/100 g/minute vs 50 to 60 mL/100 g/minute).[21] The neonatal brain has little autoregulatory capability, so it is much more vulnerable to falls or elevations in blood pressure. Neonatal ischemia is often caused by cardiac disease, sepsis with vascular collapse, and hypertension. Genetic and acquired coagulation abnormalities also may contribute to the development of neonatal strokes and brain ischemia.[14,16,20,22,23]

The most vulnerable areas for hypoxic-ischemic injury are the cerebral white matter and the cerebral cortex, especially the hippocampus; Purkinje cells of the cerebellar cortex; and the pontine nuclei in the brainstem.[17-21] Perinatal asphyxia also often causes severe damage to the putamen and thalamus on both sides. In addition, more severe hypoxic-ischemic insults damage the caudate nuclei and sensorimotor cortex around the central fissure.[18,24,25]

Three particularly common distributions of hypoxic-ischemic lesions exist in neonates—the parasagittal regions, deep periventricular white matter, and basal ganglia-thalami.[17-29] The parasagittal cortex between the anterior cerebral artery and MCA, and between the MCA and posterior cerebral artery territories are watershed zones, frequently selectively damaged by hypotension in the full-term newborn infant.[17,26,27] The most frequent resulting clinical picture is weakness of the proximal limbs, especially the arms. Spastic quadriparesis, which is worse in the arms, is the most characteristic clinical picture.[17,26,27] Computed tomography (CT), magnetic resonance imaging (MRI), radionuclide studies, and positron-emission tomography scanning can show the parasagittal distribution of ischemic damage.[17,26,27,30]

In premature infants, hypoxic-ischemic injury is often reflected in damage to the white matter around the ventricles, a process usually termed periventricular leukomalacia.[16,21,28,29,31-34] Sometimes, small isolated foci of necrosis exist at the angles of the ventricles. Often, the lesions are extensive and spread out from the ventricles toward the cortex. The periventricular lesions can be hemorrhagic and are often associated with enlargement of the ventricular system. The predominant clinical finding is spastic weakness of the legs (diplegia), with lesser involvement of the upper limbs. The white matter lesions near the anterior horns intercept the fibers coming from the parasagittal motor cortex, subserving control of the thighs, legs, and feet. CT, MRI, and ultrasound allow diagnosis during the neonatal period and sequential evaluation of the lesions. Figure 14-1 is an MRI that shows periventricular leukomalacia lesions.

Severe, acute hypoxic-ischemic insults during the perinatal period can cause severe damage to the basal ganglia and thalami.[18,24,28,29] The MRI in Figure 14-2 shows these lesions. The clinical findings during the neonatal period include tongue fasciculations and feeding problems, with impaired swallowing, irritability, and tonic posturing of the arms and legs.[18] Many individuals with these lesions die during the neonatal period. Survivors often have spastic quadriparesis, chorea-athetosis, dystonic postures, and feeding problems with recurrent aspiration and pulmonary infections.[18,29]

Focal arterial and venous infarcts are also often found in neonates, with seizures or hemiparesis.[17,28,35-38] Most of these lesions are in the territories of the major cerebral arterial distribution, most often affecting the MCA. The lesions may be

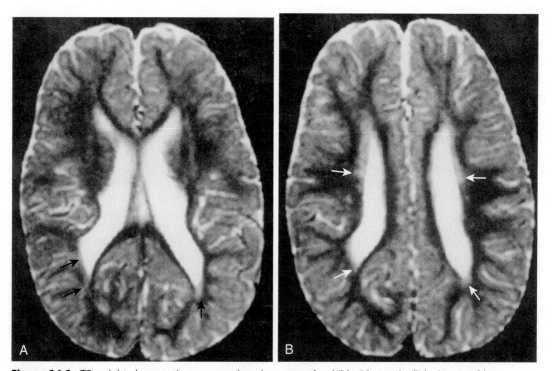

Figure 14-1. T2-weighted magnetic resonance imaging scans of a child with spastic diplegia caused by periventricular leukomalacia. The scans were taken at 15 months and show irregularity of the ventricular walls, loss of white matter, and T2 prolongation in the periventricular white matter. *Arrows* point to periventricular abnormalities. (From Aida N, Nishimura NA, Hachiya Y, et al: Magnetic resonance imaging of perinatal brain damage: Comparison of clinical outcome with initial and follow-up magnetic resonance findings. AJNR Am J Neuroradiol 1998;19:1909-1921, with permission.)

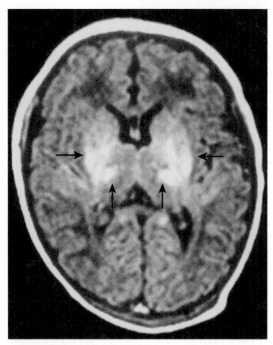

Figure 14-2. T1-weighted magnetic resonance imaging scan at 10 days shows abnormal signal intensities *(black arrows)* in the lenticular nuclei and thalamus in a child who had spastic quadriparesis, seizures, athetoid movements, and developmental delay. (From Aida N, Nishimura NA, Hachiya Y, et al: Magnetic resonance imaging of perinatal brain damage: Comparison of clinical outcome with initial and follow-up magnetic resonance findings. Am J Neuroradiol 1998;19:1909-1921, with permission.)

large and cystic and on occasion communicate with the ventricular system, forming porence-phalic cysts. Many are in the distribution of the lenticulo-striate branches of the MCAs.[16a] Obstruction of an MCA in these neonates could lead to infarction that predominates in the penetrating artery supply regions with good collaterals preserving the remainder of the cerebral cortex and white matter supplied by the MCA. For reasons that are unclear, focal asymmetric infarcts are sometimes found in asphyxiated infants with generalized hypoxia and ischemia. Focal infarcts are clearly more common than are presently diagnosed. In an autopsy study of 592 neonates, 32 (5.4%) had focal infarcts in a recognized arterial distribution.[35] Full-term neonates more often had focal infarcts than premature infants. Some children with congenital hemiplegia have focal unilateral infarcts on MRI scans in the corona radiata that are posited to be caused by compression of periventricular veins.[16a,38] These periventricular venous infarcts (PVIs) are unilateral and show evidence of hemosiderin deposition related to bleeding into the infarcted territory.[16a] Figure 14-3

from Kirton et al[16a] shows MRI scans of 10 infants with PVIs.

Arterial embolization with sepsis and disseminated intravascular coagulation are also common causes of unilateral arterial territorial infarcts. Focal arterial territory infarcts in infants can also result from drugs, especially cocaine use, by the mother.[39] Traumatic occlusions of the cervical, carotid, and vertebral arteries and intracranial vessels during delivery are another important cause of stroke in neonates.[40,41]

Arterial thromboembolism also can occur in the neonatal period, is often due to cardiac disease and/or hypercoagulability, and on rare occasions can recur during childhood especially when a cause is identified.[23] In one series among 55 infants with presumed perinatal ischemic strokes, 43 were considered arterial (26 main MCA cortical and subcortical, 8 superior division MCA, 5 inferior division MCA, and 4 lenticulo-striate), and 12 were thought to represent periventricular venous infarcts.[16a]

Dural sinus thrombosis also occurs in neonates.[42,43] Abnormalities are often evident at birth or during the first week of life, and most often include seizures, apnea, or weight loss. The sagittal sinus is most often involved. Hypoxia at birth, premature rupture of maternal membranes, abruptio placenta, maternal infections, and dehydration and infections in the neonate were common associated conditions. Some neonates had prothrombotic findings on laboratory evaluation. The resultant infarcts were often hemorrhagic. Sinovenous occlusions in neonates is a very serious disorder with a high mortality rate and a high rate of severe neurologic disability.[42,43]

Brain hemorrhages are an even more frequent and important cause of stroke in the perinatal period. Premature infants are especially susceptible to developing hemorrhages in the periventricular region, spreading into the ventricles.[17,21,44-46] These hemorrhages originate in the subependymal germinal matrix, a structure located over the head and body of the caudate nuclei at the level of the intraventricular foramina. The matrix contains fragile capillaries and loose supporting tissue. By full term, the germinal matrix is no longer visible. In the absence of effective autoregulation, increase in blood pressure or blood volume can lead to breakage of these fragile vessels and resultant intracerebral hemorrhage. An increase in venous pressure, as might be found in asphyxia or hyaline-membrane disease, might also promote hematoma formation. Hemorrhages usually extend into the adjacent ventricle. Regions of necrosis often surround the hematomas. In full-term infants, periventricular and intraventricular

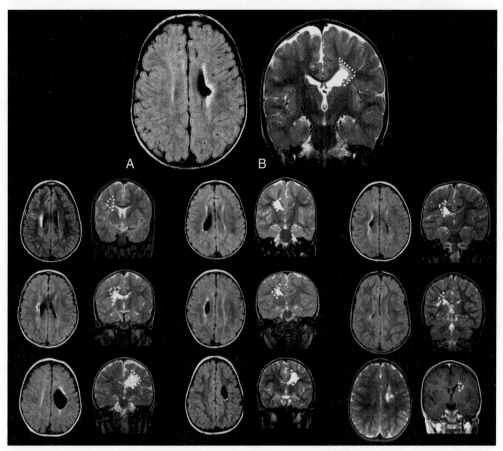

Figure 14-3. Representative pairs of axial fluid-attenuated inversion recovery *(left)* and coronal T2 *(right)* MRI images from 10 patients with periventricular venous infarction. Consistent lesion features include focal cystic softening in the periventricular white matter and T2 prolongation in the posterior limb of the internal capsule. A "caudal triangle" in which periventricular white matter is more affected than basal ganglia is diagrammed in the coronal images. (Courtesy of Adam Kirton, MD, from Kirton A, deVeber G, Pontigon A-M, et al: Presumed perinatal ischemic stroke: Vascular classification predicts outcome. Ann Neurol 2008;63:436-443, with permission.)

hemorrhages arise from residual matrix tissue or directly from the choroid plexus vasculature.

Most germinal matrix hemorrhages occur during the first 3 postnatal days, especially during the first postpartum hours, but some develop in utero.[46] Clinically, infants with germinal-matrix hemorrhages may appear very ill with coma, respiratory abnormalities, and poor muscle tone, or they may appear to be faring normally. At times, a gradual deterioration of function occurs. Ultrasound and CT are effective ways to diagnose and follow children with hemorrhages. Intraventricular hemorrhages can cause temporary hydrocephalus, which resolves itself, or progressive hydrocephalus, requiring ventricular drainage or shunting. Lumbar puncture, with removal of cerebrospinal fluid, is another effective treatment. Ventricular size should be carefully followed by ultrasound or CT.

Since the mid-1970s, cerebellar hemorrhage has been recognized more often during the early neonatal period, especially in premature infants.[21,41,47,48] Cerebellar hemorrhage occurs in an estimated 15% to 25% of preterm infants.[41,49] In the late stages of gestation, a cerebellar germinal matrix is present. This probably accounts for the high risk of bleeding in preterm babies. Asphyxia and hyaline-membrane disease are contributing factors. Trauma is the principal cause of parenchymatous cerebellar bleeding in full-term babies. Often, cerebellar hemorrhage causes catastrophic loss of function. Seizures; falling hematocrit; signs of brainstem compression, such as ocular bobbing or skew deviation; and acute hydrocephalus may result. Ultrasound, CT, and MRI allow diagnosis. Surgical decompression is often required and can be lifesaving.[41]

Subarachnoid bleeding is extremely common, and some red blood cells are found in the cerebrospinal fluid of nearly every baby delivered vaginally. Bleeding is most often trivial. More severe

14

birth trauma or coagulation abnormalities can lead to more severe subarachnoid bleeding and diminished alertness in the neonate.[21] Trauma can also cause significant subdural collections of blood.

STROKES IN CHILDREN (1 TO 18 YEARS OF AGE)

Infantile hemiplegia and childhood stroke have been recognized for centuries. In his 1888 textbook, *Neurology*, Gowers commented, "Hemiplegia of sudden onset is not uncommon in children, especially in young children."[50] Despite considerable interest, information about etiology did not come about until the report of Ford and Schaffer on acquired hemiplegia in children was published in 1927.[51] During the past 2 decades there has been important advances in knowledge about pediatric stroke. The advent of modern brain imaging, and especially vascular imaging, has identified frequent abnormalities within the intracranial arteries, now labeled with a nondescript general term, *arteriopathy*.[52-56] The present availability of safe, rapid diagnostic technology that provides brain and vascular imaging gives promise for unlocking many aspects of strokes in children concerning etiology, prognosis, and treatment that had been unattainable in the past. Another important recent advance has been the development of registries and data bases that are accruing data about childhood stroke. The largest to date is the Canadian Pediatric Ischemic Stoke Registry.[14,43] An urgent telephone consultation service, 1-800 NOCLOTS, has been active since 1994 and has accumulated information about more than 1000 children with strokes in the United States and Canada.[57] Finally, pediatric stroke neurology specialists, a new breed, have sprung up, especially in Toronto, London, and San Francisco, and have begun to collaborate in research, accumulate data, and disseminate information to pediatricians and neurologists who care for children with strokes.

Estimates of the frequency of strokes in neonates and children vary from about 2[14,58,59] to 5.5[60] per 100,000 children-years. Blacks and Hispanic children may have a higher incidence of stroke in North America,[60] and the frequency of strokes may be higher in Asia, although definitive estimates are not available. Between 1979 and 1998, mortality from stroke in children under 20 years of age declined by 58%.[61] The decline in mortality was noted among all ischemic and hemorrhagic stroke types. Mortality was higher in blacks and boys.[61] Although most strokes in children are ischemic, the ratio of ischemia to hemorrhage is lower in children than in adults.

Hemorrhagic Stroke in Children

In preadolescent children, vascular malformations are the most common cause of intracranial bleeding.[40,62-64] If all individuals younger than 20 years are included, however, subarachnoid hemorrhages are as common or more common than intracerebral bleeds and aneurysms are a more common cause of bleeding than vascular malformations. Among 124 young patients with SAH in a 1973 series, 50 patients had aneurysms and 33 had arteriovenous malformations (AVMs).[65] Among three series published before 1973, 36% of young patients had aneurysmal bleeding, whereas 27% bled from AVMs.[65] In a series of patients enrolled between 1993 and 2004, among 116 children with nontraumatic hemorrhagic strokes who had structural lesions that caused bleeding, 78% were AVMs, 33% aneurysms, and 37% cavernous malformations.[64]

Aneurysms generally become symptomatic before the age of 2 years or after age 10.[41,66] Aneurysms are more common in individuals with coarctation of the aorta and polycystic renal disease.[41] In childhood, bacterial endocarditis with embolism to the vasa vasorum of intracranial arteries, and mycotic aneurysm formation are especially important causes of SAH. Aneurysms that rupture in childhood have a somewhat different distribution than those found in adults. Shucart and Wolpert analyzed the site of rupture of 100 congenital intracranial aneurysms in children younger than 15 years.[67] Compared with adult series, the intracranial ICA was more often the site of anterior-circulation bleeding in children, whereas the posterior and anterior communicating arteries were less often implicated in children.[67] Posterior-circulation aneurysms were relatively more common in children (23% of the total) than in adults. They especially involved the intracranial vertebral artery and basilar artery apex.[67] Evaluation and treatment of aneurysms is similar in children and adults.

Intracranial vascular malformations are undoubtedly present at birth, but do not become symptomatic in most patients until adulthood. Although AVMs are the most frequent cause of intracranial bleeding in preadolescents, less than 10% of malformations are diagnosed before the age of 10 years.[41] Mackenzie noted in 1953 that 29 of his 50 patients (58%) with brain angiomas developed initial symptoms before age 20 years.[67] The advent of safer and more widely distributed brain imaging means that now cavernous malformations and AVMs are detected earlier and more often than in the past. In adolescents and older children, the most frequent symptoms in patients with vascular malformations are caused by hemorrhage. Most often, bleeding is into the brain (ICH), but superficial lesions and those abutting on ependymal surfaces can cause SAH or primary intraventricular bleeding. Approximately 20% of AVMs in children are infratentorial, approximately equally divided between the cerebellum and brainstem.[69] Supratentorial arteriovenous malformations are typically superficial and cone-shaped, with the base located on the cortical surface and the apex closer to the ventricle.[70] Approximately 10% are deep, involving the basal ganglia and thalamus.[70] Focal neurologic signs often develop gradually and can be associated with signs of increased intracranial pressure. Epilepsy and headache are other less frequent presentations of vascular malformations.

Neonates and young children often harbor a type of malformation that is rarely, if ever, first discovered in adulthood, a vein of Galen malformation. In this condition, the vein of Galen is greatly enlarged, forming a large varix, and the straight sinus is also large and tortuous. The malformation is usually fed by posterior choroidal arteries. The typical CT appearance is that of a round hyperdense mass behind the third ventricle, connected to a prominent torcula by the dilatated midline straight sinus. Hydrocephalus is also occasionally associated in approximately one third of patients. The most common presenting syndrome during the neonatal period and infancy is high-output congestive heart failure, caused by the large volume of shunted blood.[41] A loud cranial bruit is usually audible. Older infants and young children may present with SAH or intraventricular hemorrhage, seizures, or signs of hydrocephalus. If left untreated, these malformations can prove fatal early in life. I also discuss this malformation in Chapter 16.

Cavernous malformations have only recently become easily recognized with widespread availability of brain imaging. About one fourth of the patients in the various series of cerebral cavernomas were children.[71-73] Among 172 pediatric patients with cavernomas, Cavalheiro and Braga noted two age peaks—one during the first year of life and the other between the ages of 12 and 16 years.[74] When bleeding does occur, it is invariably within the capsule of the cavernoma.

Intracerebral and subarachnoid hemorrhages occasionally develop in children with various bleeding diatheses, and with acute hypertension as might be found in pheochromocytoma, cocaine and amphetamine use, or acute glomerulonephritis. In one series, recurrent hemorrhages developed in 11 of 116 (10%) of children.[64] Vascular malformations were associated with a high and prolonged risk of recurrent hemorrhage: bleeding diathesis were accompanied by a high

recurrence rate but mostly during the first week.[64] Head trauma is another important cause of intracranial hemorrhage in children. Trauma accounted for 24% of 116 hemorrhagic strokes in children in one study.[64]

Ischemic Strokes in Children

Differential diagnosis of brain infarcts in children is quite wide (Table 14-1), and many patients escape etiologic diagnosis, even after full evaluation. Deep basal ganglia, internal capsule, and thalamic infarcts are relatively more common in children than older age groups. Brower and colleagues described the clinical findings, imaging features, and causes among 36 children (newborn to 13 years) with striatocapsular and thalamic infarcts at their medical center during a 6-year period.[75] Most children presented with an acute hemiplegia that usually resolved within a week, leaving minor motor residual. Sensory and important cognitive abnormalities were unusual unless infarction was bilateral.[75] A wide variety of vasculopathies was responsible. The deep pattern is probably best explained by involvement of the proximal portions of the ICAs or MCAs, or both, and the posterior cerebral artery in the presence of good collateral circulation, which continues to supply adequate blood flow to the cerebral cortex.

The major causes of brain ischemia in children follow: (1) cardiac origin embolism, (2) arterial dissection, (3) sinovenous thrombosis, (4) coagulopathy, and (5) arteriopathies. The term *arteriopathy* includes a spectrum of causes that include infection, trauma, migraine, moyamoya, and genetic disorders such as sickle cell disease, Fabry disease, and mitochondrial disorders. The usual risk factors for the development of ischemic stroke in adults—hypertension, diabetes, hyperlipidemia, and smoking—are less important causes of brain ischemia in children.

About one fourth of ischemic strokes in young children are attributable to heart disease. A relatively high proportion of cardiac-related ischemic strokes occur in relation to surgery and other procedures, more than 40% in one study.[14] Brain infarcts in children with cardiac disease are most often caused by embolism. Bacterial endocarditis is an important cause. Congenital heart disease, especially with shunting of blood (atrial and ventricular septal defects and patent ductus arteriosis), and complex congenital defects are frequent.[14,76] Children with stroke and congenital heart disease are often cyanotic and have chronic hypoxia and polycythemia. They may develop venous and arterial occlusions related to the polycythemia. Brain abscess is also common in

14

Table 14-1.   Differential Diagnosis of Pediatric Brain Ischemia (Age 1 to 15 Years)

- Migraine
- Trauma: Dissection and other vascular injuries; abuse, including whiplash-shake injuries; oral foreign-body trauma to the internal carotid artery
- Cardiac: Congenital heart disease with right-to-left shunts, tetralogy of Fallot, transposition of great vessels, tricuspid atresia, atrial and ventricular septal defects, cardiomyopathies, endocarditis, pulmonary arteriovenous fistula
- Drugs, especially cocaine and heroin
- Infections: Bacterial meningitis, especially *Haemophilus influenzae,* pneumonococci, and streptococci; facial, otitic, and sinus infections; acquired immunodeficiency syndrome; dural sinus occlusion and infection; tuberculous meningitis
- Genetic and metabolic: Neurofibromatosis, hereditary disorders of connective tissue (Marfan's and Ehlers-Danlos syndromes), pseudoxanthoma elasticum, homocystinuria, Menkes' kinky hair syndrome, hypoalphalipoproteinemia, familial hyperlipidemias, methylmalonic aciduria, MELAS syndrome (mitochondrial, encephalopathy, lactic acidosis, and stroke-like episodes), cytochrome oxidase deficiency
- Hematologic and neoplastic: Sickle cell anemia, purpuras, leukemia, l-arginase and aminocaproic acid (Amicar) treatment, radiation vasculopathy, hypercoagulable states (e.g., caused by decrease in natural inhibitors, such as antithrombin III, protein C, protein S)
- Systemic disease: Rheumatic, gastrointestinal, renal, hepatic, pulmonary, moyamoya syndrome
- Others: Arteritis, collagen vascular disease, local infections, Takayasu's syndrome, Behçet's syndrome, venous sinus thrombosis, head and neck infections, dehydration, coagulopathy, paroxysmal nocturnal hemoglobinuria, puerperal or pregnancy related

this situation and must be distinguished from infarction. Rheumatic heart disease, endocarditis, cardiomyopathies, and myocarditis are important acquired heart diseases associated with brain embolism.[77] Diagnostic techniques, especially transesophageal echocardiography and transcranial Doppler sonography after intravenous injection of air bubbles, have led to the detection of small atrial shunts (atrial septal defects and patent foramen ovale) in children and young adults with otherwise unexplained brain infarcts.

Arterial composition and function in childhood are likely a bit different from that in most older adults, since the intracranial arteries are rarely subject to important degenerative atherosclerotic changes. The media is composed of smooth muscle cells, collagen, and elastin. The endothelium is a sensor that can release vasoactive substances, alter the extracellular matrix in the blood vessel wall, and trigger vascular remodeling. Increased vascular elasticity and reactivity contribute to the development of "arteriopathy" in this age group from a variety of different stimuli. Children in whom angiography shows an arteriopathy have a less abrupt, more indolent onset and course than those who do not show an arteriopathy by angiography.[77a] The presence of an angiographically confirmed arteriopathy conveys an increased risk for stroke recurrence.[52-56]

One important cause of arteriopathy in childhood is trauma. Direct trauma can lead to arterial occlusion and intense vasoconstriction. Stretching of arteries at locations where they are not anchored can lead to tearing of arterial walls (dissections). Head and neck traumas, even trivial ones, are often mentioned as a predisposing factor by the parents of children with ischemic strokes. Ten of the 54 patients (18.5%) in a Japanese series of children with ischemic strokes had head trauma in the home within the 2 days before the strokes.[78] Oral trauma by penetrating objects can cause ICA occlusions.[79,80] Young children may fall while keeping pencils and toothbrushes in their mouths. The pharynx is lacerated or contused, and the ICA is injured during its course behind the faucial pillars. Extracranial carotid and vertebral artery dissection can develop after head or neck injuries, especially involving sudden twisting movements and blunt trauma to the neck. Neck, jaw, or throat pain or headache may be the earliest symptoms. Brain infarction occurs when the blood within the arterial wall dissects into the arterial lumen and embolizes intracranially. At times, the intramural clot occludes the lumen sufficiently that a luminal thrombus forms in situ because of sluggish flow and activation of clotting factors.

I have seen several patients in whom seemingly trivial head trauma led to severe intracranial arterial dissections. A young girl developed a fatal intracranial ICA and MCA dissection after her head hit the top of a car when it hit a bump.[81] A young boy fell and hit his head while trick-or-treating on Halloween. Although he appeared uninjured to his mother, he developed a hemiplegia and bilateral motor signs the next day, later shown to be caused by an angiographically documented basilar artery dissection. Dissection was the most common cause of arteriopathy in several modern series that included frequent vascular imaging.[14,58]

Infection was cited as an important predisposing cause of hemiplegia in children in the 1927 report of Ford and Schaffer[51] and in other early writings.[41] Most often, the infections were respiratory or systemic, and the mechanism of stroke was uncertain. In a 1991 study of childhood stroke in the Tohoku district of Japan, 10 of 54 patients (18.5%) had upper respiratory tract infections or fevers of unknown origin.[78] Tonsillitis can occasionally lead to occlusive changes in the adjacent pharyngeal portion of the ICA. Influenza and *Mycoplasma pneumoniae* have been occasionally implicated as causes of brain infarction.[41,82,83]

The best studied infectious cause of arteriopathy is infection with the herpes zoster varicella (HZV) virus. In herpes zoster in adults, the virus can be detected in the vascular endothelium, often without an inflammatory response. Virions characteristic of HZV can be found in the nuclei and cytoplasm of smooth-muscle cells in involved arteries, amplification of HZV viral DNA by PCR can show viruses within the endothelium and vessel wall of cranial arteries.[84-86] The HZV virus gains access to the pial arteries by way of the meninges and through nerves that innervate the arteries. Endothelial viral infection could cause thrombosis by activating platelets and triggering the coagulation cascade. Endothelial perturbation could lead to vasoconstriction compromising distal blood flow and presenting as an "arteriopathy." Systemic infection can lead to changes in circulating globulins, with activation of serine protein coagulation factors, such as factor VIII, and acute-phase reactants such as fibrinogen, promoting thrombosis of involved arteries.

Postvaricella arteriopathy and brain infarction have now been studied extensively in children.[87-89] The course and progression of the arteriopathy was studied in 27 children who had serial vascular imaging.[89]

The children in this study acquired varicella infection at age 1 to 10.4 (median 4.4 years) and had their first episode of brain ischemia 4 to 47 weeks later (median 17 weeks). Arterial imaging abnormalities most often involved the supraclinoid ICA, the M1 and M2 segments of the MCA, and the A1 segment of the ACA.[89] Single regions of focal ring-like stenosis and gradual longer segments of stenosis and multifocal narrowings were found. Brain infarcts were predominantly deep in the basal ganglia, internal capsule, and thalamus.

In some patients stenosis was maximal on initial studies, but often later progressed to involve previously uninvolved arteries. The vascular abnormalities improved or completely regressed during follow-up during 6 to 79 months. Brain ischemic episodes recurred, either acutely or during the 1 to 33 weeks after symptom onset, often associated with progression of abnormalities on vascular imaging. Symptoms often continued despite antithrombotic treatments. Vasoconstriction may be one mechanism of brain ischemia in the patients with postvaricella brain ischemia.

Migraine is also common in children with brain infarcts. The frequency of its recognition depends on how vigorously physicians have explored the past personal and family history of headache. In 1990, I reported a 6-year-old boy who had severe headache preceding a basilar artery occlusion[90]; he also had a strong family history of migraine. In another young boy, a striatocapsular infarct associated with narrowing of the MCA was followed by the development of typical unilateral throbbing migraine headaches, with photophobia, nausea, and vomiting. Migraine probably causes brain infarcts due to prolonged vasoconstriction or the formation of local thrombi related to vascular narrowing and activation of the clotting system.[90,91] A genetically mediated predisposition to migraine may be a contributing factor to heightened vascular reactivity cause by other processes such as trauma and infection. In adults, the Call-Fleming syndrome of protracted vasoconstriction (discussed in Chapter 11) may have a counterpart in childhood and explain some instances of arteriopathy.

Sickle cell anemia is an important cause of brain infarction, especially in African-American children and young adults. In one study, three fourths of patients with cerebrovascular complications of sickle cell disease were younger than 15 years.[92] Patients with stroke often have a more severe form of the disease, with frequent sickle crises and lower hematocrits than other patients with the disease. Strokes often occur during a clinical sickle crisis.[41,93] Sickle cell disease is associated with occlusive changes in large intracranial arteries and small penetrating vessels.[94,95] The walls of intracranial arteries are thickened, and intimal and subintimal proliferation occurs. Subcortical, cortical, and border-zone infarcts are often found on CT and MRI[95]; angiography has shown intracranial occlusions of the major basal arteries. Arteries may become dilatated and ectatic even in childhood.[96] Occasionally, veins and dural sinuses thrombose.[97] TCD offers a noninvasive way to detect velocity changes related to intracranial, large-artery narrowing, and allows monitoring of patients with sickle cell disease.[98]

14

Blood transfusions for children whose TCD blood-flow velocities in the ICAs or MCAs or both exceed 200 cm per second have been shown in a trial to prevent first strokes from developing.[99] Hemoglobin sickle cell disease is also occasionally complicated by ischemic strokes.

Various other hematologic and coagulation disorders are found in evaluating children with strokes. Thrombocytosis and polycythemia are occasionally found. In a study of 212 children with acute arterial ischemic stroke, abnormalities were found on blood testing in nearly half of the patients.[52] Anemia was the most common finding (40% of children).[52] Anemia, increased platelet and white blood cell counts, are often a reflection of acute or chronic disease. Some of the coagulation abnormalities are a reflection of stimulation of acute phase reactants such as fibrinogen and factors VII and VIII during systemic disease. Congenital deficiency of antithrombin III, proteins C and S, and the C2 component of complement are also implicated among the causes of strokes in childhood.[41] Some children have high homocysteine levels often explained by being homozygous for the thermolabile variant of the methylene tetrahydrofolate reductase gene.[52] Advances in genetics have led to detection of resistance to the anticoagulant function of activated protein C, most often caused by factor V Leiden, and prothrombin gene mutations, in some children and young adults with venous thromboses and strokes.

The true incidence of coagulopathies in childhood and the frequency with which they cause ischemic stroke are unknown because coagulation factors and functions have seldom been systematically investigated in large series of children, with or without strokes. Activation of clotting factors could underlie some brain infarcts in children with systemic diseases, infections, and injuries.

In some children and young adults, mitochondrial and other metabolic disorders produce stroke-like episodes. These patients develop confusion; visual abnormalities, including hemianopia and visual neglect; and sometimes seizures and headache. Brain imaging often shows white matter abnormalities predominantly, but not exclusively, in the posterior portions of the cerebral hemispheres in the occipital-temporal and parietal regions. Vascular imaging is usually normal. The pathogenesis is related to energy depletion. MELAS syndrome (Mitochondrial, Encephalopathy, Lactic Acidosis, and Stroke-like episodes) is the best-known disorder that causes stroke-like episodes.[100-102] Autosomal recessive cytochrome oxidase deficiency is also associated with periodic acidosis and stroke-like episodes attributable to metabolic aberrations.[103] These

and other mitochondrial disorders are discussed in Chapter 11.

Moyamoya is another very important condition found in childhood. This condition is also discussed in Chapter 11. Although sometimes referred to as a disease, this condition is probably better thought of as a syndrome defined by a characteristic angiographic appearance. The intracranial ICAs show progressive tapering and progressive occlusion at their intracranial bifurcations (the so-called T portion of the ICAs). Basal penetrating branches of the ICAs, ACAs, and MCAs enlarge to provide collateral circulation. These branch arteries form large prominent anastomosing channels, basal telangiectasias, that appear on angiograms as a cloud of smoke; these arteries are especially prominent because of the paucity of MCA sylvian branches. The appearance of these basal telangiectasias led Japanese clinicians to use the term moyamoya, which means "something hazy like a puff of cigarette smoke drifting in the air."[104,105] Although first described in Japan,[104] the disease has been reported worldwide.[105-109]

Necropsy studies, although few, have shown severe vascular occlusive abnormalities characterized by endothelial hyperplasia and fibrosis, with intimal thickening and abnormalities of the internal elastic lamina.[108] In contrast, the intracerebral perforating arteries show microaneurysm formation, lipohyalinosis, focal fibrin deposition, and thinning of the elastic laminas and arterial walls.[110] These changes in the perforating arteries are probably the result of greatly increased flow through these small vessels. Inflammatory changes have universally been absent. In 1991, Ikeda studied the extracranial arteries of 13 Japanese patients with spontaneous occlusions of the circle of Willis at necropsy who met the research definition of moyamoya syndrome.[111] Extracranial arteries showed the same intimal lesions as the intracranial arteries. Characteristically, the proximal pulmonary arteries had fibrous nodular intimal thickening without inflammatory abnormalities.[111] Moyamoya changes have been found in a variety of situations, including sickle cell disease, neurofibromatosis, Takayasu's disease, Down's syndrome, atherosclerosis, and fibromuscular dysplasia, and can be found in young women, especially those who smoke cigarettes and take oral contraceptives.[108] A variety of different conditions can probably cause intimal changes, which lead to fibrosis and luminal narrowing.

Moyamoya syndrome is approximately 50 times more common in girls and women than in boys and men.[112] Clinically, the disorder has a bimodal distribution, presenting most often in children younger than 15 years and in adults in their third to fifth decades of life. Children usually present with transient episodes of hemiparesis or other focal neurologic signs often precipitated by physical exercise or hyperventilation. Several of my own young patients have had intermittent choreoathetosis. Other patients have sudden-onset deficits, such as hemiplegia, or the gradual development of intellectual deterioration. Headaches and seizures are common.[104,105] These symptoms are often accompanied by CT and MRI evidence of brain infarction and cerebral blood flow studies that show regions of hypoperfusion. The abnormal vasculature is often visible on MRI and MRA. A variety of surgical procedures have been performed in Moyamoya patients to attempt to enhance brain perfusion but surgery has not been studied in randomized therapeutic trials.[112-114]

Dural Sinus and Venous Occlusions in Children

Cerebral venous occlusive disease is another important consideration in children with acute or subacute brain dysfunction.[115,116,116a,116b] The ratio of venous to arterial causes of brain injury is higher in childhood than in adults. The frequency of cerebral venous thrombosis in children is estimated to be 0.4 to 0.7 per 100,000 children per year.[43,115-116a] Many children are under 1 year of age[43]; the median age of occurrence was 6 years in a large German study and boys were involved more than girls.[116]

Most instances, as in adults, involve the superior sagittal or lateral sinus or multiple dural sinuses.[43,115] The deep venous structures—the internal cerebral vein, vein of Galen, and straight sinus—are involved more often in children than in adults. Among 91 children (non-neonates), the most frequent symptoms or signs were headache (59%), focal neurologic signs (53%), decreased consciousness (49%), and seizures (48%).[43] Papilledema was detected in 22%.[43] Acute and chronic systemic illnesses and prothrombotic conditions were common causes. The causes were quite varied and included: cancer, dehydration, the use of drugs that had pro-coagulant effects, liver disease, and nephrotic syndrome among others.[43] The nephrotic syndrome is an important cause of childhood sinovenous thrombosis. Trauma is also an important cause of dural sinus thrombosis in children.[116a]

Fourteen of 91 patients had recurrent cerebral venous thromboses. The outcome depends on the associated systemic illness; more than a third of children have residual neurologic abnormalities. The frequency of detecting an underlying

coagulopathy varies.[116a] In a Canadian registry of children with sinovenous thrombosis, 39 of 123 patients tested had a prothrombotic risk factor, the most common of which was anticardiolipin antibodies.[43]

Fewer children with dural sinus thrombosis have been anticoagulated than adults, although preliminary retrospective analyses indicates that anticoagulation is probably safe in children even when a hemorrhagic lesion is shown by brain imaging.[116a,116b] Recurrent cerebral sinovenous thrombosis occurs in about 2% to 8% of pediatric patients.[43,116a,116b]

There is considerably less information about the treatment of strokes in children compared to the data in adults. The only randomized trials concern management of sickle cell disease with transfusions.[99] The available data about treatment of stroke in children has recently been compiled and published.[116c]

STROKES IN YOUNG ADULTS (18 TO 45 YEARS OF AGE)

Causes of brain hemorrhage and infarction change as individuals progress from childhood to adulthood. The differential diagnosis of ischemic stroke in this age group is listed in Table 14-2. The topic of stroke in young adults has received increasing attention, and many series report the relative frequencies of various conditions.[1,6,15,117-142] The various series, however, are not comparable because of the wide variation in socioeconomic-environmental factors, including the age, sex, and race/ethnicity of patients; the time of accrual of the series data, with widely varying available technologies for investigation; and the investigations performed to arrive at the stroke etiology. Drug use, tuberculosis, and oral contraceptive use, for example, vary widely among the United States, India, and Japan, accounting for the variability of these specific etiologies. Some compilations focus on risk factors, many on etiologies, and others on outcome. Some lump all patients who are between adolescence and mid-40s together while others consider younger adults (<30 years) separately from those between 30 and 45 years of age. Cardiac disease was assiduously sought by some authors using modern echocardiography,[125,126,130,132,135,138-142] but in other series, this technology was not available or was not systematically used. In some series, few patients had angiography, whereas in one series of 148 patients, all patients had angiography.[129] In another series, 234 out of 300 patients (78%) had angiography with abnormalities detected in 130 (56%).[137]

Table 14-2. Differential Diagnosis of Ischemia in Young Adults (Age 15 to 40 Years)

- Migraine
- Arterial dissection
- Drugs, especially cocaine and heroin
- Premature atherosclerosis, hyperlipidemias, hypertension, diabetes, smoking, homocystinuria
- Female hormone-related (oral contraceptives, pregnancy, puerperium): eclampsia, dural sinus occlusion, arterial and venous infarcts, peripartum cardiomyopathy
- Hematologic: Deficiency of antithrombin III, protein C, protein S, factor V Leiden, prothrombin gene mutations, fibrinolytic system disorders, deficiency of plasminogen activator, antiphospholipid antibody syndrome, increased factor VIII, cancer, thrombocytosis, polycythemia, thrombotic thrombocytopenic purpura, disseminated intravascular coagulation
- Rheumatic and inflammatory: Systemic lupus erythematosus, rheumatoid arthritis, sarcoidosis, Sjögren's syndrome, scleroderma, polyarteritis nodosa, cryoglobulinemia, Crohn's disease, ulcerative colitis
- Cardiac: Intra-atrial septal defect, patent foramen ovale, mitral valve prolapse, mitral annulus calcification, myocardiopathies, arrhythmias, endocarditis
- Penetrating artery disease (lacunes): Hypertension, diabetes
- Others: moyamoya syndrome, Behçet's syndrome, neurosyphilis, Takayasu's syndrome, Sneddon's syndrome, fibromuscular dysplasia, Fabry's disease, Cogan's disease

In some diagnoses, the key data come from the history (e.g., history of the use of illicit drugs and oral contraceptive agents, historical features suggestive of migraine, and the presence of preceding head trauma). The frequency of detection of these causes varies, depending on the preliminary hypotheses and biases of the investigators and on whether the series was prospective, allowing the authors to collect the history, or retrospective, gleaned from the charts. Medical records are notoriously poor in historical detail, especially in terms of negative factors. The history in the medical record may not note that the patient did not have migraine, head or neck trauma, a recent infection, and so forth. In some series, various etiologies such as arterial dissections were not considered. In other series, factors, such as oral contraceptive use, migraine, and trauma, were only noted when they were considered etiologically related to the stroke, whereas others simply noted the percentage of subjects in which these risk factors were present.

Table 14-3 displays the relative frequency of diagnoses among 20 reports of series of young stroke patients. In some series, premature atherosclerosis was an important cause of stroke in individuals older than 30 years. Large artery extracranial and intracranial atherosclerosis was a much more common cause in those over 40 than those who were younger. But in all of the series, large-artery atherosclerosis was a much less frequent cause of stroke than that found in series of older adults. Among 287 young adults with ischemic stroke in a recent French study, the most frequent risk factors were smoking (38%), hypertension (26%), high cholesterol (24%), excessive alcohol use (20%), and oral contraceptives

(16%).[139] Diabetes was present in only 8% of patients.[139] In two large series of young Mexican stroke patients, only 10% of men and 5% of women were hypertensive, and 10% of men and 2% of women had hyperlipidemia.[132,137] In one series of patients younger than 30 years who were predominately female, only 5% of ischemic strokes were attributed to premature atherosclerosis.[125] Although premature strokes and coronary artery disease are prevalent in series of patients with severe familial hyperlipidemia, hyperlipidemia was not a major risk factor among the series of young stroke patients reviewed. Similarly penetrating artery disease is much less often found under the age of 45 than in the geriatric years. Small artery disease accounted for 20% of ischemic strokes among 264 young (18 to 45 years) Taiwanese patients,[138] but represented less than 10% of strokes in other series.

Because angiography or other vascular imaging was not consistently performed in most series, the diagnosis of premature atherosclerosis was often based on the presence of risk factors. Few studies included pervasive vascular imaging. Among 148 patients studied by angiography in one series, atherosclerotic lesions were found in 22% of patients, and 19% had thrombotic occlusions (three fourths involving the carotid circulation and one fourth being vertebrobasilar).[129]

Cardiac-origin embolism is a very important cause of stroke in young adults. The cardiac disorders responsible are, however, somewhat different than those found in childhood and older adult series. Congenital cardiac disease (other than cardiac septal abnormalities), and atrial fibrillation, congestive heart failure, and coronary artery disease–related myocardial dysfunction

Table 14-3. Series of Strokes in Young Adults

References	Number	Age/Sex	Hemorrhage	Premature Atherosclerosis (%)	Cardiac Emboli (%)	Trauma (%)	Dissection (%)	Oral Contraceptive Use Peripartum (%)	Migraine (%)	Other[a] Unknown[b] (%)
Hart, Miller,[119] 1983: United States	100 Ischemia	<40/NM	—	18	31	2	2	9/5	12	15
Snyder, et al,[118] 1980: United States	61 Ischemia	16 to 49/ 62% M	—	47	11	NM	NM	11/1	NM	8
Bougousslavsky, Regli,[125] 1987: Switzerland	41 Ischemia	<30/ 27% M	—	5	29/MVP	NM	21	65 NM	15	20
Gautier, et al,[126] 1989: France	133 All strokes	9 to 45/ 51% M	9	15	12	13	21	34?NM	14	14
Adams, et al,[123] 1986: United States	144 Ischemia	15 to 45/ 51% M	—	27	24	NM	6	4/5	14	42
Hilton-Jones, Warlow,[121] 1985: United Kingdom	75 All strokes	<45/ 66% M	20	9	7	17	NM	9/NM	13	7
Berlit,[127] 1990: Germany	168 Ischemia	<40/46% M	—	32	9	4	2	12/4	10	18
Lisovoski, Rousseaux,[129] 1991: ?	148 Ischemia	5 to 40/ 51% M	—	22	13	NM	10	11	17	—
Baringarrementaria, et al,[137] 1996: Mexico	300 Ischemia	11 to 40/ 46% M	—	4	24	NM	15	NM	3	22
Baringarrementaria, et al,[132] 1998: Mexico	130 Ischemia	11 to 40/ all F	—	0	36	NM	11	12/2	7	22
Giovannoni, Fritz,[134] 1993: South Africa	75 Ischemia	<45/ 44% M	—	37	38	NM	0	5/NM	9	24
Williams, et al,[130] 1997: United States	75 TIA	18 to 45/ 52% M	—	16	14	NM	15	NM	NM	32
Kristensen, et al,[136] 1997: North Sweden	116 Ischemia	11 to 44/ 59% M	—	12	33	NM	NM	3/NM	1	30
Carolei, et al,[135] 1993: Italy	107 Ischemia	15 to 44/ 52% M	—	34	24	NM	0.3	4/NM	1	8
Kappelle, et al,[15] 1994: United States	333 Ischemia	15 to 45/ 53% M	—	22	21	NM	NM	5 out of 10 patients/ NM	NM	42

Note: The percentages in every study do not add to 100. Some authors cite oral contraceptive use, migraine, and trauma, only when thought to cause stroke. Others list all patients with these factors. Some patients have more than one condition (e.g., migraine and oral contraceptives, trauma and dissection).

[a]Other includes known or probable cause other than those specified in this chart (e.g., moyamoya syndrome, inflammatory diseases, coagulopathy).

[b]Unknown usually meant the cause was not determined.

F, females; M, males; MVP, mitral valve prolapse; NM, not mentioned; TIA, transient ischemic attack.

14

are not frequent cardiac sources in patients aged 15 to 45. Rheumatic heart disease, prosthetic valves, and various cardiomyopathies are often mentioned cardiac sources of emboli in this age group. In some recent series, atrial septal defects and patent foramen ovale with or without atrial septal aneurysms are mentioned as the predominant cardiac source of embolism.[138,140-142]

Lechat and his French colleagues found that 40% of young patients with ischemic stroke had patent foramen ovale, compared with 10% of controls the same age without stroke.[143,144] Intracardiac shunts can be detected readily by using bubbles introduced intravenously while studying patients with transesophageal echocardiography or transcranial Doppler ultrasound. Few of the series cited routinely used these techniques. Mitral valve prolapse was common in several series[125,126,138] but was infrequently identified in others. In the series studied by Gautier et al, five of the eight patients with mitral valve prolapse also had a patent foramen ovale.[126]

Trauma and arterial dissections are common causes of brain ischemia in young adults. In the series studied by Hilton-Jones and Warlow, 13 of 75 patients had head or neck trauma at varying intervals before stroke.[121] Few of these patients had other stroke risk factors. Trauma is infrequently mentioned in other series. Arterial dissections were common in some series; the frequency of its detection varied with the extent of angiography. Gautier et al identified 23 cases of dissection among their 112 (20%) arterial infarcts. One third of patients with dissection gave a history of recent trauma.[126] In their angiography series, Lisovoski and Rousseaux found that 15 of 148 patients (10.1%) had arterial dissections.[129] Arterial dissections were found in 17/116 (14.5%),[130] 45/300 (15%),[137] 35/273 (13%),[141] 48/203 (24%),[142] and 54/287 (19%)[139] in other series. In an Italian series, only 1 out of 333 patients had dissections, despite the fact that 72% of patients had angiography.[135] The authors of this series posited that the low frequency of dissection might be explained by the admission of all patients with head and neck trauma to surgical services. I believe that cervical and intracranial dissections are much more common than are appreciated. This entity is greatly underdiagnosed. Dissections are discussed in detail in Chapters 6, 7, and 11.

Many strokes in young women were related to pregnancy, the puerperium, or use of oral contraceptive agents. In India especially, puerperal stroke, usually caused by dural venous sinus occlusion, is very important.[1,120] Srinivasan reviewed the experience in Madurai, India,[120] where puerperal stroke accounted for 15% to 20% of strokes in young adults. A total of 145 cases had been seen in a decade. Usually, symptoms began during the first 3 weeks after normal childbirth in multiparous women. Common early findings included seizures (80%); reduced alertness (50%); transient focal signs, such as unilateral weakness (60%); and raised intracranial pressure (18%).[120] The vast majority of patients had dural-sinus occlusion. Fibrinogen levels were considerably raised in 104 out of 120 patients in which it was measured (86%). Mortality was high. Pulmonary embolism and puerperal cardiomyopathy were also problems in these patients.[120] Series of young women who develop dural and venous sinus thrombosis always include a large number of patients who develop the occlusions during pregnancy or the puerperium. A high rate of puerperal cerebral venous thrombosis has also been noted in Mexico.[132,137] Puerperal patients in India and Mexico who developed dural sinus thrombosis were often multiparous, relatively poor, sometimes vegetarians in India, and had significant anemia and high homocysteine blood levels.

Oral contraceptive use was common among young women with strokes, although the relationship to etiology was usually uncertain. Although 34% of young women in the series of Gautier et al used oral contraceptives, this was not significantly different from the estimated rate of use in the population of the same age (32%).[126] Lower-dose oral contraceptive agents have less risk of stroke. Published series antedate the widespread use of lower-dose contraceptives or do not report the strength of estrogen and progesterone used.

In some series, oral contraceptive use and migraine were combined risk factors. Migraine was mentioned prominently in many series,* but the mechanism by which it related to stroke was most often not identified or posited. Some series tabulated all patients that gave a history of migraine, whereas other series listed only patients in whom the authors considered that migraine was the etiology of the brain infarct.

Infections seem to be less important as an etiology of stroke in young adults than in children. Neurosyphilis is an important cause of stroke in young adults in India, as is tuberculous meningitis.[120] Neurocysticercosis was an important cause of stroke in Mexican young adults, accounting for 14 of the 80 cases of nonatherosclerotic vasculopathies found among 300 patients.[137]

An important factor that may have been unrecognized in the past is the use of drugs. Illicit

---

*See references 121, 123, 125, 126, 128, 132, 135, 137, 140, 142.

drugs, especially cocaine, have become an important and frequent cause of ischemia and hemorrhage in young adults.[6] A history of drug use was seldom mentioned in the series reviewed, and was seldom pursued vigorously as a possible etiology. In a case–control study of individuals aged 15 to 44 years, the estimated overall relative risk for stroke was 6.5 and was 11.2 for patients younger than 35 years.[145] The Baltimore-Washington Young Stroke Study investigators specifically sought data regarding stroke among 422 patients with first ischemic strokes (age range, 17 to 44 ye0ars).[146] Drug use was acknowledged in 94 patients (22%), and 51 individuals (12%) used drugs within the 48 hours before stroke onset.[146] In 20 of these 51 patients (39%) with recent drug use, no other cause of stroke was identified. Strokes were attributed directly to the drug use.[146] Cocaine was the most commonly used drug in this and other series. I discuss drug-related stroke in more detail in Chapters 11 and 13.

Few reports analyze the causes of hemorrhagic stroke in young adults.[124,131] Because hemorrhagic stroke patients are often cared for on neurosurgical services and ischemia is usually treated on neurologic units, the relative frequencies of the two types of stroke are difficult to determine. Hemorrhagic strokes probably make up a smaller proportion of strokes in the ages 15 to 45 years than before age 15 years, and during the geriatric years. The ratio of hemorrhage to ischemia varies considerably with the race/ethnicity, sex, and location of stroke patients. In Osaka, Japan, for example, among 252 young stroke patients aged 16 to 40 years, 175 had hemorrhagic strokes (70%),[128] whereas in a British series of patients younger than 45 years, only 20% had hemorrhages.[121] In a French series, only 9% of 133 patients had intracranial hemorrhages.[126]

In general, the etiology of ICH in patients younger than 45 years is similar to those older than 45 years, except for an overrepresentation of AVMs, cavernomas, drug abuse, and early-life bleeding disorders such as hemophilia.[137] Amyloid angiopathy is not encountered in young adults, and warfarin-related hemorrhages are less frequent than in older patients. Hypertension remains a frequent cause of intraparenchymatous bleeding in both age groups. Toffol and colleagues reviewed the Iowa experience with nontraumatic ICH in patients 15 to 45 years of age.[124] The most common location was lobar (41 out of 72, 57%); 11 were putaminal (15%), and four were intraventricular. Etiologies included AVMs (21 out of 55, 39%), hypertension (11 out of 72, 15%), aneurysm (7 out of 72, 10%), and drug use with amphetamines or phenylpropanolamine, or both (5 out of 72, 7%).[124] Among the 15 patients with ICH included in the British series, six were caused by AVMs and two by hypertension.[121] In a Japanese neurologic series among 25 young patients with ICH, seven had AVMs. In 16 patients, hemorrhages were attributed to hypertension.[128] Aneurysms (51%) accounted for more ICHs than AVMs (19%) among Japanese patients treated on a neurosurgical service.[128] In a Mexican study of 200 patients younger than 40 years with ICHs, AVMs and cavernous angiomas were the most common causes.[131] In this series, only 22 (11%) of hemorrhages were attributed to hypertension. The majority of hemorrhages (55%) were lobar.[131]

Aneurysms in young adults have the same locations and clinical findings as in older patients. SAHs before and after age 40 years are diagnosed and managed in the same fashion.

DIFFERENCES IN EVALUATION

In young adults and children, clinicians face a dilemma regarding the extensiveness of the evaluation. A patient's youth, with nearly a lifetime remaining of potential risks of future stroke and other vascular diseases and the vast number of diagnostic possibilities are factors that argue for extensive evaluation. On the other hand, the tendency for young patients to improve dramatically irrespective of treatment, the knowledge that a high proportion of cases go undiagnosed despite intensive testing, and the high cost of technology and testing argue for conservatism when ordering tests. Recent information from series that have included vascular imaging show that the presence and nature of arteriopathy impacts greatly on the future course, outcome, and treatment.[14,52-56,59,60] Certainly the finding of cerebral venous occlusive disease also directs evaluation, treatment, prognosis, and outcome. The frequency and importance of cardiac disease and arteriopathy and venous occlusive disease means that all young patients with strokes and TIAs should have cardiac investigations and imaging of the arteries and veins that supply the brain.

In my opinion, clinicians should spend more time with the clinical encounter. The history should include questions about smoking, headache, trauma, cardiac symptoms, past bleeding, miscarriages, thrombophlebitis, and prior strokes and ischemic attacks. The use of medicines and drugs of any kind (especially cocaine, amphetamines, and other illicit drugs) and oral contraceptive agents is particularly important. The history should include a thorough review of systems, searching for symptoms that might indicate systemic disease. Family history is important. Information about premature atherosclerosis, hypertension, hyperlipidemia, migraine,

14

and metabolic and hereditary diseases in family members should be sought.

The general physical examination should include careful inspection of the skin for rashes and other lesions. Palpation of pulses and cardiac, neck, and cranial auscultation are especially important. Blood tests, including coagulation studies; brain and vascular imaging; and cardiac evaluation are needed in every young person with stroke. Ultrasound and angiography may be indicated, depending on the findings from the clinical encounter and early investigations. The yield of angiography is high. In one series, two thirds of angiograms were abnormal, often allowing an etiologic diagnosis.[129] Magnetic resonance and CT angiography and extracranial and intracranial ultrasound may allow clinicians to noninvasively acquire enough data about the vasculature without risk to the patients. Physicians should order contrast angiography only when preliminary screening vascular imaging suggests a vascular lesion, but does not define it sufficiently to select and monitor treatment.

References

1. Chopra JS, Prabhakar S: Clinical features and risk factors in stroke in young. Acta Neurol Scand 1979;60:289-300.
2. Katrak S: Vasculitis and stroke due to tuberculosis. In Caplan LR (ed): Uncommon Causes of Stroke, 2nd ed. Cambridge: Cambridge University Press, 2008, pp 41-45.
3. Del Bruto O: Stroke and vasculitis in patients with cysticercosis. In Caplan LR (ed): Uncommon Causes of Stroke, 2nd ed. Cambridge: Cambridge University Press, 2008, pp 53-58.
4. Caplan LR, Estanol B, Mitchell WG: How to manage patients with neurocysticercosis. Eur Neurol 1997;37:124-131.
5. Nencini P, Inzitari D, Baruffi MC, et al: Incidence of stroke in young adults in Florence, Italy. Stroke 1988;19:977-981.
6. Stern B, Kittner S, Sloan M, et al: Stroke in the young. Maryland Med J 1991;40:453-462,565-571.
7. Walsh LE, Garg B: Isolated acute subcortical infarctions in children: Clinical description and radiographic correlation. Ann Neurol 1990;28:458-459.
8. Caplan LR, Babikian V, Helgason C, et al: Occlusive disease of the middle cerebral artery. Neurology 1985;35:975-982.
9. Caplan LR, DeWitt LD, Pessin MS, et al: Lateral thalamic infarcts. Arch Neurol 1988;45:959-964.
10. Caplan LR: Posterior cerebral artery disease. In Caplan LR : Posterior Circulation Disease. Boston: Blackwell, 1996, pp 444-491.
11. Ferro JM, Crespo M: Young adult stroke: Neuropsychological dysfunction and recovery. Stroke 1988;19:982-986.
12. Dooling EC, Adams RD: The pathological anatomy of posthemiplegic athetosis. Brain 1975;98:29-48.
13. Malamud N: Status marmoratus: A form of cerebral palsy following either birth injury or inflammation of the central nervous system. J Pediatr 1950;37:610-619.
14. deVeber G, et al: Arterial ischemic stroke in children: Results from the Canadian Pediatric Ischemic Stroke Registry. Personal communication/In press.
15. Kappelle LJ, Adams HP, Heffner ML, et al: Prognosis of young adults with ischemic stroke. A long-term follow-up study assessing recurrent vascular events and functional outcome in the Iowa Registry of Stroke in Young Adults. Stroke 1994;25:1360-1365.
16. Ferriero DM: Neonatal brain injury. N Engl J Med 2004;351:1985-1995.
16a. Kirton A, deVeber G, Pontigon A-M, et al: Presumed perinatal ischemic stroke: Vascular classification predicts outcome. Ann Neurol 2008;63:436-443.
16b. Back SA, Riddle A, McClure MM: Maturation-dependent vulnerability of perinatal white matter in premature birth. Stroke 2007;38(part 2):724-730.
17. Hill A, Volpe JJ: Stroke and hemorrhage in the premature and term neonate. In Edwards MB, Hoffman HJ (eds): Cerebral Vascular Diseases in Children and Adolescents. Baltimore: Williams & Wilkins, 1989, pp 179-194.
18. Roland E, Poskitt K, Rodriguez E, et al: Perinatal hypoxic-ischemic thalamic injury: Clinical features and neuroimaging. Ann Neurol 1998;44:161-166.
19. Leech RW, Alvord EC Jr: Anoxic-ischemic encephalopathy in the human neonatal period: The significance of brain stem involvement. Arch Neurol 1977;34:109-113.
20. Golomb MR, MacGregor DL, Domi T, et al: Presumed pre- or perinatal arterial ischemic stroke: Risk factors and outcomes. Ann Neurol 2001;50:163-168.
20a. Benders MJNL, Groenendaal F, Uiterwaal CSPM, et al: Maternal and infant characteristics associated with perinatal arterial stroke in the preterm infant. Stroke 2007;38:1759-1765.
21. Rorke LB, Zimmerman RA: Prematurity, postmaturity, and destructive lesions in utero. AJNR Am J Neuroradiol 1992;13:517-536.
22. Nelson KB, Dambrosia JM, Grether JK, Phillips TM: Neonatal cytokines and coagulation factors in children with cerebral palsy. Ann Neurol 1998;44:665-675.
23. Kurnik K, Kosch A, Strater R: Childhood Stroke Study Group. Recurrent thromboembolism in infants and children suffering from symptomatic neonatal arterial stroke. A prospective follow-up study. Stroke 2003;34:2887-2893.
24. Johnston MV: Selective vulnerability in the neonatal brain. Ann Neurol 1998;44:155-156.
25. Martin LJ, Brambrink A, Koehler RC, Traystman RJ: Primary sensory and forebrain motor systems in the newborn brain are preferentially damaged by hypoxia-ischemia. J Comp Neurol 1997;377:262-285.

26. Volpe JJ: Value of MR in definition of the neuropathology of cerebral palsy in vivo. AJNR Am J Neuroradiol 1992;13:79-83.

27. Volpe JJ, Pasternak JF: Parasagittal cerebral injury in neonatal hypoxic-ischemic encephalopathy: Clinical and neuroradiologic features. J Pediatr 1977;91:472-476.

28. Aida N, Nishimura NA, Hachiya Y, et al: MR imaging of perinatal brain damage: Comparison of clinical outcome with initial and follow-up MR findings. AJNR Am J Neuroradiol 1998;19: 1909-1921.

29. Bax M, Tydeman C, Flodmark O: Clinical and MRI correlates of cerebral palsy. The European Cerebral Palsy Study. JAMA 2006;296:1601-1608.

30. Volpe JJ, Herscovitch P, Perlman JM, et al: Positron emission tomography in the asphyxiated term newborn: Parasagittal impairment of cerebral blood flow. Ann Neurol 1985;17:287-296.

31. Banker BQ, Larroch JC: Periventricular leukomalacia of infancy: A form of neonatal anoxic encephalopathy. Arch Neurol 1962;7:386-410.

32. DeReuck J, Chattha AS, Richardson Jr EP: Pathogenesis and evolution of periventricular leukomalacia in infancy. Arch Neurol 1972;27:229-236.

33. Truwit CL, Barkovich AJ, Koch TK, Ferriero DM: Cerebral palsy: MR findings in 40 patients. AJNR Am J Neuroradiol 1992;13:67-78.

34. Kuban KC, Leviton A: Cerebral palsy. N Engl J Med 1994;330:188-195.

35. Barmada MA, Moossy J, Shuman RM: Cerebral infarcts with arterial occlusion in neonates. Ann Neurol 1979;6:495-502.

36. Mantovani JF, Gerber GJ: "Idiopathic" neonatal cerebral infarction. Am J Dis Child 1984;138: 359-362.

37. Rollins NK, Morris MC, Evans D, et al: The role of early MR in the evaluation of the term infant with seizures. AJNR Am J Neuroradiol 1994;15: 239-248.

38. Takanashi J, Barkovich AJ, Ferriero DM, et al: Widening spectrum of congenital hemiplegia. Periventricular venous infarction in term neonates. Neurology 2003;61:531-533.

39. Chasnoff IJ, Bussey ME, Savich R, et al: Perinatal cerebral infarction and maternal cocaine use. J Pediatr 1986;108:456-459.

40. Roessmann CC, Miller RT: Thrombus of the middle cerebral artery associated with birth trauma. Neurology 1980;30:889-892.

41. Roach ES, Riela AR: Pediatric Cerebrovascular Disorders. Mount Kisco, NY: Futura, 1988.

42. Fitzgerald KC, Williams LS, Garg BP, et al: Cerebral sinovenous thrombosis in the neonate. Arch Neurol 2006;63:405-409.

43. deVeber G, Andrew M, Adams C et al: Canadian Pediatric Ischemic Stroke Study Group. Cerebral sinovenous thrombosis in children. N Engl J Med 2001;345:417-423.

44. Ahmann PA, Lazzara A, Dykes FD, et al: Intraventricular hemorrhage in the high-risk preterm infant: Incidence and outcome. Ann Neurol 1980;7:118-124.

45. Papile LA, Burstein J, Burstein R, et al: Incidence and evolution of subependymal and intraventricular hemorrhage: A study of infants with birth weights of less than 1500 gm. Pediatrics 1978; 92:529-534.

46. Garcia JH, Pantoni L: Strokes in childhood. Semin Pediatr Neurol 1995;2:180-191.

47. Grunnet ML, Shields WD: Cerebellar hemorrhage in the premature infants. J Pediatr 1976;88: 605-608.

48. Martin R, Roessmann U, Fanaroff A: Massive intracerebellar hemorrhage in low birth-weight infants. J Pediatr 1976;89:290-293.

49. Volpe JJ: Neonatal periventricular hemorrhage: Past, present and future. J Pediatr 1978;92: 693-696.

50. Gowers WR: A Manual of Diseases of the Nervous System. Philadelphia: P Blakiston, 1888.

51. Ford FR, Schaffer AJ: The etiology of infantile acquired hemiplegia. AMA Arch Neurol Psychiatry 1927;18:323-347.

52. Ganesan V, Prengler M, McShane MA, et al: Investigation of risk factors in children with arterial ischemic stroke. Ann Neurol 2003;53:167-173.

53. Lanthier S, Armstrong D, Donni T, deVeber G: Post-varicella arteriopathy of childhood. Natural history of vascular stenosis. Neurology 2005; 64:660-663.

54. Danchaivijitr N, Cox TC, Saunders D, Ganesan V: Evolution of cerebral arteriopathies in childhood arterial ischemic stroke. Ann Neurol 2006;59: 620-626.

55. Kirkham F: Improvement or progression in childhood cerebral arteriopathies: Current difficulties in prediction and suggestions for research. Ann Neurol 2006;580-582.

56. Sebire G, Fullerton H, Riou E, deVeber G: Toward the definition of cerebral arteriopathies of childhood. Curr Opin Pediatr 2004;16:617-622.

57. Kuhle S, Mitchell L, Andrew M, et al: Urgent clinical challenges in children with ischemic stroke. Analysis of 1065 patients from the 1-800-NOCLOTS Pediatric Stroke Telephone Consultation Service. Stroke 2006;37:116-122.

58. Schoenberg BS, Mellinger JF, Schoenberg DG: Cerebrovascular disease in infants and children: A study of incidence, clinical features, and survival. Neurology 1978;28:763-768.

59. Fullerton HJ, Wu YW, Sydney S, Johnstone SC: Risk of recurrent stroke in a population-based cohort: The importance of cerebrovascular imaging. Stroke 2007;38:485.

60. Fullerton HJ, Wu YW, Sydney S, Johnstone SC: Excess stroke risk in black and Hispanic children: A population-based study. Stroke 2007;38:460.

61. Fullerton HJ, Chetkovich DM, Wu YW, et al: Deaths from strokes in US children 1979-1998. Neurology 2002;59:34-39.

62. So SC: Cerebral arteriovenous malformations in children. Childs Brain 1978;4:242-250.

63. Ventureyra EC, Herder S: Arteriovenous malformations in children. Childs Nerv Syst 1987;3:12-18.

14

64. Fullerton HJ, Wu YW, Sidney S, Johnston SC: Recurrent hemorrhagic stroke in children. A population-based cohort study. Stroke 2007; 38:2658-2662.

65. Sedzimir CB, Robinson J: Intracranial hemorrhages in children and adolescents. J Neurosurg 1973;38:269-281.

66. Orozco M, Trigueros F, Quintana F, et al: Intracranial aneurysms in early childhood. Surg Neurol 1978;9:247-252.

67. Shucart WA, Wolpert SM: Intracranial arterial aneurysms in childhood. Am J Dis Child 1974; 127:288-293.

68. Mackenzie I: The clinical presentation of the cerebral angioma. Brain 1953;76:184-213.

69. Humphreys RP: Infratentorial arteriovenous malformations. In Edwards MS, Hoffman HJ (eds): Cerebral Vascular Disease in Children and Adolescents. Baltimore: Williams & Wilkins, 1989, pp 309-320.

70. Martin NA, Edwards MS: Supratentorial arteriovenous malformations. In Edwards MS, Hoffman HJ (eds): Cerebral Vascular Diseases in Children and Adolescents. Baltimore: Williams & Wilkins, 1989, pp 283-308.

71. Metellus P, Kharkar S, Lin D, et al: Cerebral cavernous malformations and developmental venous anomalies. In Caplan LR (ed): Uncommon Causes of Stroke, 2nd ed. Cambridge: Cambridge University Press, 2008.

72. Maraire JN, Awad IA: Intracranial cavernous malformations: Lesion behavior and management strategies. Neurosurgery 1995;37:591-605.

73. Mottolese C, Hermier M, Stan H, et al: Central nervous system cavernomas in the pediatric age group. Neurosurg Rev 2001;24:55-71;discussion 72-73.

74. Cavalheiro S, Braga FM: Cavernous hemangiomas. In Choux M, Di Rocco C, Hockley AD, Walker ML (eds): Pediatric Neurosurgery. London: Churchill Livingstone, 1999, pp 691-701.

75. Brower MC, Rollins N, Roach ES: Basal ganglia and thalamic infarction in children. Cause and clinical features. Arch Neurol 1996;53:1252-1256.

76. Terplan AK: Patterns of brain damage in infants and children with congenital heart disease. Am J Dis Child 1973;125:176-185.

77. Caplan LR, Manning WJ: Brain Embolism. New York: Informa Healthcare, 2006.

77a. Braun KPJ, Rafay M, Uiterwaal CS, Pontigon A-M, De Veber G: Mode of onset predicts etiological diagnosis of arterial ischemic stroke in children. Stroke 2007;38:298-302.

78. Satoh S, Shirane R, Yoshimoto T: Clinical survey of ischemic cerebrovascular disease in children in a district of Japan. Stroke 1991;22:586-589.

79. Pitner SE: Carotid thrombosis due to intraoral trauma—an unusual complication of a common childhood accident. N Engl J Med 1966;274: 764-767.

80. Pearl PL: Childhood stroke following intraoral trauma. J Pediatr 1987;110:574-575.

81. Duncan A, Rumbaugh C, Caplan LR: Cerebral embolic disease: A complication of carotid aneurysms. Radiology 1979;133:379-384.

82. Zilkha A, Mendelsohn F, Borofsky LG: Acute hemiplegia in children complicating upper respiratory infections. Clin Pediatr 1976;15: 1137-1142.

83. Parker P, Puck J, Fernandez F: Cerebral infarction associated with Mycoplasma pneumoniae. Pediatrics 1981;67:373-375.

84. Doyle PW, Gibson G, Dolman C: Herpes zoster ophthalmicus with contralateral hemiplegia: Identification of cause. Ann Neurol 1983;14:84-85.

85. Melanson M, Chalk C, Georgevich L, et al: Varicella-zoster virus DNA in CSF and arteries in delayed contralateral hemiplegia: Evidence for viral invasion of cerebral arteries. Neurology 1996;47:569-570.

86. Ross MH, Abend WK, Schwartz RB, Samuels MA: A case of C2 herpes zoster with delayed bilateral pontine infarction. Neurology 1991;41:1685-1686.

87. Askalan R, Laughlin S, Mayank S, et al: Chickenpox and stroke in childhood: A study of frequency and causation. Stroke 2001;32:1257-1262.

88. Hausler MG, Ramaekers VT, Reul J, et al: Early and late onset manifestations of cerebral vasculitis related to varicella zoster. Neuropediatrics 1998; 29:202-207.

89. Lanthier S, Armstrong D, Domi T, deVeber G: Post-varicella arteriopathy of childhood. Neurology 2005;64:660-663.

90. Caplan LR: Migraine and vertebrobasilar ischemia. Neurology 1990;41:55-61.

91. Caplan LR: Migraine and posterior circulation stroke. In Caplan LR (ed): Posterior Circulation Disease: Clinical Findings, Diagnosis, and Management. Boston: Blackwell Science, 1996, pp 544-568.

92. Wood DH: Cerebrovascular complications of sickle-cell anemia. Stroke 1978;9:73-75.

93. Grotta JC, Manner C, Pettigrew LC, et al: Red blood cell disorders and stroke. Stroke 1986;17: 811-816.

94. Rothman SM, Fulling KH, Nelson JS: Sickle cell anemia and central nervous system infarction: A neuropathological study. Ann Neurol 1986;20: 684-690.

95. Adams RJ, Nichols FT, McKie V, et al: Cerebral infarction in sickle cell anemia: mechanisms based on CT and MRI. Neurology 1988;38:1012-1017.

96. Steen RG, Langston JW, Ogg RJ, et al: Ectasia of the basilar artery in children with sickle cell disease: Relationship to hematocrit and psychometric measures. J Stroke Cerebrovasc Dis 1998;7:32-43.

97. Oguz M, Aksungur EH, Soyupak SK, Yildirim AU: Vein of Galen and sinus thrombosis with bilateral thalamic infarcts in sickle cell anemia: CT follow-up and angiographic demonstration. Neuroradiology 1994;36:155-156.

98. Adams RJ, McKie VC, Nichols F, et al: The use of transcranial ultrasonography to predict stroke in sickle cell disease. N Engl J Med 1992;326: 605-610.

99. Adams RJ, McKie VC, Hsu L, et al: Prevention of a first stroke by transfusions in children with sickle cell anemia and abnormal results on transcranial Doppler ultrasonography. N Engl J Med 1998;339:5-11.

100. Koo B, Becker LE, Chuang S, et al: Mitochondrial encephalomyopathy, lactic acidosis, stroke like episodes (MELAS): Clinical, radiological, and genetic observations. Ann Neurol 1993;34:25-32.

101. Matthews PM, Tampieri D, Berkovic SF, et al: Magnetic resonance imaging shows specific abnormalities in the MELAS syndrome. Neurology 1991;41:1043-1046.

102. Clark JM, Marks MP, Adalsteinsson E, et al: MELAS: Clinical and pathological correlations with MRI, xenon/CT, and MR spectroscopy. Neurology 1996;46:223-227.

103. Morin C, Dube J, Robinson B, et al: Stroke-like episodes in autosomal recessive cytochrome oxidase deficiency. Ann Neurol 1999;45:389-392.

104. Suzuki J, Kodama N: Moyamoya disease—A review. Stroke 1983;14:104-109.

105. Suzuki J: Moyamoya Disease. Berlin: Springer, 1986.

106. Chiu D, Shedden P, Bratina P, Grotta JC: Clinical features of Moyamoya disease in the United States. Stroke 1998;29:1347-1351.

107. Taveras JM: Multiple progressive intracranial arterial occlusions: A syndrome of children and young adults. AJR Am J Roentgenol 1969;106:235-268.

108. Bruno A, Adams HOP, Bilbe J, et al: Cerebral infarction due to moyamoya disease in young adults. Stroke 1988;19:826-833.

109. Ganesan V, Saunders D, Kirkham R, et al: Clinical and radiological features of moyamoya syndrome in British children: Relationship with outcome. Ann Neurol 2004; 54(suppl 7):5-12.

110. Mauro AJ, Johnson ES, Chikos PM, Alvord EC: Lipohyalinosis and miliary microaneurysms causing cerebral hemorrhage in a patient with moyamoya. A clinicopathological study. Stroke 1980;11:405-412.

111. Ikeda E: Systemic vascular changes in spontaneous occlusion of the circle of Willis. Stroke 1991;22:1358-1362.

112. Ueki K, Meyer FB, Mellinger JF: Moyamoya disease: The disorder and surgical treatment. Mayo Clin Proc 1994;69:749-757.

113. Smith ER, Scott RM: Surgical management of moyamoya syndrome. Skull Base 2005; 15:15-26.

114. Scott RM, Smith JL, Roberson RL, et al: Long-term outcome in children with moyamoya syndrome after cranial revascularization by pial synangiosis. J Neurosurg 2004;100(2 suppl Pediatrics):142-149.

115. Lynch JK: Cerebrovascular disorders in children. Curr Neurol Neurosurg Reports 2004;4:129-138.

116. Heller C, Heinecke A, Junker R, et al: Cerebral venous thrombosis in children: A multifactorial origin. Circulation 2003;108:1362-1367.

116a. Carpenter J, Tsuchida T: Cerebral sinovenous thrombosis in children. Curr Neurol Neurosci Rep 2007;7:139-146.

116b. Sebire G, Tabarki B, Saunders DE, et al: Cerebral venous sinus thrombosis in children: Risk factors, presentation, diagnosis, and outcome. Brain 2005;128:477-489.

116c. Bernard TJ, Goldenberg NA, Armstrong-Wells J, et al: Treatment of childhood arterial ischemic stroke. Ann Neurol 2008;63:679-696.

117. Louis S, McDowell F: Stroke in young adults. Ann Intern Med 1967;66:932-938.

118. Snyder BD, Ramirez-Lassepas M: Cerebral infarction in young adults: Long term prognosis. Stroke 1980;11:149-153.

119. Hart RG, Miller VT: Cerebral infarction in young adults: A practical approach. Stroke 1983;14:110-114.

120. Srinivasan K: Ischemic cerebrovascular disease in the young: Two common causes in India. Stroke 1984;15:733-735.

121. Hilton-Jones D, Warlow CP: The causes of stroke in the young. J Neurol 1985;232: 137-143.

122. Radhakrishnan K, Ashek PP, Sridharan R, Mousa ME: Stroke in the young: Incidence and pattern in Benghazi, Libya. Acta Neurol Scand 1986;73: 434-438.

123. Adams HP, Butler MJ, Biller J, Toffol GJ: Nonhemorrhagic cerebral infarction in young adults. Arch Neurol 1986;43:793-796.

124. Toffol GJ, Biller J, Adams HP: Nontraumatic intracerebral hemorrhage in young adults. Arch Neurol 1987;44:483-485.

125. Bogousslavsky J, Regli F: Ischemic stroke in adults younger than 30 years of age. Arch Neurol 1987;44:479-482.

126. Gautier JC, Pradat-Diehl P, Loron PL, et al: Accidents vasculaires cérébraux des sujets jeunes. Une etude de 133 patients ages de 9 à 45 ans. Rev Neurol 1989;145:437-442.

127. Berlit P: Cerebral ischemia in young adults. Ann Neurol 1990;28:258.

128. Yamaguchi T, Yoshinaga M, Yonekawa Y: Stroke in the young—Japanese perspective. Abstracts International Conference on Stroke. Geneva, May 30-June 1, 1991.

129. Lisovoski F, Rousseaux P: Cerebral infarction in young people: A study of 148 patients with early angiography. J Neurol Neurosurg Psychiatry 1991;54:576-579.

130. Williams LS, Garg BP, Cohen M, et al: Subtypes of ischemic stroke in children and young adults. Neurology 1997;49: 1541-1545.

131. Ruiz-Sandoval JL, Cantu C, Baringarrementaria F: Intracerebral hemorrhage in young people. Analysis of risk factors, locations, causes, and prognosis. Stroke 1999;30:537-541.

132. Baringarrementaria F, Gonzalez-Duarte A, Miranda L, Cantu C: Cerebral infarction in young women: Analysis of 130 cases. Eur Neurol 1998;40:228-233.

133. Kittner SJ, Stern BJ, Wozniak M, et al: Cerebral infarction in young adults. The Baltimore-Washington Cooperative Young Stroke Study. Neurology 1998;50:890-894.

134. Giovannoni G, Fritz VU: Transient ischemic attacks in younger and older patients. A comparative study of 798 patients in South Africa. Stroke 1993;24:947-953.

135. Carolei A, Marini C, Ferranti E, et al: A prospective study of cerebral ischemia in the young. Analysis of pathogenic determinants. Stroke 1993;24:362-367.

136. Kristensen B, Malm J, Carlberg B, et al: Epidemiology and etiology of ischemic stroke in young adults aged 18 to 44 years in Northern Sweden. Stroke 1997;28:1702-1709.

137. Baringarrementaria F, Figueroa T, Huebe J, Cantu C: Cerebral infarction in people under 40 years. Etiologic analysis of 300 cases prospectively evaluated. Cerebrovasc Dis 1996;6:75-79.

138. Lee T-H, Hsu W-C, Chen C-J, Chen S-T: Etiologic study of young ischemic stroke in Taiwan. Stroke 2002;33:1950-1955.

139. Leys D, Bandu L, Henon H, et al: Clinical outcome in 287 consecutive young adults (15-45 years) with ischemic stroke. Neurology 2002;59:26-33.

140. Musolino R, La Spina P, Granata A, et al: Ischaemic stroke in young people: A prospective and long-term follow-up study. Cerebrovasc Dis 2003;15:121-128.

141. Cerrato P, Grasso M, Imperiale D, et al: Stroke in young patients: Etiopathogenesis and risk factors in different age classes. Cerebrovasc Dis 2004;18:154-159.

142. Nedeltchev K, der Maur TA, Georgiadis D, et al: Ischaemic stroke in young adults: Predictors of outcome and recurrence. J Neurol Neurosurg Psychiatry 2005;76:191-195.

143. Lechat P, Mas JL, Lescault G, et al: Prevalence of patent foramen ovale in patients with strokes. N Engl J Med 1988;318:1148-1152.

144. Lechat P, Lascault G, Thomas D, et al: Patent foramen ovale and cerebral embolism. Circulation 1985;72(suppl 3):134.

145. Kaku DA, Lowenstein DH: Emergence of recreational drug abuse as a major risk factor for stroke in young adults. Ann Intern Med 1990;113:821-827.

146. Sloan MA, Kittner SJ, Feeser BR, et al: Illicit drug-associated ischemic stroke in the Baltimore-Washington Young Stroke Study. Neurology 1998;49:1688-1693.

Spinal Cord Vascular Disease   15

Strokes affect the human spinal cord, but spinal cord strokes represent a minute fraction of all patients with central nervous system vascular disease. The rarity of spinal cord strokes and lack of accessibility to study the spinal cord vascular system during life have prevented a thorough understanding of spinal cord vascular disease. In addition, the spinal cord and its vascular system are seldom examined in detail at necropsy. Nonetheless, when sought, spinal ischemic lesions are found. In London, Ontario, Canada, a systematic search for examples of hypoxic myelopathy uncovered 52 cases among 1200 consecutive necropsies (4%).[1,2]

UNIQUE ANATOMY OF THE SPINAL CORD

The unique anatomy of the spinal cord makes the clinician's approach to spinal lesions quite different from brain lesions. Anatomic definition requires placing the lesion in two planes, longitudinally (rostrocaudally) and in depth. Imaging the lesion with magnetic resonance imaging (MRI) or standard angiography requires localization to the craniospinal junction region, cervical cord, thoracic cord, lumbar cord, or cauda equina. Lesions at different rostrocaudal levels have different likely etiologies.

The three depths of lesions with clinical importance are (1) within the epidural space; (2) inside the dura, but outside the spinal cord (intradural extramedullary); and (3) intramedullary. Most epidural lesions reflect disease of the bony fortress and its connective tissue elements that surround the spinal cord. Lesions inside the dura but outside of the spinal cord are most often benign tumors, hematomas, or abscesses. Intramedullary lesions have a wide differential diagnosis that includes infarcts and hematomas.

Rostrocaudal localization depends on the level of findings affecting the long motor (pyramidal) and sensory (spinothalamic and posterior column proprioceptive) tracts, and the presence of local segmental signs.[3] Root or dermatomal distribution of sensory, reflex, or lower motor neuron loss accurately identifies the rostrocaudal level of the process. Local bone tenderness and

pain are also usually reliable in pointing to the segment involved.

Depth localization is more difficult. Epidural processes usually involve the vertebral column, and bone and root pain usually precede symptoms related to dysfunction of the spinal cord. Intradural lesions cause root pain, but bony findings are absent clinically and by imaging. Intramedullary lesions are most often, but not always, painless. Asymmetric signs, sparing of distal sensory fibers, and dissociated sensory loss are other clues to an intramedullary localization. This subject is discussed in more depth elsewhere.[3]

Spinal Cord Vascular System

I did not include diagnosis or discussion of the spinal vascular system in the general discussion of anatomy in Chapter 2. I find it easier to understand and visualize the system by first focusing on a spinal cord segment in axial section (Figure 15-1). A large, single, anterior spinal artery runs in the ventral midline rostrally from the spinomedullary junction at the foramen magnum and caudally to the tip of the spinal cord, the filum terminale. In contrast, paired smaller posterior spinal arteries are located on the dorsal surface, which often form a plexus of small vessels. The anterior spinal artery gives off deep branches, which course along the ventral sulcus and then branch as they reach the central gray to supply left and right branches to the anterior horn regions on each side.[4,5] Lateral circumferential arteries and their penetrators course laterally from the midline anterior spinal artery to supply the ventral white matter, tips of the anterior horns, and pyramidal tracts.[4,5] This pattern is similar to that found in the brainstem, in which paramedian penetrators and short and long circumferential arteries branch from the vertebral and basilar arteries (see Fig. 2-21). The posterior spinal artery plexus also gives off penetrating branches to the posterior columns and posterior gray horns.[1,4,5] The central area of the cord is a watershed region between the anterior and posterior spinal artery supply. The area between the two zones of supply in the central portion

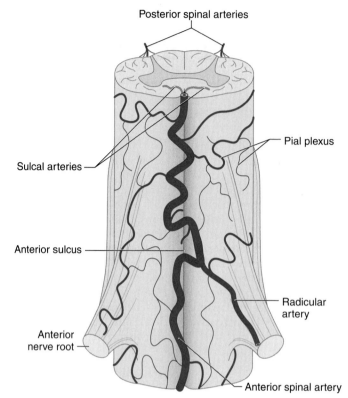

Figure 15-1. Cross-section of spinal cord, showing arterial patterns of supply. The anterior spinal artery is a single midline artery that courses in the anterior fissure. This artery divides into left and right sulcal arteries, which supply the anterior horns and white matter. There are usually two posterior spinal arteries, one on each side, which form an anastomotic rete from which branches emerge to supply the posterior gray horns and the posterior columns.

of the cord has often been called the *border zone* or *watershed region of supply.*[6]

The anterior spinal supply comes from five to 10 usually single, unpaired radicular arteries, which feed into the anterior spinal artery at various levels (Figure 15-2). The most rostral supply comes from the intracranial vertebral artery. Each intracranial vertebral artery in its distal segment gives off a ramus, which joins with that of the contralateral vertebral artery to form a midline anterior spinal artery. The midline anterior spinal artery feeds the medulla and descends in the midline through the foramen magnum to supply the cervical spinal cord. Branches from the thyrocervical and costocervical branches of the subclavian arteries and branches of the nuchal vertebral artery feed into the spinal cord at the cervical enlargement. One radicular artery arises from the vertebral arteries and supplies the spinal cord at C3 and another anterior radicular artery originates from ascending cervical arteries supplying the C6, C7 regions.

The thoracic portion of the anterior spinal artery is fed by radicular branches of the deep cervical and intercostal arteries and by branches of the aorta. Blood supply is most marginal in the upper thoracic region (T2-T4). This has been referred to as a *longitudinal spinal cord watershed region*. The largest artery usually arises in the lower thoracic or upper lumbar segments, most often between T9 and T12, but can arise as low as L2. This artery is usually referred to as the *artery of Adamkiewicz*; it usually comes from the left and supplies the lumbar enlargement of the cord. The conus medullaris and cauda equina are nourished anteriorly from the hypogastric or obturator arteries.

In contrast, there are many more posterior radicular arteries that enter along nerve roots from each side at nearly every spinal level to supply the plexus of vessels that lie on the posterior cord surface.[4] Some additional segmental arteries arise from the vertebral, aorta, and iliac arteries to supply the paraspinous structures and then end on the anterior and posterior nerve roots without

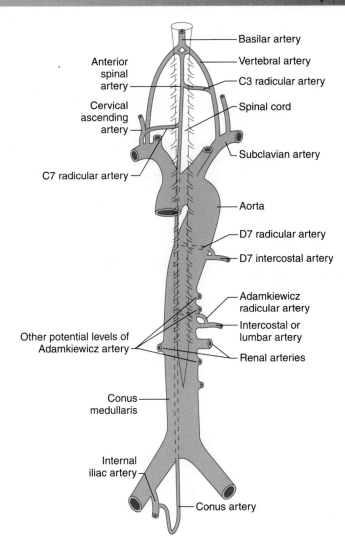

Figure 15-2. Aorta and its branches, showing important feeders at various levels. The cervical feeders come from the vertebral arteries; the others come from the aorta.

Labels in figure:
- Basilar artery
- Vertebral artery
- C3 radicular artery
- Spinal cord
- Subclavian artery
- Aorta
- D7 radicular artery
- D7 intercostal artery
- Adamkiewicz radicular artery
- Intercostal or lumbar artery
- Renal arteries
- Conus artery
- Anterior spinal artery
- Cervical ascending artery
- C7 radicular artery
- Other potential levels of Adamkiewicz artery
- Conus medullaris
- Internal iliac artery

supplying the spinal cord or penetrating the dura. These vessels are often the origin of spinal arteriovenous malformations (AVMs).[7]

The venous spinal cord anatomy has also been well worked out and studied.[8] Similar to the arterial supply, anterior and posterior venous drainage systems exist. Radicular veins are plentiful and drain into the paravertebral and intravertebral plexus into the pelvic veins. The posterior portions of the cord drain into a large midline posterior vein. The anterior and posterior venous system forms an extensive network, virtually encircling the spinal cord. Venous spinal cord infarction is probably more common than venous brain infarcts. This kind of infarction is most often caused by mechanical compression, infection, and inflammation, which obliterate the veins, and to vascular malformations, which cause increased venous pressure. Venous hypertension is an important

contributor to spinal cord infarction in patients with spinal dural fistulas.

SPINAL CORD ISCHEMIA AND INFARCTION

The history of the development of ideas about spinal cord infarction parallels the evolution of knowledge about the mechanism of brain infarcts. Most of the details of the vascular anatomy of the spinal cord were worked out by Düret, Adamkiewicz, and others in the late 19th century.[1,6] Early in the 20th century, clinicians recognized that most spinal cord infarcts involved the anterior portion of the spinal cord. Clinicians attributed spinal cord infarcts to anterior spinal artery occlusion. The putative cause was intrinsic disease of this artery, especially due to syphilis, diabetes, or atherosclerosis. Recall that during this same era, intracranial anterior circulation infarcts were invariably diagnosed as middle cerebral artery occlusions. Later, it was shown that intracranial arteries were less often the seat of disease than extracranial arteries. Embolism was a more frequent explanation for intracranial arterial occlusion than in situ atherothrombosis. Similarly, it has become clear that infarction in the distribution of the anterior spinal artery is most often caused by disease of the parent artery (usually the aorta), and less often to embolism. Intrinsic disease of intraspinal arteries is much less common.

Disease of the aorta is undoubtedly the most commonly recognized cause of spinal cord infarction. Interestingly two of the earliest reported examples of spinal cord infarction were related to aortic aneurysms.[9] Sir Astley Cooper in 1825 reported the case of a 38-year-old porter who acquired a very large traumatic aneurysm of his iliac artery that extended into the distal aorta.[9,10] Cooper ligated the aorta above the aneurysm, and the patient developed urinary retention, fecal incontinence, and loss of sensation below the abdomen and soon died. Necropsy showed that a thrombus had extended above the ligature and blocked much of the distal aorta. Gull, a surgeon at Guy's Hospital in London in 1857 described a patient who developed loss of power and sensation in the lower extremities attributable to an aortic aneurysm.[9,11] When operations on the aorta became common during the last half of the 20th century, spinal cord infarcts became well known as a complication of the surgery.[9] Surgeons recognized that operations on the aorta both above and below the renal arteries was sometimes associated with spinal paraplegia.[9,12,13]

Most often, paraplegia is recognized after repair of thoracic and abdominal aortic aneurysms.[5,6,14-16] During repair, flow through radicular supply arteries to the anterior spinal artery is compromised. When the thoracic cord is involved, usually a flaccid paraplegia is noted directly after surgery, with incontinence and a thoracic sensory level. Later, the lower limbs become spastic. When the lumbar cord is involved, a conus medullaris infarct develops, with hypotonia; wasting and areflexia of the legs; loss of sphincter function; and variable loss of touch and pinprick sensation in the lower limbs, perineum, and lower abdomen.

Similar findings are noted in unruptured aneurysms, dissections of the aorta, traumatic rupture of the aorta, thromboembolic aortic occlusions, and ulcerative aortic plaque disease. Thrombi and plaques can obstruct the orifices of radicular spinal arteries. Dissections can tear or interrupt the orifices of spinal cord feeding arteries, sometimes over a long area. Cholesterol crystals and other plaque materials can embolize into spinal arteries and block branches. In some patients, spinal ischemia develops gradually and insidiously. Spinal ischemia can be misdiagnosed as motor neuron disease or diabetic amyotrophy because of selective ischemia involving the anterior horns and, sometimes, the pyramidal tracts.[17]

In contrast to brain ischemic strokes, spinal transient ischemic attacks are quite unusual, but they do occur.[16,18] Infarcts tend to occur in different patterns.[18,19] The regions of spinal cord softening can sometimes be imaged on newer-generation MRI scanners, especially when diffusion-weighted images are included.[18-20] In a French study of 28 consecutive patients with spinal cord infarcts, 15 were thoracolumbar, 7 cervical, 3 thoracic, and 3 conus medullaris.[19] Infarcts can be classified as follows[18]:

- Bilateral, predominantly anterior (Fig. 15-3A). These patients have bilateral motor and spinothalamic type sensory deficits. Posterior column sensory functions (vibration and position sense) are spared.
- Unilateral, predominantly anterior (Fig. 15-3B). The motor deficit is a hemiparesis below the lesion and a contralateral spinothalamic tract sensory loss—a Brown-Séquard syndrome.
- Bilateral, predominantly posterior (Fig. 15-3C). Posterior column type of sensory loss below the lesion with variably severe bilateral pyramidal tract signs.
- Unilateral, mostly posterior (Fig. 15-3D). Ipsilateral hemiparesis and posterior column sensory loss.
- Central (Fig. 15-3E). Bilateral pain and temperature loss with spared posterior column and motor functions. Similar to a syrinx.
- Transverse. Loss of motor, sensory, and sphincter functions below the level of the lesion.

Anterior patterns are more common than posterior especially after aortic surgery.

Transesophageal echocardiography may show aortic plaques in patients who present with acute paraplegia.[21] Other means of imaging the aorta, including MRI are being actively explored.[22,23] Imaging signs of vertebral bone infarction may accompany spinal cord infarction caused by aortic disease.[3,18,24,25]

Embolism can and does cause spinal cord infarction. I have seen several patients with bacterial endocarditis with spinal and brain embolic infarcts, and such have been reported by others.[1,16] Atrial myxoma and nonbacterial thrombotic (marantic) endocarditis are other disorders in which small particles can embolize to the spinal cord.

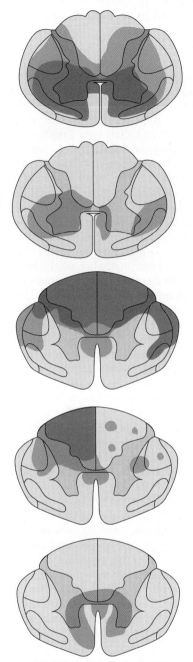

Figure 15-3. Cartoon of patterns of spinal cord infarction. Dark gray indicates usual extent, while light gray indicates potentially larger area of ischemia. **A,** Anterior bilateral infarction. **B,** Anterior predominantly unilateral infarction. **C,** Posterior bilateral infarction. **D,** Posterior predominantly unilateral infarction. **E,** Central spinal cord infarction.

Since the early 1980s, pathologists and clinicians have become aware that cartilaginous material from intervertebral disks can somehow invade the spinal arteries and veins and cause devastating spinal cord strokes.[3,26-28] Most reported cases are

cervical and involve young women. Some patients have been pregnant, puerperal, or on oral contraceptives. Minor trauma, sudden neck motion, or lifting was often mentioned as an immediate precipitant. The first symptoms are usually pain in the neck or upper back, or radicular pain. Then, a rapidly progressive, sometimes asymmetric, spinal cord syndrome with quadriparesis develops. Syringomyelia-like dissociated sensory loss, with loss of pain and temperature (but preserved touch sensation), may be found in the upper limbs or cape region. I have not seen or read of reversal of symptoms once paralysis developed. The same syndrome can affect the lumbar spinal cord and cause conus medullaris infarction.[3] MRI, contrast myelography, and other studies usually fail to show herniated disks with compression of the cord or nerve roots. Infarction is usually bland, but can be hemorrhagic.[3] Undoubtedly, this syndrome occurs more often than is now diagnosed.

Back or neck pain, often with radicular distribution paresthesias may be noted minutes before signs of spinal cord dysfunction develop. Among 27 spinal cord infarct patients in one series, 16 (59%) had such an onset.[18] The level of spinal cord ischemia was at the level of the pain and paresthesia in these patients. In 13 of these patients, ischemic symptoms developed immediately after a movement of the back, or arm, or after beginning to walk.[18] The spinal infarcts were either anterior or posterior and not central, and were predominantly at the level of acute and chronic vertebral and disc disease. Mechanical stress is posited to impinge on a spinal radicular artery causing localized spinal cord ischemia, although some cases are likely related to cartilaginous disc emboli.

Infarction and inflammation of the meningeal coverings of the spinal cord can spread to the spinal arteries, causing acute spinal cord strokes. The phenomenon is similar to Heubner's arteritis found in the brain in the presence of tuberculosis and syphilis. These two disorders, as well as fungal infections and Lyme borreliosis, probably account for the vast majority of infectious spinal arteritis. Almost invariably, the spinal fluid provides the clue to this problem.

Chronic adhesive arachnoiditis from any cause can also lead to scarring and obliteration of spinal penetrating arteries and ischemic necrosis of the central portion of the spinal cord.[29] The clinical findings are similar to syringomyelia, except that any level of the spinal cord can be involved. Arachnoidal scarring can be caused by trauma, hemorrhage, or infection. The signs and symptoms develop gradually, sometimes years after the spinal injury, bleed, or meningitis.[29] Schistosomiasis, especially *Schistosoma mansoni*, is well known to affect the spinal cord.[30,31] This parasite reaches the spinal cord through the blood vessel supply and can cause spinal cord infarction or granulomatous inflammation, most often involving the conus medullaris and the cauda equina. Spinal cord infarcts are occasionally explained by varicella-zoster virus infection.[32] Rare patients with central nervous system vasculitis develop spinal cord as well as brain infarcts.[33]

Spinal cord ischemia may also develop during severe hypotension, clinical shock, and cardiac arrest.[9,16,34-36] Damage is most likely to affect the thoracic spinal cord between the T4 and T8 segments, the most vulnerable region of the spinal cord.[16] Infarcts predominantly affect the central portion of the cord.[18] Spinal cord signs and symptoms are nearly always overshadowed by brain hypoxic-ischemic injury. The deeply comatose patient remains hypotonic and areflexic because of accompanying spinal ischemia. A pure spinal syndrome rarely complicates systemic hypoperfusion.

Spinal cord ischemia has also been reported after injection of heroin[37] and inhalation of cocaine.[38] In the case of heroin myelopathy, the spinal cord signs are usually noted after the patient awakens from a stupor. Most often the myelopathy develops when heroin is reintroduced after a period of abstinence. The mechanism of cord damage after drug abuse is most likely prolonged vasoconstriction.

Venous infarction is an important cause of cord ischemia. The infarcts may remain bland[36] or become frankly hemorrhagic.[3,39] Venous infarcts can be attributed to one of three different mechanisms (spinal dural AVMs),[3,7,38-43] coagulopathies with venous thrombosis, or mechanical compression of veins by epidural mass lesions or herniated discs.[36,42] Some patients with acute disc herniations develop the acute onset of severe spinal cord dysfunction, and MRI shows a spinal cord lesion at the site of disc herniation. These patients may not show good improvement after decompressive surgery. The spinal cord lesion in these patients is most likely an infarct caused by disc compression of the veins along the surface of the spinal cord.

SPINAL VASCULAR MALFORMATIONS

Contrary to the situation within the cranium, spinal vascular malformations often present with ischemia rather than hemorrhage, and some malformations cause bleeding and ischemia. Because of their distinctive characteristics and the fact that many neurologists and stroke experts are inexperienced with the usual findings

and diagnosis in such cases, I believe it best to consider spinal vascular malformations separately rather than in relation to the topics of ischemia or hemorrhage.

Spinal malformations should be divided into two large groups, which have differing blood supplies, presentations, and clinical findings (the dural [type I] and intradural [type II]) groups.[7,45,46] So-called type I malformations, often referred to as dural, derive their blood supply from arteries located in the dural sleeves of spinal roots.[7,41] The small nidus of arteriovenous communication is fed by dural branches of a radicular artery. These arteriovenous fistulas drain intradurally by one or more arterialized, enlarged, usually tortuous veins, which course on the dorsal surface of the spinal cord, usually above, but occasionally below, the feeding arteries. The dural feeding arteries do not participate in the blood supply of the spinal cord. Spinal dural fistulas occur predominantly in men (4-to-1 ratio) between 40 and 70 years of age, most often in the mid 50s, and involve mostly the lower thoracic and lumbosacral segments.

In one series, 26 of 27 type I malformations were fed by arteries in the thoracic or lumbar regions, and the remaining one malformation was sacral.[46] In another series of 13 dural fistulas, eight were located between T8 and T12, two were at S1, and one each was at L1 and L5.[39] Among 80 patients in a recent Dutch series, 49/80 were between T5 and T8. Figure 15-4 is a graph that shows the distribution of 146 arteriovenous fistulas in two large series.[47,48] Most often, one feeder exists, but, at times, two or three arterial feeders have been found.[7] Among a series of 27 such lesions, 24 had one feeder and three had two feeders.[46] Usually, this type of AVM is referred to as low-flow because angiography results only in slow, low-volume filling of the lesions. These lesions are not associated with arterial or venous aneurysms.[7,41] Cutaneous angiomas are not seen, and bruits are not audible.

The most frequent presentation of spinal dural fistulas is that of progressive neurologic worsening, often with acute deteriorations.[41] Among a series of 80 patients with documented spinal dural fistulas, 63% had a gradually progressive course.[47] In 21 patients, there were episodes of acute transient deterioration superimposed on the gradually progressive loss of function.[47] Five patients had a stepwise deterioration.

These fistulas usually do not cause subarachnoid bleeding, except when the lesions are cervical.[43,49] The cervical fistulas that cause subarachnoid hemorrhage (SAH) are fed by the vertebral artery and are often located near the cervicomedullary junction. Thoracic, lumbar, and sacral

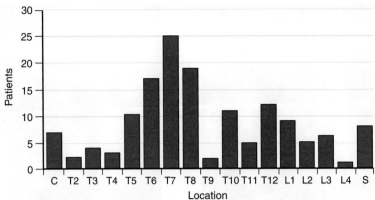

Figure 15-4. Location of spinal dural arteriovenous fistulas among 146 patients. C, cranial; T, thoracic; L, lumbar; S, sacral. (Data from Rosenblum B, Oldfield EH, Doppman JL, DiChiro G: Spinal arteriovenous malformations: A comparison of dural arteriovenous fistulas and intradural AVMs in 81 patients. J Neurosurg 1987;67:795-802; and Jellema K, Canta LR, Tijssen CC, et al: Spinal dural arterio-venous fistulas: clinical features in 80 patients. J Neurol Neurosurg Psychiatry 2003;74:1438-1440.)

fistulas rarely, if ever, present with SAH, but epidural hemorrhage occasionally develops. Pain is present in approximately 40% of patients. Pain can be radicular, sometimes mimicking sciatic pain. Symptoms often worsen after exercise. The most frequent symptoms involve gait, sensory abnormalities in the lower extremities and/or perineum, and lower extremity weakness. Most patients by the time a diagnosis is made have important symptoms and signs that indicate dysfunction of sacral cord segments—loss of sensation in the perineum, and abnormalities of micturition, defecation, and sexual function.[47,50]

Spinal TIAs do occur and are more frequent in patients with spinal dural fistulas than other spinal vascular lesions. One of my patients had two episodes of leg paralysis and numbness that occurred while she was driving a car.[51] Her husband had to grab the wheel and foot controls to avert a crash. Soon, strength and feeling returned. Another patient had a Brown-Séquard distribution attack while in hospital that lasted several hours.[51] Exercise and physical activity worsened symptoms in 19 of 27 patients (27%) in the National Institutes of Health series,[46] and often in another large series of patients.[47] Signs usually progress if the lesion is untreated, and most patients become unable to walk within 5 years of the onset of weakness. These lesions probably cause symptoms because of venous hypertension and occasional thrombosis of the venous drainage system.[7,40-42]

Type I dural lesions are often not well seen in early generation MRI scanning, but newer generation scanners now often do show abnormalities. DWI often shows spinal cord infarction and increased T2 signal, and spinal cord edema is common.[48,52-54] The key finding that suggests the possibility of a fistula are serpiginous dilated veins on the surface of the spinal cord. These are often now seen on T2-weighted and gadolinium-enhanced images and on contrast-enhanced MR angiography.[53-57] Figure 15-5 is an MR that shows these veins. Using MR angiography techniques, phase display after contrast injection can show the direction of flow within the epidural veins to indicate the likely location of arterial feeders.[54] These coiled, enlarged serpiginous veins are usually visible along the dorsal cord surface during myelography which still has a place in diagnosis.[45,46,48,52] Figure 15-6 is an intraoperative photo that shows these enlarged veins on the surface of the spinal cord. Myelographic films should be taken with the patients lying supine on their backs to show the abnormal veins. MR angiography[53-57] and CT angiography[57] sometimes show the supply arteries. Selective spinal angiography in expert, experienced hands often shows the feeding arteries, but occasionally the feeding arteries cannot be opacified.[48] I urge surgical exploration when the clinical findings are typical and abnormal veins are clearly present on myelography or magnetic resonance angiography examinations. Ligation of arterial feeders usually prevents worsening, so the venous structures need not be removed.[7] In most patients in whom the fistula has been treated effectively, muscle strength and gait improve, although sacral spinal cord dysfunction (urination, defecation, sexual function) often remain unchanged.[58]

Some dural fistulas are located in the spine or paravertebral region, but drain into epidural veins and often into the intradural venous system.[59]

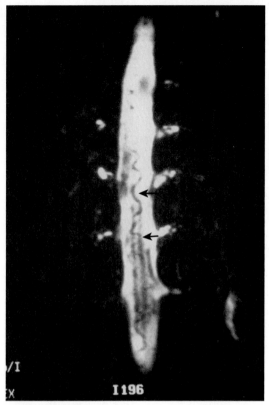

Figure 15-5. Coronal heavily T2-weighted MRI scan of the thoracolumbar spine showing serpiginous vessels *(arrows)* along the dorsal surface of the spinal cord. (From Kleefield J: Magnetic resonance and radiological imaging in the evaluation of back pain. In Aranoff GM (ed): Evaluation and treatment of chronic pain, 3rd ed. Baltimore: Williams & Wilkins, 1998, pp 477-504, with permission.)

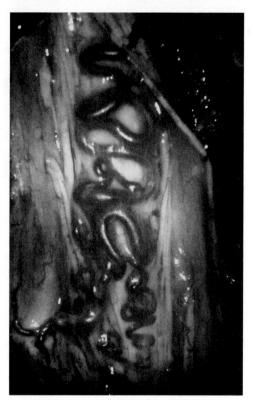

Figure 15-6. Intraoperative view of the surface of the spinal cord after the dura has been opened. Tortuous dilated veins can be seen along the surface of the cord. (Courtesy of Roberto Heros, MD, University of Miami.)

The enlarged epidural veins can cause a compressive myelopathy. The venous hypertension that results from these paravertebral fistulas can cause venous hypertension and a congestive myelopathy in the same way as dural AVMs.[56] MRI may show hyperintensity on T2-weighted sequences, spinal cord edema, and prominent perimedullary vessels. Dilatated tortuous epidural veins are often visible on magnetic resonance sequences and angiography.[59]

Remaining spinal AVMs are intradural. Type II malformations are usually intramedullary, but can be partially intramedullary, and partially between the dura and the cord. Intradural malformations are divided into various types: (1) glomus, referring to a tightly packed localized nidus of abnormal vessels within the cord; (2) juvenile, in which abnormal vessels occupy the entire spinal cord and are fed by numerous arterial feeding vessels at different levels; (3) direct arteriovenous fistulas, involving branches of arteries feeding the spinal cord; and (4) cavernous angiomas, which have no major feeding arteries and resemble cavernous angiomas of the brain. Increased availability of MRI leads frequently to identification of spinal cavernous malformations.

Usually, patients with intradural lesions are younger than those with dural lesions, but again, most patients are men. In one series, 65% of patients were younger than 25 years at first presentation.[46] These lesions have high flow, and hemorrhage is relatively common.[7,46] Intradural lesions are more widely distributed along the spinal axis and are often cervical. Spinal aneurysms, extraspinal aneurysms, other AVMs, and arterial bruits are common in patients with intradural AVMs. Most lesions are intramedullary (80% in the National Institutes of Health series)[46] and symptoms and signs are progressive.

Intradural AVMs are usually well-imaged and diagnosed by MRI. Glomus and juvenile lesions and cavernous angiomas have a nidus in the spinal cord parenchyma. The spinal cord is usually enlarged, and multiple serpiginous signal voids are seen.[52] Increased signal on T1-weighted images may represent methemoglobin from a prior hemorrhage. Low, dark signals on T1- and T2-weighted images can represent hemosiderin.[52] Spinal angiography usually readily shows intradural AVMs. Surgical treatment is not as successful for intradural AVMs as for dural ones, but glomus lesions and cavernous angiomas can be removed.

Cavernous angiomas are shown well by MRI.[60-63] Spinal cavernous angiomas usually present during the second to sixth decades and are slightly more common in women.[62] Symptoms can begin abruptly or progress gradually.[62,63] Symptoms may worsen with pregnancy, in the puerperium, and after trauma. As in the cranium, these lesions are angiographically occult. Appearance on MRI is similar to that of brain angiomas—heterogeneous, well-circumscribed, discrete lesions. Cavernous angiomas are well circumscribed and can be removed surgically.[63] When removed surgically, cavernomas appear as well-circumscribed, dark blue-brown, intramedullary, mulberry-shaped lesions that are surrounded by gliosis and hemosiderin staining.[61]

Intradural AVMs can cause chronic arachnoiditis due to bleeding, with subsequent scarring of small cord-feeding arteries and cord ischemia. Veins can thrombose. The so-called Foix-Alajouanine syndrome,[64] a subacute necrotizing ascending myelopathy, probably was, in retrospect, caused by such thrombosed vascular malformations of the dural or intradural variety.[65]

SPINAL HEMORRHAGES

Hematomyelia describes bleeding into the substance of the spinal cord parenchyma. The most common cause is trauma. Onset can be immediate or delayed. Usually, the area around the central canal and gray matter are involved, most often in the cervical region. The usual signs are neck pain; weakness; and areflexia in the arms, associated with a cape-like distribution of pain and temperature loss. Other causes include AVMs, anticoagulation, hemophilia and other bleeding disorders, and hemorrhage into spinal cord tumors, as well as (rarely) syrinxes. The spinal fluid is bloody, and MRI and myelography reveal a swollen blood-filled cord.

Spinal SAH is unusual. Unlike intracranial SAH, the most common causative lesions are AVMs. Aneurysms on spinal arteries rarely rupture.[66] Localized back pain is often followed by a stiff neck and pain that radiates along a root distribution or down the back or legs. Often, headache ensues, caused by spillage of blood intracranially. Bleeding diatheses and anticoagulants may cause spinal SAH.

Spinal epidural and subdural hematomas are rarer than intracranial hemorrhages in these compartments. Epidural hematomas are approximately four times more common than subdural hematomas. Each most often occurs in patients who are on anticoagulants.[67-70] Some patients have had liver disease and portal hypertension.[67] Lumbar punctures have been known to precipitate these bleeds in patients on anticoagulants. At times, these hemorrhages begin after exertion or straining, and, in some patients, no cause is found, even after full evaluation. Degenerative disk disease could be an etiologic factor.[71] The earliest symptom is pain in the back, usually in the neck. This is followed by radicular pain, usually in one or both arms. The earliest symptoms closely mimic disk herniation syndromes. Within hours, or rarely, days, sensory and motor signs develop in the legs, bowel, and bladder, and sexual dysfunction ensues. Usually, weakness and sensory loss are symmetric, but a Brown-Séquard distribution may be found.[67,72]

Diagnosis of spinal epidural or subdural hematoma has in the past usually been made by myelography. A block is most likely found. Computed tomography and MRI show the blood. MRI is superior in defining the location and extent of hematomas. Sagittal T1-weighted and T2-weighted images are usually reliable for diagnosis but hemorrhages and abscesses are difficult to reliably separate by imaging alone. Signs are almost invariably progressive, unless the lesions are decompressed. Anticoagulation should be reversed, using vitamin K, fresh frozen plasma, or prothrombin complex concentrates particularly those enriched with factor VII, factor X, and prothrombin. Decompression is urgent and should be pursued as soon as feasible considering the INR. Outcome depends on the severity of the deficit before surgery, the duration of spinal cord compression, and the rapidity of onset of the paraplegia. Chronic spinal subdural hematomas or hygromas are rare and are usually related to prior trauma or small bleeds.[73]

References

1. Buchan AM, Barnett HJM: Infarction of the spinal cord. In Barnett HJM, Mohr JP, Stern B, Yatsu F (eds): Stroke: Pathophysiology, Diagnosis and Management. New York: Churchill Livingstone, 1986, pp 707-719.
2. Vinters HV, Gilbert JJ: Hypoxic myelopathy. Can J Neurol Sci 1979;6:380.
3. Caplan LR: Case records of the Massachusetts General Hospital: Case 5-1991. N Engl J Med 1991;324:322-332.
4. Gillilan L: The arterial blood supply of the human spinal cord. J Comp Neurol 1958;110:75-103.

5. Mawad ME, Rivera V, Crawford S, et al: Spinal cord ischemia after resection of thoracoabdominal aortic aneurysms: MR findings in 24 patients. AJNR Am J Neuroradiol 1990;11:987-991.

6. Hogan EL, Romanul FCA: Spinal cord infarction occurring during insertion of aortic graft. Neurology 1966;16:67-74.

7. Heros R: Arteriovenous malformations of the spinal cord. In Ojemann RG, Heros RC, Crowell RM (eds): Surgical Management of Cerebrovascular Disease, 2nd ed. Baltimore: Williams & Wilkins, 1988, pp 451-466.

8. Gillilan L: Veins of the spinal cord: Anatomic details-suggested clinical applications. Neurology 1970;20:860-868.

9. Silver JR: History of infarction of the spinal cord. J History Neurosci 2003;12:144-153.

10. Cooper A: The Lectures of Sir Astley Cooper on the Principles and Practices of Surgery, vol II. London: Thomas and George Underwood, 1825.

11. Gull W: Paraplegia from obstruction of the abdominal aorta. In Wilks S, Poland A (eds): Guy's Hospital Reports, vol III. London: John Churchill.

12. DeBakey ME, Simeone FA: Battle injuries of the arteries in World War II. Ann Surg 1946;123:534-536.

13. Picone AL, Green RM, Ricotta JR, et al: Spinal cord ischemia following operations on the abdominal aorta. J Vasc Surg 1986;3:94-103.

14. Dodson WE, Landau W: Motor neuron loss due to aortic clamping in repair of coarctation. Neurology 1973;23:539-542.

15. Ross RT: Spinal cord infarction in diseases and surgery of the aorta. Can J Neurol Sci 1985;12:289-295.

16. Cheshire WP, Santos CC, Massey EW, Howard Jr JF: Spinal cord infarction: etiology and outcome. Neurology 1996;47:321-330.

17. Herrick MK, Mills PE: Infarction of spinal cord: Two cases of selective grey matter involvement secondary to asymptomatic aortic disease. Arch Neurol 1971;24:228-241.

18. Novy J, Carruzzo A, Maeder P, Bogousslavsky J: Spinal cord ischemia. Clinical and imaging patterns, pathogenesis, and outcomes in 27 patients. Arch Neurol 2006;63:1113-1120.

19. Masson C, Pruvo JP, Meder JF, et al: Study Group on Spinal Cord Infarction of the French neurovascular Society. Spinal cord infarction: Clinical and magnetic resonance imaging and short-term outcome. J Neurol Neurosurg Psychiatry 2004;75:1431-1435.

20. Shinoyama M, Takahashi T, Shimizu H, et al: Spinal cord infarction demonstrated by diffusion-weighted magnetic resonance imaging. J Clin Neurosci 2005;12:466-468.

21. Walsh DV, Uppal JA, Karalis DG, Chandrasekaran K: The role of transesophageal echocardiography in the acute onset of paraplegia. Stroke 1992;23:1660-1661.

22. Caplan LR: The aorta as a donor source of brain embolism. In Caplan LR, Manning WJ (eds): Brain Embolism. New York: Informa Healthcare, 2006, pp 187-201.

23. Amarenco P, Cohen A: Update on imaging aortic atherosclerosis. In Barnett HJM, Bogousslavsky J, Meldrum H (eds): Ischemic Stroke: Advances in Neurology, vol 92. Philadelphia: Lippincott, Williams & Wilkins, 2003, pp 75-89.

24. Yuh WT, Marsh EE III, Wang AK, et al: Imaging of spinal cord and vertebral body infarction. AJNR Am J Neuroradiol 1992;13:145-154.

25. Faig J, Busse O, Selbeck R: Vertebral body infarction as a confirmatory sign of spinal cord ischemic stroke: Report of three cases and review of the literature. Stroke 1998;29:239-243.

26. Srigley JR, Lambert CD, Bilbao JM, Pritzker KP: Spinal cord infarction secondary to intervertebral disc embolism. Ann Neurol 1981;9:296-301.

27. Raghavan A, Onikul E, Ryan MM, et al: Anterior spinal cord infarction owing to possible fibrocartilaginous embolism. Pediatr Radiol 2004;34:503-506.

28. Duprez TP, Danvoye L, Hernalsteen D, et al: Fibrocartilaginous embolization to the spinal cord: Serial MR imaging monitoring and pathologic study. AJNR Am J Neuroradiol 2005;26:496-501.

29. Caplan LR, Noronha A, Amico L: Syringomyelia and arachnoiditis. J Neurol Neurosurg Psychiatry 1990;53:106-113.

30. Haribhai HC, Bhigjee AI, Bill PL, et al: Spinal cord schistosomiasis. A clinical, laboratory and radiological study, with a note on therapeutic aspects. Brain 1991;114:709-726.

31. Saleem S, Belal AI, el-Ghandour NM: Spinal cord schistosomiasis: MR imaging appearance with surgical and pathologic correlation. AJNR Am J Neuroradiol 2005;26:1646-1654.

32. Orme HT, Smith AG, Nagel MA, et al: VZV spinal cord infarction identified by diffusion-weighted MRI (DWI). Neurology 2007;69:398-400.

33. Salvarini C, Brown Jr RD, Calamia KT, et al: Primary CNS vasculitis with spinal cord involvement. Neurology 2008;70:2394-2400.

34. Silver JR, Buxton PH: Spinal stroke. Brain 1974;97:539-550.

35. Satran R: Spinal cord infarction. Curr Concepts Cerebrovasc Dis Stroke 1987;22:13-17.

36. Singh U, Diplomate NB, Silver JR, Weply NC: Hypotensive infarction of the spinal cord. Paraplegia 1994;32:314-322.

37. Brust JCM: Stroke and substance abuse. In Bogousslavsky J, Caplan LR (eds): Uncommon Causes of Stroke. Cambridge: Cambridge University Press, 2001, pp 132-138.

38. Kim RC, Smith HR, Henbest ML, Choi BH: Non-hemorrhagic venous infarction of the spinal cord. Ann Neurol 1984;15:379-385.

39. Hughes JT: Venous infarction of the spinal cord. Neurology 1971;21:794-800.

40. Larsson EM, Desai P, Hardin CW, et al: Venous infarction of the spinal cord resulting from dural arteriovenous fistula: MR imaging findings. AJNR Am J Neuroradiol 1991;12:739-743.

41. Bradac GB, Daniele D, Riva A, et al: Spinal dural arteriovenous fistulas: An underestimated cause of myelopathy. Eur Neurol 1993;34:87-94.

42. Hurst RW, Kenyon LC, Lavi E, et al: Spinal dural arteriovenous fistula: The pathology of venous hypertensive myelopathy. Neurology 1995;45:1309-1313.

43. Hemphill III JC, Smith WS, Halbach VV: Neurologic manifestations of spinal epidural arteriovenous malformations. Neurology 1998;50:817-819.

44. Roa KR, Donnenfeld H, Chusid JG, Valdez S: Acute myelopathy secondary to spinal venous thrombosis. J Neurol Sci 1982;56:107-113.

45. DeChiro G, Doppman JL, Ommaya AK: Radiology of spinal cord arteriovenous malformations. Prog Neurol Surg 1971;4:329-354.

46. Rosenblum B, Oldfield EH, Doppman JL, DiChiro G: Spinal arteriovenous malformations: A comparison of dural arteriovenous fistulas and intradural AVMs in 81 patients. J Neurosurg 1987;67: 795-802.

47. Jellema K, Canta LR, Tijssen CC, et al: Spinal dural arteriovenous fistulas: Clinical features in 80 patients. J Neurol Neurosurg Psychiatry 2003; 74:1438-1440.

48. Gilbertson JR, Miller GM, Goldman MS, Marsh WR: Spinal dural arteriovenous fistulas: MR and myelographic findings. AJNR Am J Neuroradiol 1995;16:2049-2057.

49. Do HM, Jensen ME, Cloft HJ, et al: Dural arteriovenous fistula of the cervical spine presenting with subarachnoid hemorrhage. AJNR Am J Neuroradiol 1999;20:348-350.

50. Strom RG, Derdeyn CP, Moran CJ, et al: Frequency of spinal arteriovenous malformations in patients with unexplained myelopathy. Neurology 2006;66: 928-931.

51. Teal PA, Wityk RJ, Rosengart A, Caplan LR: Spinal TIAs—A clue to the presence of spinal dural AVMs. Neurology 1992;42(suppl 3):341.

52. Greenberg J: Neuroimaging of the spinal cord. Neurol Clin 1991;9:696-698.

53. Bowen BC, Fraser K, Kochan JP, et al: Spinal dural arteriovenous fistulas:evaluation with MR angiography. AJNR Am J Neuroradiol 1995;16: 2029-2043.

54. Mascalchi M, Quillici N, Ferrito G, et al: Identification of the feeding arteries of spinal vascular lesions via phase-contrast MR angiography with three-dimensional acquisition and phase display. AJNR Am J Neuroradiol 1997;18:351-358.

55. Saraf-Lavi E, Bowen BC, Quencer RM, et al: Detection of spinal dural arteriovenous fistulae with MR imaging and contrast-enhanced MR angiography: Sensitivity, specificity, and prediction of vertebral level. AJNR Am J Neuroradiol 2002;23: 858-867.

56. Luetmer PH, Lane JI, Gilbertson JR, et al: Preangiographic evaluation of spinal dural arteriovenous fistulas with elliptic centric contrast-enhanced MR angiography and effect on radiation dose and volume of iodinated contrast material. AJNR Am J Neuroradiol 2005;26:711-718.

57. Zampakis P, Santosh C, Taylor W, Teasdale E: The role of non-invasive computed tomography in patients with suspected dural fistulas with spinal drainage. Neurosurgery 2006;58:686-694.

58. Jellema K, Tijssen CC, van Rooiji WJJ, et al: Spinal dural arteriovenous fistulas: Long-term follow-up of 44 treated patients. Neurology 2004;62: 1839-1841.

59. Goyal M, Willinsky R, Montanera W, terBrugge K: Paravertebral arteriovenous malformations with epidural drainage: Clinical spectrum, imaging features, and results of treatment. AJNR Am J Neuroradiol 1999;20:749-755.

60. Lopate G, Black JT, Grubb RL: Cavernous hemangioma of the spinal cord: Report of two unusual cases. Neurology 1990;40:1791-1793.

61. Cosgrove GR, Bertrand G, Fontaine S, et al: Cavernous angiomas of the spinal cord. J Neurosurg 1988;68:31-36.

62. McCormick PC, Michelson WJ, Post KD, et al: Cavernous malformations of the spinal cord. Neurosurgery 1988;23:459-463.

63. Ogilvy CS, Louis DN, Ojemann RG: Intramedullary cavernous angiomas of the spinal cord: Clinical presentation, pathological features, and surgical management. Neurosurgery 1992;31: 219-230.

64. Foix C, Alajouanime T: La myelite necrotique subaique. Rev Neurol 1926;2:1-42.

65. Criscuolo GR, Oldfield EH, Doppman JL: Reversible acute and subacute myelopathy in patients with dural arteriovenous fistulas. J Neurosurg 1989;70:354-359.

66. Garcia C, Dulcey S, Dulcey J: Ruptured aneurysm of the spinal artery of Adamkiewicz during pregnancy. Neurology 1979;29:394-398.

67. Mattle H, Sieb JP, Rohner M, Mumenthaler M: Nontraumatic spinal epidural and subdural hematomas. Neurology 1987;37:1351-1356.

68. Post MJD, Becerra JL, Madsen PW, et al: Acute spinal subdural hematoma: MR and CT findings with pathological correlates. AJNR Am J Neuroradiol 1994;15:1895-1905.

69. Morandi X, Riffaud L, Chabert E, Brassier G: Acute nontraumatic spinal subdural hematomas in three patients. Spine 2001;26:E547-551.

70. Cha YH, Chi JH, Barbaro NM: Spontaneous spinal subdural hematoma associated with low-molecular-weight heparin. Case report. Neurosurg Spine 2005;2:612-613.

71. Gundry CR, Heithoff KB: Epidural hematoma of the lumbar spine: 18 surgically confirmed cases. Radiology 1993;187:427-431.

72. Russman BS, Kazi K: Spinal epidural hematoma and the Brown-Séquard syndrome. Neurology 1971;21:1066-1068.

73. Black P, Zervas N, Caplan LR, Ramirez L: Subdural hygroma of the spinal meninges: A case report. Neurosurgery 1978;2:52-54.

Most brain ischemia is caused by thromboembolism and occlusive arterial disease. However, brain infarcts and brain edema are sometimes caused by thrombosis of dural sinuses and cerebral and cerebellar veins. Since the advent of magnetic resonance imaging (MRI), computed tomography angiography (CTA), magnetic resonance angiography (MRA), and magnetic resonance venography (MRV), the diagnosis of venous occlusive disease has been made much more often than in the past. I discuss the anatomy of the venous system in Chapter 2.

DEVELOPMENT OF IDEAS

Occlusions of the veins that drain the brain were first reported in the 1820s. In 1825, Ribes described the first case of dural sinus thrombosis.[1-3] Ribes's patient was a 45-year-old man who developed epilepsy, severe headaches, and delirium. The delirium improved within a month, but headaches persisted and seizures increased in frequency. He died 6 months later. At necropsy, the superior sagittal and left lateral sinuses were thrombosed. Carcinomatous metastases were present in the brain. Three years later, John Abercrombie described the first case of puerperal sinus thrombosis.[4] A 24-year-old woman developed a severe headache after the delivery of her second child. Later, a sense of uneasiness in her head and numb feelings in her occiput and neck were followed by sudden weakness and numbness of her right hand, loss of speech, and twisting of her mouth. Frequent seizures were followed by coma and death. At necropsy, the sagittal sinus was occluded and the draining veins were distended and turgid. The brain showed softening and hemorrhage.

Tonnelle[5] published a review of thrombosis of the dural sinuses in 1829 and Cruveilhier[6] included a chapter on inflammation of the dural sinuses in his popular pathologic anatomy atlas. These authors noted that dural sinus thrombosis was common in children, especially those with fever and infections. Tonnelle and Cruveilhier noted that dural sinus thrombosis also tended to develop during the puerperium and in older, ill individuals, so-called "senile cases." At the end of the 19th century, Quinke, the clinician usually given credit for originating lumbar puncture, described patients who had headache, visual symptoms, papilledema, and evidence of raised intracranial pressure who often recovered and did not have brain tumors.[7,8] At necropsy, one of Quinke's patients had occlusion of both transverse sinuses and the vein of Galen.

Sir Charles Symonds brought the phenomena of benign intracranial hypertension and its relation to dural sinus occlusion and cerebral venous thrombophlebitis to the attention of clinicians. Symonds, in a series of key papers that spanned a quarter of a century, described the phenomenology of so-called *otitic hydrocephalus* and its relation to lateral sinus thrombosis and disease of the ears and mastoid air cells.[9-12]

In 1967, Kalbag, a neurosurgeon, and Woolf, a neuropathologist, wrote a monograph on the topic of cerebral venous thrombosis.[1] These physicians reviewed the history of recognition of this disorder, ideas about pathogenesis, and past contributions. The increased ability to recognize dural sinus and venous occlusions using magnetic resonance technology has led to a dramatic increase in knowledge about venous occlusive disease during the past two decades. This increased knowledge has led investigators and clinicians to publish comprehensive reviews and monographs on the topic of venous and dural sinus occlusions.[2,13-21]

ETIOLOGIES AND DEMOGRAPHY

Infections

In the pre-antibiotic era and until the 1970s, infections were the most common cause of dural sinus occlusions. Otitic and mastoid infections were a common cause of lateral sinus thrombosis, and facial and paranasal sinus infections could lead to septic cavernous sinus infection. In the past, authors divided the causes of venous occlusive disease into infective and noninfective causes. In the pre-antibiotic era, occlusion of the lateral and sigmoid sinuses was almost exclusively caused by spread of infection from the mastoid air cells through emissary veins or directly into the adjacent lateral sinuses. The infectious process sometimes spread from the lateral sinus to the inferior petrosal sinus and then to the cavernous sinus. Lateral sinus occlusion was found predominantly in young patients with acute and chronic otitis media and those with inflammatory cholesteatomas. Most infections were pyogenic, but tuberculosis also involved the ear structures and mastoid cells and often spread to the meninges and dural sinuses. Facial infections were the most common cause of septic cavernous sinus thrombosis before the introduction of antibiotics. Ethmoid and sphenoid sinusitis could spread into the adjacent cavernous sinus.[22] During infections of the structures of the middle third of the face, including the nose, paranasal sinuses, orbits, tonsils, and palate, bacteria entered the facial veins and pterygoid venous plexus to drain into the cavernous sinus via the superior and inferior ophthalmic veins.[22,23]

Dural sinus infection may follow open, direct traumatic injuries when bacteria are introduced into the cranial cavity and after brain and epidural abscesses. Meningitis is also occasionally complicated by dural sinus occlusion. High fever and dehydration, especially in children and the elderly, can also precipitate dural sinus thrombosis. Infections are known to increase the concentrations of acute phase reactants, including serine proteins involved in the coagulation process. The increased coagulability that results also promotes venous and dural sinus occlusion.

Infectious causes were found in 77 (12.3%) of patients aged more than 15 years included in the large International Study on Cerebral Vein and Dural Sinus Thrombosis (ISCVT).[24] Infections involving the ears, face, mouth, and neck accounted for 51 of 77, and infections involving the central nervous system were present in 13 patients.[24] An uncommon but important syndrome of tonsillopharyngitis with subsequent thrombophlebitis of the jugular vein was first described by Lemierre and is known as Lemierre's syndrome.[25,26]

Hormonal Factors and Pregnancy and the Puerperium in Women

Since Abercrombie, physicians have recognized that hormonal factors in women are important in patients with dural sinus and venous occlusions. The most common such circumstance is the puerperium, but dural sinus occlusions also occur more often than expected during pregnancy and in women who take oral contraceptive pills.[24,27-33] The U.S. National Hospital Discharge Survey (1979-1991) reported that 5723 cases of intracranial venous thrombosis were found in 50,264,631 deliveries, yielding a frequency of 11.4 per 100,000 deliveries.[33] Dural sinus occlusion during pregnancy and the puerperium is especially common, or at least often reported, in India[30-32] and Mexico.[28,29]

Venous occlusions are more common in the postpartum period than during pregnancy. Among 135 patients with cerebral venous thrombosis collected by Bousser during a 20-year period in Paris, four occurred in women during pregnancy and 17 occurred during the puerperium.[16] In the ICVST study, 53 women developed venous occlusions during the puerperium while 24 had onset during pregnancy.[24] Among a series of 113 patients with nonseptic cranial venous thromboses studied in Mexico, 67 women were diagnosed during the puerperium, five during pregnancy, and one after an abortion.[28] Among another series of 20 Mexican women with intracranial sinus thrombosis, 13 were puerperal.[29] Six women took oral contraceptive pills. Most postpartum cases occurred during the first 3 weeks after delivery, but venous thromboses also developed at any time during pregnancy. Postpartum cerebral venous thrombosis is more common in patients who have had venous thromboses outside the nervous system during previous pregnancies (pelvic or lower extremity phlebothrombosis and pulmonary embolism). Puerperal intracranial venous thrombosis is also commonly found in multiparous women, women from lower socioeconomic strata who have had less prenatal care, and after deliveries at home. Explanations for the frequency of intracranial venous thrombosis in pregnancy and the puerperium include poverty, vegetarian and vitamin-deficient food intake and depletion of vitamin and protein stores by multiple pregnancies, and anemia. These factors may cause hyperhomocysteinemia and hypercoagulability, increasing the risk of venous occlusions.[21]

Prescription of female hormones is also an important risk factor for venous occlusive disease both intracranial and extracranial. In the ICVST, 54.3% of the 381 women aged less than 50 years old were taking oral contraceptives and 27 were on hormone replacement therapy.[24] Hormonal changes might also be important in males. A healthy 31-year-old man was reported to develop extensive dural sinus occlusions after taking intramuscular injections of androgens for body building.[34] Among 27 patients with anemia treated with androgen therapy in one series, three patients developed sagittal sinus thrombosis.[35]

Neoplasms

Cancer, with its increase in acute-phase reactants and enhanced coagulability, is another common cause of thrombosis. Adenocarcinomas, especially from the pancreas and gastrointestinal tract, are especially likely to be accompanied by thrombotic complications. Hickey et al reported three patients with cancer (two with breast cancer and one with lung adenocarcinoma) who had intracranial venous sinus thrombosis.[36] They also reviewed 13 prior case reports. All patients had breast cancer, lung cancer, or hematologic malignancies, including lymphoma and leukemia. The clinical syndromes related to the intracranial venous thrombosis were indistinguishable from non-cancer patients, but coexisting limb venous thromboses and pulmonary emboli were often present. In some cancer patients, the sinovenous occlusive disease was extensive. One patient with lung cancer at necropsy had occlusion of both renal arteries and veins, both internal carotid arteries, the splenic and portal veins, the pulmonary artery, the superior sagittal sinus, vein of Galen, and numerous cortical veins.[36] In two patients, dural sinus thrombosis was the presenting problem occurring before the diagnosis of cancer. Migratory thrombophlebitis, Trousseau's sign, was first described in patients with pancreatic cancer. Trousseau's sign is common, especially in patients with mucinous adenocarcinomas.[37-39]

Cranial neoplasms can invade the dura matter and cause occlusions of the adjacent dural sinuses. This probably occurs most often in patients with meningiomas. Metastatic tumors that invade the skull, such as breast cancer and myeloma, may spread to the subjacent dura and dural sinuses and cause thrombosis. Six of the 135 patients (4.5%) in the series of Bousser had cancer, including two with carcinomatous meningitis.[16] Neck tumors and abscesses, which involve the pharynx that blocks the jugular veins, can also cause propagation of clots into the lateral sinuses.[25,26,40]

Abnormalities of Blood and Coagulation System

Acquired and congenital abnormalities of the blood and coagulation system are also important causes of dural sinus and cerebral venous thrombosis. Thrombocytosis,[41] polycythemia vera,[42-44] paroxysmal nocturnal hemoglobinuria,[45] and antiphospholipid antibody syndrome[46,47] have all been reported to cause dural sinus and cerebral venous occlusions. Some reported patients with dural sinus thrombosis have had severe anemia as the only predisposing cause.[16,24] Patients with systemic lupus erythematosus and lupus anticoagulant have also been reported to develop dural sinus occlusions, presumably because of hypercoagulability.[48,49] Sickle cell disease, protein C and protein S deficiencies, antithrombin III deficiency, plasminogen deficiency,[50] elevated levels of factor VIII,[51] disseminated intravascular coagulation, and thrombosis associated with heparin-induced thrombocytopenia have all been reported to cause dural sinus occlusions.

Resistance to activated protein C caused most often by the presence of factor V Leiden is an important cause of cerebral venous thrombosis, especially if patients with this genetic mutation take oral contraceptives or become pregnant.[21,52-54] Among 624 patients in the ISCST study, 140 (22.4%) were found to have a genetic cause of thrombophilia.[24] Among 40 patients with cerebral venous thrombosis studied for coagulation abnormalities, 3 had increased antiphospholipid antibodies; 6 had thrombophilia, including 1 with protein C deficiency, 1 with protein S deficiency, and 4 with factor V Leiden.[55]

In a recent series, among 163 patients with sinovenous thrombosis, the prothrombin G20210A gene mutation was one of the most common causes of thrombophilia and was more than twice as common in these patients than among 163 patients with lower-extremity deep venous thromboses.[55a] Activated protein C resistance, factor V Leiden, and protein C deficiency were more common among the patients with peripheral vein occlusions.[55a] Two other genetically mediated causes of thrombophilia among individuals with cerebral venous thrombosis have recently been uncovered and are being explored further—promoter polymorphisms in the plasma glutathione peroxidase (GPx-3) gene[55b] and the factor XII C46T gene polymorphism.[55c] The GPx-3 gene is posited to affect coagulation by its antioxidant functions and its relationship to nitric oxide.[55b] The FXII (C46T) polymorphism affects the function of an important component of the coagulation cascade-factor XII.[55c]

Systemic Conditions

Some systemic illnesses predispose to venous and dural sinus occlusions. Patients with the nephrotic syndrome may have renal vein and dural sinus occlusions that are probably related to deficiencies in coagulation proteins caused by the heavy proteinuria.[56,57] Dehydrated patients probably develop thrombosis because of a relatively high hematocrit and increase in viscosity and coagulability. In ill, cachectic elderly patients, a combination of dehydration and activation of coagulation factors probably cause so-called *senile marantic* venous sinus thrombosis. Congestive heart failure is also an important cause of cerebral venous thrombosis, presumably because of elevated venous pressure.

Systemic inflammatory diseases, especially ulcerative colitis,[16,58-61] Crohn's disease,[16,61-63] and Behçet's disease,[16,64-69] are known causes of dural sinus and cerebral venous occlusions. Behçet's disease may cause a pseudotumor syndrome with papilledema,[64] and is an important cause of intracranial venous occlusive disease, especially in Turkey and Mediterranean countries. Among 250 patients with Behçet's disease followed in Paris, 25 patients (10%) had angiographically confirmed cerebral venous thromboses.[67] The outcome in the Paris series of patients with Behçet's disease and venous occlusions was quite good when the patients were treated with heparin and corticosteroids. In a series of patients with dural sinus thrombosis studied in Saudi Arabia, Behçet's disease accounted for one fourth of the cases.[68]

Other Causes

Patients with dural arteriovenous fistulas may have accompanying thrombosis of dural venous sinuses and draining veins. The venous thrombosis can predispose to the development of a fistula, and fistulas can be the cause of subsequent venous thrombosis. This topic is discussed in Chapter 12. Head trauma can also lead to dural sinus thrombosis, and dural sinus occlusion occasionally develops after lumbar puncture, after cranial and systemic surgery, and in patients with thyroid disease.[16,24]

The cause of intracranial venous thrombosis is undetermined in many patients despite extensive investigations. Among the 624 patients in the ISCVT study, no identifiable cause was found in 78 (12.5%).[24] In the initial series of 76 patients reported by Bousser, 17 patients (22%) were idiopathic.[70] In the later Bousser series, 29 of 135 patients (21%) had no recognized etiology.[16] Twenty-five of 113 (22%) cases studied by Cantu and Barinagarrementeria could not be assigned an etiology.[28] In the series of cases from Saudi Arabia, 10 of 40 patients (25%) were idiopathic even after thorough evaluation.[68] Table 16-1 tabulates the etiologies of cerebral venous thromboses in two large series of patients.[16,24]

DEMOGRAPHY

Intracranial venous occlusive disease predominantly affects women and relatively young individuals. Among six series of patients,[24,28,68,71-73] 987 individuals were studied, including 706 girls or women (71.5%) and 281 boys or men (28.5%). Ages spanned 6 days to 86 years, with an average age of 36.8 years. The average age in all of the series was quite young: age 26 years in puerperal women with venous sinus thrombosis[24]; age 36 years in nonpuerperal men and women; and 38.7 years, 39.1 years, 34.3 years, 27.8 years, and

Table 16-1. Frequencies of Various Causes among Two Large Series of Patients with Cerebral Venous Occlusions

	Bousser et al[16]	Ferro et al[24]
Thrombophilia	10 (7.5%)	213 (34.1%)
Female hormones	31 (23%)	234 (37.5%)
Puerperium	13 (9.6%)	77 (12.3%)
Pregnancy	4 (3%)	24 (4.3%)
Infections	8 (6%)	77 (12.3%)
Anemia	2 (1.5%)	58 (9.2%)
Malignancy	6 (4.5%)	46 (7.4%)
Surgery	1 (0.75%)	21 (3.3%)
Corticosteroids	3 (2.2%)	10 (1.6%)
Dural fistulas	3 (2.2%)	10 (1.6%)
Behçet's disease	18 (13%)	6 (1%)
Head injury	7 (5%)	7 (1.1%)
Polycythemia	1 (0.75%)	18 (2.8%)
Inflammatory bowel disease	1 (0.75%)	10 (1.6%)
Dehydration	–	12 (1.9%)
Thyroid disease	–	11 (1.7%)
Lumbar puncture	–	12 (1.9%)
Undefined	29 (21%)	78 (12.5%)
Total number of patients	135	624

33.3 years of age in series that included both sexes.[24,68,71,73] All reviewed series showed female predominance except Bousser et al, which included 21 men (55%) and 17 women,[13] and Daif et al,[68] which included 20 men and 20 women. The sex and age predominance of patients with cerebral venous thrombosis contrasts dramatically with that found in patients with thromboembolic arterial disease, which has a male predominance and an average age at least three decades older.

PATHOPHYSIOLOGY

The development of brain pathology in patients with venous occlusions is quite different from arterial occlusive disease.[16,18,75] In arterial disease, the delivery of nutrients is directly compromised and brain ischemia and infarction develop. When elements of the venous system are occluded, drainage of blood is compromised. Pressure increases in the brain tissue drained by the obstructed veins and dural sinuses. Brain edema develops in the involved territory. If tissue pressure increases enough, capillaries and arterioles break and brain hemorrhage occurs. A useful analogy is to visualize draining systems on city streets. When drains become clogged during a rainstorm, water accumulates on the street and may flood nearby land. The major initial findings in patients with occluded cerebral veins and dural sinuses are localized brain edema and brain hemorrhage. Bleeding can spill out into the nearby subarachnoid space.

In order to perfuse brain tissue adequately, the blood pressure in the feeding artery must exceed the pressure in the tissue and draining veins. When the venous pressure and intracranial pressure become high enough, arterial perfusion may become inadequate and brain infarction can ensue.

Brain edema is potentially reversible, while brain infarction is not.

CLINICAL FINDINGS

Some clinical findings relate to occlusion of intracranial venous structures in general, whereas others are relatively specific for the location of thrombosis. General symptoms are reviewed first. Focal symptoms are discussed when various locations of venous thrombosis are analyzed.

> CD, a 57-year-old man, worked in the anatomy department of a medical school as a repairman. One day, a neuroanatomist working in the laboratory saw him suddenly stop speaking in the midst of a conversation. He repeated, "I can't, I can't" and his right arm briefly shook. He was brought to the emergency room where he was noted to have difficulty speaking. While being examined, he had a grand mal seizure heralded by turning of his head to the right. Blood pressure was 160/100 mm Hg, but gradually returned to normal (125/80 mm Hg). Postictal agitation and aphasia were present. The aphasia was fluent and consisted of paraphasic errors and difficulty naming. He had a right superior quadrantanopia. Comprehension and repetition of speech were relatively spared. When he was able to discuss his symptoms, he reported that he had awakened that morning with a headache. He felt well the day before his attack. During the preceding weeks, he had intense headaches. He was being treated for hypertension. A year ago, he had an episode of thrombophlebitis and was treated with warfarin for 4 months. He was not taking coumadin or aspirin at the time of his attack.

Onset and Course

The presentation of patients with dural sinus thrombosis may be acute, as in CD, but, in general, venous occlusions seem to develop and propagate much more slowly than arterial occlusions. In most series, a gradual or stepwise development of symptoms and signs is more common than sudden abrupt onset.[2,16,18] Progression of symptoms after onset is also common and observed more often than in patients with arterial infarcts. The onset can be characterized as acute (sudden onset or development within 48 hours), subacute (between 2 days and a month), and chronic (>30 days to evolve).[16]

In the Cantu and Barinagarrementeria series, acute onset was found more often in women who had puerperal venous thromboses when compared with nonpuerperal patients (82% vs 54%).[28] Subsequent progression was also more common in puerperal thromboses (72% vs 52%).[28] Puerperal and infectious cases tend to present acutely. Gradual increase in symptoms and a fluctuating course are the rule in patients with other causes of venous thromboses.[2,16] Acute onset patients often present with focal signs while chronic cases more often present with headaches. Ameri and Bousser found that the onset of symptoms was acute (<48 hours) in 31 (28%) patients, subacute in 46 (42%) patients, and chronic in 33 (30%) patients.[71] Insidious onset, usually without focal neurological signs, has often led to delays in admission to the hospital and presentation to doctors.

In some patients, symptoms are present for longer than 6 months when the diagnosis is made. Among 102 patients with angiographically proven intracranial venous thromboses in one series, the mean day of admission after symptom onset was the 5th day, whereas the average was the 14th day.[75] Eleven patients in this series came to the hospital more than 1 month after symptom onset.[74] Gutschera-Wang noted that 10% of patients with cerebral venous thromboses had a history of headache for longer than 6 months before the diagnosis of venous thrombosis was made.[76]

Necropsy studies sometimes document venous thrombi at different stages of formation and organization.[75,77] Radiologically confirmed extension of thrombosis within the dural sinuses and veins has been noted after anticoagulants are stopped. The slow and gradual onset of symptoms and signs can be explained by the slow evolution and propagation of thrombosis and the potentially broad collateralization potential of the cranial venous and sinus drainage patterns. Collateralization of venous drainage patterns is more likely when thrombosis is gradual rather than when the occlusion is abrupt.

Headache

Head discomfort or pain is an extremely common symptom in patients with intracranial venous occlusive disease. CD had headaches before and at the onset of his neurological symptoms. Headache is the only symptom in some patients, but is a major symptom in most patients. Cumurciuc and colleagues reported 17 patients (among a series of 123 consecutive patients with cerebral venous and dural sinus occlusions whose only presenting symptom was headache.[78] These 17 patients had neither papilledema nor raised intracranial pressure on lumbar puncture and no parenchymal lesions or subarachnoid blood on CT scans.[78] Three of these patients had "thunderclap headache"—the sudden onset of excruciating severe headache and three had severe headache that developed within 1 day. Headache is much more common in patients with venous thromboses than in patients with arterial thromboembolic disease. Table 16-2 lists the symptoms that occurred during the course of illness among various reported series of patients with cerebral venous thromboses.[24,28,68,71-73,79,80]

In the series of Cantu and Barinagarrementeria, headache was the most common presenting symptom in the puerperal group. Headache was also the most common symptom in the group of patients who did not have venous thrombosis in relation to pregnancy or the postpartum period.[28] Headache was an important symptom present in at least 949 of the total 1122 patients (85%) in these various series. This frequency of headache is most likely a minimal figure because some obtunded and confused or aphasic patients might not have been able to report the presence of headache.

The presence of headache is best explained by two major factors: (1) the local process within the veins and dural sinuses, and (2) the development of increased intracranial pressure. Unlike the brain itself, the dura and overlying skull and venous sinuses are invested with pain-sensitive fibers. Distension of the sinuses, especially when caused by inflammation, activates these pain-sensitive fibers. Thrombosis causes obstruction (at least temporarily) to venous drainage from intracranial structures. The resulting increased venous pressure causes increased intracranial pressure, brain edema, brain hemorrhage and infarction, and decreased absorption of cerebrospinal fluid. These findings cause increased intracranial pressure, often with papilledema. Papilledema was noted in 393 of 1122 (35%) patients in which this sign was sought (see Table 16-2). In the series of 76 patients reported by Bousser and Barnett, 38% had a pseudotumor syndrome characterized by headache, papilledema, and sixth nerve palsy.[79] The pseudotumor syndrome, also often called *benign intracranial hypertension,* is characterized by headache, transient visual obscuration, papilledema, and raised intracranial pressure (as measured by lumbar puncture) without important neurologic signs. Sixth nerve palsies and vision loss can result from the increased intracranial pressure. A pseudotumor syndrome was the most common clinical syndrome in the

Table 16-2. The Frequency of Various Clinical Findings in Patients with Intracranial Venous Thromboses in Selected Series

Clinical Finding	Cantu and Barinagarrementeria[28] Puerperium $n = 67$	Cantu and Barinagarrementeria[28] Nonpuerperium $n = 46$	Ameri and Bousser[71] $n = 110$	Einhaupl et al[72] $n = 71$
Headache	59 (88%)	32 (70%)	83 (75%)	63/69 (91%)
Seizures	40 (60%)	29 (63%)	41 (37%)	34 (48%)
Focal findings	53 (79%)	35 (76%)	57 (52%)	47 (66%)
Altered consciousness	42 (63%)	27 (59%)	33 (30%)	40 (56%)
Pappilledema	27 (40%)	24 (52%)	54 (49%)	19 (27%)

Clinical Finding	Tsai et al[73] $n = 29$	B&B[79] $n = 76$	Daif et al[68] $n = 40$	de Bruijn et al[80] $n = 59$	Ferro et al[24] $n = 624$
Headache	9 (31%)	61 (80%)	33 (82%)	56 (95%)	553 (88.1%)
Seizures	3 (10%)	22 (29%)	4 (10%)	28 (47%)	245 (39.3)
Focal findings	9 (31%)	34 (48%)	11 (27%)	27 (46%)	Not available
Altered consciousness	27 (93%)	18 (27%)	4 (10%)	32 (54%)	87 (13.9)
Pappilledema	2 (7%)	38 (50%)	32 (80%)	23 (41%)	174 (28.3)

series of Bousser and Barnett,[79] and is the usual presentation in patients with lateral sinus thrombosis caused by otologic infection.[12]

Focal Neurologic Signs and Symptoms

Venous occlusive disease leads to focal parenchymal abnormalities, including edema, hemorrhage, ischemia, and infarction, which cause focal neurological signs and symptoms. A focal neurologic sign, aphasia, was the presenting symptom in patient CD. Edema is probably the most common brain abnormality. Edema may be localized to the region drained by the occluded venous channel or be more generalized. Bilateral symmetric brain edema can produce a picture of small, slit-like ventricles on neuroimaging scans. When draining venous sinuses are occluded, the intravascular pressure in the feeding arteries must increase to a level above venous pressure to achieve an arterial-venous gradient sufficient for brain perfusion. Increased pressure at a capillary level leads to capillary leakage and edema in the interstitial spaces. Edema can also form around infarcts and hemorrhages.

A relatively abrupt increase in intravascular pressure in smaller arteries and arterioles often causes brain hemorrhages. Petechiae, hemorrhagic infarction, and frank hematoma formation are common in patients with cerebral venous and dural sinus occlusions. Hemorrhages may be bilateral when the superior sagittal sinus or bilateral sinuses are occluded. Some hemorrhages are subcortical and multifocal; in other patients, multiple petechiae are present amid regions of ischemia. In the series of Tsai et al, 26 of 29 patients (90%) had some degree of mass effect, nine patients had hemorrhages, and five patients had infarcts.[73] Among 102 patients studied by Villringer et al, 43 patients (42%) had some degree of intracranial hemorrhage.[75] In the series of Bousser et al among 38 patients, three had hemorrhages, seven had infarcts, seven had significant edema, two localized, and five had diffuse brain edema.[13] Infarction is most often precipitated and related to propagation and spread of thrombi to draining superficial and deep draining veins.

Focal neurologic symptoms and signs are present in approximately one-half of patients with dural sinus occlusions. Focal findings were appreciated in 273 of 498 (55%) of patients included in Table 16-2. The signs vary considerably, depending on which dural sinuses are involved and whether the deep venous system is also occluded. Most large series of patients do not divide signs according to the sinus involved. Hemiparesis is probably the most common sign. Hemianopia, ataxia, neglect, and aphasia are particularly common when the posterior dural sinuses are occluded. Aphasia was the first sign in patient CD. The aphasia and agitation were caused by focal dysfunction of the left temporal lobe.

Seizures

A grand mal seizure developed in CD shortly after onset of aphasia. In contrast to thromboembolic arterial disease in which seizures are rare during the acute period, seizures are quite common in patients with venous occlusive disease. Seizures are the presenting symptom in about 7% to 15% of patients, and often occur during the early course of the illness.[80a] Seizures were present in 446 of 1122 patients (40%) with intracranial venous thrombosis at some time during the course of illness (see Table 16-2). Seizures are approximately equally divided between focal and generalized. Often, the onset of focal seizures or generalized seizures with focal onset is followed by the appearance of residual focal neurological signs. Edematous or partially ischemic nerve cells may have more potential for discharge than cells rendered nonfunctional by ischemia. Reversibly injured neurons must be quite common, judging by the high frequency of reversible neurologic signs and reversible brain-imaging abnormalities.[75]

Decreased Level of Consciousness

Although diminished consciousness is not a common presenting symptom, 310 of 1122 (28%) reported patients included in Table 16-2 with cerebral venous occlusive disease had an alteration in their level of alertness at some time during the course of their illness. In one series of patients with intracranial venous thromboses diagnosed by neuroimaging techniques, 27 of 29 patients (93%) had some reduction in mentation or level of alertness.[73] This frequency of altered consciousness is much higher than any series of patients with arterial disease except cases of extensive basilar artery thrombosis and pseudotumoral cerebellar infarcts. In patients with intracranial venous occlusive disease, the alteration in level of consciousness is usually reversible (as contrasted to the other two situations). Brain edema and raised intracranial pressure probably account for the decreased level of consciousness found in patients who have dural sinus occlusive disease. In patients with deep venous occlusions, bilateral involvement of the medial thalami also contributes to the occurrence of drowsiness, stupor, and coma. Extensive dural sinus occlusion with involvement of both internal jugular veins is associated with increased intracranial pressure, reduced consciousness, and poor outcomes despite anticoagulation.[81,82]

DISTRIBUTION OF VENOUS STRUCTURE INVOLVEMENT AND FINDINGS RELATED TO SPECIFIC LOCATIONS

Figures 2-24 and 2-25 show the important intracranial dural sinuses. Figure 2.26 shows the major venous structures as they appear in the venous phase of a normal angiogram. In this chapter, I use the term *lateral sinus* to include the transverse and sigmoid sinuses. Some authors use the terms lateral sinus and transverse sinus interchangeably. I list in Table 16-3 the distribution of involvement of the various venous structures among reported series of patients.[22,24,28,68,71,79] Determination of the sinuses involved should be viewed as approximate estimates because many of the studies are based on incomplete neuroradiologic studies. Cerebral and cortical vein involvement were sometimes not sought specifically and probably were often missed by the brain and vascular imaging performed in these series.

The superior sagittal sinus (SSS) and the lateral sinuses were the most commonly involved venous structure in all of the studies cited. The SSS was involved in 626 of 1171 cases (54%), and the lateral sinuses in 804 of 1171 (69%) (Table 16-3). The frequency of isolated lateral sinus thrombosis was, however, less than that found of isolated SSS thrombosis in series in which this was commented on. It is my impression that lateral sinus thrombosis is becoming more common and likely now is more frequently seen than isolated SSS thrombosis.

Occlusions of the deep venous system are much less common than dural sinus occlusions. Cerebral cortical veins were often involved, but almost never in isolation. Cerebellar cortical veins are rarely involved. The incidence of multiple venous channel involvement was high. Approximately two thirds of patients had thrombosis of more than one venous channel (237 of 368 patients, 64.5%) among the series that tabulated multiple channel involvement.[28,68,71,73,79] Patency of the jugular veins is not commented on in any of the large series tabulated. Yet the bulk of blood drained from the cranium exits through the two jugular veins in the neck. When these are occluded bilaterally, increased intracranial pressure becomes a major problem, and I believe

contributes heavily to morbidity and mortality. In occasional patients, thrombosis begins in a jugular vein, usually caused by nearby septic lesions (Lemmierre's syndrome).[26,40]

The studies cited in Table 16-3 include patients who have had many different etiologies. In puerperal patients, the SSS seems to be involved much more often than in patients with thrombosis unrelated to female hormonal changes. Septic thrombosis involves preferentially the lateral and cavernous sinuses because of the drainage of the ear and paranasal sinus structures into these dural sinuses.

Cavernous Sinus Thrombosis

Thrombosis of the cavernous sinus is usually caused by sepsis and is a serious disease with high mortality. The veins draining the medial portions of the face, orbit, nose, and nasal sinuses lead into the cavernous sinus. The cavernous sinus, in turn, drains via the petrosal sinuses into the lateral sinus and ultimately into the jugular vein.

The most common organism implicated in septic cavernous sinus thromboses is *Staphylococcus aureus*.[22,83] *Pneumococci*, streptococcal species, gram-negative bacteria, and fungi, especially *Aspergillus* species, account for the remainder of cases.[16] The earliest symptoms of septic cavernous sinus thrombosis are headache, facial pain, and fever. The eyelid and eye become red. The eye becomes proptotic. The face may become edematous and red. Orbital and retinal congestion develop, and ophthalmoplegia is found on examination. The oculomotor and trochlear nerves and the ophthalmic and maxillary branches of V course along the lateral wall of the cavernous sinus. The abducens nerve and internal carotid artery with its surrounding sympathetic nerve fibers are located more in the center of the sinus. Any and all of these structures may be involved. Ophthalmoplegia may be complete or partial and is often accompanied by sensory abnormalities in the distribution of V1 and V2.

Head trauma, surgery on facial structures, prothrombotic states, and thrombosis of dural arteriovenous fistulas can cause nonseptic cavernous sinus thrombosis.[16] The onset of symptoms and signs in nonseptic patients may be gradual and indolent. Proptosis and redness of the eye may be only moderate in severity.

Sagittal Sinus Thrombosis

The SSS is a very common location of dural venous sinus thrombosis. The sagittal sinus is the favorite location for occlusion during

Table 16-3. Distribution of Venous Structures Involved in Various Studies

Vein	Cantu and Barinagarrementeria[28] Puerperium n = 67	Cantu and Barinagarrementeria[28] Nonpuerperium n = 46	Ameri and Barinagarrementeria[71] n = 110	Southwick et al[22] Septic n = 179	Tsai et al[73] n = 29	Bousser and Barnett[79] n = 76	Daif et al[68] n = 40	Ferro et al[24] n = 624
Superior sagittal sinus	60 (22)	45 (11)	79 (14)	23 (7)[a]	19 (11)	53	34 (22)	313
Lateral sinus	23 (1)	20 (1)	78 (10)	64 (4)[a]	15 (8)	55	13 (4)	536
Straight sinus	0	0	3 (1)		3	10	3	112
Cavernous sinus	0	0	3	92 (8)[a]	0	2	0	8
Deep venous system	17 (4)	10	9 (1)		1	3	4 (1)	68
Cortical or cerebellar superficial veins	13	14	30 (2)		0	29	0	110
>1 venous structure involved	39	34	85		9	56	14	

Note: Numbers in parentheses represent cases that involved structure alone.

[a] Numbers in parentheses represent personally studied cases. (The remainder derive from from literature review.)

the puerperium. Parasagittal meningiomas, neo-plastic disease of the meninges, head trauma, Behçet's disease, and prothrombotic states are other frequent causes. Symptoms and signs de-pend greatly on the involvement of cerebral veins that drain into the sinus and on involve-ment of the lateral and other dural sinuses.

When thrombosis is limited to the sagittal sinus, the presentation may be that of pseudo-tumor cerebri with isolated increased intracra-nial pressure as the only clinical manifesta-tion.[16] Extension of thrombus into rolandic and parietal veins is common and is often associated with the development of focal motor or sensory signs, or both, and focal or generalized sei-zures.[16] Sometimes, the neurological signs are transient and closely resemble transient isch-emic attacks of arterial origin. The neurological signs are often bilateral, an occurrence that should always bring to mind the possibility of sagittal sinus thrombosis. Edema and hemor-rhages are often found on brain imaging in the medial and dorsal portions of the cerebral hemi-spheres. Reduced consciousness and coma are common when the brain becomes severely edematous and bilateral hemorrhages and hem-orrhagic infarcts are present. Papilledema is common.

Lateral Sinus Thrombosis

The frequency of lateral sinus occlusions equals or now exceeds that of SSS occlusions. One or both lateral sinuses were thrombosed in 69% of 1171 cases included in Table 16-3. Within the posterior circulation, the lateral sinus is by far the most commonly occluded dural sinus. Lateral sinus thrombosis is caused by coagu-lopathies and other systemic conditions; how-ever, a much higher proportion of patients with lateral sinus thrombosis than sagittal sinus oc-clusions have an infectious etiology almost en-tirely caused by spread of infection from acute or chronic ear and mastoid infections. The in-fective process within the otologic structures often leads to a local thrombophlebitis. Infec-tions spread through emissary veins or directly through a thin sinus plate into the lateral sinus. The sigmoid portion of the lateral sinus lies adjacent to the mastoid air cells from its origin to the jugular bulb. Infection can spread from the lateral sinus into the jugular vein.

Lateral sinus thrombosis caused by otologic in-fections and mastoiditis have undoubtedly become less common because of the widespread use of antibiotics. In the past, otitis media was also often complicated by other septic intracranial complica-tions. The clinical findings in patients with lateral sinus thrombosis caused by otitic infections are quite characteristic.[22,84-87] Boys and men are more often affected than girls and women. Nearly all patients have had chronically draining ears and show acute infection or perforations of the ear-drum. Fever, headache, neck pain, and neck ten-derness are important and frequent signs. Pain and tenderness are usually centered along the anterior border of the sternocleidomastoid muscle on one side. The mastoid region is often sensitive and uncomfortable to finger percussion. Pain is usually also felt behind the ear. Headache is common and usually described as severe, persistent, and rather diffuse, located mostly in the frontotemporal and occipital areas of one or both sides.[22] If menin-gitis develops, bilateral neck stiffness and rigidity develop.

Vertigo, nausea, and vomiting are also often present. Diplopia caused by sixth nerve palsy and signs of fifth nerve irritation in the form of temporal and retro-orbital pain are often pres-ent. The combination of fifth and sixth nerve involvement, called the Gradenigo's syndrome, indicates involvement of these nerves at the petrous apex in or near Dorello's canal. De-creased alertness may be present and is ex-plained by the elevated intracranial pressure. Elevated intracranial pressure and papilledema are more common after right-sided lateral sinus thrombosis, perhaps because of the observation that the left lateral sinus is often hypoplastic. In patients with poorly developed left-sided lateral sinuses, right lateral sinus occlusion effectively causes a bilateral drainage problem.

Structures on either side of the tentorium may be involved because both the inferior portions of the temporal lobe and cerebellum drain into the lateral sinuses. Combined tempo-ral lobe and cerebellar involvement on one side suggests lateral sinus thrombosis. Aphasia, agitation, and a right hemianopia or superior quadrantanopia are the most common signs in left temporal lobe involvement. These signs were all present in patient CD, who was found to have left temporal lobe dysfunction related to a left lateral sinus occlusion. Right temporal lobe involvement usually causes an agitated state with a left visual field defect. Nystagmus and gait ataxia are the most common signs of cerebellar involvement. Spread of thrombus into the jugular vein can be accompanied by pulmonary embolism, a serious, but infrequent, complication.[88]

Plain x-rays and CT scans of the mastoid regions usually show abnormalities, including increased density with loss of the mastoid air cell trabeculae, bony sclerosis, or lytic lesions of the temporal and parietal bones.[22] Cholesteatomas are common and have sometimes eroded through the temporal bone.[22,87] Spread of the occlusive process to other adjacent dural sinuses and jugular vein is common.

Deep Venous System Occlusions

Occlusion of the deep venous system, including the internal cerebral veins and vein of Galen, is much less common than dural sinus thrombosis. Among the series included in Table 16-3, the deep venous system was occluded in 112 of 1171 (9.6%) of patients. The straight sinus is also occluded in some patients with deep venous occlusions. The straight sinus and vein of Galen receive venous inflow from both thalami, the basal ganglia, midbrain, geniculate bodies, and the cerebellum. In the past, thrombosis of the deep venous system was thought to be almost exclusively a disorder of babies and young children and uniformly fatal. Since the 1980s, the condition has become recognized in adults, and the course is often much more benign than previously thought.[89-92]

Necropsy studies of patients dying of deep vein thrombosis usually show bilateral thalamic and, often, basal ganglionic hemorrhagic infarcts.[89,90] Figure 16-1 is an MRI that shows bilateral basal ganglia and thalamic lesions in a patient with extensive thrombosis of deep veins. The causes of deep vein thrombosis are similar to dural sinus occlusion. Sepsis; dehydration, especially in babies; sickle cell disease; ulcerative colitis[92]; and oral contraceptives have been reported as etiologic factors. In some patients, the cause is not discovered.

Patients with internal cerebral vein and vein of Galen thrombosis usually have reduced consciousness and often become stuporous or comatose. Headache may precede other symptoms and may be severe. Stiffness of the limbs with decerebrate postures, coma, and vertical gaze palsy are the most common clinical findings in patients with extensive basal ganglionic and thalamic hemorrhagic infarcts and edema.[2,16] Some patients present with apathy and are found on examination to be abulic. Poor memory is a predominant sign. When patients who present with stupor or coma recover, they often show residual signs of lack of initiative and spontaneity (abulia) and may also have poor memory.

Cortical Cerebral and Cerebellar Vein Thrombosis

Isolated thrombosis of cortical veins without associated dural sinus occlusion has long been recognized as an entity, but before MRI, this diagnosis was seldom made except at surgery or necropsy.

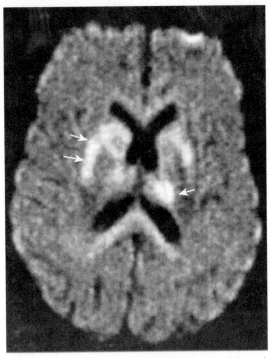

Figure 16-1. Diffusion-weighted MRI showing bilateral basal ganglionic and thalamic abnormalities. The two *small white arrows* point to the lesion in the putamen on the left of the figure and the *small white arrow* on the right of the figure points to the lesion in the right thalamus. (Courtesy of Rafael Linas, MD.)

Modern neuroimaging allows diagnosis and suspicion of this diagnosis.[93-98] Most reported patients have had seizures as a presenting or major symptom. The seizures have most often been focal or have had focal onsets with secondary generalization. Focal neurologic signs, such as hemiparesis and aphasia, are common. Headache is also a common sign. Reduced consciousness and increased intracranial pressure are less common than in patients who have dural sinus occlusions. Brain imaging shows a focal region of brain edema often with hemorrhage located along the pial surface of one cerebral hemisphere. In reported cases, occlusion has often involved the vein of Labbe.[95-98] Figure 16-2 is a digital subtraction angiogram that shows an occluded vein of Labbe.[97]

Cerebellar venous occlusions with cerebellar infarction have only rarely been described.[13,16,99,100] One reported patient had a sudden, severe headache mimicking subarachnoid hemorrhage, and another patient had multiple cranial nerve palsies, cerebellar-type incoordination, and papilledema, a syndrome that mimicked a posterior fossa tumor.[13,16] Another patient has been described who also had a pseudotumoral syndrome.[99] One reported diabetic patient presented with seizures and coma during a severe hyperosmolar state.[100]

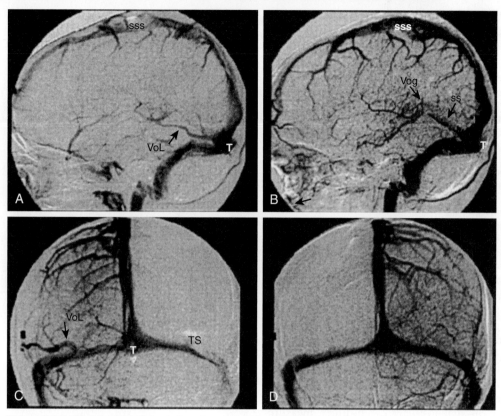

Figure 16-2. Digital subtraction angiogram, venous phase. **A** and **C** are shown after right carotid artery injection while **B** and **D** are shown after left carotid artery injection. The left vein of Labbe is not opacified. SSS, superior sagittal sinus; SS, straight sinus; TS, transverse sinus; VoL, vein of Labbe; VoG, vein of Galen. (From Thomas B, Krishnamurthy T, Purkayastha G: Isolated left vein of Labbe thrombosis. Neurology 2005; 65:1135, with permission.)

He was found to have occlusion of the straight sinus and presumed occlusion of draining cerebellar veins. He also had bilateral large cerebellar hemorrhagic infarcts and hematomas. He died of brainstem compression caused by cerebellar lesions.[100] The clinical findings in patients with arterial and venous cerebellar infarcts are probably quite similar.

DIAGNOSIS

Recognition of the presence of occlusion of the dural sinuses or intracranial venous system depends on a combination of clinical and neuroradiologic findings. The demographics and risk factors for intracranial venous occlusive disease are quite different from those found in patients with arterial occlusions. Patients with venous occlusions are younger, usually female, and have low frequencies of hypertension, coronary artery disease, diabetes, and smoking when compared with patients with arterial occlusive disease. The conditions, risk factors, and circumstances that should alert clinicians to the

possibility of venous occlusive disease are listed in Table 16-4.

Clinical symptoms and signs are also helpful in diagnosis. Headache is usually the earliest clinical symptom and often antedates any neurological symptoms or signs. Seizures and decreased alertness are much more common in sinovenous occlusive disease than in patients with arterial occlusion-related infarcts. Increased intracranial pressure, especially in the absence of severe neurological deficits, is also helpful in suggesting the possibility of venous occlusive disease. Usually, the evolution of the clinical course in patients with venous occlusive disease is slower and more indolent than in patients with arterial occlusions. The absence of cardiac and vascular abnormalities on echocardiography, MRA and computed tomography (CT) angiography, and extracranial and transcranial ultrasound in patients with clinical and imaging-documented brain infarcts should also raise the possibility of venous thrombosis. The clinical findings in patients with dural and cerebral venous occlusions are often indistinguishable from patients with

Table 16-4.   Situations or Findings Suggesting That Cerebral Venous or Dural Sinus Occlusion Be Strongly Considered in Differential Diagnosis of Stroke

Infants and babies with dehydration and sepsis
Puerperal and pregnant women and those taking oral contraceptives
Patients with known cancers, especially adenocarcinomas, leukemias, and lymphomas
Meningitis and other intracranial infections
Acute and chronic otitis media and mastoid infections
Acute sinusitis
Presence of inflammatory diseases, such as Behçet's disease, ulcerative colitis, and Crohn's disease
Nephrotic syndrome
Sepsis
Cachexia, malnutrition, and dehydration, especially in the young and old
Known hematologic disorders, which predispose to hypercoagulability
Severe anemia
Elevated homocysteine level
Presence of past recurrent leg or other systemic venous thrombosis with or without pulmonary embolism
Intracranial tumors such as meningiomas that involve or abut on dural venous sinuses
Presence of dural arteriovenous fistulas
Penetrating cranial traumatic injuries

intracranial infections, such as encephalitis, brain abscess, subdural empyema, and brain tumors, all of which are important differential diagnostic considerations.

Measurement of D-dimer levels also can be helpful in diagnosis.[21,101-104] D-dimer measurements have proven helpful in diagnosis of peripheral venous occlusions. Low levels of D-dimer (<500 ng/mL) have a high negative predictive value. Negative D-dimer studies make the diagnosis of dural and cerebral venous thrombosis less likely.[21] Patients with isolated headache often have normal values. Among 73 patients with symptoms of less than 30 days, 26% of those that presented first with headache had normal D-dimer concentrations.[104] A normal D-dimer level does not exclude the diagnosis.

Imaging and neuroradiologic investigations have dramatically improved the ability of clinicians to confirm the diagnosis of intracranial venous thrombosis. Although plain x-rays of the skull, paranasal sinuses, and mastoid air cells can show important abnormalities, CT allows for better definition of bony abnormalities and sinus disease. CT is probably the most common initial brain imaging test ordered. CT can show abnormalities within the bony structures of the skull, such as evidence of paranasal sinus infection, erosion of the middle ear structures, and changes in the mastoid regions. Infection-related erosion and thinning of the sinus plate are also sometimes evident. CT also effectively shows parenchymatous brain lesions, especially hemorrhages, and may even show abnormalities within the veins and dural sinuses.

In patient CD, the CT scan showed a hemorrhage in the inferior portion of the left temporal lobe, which extended from the pial surface nearly to the sylvian fissure (Figure 16-3A). The hematoma was surrounded by a rim of lucent brain. A focal region of hyperdensity in the left transverse sinus region was also present. A later CT scan (Figure 16-3B) showed that a large hemorrhagic infarct had developed above the hemorrhage that was previously seen. MRI was unsatisfactory because of motion, but confirmed the temporal lobe hemorrhage, edema, and infarction. Angiography showed early filling of the left basal vein of Rosenthal, nonfilling of the left vein of Labbe, and no opacification of the left transverse and sigmoid portions of the left lateral sinus (Figure 16-4). The left jugular vein was not filled.

In patient CD, the vein of Labbe was occluded in addition to thrombosis of the lateral sinus and may have been most responsible for his temporal lobe hemorrhagic infarction. Most patients with lateral sinus thrombosis without cortical vein involvement have only a pseudotumor syndrome.

Evidence for venous and dural sinus occlusion on CT can derive from direct evidence of a sinus or vein abnormality or by parenchymatous abnormalities.[2,16,105-110] The dural sinuses or deep veins can appear as hyperdense, round, or triangular ("dense triangle" sign) structures on noncontrast axial CT scan sections, indicating the presence of a thrombus within a venous channel. This sign is rarely found. The so-called "cord sign," in which a cerebral cortical vein is imaged as a high-density, linear, thin, cylindric structure that contains thrombus, is rare. When present, however, the cord sign is specific for venous

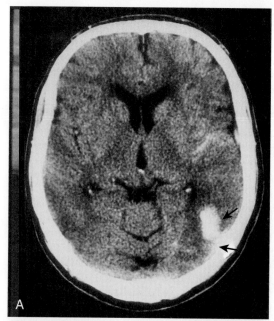

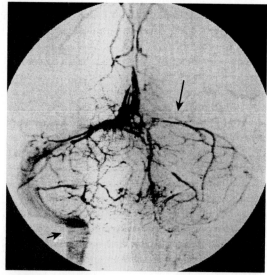

Figure 16-4. Angiogram, venous phase in patient CD. The right lateral sinus is well opacified and drains into the right jugular vein (*black arrow* at bottom left of figure). The left lateral sinus (*arrow*) does not fill, and there is no opacification of the left jugular vein. The left vein of Labbe also did not fill. (From Caplan LR: Posterior Circulation Disease: Clinical Findings, Diagnosis, and Management. Boston: Blackwell Science, with permission.)

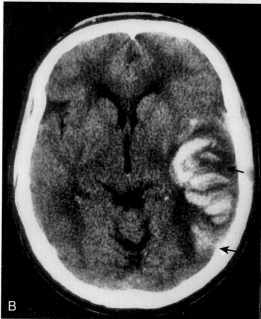

Figure 16-3. CT scans of patient CD. **A,** Left temporal-lobe hemorrhage (*upper black arrow*). Near the surface, the thrombosed lateral sinus images as a hyperdensity (*lower black arrow*). **B,** CT scan taken days later shows that a large hemorrhagic zone of infarction (*upper black arrow*) has developed above the area of hemorrhage that is still seen below (*lower black arrow*).

occlusive disease. These direct evidences of venous occlusion are not common on plain CT scans. Parenchymatous changes include regions of hypodensity, representing infarction and edema; hemorrhages; and brain edema with small, compressed ventricles. Often, the distribution of the parenchymal abnormalities, including

diffuse edema, bilaterality of infarcts and hemorrhages, predominance of hemorrhagic changes, and the presence of a lesion, which does not conform to a typical arterial distribution, suggests venous occlusive disease.

More information is usually obtained from contrast-enhanced CT scans than from plain scans.[107] Perhaps most important is the so-called "empty delta sign," a finding that has only been described in patients with sagittal sinus thrombosis.[2,16,105-110] Contrast enhances the smaller collateral veins and walls of the sinus, but the middle region representing the thrombosed lumen does not enhance. In other patients after contrast, a filling defect is present within opacified sinuses. Cortical and medullary veins may appear dilatated on contrast-enhanced scans because of dilatation of collateral draining channels.[107] Contrast enhancement in a gyral pattern may also occur as it does in arterial disease-related infarcts. The tentorium or other dural structures may enhance in the region of a thrombosed dural sinus.

Evidence of brain infarction and edema are more often found on CT scans than direct evidence of venous occlusion. In some patients, focal regions of subarachnoid bleeding are found in the vicinity of the venous occlusion. In patients with cerebellar venous infarction, hydrocephalus and compression of the fourth ventricle may be found. CT venography is a reliable means of opacifying the normal venous structures and often can show evidence of venous occlusive disease.[105,111]

CT scans are helpful in the diagnosis of occlusion of the deep venous system. The characteristic finding is bilateral hypodensity, involving the thalami and basal ganglia. Hyperdensities in these same regions representing hemorrhages or hemorrhagic infarction also suggest the diagnosis of deep vein occlusions.[90,91] Severe edema with compression of the third ventricle may occur. The occluded sinuses and deep veins may appear as hyperdense structures on unenhanced CT scans. After contrast, nonopacification of the vein of Galen, straight sinus, and retention of contrast for a prolonged period in the usual draining veins, such as the thalamostriate veins and basal vein of Rosenthal, suggest occlusion of the deep venous system.

Magnetic resonance scans are more likely than CT to provide definitive evidence of intracranial sinus or venous thrombosis.[2,16,21,105,106,112-118] MRI shows a variety of parenchymatous changes, including early infarction, hemorrhage, hemorrhagic infarction, focal edema, and diffuse edema. Gyral enhancement may be shown after gadolinium enhancement. In some patients, mass effect is found without any abnormalities of signal within the edematous regions.[116] Susceptibility-weighted (T2*) images may show small areas of hemorrhage containing hemosiderin in late stages of evolution.

Direct evidence of abnormal flow in the dural venous sinuses is more often found on MRI scans than on CT. The findings, however, depend heavily on the MRI sequences used and the stage of the thrombosis. Dormont and colleagues studied 53 patients with cerebral venous thromboses imaged at various clinical stages.[115] During the first week after thrombosis, the occluded sinuses appear as iso-signals on T1-weighted scans and a low-intensity signal on T2-weighted images. Flow-sensitive gradient echo images at this time show an iso-signal within the sinus instead of the normal high signal appearance, indicating a lack of flow in the sinus. In patients with cortical vein thrombosis, the lumens of the thrombosed veins may appear hyperintense on T1-weighted images.[94] During the next few weeks when most images are obtained, the dural sinus thrombi appear as high-signal intensity structures on all images. During the chronic stages longer than a month after onset, the sinuses most often appear as iso-signals on T1-weighted and flow-sensitive images and have an increased signal on T2-weighted images.[112,113,117] Isensee et al studied 23 patients with dural sinus thrombosis using multiplanar spin-echo and flow-sensitive

sequences.[113] They described similar signal intensities on various magnetic resonance sequences, but also noted that during the first 5 days after thrombosis, the thrombus signal was always homogeneous and the sinus itself appeared expanded by the thrombus.[113] During days 6 through 15, the signal from the thrombus was always hyperintense, irrespective of the magnetic resonance sequence used. Figure 16-5 is an MRI that shows increased signal in the sagittal sinus on a T2-weighted scan. Sometimes, a *target sign*, consisting of a central isointensity surrounded by peripheral circumferential hyperintensity, is seen.

The absence of cardiac and vascular abnormalities on echocardiography, MRA and computed tomography angiography, and extracranial and transcranial ultrasound in patients with clinical and imaging-documented brain infarcts should also raise the possibility of venous thrombosis. Later, depending on recanalization, the thrombus signal is decreased on all sequences. The signal becomes inhomogeneous in the late stages. When the sinus completely recanalizes, the signals become normal. Mas and colleagues showed that some patients with dural sinus thrombosis continued to have hyperintensity on T2-weighted images when studied 6 months after symptom onset.[114] The signal changes within the dural sinuses depend on the presence or absence of flow; presence of deoxyhemoglobin, which produces hypointensity on T2-weighted images; and extracellular methemoglobin. The signal changes related to chemical transformation of hemoglobin

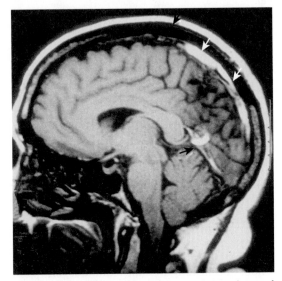

Figure 16-5. MRI of patient with multiple thromboses of dural sinuses. The superior sagittal sinus thrombosis is shown as a hyperintense signal *(two small white arrows)*. The straight sinus is also occluded and shows a hyperintense signal *(lower black arrow)*. The non-thrombosed portion of the sagittal sinus appears dark *(upper black arrow)*.

within the thrombus proceed from the periphery to the center of the thrombus, explaining the occurrence of a target sign.[113]

Decreased blood flow in veins and dural sinuses promotes a local shift in the hemoglobin oxygenation curve toward the formation of deoxyhemoglobin. Deoxyhemoglobin produces a "magnetic susceptibility effect" that images as signal loss (darkening), which is best seen on Echo-planar T2*-weighted (susceptibility) images. The T2* MRI sequence can detect the presence of intravenous clot during the acute and subacute phase of venous occlusive disease, shown as an area of hypointensity within the affected sinus.[119,120] The T2* sequence also allows direct visualization of associated venous infarcts that are often hemorrhagic, and small petechial hemorrhages.

The lateral sinuses are often of unequal size; the larger sinus is the one with a more direct connection to the SSS. The right lateral sinus usually drains the SSS. The straight sinus usually drains into the left lateral sinus. The left lateral sinus is sometimes hypoplastic and in one study did not opacify in 14% of normal angiograms.[114] Mas et al used MRI to study patients in whom angiography had shown nonvisualization or poor visualization of one or both lateral sinuses at angiography to determine if magnetic resonance studies could distinguish between hypoplastic and thrombosed lateral sinuses.[114] Hypoplastic sinuses were smaller, asymmetric structures on parasagittal MRI images without abnormal signal intensities along the course of the sinus. In contrast, occluded sinuses had increased intraluminal signals on all pulse sequences.[114]

In the chronic phase of dural sinus thrombosis, enhancement of chronic thromboses often occurs after the injection of gadolinium dimeglumine.[115,116] This enhancement is explained by organization of the thrombus, which is changed to vascularized connective tissue. On three-dimensional time-of-flight MRA images taken after enhancement, the thrombosed sinuses may be indistinguishable from normal sinuses because of this organized thrombus enhancement and may give a false-negative result on MRA. Hyperemia of dural structures that lie adjacent to thrombosed sinuses may appear on gadolinium-enhanced images as thickened and enhanced meninges, including the tentorium.[110]

MRA techniques, especially magnetic resonance venography, are particularly useful in defining dural sinus and cerebral and cerebellar venous occlusions by abnormalities in the normal flow signals, nonopacification of sinuses, and by showing collateral venous channels. Figure 16-6 illustrates the absence of the deep venous structures on magnetic resonance venography, confirming the diagnosis of deep vein occlusion. MRV has now become the imaging modality most widely used to establish the diagnosis of cerebral venous occlusive disease. MRV can be performed with time-of-flight or phase-contrast techniques.[117,121,122] Time-of-flight relies mainly on flow-related enhancement to produce images of the blood vessels, whereas phase contrast techniques use velocity-induced phase shifts to separate moving blood flow from surrounding stationary tissue. Time-of-flight technique has shorter acquisition times and covers more regions. Absence of flow signal within a sinus and its nonopacification suggest intraluminal thrombosis. The occluding thrombus

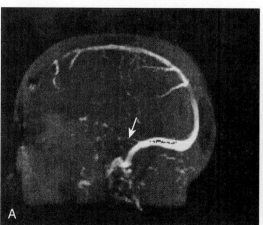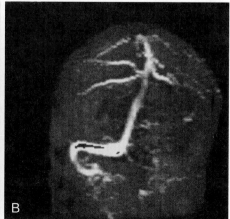

Figure 16-6. Magnetic resonance venogram (MRV) in patient whose MRI is shown in Figure 16-1. **A,** Sagittal view. The vein of Galen and the straight sinus are not seen. The *small white arrow* points to their usual location. **B,** Axial view. The deep veins, straight sinus, and lateral sinus on the right of the figure are not seen. (Courtesy of Rafael Linas, MD.)

often appears hyperintense. However, flow gaps in the nondominant (hypoplastic) transverse sinuses are seen in up to 30% of normal individuals when using time-of-flight MRV, leading to an erroneous diagnosis of sinus thrombosis.[105,121] These artifactual flow gaps are attributed to slow intra-sinus blood flow, in-plane flow, or complex blood flow patterns which can result in intra-sinus signal loss mimicking occlusion. Saturation of blood flow when images are parallel to a sinus, especially the anterior portion of the superior sagittal sinus, can result in loss of signal intensity and false diagnosis of sinus occlusion.[98,117,121]

With the advent of CT angiography and venography and newer magnetic resonance techniques, that allow dural sinus and venous imaging, catheter angiography, once considered the "gold standard," is used much less often than in the past. Conventional catheterization angiography, when necessary, can be performed using conventional filming or by digitalized intra-arterial filming techniques. Anteroposterior and lateral films are required with opacification of the entire venous system. Sometimes, oblique films are also useful, but are most helpful in patients with suspected sagittal sinus thrombosis. The partial or complete lack of opacification of venous channels is the primary angiographic evidence of venous occlusion. In patient CD, nonfilling of the left lateral sinus confirmed the clinical diagnosis (see Figure 16-6). Delayed emptying and dilatation of collateral venous channels are other signs that are often present.[13,110,123] Because of wide variability in the development of the lateral sinuses, the entire lateral sinus, especially the sigmoid portion, should fail to opacify to be certain of occlusion. Neck films help to show whether the jugular bulb and vein are thrombosed. Delayed venous filling and emptying are common and are found in one half of the patients with dural sinus occlusions.[13] Dilated and tortuous cortical veins are more often seen at angiography than transcerebral collaterals.

Images of the dural sinuses can also be obtained by introducing catheters into the venous system and injecting contrast. Retrograde jugular catheterization with installation of contrast and dural sinus venography are usually done only when the angiographer intends to instill local fibrinolytic agents into the thrombosed venous sinuses.

Transcranial Doppler (TCD) ultrasonography has been used to diagnose and follow patients with dural sinus thrombosis.[124-127] In normal individuals and in patients, venous signals can be detected and displayed from the region of the basal vein of Galen, which lies adjacent to the P2 portion of the posterior cerebral artery, and from the straight sinus and superior and inferior

portions of the sagittal sinus. In patients with dural sinus occlusions, the veins of Labbe and Rosenthal often serve as collateral channels. Increased blood flow in these veins increases the blood-flow velocities measured by TCD. Intravenous instillation of echo-contrast material helps to image the sinuses, using transcranial color-coded real-time sonography.[124,127] The mean blood-flow velocities in the region of the basal vein of Rosenthal are elevated acutely and later return to normal after treatment and presumed recanalization of the original dural sinus occlusion.[125,126] TCD may be most useful in monitoring changes in venous flow and showing the effect of treatment. Data about the use of TCD is preliminary. Too few patients have been studied to know the effect of the location of the dural sinus occlusion on the frequency and reliability of the TCD results.

TREATMENT

Antibiotics and surgical drainage of paranasal sinus infections and middle ear and mastoid infections remain the most important treatments in patients with septic dural sinus thrombosis. Anticonvulsants for seizure control are important in patients who have seizures. Raised intracranial pressure can be managed with osmotic diuretics, such as mannitol, glycerol, acetazolamide, and lumbar punctures.[21,128,129] In patients with pseudotumor syndromes, the intracranial pressure can usually be managed using lumbar punctures and acetazolamide. Temporary ventricular drains and shunts are seldom necessary. Among 110 patients in the series of Ameri and Bousser, only two required shunting procedures.[71] Mannitol and steroids might be useful in patients who have severe brain edema with small, slit-like ventricles as long as sepsis, when present, is appropriately treated with antibiotics. However in one large series, among 624 patients with cerebral sinovenous occlusions, 150 (24%) were treated with corticosteroids; steroids had no beneficial effect on the frequency of poor outcomes.[129a] Patients who had no parenchymal lesions seemed to have worse outcomes when treated with steroids.[129a]

> CD was treated with anticonvulsants. Heparin was begun on the 6th hospital day despite the large temporal lobe hematoma. Lupus anticoagulant studies were positive. The platelet count was slightly reduced and the prothrombin time was slightly accelerated. A new phlebothrombosis in the leg was identified and an inferior vena cava filter was placed. CD gradually improved, but remained aphasic.

The use of anticoagulants was once controversial in patients with dural sinus thrombosis, especially in patients with hemorrhagic infarcts and frank hematomas. However now the great majority of clinicians use anticoagulants acutely in patients with dural sinus and venous occlusions unless there are strong contraindications. Convinced by the available data, the European Federation of Neurological Societies guidelines, published in 2005, stated that when there are "no contraindications for anticoagulants—body-weighted subcutaneous low-molecular-weight heparin in full therapeutic dosage or APPT (two times above normal values) dose-adjusted intravenous heparin—be given."[21,129]

Anticoagulants were first used to treat patients with puerperal intracranial venous thrombosis by Stansfield[130] and by Martin and Sheenan[131] in the early 1940s. In their monograph on cerebral venous thrombosis published in 1967, Kalbag and Woolf favored early anticoagulation before thrombosis spread to cortical veins.[1] In the same year, Krayenbuhl noted that patients treated with anticoagulants and antibiotics had a 7% mortality compared with 37% mortality in those treated only with antibiotics and compared with 70% mortality in those not given antibiotics or anticoagulants.[132] Krayenbuhl wrote that he never had a patient who developed intracranial hemorrhage during well-controlled anticoagulant treatment of intracranial venous thrombosis.[132] Despite the opinions of these authorities, most clinicians considered anticoagulants to be too dangerous because of the risk of further brain hemorrhage. The known tendency for intracranial venous thrombosis to be associated with hemorrhage persuaded many that anticoagulants were risky.

An important reason to use anticoagulants was to prevent pulmonary embolism from the venous clots, which often extended into the jugular vein. Like any other peripheral venous occlusion, venous clots can extend to the heart. Diaz and colleagues reported a patient with SSS thrombosis who died of a fatal pulmonary embolus.[133] They reviewed the available literature on patients with dural sinus occlusion studied between 1942 and 1990 and found that in 23 of 203 patients (11%), dural sinus thrombosis was complicated by pulmonary embolism. All but 1 of these 23 patients died.[133]

More recently, Cakmak et al reported pulmonary embolism in a 22-year-old man with lateral sinus thrombosis.[88] Case reports and retrospective reviews showed that patients did not seem to worsen or have new hemorrhagic changes after institution of heparin or other anticoagulants.[134,135] Ameri and Bousser noted that among 82 patients treated with heparin, no deaths occurred, and 77% of patients had a complete recovery.[71] Austrian clinicians published the results of 42 patients with dural sinus thrombosis treated with heparin followed by oral anticoagulants.[136] Partial or complete recanalization of the thrombosed sinus was achieved in 36 of 40 (90%) patients; 40 patients improved clinically, among whom 26 recovered completely. Only one patient had a hemorrhagic transformation, but this patient did not worsen clinically.[136] Table 16-5 reviews retrospective, nonrandomized results accumulated in 1990 from other case reports and series of patients with intracranial venous thromboses treated or not treated with anticoagulants.[135] In these series, among 79 patients given anticoagulants, 94% improved and survived, whereas only approximately one half of the 157 patients not given anticoagulants survived.[135] In a retrospective review published in

---

Table 16-5.   Retrospective Nonrandomized Studies of Anticoagulation Effects in Patients with Intracranial Venous Thrombosis

	Anticoagulated		Not Anticoagulated	
	Survived/Improved	*Died*	*Survived/Improved*	*Died*
Krayenbuhl (1954)[123]	16	1	32	24
Bousser et al (1985)[13]	23	0	11	4
*Case reports 1942-1987	25	3 bled	25	44
*Walker (unpublished)	6	0	7	1
Jacewicz and Plum (1990)[135]	4	1 (veg)	4	5
Totals	74 (94%)	5 (6%)	79 (50%)	78 (50%)

* Data from Jacewicz M, Plum F: Aseptic cerebral venous thrombosis. In Einhaupl K, Kempski O, Baethmann A (eds): Cerebral Sinus Thrombosis: Experimental and Clinical Aspects. New York: Plenum, 1990, pp 157-170.

2004 of outcomes in the International Study on Cerebral Vein and Dural Sinus Thrombosis, 66 of the 520 patients anticoagulated acutely were dead or dependent at follow-up (12.7%), while 19 of the 104 patients who were not anticoagulated became dependent or died (18.3%).[24] Although these studies cannot prove effectiveness, they show that anticoagulants are probably seldom harmful.

Although anecdotal data on the effectiveness of anticoagulants are persuasive, there are scant definitive data from randomized trials. A small, randomized, double-blind, prospective trial of heparin use in patients with intracranial venous thrombosis was reported by Einhaupl and colleagues.[137] During 1982-1984, they studied 28 patients with angiographically proven dural sinus thrombosis. Ten of the 20 patients were heparinized while the other 10 were given placebo. At the start of treatment, three patients in the heparin-treated group and two patients in the placebo group had hemorrhages on CT scans.[137] The investigators planned to admit 60 patients with an interim analysis after the first 20 patients. The interim analysis was considered so positive for anticoagulation that the study was terminated after the first 20 patients were entered. One patient in the placebo group died after pulmonary embolism. No patient in the heparin-treated group had a new brain hematoma. In the placebo group, three patients with new brain hemorrhages were present, two of whom did not have a hemorrhage at onset. In the three patients with brain hemorrhages present before heparin treatment, two had a complete recovery.[137]

Einhaupl et al also retrospectively analyzed their data from 102 patients with angiographically proven intracranial dural sinus and venous occlusions studied between 1977 and 1991.[137,138] Among the 102 patients, 43 had an ICH. Two patients had their first ICH after heparin treatment. One patient who had an ICH before treatment had another while receiving heparin. Altogether, six patients had ICH after heparin. Thirty-three patients not treated with heparin had new hemorrhages. They also analyzed data from 40 patients who had known ICH before heparin treatment (27 patients) and before no heparin treatment (13 patients). The patients not treated with heparin fared worse and had a higher mortality.[137,138]

Another randomized trial studied the use of low-molecular-weight heparin in patients with dural sinus thrombosis.[139] No statistically significant difference existed in outcome between the 30 patients treated with low-molecular-weight heparin and the 30 patients given placebo. No patient had a new symptomatic hemorrhage. One patient treated with low-molecular-weight heparin had a major gastrointestinal hemorrhage, and one patient in the placebo-treated group died of pulmonary embolism.[138]

I find the data quite convincing that heparin and low-molecular-weight heparin are not associated with clinical worsening and do not predispose to ICH. Heparin should be given to patients with intracranial dural and venous thrombosis, "whatever the clinical or neuroimaging pattern,"[140] unless a strong contraindication is present. Heparin is customarily administered during acute hospitalization and is followed by coumadin, which is usually given for a period of months. Longer-term coumadin is used in patients with important prothrombotic conditions.

Thrombolytic agents have also been used to treat patients with dural sinus thrombosis. The results, however, are still quite preliminary.[73,141-149] Canhao et al performed a systematic review of published cases.[149] Among 169 patients treated with thrombolytics: Urokinase was the commonest agent used; in 88% the thrombolytic was infused locally directly into a sinus; dosages of urokinase and tPA were far higher than those used systemically or intra-arterially to treat arterially related brain ischemia; and duration of treatment was much longer range, at 1 to 244 hours (mean 41 to 49 hours).[149] Dural sinus venography was performed before infusion of thrombolytic agents. Infusion of the thrombolytic drug was then given locally through catheters introduced into the regions of the occluded sinuses. When follow-up imaging was performed and reported, the treated sinuses were usually recanalized. Heparin was usually given with and after thrombolytic treatment. These studies were all uncontrolled. They show that dural sinus venography is feasible. Thrombi can be lysed, but the dose of thrombolytic drugs used and the infusion times are much higher than those used to treat patients with arterial thromboses.

Studies of patients with dural sinus thrombosis who die despite acute anticoagulation treatment reveals that a very common cause of failure is occlusion of multiple sinuses and cerebral veins.[81,82] In a retrospective analysis of 79 patients treated with intravenous heparin, all 8 patients who died had stupor and coma and all had a severe restriction of venous outflow shown angiographically.[81,82] In these patients, increased intracranial pressure and poor brain perfusion proved fatal. Opening of occluded jugular veins and dural sinuses mechanically or chemically makes sense in patients with very restricted venous outflow, often characterized by bilateral jugular vein occlusions.

Direct surgery on the dural sinuses has been occasionally performed.[150] In the late 1960s and early 1970s, Yasargil[151] and Donaghy,[152] pioneers in the field of microneurosurgery for intracranial vascular disease, performed a number of reparative surgeries on the dural sinuses mostly for repair of traumatic injuries. Since then, a handful of surgeons have performed various procedures, including venous bypass and disobliteration of an occluded sinus in patients with dural sinus thrombosis. Surgery has most often been performed in patients with dural arteriovenous fistulas and sinus thrombosis.[153,154] Jugular vein ligation was at one time a popular surgical procedure in patients with lateral sinus thrombosis due to ear and mastoid infections. Tying of the jugular vein was thought to effectively isolate the septic source in the lateral sinus from the general circulation and prevent pulmonary embolism. This procedure was often followed by septic complications and could promote retrograde thrombosis and interrupt drainage of venous blood from the head. Internal jugular vein ligation is seldom performed today. Most neurologists and neurosurgeons agree that the treatment of dural sinus thrombosis is medical except for patients with dural sinus thrombosis related to dural fistulas. Occasionally, patients with pseudotumoral cerebellar infarcts may need decompressive surgery. Hydrocephalus may require a ventricular shunt procedure in some patients.

OUTCOME

Unlike the situation in patients with brain infarction caused by arterial disease, patients with venous occlusive disease usually have complete recovery or become dependent or die. In the large International Study on Cerebral Vein and Dural Sinus Thrombosis, among 624 patients, at last follow-up (median follow-up length 16 months), 493 (79%) had a complete recovery while 84 (13.4%) were dead or dependent.[24]

Outcome depends on the following factors:

- Extent of thrombosis within the dural venous sinuses
- Occlusion of the jugular veins
- Spread to cortical and deep veins
- Nature of the underlying causative disease
- Presence and extent of parenchymal infarcts and hemorrhages
- State of consciousness at presentation and during the early course
- Use of anticoagulants and thrombolytic agents
- Treatment of raised intracranial pressure

References

1. Kalbag RM, Woolf AL: Cerebral Venous Thrombosis. London: Oxford University Press, 1967.
2. Caplan LR: Posterior Circulation Disease: Clinical Findings, Diagnosis, and Management. Boston: Blackwell Science 1996.
3. Ribes MF: Des recherches faites sur la phlebite. Revue Medicale Francaise et etrangere et Jornal de clinique de l'Hotal-Dieu et de la Charite de Paris 1825;3:5-41.
4. Abercrombie J: Pathological and practical researches on diseases of the brain and spinal cord. Edinburgh: Waugh and Innes, 1828;83-85.
5. Tonnelle M-L: Memoire sur les maladies des sinus veineux de la dure-mere. J Hebd Med 1829;5: 337-403.
6. Cruveilhier J: Anatomie pathologique du corps humain: Descriptions avec figures lithographiées et caloriées des diverses alterations morbides dont le corps humain est susceptible. Paris: J.B. Bailliere, 1835-1842.
7. Quinke H: Ueber meningitis serosa. Inn Med Nr 1891;23:655-694.
8. Quinke H: Ueber meningitis serosa und verwandte Zustande. Dtsch Z Nervenheilk 1896;9:149-168.
9. Symonds CP: Otitic hydrocephalus. Brain 1931; 54:55-71.
10. Symonds CP: Hydrocephalus and focal cerebral symptoms in relation to thrombophlebitis of dural sinuses and cerebral veins. Brain 1937;60:531-550.
11. Symonds CP: Cerebral thrombophlebitis. BMJ 1940;2:348-352.
12. Symonds CP: Otitic hydrocephalus. Neurology 1956;6:681-685.
13. Bousser M-G, Chiras J, Bories J, Castaigne P: Cerebral venous thrombosis—A review of 38 cases. Stroke 1985;16:199-213.
14. Einhaupl KM, Kempski O, Baethman A: Cerebral Sinus Thrombosis: Experimental and Clinical Aspects. New York: Plenum, 1990.
15. Einhaupl KM, Masuhr F: Cerebral venous and sinus thrombosis. An update. Eur J Neurol 1994;1:109-126.
16. Bousser M-G, Ross Russell R: Cerebral Venous Thrombosis. London: Saunders, 1997.
17. Biousse V, Bousser MG: Cerebral venous thrombosis. Neurologist 1999;5:326-349.
18. Stam J: Thrombosis of cerebral veins and sinuses. N Engl J Med 2005;352:1791-1798.
19. Ehtisham A, Stern BJ: Cerebral venous thrombosis: A review. Neurologist 2006;12:32-38.
20. Mehdiratta M, Kumar S, Selim M, Caplan LR: Cerebral venous sinus thrombosis: Clinical features, diagnosis and treatment. In Caplan LR (ed): Uncommon Causes of Stroke, 2nd ed. Cambridge: Cambridge University Press, 2008, pp ..
21. Bousser M-G, Ferro JM: Cerebral venous thrombosis: An update. Lancet Neurol 2007;6: 162-170.
22. Southwick FS, Richardson EP, Swartz MN: Septic thrombosis of the dural venous sinuses. Medicine (Baltimore) 1986;65:82-106.
23. Tveteras K, Kristensen S, Dommerby H: Septic cavernous and lateral sinus thrombosis. J Laryngol Otol 1988;102:877-882.
24. Ferro JM, Canhao P, Stam J, et al: Prognosis of cerebral vein and dural sinus thrombosis. Stroke 2004;35:664-670.

25. Chirinos JA, Lichstein DM, Garcia J, Tamariz IJ: The evolution of Lemierre syndrome: Report of 2 cases and review of the literature. Medicine 2002;81:458-465.

26. Bliss SJ, Flanders SA, Saint S: A pain in the neck. N Engl J Med 2004;350:1037-1042.

27. Donaldson JO: Neurology of pregnancy. Philadelphia: Saunders, 1978.

28. Cantu C, Barinagarrementeria F: Cerebral venous thrombosis associated with pregnancy and puerperium. Review of 67 cases. Stroke 1993;24: 1880-1884.

29. Estanol B, Rodriguez A, Conte G, et al: Intracranial venous thrombosis in young women. Stroke 1979;10:680-684.

30. Srinivasan K: Cerebral venous and arterial thrombosis in pregnancy and puerperium, a study of 135 patients. Angiology 1983;34:733-746.

31. Chopra JS, Banerjee AK: Primary intracranial sinovenous occlusions in youth and pregnancy. In Vinken PJ, Bruyn GW, Klawans HL (eds): Handbook of Clinical Neurology, vol 10. Amsterdam: Elsevier, 1989, pp 425-452.

32. Srinivasan K: Puerperial cerebral venous and arterial thrombosis. Semin Neurol 1988;8:222-225.

33. Lanska DJ, Kryscio R: Stroke and intracranial venous thrombosis during pregnancy and puerperium. Neurology 1998;51:1622-1628.

34. Jaillard AS, Hommel M, Mallaret M: Venous sinus thrombosis associated with androgens in a healthy young man. Stroke 1994;25:212-213.

35. Shiozawa Z, Yamada H, Mabuchi C, et al: Superior sagittal sinus thrombosis associated with androgen therapy for hypoplastic anemia. Ann Neurol 1982; 12:578-580.

36. Hickey WF, Carnick MB, Henderson IC, Dawson DM: Primary cerebral venous thrombosis in patients with cancer—A rarely diagnosed paraneoplastic syndrome. Report of three cases and review of the literature. Am J Med 1982;73:740-750.

37. Sproul EE: Carcinoma and venous thrombosis: The frequency of association of carcinoma in the body or tail of the pancreas with multiple venous thrombosis. Am J Cancer 1938;34: 566-585.

38. Miller SP, Sanchez-Avalos J, Stefanski T, Zuckerman L: Coagulation disorders in cancer: I. Clinical and laboratory studies. Cancer 1967;20:1452-1465.

39. Amico L, Caplan LR, Thomas C: Cerebrovascular complications of mucinous cancers. Neurology 1989;39:523-526.

40. Poe LB, Manzione JV, Wasenko JJ, Kellman RM: Acute internal jugular vein thrombosis associated with pseudoabscess of the retropharyngeal space. AJNR Am J Neuroradiol 1995;16:892-896.

41. Mitchell D, Fisher J, Irving D, et al: Lateral sinus thrombosis and intracranial hypertension in essential thrombocythaemia. J Neurol Neurosurg Psychiatry 1986;49:218-219.

42. Haan J, Caebeke JFV, van der Meer FJM, Wintzen AR: Cerebral venous thrombosis as a presenting sign of myeloproliferative disorders. J Neurol Neurosurg Psychiatry 1988;51:1219-1220.

43. Pouillot B, Pecker J, Guegan Y, et al: Benign intracranial hypertension in polycythemia which had caused a lateral sinus thrombosis. Neurochirurgie 1984;30:131-134.

44. Lauvin R, Lore P, Pinel JF, et al: Intracranial hypertension caused by lateral sinus thrombosis in Vaquez's disease. Rev Med Interne 1985;6: 158-161.

45. Johnson RV, Kaplan SR, Blailock Z: Cerebral venous thrombosis in paroxysmal nocturnal hemoglobinuria. Neurology 1970;20:681-686.

46. Mokri B, Jack Jr CR, Petty GW: Pseudotumor syndrome associated with venous sinus occlusion and antiphospholipid antibodies. Stroke 1993;24: 469-472.

47. Agah R, Rice L, Winikates J: Fatal cerebral venous thrombosis as the initial manifestation of the antiphospholipid syndrome. J Neurol Neurosurg Psychiatry 1996;98:189-191.

48. Vidailhet M, Piette J-C, Wechsler B, et al: Cerebral venous thrombosis in systemic lupus erythematosis. Stroke 1990;21:1226-1231.

49. Levine SR, Kieran S, Puzio K, et al: Cerebral venous thrombosis with lupus anticoagulants: Report of two cases. Stroke 1987;18:801-804.

50. Schutta HS, Williams EC, Baranski BG, Sutula TP: Cerebral venous thrombosis with plasminogen deficiency. Stroke 1991;22:401-405.

51. Kim MJ, Cho A-H, No Y-J, et al: Recurrent cerebral venous thrombosis associated with elevated factor VIII. J Clin Neurol 2006;2:286-289.

52. Zuber M, Toulon P, Marnet L, et al: Leiden mutation in cerebral venous thrombosis. Stroke 1996;27:1721-1723.

53. Dulli D, Luzzio CC, Williams EC, Schutta HS: Cerebral venous thrombosis and activated protein C resistance. Stroke 1996;27:1731-1733.

54. Brey RL, Coull BM: Cerebral venous thrombosis. Role of activated protein C resistance and factor V gene mutation. Stroke 1996;27:1719-1720.

55. Deschiens M-A, Conard J, Horellou MH, et al: Coagulation studies, factor V Leiden, and anticardiolipin antibodies in 40 cases of cerebral venous thrombosis. Stroke 1996;27:1724-1730.

55a. Wysokinska EM, Wysokinska WE, Brown RD, et al: Thrombophilia differences in cerebral venous sinus and lower extremity deep venous thrombosis. Neurology 2008;70:627-633.

55b. Voetsch B, Jin RC, Bierl C, et al: Role of promotor polymorphisms in the plasma glutathione peroxidase (GPx-3) gene as a risk factor for cerebral venous thrombosis. Stroke 2008;39: 303-307.

55c. Reuenr KH, Jenetzky E, Aleu A, et al: Factor XII C46T gene polymorphism and the risk of cerebral venous thrombosis. Neurology 2008;70:129-132.

56. Barthelemy M, Bousser M-G, Jacobs C: Thrombose veineuse cerebrale au cours d'un syndrome nephrotique. Nouv Presse Med 1980;9:367-369.

57. Lau SU, Bock GH, Edson JR, Michael AF: Sagittal sinus thrombosis in the nephrotic syndrome. J Pediatr 1980;97:948-950.

58. Harrison MJG, Truelove SC: Cerebral venous thrombosis as a complication of ulcerative colitis. Am J Digest Dis 1967;12:1025-1028.

59. Das R, Vasishta RK, Banerjee AK: Aseptic cerebral venous thrombosis associated with idiopathic ulcerative colitis: A report of two cases. Clin Neurol Neurosurg 1996;98:179-182.

60. Silburn PA, Sandstrom PA, Staples C, et al: Deep cerebral venous thrombosis presenting as an encephalitic illness. Postgrad Med J 1996;72:355-357.

61. De Georgia MA, Rose DZ: Stroke in patients who have inflammatory bowel disease. In Uncommon Causes of Stroke, 2nd ed, Caplan LR (ed): Cambridge: Cambridge University Press, 2008.

62. Sigsbee B, Rotenberg DA: Sagittal sinus thrombosis as a complication of regional enteritis. Ann Neurol 1978;3:450-452.

63. Motte S, Flamme F, Depianeux M, Wantrecht JC, et al: Venous thromboangiitis associated with regional enteritis. Intern Angiol 1992;11:237-240.

64. Pamir MN, Kansu T, Erbengi A, Zileli T: Papilledema in Behçet's syndrome. Arch Neurol 1981;38:643-645.

65. Bousser M-G, Bletry O, Launay M, et al: Thrombose veineuse cerebrale au cours de la maladie de Behcet. A propos deux cas. Rev Neurol 1980;136:753-762.

66. Rougemont D, Bousser M-G, Wechsler B, et al: Manifestations neurologiques de la maladie de Behcet: 24 observations. Rev Neurol (Paris) 1982;138:493-505.

67. Wechsler B, Vidailhet M, Piette JC, et al: Cerebral venous thrombosis in Behçet's disease: Clinical study and long-term follow-up of 25 cases. Neurology 1992;42:614-618.

68. Daif A, Awada A, Al-Rajeh S, et al: Cerebral venous thrombosis in adults. A study of 40 cases from Saudi Arabia. Stroke 1995;26:1193-1195.

69. Kumral E: Behçet's disease. In Caplan LR (ed): Uncommon Causes of Stroke, 2nd ed. Cambridge: Cambridge University Press, 2008.

70. Bousser M-G: Thromboses veineuses cerebrales. A propos de 76 cas. J Mal Vasc 1991;16:249-255.

71. Ameri A, Bousser M-G: Cerebral venous thrombosis. Neurol Clin 1992;10:87-111.

72. Einhaupl K, Villringer A, Haberl RL, et al: Clinical spectrum of sinus venous thrombosis. In Einhaupl K, Kemski O, Baethmann A (eds): Cerebral Sinus Thrombosis, Experimental and Clinical Aspects. New York: Plenum, 1990, pp 149-155.

73. Tsai F, Wang A-M, Matovich VB, et al: MR staging of acute dural sinus thrombosis: Correlation with venous pressure measurements and implications for treatment and prognosis. AJNR Am J Neuroradiol 1995;16:1021-1029.

74. Schaller B, Graf R: Cerebral venous infarction: The pathophysiological concept. Cerebrovasc Dis 2004;18:179-188.

75. Villringer A, Mehraein S, Einhaupl KM: Pathophysiological aspects of cerebral sinus venous thrombosis (SVT). J Neuroradiol 1994;21:72-80.

76. Gutschera-Wang L: Zur klinik von letalen hirnvenen-und sinus thrombosen anhand von 102 fallen. Erwachsener in der literatur. Munich, 1982.

77. Cervos-Navarro J, Kannuki S: Neuropathological findings in the thromboses of cerebral veins and sinuses: Vascular aspects. In Einhaupl K, Kempski O, Baethmann O (eds): Cerebral Sinus Thrombosis: Experimental and Clinical Aspects. New York: Plenum, 1990, pp 15-25.

78. Cumurciuc R, Crassard I, Sarov M, et al: Headache as the only neurological sign of cerebral venous thrombosis: A series of 17 cases. J Neurol Neurosurg Psychiatry 2005;76:1084-1087.

79. Bousser M-G, Barnett HJM: Cerebral venous thrombosis. In Barnett HJM, Mohr JP, Stein BM, Yatsu F (eds): Stroke Pathophysiology, Diagnosis, and Management, 2nd ed. New York: Churchill Livingstone, 1992, pp 517-537.

80. de Bruijn SF, de haan RJ, Stam J: F Clinical features and prognostic factors of cerebral venous sinus thrombosis in a prospective series of 59 patients. Cerebral Venous Sinus Thrombosis Study Group. J Neurol Neurosurg Psychiatry 2001;70:105-108.

80a. Ferro JM, Canhao P, Bousser M-G, et al: Early seizures in cerebral vein and dural sinus thrombosis. Risk factors and role of antiepileptics. Stroke 2008;39:1152-1158.

81. Mehraein S, Schmidtke K, Villringer A, et al: Heparin treatment in cerebral sinus and venous thrombosis: Patients at risk of fatal outcome. Cerebrovasc Dis 2003;15:17-21.

82. Masuhr F, Mehraein S: Cerebral venous and sinus thrombosis. Patients with a fatal outcome during intravenous dose-adjusted heparin treatment. Neurocrit Care 2004;1:355-361.

83. DiNubile MJ: Septic thrombosis of the cavernous sinus. Arch Neurol 1988;45:567-572.

84. Samuel J, Fernandes CM: Lateral sinus thrombosis: A review of 45 cases. J Laryngol Otol 1987; 101:1227-1229.

85. Mathews TJ: Lateral sinus pathology: 22 cases managed at Groote Schuur hospital. J Laryngol Otol 1988;102:118-120.

86. Tveteras K, Kristensen S, Dommerby H: Septic cavernous and lateral sinus thrombosis; modern diagnostic and therapeutic principles. J Laryngol Otol 1988;102:877-882.

87. Singh B: The management of lateral sinus thrombosis. J Laryngol Otol 1993;107:803-808.

88. Cakmak S, Nighoghossian N, Desestret V, et al: Pulmonary embolism: An unusual complication of cerebral venous thrombosis. Neurology 2005;65:1136-1137.

89. Bots GAM: Thrombosis of the Galenic system veins in the adult. Acta Neuropathol 1971;17:227-233.

90. Haley EC, Brashear R, Barth JT, et al: Deep cerebral venous thrombosis: Clinical, neuroradiological, and neuropsychological correlates. Arch Neurol 1989;46:337-340.

91. Johnsen S, Greenwood R, Fishman MA: Internal cerebral vein thrombosis. Arch Neurol 1973;28: 205-207.

92. Averback P: Primary cerebral venous thrombosis in young adults: The diverse manifestations of an underrecognized disease. Ann Neurol 1978; 3:81-86.

93. Jacobs K, Moulin T, Bogousslavsky J, et al: The stroke syndrome of cortical vein thrombosis. Neurology 1996;47:376-382.

94. Leach JL, Bulas RV, Ernst RJ, Cornelius RS: MR imaging of isolated cortical vein thrombosis: The hyperintense vein sign. J Neurovasc Dis 1996; 1:32-38.

95. Dorndorf D, Wessel K, Kessler C, Kompf D: Thrombosis of the right vein of Labbe: Radiological and clinical findings. Neuroradiology 1993;35: 202-204.

96. Cambria S: Infarctus cerebral hemorrhagique par thrombose de la veine de Labbe. Rev Neurol (Paris) 1980;136:321-326.

97. Thomas B, Krishnamurthy T, Purkayastha G. Isolated left vein of Labbe thrombosis. Neurology 2005;65:1135.

98. Jones BV: Case 62. Lobar hemorrhage from thrombosis of the vein of Labbe. Radiology 2003;228:693-696.

99. Rousseaux P, Lesoin F, Barbaste P, Jomin M: Infarctus cerebelleux pseudotumoral d'origine veineuse. Rev Neurol (Paris) 1987;144:209-211.

100. Eng LJ, Longstreth WT, Shaw CM, et al: Cerebellar venous infarction: Case report with clinicopathologic correlation. Neurology 1990; 40:837-838.

101. Lalive PH, de Moerloose P, Lovblad K, et al: Is measurement of D-dimer useful in the diagnosis of cerebral venous thrombosis. Neurology 2003;61:1057-1060.

102. Tardy B, Tardy-Poncet B, Viallon A, et al: D-dimer levels in patients with suspected acute cerebral venous thrombosis. Am J Med 2002;113:238-241.

103. Kosinski CM, Mull M, Schwartz M, et al: Do normal D-dimer levels reliably exclude cerebral sinus thrombosis? Stroke 2004;35: 2820-2825.

104. Crassard J, Soria C, Tzourio Ch, et al: A negative D-dimer assay does not rule out cerebral venous thrombosis: A series of 73 patients. Stroke 2005; 36:1716-1719.

105. Selim M, Caplan LR: Radiological Diagnosis of Cerebral Venous Thrombosis.

106. Singh V, Gress DR: Cerebral venous thrombosis. In Babikian VL, Wechsler LR, Higashida RT (eds): Imaging Cerebrovascular Disease. Philadelphia: Butterworth-Heinemann, 2003, pp 209-221.

107. Rao CV, Knipp HC, Wagner EJ: Computed tomographic findings in cerebral sinus and venous thrombosis. Radiology 1981;140:391-398.

108. Tovi F, Hirsch M: Computed tomographic diagnosis of septic lateral sinus thrombosis. Ann Otol Rhinol Laryngol 1991;100:79-81.

109. De Slegte RGM, Kaiser MC, van der Baan S, Smit L: Computed tomographic diagnosis of

septic sinus thromboses and their complications. Neuroradiology 1988;30:160-165.

110. Bousser M-G, Goujon C, Ribeiro V, Chiras J: Diagnostic strategies in cerebral sinus vein thrombosis. In Einhaupl K, Kempski O, Baethmann O (eds): Cerebral Sinus Thrombosis, Experimental and Clinical Aspects. New York: Plenum, 1990, pp 187-197.

111. Wetzel SG, Kirsch E, Stock KW, et al: Cerebral veins: Comparative study of CT venography with intraarterial digital subtraction angiography. AJNR Am J Neuroradiol 1999;20:249-255.

112. Dormont D, Axionnat R, Evrard S, et al: IRM des thromboses veineuses cerebrales. J Neuroradiol 1994;21:81-99.

113. Isensee Ch, Reul J, Thron A: Magnetic resonance imaging of thrombosed dural sinuses. Stroke 1994;25:29-34.

114. Mas J-L, Meder J-F, Meary E, Bousser M-G: Magnetic resonance imaging in lateral sinus hypoplasia and thrombosis. Stroke 1990;21: 1350-1356.

115. Dormont D, Sag K, Biondi A, et al: Gadolinium-enhanced MR of chronic dural sinus thrombosis. AJNR Am J Neuroradiol 1995;16:1347-1352.

116. Yuh WTC, Simonson TM, Wang A-M, et al: Venous sinus occlusive disease: MR findings. AJNR Am J Neuroradiol 1994;15:309-316.

117. Bianchi D, Maeder P, Bogousslavsky J, et al: Diagnosis of cerebral venous thrombosis with routine magnetic resonance: An update. Eur Neurol 1998;40:179-190.

118. Mas J-L, Meder JF, Meary E: Dural sinus thrombosis: Long-term follow-up by magnetic resonance imaging. Cerebrovasc Dis 1992;2: 137-144.

119. Selim M, Fink J, Linfante I, et al: Diagnosis of cerebral venous thrombosis with echo-planar T2*-weighted magnetic resonance imaging. Arch Neurol 2002;59:1021-1026.

120. Idbaih A, Boukobza M, Crassard I, et al: MRI of clot in cerebral venous thrombosis: High diagnostic value of susceptibility-weighted images. Stroke 2006;37(4):991-995.

121. Ayanzen RH, Bird CR, Keller PJ, et al: Cerebral MR venography: Normal anatomy and potential diagnostic pitfalls. AJNR Am J Neuroradiol 2000;21:74-78.

122. Ko SB, Kim D-E, Kim SH, Roh J-K: Visualization of venous system by time-of-flight magnetic resonance angiography. J Neuroimaging 2006;16:353-356.

123. Krayenbuhl H: Cerebral venous thrombosis. The diagnostic value of cerebral angiography. Schweiz Arch Neurol Neurochir Psychiatry 1954;74: 261-287.

124. Becker G, Bogdahn U, Gehlberg C, et al: Transcranial color-coded real-time sonography of intracranial veins. J Neuroimaging 1994; 5:87-94.

125. Wardlaw JM, Vaughan GT, Steers AJW, Sellar RJ: Transcranial Doppler ultrasound findings in venous sinus thrombosis. J Neurosurg 1994;80:332-335.

126. Valdueza JM, Schultz M, Harms L, Einhaupl KM: Venous transcranial Doppler ultrasound monitoring in acute dural sinus thrombosis. Report of two cases. Stroke 1995;26:1196-1199.

127. Ries S, Steinke W, Neff KW, Hennerici M: Echocontrast-enhanced transcranial color-coded sonography for the diagnosis of transverse sinus venous thrombosis. Stroke 1997;28:696-700.

128. Hanley DF, Feldman E, Borel CO, et al: Treatment of sagittal sinus thrombosis associated with cerebral hemorrhage and intracranial hypertension. Stroke 1988;19:903-909.

129. Einhaupl K, Bousser M-G, de Bruijn SFTM, et al: EFNS Guideline on the treatment of cerebral venous and sinus thrombosis. Eur J Neurol 2006;13:553-559.

129a. Canhao P, Cortesao A, Cabral M, et al: Stroke 2008;39:105-110.

130. Stansfield FR: Puerperial cerebral thrombophlebitis treated by heparin. BMJ 1942;1:436-438.

131. Martin JP, Sheenan HL: Primary thrombosis of cerebral veins (following childbirth). BMJ 1941;1:349.

132. Krayenbuhl H: Cerebral venous and sinus thrombosis. Clin Neurosurg 1967;14:1-24.

133. Diaz JM, Schiffman JS, Urban ES: Superior sagittal sinus thrombosis and pulmonary embolism: A syndrome rediscovered. Acta Neurol Scand 1992;86:390-396.

134. Levine SR, Twyman RE, Gilman S: The role of anticoagulation in cavernous sinus thrombosis. Neurology 1988;38:517-522.

135. Jacewicz M, Plum F: Aseptic cerebral venous thrombosis. In Einhaupl K, Kempski O, Baethmann A (eds): Cerebral Sinus Thrombosis: Experimental and Clinical Aspects. New York: Plenum, 1990, pp 157-170.

136. Brucker AB, Vollert-Rogenhofer H, Wagner M, et al: Heparin treatment in acute cerebral sinus venous thrombosis: A retrospective clinical and MR analysis of 42 cases. Cerebrovasc Dis 1998; 8:331-337.

137. Einhaupl KM, Villringer A, Meister W, et al: Heparin treatment in sinus venous thrombosis. Lancet 1991;338:597-600.

138. Meister W, Einhaupl K, Villringer A, et al: Treatment of patients with cerebral sinus and vein thrombosis with heparin. In Einhaupl K, Kempski O, Baethmann A (eds): Cerebral Sinus Thrombosis: Experimental and Clinical Aspects. New York: Plenum, 1990, pp 225-230.

139. de Bruijn SF, Stam J: Randomized, placebo-controlled trial of anticoagulant treatment with low-molecular-weight heparin for cerebral sinus thrombosis. Stroke 1999;30:484-488.

140. Bousser M-G: Cerebral venous thrombosis. Nothing, heparin or local thrombolysis? Stroke 1999;30:481-483.

141. Scott JA, Pascuzzi RM, Hall PV, Becker GJ: Treatment of dural sinus thrombosis with local urokinase infusion. J Neurosurg 1988;68: 284-287.

142. Higashida RT, Helmer E, Halbach VV, Heishima G: Direct thrombolytic therapy for superior sagittal sinus thrombosis. AJNR Am J Neuroradiol 1989;10:S4-S6.

143. Tsai F, Higashida R, Matovich V, Alfieri K: Acute thrombosis of the intracranial dural sinus: Direct thrombolytic treatment. AJNR Am J Neuroradiol 1992;13:1137-1141.

144. Smith TP, Higashida R, Barnwell S, et al: Treatment of dural sinus thrombosis by urokinase infusion. AJNR Am J Neuroradiol 1994;15: 801-807.

145. Griesmer DA, Theodorou A, Berg RA, Spera TD: Local fibrinolysis in cerebral venous thrombosis. Pediatr Neurol 1994;10:78-80.

146. Horowitz M, Purdy P, Unwin H, et al: Treatment of dural sinus thrombosis using selective catheterization and urokinase. Ann Neurol 1995;38:58-67.

147. Kim SY, Suh JH: Direct endovascular thrombolytic therapy for dural sinus thrombosis: infusion of alteplase. AJNR Am J Neuroradiol 1997;18:639-645.

148. Frey JL, Muro GJ, McDougall CG, et al: Cerebral venous thrombosis. Combined intrathrombus rtPA and intravenous heparin. Stroke 1999;30: 489-494.

149. Canhao P, Falcao F, Ferro JM: Thrombolysis for cerebral sinus thrombosis. A systematic review. Cerebrovasc Dis 2003;15:159-166.

150. Gratzl O: Neurosurgery of the cerebral venous and sinus system. In Einhaupl K, Kempski O, Baethmann A (eds): Cerebral Sinus Thrombosis: Experimental and Clinical Aspects. New York: Plenum, 1990, pp 219-224.

151. Yasargil MG: Microsurgery. Stuttgart: Thieme, 1969.

152. Donaghy P, Wallman LJ, Flanagan MJ, Numoto M: Sagittal sinus repair. J Neurosurg 1973;38: 244-248.

153. Sundt T, Piepgras DG: The surgical approach to arterio-venous malformations of the lateral and sigmoid dural sinuses. J Neurosurg 1983; 59:32-39.

154. Awad IA, Barrow DL (eds): Dural Arteriovenous Malformations. Park Ridge, Ill: American Association of Neurological Surgeons, 1993.

Prevention, Complications, and Recovery–Rehabilitation

III

When meditating over a disease, I never think of finding a remedy for it, but instead a means of preventing it.

Louis Pasteur[1]

Prevention of stroke is much more likely to have a major impact on the health and welfare of the population than even the most effective treatment after stroke has occurred. For this cogent reason, much effort is aimed at identifying and modifying, whenever possible, risk factors for cerebrovascular disease and cardiovascular disease in general.

Despite these efforts, much of the population is still woefully ignorant about stroke. The medical profession and media have been relatively successful in educating the public about heart attacks, cancer, and acquired immunodeficiency syndrome. Stroke, although the third leading cause of death in the United States, has received much less public attention and remains poorly understood by most Americans, and most of the public around the world. Publicity about thrombolysis has increased public awareness about stroke and may increase general knowledge. Surveys and studies show that many individuals throughout the world do not know any of the major symptoms or warning signs of stroke or important stroke risk factors.[2-7] Some do not even know that stroke involves the brain. Many respondents think that strokes are almost invariably permanently disabling. In the United States, efforts are made to educate the public to call 911 or another specified number if they suspect that they or another person is having a stroke. Sadly, many operators who pick up the phone when 911 is called know little about stroke and do not triage the call as urgent.

Kothari and colleagues interviewed patients admitted to the emergency room with possible strokes at the University of Cincinnati Medical Center.[4] Their interviews consisted of open-ended questions and were conducted during the first 48 hours after hospital admission. Among 163 patients, 63 (39%) did not know a single symptom or sign of stroke. Unilateral weakness (26%) and numbness (22%) were the most often mentioned symptoms.[4] Persons older than 65 years were less knowledgeable than younger patients.[4] In one study, even when attempts were made to educate patients with TIA or minor stroke about these conditions, when queried 3 months later, only 15 of 57 (26%) correctly identified the brain as the affected organ and only 21 of 57 (37%) could give a correct description of a TIA or stroke.[6] One study did suggest that gains are being made in public knowledge about stroke. Among 2173 individuals that responded to a survey in Cincinnati, knowledge about stroke warning signs and risk factors improved appreciably between the 1995 and 2000 surveys.[3]

Despite the lack of public knowledge about stroke, an important decline in stroke incidence and mortality occurred during the second half of the 20th century.[8-10] This fact is probably explained by a number of factors. The public has definitely become more health conscious. Good eating habits; regular exercise; and avoidance of cigarettes, alcohol, and dietary excesses have been an educational and media theme. Reduction in risk factors perceived in the public mind as related to heart attacks has reduced cerebrovascular disease as well. Emphasis on check-ups and screenings for high blood pressure, diabetes, and high cholesterol has also had an impact. Physicians' aggressive treatment of hypertension and better technology for assessing vascular disease have also played a role. I have tried to do my part by publishing three books for the public.[11-13] Clearly, much more public and physician education are needed for further gains to be made in stroke prevention.

Prevention of stroke is a vast subject. I cannot even attempt to do justice to it in this short chapter. Herein I will try to emphasize key topics but will not discuss in any detail specific therapies and treatments. Antithrombotic and other treatments are discussed in detail in Chapter 5.

NEW PREVENTION STRATEGIES

In his 2006 Feinberg lecture, Sacco outlined a shift in physician strategy for preventing cerebrovascular disease.[14] Since cardiovascular disease shares most risk factors with cerebrovascular disease, and since cardiac disease poses a risk for brain embolism and hypoperfusion, doctors should evaluate patients for the presence of both

17

cardiovascular and cerebrovascular abnormalities, as well as emphasizing management of treatable risk factors. Optimally the evaluation might include the following:

- Illnesses and behaviors known to increase the risk of vascular disease (for example, smoking, physical inactivity, hypertension, diabetes etc). These are the customary "risk factors" that have long been discussed.
- Subclinical brain lesions (e.g., unexpected infarcts, white matter hyperintensities, microbleeds, etc.)
- Subclinical vascular disease (e.g., carotid artery plaques, arterial intima-media thickness, etc.)
- Biomarkers and genetic findings and conditions known to relate to vascular disease (e.g., fibrinogen, C-reactive protein (CRP), homocysteine levels, etc.)

Extensive information has been accumulated and analyzed regarding risk factors for the general category of stroke[15-24] and brain ischemia.[25-32] With regard to some stroke mechanisms, such as subarachnoid hemorrhage (SAH),[33-37] intracerebral hemorrhage (ICH),[38-41] and brain embolism,[42,43] ample data exist. I discuss causes of hemorrhage in detail in Chapters 12 and 13. The major risk factors for cardiac-origin embolism are those that predispose to the various cardiac conditions. These are described in Chapter 9. Relatively less information is available about other specific stroke mechanisms, especially within the broad group of patients with brain ischemia. Most analyses of risk factors do not differentiate among patients with stenotic lesions of the extracranial arteries, those with stenosis of the large intracranial vessels, such as the middle cerebral and intracranial vertebral arteries, and those with disease of penetrating arteries, such as the lenticulostriate arteries. Evidence exists that various risk factors, such as race/ethnicity and sex, have a differential effect on various pathologic lesions and on lesions at various loci within the vasculature.[29,44-49] Further data, especially in patients with specific stroke subtypes studied prospectively, are needed.

Despite these limitations, the currently identified risk factors are of great significance. These risk factors help identify individuals at risk for stroke in whom modification of lifestyle might reduce the chance of stroke and other cardiovascular diseases. In this section, I only briefly discuss these risk factors. Larger, more detailed reviews of the subject are available.[14,15,17-24] When risk factors are identified, the evidence usually consists of an epidemiologic relationship between the factor and the occurrence of

stroke; correlation does not necessarily indicate causation. For example, being female is strikingly associated with becoming pregnant, but clearly this does not cause the condition.

A relatively new concept that Sacco also emphasized in his 2006 Feinberg lecture is the idea of "vascular risk modulators."[14] Doctors and epidemiologists have been accustomed to analyzing various risks as binary variables. For example, an individual is considered to have or not have hypertension if their blood pressure exceeds or falls below a set number such as 140/90. Similarly, they are defined as diabetic, or to have hypercholesterolemia if their blood sugar and blood cholesterol levels are above or below arbitrarily designated values. Studies have shown, however, that risk factors are all continuous rather than categorical (yes or no) variables. A systolic blood pressure of 160 carries more risk than 150, and in turn 150 has more risk than 140, and 140 more risk than 130.[14,50] It is simple for clinicians to characterize an individual as hypertensive or not, or obese or not, but this categorization loses a great deal of information. Risk can often be modulated by reducing blood pressure, blood sugar, weight, and cholesterol levels, even if the present values are considered "within the normal range."

Nonmodifiable Demographic Risk Factors

Parents cannot be selected, nor can race/ethnicity and sex. Time cannot be turned back to reverse the aging process. Age, race/ethnicity, sex, and family history of cardiovascular risk factors and disease are among the most important risk factors for stroke.

Age is probably the risk factor best correlated with stroke. The Framingham Study showed that as a person ages, his or her risk of stroke increases, with incidence rates per 10,000 increasing from 22% to 32% to 83% in the age groups 45 to 55, 55 to 64, and 65 to 74 years, respectively.[51] With increasing age, an exponential increase occurs in the frequency of stroke. The great majority of ischemic strokes occur in individuals older than 65 years.[29] The incidence of SAH also rises steadily with age.[34] Data on age in patients with ICH also show high frequency in the elderly. Despite the best efforts, aging is inevitable; all of us strive to eventually join the "old age club." Stroke also occurs in younger patients. Ischemic stroke in patients younger than 45 years is correlated with more frequent cardiac-origin embolism and less common occlusive lesions, whereas in stroke patients older than

65 years, intrinsic large- and small-artery diseases are most common, closely followed by cardiac-origin embolism.

Race/ethnicity and sex also influence the occurrence and subtypes of stroke.[29,44-49] African Americans and Asians have a higher risk of intracerebral hemorrhage than whites.[38,52] African Americans, persons of Asian descent, and women have more intracranial occlusive disease and less extracranial occlusive disease than white men.[44-49] Men have a greater frequency of stroke than women, but because life expectancy is higher in women, women often outnumber men in many stroke studies.[29] During the premenopausal years, women have fewer strokes than men, but incidence levels off after age 60 years.

The Importance of Beginning Prevention at an Early Age

A history of stroke or other important cardiovascular disease among first-degree relatives, including coronary artery disease, peripheral vascular disease, and hypertension, is an important risk factor for stroke even after adjustment for other personal stroke risk factors.[53-57] Atherosclerotic lesions often begin at a very young age. Autopsy studies among individuals of varied racial geographical backgrounds have shown that fatty streaks (yellow lipid deposits that elevate the intima only slightly) are found in the aorta of all groups during infancy and reach a peak in puberty.[58,59] These deposits develop into raised lesions and fibrous plaques in subsequent decades.[58,59] Since familial and genetic factors are quite individual and very important, knowledge of risks and prevention should begin in the young.

I once heard an informal presentation by a seventh-grade school teacher from the southern part of the United States. During a discussion about health in her classroom, this teacher discovered that few of her students knew about illnesses within their own families. She then gave her students a homework assignment to inquire in detail about the medical conditions that affected close relatives. Doctors volunteered to test the students who were about 12 to 13 years old for various conditions. Children whose parents both had hypertension had a high frequency of elevated blood pressure themselves. Those with a strong family history of diabetes often had high blood sugars. Children whose family members were overweight, were themselves often far overweight for age and height. Students whose family history included elevated cholesterol levels, frequently had high serum cholesterol levels when tested. A routine examination 25 years ago showed that my cholesterol level was quite high—over 300. When I later tested my six children (ages 6 to 18 years at the time), five of them also had abnormally high cholesterol levels. My wife and I then made sure to pay careful attention to the children's diets and nutritional behavior.

When neurologists and other physicians care for patients with risk factors, such as high cholesterol, severe hypertension, and diabetes, they should urge patients to test their children, especially if risk factors have been prevalent in their family histories. It is known that some risk factors are found at relatively early ages, even in children and young adults. Finding and modifying risk factors at an early age is far superior to modification only after an index cardiac or cerebrovascular event.

Hypertension

After age, hypertension is the single risk factor that most significantly correlates with stroke. Hypertension plays a role in numerous mechanisms of stroke. Without a prior history of hypertension or cardiomegaly, lacunar infarcts are rarely found at necropsy. The association among hypertension, cardiac disease, and kidney disease is well known. Cardiac and renal pathology contribute to many stroke subtypes. Hypertension plays a role in the atherodegenerative process in large blood vessels, resulting in occlusive and artery-to-artery embolic strokes. Hypertension plays a role in the rupture of cerebral aneurysms. Intracerebral hemorrhage in the basal ganglia, thalamus, pons, and cerebellum is more commonly found in the setting of acute and chronic hypertension.

The literature on hypertension is vast. I hope that some information-opinion short "bites," along with key references that discuss the data in detail, will serve to summarize key points.

Hypertension is extremely common. Nearly one in four individuals in the United States are estimated to be hypertensive.[60,61] The prevalence of hypertension increases with age and is more common in blacks than whites, and in women over 55 than in men.[60-62] Figure 17-1 from American Heart Association statistics displays the prevalence of high blood pressure in men and women by age deciles.[62]

Many individuals with high blood pressure are unaware that they have it; many who are aware are untreated or undertreated. Awareness and treatment of hypertension are woefully inadequate. The seventh report of the Joint National Committee on Prevention, Detection, Evaluation, and Treatment of High Blood Pressure, issued in 2003, contained the following estimates about individuals in the United States: 30% were unaware of

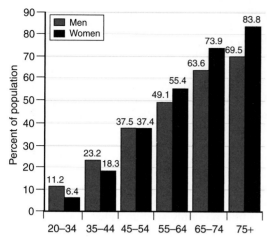

Figure 17-1. Prevalence of high blood pressure in adults by age and sex (NHANES: 1999-2004). (Data from American Heart Association: Heart Disease and Stroke Statistics 2006 Update. Available at http://www.americanheart.org/presenter.jhtml. Identifier=3018163.)

hypertension and were untreated, 11% were aware but untreated, 24% were treated but inadequately, and only 35% had blood pressures below the 140/90 cut-off range.[63] Figure 17-2 has updated figures about hypertension awareness and treatment by age range supplied by the American Heart Association in 2006.[62]

Blood pressure reduction is effective along a range of systolic and diastolic blood pressures, and at all ages, including the elderly. Figure 17-3 shows the effect of various blood pressures on stroke mortality at various ages.[64] Antihypertensive treatment reduces stroke incidence and mortality in individuals

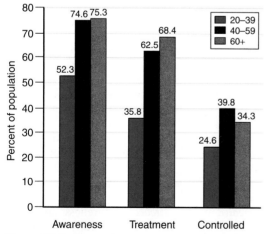

Figure 17-2. Extent of awareness, treatment, and control of high blood pressure by age (NHANES: 1999-2004). (Data from American Heart Association: Heart Disease and Stroke Statistics 2006 Update. Available at http://www.americanheart.org/presenter.jhtml. Identifier=3018163.)

aged over 80 who have high blood pressures.[65,66,66a] In a recent randomized trial, during a mean follow-up period of 1.8 years, among 3845 patients aged 80 or more years (average age 83.6 years), active treatment of hypertension was accompanied by a 30% reduction in the rate of fatal and non-fatal strokes.[66a] The degree of elevation of systolic and diastolic pressure is correlated with the risk of stroke. The risk curve is a continuum without any clear point separating the stroke-prone from the non–stroke-prone individual.

Systolic blood pressure is at least as important and may be more important in promoting stroke and other manifestations of cardiovascular disease as diastolic pressure. In the Framingham study, average systolic blood pressure increased by 20 mm Hg between ages 30 and 65. Systolic blood pressure continued to rise into the 80s in women and 70s in men.[60] Numerous studies, especially the Systolic Hypertension in the Elderly Program (SHEP)[67-71] show that isolated systolic blood pressure in the elderly is a very important stroke risk factor, and that optimizing systolic blood pressure reduction decreases the risk of stroke.[67-73] An analysis of data from 11,466 men in the Physicians' Health Study concluded that although diastolic blood pressure, pulse pressure, and mean arterial pressure were all significant predictors of stroke risk, none was a significantly better predictor than systolic blood pressure alone.[72]

Blood pressure reduction is as (or more) important in women as it is in men. For stroke in general and atherothrombotic brain infarction, no evidence exists that shows that women tolerate hypertension better than men. Hypertension is more prevalent in women after age 65 years than in men.[60,74] Women incur as many, if not more, complications of hypertension than men. In women over 65, stroke is the most common vascular event, exceeding myocardial infarction.[75]

Pulse pressure is also very important. Systolic hypertension is accompanied by increased arterial stiffness and decreased compliance, and as a result diastolic blood pressure often decreases. Pulse pressure is the difference between systolic and diastolic pressure. A large pulse pressure may exert its own additional stress on arterial walls. Pulse pressure was an important risk factor for the development of atrial fibrillation in the Framingham study.[75a] In one study, mean arterial pressure and pulse pressure were independent predictors of stroke mortality.[76] In other studies pulse pressure was the best predictor of stroke mortality outperforming systolic, diastolic, and mean arterial pressures,[77] and pulse pressure during an acute stroke was an independent predictor of long-term mortality.[78]

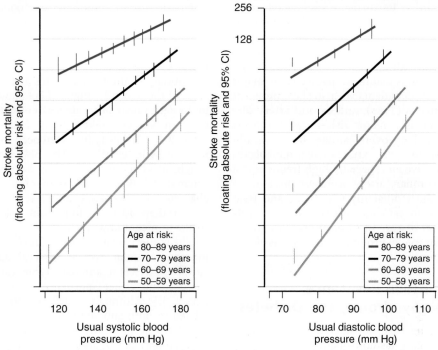

Figure 17-3. The effect of systolic and diastolic blood pressure on mortality from stroke at various ages. (Data from Lewington S, Clarke R, Qizilbash N, et al: Prospective Studies Collaboration. Age-specific relevance of usual blood pressure to vascular mortality: A meta-analysis of individual data for one million adults in 61 prospective studies. Lancet 2002;360:1903-1913.)

Casual blood pressure measurement in a doctor's office are inadequate to quantify the severity of hypertension. Digital techniques to measure and record blood pressures at home, and at various times and after various circumstances are helpful. The effect of blood pressure on target organs, especially the heart, retina, and kidney are also important in judging the severity and effects of hypertension. Electrocardiograms, echocardiography, measures of renal function, and a careful look at retinal arteries and veins should be part of the evaluation of hypertensive patients.

Twenty-four-hour blood pressure monitoring yields more useful information than casual or even multiple daytime blood pressures. Blood pressure often dips at night. Studies using ambulatory 24-hour blood pressure monitoring have shown that patients with excessively high and abnormally low nocturnal blood pressures and high pulse pressures have a higher frequency of new strokes and hypertension-related white matter damage than patients who have normal nocturnal blood pressures.[79-84]

The type of antihypertensive agent is important. A variety of different types of antihypertensive agents—diuretics, alpha-blockers, beta-blockers, calcium channel blockers, angiotensin-converting enzyme (ACE) inhibitors, and angiotensin receptor binding (ARB) agents—have all proved effective in reducing blood pressure and cardiovascular

mortality.[63,85-87] Diuretics are quite effective, especially in African Americans.[88] Some evidence suggests that ACE inhibitors and ARBs are effective in reversing endothelial dysfunction associated with hypertension and may be more effective in stroke reduction than other agents.[89-94] Choice of agent also should consider other comorbidities such as bradycardia, coronary artery disease, renal disease, migraine, and so on because many of the agents that reduce blood pressure also have other cardiovascular effects.

Heart Disease

The incidence of various cardiac diseases is highly correlated with stroke risk. Cardiac disease is a direct cause of stroke when the heart is a donor source of emboli to the brain. Heart disease, usually related to hypertension or coronary artery disease, coexists with hypertensive and atherosclerotic disease of the cervicocranial arteries in other patients. Cardioembolic stroke occurs in the setting of mitral or aortic valve disease, atrial fibrillation of any cause, prosthetic heart valves, endocarditis, myocardiopathies, akinetic myocardial segments, and ventricular aneurysms. Embolism from cardiac sources is discussed in Chapter 9. Atrial fibrillation is the most common cardiac source of brain embolism.

17

Indices of cardiac impairment, such as coronary artery disease, congestive heart failure, and left ventricular hypertrophy as measured by electrocardiography, chest x-ray, and echocardiography, are associated with increased stroke risk. Particularly important is that heart disease is the major cause of death in patients with strokes, transient ischemic attacks (TIAs), and carotid artery disease.[95] Stroke is a major risk factor for heart disease even if no overt cardiac disease is observed. Patients with extracranial artery occlusive disease have an especially high frequency of coexistent coronary artery occlusive disease.[96,97] Physicians must diligently search for and treat heart disease in patients with stroke. The treatment of heart disease in association with stroke plays a major role in prolonging life and avoiding significant morbidity.

Obesity, Insulin Resistance, Metabolic Syndrome, and Diabetes

Doctors, in the past, considered blood glucose levels in a binary fashion—patients were either diabetic or not, and some might be "prediabetic." Now studies show clearly that risk in relation to glucose utilization, like blood pressures, should be considered over a continuum.[98] Glucose metabolism is heavily linked to the secretion and effectiveness of insulin, and to body fat and inflammation. Adipose tissue releases substances that relate to body energy, glucose levels, and insulin effectiveness in controlling glucose utilization. These substances include nonesterified fatty acids, cytokines, and adiponectin.[99] Knowledge of the interrelationship of abdominal obesity to glucose metabolism, insulin resistance, and hypertension has led to definition of a "metabolic syndrome" that represents a very important risk factor for stroke as well as other cardiovascular conditions.[99-104,104a,104b] The components of the metabolic syndrome are listed in Table 17-1.

Table 17-1.	**Components of Metabolic Syndrome as Defined by Proceedings of National Heart, Lung, and Blood Institute and American Heart Association Conference[99]**
Abdominal obesity	
Atherogenic dyslipidemia	
Raised blood pressure	
Insulin resistance with or without glucose intolerance	
Proinflammatory state	
Prothrombotic state	

Obesity is an important component of the metabolic syndrome, and data now clearly identifies obesity as a major risk factor for all forms of cardiovascular disease including stroke. Furthermore, there is a major epidemic of weight gain and obesity in the United States and many other parts of the world.[105] Figure 17-4 shows changes in the age-adjusted prevalence of obesity in adults between surveys taken from 1960-1962 and 2001-2004.[62] Obesity has often been measured by body mass index (BMI). The BMI is defined as weight in kilograms divided by height in meters squared.[106] A BMI of 30 or higher is a criterion for characterizing someone as obese,[62] and a BMI greater than 30 is an important risk factor for stroke in men and women.[106-108]

The major obesity-related culprit contributing to cardiovascular risk is visceral adipose tissue.[109-111] Visceral adipose tissue can be measured using either modern CT or MRI scanners.[109-111] Although waist circumference is related to both subcutaneous and visceral fat, it correlates quite highly with the amount of visceral fat and can be used as a convenient surrogate measure of visceral adipose tissue.[109] I have heard some epidemiologists argue that waist circumference should be another vital sign, measured often in those suspected of being overweight. Abdominal obesity as measured by waist circumference is highly associated with an increased risk of developing atherosclerosis and having an ischemic stroke.[108,109,112]

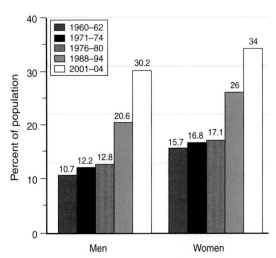

Figure 17-4. Age-adjusted prevalence of obesity in adults ages 20-74 by sex and survey (NHES 1960-1962; NHANES 1971-1974, 1976-1980, 1988-1994, and 2001-2004). (Data from American Heart Association: Heart Disease and Stroke Statistics 2006 Update. Available at http://www.americanheart.org/presenter.jhtml. Identifier=3018163.)

A strong correlation exists between abdominal obesity and insulin resistance. Most obese individuals have postprandial hyperinsulinemia and relatively low insulin sensitivity, although variations are often present within the obese population, and an individual can be insulin resistant and not be obese.[99,100,113,114] Clearly both genetic and fat accumulation contribute to insulin resistance. Obesity also predisposes to an increase in blood markers of inflammation. I discuss inflammatory markers later in this chapter.

Frank diabetes mellitus has long been known to be associated with an increased risk of atherosclerosis, cardiovascular disease, and ischemic stroke and increased mortality in patients with stroke.[20-30,115-119]

Hypertension is more common among patients with diabetes, and in overweight individuals, so some of the effects attributed to diabetes may be related to accompanying obesity, hypertension, and dyslipidemia. The increased risk of stroke is present in insulin-dependent and non–insulin-dependent diabetic patients and does not diminish with advancing age in either men or women. Diabetes is a risk factor for intracranial and extracranial large artery occlusive disease and penetrating artery disease. Intracranial branch artery atheromatous disease is particularly common among diabetic patients.[120,121] Atheromatous branch disease affects predominantly the paramedian pontine penetrating arteries, anterior choroidal arteries, and anterior inferior cerebellar arteries.

Optimizing body weight and glucose metabolism are clearly very important strategies to reduce the risk of stroke. Recent research has identified the endocannabinoid system and the cannabinoid CB_1 receptor as important in determining energy balance and body composition. The CB_1 receptor is an important target for blockade in an attempt to reduce body weight and waist circumference.[122]

Smoking

Convincing epidemiologic data strongly relate cigarettes to an increased risk of stroke and extracranial and intracranial atherosclerosis.[123-128] Like blood pressure and blood sugar levels, the titer of smoking (number of cigarettes/day, number of years of smoking, and present smoking) represents a continuum of risk. The increased stroke risk applies to middle-aged and older individuals and men and women, but is especially important in the young. In the Framingham study, smoking was a significant risk factor for atherothrombotic brain infarction only in men younger than 65 years.[129] Paffenbarger and Williams found that smoking was one of the most important risk factors among college students who later had ischemic strokes.[130] In a series of patients with extracranial carotid artery disease studied at the Mayo Clinic, the total years of cigarette smoking was the single, most significant, independent predictor of the presence of severe occlusive disease.[125] Duration of cigarette smoking and hypertension were the most important predictors of intracranial internal carotid artery disease in another study.[126] Stopping smoking mitigates the risk of stroke[131] as it does with other conditions. In a study of Korean men, low cholesterol levels did not confer any lowering of risk against smoking-related atherosclerotic disease.[132] In regard to SAH, cigarette smoking seems to be a risk factor in men,[33-37,133] and in women when combined with the use of high-dose estrogen and contraceptive pill use.[34,134] Smoking conveyed the same magnitude of risk for intracerebral hemorrhage as for ischemic stroke among 22,022 men in the Physicians' Health Study.[133] Genetic factors have recently been found to impact the tendency for tobacco addiction,[135] and the adverse effects of smoking on cardiovascular risks.[136]

Elevated Blood Lipids

Abnormalities of blood lipids, especially cholesterol, triglycerides, and high- and low-density lipoproteins, are less closely correlated with stroke than with coronary heart disease. Studies do confirm, however, that elevated low-density lipoprotein cholesterol and low high-density lipoprotein cholesterol levels do increase the risk of stroke.[137,137a,137b] Elevated levels of triglycerides are a risk factor for large-artery atherosclerotic stroke.[137b] In the Framingham study and others, the risk is primarily shown in patients younger than 55 years old.[138] A relationship between low cholesterol and ICH in Asians has been shown in several reports.[139,140] The risk of ICH is especially high in patients with low cholesterol levels.[141,142] The mechanism of how low cholesterol levels increase the risk for brain infarction and SAH remains obscure. The association has been demonstrated primarily among Asians who have lifelong low cholesterol levels. It may not be true for individuals whose cholesterol levels are lowered iatrogenically.

In one large series of more than 350,000 men, a significant relationship existed between morbidity from ischemic stroke and high serum cholesterol levels.[140] Among 27,937 U.S. women in the Women's Health Study total cholesterol, low-density lipoprotein cholesterol, total cholesterol/high-density lipoprotein cholesterol, and non–high-density lipoprotein cholesterol levels were significantly associated with increased risk of ischemic stroke.[143] In a study of ischemic stroke mortality among 8586 Israeli men, low high-density lipoprotein cholesterol levels were related to an increased risk of death caused by stroke.[144] Elevated levels of low-density lipoproteins, a decrease in concentrations of high-density lipoproteins, and the presence of lipoprotein(a) correlate better with coronary and extracranial atherosclerosis than do total cholesterol levels.[145,146] Patients with ischemic cerebrovascular disease have an increased frequency of elevated levels of lipoprotein(a).[147] Low levels of high-density lipoprotein cholesterol do correlate with carotid atherosclerosis in men,[148] but serum lipids and lipoprotein levels are not as powerful predictors of extracranial internal carotid artery disease as are hypertension and cigarette smoking.[149]

One of the strongest indicators that cholesterol may have an important role in extracranial and intracranial atherosclerosis and ischemic stroke is the effectiveness of hydroxyl-methylglutaryl-coenzyme A reductase inhibitors (statins) in decreasing the growth of atherosclerotic plaques in the carotid arteries and reducing the incidence of stroke.[150-153] Although these drugs may have effects on plaques and vascular endothelia in addition to their cholesterol-lowering effects, reduction of low-density lipoprotein cholesterol is their predominant action.

Alcohol Use

The amount of alcohol that an individual consumes affects his or her stroke risk.[154] Excess alcohol intake increases the risk of brain hemorrhage. Finnish studies, although not well controlled, clearly linked heavy alcohol consumption and recent alcohol use to the occurrence of SAH.[155] ICH can be caused by the hypoprothrombinemia accompanying cirrhosis of the liver. In the Honolulu Heart Study, alcohol consumption was associated with intracranial hemorrhage, not with ischemic stroke.[139,156]

Most epidemiologists describe a J-shaped curve in relation to alcohol consumption and the risk of ischemic stroke. Light-to-moderate regular consumption of alcohol seems to be inversely related to carotid artery and systemic atherosclerosis, yet acute and chronic heavy use of alcohol increases ischemic stroke risk.[157-159] The effect of alcohol as a stroke risk factor is at least partially explained by the frequent coexistence of hypertension and cigarette smoking.[160,161] The effect of the type of alcohol consumed has not been well studied. In a study performed in Copenhagen, regular wine consumption did confer a protective effect, whereas intake of beer and other spirits did not.[162] Some have attributed the salutary effects of wine to its

nonalcoholic contents, especially to antioxidant flavinoids and tannins, which are posited to have a protective effect against atherosclerosis.[162-164] Grape juice might have the same effects as alcohol, although this hypothesis has not been systematically studied. Acute alcohol intoxication may precipitate ischemic strokes.[165]

Figure 17-5 shows the relative frequency of various risk factors in the REduction of Arthrothrombosis for Continued Health (REACH) registry.

Symptomatic Atherosclerosis of Coronary and Peripheral Limb Arteries

Peripheral vascular arterial occlusive disease is a strong predictor of extracranial cerebrovascular and coronary artery disease. Patients with claudication and peripheral arterial disease have a high frequency of stroke and cardiovascular mortality.[166-168] I have already commented earlier in this chapter on the close association between coronary artery and extracranial arterial disease and stroke.

Transient Ischemic Attacks

When properly diagnosed, TIAs are an indication that occlusive cerebrovascular disease has already become established. With development of CT and MRI scanning in the 1970s and 1980s, it

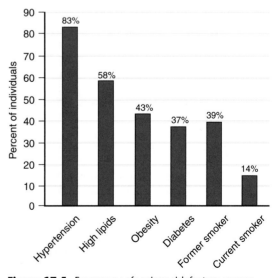

Figure 17-5. Frequency of various risk factors among 18,843 international patients with cerebrovascular disease in the REACH registry. (Data from Bhatt DL, Steg PG, Ohman EM, et al: International prevalence, recognition, and treatment of cardiovascular risk factors in outpatients with atherothrombosis. REACH Registry Investigators. JAMA 2006;295:180-189.)

became evident that many patients with clinical TIAs have brain imaging evidence of infarction in regions that correlate with the symptoms.[169-171]

When modern advanced MRI technology became available in the 1990s, the frequency of positive diffusion-weighted MRI images in patients with clinical TIAs was even higher than that seen previously.[172,173] Inatomi and colleagues studied 129 consecutive TIA patients. among whom 57 patients (44%) had positive diffusion-weighted image lesions appropriate to the neurologic symptoms.[173] When the TIAs lasted more than 30 minutes and contained a higher cortical function abnormality, the likelihood of a positive diffusion-weighted image lesion was high.

Risk factors and prognosis are similar for patients with TIAs and those with minor strokes because the underlying vascular diseases are the same.[174] Many studies in varied populations have shown that TIAs carry a very substantial risk of imminent brain infarction and should be handled emergently.[175-182] Johnston et al analyzed the outcomes among 1707 patients with TIAs who presented to emergency departments in 16 California hospitals.[175] During the 90 days after the emergency room visit, 180 patients (10.5%) returned with a stroke, occurring in half the patients within the first 2 days.[175] Daffertshofer and colleagues collected data from 82 German hospitals.[176] Among 1380 TIA patients seen during a 6-month period, stroke frequency during the hospital stay was 8% and another 5% of TIA patients had a stroke within the first half-year.[176] Kleindorfer et al performed a population-based study of 1023 TIA events among 927 individuals occurring in the Cincinnati-northern Kentucky region during 1 year.[177] Within 6 months of the index TIA, 144 patients had an ischemic stroke and 77 died. The median time for stroke to develop was 12 days.[177] Hill et al reviewed data from Alberta, Canada during a 1-year period.[178] Stroke occurred in 15.1% of TIA patients within 1 year; half of the risk at 1 year was accrued within the first 38 days.[178] Rothwell and Warlow used a different approach.[179] A retrospective review of 2146 stroke admissions in the United Kingdom showed that a preceding TIA was present in 23%; 17% of TIAs occurred on the day of the stroke, 9% on the preceding day, and 43% during the preceding week.[179] The data are quite clear and consistent. A TIA is a major risk factor for imminent stroke and is a true medical emergency.[181] Patients with clinical TIAs who have infarcts on brain imaging may have an especially high risk of stroke soon after the TIA.[182]

For the individual patient, failure to recognize that a TIA has occurred and failure to diagnose and treat potentially remediable abnormalities can be a great personal and family tragedy. All too often, patients do not understand the importance of temporary focal nervous system and ocular symptoms. Patients often do not report these transient symptoms to their physicians. In my experience, general physicians often reassure patients that the spells are not important. When the nature of the spells is correctly identified, treatment often involves automatic prescription of the latest panacea for ischemic stroke (i.e., warfarin, vasodilators, and aspirin). Thoughtful and thorough evaluation of the cause in the individual patient followed by treatment of the specific abnormalities found is the exception, not the rule.

Hormones and Oral Contraceptive Use

Most of the data that attributed a risk of stroke to the use of oral contraceptives were acquired in patients who used pills with a relatively high estrogen content (50 μg of ethinyl estradiol or estranes).[183-185,185a] In these studies, hypertension, migraine, diabetes, hyperlipidemia, cigarette smoking, age older than 35 years, and prolonged use of oral contraceptive pills compounded the risk of ischemic stroke in oral contraceptive users. Lower-dose estrogen (20 to 40 μg of ethinyl estradiol) combined with newer progestational drugs are now usually prescribed as oral contraceptive agents. Studies show that young women who take these lower-dose pills do not have an important increased risk of stroke.[186-189] Contraceptive patches that contain 35 μg of ethinyl estradiol did not increase the risk of ischemic stroke or myocardial infarction in one study.[190] Among users of low-dose contraceptives, strokes most often occur in older women who have other stroke risk factors, such as hypertension and cigarette smoking.[191] Genetics also probably play a role, but this has been inadequately explored. Patients with prothrombin gene mutations have an increased risk of stroke when they take oral contraceptives.[192] The presence of factor V Leiden; prothrombin gene mutations; other causes of resistance to activated protein C; abnormalities of antithrombin III, protein C, and protein S; and other genetic-related disorders of coagulation proteins might make women who take oral contraceptives or smoke cigarettes especially susceptible to thrombosis.

The influence of female hormones on stroke frequency and subtypes has also been explored by studies on pregnancy and stroke.[185a] Women with six or more pregnancies are at a higher risk for stroke and cerebral infarction than women who have had fewer pregnancies.[193] One study showed that the risk of stroke was not increased during pregnancy, but the risk of brain infarction and brain hemorrhage were significantly increased during the 6 weeks after delivery.[194] The risk of cerebral venous thrombosis is especially high during the puerperium.

Probably the most controversial hormone-related topic relates to the risk of stroke in postmenopausal women who were prescribed hormone replacement therapy.[185a] Four published cohort studies revealed a neutral or minor effect of hormonal replacement. One study, National Health and Nutrition Examination Survey (NHANES), showed a protective effect on stroke, a relative risk of 0.69,[195] while the others—the Nurses Health Study,[196] Danish Nurse Study,[197] and Framingham study[198]—showed a small relative risk of stroke. However, randomized controlled trials did show that hormone replacement therapy did increase the risk of stroke. The Heart and Estrogen/Progestin Replacement Study (HERS) studied women who were given conjugated equine estrogen (Premarin)/medroxyprogesterone (Provera) or placebo and had one or more cardiovascular risk factors.[199,200] Overall there was no significant difference in strokes, but a 1.6 relative risk for fatal strokes. The Women's Estrogen Stroke Trial (WEST) studied 1 mg of 17-beta estradiol (Estrace) versus placebo as hormonal replacement in postmenopausal women.[201] There was no overall difference in strokes or deaths between groups, but there was an increased incidence of strokes during the first 6 months in the Estrace replacement group (relative risk of 2.3; 95% confidence interval, 1.1 to 5.0).

The Women's Health Initiative (WHI), which included 162,000 postmenopausal women aged 50 to 79, was the largest study.[202,203] The cumulative hazards for stroke were 1.3 in an intention-to-treat analysis and 1.5 in an on-treatment analysis. Another study within the Women's Health Initiative studied 10,739 postmenopausal women who had hysterectomies and were treated with either conjugated equine estrogen (Premarin) or placebo.[204] There was no impact on heart disease, but there was an increased frequency of venous thrombosis and stroke in the Premarin-treated group.

Sedentary Lifestyle and Lack of Exercise

The effect of physical activity and exercise on health and disease has been the focus of much attention. In a study of 7735 British middle-aged men, regular, moderate-degree physical activity reduced the risk of stroke and heart attacks, but more vigorous physical activity did not confer any further protection.[205] Similarly, in the North Manhattan Stroke Study,[206] Copenhagen City Heart Study,[207] Reykjavik (Iceland) Study,[208] and

in patients in Seoul, Korea,[209] participation in at least moderate-degree physical activity had a protective effect against stroke when compared with individuals who did not exercise regularly. This finding was true for men and women. Lee and Paffenbarger studied the relationship between physical activity (walking, climbing stairs, sports participation, and recreational physical activities) and stroke risk among 11,130 men who were Harvard University alumni.[210] They found that decreased stroke risk was found at energy expenditures of 1000 to 1999 kcal per week, with further decrements found at 2000 to 2999 kcal per week. Higher rates of exercise did not further decrease the risk of stroke.[210] In the Physicians Health Study among 21,823 male physicians, regular exercise that was vigorous enough to produce a sweat was associated with decreased stroke risk.[211] In the Nurses Health Study, among 72,488 female nurses, physical activity including moderate-intensive exercise such as walking was associated with substantial reduction in risk of total and ischemic stroke.[212] A meta-analysis of 23 studies concluded that there was strong evidence that moderate and high levels of physical activity were associated with reduced risk of total, ischemic, and hemorrhagic stroke.[213] The mechanism by which exercise decreases stroke risk is likely multifactoral, reducing hypertension,[214-216] weight, and lipids, and increasing cerebral blood flow by a salutary effect on cerebral endothelial activity.[217]

Geographic Location

In the United States, physicians and epidemiologists have long been aware of a so-called "stroke belt." This region of high incidence of stroke and stroke mortality is located within the southeastern portion of the United States, with extreme mortality rates in Georgia and the Carolinas.[218-220] Clusters of regions with high stroke mortality rates also exist along the Mississippi and Ohio river valleys.[218] Residence in these regions conveys to men and women of all races/ethnicities a strikingly higher rate of stroke than in other locations within the United States.[219] The excess stroke risk for individuals living in the stroke belt seems limited to those who were there during childhood and not those who moved there as adults.[221] Hypertension is very common in these regions, especially among blacks.[222] The reason for the presence of such a stroke belt remains mostly obscure, but many factors, such as the genetic makeup of the people; distribution of stroke risk factors, including hypertension and cigarette smoking; dietary habits; and even constituents of the water have been posited.

Subclinical Brain, Eye, and Systemic Lesions That Indicate the Presence of Vascular Disease and Vascular Risks

Modern brain imaging often reveals abnormalities related to vascular diseases even when an individual has not had a known stroke. The most important vascular-related abnormalities are unexpected brain infarcts, white matter lesions, and microbleeds. Any of these findings indicate that a vascular process is biologically active despite the fact that there is no history of a stroke.

Unexpected Brain Infarcts

CT and MRI scans very often reveal definite brain infarcts even when the patient gives no history of stroke. In the Rotterdam Scan Study, a population-based cohort study of 1077 individuals aged 60 to 90, silent brain infarcts were five times more common than symptomatic brain infarcts.[223] Although these have traditionally been called "silent infarcts," I prefer the term *unexpected infarcts*. Often these infarcts were not truly silent but were not suspected by the individual who ordered the brain image. In my experience, even though the patient may not give a history of having had a stroke, a wife or other accompanying person will remind the patient of an incident (e.g., "Don't you remember at Ms X's house, you stumbled and had difficulty walking for a few days, and then got better."). Often symptoms had been present but were misinterpreted as arthritis, the flu, too much alcohol, and so on. In other patients, findings on neurologic examination give strong evidence of past brain vascular-related damage, but the patient and his or her family give no history of one or more acute events. Whether brain infarcts are truly silent depends very much on the zeal and time spent by the examiner in taking a detailed history from the patient and significant others and careful examination of the patient as well as the size and location of the brain infarcts.

Unexpected brain infarcts are seen more often on T2-weighted and FLAIR MRI scans than on brain CT scans.[224] These infarcts fall into two large groups with varying significance: small deep infarcts (lacunes), and cortical or cortical and subcortical infarcts. Lacunes are often accompanied by white matter hyperintensities. These lesions give evidence that the patient has a biologically active process that has already damaged the brain. Usually this means inadequately controlled hypertension, diabetes, or polycythemia. Cortical-subcortical infarcts mean that the individual must harbor a source of embolism or hypoperfusion in the cardiac-aortic-extracranial-intracranial pathway that supplies the infarct. This should lead to a search for one or more culprit vascular lesions along this pathway.

White Matter Lesions

Abnormal intensity of the white matter is often found on brain imaging scans of elderly individuals. CT often shows periventricular hypodensities. On MRI, the findings are more obvious and dramatic, with zones of periventricular increased density on T2-weighted images and patchy white matter abnormalities.[225] Often these periventricular abnormalities are related to Alzheimer disease, especially if the lesions are uniform and surround the ventricles. In some other patients, the periventricular lesions represent transependymal flow of CSF and not active vascular disease. When the white matter abnormalities are irregular and are located in the corona radiata or centrum semi-ovale and jut out from the periventricular area into these regions, then active vascular disease is present. Most often the condition is one that predisposes to penetrating artery disease—hypertension, diabetes, or hyperviscosity.[226-229] In some patients, these white matter lesions are attributable to cerebral amyloid angiopathy, especially when small hemorrhages are also evident on T2*-weighted MRI images.[230-232] White matter abnormalities are often seen before clinical symptoms in patients with CADASIL.[233-235] These white matter abnormalities and conditions that cause them are discussed in more detail in Chapter 8 on penetrating artery disease.

Microbleeds

Echo planar MRI scans often show small old lesions that image as discrete, black, usually round abnormalities. These black regions indicate that hemosiderin or blood is present. Some of these discrete black images are small blood vessels cut transversely. These abnormalities are often referred to as *microbleeds*. Some likely represent hemosiderin within or adjacent to small infarcts and are not truly bleeds in the strict sense. Others are tiny dot hemorrhages.[236-238] The two most common conditions that produce small hemorrhages are hypertension and cerebral amyloid angiopathy. Microbleeds are often accompanied by white matter abnormalities in patients with cerebral amyloid angiopathy and are likely predictive of future hemorrhages.[236] Some lesions that appear black on Echo planar MRI represent cavernous angiomas. Chapter 12 discusses these lesions in more detail.

Other Target Organ Vascular Damage

The retina provides ready access to view blood vessels, and of course, is supplied by the internal carotid artery that also supplies the brain. Old retinal infarcts, Hollenhorst plaques and other retinal emboli,[239,240] and the presence of venous stasis retinopathy[241,242] provide evidence of a potential embolic source or severe occlusive disease in the heart-aorta-carotid-ophthalmic artery pathway. These and other ocular signs of carotid artery disease are discussed in Chapter 6.

Recently my colleagues and I were surprised to find on abdominal imaging (often done for belly pain and not neurologic reasons) discrete infarcts in the spleen, kidneys, or other visceral organs. One such patient had bacterial endocarditis, and another had intermittent atrial fibrillation that was not suspected until after the abdominal scans were interpreted. We know that systemic embolisms to peripheral and visceral locations are often present but difficult to diagnose clinically. The presence of visceral infarcts gives strong evidence of a source of embolism in the heart or aorta. Abdominal imaging has often been useful in seeking such evidence of systemic embolization in puzzling cases.

Subclinical Cardio-Cervico-Cranial-Hematologic Lesions

Physicians are now able to detect many different cardio-vascular-hematologic lesions that, although not known to have caused strokes, pose risks for causing brain damage. I list some of these in Table 17-2.

Cardiac and Aortic

Many cardiac conditions pose a risk for stroke. The heart often serves as an embolic source. Furthermore, coronary artery disease often parallels extracranial vascular occlusive disease and itself poses strong health and mortality risks for patients. EKG can detect regions of myocardial hypertrophy and ischemic damage and identify arrhythmias. In patients suspected of having an arrhythmia, ambulatory cardiac rhythm monitoring can document atria fibrillation, sick-sinus syndrome, and other important rhythm disturbances. Transthoracic echocardiography yields a good image of the cardiac valves and ventricles and can show areas of akinesis, hypokinesis, and generalized cardiac dysfunction with a low ejection fraction. Transesophageal echocardiography shows the atria, and is useful in identifying cardiac septal abnormalities as well as providing a view of the aortic arch and ascending aorta. Large

Table 17-2.	Subclinical Cardiac-Cervico-Cranial-Hematologic Lesions

Cardiac valvular lesions
Myocardial infarcts
Myocardiopathies with poor ejection fractions
Atrial fibrillation
Aortic atheromas
Plaques or stenosis of carotid and/or vertebral arteries in neck
Carotid intima-media thickness
Stenosis of intracranial arteries
Dolichoectasia of intracranial arteries
Unruptured aneurysms
Polycythemia or anemia
Thrombocytosis or thrombocytopenia
Hypercoagulability

aortic plaques are readily visible on TEE. Noninvasive coronary artery imaging using modern MRI can show coronary artery calcifications that correlate well with coronary artery occlusive disease. Coronary angiography is sometimes useful even in asymptomatic patients in whom the EKG, echocardiogram, stress testing, or noninvasive vascular imaging gives rise to a strong suspicion of important coronary artery disease. Cardiac evaluation is discussed in more detail in Chapter 4 on diagnosis and Chapter 9 on brain embolism.

Abnormalities in Cervico-Cranial and Intracranial Arteries That Supply the Brain

Patients with extracranial carotid and vertebral artery plaques and thickened arterial walls have atherosclerosis, and thus have a higher risk of ischemic strokes and brain and retinal infarcts.[243-245] The risk increases proportionately to the severity of arterial stenosis and also correlates with the presence of ulcerated carotid artery plaques. Narrowing and plaques within the proximal portion of the vertebral artery also correlate with the presence of carotid artery and coronary artery disease.[244,245] The availability of duplex carotid and vertebral artery ultrasound scanning makes it possible to objectively detect and measure the severity of atherosclerotic abnormalities within the extracranial arteries. The intima-media thickness of the carotid artery is also an important parameter to study since increased thickness correlates with atherosclerotic disease. The progression or regression of these abnormalities during and after treatment gives clinicians a means of monitoring the atherosclerotic process in the arteries studied. The presence of a neck bruit should not be used as a risk factor because some bruits are not associated with carotid or vertebral artery disease. Ultrasound studies should be performed in patients who have bruits thought to indicate atherosclerotic narrowing to identify and quantify the disease. MRA and CTA are other relatively noninvasive techniques able to provide useful images of the cervical brain-supplying arteries.

The intracranial arteries can also be studied effectively using Doppler techniques (transcranial Doppler [TCD]) and CTA and MRA. Occlusive lesions, vasoconstriction, dolichoectasia can all be identified and monitored, often before a stroke develops. At times these diagnostic techniques also show aneurysms that have not ruptured, yielding an opportunity to prevent devastating subarachnoid hemorrhage. Vascular imaging is discussed in detail in Chapter 4.

Hematologic Abnormalities

Polycythemia and severe anemia both predispose to stroke and cerebral venous occlusions. Thrombocytosis and thrombocytopenia also convey important stroke risks. A complete blood count including a platelet count and a prothrombin time reported as an international normalized ratio (INR) should be part of the routine evaluation for stroke risk.

BIOMARKERS AND GENETIC FINDINGS AND CONDITIONS KNOWN TO RELATE TO VASCULAR DISEASE

Results of blood and urine tests of certain factors also correlate with the probability of an individual developing a stroke. I list these in Table 17-3. These biomarkers have also been discussed in Chapter 4. Pathologically elevated and high normal hematocrits have been associated with increased stroke and TIA risk even when hypertension and cigarette smoking are accounted for in the analysis.[246,247] High hemoglobin levels are also correlated with the

Table 17-3.	**Biomarkers That Correlate with Cardiovascular and Cerebrovascular Disease**

Hematocrit
White blood count
C-reactive protein (CRP)
Homocysteine
Erythrocyte sedimentation rate (ESR)
Fibrinogen
Albuminuria

presence of brain infarction[248] and larger brain infarcts.[249] This correlation might be partly caused by the fact that chronic hypoxemia, pulmonary disease, and smoking may have caused high hematocrits. The adverse effect of high hematocrits could also relate to increased whole-blood viscosity.[249,250] Cerebral blood flow nearly doubles when a hematocrit of 45 is lowered to 35.

The white blood cell (WBC) count is often elevated in patients with myocardial infarction and is also often slightly high in patients with brain infarcts. In the Northern Manhattan Study, there was an increased risk of ischemic stroke with each quartile of WBC even after adjusting for other stroke risk factors.[251] A high WBC count has been correlated with the severity of carotid atherosclerosis[252] and carotid[253] and aortic arch plaque[254] thickness, but interpretation of this finding is clouded by the fact that cigarette smoking is one cause of a high WBC count. A high WBC at entry into the Warfarin-Aspirin Symptomatic Intracranial Disease (WASID) trial was associated with an increased risk of stroke and vascular death when compared with patients with the lowest quartile of WBC counts.[255] Patients with elevated WBC counts also seem to have reduced endothelial reactivity.[256] A high WBC count is also a marker of inflammatory activity in the body and inflammation is an important cause of blood vessel damage.[257]

Elevated, high-sensitivity C-reactive protein levels correlate with a risk of stroke, cardiovascular disease, and carotid and intracranial large-artery atherosclerosis.[258-260] Some patients with significant atherosclerotic lesions have normal lipids but high CRP levels, indicating the likely importance of inflammation in contributing to their vascular disease.

The plasma level of fibrinogen is also an important determinant of stroke risk. Individuals with high levels of fibrinogen have an increased risk of developing myocardial infarction and stroke.[261-263] Fibrinogen levels relate to age, sex, female hormone status, smoking, body weight, alcohol intake, and the presence of vascular and inflammatory diseases.[262] Fibrinogen is an important participant in the development of red and white thrombi. Along with the hematocrit, fibrinogen is an important determinant of whole-blood viscosity.[263,264]

Elevated levels of plasma homocysteine increase the risk of developing myocardial infarction and stroke.[265-268] The risk is important especially when the homocysteine level is quite high. High plasma homocysteine levels and low concentrations of folic acid and vitamin B_6 (probably because of their role in homocysteine metabolism) are associated with increased risk of large artery atherosclerosis.[269,270] There is also an association with penetrating artery disease.[270] I have seen several patients with very high homocysteine levels (>40) that had repeated penetrating artery-related lacunar strokes.

Glycosuria and heavy proteinuria predispose to stroke. Even relatively small amounts of protein in the urine (microalbuminuria) and reduced glomerular filtration rate are risk factors for stroke.[271-273,273a] Chronic kidney disease is also associated with brain white matter hyperintensities.[273b] In a study of 186 older men and women (average age, 65 years), the presence of microalbuminuria (20 to 200 mg/L) was three times more prevalent in patients with recent stroke when compared with normal, healthy individuals and individuals with risk factors for stroke who did not have a recent stroke.[271] One study showed that intensive, multifactorial, therapeutic interventions in patients with non–insulin-dependent diabetes and microalbuminuria did decrease the incidence of macrovascular events (myocardial infarcts and stroke).[272]

Genetic Conditions

Some genetic disorders, such as Fabry's disease, homocystinuria, Ehlers-Danlos syndrome, and pseudoxanthoma elasticum, are recognized to confer increased stroke risk. Various genetically-related disorders affect blood coagulability including factor V Leiden and a prothrombin gene mutation. Research on genetic determinants of atherosclerosis, hypertension, stroke, and other vascular disease is progressing at a rapid rate. This research gives promise for unlocking some of the present mysteries and uncertainties about stroke development, especially among the young.[274-280] Genetic disorders are considered in Chapters 4 and 11.

STROKE PREVENTION

Prevention is customarily separated into primary prevention (strategies to prevent stroke in patients who have never had a stroke) and secondary prevention (strategies to prevent a stroke recurrence).

Primary Prevention

For primary prevention, public education must be improved, especially in underdeveloped countries. Improvement in general health practices in the population undoubtedly decreases modifiable stroke risk factors in many patients. Educating the public in general to implement good general health measures probably would have a large impact on the frequency of stroke and other cardiovascular disease. The public should be encouraged to stop smoking, avoid excessive alcohol intake, exercise regularly, make time for leisure activities, avoid becoming overweight, and decrease intake of foods high in fat and cholesterol.

The risk of stroke, however, varies greatly among individuals and depends heavily on individual factors present in each person. For example, some individuals can eat large quantities of eggs, milk, ice cream, and red meat and still have quite normal serum cholesterol and lipid values, whereas in others, simply smelling foods high in cholesterol seems to send their cholesterol levels skyrocketing. I have already emphasized the importance of hereditary diseases in the family and beginning awareness early in life. I believe that each individual should become aware of the cardiovascular disorders and stroke and heart disease risk factors prevalent in their families. Periodic check-ups with physicians who monitor blood pressure, weight, blood sugar and lipid levels, and who inquire about habits and health practices are important. This strategy is especially important for the children of patients who have had a myocardial infarct, stroke, or important stroke risk factors, such as hypertension, diabetes, and hypercholesterolemia.

When multiple risk factors are considered together, patients at particular risk for stroke can be identified. When systolic hypertension, elevated serum cholesterol, glucose intolerance, cigarette smoking, and electrocardiogram findings of left ventricular hypertrophy are combined, a population accounting for one third of all strokes can be identified.[129] Wolf and his colleagues created a stroke risk-factor score based on data obtained from the Framingham Study, which reflects an individual's 10-year probability of having a stroke.[281,282]

Secondary Prevention

For secondary stroke prevention, identification of the mechanism of the initial stroke is most important. In patients who have lacunar infarcts caused by penetrating artery disease due to hypertension and in patients who have hypertensive ICHs, control of blood pressure is the most important strategy. In patients with severe carotid artery stenosis, surgery or angioplasty of the involved carotid artery may be the best strategy for secondary prevention. In patients with non-stenosing plaques, statins, and an agent that decreases platelet functions, such as aspirin, clopidogrel, or combined low-dose aspirin and modified-release dipyridamole, are probably most effective. In patients who have had brain embolism caused by atrial fibrillation, anticoagulation with coumadin represents the best strategy for secondary stroke prevention unless contraindications to the use of coumadin are present.

In most patients, recurrent strokes are caused by the same mechanism as the initial stroke.[283] Sometimes, second and third strokes, however, have a different stroke mechanism than the initial stroke.[283,284] For example, some patients with atrial fibrillation also have hypertension and carotid artery disease. Their initial stroke may have been caused by their carotid artery disease, but atrial fibrillation poses a threat for brain embolism. The results of the North American Symptomatic Carotid Endarterectomy Trial, which included patients with various severities of carotid artery occlusive disease and excluded patients with cardiac lesions thought to carry high risk of cardioembolism, found that a significant number of strokes were caused by cardioembolism and penetrating artery disease.[285] Identification of all stroke risk factors by thorough cardiac, cerebrovascular, and blood evaluations at the time of the initial stroke allows factors and lesions present in the individual to be recognized and creates a database for the logical selection of strategies for secondary prevention of stroke and myocardial infarction.[284] Even when stroke has already occurred, treatment of identifiable stroke risk factors, such as hypertension, was shown in one study to decrease the expected mortality and stroke recurrence rate during the 5 years after the first stroke.[286] Several studies document that the optimal opportunity to begin secondary stroke prevention is when the patient is still in the hospital.[287,288] Computerized programs can ensure that, upon discharge, key preventive strategies are addressed and appropriate follow-up care is arranged. Doctors who have treated the patient in the hospital must communicate with the patient's primary physician the findings, recommendations, medications, instructions, and treatment plan.

The incidence of stroke is declining, but much more can be done. Advances will probably involve the following:

- Improved general health measures initiated by individuals concerned about their bodies.
- Education for patients regarding the symptoms and significance of hypertension, excess weight, exercise, and TIAs. Patients should become educated consumers who recognize and seek the most competent care.
- Education for the public about the brain and symptoms that might indicate stroke and other brain diseases.

- Education of general physicians. Physicians should know about the warning signs of stroke, stroke risk factors, and how to manage patients with cerebrovascular disease.
- Education of neurologists, vascular surgeons, neurosurgeons, and other stroke specialists. These specialists should know when and how to manage risk factors, as well as how to treat the presenting stroke problem.
- Basic and clinical research. This will surely advance the present capabilities for diagnosing and treating stroke patients and stroke-prone individuals.

References

1. Pasteur L: Address to the Fraternal Association of former students of the École Centrale des Arts et Manufactures, Paris, May 15, 1884.
2. Sug YS, Heller RF, Levi C, et al: Knowledge of stroke risk factors, warning symptoms, and treatment among an Australian urban population. Stroke 2001;32:1926-1930.
3. Schneider AT, Pancioli AM, Khoury JC, et al: Trends in community knowledge of the warning signs and risk factors for stroke. JAMA 2003;289: 343-346.
4. Kothari R, Sauerbeck L, Jauch E, et al: Patients' awareness of stroke signs, symptoms, and risk factors. Stroke 1997;28:1871-1875.
5. Pandian JD, Jaison A, Deepak SS, et al: Public awareness of warning symptoms, risk factors, and treatment of stroke in northwest India. Stroke 2005;36:644-648.
6. Maasland L, Koudstaal PJ, Habbema JD, Dippel DW: Knowledge and understanding of disease process, risk factors and treatment modalities in patients with a recent TIA or minor ischemic stroke. Cerebrovasc Dis 2007;23:435-440.
7. Nedeltchev K, Fischer U, Arnold M, et al: Low awareness of transient ischemic attacks and risk factors for stroke in a Swiss urban community. J Neurol 2007;254:179-184.
8. Garraway WM, Whisnant JP, Furlan AJ, et al: The declining incidence of stroke. N Engl J Med 1979;300:449-452.
9. Bonita R, Stewart A, Beaglehole R: International trends in stroke mortality: 1970-1985. Stroke 1990;21:989-992.
10. Sytkowski PA, Kannel WB, D'Agostino RB: Changes in risk factors and the decline in mortality from cardiovascular disease. N Engl J Med 1990;322:1635-1641.
11. Caplan LR, Dyken ML, Easton JD: American Heart Association Family Guide to Stroke Treatment, Recovery, and Prevention. New York: Random House-Times Books, 1994.
12. Hutton C, Caplan LR: Striking Back at Stroke: A Doctor-Patient Journal. New York: Dana Press, 2003.
13. Caplan LR: Stroke. New York: Demos-American Academy of Neurology, 2005.

17

14. Sacco RL: The 2006 William Feinberg lecture. Shifting the paradigm from stroke to global vascular risk estimation. Stroke 2007;38:1980-1987.

15. Wolf P, Dyken M, Barnett HJM, et al: Risk factors in stroke. Stroke 1984;15:1105-1111.

16. Shaper AG, Phillips AN, Pocock SJ, et al: Risk factors for stroke in middle-aged British men. BMJ 1991;302:1111-1115.

17. Matchar DB, McCrory DC, Barnett HJM, Feussner JR: Medical treatment for stroke prevention. Ann Intern Med 1994;121:41-53.

18. Bronner LL, Kanter DS, Manson JE: Primary prevention of stroke. N Engl J Med 1995;333: 1392-1400.

19. Kalra L, Perez I, Melbourn A: Stroke risk management. Change in mainstream practice. Stroke 1998;29:53-57.

20. Gorelick PB, Sacco RL, Smith DB, et al: Prevention of a first stroke. A review of guidelines and a multidisciplinary consensus statement from the National Stroke Association. JAMA 1999;281:1112-1120.

21. Whisnant JP: Stroke Populations, Cohorts, and Clinical Trials. Boston: Butterworth-Heinemann, 1993.

22. Dorndorf W, Marx P: Stroke Prevention. Basel: Karger, 1994.

23. Norris JW, Hachinski VC: Prevention of Stroke. New York: Springer, 1991.

24. Gorelick PB, Alter M: The Prevention of Stroke. Boca Raton, Fla: Parthenon Publishing Group, 2002.

25. Sobel E, Altu M, Davanipour Z, et al: Stroke in the Lehigh Valley: Combined risk factors for recurrent ischemic stroke. Neurology 1989;39:669-672.

26. Davis PH, Dambrosia JM, Schoenberg BS, et al: Risk factors for ischemic stroke: A prospective study in Rochester, Minnesota. Ann Neurol 1987;22:319-327.

27. Simons LA, McCallum J, Friedlander Y, Simons J: Risk factors for ischemic stroke. Dubbo study of the elderly. Stroke 1998;29:1341-1346.

28. Whisnant JP, Wiebers DO, O'Fallon WM, et al: A population-based model of risk factors for ischemic stroke: Rochester, Minnesota. Neurology 1996;47:1420-1428.

29. Sacco RL: Risk factors, outcomes, and stroke subtypes for ischemic stroke. Neurology 1997; 49 (suppl 4):S39-S44.

30. Goldstein LB, Adams R, Becker K, et al: Primary prevention of ischemic stroke: A statement for healthcare professionals from the Stroke Council of the American Heart Association. Stroke 2001;32: 280-299.

31. Johnson P, Rosewell M, James MA: How good is the management of vascular risk after stroke, transient ischemic attack, or carotid endarterectomy? Cerebrovasc Dis 2007;32:156-161.

32. Romero JR: Prevention of ischemic stroke: overview of traditional risk factors. Curr Drug Targets 2007;8:794-801.

33. Longstreth WT, Koepsell T, Yerby M, et al: Risk factors for subarachnoid hemorrhage. Stroke 1985;16:377-385.

34. Teunissen LL, Rinkel GJE, Algra A, van Gijn J: Risk factors for subarachnoid hemorrhage. A systematic review. Stroke 1996;27:544-549.

35. Qureshi AI, Suri MF, Yahia AM, et al: Risk factors for subarachnoid hemorrhage. Neurosurgery 2001;49:607-612.

36. Isaksen J, Egge A, Waterloo K, et al: Risk factors for aneurysmal subarachnoid haemorrhage: The Tromso study. J Neurol Neurosurg Psychiatry 2002;73:185-187.

37. Ohkuma H, Tabata H, Suzuki S, Islam S: Risk factors for aneurysmal subarachnoid hemorrhage in Aomori, Japan. Stroke 2003;34:96-100.

38. Broderick JP: Intracerebral hemorrhage. In Gorelick PB, Alter M (eds): Handbook of Neuroepidemiology. New York: Marcel Dekker, 1994, pp 141-167.

39. Qureshi AI, Suri MA, Safdar K, et al: Intracerebral hemorrhage in blacks: Risk factors, subtypes, and outcome. Stroke 1997;28:961-964.

40. Bateman BT, Schumacher HC, Bushnell CD, et al: Intracerebral hemorrhage in pregnancy: Frequency, risk factors, and outcome. Neurology 2006;67: 424-429.

41. Mitchell P, Mitra D, Gregson BA, Mendelow AD: Prevention of intracerebral haemorrhage. Curr Drug Targets 2007;8:832-838.

42. Caplan LR: Brain embolism. In Caplan LR, Hurst JW, Chimowitz M (eds): Clinical Neuro-cardiology. New York: Marcel Dekker, 1999, pp 35-185.

43. Caplan LR, Manning WJ: Brain Embolism. New York: Informa Healthcare, 2006.

44. Gorelick PB, Caplan LR, Hier DB, et al: Racial differences in the distribution of anterior circulation occlusive cerebrovascular disease. Neurology 1984;34:54-59.

45. Gorelick PB, Caplan LR, Hier DB, et al: Racial differences in the distribution of posterior circulation occlusive disease. Stroke 1985;16:785-790.

46. Caplan LR: Race, sex, and occlusive cerebrovascular disease: A review. Stroke 1986;17:648-655.

47. Caplan LR: Cerebral ischemia and infarction in blacks. Clinical, autopsy, and angiographic studies. In Gillum RF, Gorelick PB, Cooper ES (eds): Stroke in Blacks. Basel: Karger, 1999, pp 7-18.

48. White H, Boden-Albala B, Wang C, et al: Ischemic stroke subtype incidence among whites, blacks, and Hispanics: The Northern Manhattan Study. Circulation 2005;111:1327-1331.

49. Sacco RL, Kargman DE, Gu Q, Zamanillo MC: Race-ethnicity and determinants of intracranial atherosclerotic cerebral infarction. The Northern Manhattan Stroke Study. Stroke 1995;26:14-20.

50. Lewington S, Clarke R, Qizilbash N, et al: Age-specific relevance of usual blood pressure to vascular mortality: A meta-analysis of individual data for one million adults in 61 prospective studies. Lancet 2002;360:1903-1913.

51. Kannel WB: Current status of the epidemiology of brain infarction associated with occlusive vascular disease. Stroke 1971;2:295-318.

52. Gebel J, Broderick J: Primary intracerebral hemorrhage and subarachnoid hemorrhage in black patients: Risk factors, diagnosis, and prognosis. In Gillum RF, Gorelick PB, Cooper ES (eds): Stroke in Blacks. Basel: Karger, 1999, pp 29-35.

53. Kiely DK, Wolf PA, Cupples LA, et al: Family aggregation of stroke: The Framingham Study. Stroke 1993;24:1366-1371.

54. Liao D, Myers R, Hunt S, et al: Family history of stroke and stroke risk. The Family Heart Study. Stroke 1997;28:1908-1912.

55. Wannamethee SG, Shaper AG, Ebrahim S: History of parental death from stroke or heart trouble and the risk of stroke in middle-aged men. Stroke 1996;27:1492-1498.

56. Jousilahri P, Rastenyte D, Tuomilehto J, et al: Parental history of cardiovascular disease and risk of stroke. A prospective follow-up of 14,371 middle-aged men and women in Finland. Stroke 1997;28:1361-1366.

57. Meschia JF, Case LD, Worrall BB, et al: Ischemic Stroke Genetics Study Group. Family history of stroke and severity of neurologic deficit after stroke. Neurology 2006;67:1396-1402.

58. McGill HC, Arias-Stella J, Carbonell LM, et al: General findings of the International Atherosclerosis Project. Lab Invest 1968;18:498-502.

59. Solberg LA, McGarry PA, Moosy J, et al: Distribution of cerebral atherosclerosis by geographic location, race, and sex. Lab Invest 1968;158:604-612.

60. Kannel WB: Blood pressure as a cardiovascular risk factor. JAMA 1996;275:1571-1576.

61. National Heart, Lung, and Blood Institute: Working Group Report on Primary Prevention of Hypertension: National High Blood Pressure Education program. NHLBI doc 93-2669. Bethesda, Md: National Institutes of Health, 1993.

62. American Heart Association: Heart Disease and Stroke Statistics 2006 Update. Available at http://www.americanheart.org/presenter.jhtml.

63. Chobanian AV, Bakris GL, Black HR, et al: The seventh report of the Joint National Committee on Prevention, Detection, Evaluation, and Treatment of High Blood Pressure. JAMA 2003;289:2560-2572.

64. Prospective Studies Collaboration: Age-specific relevance of usual blood pressure to vascular mortality: A meta-analysis of individual data for one million adults in 61 prospective studies. Lancet 2002;360:1903-1913.

65. Gueyffier F, Bulpitt C, Boissel J-P, et al: Antihypertensive drugs in very old people: A subgroup meta-analysis of randomized controlled trials. Lancet 1999;353:793-796.

66. Howard G, Manolio TA, Burke GL, et al: Does the association of risk factors and atherosclerosis change with age? Stroke 1997;28:1693-1701.

66a. Beckett NS, Peters R, Fletcher AE, et al: Treatment of hypertension in patients 80 years of age or older. HYVET Study Group. N Engl J Med 2008;358:1887-1898.

67. SHEP Cooperative Research Group: Prevention of stroke by antihypertensive drug treatment in older persons with isolated systolic hypertension. JAMA 1991;265:3255-3264.

68. Sutton-Tyrrell K, Alcorn HG, Herzog H, et al: Morbidity, mortality, and antihypertensive treatment effects by extent of atherosclerosis in older adults with isolated systolic hypertension. Stroke 1995;26:1319-1324.

69. Davis BR, Vogt T, Frost PH, et al: Risk factors for stroke and type of stroke in persons with isolated systolic hypertension. The Systolic Hypertension in the Elderly Program (SHEP) Research Group. Stroke 1998;29:1333-1340.

70. Perry HM, Davis BR, Price TR, et al: Effect of treating isolated systolic hypertension on the risk of developing various types and subtypes of stroke. Systolic Hypertension in the Elderly Program (SHEP) Cooperative Research Group. JAMA 2000;284:465-471.

71. Staessen JA, Gasowski J, Wang JG, et al: Risks of untreated and treated isolated systolic hypertension in the elderly: Meta-analysis of outcome trials. Lancet 2000;355:865-872.

72. Bowman TS, Gaziano JM, Kase CS, et al: Blood pressure measures and risk of total, ischemic, and hemorrhagic stroke in men. Neurology 2006;67:820-823.

73. Chobanian AV: Isolated systolic hypertension in the elderly. N Engl J Med 2007;357:789-796.

74. Wenger NK: Hypertension and other cardiovascular risk factors in women. Am J Hypertens 1995;8:94S-99S.

75. Rothwell PM, Coull AJ, Silver LE, et al: Population-based study of event-rate, incidence, case fatality, and mortality for all acute vascular events in all arterial territories (Oxford Vascular Study). Lancet 2005;366:1773-1783.

75a. Mitchell GF, Ramachandran SV, Keyes MJ, et al: Pulse-pressure and risk of new-onset atrial fibrillation. JAMA 2007;297:709-715.

76. Weitzman D, Goldbourt U: The significance of various blood pressure indices for long-term stroke, coronary heart disease, and all-cause mortality in men. The Israeli Ischemic Heart Disease Study. Stroke 2006;37:358-363.

77. Paultre F, Mosca L: Association of blood pressure indices and stroke mortality in isolated systolic hypertension. Stroke 2005;36:1288-1290.

78. Vemmos KN, Tsivgoulis G, Spengos K, et al: Pulse pressure in acute stroke is an independent predictor of long-term mortality. Cerebrovasc Dis 2004;18:30-36.

79. Watanabe N, Imai Y, Nagai K, et al: Nocturnal blood pressure and silent cerebrovascular lesions in elderly Japanese. Stroke 1996;27:1319-1327.

80. Yamamoto Y, Akiguchi I, Oiwa K, et al: Adverse effect of nighttime blood pressure on the outcome of lacunar infarct patients. Stroke 1998;29:570-576.

81. Lip GY, Zarifis J, Farooqi S, et al: Ambulatory blood pressure monitoring in acute stroke. The West Birmingham Stroke Project. Stroke 1997;28:31-35.

82. Staessen JA, Thijs L, Fagard R, et al: Predicting cardiovascular risk using conventional vs ambulatory blood pressure in older patients with systolic hypertension. Systolic Hypertension in the Europe Trial Investigators. JAMA 1999;282:539-546.

83. Goldstein IB, Bartzokis G, Guthrie D, Shapiro D: Ambulatory blood pressure and the brain. A 5-year follow-up. Neurology 2005;64:1846-1852.

84. Tsivgoulis G, Spengos K, Zakopoulos N, et al: Twenty-four-hour pulse pressure predicts long-term recurrence in acute stroke patients. J Neurol Neurosurg Psychiatry 2005;76: 1360-1365.

85. Rashid P, Leonardi-Bee J, Bath P: Blood pressure reduction and secondary prevention of stroke and other vascular events. A systematic review. Stroke 2003;34:2741-2749.

86. Psaty BM, Lumley T, Furberg CD, et al: Health outcomes associated with various antihypertensive therapies used as first-line agents. JAMA 2003;289:2534-2544.

87. Blood Pressure Lowering Treatment Trialists' Collaboration: Effects of different blood-pressure-lowering regimens on major cardiovascular events: Results of prospectively-designed overviews of randomized trials. Lancet 2003;362: 1527-1535.

88. Hall WD, Kong W: Hypertension in blacks: nonpharmacologic and pharmacologic therapy. In Saunders E (ed): Cardiovascular Disease in Blacks. Philadelphia: FA Davis, 1991, pp 157-169.

89. Rajagopalan S, Harrison D: Reversing endothelial dysfunction with ACE inhibitors. A new trend? Circulation 1996;94:240-243.

90. Bosch J, Yusuf S, Pogue J, et al: Use of ramipril in preventing stroke: Double blind randomized trial. HOPE Investigators. BMJ 2002;324:1-5.

91. van Gijn J: The PROGRESS Trial: Preventing strokes by lowering blood pressure in patients with cerebral ischemia. Stroke 2002;33:319-320.

92. Hankey GJ: Angiotensin-converting enzyme inhibitors for stroke prevention. Is there HOPE for PROGRESS after LIFE? Stroke 2003;34:354-356.

93. Chapman N, Huxley R, Anderson C, et al: Effects of a perendopril-based blood pressure-lowering regimen on the risk of recurrent stroke according to stroke subtype and medical history. The PROGRESS Trial. Stroke 2004;35: 116-121.

94. Iadecola C, Gorelick PB: Hypertension, angiotensin, and stroke: Beyond blood pressure. Stroke 2004;35:348-350.

95. Toole JF, Janeway R, Choi K, et al: Transient ischemic attacks due to atherosclerosis: A prospective study of 160 patients. Arch Neurol 1975;32:5-12.

96. Chimowitz MI, Weiss DG, Cohen SL, et al: Veterans Affairs Cooperative Study Group 167. Cardiac prognosis of patients with carotid stenosis and no history of coronary artery disease. Stroke 1994;25:759-765.

97. Chimowitz MI: Asymptomatic coronary artery disease in patients with carotid artery stenosis: Incidence, prognosis, and treatment. In Caplan LR, Hurst JW, Chimowitz M (eds): Clinical Neurocardiology. New York: Marcel Dekker, 1999, pp 287-295.

98. DECODE Study Group, European Diabetes Epidemiology Group: Glucose tolerance and mortality: Comparison of WHO and American Diabetes Association diagnostic criteria. Lancet 1999;354:617-621.

99. Grundy SM, Brewer Jr B, Cleeman JI, et al: NHLBI/AHA Conference proceedings. Definition of metabolic syndrome. Circulation 2004;109: 433-438.

100. Grundy S, Cleeman JI, Daniels SR, et al: Diagnosis and management of the metabolic syndrome. An American Heart Association/National Heart Lung, and Blood Institute Scientific Statement. Circulation 2005;112: 2735-2752.

101. Bang OY, Kim JW, Lee JH, et al: Association of the metabolic syndrome with intracranial atherosclerotic stroke. Neurology 2005;65: 296-298.

102. Mak KH, Ma S, Heng D, et al: Impact of sex, metabolic syndrome, and diabetes mellitus on cardiovascular events. Am J Cardiol 2007;100: 227-233.

103. Arenillas JF, Moro MA, Dávalos A: The metabolic syndrome and stroke: Potential treatment approaches. Stroke 2007;38:2196-2203.

104. Kurl S, Laukkanen JA, Niskanen L, et al: Metabolic syndrome and the risk of stroke in middle-aged men. Stroke 2006;37:806-811.

104a. Boden-Albala B, Sacco RL, Lee H-S, et al: Metabolic syndrome and ischemic stroke risk. Northern Manhattan Study. Stroke 2008;39:30-35.

104b. Li W, Ma D, Liu M, et al: Association between metabolic syndrome and risk of stroke: A meta-analysis of cohort studies. Cerebrovasc Dis 2008;25:539-547.

105. Mokdad AH, Bowman BA, Ford ES, et al: The continuing epidemics of obesity and diabetes in the United States. JAMA 2001;286: 1195-1200.

106. Kurth T, Gaziano JM, Berger K, et al: Body mass index and the risk of stroke in men. Arch Intern Med 2002;162:2557-2562.

107. Kurth T, Gaziano JM, Rexrode KM, et al: Prospective study of body mass index and risk of stroke in apparently healthy women. Circulation 2005;111:1992-1998.

108. Hu G, Tuomilehto J, Silventoinen K, et al: Body mass index, waist circumference, and waist-hip ratio on the risk of total and type-specific stroke. Arch Intern Med 2007;167: 1420-1427.

109. Depres J-P, Lemieux I, Prud'homme D: Treatment of obesity: need to focus on high risk abdominally obese subjects. BMJ 2001;322: 716-720.

110. Fox CS, Massaro JM, Hoffmann U, et al: Abdominal visceral and subcutaneous adipose tissue compartments: Association with metabolic risk factors in the Framingham Heart Study. Circulation 2007;116:39-48.

111. Lear SA, Humphries KH, Kohli S, et al: Visceral adipose tissue, a potential risk factor for carotid atherosclerosis. Results of the Multicultural Community Health Assessment Trial (M-CHAT). Stroke 2007;38:2422-2429.

112. Suk SH, Sacco RL, Boden-Albala B, et al: Abdominal obesity and risk of ischemic stroke: The Northern Manhattan Stroke Study. Stroke 2003;34:1586-1592.

113. Ruderman N, Chisholm D, Pi-Sunyer X, Schneider S: The metabolically obese, normal weight individual revisited. Diabetes 1998;47: 699-713.

114. McLaughlin T, Allison G, Abbasi F, et al: Prevalence of insulin resistance and associated cardiovascular risk factors among normal weight, overweight, and obese individuals. Metabolism 2004;53:495-499.

115. Schoenberg BS, Schoenberg DG, Pritchard DA, et al: Differential risk factors for completed stroke and transient ischemic attack (TIA): Study of vascular disease (hypertension, cardiac disease, peripheral vascular disease) and diabetes mellitus. Trans Am Neurol Assoc 1980;105: 165-167.

116. Burchfiel CM, Curb D, Rodriguez B, et al: Glucose intolerance and 22-year stroke incidence. The Honolulu Heart Program. Stroke 1994;25:951-957.

117. Jorgenson H, Nakayama H, Raaschou HO, Olsen TS: Stroke in patients with diabetes. The Copenhagen Stroke Study. Stroke 1994;25: 1977-1984.

118. Karapanayiotides TH, Piechowski-Jozwiak B, van Melle G, et al: Stroke patterns, etiology, and prognosis in patients with diabetes mellitus. Neurology 2004;62:1558-1562.

119. Fox C, Coady S, Sorlie P, et al: Increased cardiovascular disease burden due to diabetes mellitus. The Framingham Heart Study. Circulation 2007; 115:1544-1550.

120. Caplan LR: Intracranial branch atheromatous disease: A neglected, understudied, and underused concept. Neurology 1989;39: 1246-1250.

121. Caplan LR: Diabetes and brain ischemia. Diabetes 1996;45 (suppl 3):595-597.

122. Depres J-P, Golay A, Sjostrom L: Effects of rimonabant on metabolic risk factors in overweight patients with dyslipidemia. Rimonabant in Obesity-Lipids Study Group. N Engl J Med 353:2121-2134.

123. Higa M, Davanipour Z: Smoking and stroke. Neuroepidemiology 1991;10:211-222.

124. Love BB, Biller J, Jones MP, et al: Cigarette smoking: A risk factor for cerebral infarction in young adults. Arch Neurol 1990;47: 693-698.

125. Whisnant JP, Homer D, Ingall TJ, et al: Duration of cigarette smoking is the strongest predictor of severe extracranial carotid artery atherosclerosis. Stroke 1990;21:707-714.

126. Ingall TJ, Homer D, Baker HL, et al: Predictors of intracranial carotid artery atherosclerosis: Duration of cigarette smoking and hypertension are more powerful than serum lipid levels. Arch Neurol 1991;48:687-691.

127. Colditz GA, Bonita R, Stampfer MJ, et al: Cigarette smoking and risk of stroke in middle-aged women. N Engl J Med 1988;318:937-941.

128. Donnan GA, You R, Thrift A, McNeil JJ: Smoking as a risk factor for stroke. Cerebrovasc Dis 1993;3:129-138.

129. Wolf P, Kannel WB, Verter J: Current status of risk factors for stroke. In Barnett HJM (ed): Neurologic Clinics, vol 1. Cerebrovascular Disease. Philadelphia: Saunders, 1983, pp 317-343.

130. Paffenbarger R, Williams J: Chronic disease in former college students: V. Early precursors of fatal stroke. Am J Public Health 1967;57: 1290-1299.

131. Kawachi I, Colditz GA: Smoking cessation and decreased risk of stroke in women. JAMA 1993; 269:232-236.

132. Jee SH, Suh I, Kim IS, Appel LJ: Smoking and atherosclerotic cardiovascular disease in men with low levels of serum cholesterol. JAMA 1999;282:2149-2155.

133. Kurth T, Kase CS, Berger K, et al: Smoking and the risk of hemorrhagic stroke in men. Stroke 2003;34:1151-1155.

134. Collaborative Group for the Study of Stroke in Young Women: Oral contraceptives and stroke in young women: Associated risk factors. JAMA 1975;231:718-722.

135. Fust G, Arason GJ, Kramer J, et al: Genetic basis of tobacco smoking: Strong association of a specific major histocompatibility complex haplotype on chromosome 6 with smoking behavior. Int Immunol 2004;16:1507-1514.

136. Arason GJ, Kramer J, Blasko B, et al: Smoking and a complement gene polymorphism interact in promoting cardiovascular disease morbidity and mortality. Clin Exp Immunol 2007;149: 132-138.

137. Tell GS, Crouse JR, Furberg CD: Relation between blood lipids, lipoproteins, and cerebrovascular atherosclerosis. A review. Stroke 1988;19:423-430.

137a. Kurth T, Everett BM, Buring JE, et al: Lipid levels and the risk of ischemic stroke in women. Neurology 2007;68:556-562.

137b. Bang OY, Saver JL, Liebeskind DS, et al: Association of serum lipid indices with large artery atherosclerotic stroke. Neurology 2008; 70:841-847.

138. Kannel WB: Epidemiology of cerebrovascular disease. In Ross-Russel RW (ed): Cerebral Arterial Disease. New York: Churchill Livingstone, 1976, pp 1-23.

139. Kagan A, Popper J, Rhoads G: Factors related to stroke incidence in Hawaiian Japanese men: The Honolulu Heart Study. Stroke 1980; 11:14-21.

140. Stemmerman G, Hayashi T, Resch J, et al: Risk factors related to ischemic and hemorrhagic cerebrovascular disease at autopsy: The Honolulu Heart Study. Stroke 1984;15:23-28.

141. Iso H, Jacobs DR, Wentworth D, et al: Serum cholesterol levels and six year mortality from stroke in 350,977 men screened for the Multiple Risk Factor Intervention Trial. N Engl J Med 1989;320:904-910.

142. Yano K, Reed DM, Maclean CJ: Serum cholesterol and hemorrhagic stroke in the Honolulu Heart Program. Stroke 1989;20:1460-1465.

143. Kurth T, Everett BM, Buring JE, et al: Lipid levels and the risk of ischemic stroke in women. Neurology 2007;68:556-562.

144. Tanne D, Yaari S, Goldbourt U: High-density lipoprotein cholesterol and risk of ischemic stroke mortality. A 21-year follow-up of 8586 men from Israeli Ischemic Heart Disease Study. Stroke 1997;28:83-87.

145. Steinberg D, Parthasarthy S, Carcio TE, et al: Beyond cholesterol: Modification of low-density lipoprotein that increases its atherogenicity. N Engl J Med 1989;320:915.

146. Scanu A, Lawn RM, Berg K: Lipoprotein (a) and atherosclerosis. Ann Intern Med 1991;115:209-218.

147. Pedro-Botet J, Senti M, Nogues X, et al: Lipoprotein and apolipoprotein profile in men with ischemic stroke. Role of lipoprotein (a), triglyceride-rich lipoproteins, and apolipoprotein E polymorphism. Stroke 1992;23:1556-1562.

148. Wilt TJ, Rubins HB, Robins SJ, et al: Carotid atherosclerosis in men with low levels of HDL cholesterol. Stroke 1997;28:1919-1925.

149. Homer D, Ingall TJ, Baber HL, et al: Serum lipids and lipoproteins are less powerful predictors of extracranial carotid artery atherosclerosis than are cigarette smoking and hypertension. Mayo Clin Proc 1991;66:259-267.

150. Bucher HC, Griffith LE, Guyatt GH: Effect of HMGCoA reductase inhibitors on stroke. A meta-analysis of randomized controlled trials. Ann Intern Med 1998;128:89-95.

151. Amarenco P, Lavallee P, Touboul P-J: Stroke prevention, blood cholesterol, and statins. Lancet Neurol 2004;3:271-278.

152. SPARCL Investigators: High-dose atorvastatin after stroke or transient ischemic attack. N Engl J Med 2006;355:549-559.

153. Paciaroni M, Hennerici M, Agnelli G, Bogousslavsky J: Statins and stroke prevention. Cerebrovasc Dis 2007;24:170-182.

154. Gorelick PB: The status of alcohol as a risk factor for stroke. Stroke 1989;20:1607-1610.

155. Hillborn M, Kaste M: Alcohol intoxication: A risk factor for primary subarachnoid hemorrhage. Neurology 1982;32:706-711.

156. Kagan A, Yano K, Rhoads G, et al: Alcohol and cardiovascular disease: The Hawaiian experience. Circulation 1981;64(suppl 3):27-31.

157. Bogousslausky J, Van Melle G, Despland PA, Regli F: Alcohol consumption and carotid atherosclerosis in the Lausanne stroke registry. Stroke 1990;21:715-720.

158. Palomaki H, Kaste M: Regular light-to-moderate intake of alcohol and the risk of ischemic stroke. Stroke 1993;24:1828-1832.

159. Kiechi S, Willeit J, Rungger G, et al: Alcohol consumption and atherosclerosis: What is the relation. Prospective results from the Bruneck Study. Stroke 1998;29:900-907.

160. Gorelick PB, Rodin MB, Langenberg P, et al: Is acute alcohol ingestion a risk factor for ischemic stroke? Stroke 1987;18:359-364.

161. Gorelick PB, Rodin MB, Langengerg P, et al: Weekly alcohol consumption, cigarette smoking, and the risk of ischemic stroke. Neurology 1989;39:339-343.

162. Truelsen T, Gronbaek M, Schnohr P, Boysen G: Intake of beer, wine, and spirits and risk of stroke. The Copenhagen Heart Study. Stroke 1998;29:2467-2472.

163. Hertog MG, Feskens EJ, Hollman PC, et al: Dietary antioxidant flavonoids and risk of coronary heart disease. Lancet 1993;342:1007-1011.

164. Frankel EN, Kanner J, German JB, et al: Inhibition of oxidation of human low-density lipoproteins by phenolic substances in red wine. Lancet 1993;341:454-457.

165. Hillbom M, Haapaniemi H, Juvela S, et al: Recent alcohol consumption, cigarette smoking, and cerebral infarction in young adults. Stroke 1995;26:40-45.

166. Criqui MH: Peripheral arterial disease and subsequent cardiovascular mortality: A strong and consistent association. Circulation 1990;82:2246-2247.

167. Criqui MH, Langer RD, Fronek A, et al: Mortality over a period of 10 years in patients with peripheral arterial disease. N Engl J Med 1992;326:381-386.

168. Bhatt DL, Steg PG, Ohman EM, et al: International prevalence, recognition, and treatment of cardiovascular risk factors in outpatients with atherothrombosis. REACH Registry Investigators. JAMA 2006;295:180-189.

169. Bogousslavsky J, Regli F: Cerebral infarct in apparent transient ischemic attack. Neurology 1985;35:1501-1503.

170. Awad I, Modic M, Little JR, et al: Focal parenchymal lesions in transient ischemic attacks: Correlation of computed tomography and magnetic resonance imaging. Stroke 1986;17:399-403.

171. Caplan LR: TIAs: We need to return to the question, "What is wrong with Mr Jones?" Neurology 1988;39:791-793.

172. Fazekas F, Fazekas G, Schmidt R, et al: Magnetic resonance imaging correlates of transient cerebral ischemic attacks. Stroke 1996;27:607-611.

173. Inatomi Y, Kimura K, Yonehara T, et al: DWI abnormlities and clinical characteristics in TIA patients. Neurology 2004;62:376-380.

174. Dennis MS, Bamford JM, Sandercock PA, Warlow CD: A comparison of risk factors and prognosis for transient ischemic attacks and minor ischemic strokes. Stroke 1989;20:1494-1499.

175. Johnston SC, Gress DR, Browner WS, Sidney S: Short-term prognosis after emergency department diagnosis of TIA. JAMA 2000;284:2901-2906.

176. Daffertshofer M, Mielke O, Pullwitt A, et al: Transient ischemic attacks are more than "ministrokes." Stroke 2004;35:2453-2458.

177. Kleindorfer D, Pangos P, Pancoli A, et al: Incidence and short-term prognosis of transient ischemic attack in a population-based study. Stroke 2005;36:720-724.

178. Hill MD, Yiannakoulias N, Jeerakathil T, et al: The high risk of stroke immediately after transient ischemic attack. A population-based study. Neurology 2004;62:2015-2020.

179. Rothwell PM, Warlow CP: Timing of TIAs preceding stroke. Time window for prevention is very short. Neurology 2005;64;817-820.

180. Touze E, Varenne O, Chatellier G, et al: Risk of myocardial infarction and vascular death after transient ischemic attack and ischemic stroke. Stroke 2005;36:2748-2755.

181. Nguyen-Huynh MN, Johnston SC: Transient ischemic attack: A neurologic emergency. Curr Neurol Neurosci Rep 2005;5:13-20.

182. Ay H, Koroshetz WJ, Benner T, et al: Transient ischemic attack with infarction: A unique syndrome. Ann Neurol 2005;57:679-686.

183. Collaborative Group for the Study of Stroke in Young Women: Oral contraception and increased risk of cerebral ischemia or thrombosis. N Engl J Med 1973;288:871-878.

184. Handin R: Thromboembolic complications of pregnancy and oral contraceptives. Prog Cardiovasc Dis 1974;16:395-405.

185. Layde P, Beral V, Kay C: Further analyses of mortality in oral contraceptive users. Lancet 1981;1:541-546.

185a. Bushnell CD: Stroke and the female brain. Nat Clin Pract Neurol 2008;4:22-33.

186. Lidegaard O, Kreiner S: Cerebral thrombosis and oral contraceptives: A case-control study. Contraception 1998;57:303-314.

187. Schwartz SM, Siscovick DS, Longstreth WT Jr, et al: Use of low-dose oral contraceptives and stroke in young women. Ann Intern Med 1997;127:596-603.

188. Schwartz SM, Petitti DB, Siscovick DS, et al: Stroke and use of low-dose oral contraceptives in young women. A pooled analysis of two U.S. studies. Stroke 1998;29:2277-2284.

189. Siritho S, Thrift A, McNeil JJ, et al: Risk of ischemic stroke among users of the oral contracveptive pill. The Melbourne Risk Factor Study (MERFS) Group. Stroke 2003;34:1575-1580.

190. Jick SS, Jick H: The contraceptive patch in relation to ischemic stroke and acute myocardial infarction. Pharmacotherapy 2007;27:218-220.

191. Chasan-Taber L, Stampfer MJ: Epidemiology of oral contraceptives and cardiovascular disease. Ann Intern Med 1998;128:467-477.

192. Martinelli I, Sacchi E, Landi G, et al: High risk of cerebral-vein thrombosis in carriers of a prothrombin-gene mutation and in users of oral contraceptives. N Engl J Med 1998;338:1793-1797.

193. Qureshi A, Giles WH, Croft JB, Stern BJ: Number of pregnancies and risk for stroke and stroke subtypes. Arch Neurol 1997;54:203-206.

194. Kittner SJ, Stern BJ, Feeser BR, et al: Pregnancy and the risk of stroke. N Engl J Med 1996;335:768-774.

195. Finucane FF, Madans JH, Bush TL, et al: Decreased risk of stroke among postmenopausal hormone users. Arch Intern Med 1993;153:73-79.

196. Grodstein F, Manson JE, Colditz GA, et al: A prospective observational study of postmenopausal hormone therapy and primary prevention of cardiovascular disease. Ann Intern Med 2000;133:933-941.

197. Lokkegaard E, Jovanovic Z, Heitemann BL, et al: Increased risk of stroke in hypertensive women using hormone therapy. Analysis based on the Danish Nurse Study. Arch Neurol 2003;60:1379-1384.

198. Wilson PW, Garrison RJ, Castelli WP: Postmenopausal estrogen use, cigarette smoking, and cardiovascular morbidity in women over 50. The Framingham Study. N Engl J Med 1985;313:1038-1043.

199. Simon JA, Hsia J, Cawley JA, et al: Postmenopausal hormone therapy and risk of stroke. The Heart and Estrogen/Progestin Replacement Study (HERS). Circulation 2001;103:638-642.

200. Grady D, Harrington D, Bittner V, et al: For the HERS Research Group. Cardiovascular disease outcomes during 6-8 years of hormone therapy. The Heart and Estrogen/Progestin Replacement Study (HERS II). JAMA 2002;288:49-57.

201. Viscoli CM, Brass LM, Kernan WN, et al: A clinical trial of estrogen-replacement therapy after ischemic stroke. N Engl J Med 2001;345:1243-1249.

202. Rossouw JE, Anderson GL, Prentice RL, et al: Risks and benefits of estrogen plus progestin in healthy postmenopausal women: Principal results from the Women's Health Initiative randomized controlled trial. JAMA 2002;288:321-333.

203. Wassertheil-Smoller S, Hendrix SL, Mimacher M, et al: Effect of estrogen plus progestins on stroke in postmenopausal women. The Women's Health Initiative: A randomized controlled trial. JAMA 2003;289:2673-2684.

204. The Women's Health Initiative Steering Committee: Effects of conjugated equine estrogen in postmenopausal women with hysterectomy. The Women's Health Initiative: A randomized controlled trial. JAMA 2004;291:1701-1712.

17

205. Wannamethee G, Shaper AG: Physical activity and stroke in middle-aged men. BMJ 1992;304: 597-601.

206. Sacco RL, Gan R, Boden-Albala B, et al: Leisure-time physical activity and ischemic stroke risk. The Northern Manhattan Stroke Study. Stroke 1998;29:380-387.

207. Lindenstrom E, Boysen G, Nyboe J: Lifestyle factors and risk of cerebrovascular disease in women. The Copenhagen City Heart Study. Stroke 1993;24:1468-1472.

208. Agnarsson U, Thorgeirsson G, Sigvaldson H, Sigfusson N: Effects of leisure-time physical activity and ventilatory function on risk for stroke in men: The Reykjavik Study. Ann Intern Med 1999;130:987-990.

209. Choi-Kwon S, Kim JS: Lifestyle factors and risk of stroke in Seoul, South Korea. J Stroke Cerebrovasc Dis 1998;7:414-420.

210. Lee I-M, Paffenbarger Jr RS: Physical activity and stroke incidence. The Harvard Alumni Health Study. Stroke 1998;29:2049-2054.

211. Lee I-M, Hennekens CH, Berger K, et al: Exercise and risk of stroke in male physicians. Stroke 1999;30:1-6.

212. Hu FB, Stampfer MJ, Colditz G, et al: Physical activity and risk of stroke in women. JAMA 2000;283:2961-2967.

213. Lee CD, Folsom AR, Blair SN: Physical activity and stroke risk. A meta-analysis. Stroke 2003;34: 2475-2482.

214. Paffenbarger Jr RS, Wing AL, Hyde RT, Jung DL: Physical activity and incidence of hypertension in college alumni. Am J Epidemiol 1983;117: 245-257.

215. Paffenbarger Jr RS, Jung DL, Leung RW, Hyde RT: Physical activity and hypertension: An epidemiological view. Ann Med 1991;23:319-327.

216. Hayashi T, Tsumura K, Suematsu C, et al: Walking to work and the risk of hypertension in men: The Osaka Health Survey. Ann Intern Med 1999; 130:21-26.

217. Endres M, Gertz K, Lindauer U, et al: Mechanisms of stroke protection by physical activity. Ann Neurol 2003;54:582-590.

218. Wing S, Casper M, Davis WB, et al: Stroke mortality maps. Stroke 1988;19:1507-1513.

219. Lanska DJ: Geographic distribution of stroke mortality in the United States: 1939-1941 to 1979-1981. Neurology 1993;43:1839-1851.

220. Lanska DJ, Kryscio R: Geographic distribution of hospitalizatioon rates, case fatality, and mortality from stroke in the United States. Neurology 1994; 44:1541-1550.

221. Glymour WM, Avendano M, Berkman LF: Is the "stroke belt" worn from childhood? Risk of first stroke and state of residence in childhood and adulthood. Stroke 2007;38:2415-2421.

222. Howard G, Prineas R, Moy C, et al: Racial and geographic differences in awareness, treatment, and control of hypertension: The Reasons for Geographic and Racial Differences in Stroke Study. Stroke 2006;37:1171-1178.

223. Vermeer SE, Koudstaal PJ, Oudkerk M, et al: Prevalence and risk factors of silent brain infarcts in the population-based Rotterdam Scan Study. Stroke 2002;33:21-25.

224. Caplan LR: Significance of unexpected (silent) brain infarcts. In Caplan LR, Shifrin EG, Nicolaides AN, Moore WS (eds): Cerebrovascular Ischaemia. Investigation and Management. London: Med-Orion, 1996, pp 423-433.

225. Ward NS, Brown MM: Leukoaraiosis in subcortical stroke, 2nd ed. Donnan G, Norrving B, Bamford J, Bogousslavsky J (eds): Oxford: Oxford University Press, 2002, pp 47-66.

226. Caplan LR, Schoene WC: Clinical features of subcortical arteriosclerotic encephalopathy (Binswanger's disease). Neurology 1978;28: 1206-1215.

227. Caplan LR: Binswanger's disease—revisited. Neurology 1995;45:626-633.

228. Babikian V, Ropper AH: Binswanger disease: A review. Stroke 1987;18:1-12.

229. Fisher CM: Binswanger's encephalopathy: A review. J Neurol 1989;236:65-79.

230. Gray F, Dubas F, Roullet E, Escourolle R: Leuko-encephalopathy in diffuse hemorrhagic cerebral amyloid angiopathy. Ann Neurol 1985;18:54-59.

231. Dubas F, Gray F, Roullet E, Escourolle R: Leuko-encephalopathies arteriopathiques. Rev Neurol 1985;141:93-108.

232. Loes D, Biller J, Yuh WT, et al: Leukoencephalopathy in cerebral amyloid angiopathy: MR imaging in four cases. AJNR Am J Neuroradiol 1990;11:485-488.

233. Baudrimont M, Dubas F, Joutel A, et al: Autosomal dominant leukoencephalopathy and subcortical ischemic stroke: A clinicopathological study. Stroke 1993;24:122-125.

234. Davous P: CADASIL: A review with proposed diagnostic criteria. Eur J Neurology 1998;5: 219-233.

235. Chabriat H, Levy C, Taillia H, et al: Patterns of MRI lesions in CADACIL. Neurology 1998;51: 452-457.

236. Chen YW, Gurol ME, Rosand J, et al: Progression of white matter lesions and hemorrhages in cerebral amyloid angiopathy. Neurology 2006; 67:83-87.

237. Imaizumi T, Honma T, Horita Y, et al: Hematoma size in deep intracerebral hemorrhage and its correlation with dot-like hemosiderin spots on gradient echo T2*-weighted MRI. J Neuroimaging 2006;16:236-242.

238. Imaizumi T, Horita Y, Hashimoto Y, Niwa J: Dotlike hemosiderin spots on T2*-weighted magnetic resonance imaging as a predictor of stroke recurrence: A prospective study. J Neurosurg 2004;101:915-920.

239. Hollenhorst R: Ocular manifestations of insufficiency or thrombosis of the internal carotid artery. Am J Ophthalmol 1959;47:753-767.

240. Fisher CM: Observations of the fundus oculi in transient monocular blindness. Neurology 1959; 9:333-347.

241. Kearns T, Hollenhorst R: Venous stasis retinopathy of occlusive disease of the carotid artery. Mayo Clin Proc 1963;38:304-312.

242. Carter JE: Chronic ocular ischemia and carotid vascular disease. In Bernstein EF (ed): Amaurosis Fugax. New York: Springer, 1988, pp 118-134.

243. Nicolaides AN: Asymptomatic Carotid Stenosis and the Risk of Stroke (the ACSRS Study): Identification of a high-risk group. In Caplan LR, Shifrin EG, Nicolaides AN, Moore WS (eds): Cerebrovascular Ischaemia: Investigation and Management. London: Med-Orion, 1996, pp 435-441.

244. Wityk RJ, Chang H-M, Rosengart A, et al: Proximal extracranial vertebral artery disease in the New England Medical Center Posterior Circulation Registry. Arch Neurol 1998;55: 470-478.

245. Caplan LR: Posterior Circulation Disease: Clinical Findings, Diagnosis, and Management. Boston: Blackwell, 1996.

246. Toghi H, Yamanouchi H, Murakami M, et al: Importance of the hematocrit as a risk factor in cerebral infarction. Stroke 1978;9:369-374.

247. Harrison MJG, Pollock S, Thomas D, et al: Hematocrit, hypertension, and smoking in patients with transient ischemic attack and in age and sex matched controls. J Neurol Neurosurg Psychiatry 1982;45:550-551.

248. Di Mascio R, Marchioli R, Vitullo F, Tognoni G: A positive relation between high hemoglobin values and the risk of ischemic stroke. Progetto 3A Investigators. Eur Neurol 1996; 36:85-88.

249. Harrison MJG, Pollock S, Kendall B, et al: Effect of hematocrit on carotid stenosis and cerebral infarction. Lancet 1981;2:114-115.

250. Thomas DJ, Marshall J, Ross-Russel RW, et al: Effects of hematocrit on cerebral blood flow in man. Lancet 1977;2:940-943.

251. Elkind MS, Sciacca RR, Boden-Albala B, et al: Relative elevation in baseline leukocyte count predicts first cerebral infarction. Neurology 2005;64:2121-2125.

252. Mercuri M, Bond MG, Evans G, et al: Leukocyte count and carotid atherosclerosis. Stroke 1991: 22:134.

253. Elkind MS, Cheng I, Boden-Albala B, et al: Elevated white blood cell count and carotid plaque thickness: The Northern Manhattan Stroke Study. Stroke 2001;32:842-849.

254. Elkind MS, Sciacca R, Boden-Albala B, et al: Leukocyte count is associated with aortic arch plaque thickness. Stroke 2002;33:2587-2592.

255. Ovbiagele B, Lynn MJ, Saver JL, et al: Leukocyte count and vascular risk in symptomatic intracranial atherosclerosis. WASID Study Group. Cerebrovasc Dis 2007;24:283-288.

256. Elkind MS, Sciacca RR, Boden-Albala B, et al: Leukocyte count is associated with reduced endothelial reactivity. Atherosclerosis 2005;181: 329-338.

257. Elkind MS: Inflammation, atherosclerosis, and stroke. Neurologist 2006;12:140-148.

258. Eikelboom JW, Hankey GJ, Baker RI, et al: C-reactive protein in ischemic stroke and its etiologic subtypes. J Stroke Cerebrovasc Dis 2003;12:74-81.

259. Arenillas JF, Alvarez-Sabin J, Molina CA, et al: C-reactive protein predicts further ischemic events in first-ever transient ischemic attack or stroke patients with intracranial large-artery occlusive disease. Stroke 2003;34: 2463-2470.

260. Wakugawa Y, Kiyohara Y, Tanizaki Y, et al: C-reactive protein and risk of first-ever ischemic and hemorrhagic stroke in general Japanese population. The Hisayama Study. Stroke 2006; 37:27-32.

261. Wilhelmsen L, Svarrdsudd K, Korsan-Bengtsen K, et al: Fibrinogen as a risk factor for stroke and myocardial infarction. N Engl J Med 1984;311: 501-505.

262. Drouet L: Fibrinogen: A treatable risk factor. Cerebrovasc Dis 1996;6(suppl 1):2-6.

263. Kristensen B, Malm J, Nilsson T, et al: Increased fibrinogen levels and acquired hypofibrinolysis in young adults with ischemic stroke. Stroke 1998;29:2261-2267.

264. Grotta J, Ackerman R, Correia J, et al: Whole-blood viscosity parameters and cerebral blood flow. Stroke 1982;13:296-298.

265. Graham IM, Daly LE, Refsum HM, et al: Plasma homocysteine as a risk factor for vascular disease. The European Concerted Action Project. JAMA 1997;277:1775-1781.

266. Welch GN, Loscalzo J: Homocysteine and atherothrombosis. N Engl J Med 1998;338: 1042-1050.

267. Giles WH, Croft JB, Greenlund KJ, et al: Total homocyst(e)ine concentration and the likelihood of nonfatal stroke. Results from the Third National Health and Nutrition Examination Survey, 1988-1994. Stroke 1998;29:2473-2477.

268. Sacco RL, Ananad K, Lee H-S, et al: Homocysteine and the risk of ischemic stroke in a triethnic cohort. The Northern Manhattan Study. Stroke 2004;35:2263-2269.

269. Selhub J, Jacques PF, Bostom AG, et al: Association between plasma homocysteine concentrations and extracranial carotid-artery stenosis. N Engl J Med 1995;332:286-291.

270. Eikelboom JW, Hankey GJ, Ananad S, et al: Association between high homocyst(e)ine and ischemic stroke due to large and small-artery disease but not other etiologic subtypes of ischemic stroke. Stroke 2000;31:1069-1075.

271. Beamer NB, Coull BM, Clark WM, Wynn M: Microalbuminuria in ischemic stroke. Arch Neurol 1999;56:699-702.

272. Gaede P, Vedel P, Parving H-H, Pederson O: Intensified multifactorial intervention in patients with type 2 diabetes mellitus and micro-albuminuria: The Steno type 2 randomized study. Lancet 1999;353:617-622.

17

273. Gerstein H, Mann JFE, Yi Q, et al: F Albuminuria and risk of cardiovascular events, death, and heart failure in diabetic and nondiabetic individuals. HOPE Study Investigators. JAMA 2001;286:421-426.

273a. Ovbiagele B: Impairment in glomerular filtration rate or glomerular filtration barrier and occurrence of stroke. Arch Neurol 2008;65: 934-938.

273b. Khatri M, Wright CB, Nickolas TL, et al: Chronic kidney disease is associated with white matter hyperintensity volume. The Northern Manhattan Study (NOMAS). Stroke 2007;38:3121-3126.

274. Alberts MJ: Genetics of Cerebrovascular Disease. Armonk, NY: Futura, 1999.

275. Meschia JF, Worrall BB: New advances in identifying genetic anomalies in stroke-prone probands. Curr Neurol Neurosci Rep 2004;4: 420-426.

276. Gretarsdottir S, Thorleifsson G, Reynisdottir ST, et al: The gene encoding phosphodiesterase 4D confers risk of ischemic stroke. Nat Genet 2003;35:131-138.

277. Yee RYL, Brophy VH, Cheng S, et al: Polymorphisms of the phosphodiesterase 4D, camp-specific (PDE4D) gene and risk of ischemic stroke. A prospective, nested case-control evaluation. Stroke 2006;37:2012-2017.

278. Worrall BB, Mychaleckyj JC: PDE4D and stroke. A real advance or a case of the emperor's new clothes? Stroke 2006;37:1955-1957.

279. Ruigrok YM, Rinkel GJE, Wijmenga C: Genetics of intracranial aneurysms. Lancet Neurol 2005; 4:179-189.

280. Ruigrok YM, Rinkel GJ, Wijmenga C: The versican gene and the risk of intracranial aneurysms. Stroke 2006;37:2372-2374.

281. Wolf PA, D'Agostino RB, Belanger AJ, Kannel WB: Probability of stroke: A risk profile from the Framingham Study. Stroke 1991;22:312-318.

282. Wolf PA, Belanger AJ, D'Agostino RB: Quantifying stroke risk factors and potentials for risk reduction. Cerebrovasc Dis 1993 (suppl 1) 7-14.

283. Yamamoto H, Bogousslavsky J: Mechanisms of second and further strokes. J Neurol Neurosurg Psychiatry 1998;64:771-776.

284. Caplan LR: Editorial. J Neurol Neurosurg Psychiatry 1998;64:716.

285. Inzitari D, Eliasziw M, Gates P, et al: The causes and risk of stroke in patients with asymptomatic internal-carotid-artery stenosis. North American Symptomatic Carotid Endarterectomy Trial Collaborators. N Engl J Med 2000;342:1693-1700.

286. Leonberg SC, Elliot FA: Prevention of recurrent stroke. Stroke 1981;12:731-735.

287. Ovbiagele B, Saver JL, Fredieu A, et al: In-hospital initiation of secondary stroke prevention therapies yields high rates of adherence at follow-up. Stroke 2004;35:2879-2883.

288. Touze E, Coste J, Voicu M, et al: Importance of in-hospial initiation of therapies and therapeutic inertia in secondary stroke prevention. IMplemetation of Prevention after a Cerebrovascular evenT (IMPACT) Study. Stroke 2008; 39:1834-1843.

Sometimes, the brain injury that develops during a stroke is not the only medical problem the patient, family, and doctor must battle. Strokes, like many other serious medical illnesses, can be followed by a host of other problems. These complications can sometimes cause neurologic deterioration; in other instances, the patient feels worse and the deterioration is falsely attributed to worsening of the stroke. Most of the complications that occur after stroke are medical and not neurologic. Complications are extremely common. In the Randomized Trial of Tirilazad Mesylate in Acute Stroke, 95% of the 279 stroke patients had at least one complication.[1] Complications may occur during hospitalization for acute stroke or may develop during rehabilitation and neurologic recovery. A number of reports and reviews discuss the various complications of stroke, frequencies of occurrence, and prevention and management.[1-10] Tables 18-1 and 18-2 list the frequency of various medical complications found in four series of stroke patients.[1,7-9] Although medical errors such as giving wrong medications, omitting medications and treatments, and wrong dosing also occur all too often,[11] these problems are not unique to stroke patients and therefore will not be discussed here.

Complications can be serious and cause death. The most common causes of death in patients with stroke are shown in Table 18-3. Brain edema, cardiac abnormalities, and pulmonary embolism dominate during the first week.[12] Pneumonia, urinary tract infections, bed sores, phlebothrombosis and pulmonary embolism, gastrointestinal bleeding, contractures, falls, osteopenia, and depression also occur during the first week. These problems may continue during recovery and even after patients return home. Randomized trials, analyses, and meta-analyses have all shown that units dedicated solely to the care of stroke patients decrease mortality and morbidity among stroke patients.[13-18] One important function of stroke units and stroke teams is to systematically pursue measures to monitor complications and prevent their occurrence.

NEUROLOGIC COMPLICATIONS

Stroke Progression or Recurrence

Deterioration of neurologic functions, including a decrease in the level of consciousness or progression of focal neurological signs, develops in more than 25% of stroke patients.[6] In most patients, this progression occurs during the first 24 to 72 hours and is much less common thereafter.[6,19,20] In patients with intracerebral hemorrhages, the deterioration is often caused by continued bleeding.[21-24] In patients with aneurysmal subarachnoid hemorrhage, rebleeding and vasoconstriction with delayed brain ischemia are most often responsible for neurologic deterioration during the 2 weeks after the initial bleed. Progression of brain ischemia is most common in patients with occlusions of large extracranial and intracranial arteries and those with lacunar infarcts. In patients with ischemic strokes, progression of brain ischemia is often related to propagation of thrombi, embolism, and failure of collateral circulation to develop adequately.

A second stroke may develop in the days and weeks after the initial stroke. This may occur while the patient is still in the acute hospital or during rehabilitation. Among 1273 patients with brain infarcts entered in the Stroke Data Bank, 40 had a stroke recurrence during the 30 days after the index stroke.[25] The likelihood of recurrence depends heavily on the mechanism of the first stroke and treatment. Recurrences are most likely to be caused by the same stroke mechanism as the index stroke.[26] Patients with cardiac-origin embolism are at the highest risk for having a second stroke, but different sources of emboli have different rates of recurrence.[27,28]

Brain Edema

The most lethal complication of stroke is brain edema after large ischemic and hemorrhagic strokes. In stroke units, brain edema, pulmonary embolism, and cardiac abnormalities are the major cause of early death.[6,13,29] Brain infarcts evolve rapidly, whereas brain edema not only varies with time but also varies in severity in different areas within and surrounding the lesion.[30] The two main

18

Table 18-1. Most Frequent Important Medical Events Among 279 Stroke Patients in the Control Limb of the Randomized Trial of Tirilazad Mesylate in Acute Stroke

Event	Serious	Total
Sepsis	3(1%)	3(1%)
Cellulitis	2(1%)	5(2%)
Congestive heart failure	7(3%)	30(11%)
Cardiac arrest	5(2%)	5(2%)
Angina, myocardial infarct	4(1%)	16(6%)
Deep vein thrombosis	3(1%)	6(2%)
Pulmonary embolism	3(1%)	4(1%)
Peripheral vascular disease	2(1%)	2(1%)
Pneumonia (all)	13(5%)	27(10%)
Aspiration pneumonia	8(3%)	16(6%)
Dyspnea	3(1%)	11(4%)
Pulmonary edema	3(1%)	9(3%)
Gastrointestinal bleed	7(3%)	15(5%)
Dehydration	3(1%)	6(2%)
Hypoxia	2(1%)	8(3%)
Urinary tract infection	3(1%)	30(11%)

Modified from KC Johnston, JY Li, PD Lyden, et al: Medical and neurological complications of ischemic stroke. Experience from the RANTTAS trial. Stroke 1998;29:447-453.

Table 18-2. Number of Observed Medical Complications Among 100 Consecutive Stroke Patients during Rehabilitation

Medical Complication	Number
Urinary tract infection	44
Musculoskeletal pain	31
Urinary retention	25
Falls	25
Fungal rash	24
Hypotension	19
Diabetes mellitus	16
Hypertension	15
Cardiac arrythmia	8
Pneumonia	7
Congestive heart failure	6
Angina pectoris	4
Myocardial infarct	0
Thrombophlebitis	4
Pulmonary embolism	0
Other miscellaneous complications	135
Total	**363**

Reprinted with permission from Dromerick A, Reding M. Medical and neurological complications during in-patient stroke rehabilitation. Stroke 1994;25:358(361).

components of the edema are: (1) intracellular (cytotoxic) edema, which results from damage to the sodium-potassium pump with failure of the cell to maintain the normal osmotic gradient across its membrane; and (2) extracellular (vasogenic) edema with fluid occupying the interstitial spaces, especially at the edge of infarcts and hemorrhages.

Brain edema may begin within hours but usually does not become clinically obvious until 1 to 4 days after the stroke. Ropper and Shafran analyzed the fluctuating clinical course of patients with stroke and brain edema.[31] During the acute presentation, patients were often drowsy. Usually, a subsequent improvement in the level of consciousness occurred, and by the second or third day, patients were usually more alert. As brain edema increased, patients again became drowsy. In the series of Ropper and Shafran, drowsiness was not the only sign and was accompanied by one or more of the following[31]:

1. Pupillary asymmetry or lack of pupillary response to light. In most patients, the larger pupil was on the side ipsilateral to the brain infarct; pupillary asymmetry varied from 0.5 to 2.0 mm.
2. Periodic breathing patterns.
3. Sixth nerve paresis.
4. Extensor plantar responses on the previously spared side.
5. Papilledema.
6. Headache or vomiting.
7. Bilateral spontaneous extensor posturing.

The clinical findings clearly need not follow the typical "central" or "uncal" herniation syndromes described originally by Plum and Posner.[32]

Computed tomography and magnetic resonance imaging show mass effect from the edema with compression of the lateral ventricles and shift of midline structures. As expected, patients with the largest infarcts and most mass effect have the poorest prognosis. This does not apply, however, to patients with posterior fossa strokes. When intracranial pressure (ICP) monitoring is performed, pressures consistently greater than 15 mm Hg as determined by subarachnoid screw devices are usually fatal.[31]

Table 18-3.	**Causes of Death in Stroke Patients with Supratentorial Lesions**			
	Infarction		Hemorrhage	
Cause of Death	Week 1	Week 2-4	Week 1	Week 2-4
Transtentorial herniation	36	6	42	2
Pneumonia	0	28	1	2
Cardiac	7	17	0	2
Pulmonary embolism	0	4	0	0
Sudden death	2	8	0	0
Septicemia	1	4	0	0
Unknown	0	12	1	3
Brainstem extension of hematoma			1	1
Total	**46**	**79**	**45**	**10**

Reprinted with permission from Silver F, Norris JW, Lewis A, Hachinsky V. Early mortality following stroke: a prospective review. Stroke 1984;15:494.

In patients with large cerebellar infarcts and hemorrhages, small amounts of swelling can compress the brainstem, injure its vital structures, and cause a rapidly progressive obstructive hydrocephalus.[33,34] Computed tomography may show crowding of the perimesencephalic, ambient, and cerebellopontine-angle cisterns and lack of visibility or displacement of the fourth ventricle. The typical syndrome includes headache, vertigo, nausea, vomiting, and ataxia. Drowsiness may start almost immediately but usually develops during the next 12 hours to 4 days. It is not unusual for a patient with cerebellar infarction to be sent home from the emergency room with the diagnosis of labyrinthitis only to return in 24 to 48 hours in a coma.[35] This serious mistake can be avoided if the patient's gait is tested at the time of the initial evaluation. Patients with sizable cerebellar hemorrhages and infarcts nearly always cannot walk or have abnormal gaits with veering or leaning to one side. In the presence of increased posterior fossa pressure, suboccipital decompressive surgery or draining cerebrospinal fluid by a shunt can be life saving.[33,36]

In supratentorial lesions, the therapy for increased pressure is twofold. First, physicians avoid factors that can further increase ICP and promote fluid retention. These include unusual head and neck positions, fever, increased central venous pressure, overhydration, hypoxia, hypercapnia, increased mean airway pressure, and agitation. Second, specific measures can be attempted to decrease pressure. Hyperventilation with reduction of the arterial carbon-dioxide tension to between 20 and 34 mm Hg reduces ICP during the short term, but ICP usually returns to pretreatment levels. Infusion of mannitol and glycerol to maintain blood osmolality between 300 and 310 µOsm/liter also decreases intracranial pressure. This osmotic therapy is effective only when the cell endothelium and membranes are intact. Thus, this therapy is not effective within the core of the infarct or for cytotoxic edema, but it helps reduce the extracellular edema that surrounds infarcts.[30]

Steroids may also be tried. The effectiveness and mechanism of action of steroids in decreasing ICP is obscure. Steroids may ameliorate the extracellular edema that surrounds the infarct (as they do in brain tumors) or in areas where the cell membrane is not severely damaged. Steroids may also protect against free-radical generation. The efficacy of steroids is in doubt. Increased risk of gastrointestinal bleeding, infections, and exacerbation of diabetes are reported when steroids are used in stroke patients.[37-39] Therefore, I rarely use steroids after ischemic infarction. In occasional patients, especially young individuals, an impressive edema exists despite a relatively small zone of infarction. In this rare situation, steroids can be helpful. In patients with brain hematomas, I use steroids and osmotic agents to reduce pressure. In patients with large infarcts, although steroids occasionally allow survival for the short term, most such patients remain in disabled states and succumb later from pneumonia or other complications. Thus, I rarely use steroids in patients with massive infarcts. Craniectomy is another important consideration, especially in young patients with swollen cerebral hemispheres and incipient brain herniation. I discuss craniectomy as a decompressive strategy in Chapter 5.

Seizures

Seizures may also follow strokes. As early as 1864, Jackson recognized seizures as a complication that frequently occurred during the recovery phase of stroke.[40] Among 1000 patients in a data bank collected in Girona, Spain, 50 (5%) patients had epileptic seizures during the first 48 hours after stroke.[41] Patients with brain hemorrhages have seizures more often than those with infarcts. In the Lausanne Stroke Registry, 7% of intracerebral hemorrhage patients had seizures during acute stroke compared with less than 1% of patients with ischemic strokes.[42] In the Harvard Stroke Registry, 6% of patients with hematomas had seizures during acute hospitalization.[43] Subcortical "slit" hemorrhages are most often accompanied by seizures.[44] Among patients with brain infarcts, those patients who have large and hemorrhagic infarcts have the most likelihood of developing seizures.[41,45,46] Patients with lesions that include the cerebral cortex have a much higher frequency of seizures than those whose lesions are only subcortical.[41,45-47] Patients with embolic brain infarcts of cardiac-origin have a much higher frequency of seizures than those who have large artery occlusive disease. Among 770 patients with supratentorial brain infarcts, the presence of cardiac origin brain embolism meant that the patient had a relative risk of 5.14 of developing early seizures compared with patients without cardiac-origin embolism.[46] Post-stroke seizures can occasionally cause worsening of neurologic deficits.[48] Patients who develop early seizures after stroke have a higher in-hospital mortality than those without seizures, probably reflecting the observation that patients with large infarcts are more likely to develop seizures.[49]

Approximately 10% of patients with strokes have seizures at some time after their stroke. In the Seizures after Stroke Study, a prospective, multicenter study among university hospitals in Canada, Australia, Israel, and Italy, 8.3% of stroke patients had seizures.[50] In this series, more than one-half of seizures occurred on the first day. Eighty percent of seizures occurred by the first month.[50] Gupta and colleagues analyzed the timing of postinfarction seizures.[51] In their series of 70 patients with seizures after ischemic strokes, one-third occurred within the first 2 weeks. Ninety percent of the 30 early seizures occurred within the first 24 hours.[51] Nearly three-fourths of seizures occurred within the first year. Only 2% developed more than 2 years after stroke.[51]

The electroencephalogram may have some prognostic value concerning the likelihood of a stroke patient developing a seizure.[52] Patients with periodic, lateralizing, epileptiform discharges are particularly likely to develop seizures. Patients who have focal spikes are also at increased risk, with 78% developing seizures. In patients with focal slowing, diffuse slowing, or normal electroencephalogram records, only 20%,

10%, and 5%, respectively, had seizures.[52] Early seizures are usually focal spells with secondary generalization. Late-onset seizures are more often generalized.[41,51] Patients with cortical infarcts, especially large infarcts with persistent hemiplegia, are most susceptible to postinfarction epilepsy.[47,51] Usually, poststroke seizures are readily controlled with one anticonvulsant.[51] I do not prescribe prophylactic anticonvulsants in stroke patients. The vast minority of stroke patients develop seizures. Potential side effects and toxicity of anticonvulsants complicates the care of patients. I use anticonvulsants only after the patient has had a well-documented seizure.

MEDICAL COMPLICATIONS

Deep Vein Thrombosis and Pulmonary Embolism

Pulmonary embolism is the most feared and lethal medical complication in stroke patients. Pulmonary embolism occurs in about 1% of stroke patients and accounts for up to 15% of deaths.[8] The great majority of patients who develop pulmonary embolism have deep vein thrombi in their lower extremities. Thrombi tend to develop mostly in paretic limbs in patients who are not yet walking. Some venous thrombi are located in pelvic structures. Stasis of blood and an increase in acute phase reactants that follows brain ischemia increase blood coagulability and combines to promote venous thrombosis and thromboembolism. Among patients in eight trials that studied the effect of treatment with heparin given within the first 3 weeks after ischemic stroke, 54% of control patients developed deep vein thrombosis as detected by systematic iodine (I^{125}) fibrinogen scanning or venography.[6,53] Prophylactic administration of heparin, low-molecular-weight heparin, or heparinoids in these patients led to an 81% reduction in deep vein thrombosis as detected by I^{125} fibrinogen scanning and venography.[53]

Patients who harbor deep vein thrombi detected by noninvasive techniques and venography often do not have abnormal physical signs or symptoms.[6,54,55] Patients with severe leg weakness[56] and those with congestive heart failure and atrial fibrillation[57] are most likely to develop deep vein thrombosis. Venous occlusions most often involve the paretic leg in patients with hemiparesis. The true frequency of pulmonary emboli is unknown because many are silent. In necropsy series of patients who die during the first week after stroke, pulmonary emboli, although not always the cause of death, are frequently noted by the pathologist. Wijdicks and Scott reviewed the patient records of 33 patients who had pulmonary emboli after strokes during two decades (1976-1995) at the Mayo Clinic.[58] In three patients who died of progressive brain swelling, pulmonary emboli were found in small pulmonary arteries at necropsy. Among the remaining 30 patients, 15 patients had brain infarcts and 15 patients had intracerebral hemorrhages. None received heparin.[58] Pulmonary embolism occurred from days 3 to 120 (median day, 20) after stroke. Pulmonary embolism resulted in sudden death in 15 of the 30 patients.[58] Pleuritic chest pain, dyspnea, tachycardia, and hypoxemia were clinical clues revealing the presence of pulmonary embolism.

Physical measures such as compression stockings and devices that produce intermittent pneumatic compression are in common use to prevent the development of phlebothrombosis, but their effectiveness is marginal at best.[59-62] Unfractionated heparin and low-molecular-weight heparin are more effective than aspirin or physical measures.[63,64] Some studies indicate that relatively low doses of low-molecular-weight heparin have a better benefit/risk ratio than use of unfractionated heparin.

I consider all stroke patients at risk for the development of deep venous thrombosis. I pay particular attention to patients who are immobile. Obesity, obtundation, congestive heart failure, paralysis of one or both legs, hypercoagulability, and abulia are risk factors for phlebothrombosis. I keep some patients with acute cerebral ischemia at bed rest to maximize cerebral blood flow. I mobilize all other patients as soon as possible. Physical therapy is started at the bedside. I encourage patients to flex and extend the knees and ankles throughout the day. Support hose or special inflated stockings are often used. Patients who have not had a hemorrhagic stroke and are not on anticoagulants are given low-dose subcutaneous heparin (5000 units ["mini" heparin] twice per day) or low-molecular-weight heparin.

Patients who have sudden shortness of breath, chest pain, hypotension, hemoptysis, change in respiratory pattern, hypoxemia, agitation, confusion, or other worsening are suspected of having pulmonary embolism. Depending on the index of suspicion, evaluation should include the following tests:

1. Examination of arterial blood gases
2. Chest x-ray
3. Electrocardiogram
4. Noninvasive studies of the venous circulation in the legs[46]
5. Venography, nuclear lung ventilation, and perfusion scans

6. Pulmonary CT angiography or dye contrast angiography

Patients who develop phlebothrombosis or pulmonary embolism, or both, are treated urgently with intravenous full-dose heparin or low-molecular-weight heparin.

A recent brain hemorrhage contraindicates the acute use of full dose anticoagulation. Antifibrinolytic therapy with urokinase or streptokinase therapy is also contraindicated in the presence of a recent stroke. If the pulmonary emboli were multiple and life threatening, the patient might require placement of a venous umbrella or other procedure to occlude the venous circulation. Pulmonary embolism remains a vexing problem throughout the rehabilitation process in patients who remain paretic.

Cardiac Abnormalities

Cardiac dysfunction is another frequent accompaniment of stroke. The dysfunctioning heart may be the source of stroke, coexist with stroke, or be the result of stroke.[28,65] Cardiac-related mortality is the second most common cause of death in the acute stroke population, second only to neurologic complications.[66] In the VISTA data compilation, among 846 ischemic stroke patients, 35 (4.1%) died of cardiac causes and 161 (19%) had at least one serious cardiac adverse event.[66] Death from cardiac-related events is highest during the first month after stroke and declines in frequency thereafter.

Patients with ischemic and hemorrhagic stroke have been shown at necropsy to have subendocardial hemorrhages and focal regions of necrosis of cardiac muscle cells.[65,67-70] Electrocardiogram changes consistent with ischemia, elevated creatine-phosphokinase-myoglobin levels, troponin levels, and various cardiac arrhythmias are found in stroke patients even without known previous heart disease.[65,72,73] In some series, one-third to one-half of patients with strokes have serious cardiac rhythm disturbances, including ventricular tachycardia, salvos or couplets of premature ventricular beats greater than 10 premature beats per minute, second- or third-degree heart block, or asystole.[65,71,73,74] In control populations matched for age and history of cardiac disease, such arrhythmias are found in only 15%. Mortality has rarely been related to these arrhythmias. Atrial fibrillation can also develop as a sequel to stroke.[75]

Lesions of particular regions of the brain are most likely to be associated with cardiac abnormalities.[65] Three ways that strokes cause secondary cardiac, cardiovascular, and respiratory changes are as follows[51]:

1. Direct involvement of critical structures, such as the cortex of the insula of Reil, hypothalamus, and brainstem nuclei that make up the central autonomic network,[76] which activate autonomic descending fiber pathways to the heart, blood vessels, and lungs.
2. Mass effect with compression of the hypothalamus or brainstem, or both, also activates autonomic pathways.
3. The acute brain lesion and its stress effects stimulate the hypothalamic-pituitary axis triggering the release of catecholamines and corticosteroids.

Electrical stimulation of the anterior part of the brain, including the frontal pole, premotor and motor cortex, cingulate gyri, orbital frontal gyri, insular cortex, anterior part of the temporal lobe, amygdala, and hippocampus are all known to produce pressor or depressor effects on blood pressure or atrial and ventricular arrhythmias.[65,70,77] Stimulation of some of these regions may cause cardiovascular effects because of a nonspecific activation of limbic cortex, which has secondary effects on the hypothalamus, autonomic nervous system, and hypothalamic-pituitary endocrine axis. Stimulation of the insula has a more specific relation to cardiac and cardiovascular functions. After showing that stimulation of the posterior portions of the rat insular cortex had reproducible effects on heart rate and rhythm, Oppenheimer and colleagues stimulated the insular cortex of human epileptic patients.[78,79] They found that electrical stimulation in areas of the left human insular cortex produced bradycardia and reduced blood pressure, whereas stimulation of the right insular cortex elicited tachycardia and increased blood pressure.[79] Strokes that involve the insular cortex may be accompanied by arrhythmias and other cardiovascular effects. The insular cortex is very commonly involved in patients with acute non-lacunar middle cerebral artery territory infarcts.[80]

Projections from the cerebral cortex of the frontal lobe sometimes passing through the temporal lobes and thalami are relayed to the hypothalamus and brainstem nuclei, which then project directly to the intermediolateral cell columns of the thoracic spinal cord that control sympathetic nervous system output to the heart. Stimulation of the lateral and posterior portions of the hypothalamus cause the release of large amounts of catecholamines from the adrenal medulla.[70] Sympathetic stimulation mostly increases the rate and force of the heartbeat and dilates coronary arteries, whereas parasympathetic stimulation slows the atrial rate

and force of contractions and constricts the coronary arteries.[65] Brainstem compression and direct involvement of the medulla oblongata can lead to vagal discharges, which can cause sinus bradycardia, cardiac arrhythmias, and even cardiac arrest, as well as elevation of systolic blood pressure and a fall in diastolic blood pressure. This train of events is the likely explanation of the blood pressure and pulse changes found in patients with increased ICP and brain herniations that were discovered and emphasized by Harvey Cushing. These changes are usually called the *Cushing response.*

When these changes occur during strokes, creatine-phosphokinase and troponin elevations tend to be longer lasting than those associated with primary cardiac disease. Elevations may peak at the fifth day and persist until the twelfth day.[72] When levels of norepinephrine, epinephrine, and dopamine are measured in patients with stroke, patients with transient ischemic attacks, and non-stroke controls, the highest levels are found in stroke patients.[65] The next highest levels are found in transient disorders. Normal values occur in the control population.[65,81] Those patients with stroke and the highest cardiac enzyme values have the highest levels of norepinephrine. This information suggests that stroke causes an increase in sympathetic tone elevating levels of catecholamines, which in turn cause focal myocardial damage and subsequent arrhythmias.

Patients who have subarachnoid hemorrhage and vertebrobasilar-territory ischemia and hemorrhages sometimes develop acute pulmonary edema, which is often sudden in onset and sometimes fatal.[65,82] Pulmonary edema is most likely to develop when a sudden-onset and severe increase in ICP occurs. Weir studied the occurrence of pulmonary edema in patients with fatal subarachnoid hemorrhages.[82] The sudden onset of coma was present in 70% of his fatal cases of patients with ruptured aneurysms who developed pulmonary edema. Respiratory symptoms were noted within a short time period after the onset of headache and neurologic symptoms.[82] Weir attributed the occurrence of pulmonary edema to a sudden, severe increase in ICP, which in turn caused massive autonomic stimulation. Experimental data from studies in cats confirm this hypothesis.[83] Myocardial enzyme release and electrocardiogram changes that indicate abnormal wall motion are often accompanied by decreased left ventricular performance in patients with subarachnoid hemorrhage.[84] Decreased cardiac output often results from the impaired left ventricular function.[84]

Myocardial infarction is also common after stroke, especially in patients with preexistent ischemic heart disease. The increase in acute phase reactants that accompanies stroke can promote coronary thrombosis. Gongora-Rivera and his French colleagues examined the frequency of cardiac-related ischemic lesions among 341 stroke patients that came to necropsy at the Salpetriere hospital in Paris.[85] The frequency of coronary atherosclerotic plaques in these patients was 26.8%, while coronary artery stenosis was found in 37.5% and myocardial infarcts in 40.8%.[85] Two thirds of the myocardial infarcts were not recognized during life and were found only at autopsy.[85] Significant coronary artery disease was especially common in patients with occlusive lesions in the cervical-cranial arteries. It may be difficult in individual patients, especially those with large strokes, to differentiate the changes related to myocytolysis from those caused by coronary artery thrombosis without echocardiography and coronary angiography.

Older patients with cerebral hemispheric infarction have the highest risk for cardiac arrhythmias.[74] Heart rate variability is common in patients with cerebral hemispheric and medullary infarcts.[86] All stroke patients require careful attention to the cardiovascular system by clinical examination and laboratory tests. In addition to surveillance for symptoms, clinicians should carefully monitor vital signs, regular cardiovascular examinations, echocardiography, and routine electrocardiograms. In some patients, continuous cardiac rhythm monitoring may be needed. Although its efficacy is unproved, propranolol or other beta blockers are theoretically useful in patients with neurogenic cardiac arrhythmias, treating both the arrhythmia and its cause.[74] Propranolol could, however, worsen sinus bradycardia, heart block, and episodes of asystole. In experimental animals, the cardiac rhythm abnormalities secondary to cerebral ischemia can be effectively treated with propranolol and atropine.[87] If rhythm disturbances occur, I treat with standard antiarrhythmics according to suggestions of cardiology consultants.

Swallowing Abnormalities, Aspiration, and Pneumonia

Dysphagia and aspiration are common after stroke. Symptomatic dysphagia is noted in approximately one fourth to one third of stroke patients.[88,89] Dysphagia and aspiration are especially common in patients who have had bilateral hemispheric strokes or strokes that involve the brainstem.[90,91] Severe strokes and patients with reduced consciousness and dementia are also conditions in which dysphagia and aspiration are common. So-called silent aspiration is also common when clinicians look for it.

Clinical bedside testing of swallowing ability should be a part of the early assessment of each stroke patient. Examination of the pharynx and palate as they move on saying "ah" and watching the patient swallow some water should be part of the routine examination. Dysphonia, dysarthria, abnormal cough to extricate food from the oropharynx, and voice change after swallowing are highly predictive of a heightened risk of aspiration.[92] A change in pulse oximetry after swallowing has also been used to detect potential for aspiration.[92] Videofluoroscopic examination and fiberoptic endoscopic evaluation of swallowing detects more patients with dysphagia and aspiration than the clinical examination. Videofluoroscopic studies can detect abnormalities of swallowing in approximately 50% of stroke patients.[91-96] In one study among 128 patients hospitalized for first strokes, 65 (51%) had swallowing abnormalities detected clinically and 82 (64%) had swallowing abnormalities shown by videofluoroscopy.[95] During the next 6 months, 26 patients (20%) had pulmonary infections, among whom 24 had videofluoroscopic swallowing abnormalities when studied during their acute stroke.[95] Physical therapy with guidance in positioning of food within the oral cavity and pharynx, choice of foods, the use of thermal stimulation, and instructions to the patient can help prevent aspiration. Most patients are able to resume oral feeding within months, although feeding tubes may be needed temporarily.

Pneumonia is common after stroke during the immediate and late periods. The true frequency of this complication is unknown. In a retrospective postmortem study of patients dying with cerebrovascular disease, pneumonia was recorded as a complication in 33%.[97] Among 1455 patients enrolled in an international randomized trial of a neuroprotectant, 1.6% of patients developed pneumonia.[98] The cause of pneumonia in patients with stroke is multifactorial. Decreased alertness, severe neurologic deficits, and dysphagia are highly associated with the development of pneumonia during hospitalization.[99] In a recumbent position, atelectasis and poor mobilization of secretions often occur. Difficulty in swallowing may also lead to aspiration. Coughing and deep breathing may not be done or may be only poorly performed. Chest movements are also decreased on the hemiplegic side.[100,101] Kaldor and Berlin noted that pneumonia is more likely to exist on the hemiparetic side because of the decreased thoracic movements and impaired pulmonary circulation.[102] Respiratory drive and the function of interstitial muscles are often abnormal on the hemiplegic side.[102] Recently, investigators have found evidence that strokes create an immunodepressed state, and this also can contribute to the development of pneumonia and other infections while in the hospital and afterward.[103-105]

Although many dysphagic patients are fed through nasogastric tubes, this does not seem to prevent pneumonia.[106] Among 100 acute stroke patients given tube feedings because of dysphagia, pneumonia developed in 44.[106] Swallowing function should be tested before giving patients oral feedings. Physiotherapy or nursing techniques probably help to prevent pneumonia after stroke. I encourage deep breathing, coughing, frequent turning, and early mobilization of patients. If fever develops despite these measures, the lung should be aggressively evaluated as the potential source of infection.

Metabolic and Nutritional Disorders

Prolonged undernutrition is an important but seldom recognized complication of stroke, especially in elderly patients whose nutritional intake was poor or marginal before their stroke. Undernutrition is an important predictor of poor outcome.[107] Finestone and colleagues evaluated the nutritional state of 49 consecutive stroke patients admitted to a rehabilitation unit and found that approximately one half were malnourished.[108] In another study, the authors correlated serum albumin concentration, an index of nutritional state, and the presence of chronic disease with the frequency of medical complications and found that 79% of patients with an albumin less than 2.9 g/dl had at least one medical complication during rehabilitation.[109] A high serum albumin correlated with good gains in neurologic functional status.[109] Malnutrition can contribute to diminished immune functions, cardiac and gastrointestinal dysfunction, and abnormal bone metabolism. Malnutrition is a factor in the formation and repair of decubitus ulcers.

To help maintain an adequate nutritional state, I give multivitamins and especially thiamine orally, if the patient is able, or parenterally. If the patient is unable to eat by the fourth or fifth day, I insert a small nasogastric feeding tube through which nutritional supplements can be given. Prolonged inability to swallow may require the placement of gastric feeding tubes. The use of percutaneous endoscopic gastrostomy (PEG) tubes with maintenance of nutrition has undoubtedly helped many stroke patients maintain reasonable nutritional balance despite dysphagia. Early PEG placement can improve the outcome in stroke patients.[110] Nutrition can be better maintained using PEGs than with nasogastric tube feedings.[108] PEG placement can be managed with rare

complications, such as wound infection and gastrointestinal bleeding. In approximately 25% or more of patients, PEGs can be removed when swallowing improves.[111]

Fluid, electrolyte, and nutritional abnormalities may also occur during the acute stroke and recovery periods. Approximately 15% of patients with acute stroke develop hyponatremia. Hyponatremia can cause nausea, vomiting, weakness, confusion, and seizures. Joynt et al posited that poststroke hyponatremia is usually related to inappropriate secretion of antidiuretic hormone (ADH).[112] They showed that stroke patients often had excess ADH even in the presence of normal serum sodium levels. Although the mechanism of the inappropriate ADH secretion is unknown, Joynt et al reviewed some of the potential mechanisms, including damage to the anterior hypothalamus, effects on ADH secretion related to recumbency, resetting of osmoreceptors, damage to a more widespread vasopressin neuronal system, increased release of ADH, and secondary stroke-related elevations in serum catecholamines and cortisol.[112] Changes in the levels of atrial natriuretic factor have also been posited to cause abnormalities of serum sodium concentrations.

In hyponatremic patients, volume depletion and overload must be excluded as contributing factors. To assess this problem, remember that fluid may accumulate in the sacral regions during prolonged bed rest. If volume status is normal, the syndrome of inappropriate ADH secretion can be diagnosed if symptoms, including decreased serum osmolality, continued urinary excretion of sodium, urine less than maximally dilute, normal renal function, and normal thyroid function, exist in addition to hyponatremia. During the acute stroke period, I advise carefully following the patient's volume status by clinical examination; uniform charting of input, output, and daily weights; and monitoring of renal function and electrolytes.

Urinary Tract Infections and Urinary Incontinence

Urinary tract infections are also a common complication of stroke. In an international trial of a neuroprotectant, 17.2% of 1455 patients developed urinary infections.[98] The high frequency of urinary tract infections is probably caused by the following two factors. First, an indwelling catheter is often placed to empty the urinary bladder. This foreign body allows for the introduction and growth of bacteria. Whenever possible, continuous catheter drainage should be avoided. Intermittent catheterization using strict sterile techniques is preferable. In some men, condom catheters suffice. A Foley catheter should never be used as a convenience for the staff. Second, the functioning of the urinary bladder and external sphincter can be altered by the stroke. Urinary symptoms are common even in patients with uninfected bladders and include urinary urgency, frequency, and retention. Tsuchida et al documented these symptoms and attempted to establish their relationship to brain lesions.[113] Patients with frontal and internal-capsular lesions showed a hyperactive bladder or uninhibited sphincter relaxation with subsequent urinary frequency or incontinence. Patients with putaminal lesions had hyperactive bladders with usually normal sphincter function. Patients who had urinary retention showed an inactive or hypoactive bladder with an uncoordinated or normal sphincter; localization of the offending lesion could not be accomplished in these patients. Men in the stroke age group are often geriatric and also have large prostates, which can contribute to the obstructive uropathy.

When confronted with patients with abnormal micturition, I survey for and treat bacterial urinary tract infections when present. In addition, I attempt to define other mechanisms that may be operative in causing symptoms, such as inability to reach the commode or urinal because of gait or limb abnormalities, communication difficulty that may make it hard to signal the nurse, and unavailable nursing personnel. Measurement of post-voided residual urine may be all that is needed, but at times, cystometrics and imaging of the kidneys and urinary tract are required to define the problem. I encourage frequent voiding during the day and night in an effort to train the bladder. Pharmacotherapy can be used if these maneuvers fail to help alleviate the problem.

Gastrointestinal Bleeding

Physicians have long realized that some patients with stroke and other brain diseases develop gastrointestinal hemorrhage. This problem, usually called *Cushing's ulcers, stress ulcers,* or *hemorrhagic gastritis,* can be life threatening when severe. Davenport and colleagues reported that 18 of 607 (3%) stroke patients at their hospital in Edinburgh had gastrointestinal hemorrhages. One half of the hemorrhages were severe.[114] Most patients had hematemesis or melena, but one patient suddenly developed abdominal pain and hemodynamic shock.[114] Older patients with severe strokes and decreased levels of consciousness are most likely to develop gastrointestinal bleeding. Corticosteroids given for brain edema also increase the risk of stress ulceration in the stomach. Prophylactic use of H_2 antagonists is recommended in patients who have large strokes with reduced awareness.

IMMOBILITY AND ITS COMPLICATIONS

Pressure Decubitus Ulcers

The development of bedsores is an iatrogenic and preventable complication of stroke that significantly hinders the rehabilitation process. Patients who are immobilized, have limited ability to reposition themselves, and do not sense the need to change position are at risk of developing bedsores if they are not frequently turned and repositioned.[115] Incontinence also increases the risk for developing skin breakdown. The skin should be kept clean and dry, and the patient should be turned frequently. Adequate nutrition should be given. Pressure on anesthetic or immobilized limbs must be avoided. The use of padded heel boots can spare the heels from ulcers. Egg-crate mattresses, waterbeds, or soft cotton padding may help retard the development of sacral pressure sores. Physicians and nursing personnel should periodically examine the entire skin surface looking for any area of early breakdown. Particular attention should be paid to susceptible areas, such as the sacrum, buttocks, heels, elbows, wrists, toes, and occiput. If an ulcer develops, pressure on that area should be totally avoided, special mattresses should be used, and the wound should be dressed and, if necessary, debrided and the skin grafted.

Contractures and Shoulder Pain

Limb immobility and maintenance in fixed, usually flexed positions can lead to fixed contractures at the knees and elbows. Decreased shoulder movement can lead to shoulder pain, frozen shoulders, and the so-called shoulder-hand syndrome. In the Lund Stroke Register, 22% of over 300 patients developed significant shoulder pain within 4 months after stroke.[116] In one study, 36 of 132 (27%) hemiplegic stroke patients developed the shoulder-hand syndrome.[117] The shoulder-hand syndrome is characterized by pain and tenderness when abducting, flexing, and externally rotating the upper arm; pain and swelling over the carpal bones; and edema of the distal hand joints. Severe shoulder weakness, spasticity, and subluxation of the shoulder increase the likelihood of developing shoulder pain and swelling of the upper extremity. Early full range of movement of the shoulder joint is important in preventing this unpleasant and disabling stroke complication. Nonsteroidal anti-inflammatory drugs, such as indomethacin and low-dose corticosteroids, may be helpful in patients who develop shoulder pain. The most

18

important treatment, however, is vigorous physical therapy.[117] Subluxation of the shoulders is another complication of hemiparesis. The weak arm should not be left to hang without support.

Peripheral Nerve Injuries

Peripheral nerve compression is also a hazard in limbs with weakness and reduced sensation. The peroneal nerve is most commonly involved; its compression causes a foot drop. Ulnar palsy caused by compression of the nerve at the elbow is also common, especially in wheelchair-bound patients. Occasionally, patients compress their femoral nerve in relation to local pressure on the groin region while consciousness is reduced. The femoral nerve can also be compressed by retroperitoneal hemorrhages that involve the iliopsoas muscles. The most common cause of these hematomas is anticoagulation. The earliest sign is often a dropped knee jerk on the side of the retroperitoneal hematoma.

Osteopenia and Osteoporosis

Studies of bone mineral densities after stroke have shown that a significant reduction in bone mineral density occurs on the hemiplegic side.[118-121] The causes are multifactoral but include immobilization-induced calcium resorption from bone, sometimes with hypercalcemia; lack of sunlight exposure; poor nutrition with inadequate vitamin D stores; and osteoporosis before the stroke. The hemiosteoporosis is most severe in those patients with severe hemiplegia, especially those that have prolonged immobilization. The reduced bone density predisposes to hip and other fractures, which tend to occur predominantly on the hemiplegic side. Calcium and vitamin D supplements are important prophylactically in patients at risk for this complication.[119] Early mobilization and exposure to sunlight are also important. In one small study, Zoledronate, given within 35 days after stroke in a single intravenous infusion of 4 mg, prevented hip osteopenia on the hemiplegic side.[122]

Fatigue

Stroke patients often complain of fatigue, even long after their stroke. Fatigue is a well-known problem after other neurologic illnesses, especially multiple sclerosis. Although some causative factors are evident, they do not always explain the extreme fatigue that develops in some stroke patients. Patients with neurologic deficits may need to use more energy to do the same activities that they were able to perform easily before their strokes. The stroke and poststroke period may have led to a prolonged decrease in physical activity and deconditioning likely developed and persisted. Fatigue does correlate with the severity of the neurologic deficit.[123] Fatigue should be separated from apathy and disinterest in performing activities. Fatigue is also quite different from depression. Several studies have noted that fatigue is quite common and underappreciated after stroke, can persist for an extended and even indefinite period, and is not explained by depression.[123,124] Patients and their caregivers should be encouraged to gradually increase the physical activity level to potentially increase the stoke patients stamina.

DEPRESSION AND OTHER PSYCHOLOGICAL EFFECTS OF STROKE

One of the most important and yet frequently overlooked complications of stroke is depression. New personality traits can emerge or old ones become accentuated. The patient may become apathetic, inflexible, rigid, impulsive, insensitive, or indifferent to others; adopt a poor perception of self; or become guilt-ridden, paranoid, or suicidal.

Depression is reported to occur in 26% to 60% of stroke patients.[125-129] Approximately 20% to 25% of patients have a major depressive disorder.[128-130] Astrom and colleagues analyzed the prevalence of major depression at various time intervals after stroke and their most important correlations and determinants.[128] Approximately 25% of their stroke patients had a major depression during the acute poststroke period, and 31% were depressed at 3 months. Acute depression was most frequent in patients with anterior lesions in the left hemisphere, aphasic patients, and those who lived alone. At 1 year, 16% of patients were depressed. Two- and 3-year depression rates were 19% and 29%, respectively. Dependency and lack of social contacts were important determinants of late depression.[128] In another study, among 202 stroke patients, depressive symptoms were present in 43% at 6 months, 36% at 1 year, 24% at 2 years, and 18% at 3 years.[131]

Patients who have a history of depression before their stroke are also prone to become depressed after a stroke.[129] Others have found that at 6 months after stroke, an increased prevalence of symptoms of both major and minor depressive symptoms can be found, increasing from 23% and 20%, respectively, immediately after the stroke to 35% and 26% at 6 months.[130,132] Diagnosis of depression is often difficult because functional psychogenic reactions are hard to separate from organic behavioral changes related to the stroke, such as abulia, apathy, aprosodia, impersistence, and anosognosia.[133]

Facial expression, gestures, pauses, loudness, emphasis, and other nonlinguistic aspects give verbal communication an emotive context. Aprosodia is the inability to express or understand the emotive content of spoken language. Patients with right perisylvian strokes may be unable to communicate emotion in spoken language. Thus, an observer might erroneously believe that they are depressed. Binder noted additional factors complicating the recognition of depression.[134] An accurate history may not be available because of aphasia or slowed responses. Vegetative and autonomic signs may also be difficult to interpret. Stroke may suppress appetite, change sleep patterns, or create a pseudobulbar state with rapid shifts from laughing to crying. To complicate matters, persistent depressive symptoms are more common in patients with cognitive and behavioral abnormalities.[131] Neurologic and psychological effects often coexist and augment each other. Loss of function makes individuals sad, and depressive patients cannot perform up to their potential.

Often, sexual function in patients with stroke is ignored. For some patients, stroke may make sexual relations cumbersome and decrease their frequency. The patient and family should be reassured that for most mechanisms of stroke, sex is unlikely to cause a recurrent stroke. Sexual activity should be encouraged in those couples who were sexually active before the stroke, although it may require some creativity on the part of the participants.

Ross and Rush proposed guidelines for the diagnosis of depression.[135] Depression should be considered in patients who are not making expected recovery, are uncooperative in rehabilitation, or lose previously achieved milestones. Emotional outbursts, inflexibility, irritability, insensitivity to others, and suicidal ideations may occur. A flat affect must be distinguished from a depressed affect. Collateral history from friends and caregivers are also needed.

In some studies, depression was more common after left- than right-hemisphere strokes.[126,128,133, 136-139] In the left hemisphere, the more anteriorly placed infarctions are correlated with a higher frequency of depression.[137,138] When cortical and basal ganglia lesions, infarcts, and hemorrhages affect the left hemisphere anteriorly, they are more likely to be associated with depression than similarly placed right-cerebral lesions.

Finkelstein et al. used the dexamethasone-suppression test to assess patients with mood and vegetative disturbances after stroke.[127] An abnormal test is defined as failure to suppress cortisol secretion in response to exogenously administered dexamethasone. This test is reported to be abnormal in 60% to 80% of psychiatric patients with endogenous depression. Abnormal dexamethasone suppression tests in patients with stroke were associated with occurrence of moderate to severe mood, sleep, and appetite disturbances.[127]

The causes of late depressive reaction are often unknown. Whether it is a reaction to the loss the patient feels or a result of brain injury is unclear. Injury may result in depletion of noradrenergic neurotransmitters resulting in depression. Nortriptyline, trazodone, and serotonin re-uptake inhibitors are reported to be effective in ameliorating significantly the symptoms of depression in patients with stroke.[133,140-142]

Beyond pharmacologic therapy, clinicians should try to adopt a hopeful and fighting attitude. I encourage activity and independence for the family and patient. Physicians should attempt to promote continued affection, understanding, and respect between the family and patient. I suggest that physicians reassure all involved that efforts are intended to maximize rehabilitation and prevent recurrent stroke. I recommend that physicians promote the patient's self-confidence and emphasize the old adage, "When the going gets tough, the tough get going!"

Table 18-4 summarizes my suggestions for prevention of stroke complications.

CAREGIVERS AND THEIR REACTIONS TO THE STROKE PATIENT

Strokes and stroke patients do not live in a vacuum. Strokes cause important ramifications that affect all those who interact with the individual stroke survivor, but most of the burden falls on the family and principal caregiver. Stroke is a disease that hits the whole family constellation, not merely the stroke patient.

Stroke patients who have severe deficits often become dependent on caregivers for daily activities and physical and emotional support. Members of the family must deal with the physical handicaps and, often, new personality traits. If the patient is dependent on family members for care, the main caregiver can develop feelings of entrapment, isolation, anger, and depression. In some families, it seems as if a new dependent child has been thrust on them. Physicians should remember that caregivers are often old and sick and have their own physical and emotional problems.

Researchers have begun to analyze and quantitate burdens perceived by those caring for

Table 18-4. Prevention of Complications

1. Care for patients in Stroke Units of the hospital where physicians and nurses have protocols to protect against complications.
2. Evaluate swallowing function. The water swallow test is a useful screen. Do not give oral liquids, or foods to patients with dysphagia.
3. Consider prophylactic measures to prevent deep vein thrombosis in limbs that are not active.
4. Mobilize patients as soon as appropriate. Passive range of motion should be performed often in paralyzed upper and lower limbs.
5. Evaluate cardiac and respiratory function.
6. Pay attention to urinary function, and prevent overdistention of the bladder.
7. Monitor for infection, especially pneumonia and urinary tract infections, and treat early with appropriate antibiotics.
8. Pay attention to the nutritional state of the patient.
9. Protect pressure point on the patient's body, and turn and move patients often to avoid pressure sores.
10. Be alert for the development of depressive symptoms and treat early.
11. Involve potential caregivers early in procedures to prevent complications once the patient is home.

Source: Reprinted with permission from Silver F, Norris JW, Lewis A, Hachinski V. Early mortality following stroke: a prospective review. Stroke 1984;15:494.

stroke patients. Researchers have also begun to describe and quantify the emotional and physical consequences of caregiving.[143-147] A Dutch study analyzed the burden of caregiving among 121 partners of patients who were living at home.[145] The investigators interviewed the caregivers 3 years after stroke affected their loved ones. Caregivers reported feeling overwhelmed with responsibility, uncertainty, and worry. They found it difficult to handle the restraints placed on their own social lives and interests.[145] Analysis showed that higher levels of burden were explained by the stroke patient's degree of disability and the amount of care needed. The caregiver's emotional distress, loneliness, and perception of his or her ability to care for the stroke patient shaped the burden the caregiver felt.[145]

The emotional outcome of stroke on caregivers was analyzed in a Scottish study of 231 stroke patients and their caregivers.[146] Severe emotional distress and depression were common among caregivers. Caregivers were more likely to be depressed if the stroke patient was dependent or emotionally distressed. The caregivers' emotional state in terms of anxiety and depression highly correlated with the emotional state of the stroke patient. Women who cared for male stroke patients had more anxiety and depression than male caregivers. Older caregivers were more depressed than young caregivers.[146] In another study, the proportion of caregivers that were depressed did not diminish over time.[143]

Clearly, care, education, and concern must be addressed to the caregivers and their families, as well as the stroke patients.

References

1. Johnston KC, Li JY, Lyden PD, et al: Medical and neurological complications of ischemic stroke: experience from the RANTTAS trial. RANTTAS Investigators. Stroke 1998;29:447-453.
2. Davenport RJ, Dennis MS, Wellwood I, Warlow CP: Complications after acute stroke. Stroke 1996;27:415-420.
3. Smithard DG, O'Neill PA, Park C, et al: Complications and outcome after acute stroke. Stroke 1996;27:1200-1204.
4. Biller J, Patrick JT: Management of medical complications of stroke. J Stroke Cerebrovasc Dis 1997;6:217-220.
5. Zorowitz RD, Tietjen GE: Medical complications after stroke. J Stroke Cerebrovasc Dis 1999;8:192-196.
6. van der Worp HB, Kappelle LJ: Complications of acute ischaemic stroke. Cerebrovasc Dis 1998;8:124-132.
7. Dromerick A, Reding M: Medical and neurological complications during inpatient stroke rehabilitation. Stroke 1994;25:358-361.
8. Langhorne P, Stott DJ, Robertson L, et al: Medical complications after stroke. Stroke 2000;31:1223-1228.
9. Weimar C, Roth M, Zillessen G, et al: Complications following acute ischaemic stroke. On behalf of the German Stroke Data bank Collaborators. Eur Neurol 2002;48:133-140.
10. Kappelle LJ, van der Worp HB: Treatment and prevention of complications of acute ischemic stroke. Current Neurology Neuroscience reports 2004;4:36-41.
11. Holloway RG, Tuttle D, Baird T, Skeleton WK: The safety of hospital care. Neurology 2007;68:550-555.
12. Silver F, Norris JW, Lewis A, Hachinski V: Early mortality following stroke: a prospective review. Stroke 1984;15:494.
13. Kaste M, Palmomaki H, Sarna S: Where and how should elderly stroke patients be treated? A randomized trial. Stroke 1995;26:249-253.

14. Indredavik B, Slordahl SA, Bakke F, et al: Stroke unit treatment. Long term effects. Stroke 1997;28: 1861-1866.

15. Stroke Unit Trialists' Collaboration. Collaborative systematic review of the randomized trials of organised in-patient (stroke unit) care after stroke. BMJ 1997;314:1151-1159.

16. Stroke Unit Trialists' Collaboration. How do stroke units improve patient outcomes? A collaborative systematic review of the randomized trials. Stroke 1997;28:2139-2144.

17. Diez-Tejedor E, Fuentes B: Acute care in stroke: do stroke units make the difference? Cerebrovasc Dis 2001;11(suppl 1):31-39.

18. Birbeck GL, Zingmond DS, Cui X, Vickrey BG: Multispecialty stroke services in California hospitals are associated with reduced mortality. Neurology 2006;66:1527-1532.

19. Toni D, Fiorelli M, Gentile M, et al: Progressing neurological deficit secondary to acute ischemic stroke: a study on predictability, pathogenesis, and prognosis. Arch Neurol 1995;52:670-675.

20. Davalos A, Cendra E, Teruel J, et al: Deteriorating ischemic stroke: risk factors and prognosis. Neurology 1990;40:1865-1869.

21. Kelly R, Bryer JR, Scheinberg P, Stokes IV: Active bleeding in hypertensive intracerebral hemorrhage: computed tomography. Neurology 1982;32:852-856.

22. Broderick JP, Brott TG, Tomsick T, et al: Ultra-early evaluation of intracerebral hemorrhage. J Neurosurg 1990;72:195-199.

23. Fujii Y, Tanaka R, Takeuchi S, et al: Hematoma enlargement in spontaneous intracerebral hemorrhage. J Neurosurg 1994;80:51-57.

24. Kazui S, Naritomi H, Yamamoto H, et al: Enlargement of spontaneous intracerebral hemorrhage. Incidence and time course. Stroke 1996;27: 1783-1787.

25. Sacco RL, Foulkes MA, Mohr JP, et al: Determinants of early recurrence of cerebral infarction. The Stroke Data Bank. Stroke 1989;20:983-989.

26. Yamamoto H, Bogousslavsky J: Mechanisms of second and further strokes. J Neurol Neurosurg Psychiatry 1998;64:771-776.

27. Caplan LR: Brain Embolism. In Caplan LR, Hurst JW, Chimowitz MI (eds): Clinical Neurocardiology. New York: Marcel Dekker, 1999, pp 35-185.

28. Caplan LR, Manning W (ed): Brain embolism, New York, Informa Healthcare, 2006, 129-186.

29. White DB, Norris JW, Hachinski VC, et al: Death in early stroke: causes and mechanisms. Stroke 1979;10:743.

30. O'Brien MD: Ischemic Cerebral Edema. In LR Caplan (ed): Brain Ischemia. Basic Concepts and Clinical Relevance. London: Springer, 1995, pp 43-50.

31. Ropper AH, Shafran B: Brain edema after stroke. Arch Neurol 1984;41:26-29.

32. Plum F, Posner JB: Diagnosis of Stupor and Coma (3rd ed). Philadelphia: Davis, 1980.

33. Caplan LR: Posterior Circulation Disease. Clinical findings, diagnosis, and management. Boston: Blackwell, 1996.

34. Caplan LR: Cerebellar infarcts. Rev Neurol Dis

35. Savitz SI, Caplan LR, Edlow JA: Pitfalls in the diagnosis of cerebellar infarction. Acad Emerg Med 2007;14:63-68.

36. Rieke K, Krieger D, Adams H-P, et al: Therapeutic strategies in space-occupying cerebellar infarction based on clinical, neuroradiological, and neurophysiological data. Cerebrovasc Dis 1993;3:45-55.

37. von Rosen F, Guazzo EP: Increased intracranial pressure. In T Brandt, LR Caplan, J Dichgans, et al (eds): Neurological Disorders: Course and Treatment. San Diego: Academic, 1996, pp 521-529.

38. Norris JW: Steroid therapy in acute cerebral infarction. Arch Neurol 1976;33:69-71.

39. Ottonello GA, Primavera A: Gastrointestinal complications of high dose corticosteroid therapy in acute cerebrovascular patients. Stroke 1979;10: 208-210.

40. Taylor J: Selected writings of John Hughlings Jackson on epilepsy and epileptiform convulsions, Vol. 1. London: Hodder & Stoughton, 1931, pp 230-235.

41. Davalos A, de Cendra E, Molins A, et al: Epileptic seizures at the onset of stroke. Cerebrovasc Dis 1992;2:327-331.

42. Bogousslavsky J, van Melle G, Regli F: The Lausanne Stroke Registry: analysis of 1000 consecutive patients with first stroke. Stroke 1988; 19:1083-1092.

43. Mohr JP, Caplan LR, Melski JW, et al: The Harvard Cooperative Stroke Registry: a prospective registry. Neurology 1978;28:754-762.

44. Caplan LR: General Symptoms and Signs. In Kase CS, Caplan LR (eds): Intracerebral Hemorrhage. Boston: Butterworth-Heinemann, 1994, pp 31-43.

45. Bladin CF: Seizures after stroke. M.D. thesis. University of Melbourne, Australia, 1997.

46. Heuts-van Rank EPM: Seizures following a first cerebral infarct. Risk factors and prognosis. Thesis. Rijksuniversiteit Limberg, Maastricht, Netherlands, 1996.

47. Olsen TS, Hogenhaven H, Thage O: Epilepsy after stroke. Neurology 1987;37:1209-1211.

48. Bogousslavsky J, Martin R, Regli F, et al: Persistent worsening of stroke sequelae after delayed seizures. Arch Neurol 1992;49:385-388.

49. Arboix A, Comes E, Massons J, et al: Relevance of early seizures for in-hospital mortality in acute cerebrovascular disease. Neurology 1996;47:1429-1435.

50. Bladin CF, Johnston PJ, Smuraloska L, et al: What causes seizures after stroke? Stroke 1994;25:245.

51. Gupta SR, Naheedey MH, Elias D, Rubino F: Postinfarction seizures: a clinical study. Stroke 1988;19:1477-1481.

52. Holmes GL: The electroencephalogram as a predictor of seizures following cerebral infarction. Clin Electroencephalogr 1980;11:83-86.

53. Sandercock PAG, van den Belt AGM, Lindley RI, Slattery J: Antithrombotic therapy in acute ischaemic stroke: an overview of the completed randomised trials. J Neurol Neurosurg Psychiatry 1993;56:17-25.

54. Warlow C, Ogston D, Douglas AS: Deep venous thrombosis of the legs after stroke. BMJ 1976;1: 1178-1183.

55. Kearon C, Julian JA, Math JM, et al: Noninvasive diagnosis of deep venous thrombosis. Ann Intern Med 1998;128:663-677.

56. Landi G, D'Angelo A, Boccardi E, Candelise L, et al: Venous thromboembolism in acute stroke: prognostic importance of hypercoagulability. Arch Neurol 1992;49:279-283.

57. Noel P, Gregoire F, Capon A, Lehrert P: Atrial fibrillation as a risk factor for deep venous thrombosis and pulmonary emboli in stroke patients. Stroke 1991;22:760-762.

58. Wijdicks EFM, Scott JP: Pulmonary embolism associated with acute stroke. Mayo Clin Proc 1997;72:297-300.

59. Kamran SI, Downey D, Ruff RL: Pneumatic sequential compression reduces the risk of deep vein thrombosis in stroke patients. Neurology 1998;50:1683-1688.

60. Kamphulsen PW, Agnelli G, Sebastianelli M: Prevention of venous thromboembolism after acute ischemic stroke. J Thromb Haemost 2005;3: 1187-1194.

61. Mazzone C, Chiodo GF, Sandercock P, Miccio M, Salvi R: Physical methods for preventing deep vein thrombosis inn stroke. Cochrane Database Syst Rev 2004;18:CD001922.

62. Andre C, de Freitas GR, Fukujima MM: Prevention of deep vein thrombosis and pulmonary embolism following stroke: a systematic review of published articles. Eur J Neurol 2007;14:21-32.

63. Kamphulsen PW, Agnelli G: What is the optimal pharmacological prophylaxis for the prevention of deep-vein thrombosis and pulmonary embolism in patients with acute ischemic stroke? Thromb Res 2007;119:265-274.

64. Sherman DG, Albers GW, Bladin C et al for the PREVAIL Investigators: The efficacy and safety of enoxyparin versus unfractionated heparin for the prevention of venous thromboembolism after acute ischaemic stroke (PREVAIL Study): an open-label randomized comparison. Lancet 2007;369:1347-1355.

65. Caplan LR, Hurst JW: Cardiac and cardiovascular findings in patients with nervous system diseases-brain diseases-stroke. In Caplan LR, Hurst JW, Chimowitz MI (eds): Clinical Neurocardiology. New York: Marcel Dekker, 1999, pp 303-312.

66. Prosser J, MacGregor L, Lees KR et al on behalf of the VISTA Investigators: Predictors of early cardiac morbidity and mortality after ischemic stroke. Stroke 2007;38:2295-2302.

67. Norris JW, Kolin A, Hachinski VC: Focal myocardial lesions in stroke. Stroke 1980;11:130.

68. Connor RC: Focal myocytolysis and fuchsinophilic degeneration of the myocardium of patients dying with various brain lesions. Ann N Y Acad Sci 1969; 156:261-270.

69. Samuels M: "Voodoo" death revisited: the modern lessons of neurocardiology. Neurologist 1997;3: 293-304.

70. Ali AS, Levine SR: Heart and Brain Relationships. In Caplan LR (ed): Brain Ischemia, Basic Concepts and Clinical Relevance. London: Springer, 1995, pp 317-328.

71. Rolak LA, Rokey R: Electrocardiographic features. In Rolak LA, Rokey R (eds): Coronary and Cerebrovascular Disease. A Practical Guide. Mt Kisco, NY: Futura, 1990, pp 139-197.

72. Puleo P: Cardiac enzyme assessment. In Rolak LA, Rokey R (eds): Coronary and Cerebrovascular Disease. A Practical Guide. Mt Kisco, NY: Futura, 1990, pp 199-216.

73. Myers MG, Norris JW, Hachinski VC, et al: Cardiac sequelae of acute stroke. Stroke 1982;13: 838-842.

74. Mikolich JR, Jacobs WC, Fletcher GF: Cardiac arrhythmias in patients with acute cerebrovascular accidents. JAMA 1981;246:1314-1317.

75. Vingerhoets F, Bogousslavsky J, Regli F, Van Melle G: Atrial fibrillation after acute stroke. Stroke 1993;24:26-30.

76. Benarroch EE: The central autonomic network: functional organization, dysfunction, and perspective. Mayo Clin Proc 1993;68:988-1001.

77. Talman WT: Cardiovascular regulation and lesions of the central nervous system. Ann Neurol 1985; 18:1-12.

78. Oppenheimer SM, Cechetto DF, Hachinski VC: Cerebrogenic cardiac arrhythmias. Cerebral electrocardiographic influences and their role in sudden death. Arch Neurol 1990;47: 513-519.

79. Oppenheimer SM, Hopkins DA: Suprabulbar Neural Regulation of the Heart. In Armour JA, Ardell JL (eds): Neurocardiology. New York: Oxford University Press, 1994, pp 309-341.

80. Fink JN, Selim MH, Kumar S, Voetsch B, Fong WC, Caplan LR: Insular cortex infarction in acute middle cerebral artery territory stroke: predictor of stroke severity and vascular lesion. Arch Neurol. 2005;62: 1081-1085.

81. Myers MS, Norris JW, Hachinski VC, et al: Plasma norepinephrine in stroke. Stroke 1981; 12:200-204.

82. Weir BK: Pulmonary edema following fatal aneurysmal rupture. J Neurosurg 1978;49:502-507.

83. Hoff JT, Nishimura M: Experimental neurogenic pulmonary edema in cats. J Neurosurg 1978;18: 383-389.

84. Mayer SA, Lin J, Homma S, et al: Myocardial injury and left ventricular performance after subarachnoid hemorrhage. Stroke 1999;30: 780-786.

85. Gongora-Rivera F, Labreuche J, Jaramillo A et al: Autopsy prevalence of coronary atherosclerosis in patients with fatal stroke. Stroke 2007;38: 1203-1210.

86. Korpelainen JT, Sotaniemi KA, Makkallio A, et al: Dynamic behavior of heart rate in ischemic stroke. Stroke 1999;30:1008-1013.

87. Weidler DJ, Das SK, Sodeman TM: Cardiac arrhythmias secondary to acute cerebral ischemia: prevention by autonomic blockade. Circulation 1976;53(Suppl 2):102.

88. Horner J, Massey EW: Silent aspiration following stroke. Neurology 1988;38:317-319.

89. Groher ME, Bukatman R: The prevalence of swallowing disorders in two teaching hospitals. Dysphagia 1986;1:3-6.

90. Horner J, Massey EW, Brazer SR: Aspiration in bilateral stroke patients. Neurology 1990;40:1686-1688.

91. Alberts MJ, Horner J: Dysphagia and aspiration syndromes. In Bogousslavsky J, Caplan LR (eds): Stroke Syndromes. Cambridge: Cambridge University Press, 1995, pp 213-222.

92. Ramsey DJ, Smithard DG, Kaira L: Can pulse oximetry or a bedside swallowing assessment be used to detect aspiration after stroke? Stroke 2006;37:2984-2988.

93. Leder SB, Espinosa JF: Aspiration risk after stroke: comparison of clinical examination and fiberoptic endoscopic evaluation of swallowing. Dysphagia 2002;17:214-218.

94. Horner J, Massey EW, Risler JE, et al: Aspiration following stroke: clinical correlates and outcome. Neurology 1988;38:1359-1362.

95. Mann G, Dip PG, Hankey GJ, Cameron D: Swallowing function after stroke. Prognosis and prognostic factors at 6 months. Stroke 1999;30:744-748.

96. Ramsey DJ, Smithard DG, Kaira L: Early assessment of dysphagia and aspiration risk in acute stroke patients. Stroke 2003;34:1252-1257.

97. Mulley GP: Pneumonia, stroke, and laterality. Lancet 1981;1:1051.

98. Asianyan S, Weir CJ, Diener HC, Kaste M, Lees KR: GAIN International Steering Committee and Investigators. Eur J Neurol 2004;11:49-53.

99. Sellars C, Bowie L, Bagg J et al: Risk factors for chest infection in acute stroke: a prospective cohort study. Stroke 2007;38:2284-2291.

100. Fluck DC: Chest movements in hemiplegia. Clin Sci 1966;31:383-388.

101. Przedborski S, Brunko E, Hubert M, et al: The effect of acute hemiplegia on intercostal muscle activity. Neurology 1988;38:1882-1884.

102. Kaldor A, Berlin I: Pneumonia, stroke, and laterality. Lancet 1981;1:843.

103. Dirnagl U, Klehmet J, Braun, et al: Stroke-induced immunodepression. Experimental evidence and clinical relevance. Stroke 2007;38(part 2):770-773.

104. Chamorro A, Urra X, Planas AM: Infection after acute ischemic stroke. A manifestation of brain-induced immunodepression. Stroke 2007;38:1097-1103.

105. Emsley HCA, Hopkins SJ: Acute ischaemic stroke and infection: recent and emerging concepts. Lancet Neurol 2008;7:341-353.

106. Dziewas R, Ritter M, Schilling M, et al: Pneumonia in acute stroke patients fed by nasogastric tube. J Neurol Neurosurg Psychiatry 2004;75:852-856.

107. Yoo S-H, Kim JS, Kwon SU, et al: Undernutrition as a predictor of poor clinical outcomes in acute ischemic stroke patients. Arch Neurol 2008;65:39-43.

108. Finestone HM, Green-Finestone LS, Wilson ES, Teasell RW: Malnutrition in stroke patients on the rehabilitation service and at follow-up. Prevalence and predictors. Arch Phys Med Rehabil 1995;76:310-316.

109. Aptaker RI, Roth EJ, Reichhardt G, et al: Serum albumin level as a predictor of geriatric stroke rehabilitation outcome. Arch Phys Med Rehabil 1994;75:80-84.

110. Norton B, Homer-Ward M, Donnelly MT, et al: A randomized prospective comparisonn of percutaneous endoscopic gastrostomy and nasogastric tube feedings after acute dysphagic stroke. BMJ 1996;312:13-16.

111. Wijdicks EFM, McMahon MM: Percutaneous endoscopic gastrostomy after acute stroke: complications and outcome. Cerebrovasc Dis 1999;9:109-111.

112. Joynt RJ, Feibel JH, Sladek CM: Antidiuretic hormone levels in stroke patients. Ann Neurol 1981;9:182-184.

113. Tsuchida S, Noto H, Yamaguchi D, et al: Urodynamic studies on hemiplegia patients after cerebrovascular accident. Urology 1983;21:315-318.

114. Davenport RJ, Dennis MS, Warlow CP: Gastrointestinal hemorrhage after acute stroke. Stroke 1996;27:421-424.

115. Smith DM: Pressure ulcers in the nursing home. Ann Intern Med 1995;123:433-442.

116. Lindgren I, Jonsson A-C, Norrving B, Lindgren A: Shoulder pain after stroke. Stroke 2007;38:343-348.

117. Braus DF, Krauss JK, Strobel J: The shoulder-hand syndrome after stroke: a prospective clinical trial. Ann Neurol 1994;36:728-733.

118. Sato Y, Kuno H, Kaji M, et al: Increased bone resorption during the first year after stroke. Stroke 1998;29:1373-1377.

119. Sato Y, Maruoka H, Oizumi K: Amelioration of hemiplegia-associated osteopenia more than 4 years after stroke by 1 alpha-hydroxyvitamin D3 and calcium supplementation. Stroke 1997;28:736-739.

120. Sato Y, Fujimatsu Y, Honda Y, et al: Accelerated bone remodeling in patients with poststroke hemiplegia. J Stroke Cerebrovasc Dis 1998;7:58-62.

121. Ramnemark A, Nyberg L, Lorentzon R, et al: Hemiosteoporosis after severe stroke, independent of changes in body composition and weight. Stroke 1999;30:755-760.

122. Poole KES, Loveridge N, Rose CM, Warburton EA, Reeve J: A single infusion of Zoledronate prevents bone loss after stroke. Stroke 2007;38:1519-1525.

123. van der Werf SP, van den Broek HLP, Anten HWM, Bleijenberg G: Experience of severe fatigue long after stroke and its relation to depressive symptoms and disease characteristics. Eur Neurol 2001;45:28-33.

124. Ingles JL, Eskes GA, Phillips SJ: Fatigue after stroke. Arch Phys Med Rehabil 1999;80:173-178.

125. Feibel JH, Springer CJ: Depression and failure to resume social activities after stroke. Arch Phys Med Rehabil 1982;63:276-277.

126. Robinson RG, Szetela B: Mood change following left hemisphere brain injury. Ann Neurol 1981;9:447-453.

127. Finkelstein S, Benowitz LI, Baldessarini RJ, et al: Mood, vegetative disturbances, and dexamethasone suppression test after stroke. Ann Neurol 1982;12:463-468.

128. Astrom M, Adolfdon R, Asplund K: Major depression in stroke patients. A 3-year longitudinal study. Stroke 1993;24:976-982.

129. Pohjasvaara T, Leppavuori A, Siira I, et al: Frequency and clinical determinants of poststroke depression. Stroke 1998;29:2311-2317.

130. Robinson RG, Price TR: Poststroke depressive disorders: a follow-up study of 103 patients. Stroke 1982;13:635-641.

131. Verdelho A, Henon H, Lebert F, Pasquier F, Leys D: Depressive symptoms after stroke and relationship with dementia. A three-year follow-up study. Neurology 2004;62:905-911.

132. Robinson RG, Starr LB, Price TR: A two-year longitudinal study of mood disorders following stroke. Br J Psychiatry 1984;144:256-262.

133. Ghika-Schmid F, Bogousslavsky J: Affective disorders following stroke. Eur Neurol 1997;38:75-81.

134. Binder LM: Emotional problems after stroke. Stroke 1984;15:174-177.

135. Ross ED, Rush AJ: Diagnosis and neuroanatomical correlates of depression in brain-damaged patients. Arch Gen Psychiatry 1981;38:1344-1354.

136. Robinson RG, Starr LB, Kubos K, et al: A two-year longitudinal study of poststroke mood disorders: findings during the initial evaluation. Stroke 1983;14:736-741.

137. Robinson RG, Kubos KL, Starr LB, et al: Mood disorders in stroke patients: importance of location of lesion. Brain 1984;107:81-93.

138. Robinson RG, Kubos KL, Starr LB, et al: Mood changes in stroke patients: relationship to lesion location. Compr Psychiatry 1983;24:555-566.

139. Herrmann M, Bartels C, Schumacher M, Wallesch C-W: Poststroke depression. Is there a pathoanatomic correlate for depression in the postacute stage of stroke? Stroke 1995;26:850-856.

140. Lipsey JR, Robinson RG, Pearlson GD, et al: Nortriptyline treatment of poststroke depression: a double-blind study. Lancet 1984;1:297-300.

141. Reding JJ, Orto LA, Winter SW, et al: Antidepressant therapy after stroke: a double blind trial. Arch Neurol 1986;43:763-765.

142. Andersen G, Vestergaard K, Lauritzen L: Effective treatment of post-stroke depression with the selective reuptake inhibitor citalopram. Stroke 1994;25:1099-1104.

143. Wade DT, Legh-Smith J, Langton-Hewer R: Effects of living with and looking after survivors of a stroke. BMJ 1986;293:418-420.

144. Anderson CS, Linto J, Stewart-Wynne EG: A population-based assessment of the impact and burden of caregiving for long-term stroke survivors. Stroke 1995;26:843-849.

145. Scholte OP, Reimer WJ, de Haan RJ, Rijnders PT, Limburg M, van den Bos GA. The burden of caregiving in partners of long-term stroke survivors. Stroke 1998;29:1605-1611.

146. Dennis M, O'Rourke S, Lewis S, et al: A quantitative study of the emotional outcome of people caring for stroke survivors. Stroke 1998;29:1867-1872.

147. van Exel NJ, Koopmanschap MA, van den Berg B, Brouwer WB, van den Bos GA: Burden of informal caregiving for stroke patients. Identification of caregivers at risk of adverse health effects. Cerebrovasc Dis 2005;19:11-17.

RECOVERY

Recovery of neurologic function after stroke is complex and depends on many factors.[1,1a] Some factors relate to the nature and severity of the stroke mechanism. For example, patients with brain hemorrhages recover at a different rate and extent than patients with infarcts of comparable size and location. In many patients, ischemia is transient. Portions of the ischemic zone can return to normal without leaving permanent damage. Positron emission tomography scans and magnetic resonance imaging diffusion and perfusion scanning often show regions of brain tissue that are underperfused acutely but return to normal after reperfusion. Neuroanatomic factors play a major role. The location and size of the infarct or hemorrhage are important as are the lobes and brain regions that are spared.[1,2]

Function-related factors are also important. Limitations of some neurologic functions are easier to overcome or adapt to than other functions. Most patients adapt to a hemianopia that results from an occipital-lobe lesion by paying more attention to stimuli in their impaired field of vision, but it is more difficult for patients to overcome visual neglect from a parietal-lobe lesion. In the circumstance of an occipital-lobe lesion, the patient is aware of the visual-field deficit and can learn to adapt or compensate for it. Patients with parietal-lobe lesions have more difficulty perceiving and understanding the nature of their visual deficit and are often less able to cope. A visual-field deficit is usually less disabling than hemiparesis. Constructional apraxia is less of a handicap than aphasia.

Some neurologic functions are subserved by networks of regions that interact together, whereas other functions are more strictly localized to one or two brain sites. A lesion in the visual cortex-striate region (Brodmann's area 17) involving both banks of the calcarine fissure invariably causes a hemianopia. No other regions exist that subserve identical visual function. Attention to the contralateral side of visual space is a more complex function subserved by the frontal and parietal lobes, with strong thalamic and limbic input and also some involvement of basal-ganglionic structures.[3] A lesion that involves one of these regions might temporarily disrupt attentional functions but usually does not cause persistent neglect. Some functions seem to reside in several different regions. In case of injury to one region, the function is assumed by other spared regions. Patients with persistent lesions in Broca's area often regain excellent speech after a temporary period of mutism.[4-6]

Individual patient and character-related factors exist that heavily influence recovery. Older patients may have more difficulty adjusting to deficits and changing behaviors than younger patients. Some individuals are "survivors" and have the intelligence, determination, and character to succeed under adverse circumstances. Past personal accomplishments, flexibility, and attitudes are important determinants of functional recovery and ability to adapt to a disability. Also important are medical comorbidities. The presence of significant heart disease, obesity, pulmonary abnormalities, arthritis, and other diseases and conditions impact heavily on the patient's physical ability to pursue rehabilitation with vigor.

Social, economic, and environmental factors are also very important. Does the patient have a competent caregiver who will prod, cajole, and motivate the patient to do better? Are sufficient economic resources available? What floor does the patient live on? Is an elevator available in the building? Are stores, restaurants, movie theaters, and recreational and social activities within easy access for the patient? Are family members and friends nearby? Are they supportive and helpful? The answers to these queries are seldom noted in hospital charts but are just as important for meaningful recovery as the extent of brain injury and the nature and severity of the neurologic signs.

A New Emphasis on Scientific Aspects of Recovery

The study of recovery from brain injuries has been greatly facilitated by new technologies that can localize and quantify brain anatomy and function,[1a,7-12] by animal experiments that show cell growth and repair and molecular responses to injury,[1a,12a,12b] and by new therapeutic capabilities and strategies. The brains of stroke patients can now be studied using functional magnetic resonance imaging (fMRI), positron emission tomography (PET) scanning, and transcranial magnetic stimulation to show which regions are activated in individual patients who recover or do not recover functions after brain infarcts and hemorrhages. The ability to study white matter tracts using diffusion tensor imaging (DTI), and to analyze MRI images for Wallerian degeneration has also been helpful in assessing brain damage to motor and other CNS white matter pathways.[9,11]

Studies of motor recovery after strokes that involve the primary motor cortex show that some structures on the same side of the lesion show more activity than in controls. The supplementary motor cortex, premotor regions, and parietal cortical regions on the same side of the brain injury are activated.[9,10] The contralesional sensorimotor paracentral cortex and supplementary motor areas are also often activated.[9,10,12] The more severe the hemiparesis, the greater the extent of activation of ancillary regions. Some areas take on new functions. For example, the dorsolateral premotor cortex, in some recovering patients, assumes executive motor functions such as activation during specific tasks.[10] With time the widespread brain activation pattern during motor tasks using a paretic limb seem to become more focused on one or more regions. Clearly, some sparing of primary motor cortex on the side of the injury is very helpful in predicting recovery. At times, in some patients, the contralesional sensorimotor cortex may exert an inhibitory effect on motor function of the hemiparetic hand.[10,12-14]

Similarly, researchers are beginning to study recovery from other neurologic deficits. These baseline studies and objective evaluation techniques now provide a scientific basis for evaluating strategies to facilitate recovery. I predict that increasing emphasis in the future will be devoted to recovery and its mechanisms and augmentation.

REHABILITATION UNITS AND SERVICES

In the preceding chapters of this volume, care by physicians was centered either in outpatient facilities, or in acute care hospitals. A unique feature in relation to recovery and the after-effects of stroke is that much care occurs in rehabilitation units. I feel it important to introduce and discuss these units before launching into new ideas about recovery and rehabilitation.

Present rehabilitation services are quite different from most traditional medical and surgical units and the process is unfamiliar to many physicians. Rehabilitation has a different emphasis

and goal than traditional medicine. Rehabilitation focuses on recovery and adaptation to loss of neurologic function. In contrast, traditional medicine has a pathologic and pathophysiologic emphasis. The goal of traditional medical care is to prevent and treat disease. Rehabilitation is usually performed in buildings or units separated from acute-care hospitals and other neurologic facilities. Personnel include a much higher ratio of nonphysician to physician staff members. Although a physician usually captains the team, the role of other paramedical personnel is more important than in most acute-care units. The physician in-charge is often a physical medicine specialist. Internists, cardiologists, geriatricians, and orthopedists are also often involved since rehabilitation facilities typically house patients recovering from a variety of medical and orthopedic conditions and surgeries. In the past and at present, few neurologists in the United States have chosen to specialize in rehabilitation or to work full time in rehabilitation units. Rehabilitation units have a slower pace, longer patient stays, and, at times, different reimbursement rules for third-party payers.

Rehabilitation encourages and relies heavily on family involvement and the education of patients, families, and caregivers. Rehabilitation uses a lot of equipment, such as braces, walking aids, and parallel bars, which are foreign to most medical units. Parts of rehabilitation units look more like gymnasiums, exercise areas, workshops, or schools than standard medical wards.

Because of this perceived strangeness, and because they feel that they have little input or control while their patients are in rehabilitation units, some physicians are reluctant to refer their patients to rehabilitation facilities. As a result, many patients who should have rehabilitation do not receive it. Rehabilitation for stroke patients is very important but underused. In some patients, rehabilitation training can make the difference between a vegetative, bedridden existence in a nursing home and a productive life in society. Immobile patients discharged directly home or to nursing homes and not mobilized during the first months after stroke are unlikely to become more active later. A bed or bed-and-chair existence is physically and psychologically destructive. If the same immobile patients are admitted to rehabilitation units and successfully trained to sit and walk, the probability is high that they can become and remain self-reliant and increase their activities and independence during the ensuing months. Rehabilitation can also be effectively administered at home and at work sites.

Time is of the essence; training must begin in the weeks after the stroke. Major recovery from stroke takes place during the first 3 to 6 months.[1a,14a] Only small numbers of patients show dramatic improvement during the next 18 to 24 months.[15-17] The push from managed-care personnel to get patients out of acute hospitals sicker and quicker means that many patients who are transferred to rehabilitation units require more acute care than they did in the past. The high cost of in-patient rehabilitation programs has led managed-care payers to offer therapy programs in the patients' homes, nursing homes, or as outpatients instead of at rehabilitation facilities.[17]

Functioning in Rehabilitation Units

Rehabilitation should be considered in terms of the general process of stroke recovery. Rehabilitation occurs during the first weeks and months after stroke onset. Natural recovery mechanisms occur at the same time, especially if patients remain active. Much of the recovery is natural, although most patients are inclined to give complete credit for their improvement to various therapies that they receive during rehabilitation.

Strategies and methods of rehabilitation vary greatly between units and have changed over time. Descriptions of the methods, techniques, and aids used during rehabilitation are far beyond the scope of this book and beyond the knowledge and expertise of the author. Excellent chapters and monographs devoted entirely to this subject exist elsewhere.[17-22,22a,22b] Stroke units and rehabilitation services exist in different locations, some within acute-care hospitals, others in free-standing chronic care hospitals apart from acute-care facilities, and some in out-patient facilities in the community.

In excellent rehabilitation facilities, a number of goals should be pursued concurrently.[17-23] Methods used to treat acute stroke and preventive strategies emphasized at the acute-care facility should be continued. This means that physicians and nurses at the rehabilitation facility should become fully knowledgeable about the causative stroke mechanism and treatments used to minimize the deficit and prevent worsening and stroke recurrence. Many patients are sent to rehabilitation units with incomplete evaluations at acute-care facilities. Investigations of the causative cardio-cerebrovascular-hematological causes of stroke in these patients must be pursued further while the patient is being rehabilitated. Control of stroke risk factors, such as cessation of smoking and appropriate diet, should be continued at the rehabilitation unit.

Nurses and physicians in rehabilitation units must monitor the occurrence of stroke complications and use strategies to prevent them.[14-16]

Chapter 18 is devoted to stroke complications. Probably one of the major explanations for the success of stroke units is their focus on systematically watching for and treating complications that develop. Mobilization and physical therapy help prevent phlebothrombosis, contractures, and bed sores. Therapy can also ameliorate dysphagia and help prevent aspiration and pneumonia. Attention to micturition can help prevent urinary tract infections and urosepsis.

The process of evaluating the nature and severity of various neurologic, medical, and psychological dysfunctions and disabilities should begin shortly after the patient is transferred to the rehabilitation unit.[22,23] The outcome of rehabilitation can often be predicted by analysis of a number of variables related to the neurologic deficits found.[22] Motor functions of the limbs, micturition, swallowing, gait, speech, perception, cognitive and behavioral abilities, psychological reactions, and intelligence should be assessed. Recognition of impairments and disabilities is the first step in devising strategies and programs to train the stroke patient to overcome and adapt to any dysfunctions found and prevent the development of further handicaps. The terms *impairment*, *disability*, and *handicap* are in common use by rehabilitation specialists and units so that clinicians should be aware of the way that these words are used. The definitions of these terms by the World Health Organization[24] are noted in Table 19-1.

Table 19-1.	Definition of Terms by the World Health Organization (WHO)[18]
Impairment	Any loss or abnormality of psychological, physiologic, or anatomic structure or function
Disability	Any restriction or lack of ability resulting from impairment to perform an activity in the manner or within the range considered normal for a human being
Handicap	A disadvantage for a given individual resulting from an impairment or disability that limits or prevents the fulfillment of a role that is normal for that individual

Strokes do not only affect the individual stroke patient. Stroke is a disease that affects the patient's family, friends, and environment. The caregiver, family, and friends play a major role in rehabilitation. Educating and training caregivers are important tasks during the rehabilitation process. Caregivers should be instructed about the nature of the stroke patient's dysfunctions and strategies used to deal with these impairments.

During rehabilitation, strategies are devised to reintegrate the patient back to his or her home. This often entails evaluation of the home and suggestions to make the home environment safer for the patient. For example, if the patient customarily slept on the second floor and the kitchen, television, and living and dining rooms are on the first floor, it might be simpler to create a sleeping area for the patient on the first floor to facilitate eating and daily activities. Showers may need to be made safer and more readily usable. Social agencies may need to be mobilized for the care and support of the patient. Visiting nurses, therapists, homemakers, and food delivery services may need to be consulted when patients return to their homes.

The general theme of stroke rehabilitation is a disability-oriented, multidisciplinary team approach. Team members include the patient, patient's family, primary-care physician, neurologist, physical therapist, occupational therapist, speech therapist, social worker, and rehabilitation nurse. Members of the team should meet regularly to identify specific rehabilitation goals, strategies for their attainment, and methods of implementation. These team members educate and train patients and family members in their areas of expertise. Ideally, the team rehabilitation process should begin early in the course of the acute stroke so that improvement in quality of life can be achieved as early as possible.

The role of physicians differs within rehabilitation units from the traditional role of doctors in an acute-care facility.[18] Physicians direct the team. They evaluate and prognosticate. These physicians interact with the team of therapists about compensatory physical and cognitive strategies and assist devices. They try various drug interventions to treat pain, spasticity, and cognitive and mood disorders. These physicians serve as administrative brokers to gather the resources and services that the patients and their families need.

Rehabilitation nurses are key members of the team. Often, one nurse acts to coordinate physician orders and integrate the various strategies used in the rehabilitation process. Nurses must often pursue an attitude unusual in the nursing profession. A nurse is usually the provider of direct care. On a rehabilitation unit, however, the nurse must often sit back and let the patient accomplish tasks at hand, providing teaching, encouragement, and help as needed. Extreme patience is required. Nurses must synthesize the recommendations of other team members and directly apply these ideas to the everyday care of patients. Nurses also monitor and direct treatment for medical complications that might occur during rehabilitation.

The physical therapist's main function is training the patient for ambulation. Balancing, weight-shifting techniques, parallel bars, various orthotics, and quad canes are used. Severe weakness in a lower extremity does not preclude ambulation. Often, a patient is unable to lift his or her leg from the bed yet eventually becomes ambulatory. Increased extensor tone combined with minimal bracing permits walking. Even before ambulation training begins, physical therapists perform range-of-motion, strengthening, and endurance exercises. In addition, physical therapists can help provide appropriate supporting apparatus, such as lap boards, chair-arm supports, and swings. Range-of-motion exercises are passive and active and should be performed at least four times daily. Patients can use the normal arm to passively move the paralyzed extremity through a full range of motion. These exercises help prevent deconditioning, excessive spasticity, joint contractures, and peripheral edema. Range-of-motion exercises combined with upper-extremity support are the keys to preventing a painful shoulder caused by subluxation or spasticity. Both the family and nursing staff should take active roles using the recommendations of the physical therapist for remobilization throughout the day.

Occupational therapists perform upper-extremity retraining with particular attention to teaching practical activities of daily living. Patients and therapists work on improving fine-motor skills so that activities such as feeding, dressing, personal hygiene, and cooking can be accomplished. These skills allow the development of independent function. Often, special devices, including a reacher, utensil holder, specially placed rails or handles, commodes, tub benches, or hand-held showers, are used. An occupational therapist can customize these techniques and physical changes in the home to adapt to the patient's deficits.

Speech therapists work to improve communication skills. The goal is to facilitate communication early in the patient's rehabilitation. The methods may be verbal or nonverbal, using spoken or written words, gestures, or word boards. The boards may contain letters that patients point to for spelling words or may contain words or pictures to designate needs or wishes. Computer programs are often helpful for facilitating communication skills. Often, therapists can develop techniques of nonverbal communication for severely aphasic patients so their needs can be met and feelings of isolation eliminated. During the first 3 months after a stroke, much spontaneous language recovery occurs. Beyond 3 months, the therapist's role is to enhance further recovery of language function. Physicians should not accept a nihilistic attitude toward speech therapy. I advise physicians to start aphasic patients on a comprehensive program of speech therapy early during the course of treatment. Physicians should continue to pursue a vigorous course of treatment in most patients, withholding treatment only in patients who are demented or severely globally aphasic. Speech therapists also help evaluate and treat dysarthria and dysphagia, breath control, and articulation. Speech therapists can often suggest types of foods, liquids, and eating techniques that might be best tolerated by patients.

Next to the patient, family members have the most difficult task. Usually medically unsophisticated, they must learn new skills from rehabilitation team members and directly supervise the care of the stroke patient. The family's questions and concerns should be carefully addressed by each team member. It is often useful for the family member most directly involved in home care to spend a few days at the hospital to effectively acquire the necessary skills. Once patients return home, continued contact with the team is crucial so progress can be monitored, new problems identified, and solutions implemented. This contact may be in the form of visits to the home or appointments at the rehabilitation unit with individual team members.

Perhaps most important are the spirit and milieu of the unit. Personnel must possess an optimistic outlook accompanied by understanding. Planning should be practical, and goals must be realistic. The use of equipment, strategies, and programs that help patients and caregivers recognize and deal with disabilities is helpful.

Patient Selection

Although rehabilitation is important, not all stroke patients benefit from treatment within a rehabilitation unit. If every stroke patient were referred, rehabilitation facilities would be swamped and the cost to taxpayers would greatly increase, whereas effective retraining for those who may benefit most would suffer from dilution. Selection of appropriate patients is important. Patients who are already ambulatory and have only slight or temporary deficits do not need to stay in a rehabilitation unit; they do well on their own or with outpatient therapy. The patient who is stuporous, completely immobile, or has severe right-hemisphere dysfunction does not usually benefit from rehabilitation. Most observers agree that the middle group between these two extremes is the appropriate target for rehabilitative care. How should this group be identified? What factors should be considered in making the triage decision?

Patients of all ages can be offered rehabilitation. By decade, no difference in outcome has been shown; substantial recovery is noted in all age groups.[18,19,25,26] Patients who have serious cognitive impairment or severe underlying medical illness may be unable to participate in effective rehabilitation programs; these patients are either unable to learn compensatory techniques or cannot tolerate the physical activity required. Aphasia, however, does not preclude stroke rehabilitation. When outcome is measured by performance of daily activities, ability to walk, and discharge disposition, no difference has been found between aphasic and nonaphasic patients referred for rehabilitation.[26-29] Higher cortical-function abnormalities other than aphasia, such as perceptual abnormalities, anosognosia, aprosodia, neglect, impersistence, reduplicative paramnesia, and prosopagnosia, may make rehabilitation more difficult but not impossible. These cognitive abnormalities tend to improve with time, allowing the stroke rehabilitation process to proceed.[1,2]

Neurologic findings, such as limb paralysis, are prognostically important,[18,19,23,30] but neurologic disability and accompanying medical illness are not the only factors that predict outcome. A host of nonmedical social, psychological, and environmental factors are of equal or even greater importance. Two of the most accurate prognostic predictors in patients with head trauma are (1) presence of a "significant other" to help the patient, and (2) whether the patient had a job before the injury.

Similarly, a number of seemingly mundane factors apply when deciding on treatment for a stroke patient. What was the patient's prestroke level of capability? Does the patient have financial support to help with special equipment, transportation, and so forth? Does the patient have a car or access to other transportation? Does the patient have someone at home who is motivated, capable, and available to help and encourage recovery?[31] Does the home have stairs or a bathroom on every floor? Is a meals-on-wheels program or a store that delivers and takes telephone orders accessible to the patient? What community services are available? These prognostic factors and others must be considered to offer rehabilitation to those who will benefit most. I believe that when prognosis is uncertain, the patient should be given the benefit of the doubt. A trial period of rehabilitation should be offered. Some rehabilitation now takes place in specified nursing homes. Placement in these designated nursing home facilities is an alternative for those patients not able to participate fully in vigorous rehabilitation in-patient units.

Rehabilitation has been studied in a number of trials.[17,18,32-40] Some trials considered units within the hospital and others relate to separate units. These trials suggest that the milieu and greater frequency and intensity of rehabilitation services in dedicated stroke and rehabilitation units lead to better outcomes. Mortality is reduced. More patients return home and less patients are transferred to chronic hospitals and nursing homes. Short- and long-term functional outcomes are also improved. Doubt that stroke units work no longer exists. Some trials have studied the use of various techniques and strategies for specific functions, such as recovery of hemiplegic gait,[41,41a,41b] improvement in upper-extremity function,[42] recovery from aphasia,[43,44] and management of spatial neglect.[45] Other trials study the effects of specific strategies on general functional outcome (e.g., the effect of sensory stimulation on outcome of patients with severe stroke-related hemiparesis).[46]

Ottenbacher and Jannell performed a meta-analysis of trials and studies conducted between 1960 and 1990.[36] The analysis included patients who had a stroke-related hemiparesis who were given rehabilitation services in a design that compared at least two groups or conditions for change in a quantifiable functional measure. Outcomes studied included gait, hand functions, activities of daily living, response times, and visual perceptual functions. From 173 statistical evaluations performed on 3717 patients studied in these trials, the meta-analysis showed that the average patient who received a program that included focused stroke rehabilitation or a particular procedure performed better than approximately 65% of patients in the comparison groups.[17,36] Greater effects of treatment were obtained when rehabilitation was performed early. Younger patients tended to do better than older patients.

Why do stroke units perform better than non-dedicated units? The reasons are probably multifactorial and include such difficult-to-quantify ingredients as attitude, milieu, caring, education, multidisciplinary approach, and systematic attention to routines and details.

Coordination of Acute and Long-Term Care

To be optimally successful, rehabilitation should be fully integrated with traditional medical care. Therapy should begin as early as possible while the patient is still on the acute medical or neurologic unit. Physicians, nurses, and other personnel must be involved. Therapy should not be completely delegated to physical and occupational therapists. Consultations should not be limited to the 30 minutes or so that patients typically spend each day with therapists. Passive and active range-of-motion exercises and other physical therapy should be encouraged by ward personnel. If the patient goes to a rehabilitation unit, the acute-care team should continue to follow the patient whenever possible. Acute medical problems do not suddenly disappear when the patient is transferred. Subsequent strokes and medical complications are common among recuperating patients.

The patient receives mixed signals if treatment and advice begun on the acute-care unit are not followed through at the rehabilitation unit. The patient may have been persuaded by a doctor on the acute-care unit who advised the need for a low-salt, low-cholesterol diet, only to be served butter, cream, and eggs on the rehabilitation unit. Medical treatment and surveillance should be continued during rehabilitation and afterward. Similarly, when the patient leaves the rehabilitation unit, the physician must continue to emphasize the need to carry out various rehabilitation techniques. After treatment in the acute-care center and rehabilitation facilities, patients usually return to the care of their primary care physician, most likely an internist or family practitioner. The primary care physician must be kept up-to-date with the patient's findings, current treatment decisions, and recommendations so they can continue medical treatment and retraining procedures and strategies. Rehabilitation and traditional medical care should be intertwined and overlapped, not seen by the patient as unrelated phases with one consultation succeeding the other.

Pitfall of Exaggerated Emphasis on Physical Therapy

I have been impressed with the frequency after discharge of a phenomenon that I have referred to as the hyper–physical therapy syndrome. Patients affected by this syndrome continue to intensively strive to improve hand, arm, or limb function and return these functions to "normal." Instead of expending energy on readapting to their former lifestyle, which probably does not require absolutely normal function, they continue to exercise and focus excessive attention on their limb dysfunction. These patients exchange a practical, reachable goal (a return to all prior activities) for an impractical, unreachable, and relatively less important goal (a return to normal premorbid strength and function). Many patients attribute their recovery entirely to physical therapy and are fearful of stopping or decreasing it. Much of their energy and time are taken up in going to and from therapy, doing therapy at home, and resting after therapy is over. These individuals have little time and energy left for living. Patients should be gradually weaned from physical therapy at the appropriate time and be encouraged to adapt to their deficit, turning attention away from limb impairment toward enjoyment of life.

Loss of self-image and oversensitivity to minor disabilities are other common problems. Sometimes, exposure to others who have regained full prestroke activities despite unresolved neurologic deficits is of great help to patients.

Newer Concepts and Strategies for Augmenting Natural Recovery

At the beginning of this chapter, I discussed natural recovery and commented on enthusiasm within the neurologic community for using information based on new technology to guide a more scientific and rational approach to rehabilitation therapeutics than was feasible in the past. In this concluding section, I now mention some newer strategies, many still untested and unproven, that show promise. The proliferation of various studies makes it possible to provide only a glimpse of some of the various strategies being tried.

Functional neuroimaging studies clearly show dynamic changes in the brain after stroke.[1a,7-12,22b] These alterations in electrical activity and function change over time. Plasticity is the rule in the brain. Experimental studies in animals with iatrogenically induced strokes document extensive cellular and molecular alterations after brain damage.[1a,12a,12b] New pathways and circuits develop in response to injury. These changes in the brain are clearly modified by activity. Using a particular brain function and activating brain regions stimulates adaptation and has the potential to improve recovery of function.[1a,14a,22b] "Use it or lose it" and "practice makes perfect" are old wise sayings that are proving to be accurate in describing brain responsivity. Newer strategies incorporate various ways to stimulate brain regions related to functions lost.[22a,22b] Some encourage or force use of paretic limbs and of impaired functions such as speaking and reading. Others

activate brain regions by sensory or physical stimuli of the limbs. Others use physical stimulation of brain regions by electrical current or magnetic stimulation. Others use pharmacologic techniques to activate neurotransmitters involved in the defective functions. Some strategies are focused on ways to minimize or eliminate inhibitory circuits in the brain. Finally, physicians seek ways to stimulate endogenous primitive cells within the brain, or to introduce stem cells directly or indirectly into the brain that will proliferate and migrate to injured areas to enhance repair. These cells also provide important growth factors that stimulate cell growth.

Increased Use and Sensory Stimulation

Researchers have explored the effectiveness of forcing use of a hemiparetic arm by constraining the good arm. Preliminary studies investigated the effect of therapeutic interventions for the arm in both acute and chronic stroke patients with hemiparesis.[47-51] A small pilot study of forced use of the upper extremity in chronic stroke patients suggested some benefit.[47] A much larger multisite, randomized clinical trial conducted at seven U.S. academic centers between January 2001 and January 2003 entitled the Extremity Constraint Induced Therapy Evaluation (EXCITE) trial, enrolled 222 patients who mostly had ischemic strokes during the 3 to 9 months before entry.[51] In order to qualify for the study, individuals must have had some wrist and finger extension in their hemiparetic hand. Participants were assigned to receive either constraint-induced movement therapy wearing a restraining mitt on the less-affected hand while engaging in therapy on the weak arm and hand ($n = 106$) or usual and customary care that ranged from no treatment after formal acute stroke rehabilitation to pharmacologic or physiotherapeutic interventions ($n = 116$). Among patients who had a stroke within the previous 3 to 9 months, restraint with accompanying physical therapy on the hemiparetic hand produced statistically significant and clinically relevant improvements in arm motor function that persisted for at least 1 year.[51]

Others have examined the effect of sensory and sensorimotor stimulation of paretic limbs. One study examined the effect of repetitive sensorimotor training of the arm after stroke.[52] One hundred consecutive stroke patients were randomly assigned to an experimental group that received daily additional sensorimotor stimulation of the arm or to a control group. The treatment period was 6 weeks. Assessments of the patients were made before and after treatment and at 6 and 12 months after stroke, and in 62 patients, 5 years after stroke. At the 5-year follow-up, there was a statistically significant difference in function tests favoring the treatment group that received early, repetitive, and targeted stimulation of the paretic arm. Extra stimulation of the arm during the acute phase after a stroke resulted in a clinically meaningful and long-lasting salutary effect on motor function.[52] Another study showed that 100-Hz current applied to finger surfaces in patients with chronic post-stroke deficits improved the use of utensils with the involved hand.[17] Many different types of sensory input—optokinetic, neck proprioceptive, vestibular, and somatosensory—show improvement in neglect in stroke patients.[53,54]

Brain Stimulation

Another way to attempt to facilitate functional recovery is to directly stimulate the brain.[55-59,59a,59b,59c,59d] Transcranial stimulation can be performed using magnetic or direct current, and either the hemisphere ipsilateral to an infarct or the contralateral hemisphere can be stimulated. Repetitive transcranial magnetic stimulation (rTMS) has potential long-term effects on cerebral cortical excitability. Researchers have begun to explore the potential of rTMS in facilitating recovery. Both inhibitory and facilitatory effects can result from rTMS depending on the frequency range of the stimulation. When applied to the primary motor cortex (M1), low-frequency (1 Hz) stimulation inhibits excitability while high-frequency (5 to 20 Hz) stimulation increases cortical excitability. Studies show that low-frequency rTMS applied to the motor cortex on the side opposite a brain infarct can improve function in the hand that was weakened by the stroke.[14,55,56,59a] The authors posit that inhibition of activity contralateral to the infarct facilitated activity in the hemisphere harboring the brain infarct. Other studies showed that rTMS (applied at a frequency of 3 Mz[57] and 10 Mz[58]) to the motor cortex on the side of a brain infarct improved function of the contralateral weak hand. Often rTMS was applied along with routine standard physical and occupational therapy. Figure 19-1 shows a patient being stimulated using rTMS and the brain localization of the stimuli.

Direct current can also be applied transcranially. During transcranial direct current stimulation (tDCS) a constant low-amplitude DC current is transmitted to the cerebral cortex by way of surface mounted scalp electrodes (Fig. 19-2).[59c] Stimulation or inhibition depends on whether the direct current stimulation is anodal or cathodal. Anodal stimulation increases brain activity and

excitability while cathodal stimulation is inhibitory. The patient cannot tell if the current is turned on or off. Preliminary studies show that direct current stimulation can facilitate movement of paretic limbs.[59,59d,60] Direct current stimulation has been tested concurrent with other rehabilitative therapies in promoting recovery.[62] Studies show that pharmacologic therapy accompanied by physical therapy measures proved more effective than either pharmacologic or physical therapy alone.[62-64] Nair and colleagues gave patients 30 minutes of cathodal transcranial direct current stimulation during occupational therapy.[61] They compared this treatment group with a group given occupational therapy with sham stimulation. The investigators calculated a score for range of motion around 3 different upper extremity joints before and after treatment. The direct current–treated group improved 11.3% compared to 3.8% in the sham group ($P < 0.02$).[61]

Direct current stimulation has also been used to treat aphasic patients. One study analyzed the effect of direct current stimulation on aphasia recovery in patients treated with melodic intonation therapy.[44] They compared the effect of anodal transcranial direct current stimulation and sham treatment over the right inferior frontal gyrus (a region they had previously shown to be activated by therapy) during melodic intonation therapy sessions. The direct current stimulation group performed better on expressive speech tests.[44] Both direct current and TMS stimulation are modalities now being tested in treatment trials with and without concomitant therapies.

Robot-Assisted Training

Recently there has been an increased interest in using robots to assist therapy.[22a] Robotic devices can increase the amount and intensity of movement of plegic limbs. Similar to constraint-induced or forced use of paretic limbs, and stimulation of limbs, robots clearly increase the use of paretic extremities. Robot-aided, sensorimotor training can improve limb function.[65-69] A preliminary study in 20 patients showed that goal-directed, robot-assisted, sensorimotor activity of paretic upper limbs increased motor function in exercised muscles compared with controls not treated with robots.[65] Study of 12 of the original 20 patients 3 years later showed that the motor impairments in their upper limbs had decreased even further.[66] Cramer and colleagues used a hand-wrist–assisting robotic device during physical therapy sessions and showed dose-dependent improvements in hand motor function after chronic stroke.[69] Use of a limb and movement of a joint facilitates

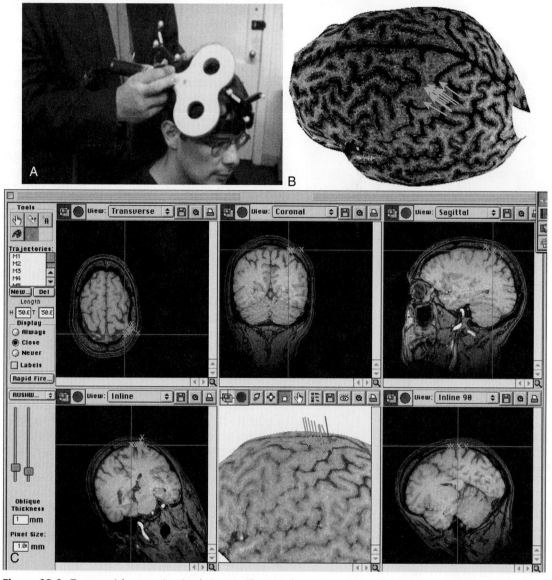

Figure 19-1. Transcranial magnetic stimulation. **A,** The stimulus equipment applied to the head. **B,** Exterior of the brain showing the region of stimulation. **C,** Magnetic resonance images showing the region of stimulation in multiple planes. (From Brainsight, Rogue Research Inc, with permission.)

recovery whether by forced use (constraint therapy) or robotic assistance.

Pharmacologic Therapies

Many drugs have been tried in the past, mostly in an attempt to enhance recovery regarding motor and cognitive and behavioral sequellae of strokes. The effectiveness of most attempts at pharmacologic manipulation have been disappointing. However, administering pharmacologic agents as an adjunct to other therapies has shown some promise. The most frequently used agents are noradrenergic or dopaminergic.[17,62-64,70-72] The most frequently reported agents used include amphetamine, methylphenidate, amantidine, memantine, bromcriptine, and carbidopa/levodopa.[70]

Some pharmacologic agents can retard recovery. Haloperidol has a definite negative effect on recovery.[73,74] Drugs that enhance gamma-aminobutyric acid transmission, such as diazepam, might increase inhibition of function and also delay recovery.[70,75] Stroke patients are often exposed to polypharmacy.[76-78] Some drugs were prescribed before the stroke and others are given after the stroke to

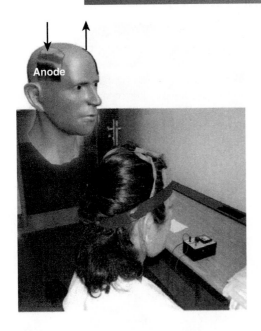

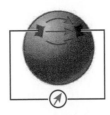

Figure 19-2. Transcranial direct current stimulation (TDCS) being applied. **A,** The DC current is transmitted by way of a pair of electrodes. **B,** Stimulation induces a current in the brain region under the electrode. (From Wagner T, Valero-Cabre A, Pascual-Leone A: Noninvasive human brain stimulation. Annu Rev Biomed Eng 2007;9: 527-565. Reprinted permission from the *Annual Review of Biomedical Engineering,* Volume 9, 2007 by Annual Reviews, www.annualreviews.org)

treat various symptoms and general medical conditions. In general, the acute and chronic effects of concurrent drugs on recovery have been poorly studied but are definitely important. Sedatives, anticonvulsants, haloperidol, and opiates should be avoided when possible.

Gait Training

The ability to walk unaided is a critical function. Especially for patients with hemiplegia, walking is the difference between becoming ambulatory and mobile without help and remaining dependent. One newer modality of treatment involves having patients walk on a treadmill at different speeds while their body is supported in a harness-type body-weight–supporting device.[22b] This technique allows patients who would otherwise be

wheelchair bound to practice gait soon after their stroke without fear of falling.[70] Animal experiments show that forced locomotion activates spinal and supraspinal automatic systems active during gait.[79] Walking is basically an automatic function that requires little direct attention to the particulars of the process. Individuals can walk and talk and perform complex acts at the same time without difficulty. In fact, once an individual obsessively watches his or her feet, and is conscious and deliberate about placing them, their gait deteriorates.

At the onset of training, one or two physical therapists usually must facilitate the appropriate movements but with time the amount of weight support and supervision usually decline.[70] During a 30-minute therapy session using body-weight–supported treadmill training, a patient could perform up to 1000 gait cycles compared to a median of 30 cycles during present regular therapy. The speed of the treadmill setting may be important in retraining automatic reflex functions used during walking.[70]

A number of studies and trials have shown the superiority of body-weight supported treadmill gait training over other methods now in standard use.[41b,79-84] The technique is even useful in chronic stroke patients with severe deficits. In one study, 34 stroke patients (average age 59) who had severe neurologic deficits who could not walk safely unaided on a treadmill were treated in a community program one to three times per week using a body-weight–support treadmill program.[84] Objective testing showed that this technique improved walking endurance, balance, and lower extremity strength. This program also used swimming pool activities and rehabilitation techniques at the home and work sites to promote recovery and reintroduction into their pre-stroke environments.

Aphasia, Other Cognitive Deficits, and Visual Field Loss

The effectiveness of various strategies on recovery from motor deficits has been easier to study than cognitive and behavioral abnormalities. Weakness and gait disorders can be quantified in a variety of ways, such as time, power, and duration of a specific activity with specific body parts. The clinical manifestations of higher cortical functions and their neuroanatomic correlations are much more diverse and less easily quantified and homogenized than weakness. Speech therapists have used various strategies and modalities to improve language function.[6,17,84,85] Recently some researchers have applied a strategy used in treating motor abnormalities—that is, combining stimulation (magnetic, direct current, pharmacologic) with physical therapy in order to augment use-related improvement. In one study, direct current stimulation with melodic intonation therapy seemed to complement each other.[44]

Visual field defects, especially if accompanied by visual neglect or difficulty reading, can be quite disabling for many stroke patients. Visual field defects most often involve one side of visual space (hemianopia) and vary considerably in their configuration—some involving only one superior or inferior quadrant, some sparing macular vision, and some involving only a hole in vision (scotoma).[86] Strokes, both ischemic and hemorrhagic, are by far the most common cause of persistent visual field defects.[87] Most physicians considered that visual field defects were usually permanent and immutable. Until recently, there was little enthusiasm for available remedial techniques to promote visual recovery.

Recently, experimentalists have shown that plasticity does occur in the human adult central nervous system, even after strokes, a recurrent theme and emphasis in this chapter.[88] Research in mammals and humans shows that the human striate and peristriate visual cortex is also plastic and able to adopt and change after injury.[89-91] Studies of patients with stroke-related hemianopia show that recovery is quite common.[92] Renewed interest and novel strategies are now being studied to restore visual function in patients with visual field defects.[93]

One of the most promising treatments involves a computer-based training program that patients with visual field defects perform at home, with periodic supervision.[94] In this visual restoration training program, while fixating on a central point, patients press keys in response to repetitive visual stimuli presented in the transition zone between their intact and damaged visual field sectors.[93-97] Their responses are monitored by a computer and stimulus patterns are sequentially changed in accord with the responses. The results show promise in enlarging the visual field, especially the parafoveal portion, allowing important practically useful gains in visual function.[93-97]

The visual field improvement persists years after the training period ends.[97] The visual restoration training program takes months of regular hour-long sessions, and thus patients must be highly motivated and compulsive enough to sustain the training. The aim of this therapy is to stimulate plasticity in neurons adjacent to the damaged visual cortex.

Others have tried to restore visual function in hemianopic visual fields by directing attention and gaze into the previously blind field.[93,98] One promising approach takes advantage of optokinetic reflexes to expand attention to visual field defects.[98] When hemianopic individuals read, they produce many more saccadic eye movements than normals, because the hemianopia diminishes their appreciation of key visual information about words that will appear next in their blind field.[98] Training patients with visual field defects by scanning moving text can train involuntary saccades and so improve reading and presumably other visual perception in the previously blind visual field.[98]

Mental Activity and Observation

A relatively new concept that is driving rehabilitation strategies is based on the discovery of so-called "mirror neurons" by Rizzolatti and colleagues.[98a,98b] These nerve cells discharge during various hand-directed actions and also while observing others performing the same actions. Mirror neurons also likely are activated during face and lower extremity goal-directed actions and almost surely in relation to emotional activities. This system is important in understanding actions, during learning to imitate novel complex actions, and in internal rehearsal of actions.[98c] Mental practice (cognitive rehearsal),[98d] and observing others performing a task,[98e] when combined with standard physical therapy in which the task is actively performed, may facilitate a patient's ability to perform.

Introducing Primitive Cells and/or Growth Factors into the Brain

Stem cell research has greatly stimulated an interest in the plasticity of the nervous system and regeneration. One of the most exciting new research strategies to promote recovery involves introducing primitive pluripotential stem cells into patients with stroke.[99-101,101a] Early transplantation experiments that involved introducing primitive cells into the brains of animals showed that grafted neurons survive and remain viable only if they are immature before they have elaborated axonal connections. Preliminary studies in humans that used postmitotic human neuron–like cells, derived originally from a human testicular germ cell tumor, showed the feasibility of implanting cells into humans after striato-capsular infarcts and hemorrhages.[102,103] Cyclosporine immunosuppression was given to the transplanted patients. Some patients seemed to improve.[102,103] There were no major complications. Transplantation of fetal porcine cells derived from the lateral ganglionic eminence have also been transplanted into five patients with basal ganglionic infarct cavities.[99,104] To prevent rejection in this study, the cells were pretreated with an anti-MHC1 antibody and the patients were not given immunosuppressive agents.[104]

Stem cell research in stroke patients is clearly very preliminary. When primitive embryonal cells are used, the transplants often also contain abundant growth factors that could stimulate endogenous proliferation of neural elements. Researchers are exploring the potential for using bone-marrow stromal cells[99,101,101a,105-107] and blood from the human umbilical cord[99,101,108,109] as potential donor sources of cells and accompanying growth factors. Endothelial progenitor cells are also potential donor type cells. Researchers are actively exploring different ways to introduce cells and growth factors: directly into or near the lesion, intra-arterially into the ipsilateral carotid artery, and intravenously. The discovery that animals and humans have a reservoir of primitive cells within brain regions has led to research into means of stimulating these endogenous cells to proliferate and migrate into injured areas.

Growth factors have recently been further categorized. They are polypeptide proteins that influence cell growth, maturation, and division.[22a] They have an important role in the response to brain injuries such as strokes. Basic fibroblastic growth factor (bFGF),[110] brain-derived neurotrophic factor (BDNF),[111] vascular endothelial growth factor (VEGF),[112] erythropoietin (EPO),[113,114] and granulocyte-colony stimulating factor (GCSF)[115] have all shown promise in experimental studies of brain ischemia. Some of the growth factors seem able to penetrate through the normal blood–brain barrier while others do not, so that the access route for their introduction will vary.

Many important questions are as yet unresolved[99,101a]: (1) When should cells be introduced? If too early, ischemia may reduce the potential for the implants to take and cytokines and leukocytes could impair implantation. In addition, prognosis is often less evident during the acute period, making it less likely that patients and physicians would accept an experimental procedure soon after stroke onset. Transplantation weeks or months after stroke may be too late. (2) Which cells should be chosen as a donor source and how many? Both neurogenesis and angiogenesis are important for recovery. (3) Should growth factors be introduced with, or instead of, cells? (4) Which strokes? Should only patients with infarcts limited to one area, such as the putamen, be chosen? Would transplants be effective if a number of divergent neuronal cells are infarcted (cortical, putaminal, hippocampal, etc.)? What about size? What if the infarct involves mostly white matter or involves important white matter tracts such as those that travel in the internal capsule? Are patients with intracerebral hemorrhages also candidates for cell or growth factor treatment? (5) What avenue should be used to introduce the cells? Intravenous, intra-arterial or directly into the brain? If into the brain, where should the cells be implanted? Directly into the infarct or in the presumed penumbra? Multisite injections or one large implant? Hopefully, ongoing research will answer these queries, if not curtailed by political and religious authorities.

References

1. Caplan LR, Hier DB: Recovery from right hemisphere stroke. In Corbier R (ed): Basis for a Classification of Cerebral Arterial Diseases. Amsterdam: Excerpta Medica, 1985, pp 163-171.
1a. Cramer S: Repairing the human brain after stroke: 1. Mechanisms of spontaneous recovery. Ann Neurol 2008;63:272-287.
2. Hier DB, Mondlock J, Caplan LR: Recovery of behavioral abnormalities after right hemisphere stroke. Neurology 1983;33:345-350.
3. Mesulam M: From sensation to cognition. Brain 1998;121:1013-1052.
4. Mohr JP, Pessin MS, Finkelstein S, et al: Broca aphasia: Pathological and clinical aspects. Neurology 1978;28:311-324.
5. Alexander M, Naeser M, Palumbo C: Broca's area aphasia. Neurology 1990;40:353-362.
6. Hillis AE: Aphasia: Progress in the last quarter of a century. Neurology 2007;69:200-213.
7. Weiler C, Chollet F, Frackowiak RSJ: Physiological aspects of recovery from stroke. In Ginsberg M, Bogousslavsky J (eds): Cerebrovascular Disease: Pathophysiology, Diagnosis, and Management. Malden, Mass: Blackwell, 1998, pp 2057-2067.
8. Binkofski F, Seitz RJ, Hacklander T, et al: Recovery of motor functions following hemiparetic stroke: A clinical and magnetic resonance—morphometric study. Cerebrovasc Dis 2001;11:273-281.
9. Feydy A, Carlier R, Roby-Brami A, et al: Longitudinal study of motor recovery after stroke. Recruitment and focusing of brain activation. Stroke 2002;33:1610-1617.
10. Ward NS, Cohen LG: Mechanisms underlying recovery of motor function after stroke. Arch Neurol 2004;61:1844-1848.
11. Han BS, Kim SH, Kim OL, et al: Recovery of corticospinal tract with diffuse axonal injury: A diffusion tensor image study. NeuroRehabilitation 2007;22:151-155.
12. Cramer SC: Functional imaging in stroke recovery. Stroke 2004;35:2695.

12a. Dancause N, Barbay S, Frost S, et al: Extensive cortical rewiring after brain injury. J Neurosci 2005;25:10167-10179.

12b. Nudo RJ: Postinfarct cortical plasticity and behavioral recovery. Stroke 2007;38(part 2): 840-845.

13. Murase N, Duque J, Mazzocchio R, Cohen LG: Influence of interhemispheric interactions on motor function in chronic stroke. Ann Neurol 2004;55:400-409.

14. Fregni F, Boggio PS, Valle AC, et al: A sham-controlled trial of a 5-day course of repetitive transcranial magnetic stimulation of the unaffected hemisphere in stroke patients. Stroke 2006;37:2115-2122.

14a. Kreisel SH, Hennerici MG, Bazner H: Pathophysiology of stroke rehabilitation: The natural course of clinical recovery, use-dependent plasticity and rehabilitative outcome. Cerebrovasc Dis 2007;23: 243-255.

15. Andrew K, Brocklehurst JC, Richard B, et al: The rate of recovery from stroke and its measurement. Rehab Med 1981;3:155-161.

16. Katz S, Ford AB, Chinn AB, et al: Prognosis after stroke: II. Long-term course of 159 patients. Medicine (Baltimore) 1966;45:236-246.

17. Dobkin BH: Neurologic Rehabilitation. Philadelphia: Davis, 1996.

18. Dobkin BH: Rehabilitation after stroke. N Engl J Med 2005;352:1677-1684.

19. U.S. Department of Health and Human Services: Post-Stroke Rehabilitation. Clinical Practice Guideline, number 16. Rockville, Md: U.S. Public Health Service, Agency for Health Care Policy and Research, 1995.

20. Bates B, Choi JY, Duncan PW, et al: Veterans Affairs/Department of Defense clinical practice guideline for the management of adult stroke rehabilitation care. Executive summary. Stroke 2005;36:2049-2056.

21. Miyai I, Reding MJ: Stroke recovery and rehabilitation. In Ginsberg M, Bogousslavsky J (eds): Cerebrovascular Disease: Pathophysiology, Diagnosis, and Management, vol 2. Malden, Mass: Blackwell, 1998, pp 2043-2056.

22. Ozer MN, Materson RS, Caplan LR: Management of Persons with Stroke. St Louis: Mosby, 1994.

22a. Cramer SC: Repairing the human brain after stroke. II. Restorative therapies. Ann Neurol 2008;63:549-560.

22b. Dobkin BH: Training and exercise to drive poststroke recovery. Nat Clin Pract Neurol 2008;4:76-85.

23. Alexander M: Stroke rehabilitation outcome: A potential use of predictive variables to establish levels of care. Stroke 1994;25:128-134.

24. World Health Organization: WHO International Classification of Impairments, Disabilities, and Handicaps: A Manual of Classification Relating to the Consequences of Disease. Geneva: World Health Organization, 1980.

25. Feigenson JS: Neurological rehabilitation. In Baker AB (ed): Clinical Neurology. New York: Harper and Row, 1983, pp 1-66.

26. Feigenson JS, McDowell FH, Meese P, et al: Factors influencing outcome and length of stay in a stroke rehabilitation unit: I. Analysis of 248 unscreened patients-medical and function prognostic indication. Stroke 1977;8: 651-656.

27. Feigenson JS, McCarthy ML, Greenberg SD, et al: Factors influencing outcome and length of stay in a stroke rehabilitation unit: II. Comparison of 318 screened and 248 unscreened patients. Stroke 1977;8:657-662.

28. Feigenson JS, McCarthy ML, Meese P, et al: Stroke rehabilitation: Factors predicting outcome and length of stay—an overview. N Y State J Med 1977;77:1426-1430.

29. Nicholas M, Helm-Estabrooks N, Ward-Lonergan J, et al: Evolution of severe aphasia in the first two years post onset. Arch Phys Med Rehabil 1993;74:830-836.

30. Taub N, Wolfe C, Richardson E, et al: Predicting the disability of first-time stroke sufferers at 1 year. Stroke 1994;25:352-357.

31. DeJong G, Branch LG: Predicting the stroke patient's ability to live independently. Stroke 1982;13:648-655.

32. Wood-Dauphinee S, Shapiro S, Bass E, et al: A randomized trial of team care following stroke. Stroke 1984;15:864-872.

33. Strand T, Asplund K, Eriksson S, et al: A non-intensive stroke unit reduces functional disability and the need for long-term hospitalization. Stroke 1985;17:377-381.

34. Indredavik B, Bakke F, Solberg R, et al: Benefit of a stroke unit: A randomized controlled trial. Stroke 1991;22:1026-1031.

35. Kalra L, Dale P, Crome P: Improving stroke rehabilitation: A controlled trial. Stroke 1993;24: 1462-1467.

36. Ottenbacher KJ, Jannell S: The results of clinical trials in stroke rehabilitation research. Arch Neurol 1993;50:37-44.

37. Kaste M, Palmomaki H, Sarna S: Where and how should elderly stroke patients be treated? A randomized trial. Stroke 1995;26:249-253.

38. Indredavik B, Slordahl SA, Bakke F, et al: Stroke unit treatment. Long-term effects. Stroke 1997;28: 1861-1866.

39. Stroke Unit Trialists' Collaboration: Collaborative systematic review of the randomized trials of organized in-patient (stroke unit) care after stroke. BMJ 1997;314:1151-1159.

40. Stroke Unit Trialists' Collaboration: How do stroke units improve patient outcomes? A collaborative systematic review of the ramdomized trials. Stroke 1997;28:2139-2144.

41. Colborne G, Olney S, Griffin M: Feedback of ankle and soleus electromyography in the rehabilitation of hemiplegic gait. Arch Phys Med Rehabil 1993;74:1100-1106.

41a. da Cunha-Filho TI, Lim PA, Qureshy H, et al: Gait outcomes after acute stroke rehabilitation with supported treadmill ambulation training: A randomized controlled pilot study. Arch Phys Med Rehabil 2002;83:1258-1265.

41b. Maple FW, Tong RKY, Li LSW: A pilot study of randomized clinical controlled trial of gait training in subacute stroke patients with partial body-weight support electromechanical gait trainer and functional electrical stimulation. Stroke 2008;39:154-160.

42. Nakayama H, Jorgenson H, Raaschou H, et al: Recovery of upper extremity function in stroke patients. The Copenhagen Stroke Study. Arch Phys Med Rehabil 1994;75;394-398.

43. Shewan C, Kertesz A: Effects of speech and language treatment on recovery from aphasia. Brain Lang 1984;23:272-299.

44. Vines BW, Norton AC, Schlaug G: Applying transcranial direct current stimulation in combination with melodic intonation therapy facilitates language recover for Broca's aphasic patients. Stroke 2007;38:519.

45. Halligan P, Marshall J: Spatial neglect. Position papers on theory and practise. Neuropsych Rehabil 1994;4:103-230.

46. Johansson K, Lindgren I, Widner H, et al: Can sensory stimulation improve the functional outcome in stroke patients? Neurology 1993;43:2189-2192.

47. van der Lee JH, Wagenaar RC, Lankhorst GJ, et al: Forced use of the upper extremity in chronic stroke patients: Results from a single-blind randomized clinical trial. Stroke 1999;30:2369-2375.

48. Pierce SR, Gallagher KG, Schaumburg SW, et al: Home forced use in an outpatient rehabilitation program for adults with hemiplegia: A pilot study. Neurorehab Neural Repair 2003;17:214-219.

49. Miltner WH, Bauder H, Sommer M, et al: Effects of constraint-induced movement therapy on patients with chronic motor deficits after stroke: A replication. Stroke 1999;30:586-592.

50. Fritz SL, Light KE, Patterson TS, et al: Active finger extention predicts outcome after constraint-induced movement therapy for individuals with hemiparesis after stroke. Stroke 2005;36:1172-1177.

51. Wolf SL, Winstein CJ, Miller JP, et al: Effect of constraint-induced movement therapy on upper extremity function 3 to 9 months after stroke: The EXCITE randomized clinical trial. EXCITE Investigators. JAMA 2006;296:2095-2104.

52. Feys H, De Weerdt, Verbeke G, et al: Early and repetitive stimulation of the arm can substantially improve the long-term outcome after stroke: A 5-year follow-up study of a randomized trial. Stroke 2004;35:924-929.

53. Teasell RW, Kalra L: What's new in stroke rehabilitation. Stroke 2004;35:383-385.

54. Kerkhoff G: Modulation and rehabilitation of spatial neglect by sensory stimulation. Prog Brain Res 2003;142:257-271.

55. Takeuchi N, Chuma T, Matsuo Y, et al: Repetitive transcranial magnetic stimulation of contralesional primary motor cortex improves hand function after stroke. Stroke 2005;36:2681-2686.

56. Kobayashi M, Hutchinson S, Theoret H, et al: Repetitive transcranial magnetic stimulation of the motor cortex improves ipsilateral sequential simple finger movements. Neurology 2004;62:91-98.

57. Khedr EM, Ahmed MA, Fathy N, Rothwell JC: Therapeutic trial of repetitive transcranial magnetic stimulation after acute ischemic stroke. Neurology 2005;65:466-468.

58. Kim Y-H, You SH, Ko M-H, et al: Repetitive transcranial magnetic stimulation-induced cortico-motor excitability and associated motor skill acquisition in chronic stroke. Stroke 2006;37:1471-1476.

59. Hummel F, Cohen LG: Improvement of motor function with noninvasive cortical stimulation in a patient with chronic stroke. Neurorehab Neural Repair 2005;19:14-19.

59a. Nowak DA, Grefkes C, Dafotakis M, et al: Effects of low-frequency repetitive transcranial magnetic stimulation of the contralesional primary motor cortex on movement kinematics and neural activity in subcortical stroke. Arch Neurol 2008;65:741-747.

59b. Rossini P, Rossi S: Transcranial magnetic stimulation. Diagnostic, therapeutic, and research potential. Neurology 2007;68:484-488.

59c. Wagner T, Valero-Cabre A, Pascual-Leone A: Noninvasive human brain stimulation. Annu Rev Biomed Eng 2007;9:527-565.

59d. Alonso-Alonso M, Fregni F, Pascuazl-Leone A: Brain stimulation in post-stroke rehabilitation. Cerebrovasc Dis 2007;24(suppl 1):157-166.

60. Hummel F, Celnik P, Giraux P, et al: Effects of non-invasive cortical stimulation on skilled motor function in chronic stroke. Brain 2005;128:490-499.

61. Nair DG, Pascual-Leone A, Schlaug G: Transcranial direct current stimulation in combination with occupational therapy for 5 consecutive days improves motor function in chronic stroke patients. Stroke 2007;38:518.

62. Davis JN, Crisostomo EA, Duncan P, et al: Amphetamine and physical therapy facilitate recovery of function from stroke: Correlative animal and human studies. In Raichle ME, Powers W (eds): Cerebrovascular Diseases. New York: Raven Press, 1987, pp 297-304.

63. Goldstein LB: Amphetamine-facilitated functional recovery after stroke. In Ginsberg MD, Dietrich WD (eds): Cerebrovascular Diseases. New York: Raven Press, 1989, pp 303-308.

64. Sawaki L, Cohen LG, Classen J, et al: Enhancement of use-dependent plasticity by d-amphetamine. Neurology 2002;59:1262-1264.

65. Aisen ML, Krebs HI, Hogan N, et al: The effect of robot assisted therapy and rehabilitative training on motor recovery following stroke. Arch Neurol 1997;54:443-446.

66. Volpe BT, Krebs HI, Hogan N, et al: Robot training enhanced motor outcome in patients with stroke maintained over 3 years. Neurology 1999;53:1874-1876.

67. Volpe BT, Krebs HL, Hogan N: Robot-aided sensorimotor training in stroke rehabilitation. Adv Neurol 2003;92:429-433.

68. Krebs HI, Volpe BT, Ferraro M, et al: Robot-assisted neurorehabilitation from evidence-based to science-based rehabilitation. Top Stroke Rehabil 2002;8:54-70.

69. Cramer SC, Der-Yeghiaian L, See J, et al: Robot-based hand motor therapy after stroke. Stroke 2007;38:518.

70. Dombovy ML: Understanding stroke recovery and rehabilitation: Current and emerging approaches. Curr Neurol Neurosci Rep 2004; 4:31-35.

71. Cristostomo EA, Duncan PW, Propst MA, et al: Evidence that amphetamine with physical therapy promotes motor function in stroke patients. Ann Neurol 1988;23:94-97.

72. Goldstein LB: Effects of amphetamines and small related molecules on recovery after stroke in animals and man. Neuropharmacology 2000;39: 852-859.

73. Feeney DM, Gonzalez A, Law WA: Amphetamine, haloperidol and experience interact to affect the rate of recovery after motor cortex injury. Science 1982;217:855-857.

74. Houda DA, Feeney DM: Haldoperidol blocks amphetamine induced recovery of binocular depth perception after bilateral visual cortex abilities in the cat. Proc West Pharmacol Soc 1985;28:209-211.

75. Schallert T, Hernandez T: GABAnergic drugs and neuroplasticity after brain injury. In Goldstein LB, Ammon K (eds): Restorative Neurology: Advances in Pharmacotherapy for Recovery after Stroke. New York: Futura, 1998, pp 91-120.

76. Goldstein LB, Davis JN: Physician prescribing patterns following hospital admission for ischemic cerebrovascular disease. Neurology 1988;38: 1806-1809.

77. Goldstein LB: Potential effects of common drugs on stroke recovery. Arch Neurol 1998;55: 454-456.

78. Goldstein LB: Common drugs may influence motor recovery after stroke. The Sygen in Acute Stroke Study Investigators. Neurology 1995;45: 865-871.

79. Lovely RG, Gregor RJ, Ray RR, et al: Effects of training on the recovery of full weight-bearing stepping in the adult spinal cat. Exp Neurol 1986;92:421-435.

80. Hesse S, Bertelt C, Jahnke MT, et al: Treadmill training with partial body-weight support as compared to physiotherapy in non-ambulatory hemiparetic patients. Stroke 1995;26:976-981.

81. Visintin M, Barbeau H, Korner-Bitensky N, et al: A new approach to retrain gait in stroke patients through body-weight support and treadmill stimulation. Stroke 1998;29:1122-1128.

82. Kosak MC, Reding MJ: Comparison of partial body-weight supported treadmill training versus aggressive bracing assisted walking post stroke. Neurorehabil Neural Repair 2000;14:13-19.

83. daCunha Filho IT, Lim PA, Qurey H, et al: A comparison of regular rehabilitation and regular rehabilitation with supported treadmill ambulation training for acute stroke patients. J Rehabil Res Develop 2001;3:37-47.

84. Breen JC, Baker B, Thibault K, Snyder DE: Body weight support treadmill training improves walking in subacute and chronic severely disabled stroke patients. Stroke 2007; 38:571.

85. Hillis AE: Pharmacological, surgical, and neurovascular interventions to augment acute aphasia recovery. Am J Phys Med Rehabil 2007;86: 426-434.

86. Zhang X, Kedar S, Lynn MJ, et al: Homonymous hemianopias: Clinical-anatomic correlations in 904 cases. Neurology 2006;66:906-910.

87. Zhang X, Kedar S, Lynn MJ, et al: Homonymous hemianopia in stroke. J Neuro-Ophthalmol 2006; 26:180-183.

88. Carmichael ST: Cellular and molecular mechanisms of neural repair after stroke: Making waves. Ann Neurol 2006;59:735-742.

89. Gilbert CD, Wiesel TN: Intrinsic connectivity and receptive field properties in visual cortex. Vision Res 1985;365-374.

90. Gilbert CD, Wiesel TN: Receptive field dynamics in adult primary visual cortex. Nature 1992;356: 150-152.

91. Kaas JH, Krubitzer LA, Chino YM, et al: Reorganization of retinotopic cortical maps in adult mammals after lesions of the retina. Science 1990;248:229-231.

92. Zhang X, Kedar S, Lynn MJ, et al: Natural history of homonymous hemianopia. Neurology 2006;66:901-905.

93. Pambakien A, Currie J, Kennard C: Rehabilitation strategies for patients with homonymous visual field defects. J Neuro-Ophthalmol 2005; 25:136-142.

94. Kasten E, Behrens-Baumann, Sabel BA: Computer-based training for the treatment of partial blindness. Nature Med 1998;4:1083-1087.

95. Kasten E, Poggel DA, Sabel BA: Computer-based training of stimulus detection improves color and simple pattern recognition in the defective field of hemianopic subjects. J Cognitive Neurosci 2000;12:1001-1012.

96. Poggel DA, Kasten E, Sabel BA: Attentional cueing improves vision restoration therapy in patients with visual field defects. Neurology 2004;63:2069-2076.

97. Kasten E, Muller-Oehring E, Sabel BA: Stability of visual field enlargements following computer-based restitution training—Results of a follow-up. J Clin Exp Neuropsychol 2001;23:297-305.

98. Spitzyna GA, Wise RJS, McDonald SA, et al: Optokinetic therapy improves text reading in patients with hemianopic alexia. Neurology 2007;68:1922-1930.

98a. Gallese V, Fadiga L, Fogassi L, Rizzolatti G: Action recognition in the premotor cortex. Brain 1996; 119:593-609.

19

98b. Fogassi L, Ferrari PF, Gesierich B, et al: Parietal lobe: From action organization to intention understanding. Science 2005;308:662-667.

98c. Kalra L, Ratan R: Recent advances in stroke rehabilitation 2006. Stroke 2007;38:235-237.

98d. Page SJ, Levine P, Leonard A: Mental practice in chronic stroke. Results of a randomized, placebo-controlled trial. Stroke 2007;38:1293-1297.

98e. Celnik P, Webster B, Glasser DM, Cohen LG: Effects of action observation on physical training after stroke. Stroke 2008;39:1814-1820.

99. Savitz SI, Rosenbaum DM, Dinsmore JH, et al: Cell transplantation for stroke. Ann Neurol 2002;52:266-275.

100. Roitberg B: Transplantation for stroke. Neurol Res 2004;26:256-264.

101. Bliss T, Guzman R, Daadi M, Steinberg GK: Cell transplantation therapy for stroke. Stroke 2007;38:817-826.

101a. Savitz SI, Rosenbaum DM: Stroke Recovery with Cellular Therapies. Totowa, NJ: Humana Press, 2008.

102. Kodziolka D, Wechsler L, Goldstein S, et al: Transplantation of cultured human neuronal cells for patients with stroke. Neurology 2000;55:565-569.

103. Kondziolka D, Steinberg GK, Wechsler L, et al: Neurotransplantation for patients with subcortical motor stroke: A phase 2 randomized trial. J Neurosurg 2005;103:38-45.

104. Savitz SI, Dinsmore J, Wu J, et al: Neurotransplantation of fetal porcine cells in patients with basal ganglia infarcts: A preliminary safety and feasibility study. Cerebrovasc Dis 2005;20:101-107.

105. Chen J, Li Y, Wang L, et al: Therapeutic benefit of intravenous administration of bone marrow stromal cells after cerebral ischemia in rats. Stroke 2001;32:1005-1011.

106. Chopp M, Li Y: Transplantation of bone marrow stromal cells for treatment of central nervous system diseases. Adv Exp Med Biol 2006;585:49-64.

107. Tang Y, Yasuhara T, Hara K, et al: Transplantation of bone marrow–derived stem cell: A promising therapy for stroke. Cell Transpl 2007;16:159-169.

108. Chen J, Sanberg PR, Li Y, et al: Intravenous administration of human umbilical cord blood reduces behavioral deficits after stroke in rats. Stroke 2001;32:2682-2688.

109. Newman MB, Emerich DF, Borlongan CV, et al: Use of human umbilical cord blood (HUBC) to repair the damaged brain. Cur Neurovasc Res 2004;1:269-281.

110. Kawamata T, Dietrich W, Schallert T, et al: Intracisternal basic fibroblast growth factor (bFGF) enhances functional recovery and upregulates the expression of a molecular marker of neuronal sprouting following focal cerebral infarction. Proc Natl Acad Sci U S A 1997;94:8179-8184.

111. Schabitz WR, Berger C, Kollmar R, et al: Effect of brain derived neurotrophic factor treatment and forced arm use on functional motor recovery after small cortical ischemia. Stroke 2004;35:992-997.

112. Zheng GZ, Li Z, Quan J, et al: VEGF enhances angiogenesis and promotes blood–brain barrier leakage in the ischemic brain. J Clin Invest 106;829-838.

113. Wang L, Zhang Z, Wang Y, et al: Treatment of stroke with erythropoietin enhances neurogenesis and angiogenesis and improves neurological function in rats. Stroke 2004;35:1732-1737.

114. Tsai PT, Ohab JJ, Kertesz N, et al: A critical role of erythropoietin receptor in neurogenesis and post-stroke recovery. J Neurosci 2006;26:1269-1274.

115. Schneider UC, Schilling L, Schroeck H, et al: Granulocyte-macrophage colony stimulating factor-induced vessel growth restores cerebral blood supply after bilateral carotid artery occlusion. Stroke 2007;238:1320-1328.

Index

Page numbers followed by f indicate figures; and page numbers followed by t indicate tables.

A